Swanson's
Family Medicine
Review

Swanson's
Family Medicine
Review
A Problem-Oriented Approach
6TH EDITION

Alfred F. Tallia, MD, MPH

Editor-in-Chief
Professor and Chair
Department of Family Medicine
Robert Wood Johnson Medical School
University of Medicine and Dentistry of New Jersey
New Brunswick, New Jersey

Joseph E. Scherger, MD, MPH

Co-Editor
Clinical Professor
Department of Family and Preventive Medicine
University of California, San Diego School of Medicine
Medical Director, AmeriChoice
San Diego, California

Nancy W. Dickey, MD

Co-Editor
President
Texas A&M Health Science Center
College Station, Texas

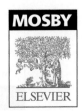

MOSBY

ELSEVIER

MOSBY
ELSEVIER

1600 John F. Kennedy Blvd.
Ste 1800
Philadelphia, PA 19103-2899

SWANSON'S FAMILY MEDICINE REVIEW: ISBN: 978-0-323-05554-3
A PROBLEM-ORIENTED APPROACH,
SIXTH EDITION

Previous editions copyrighted 2005, 2001, 1996, 1991.

Library of Congress Cataloging-in-Publication Data
Swanson's family medicine review : a problem-oriented approach.—6th ed. / Alfred F. Tallia, editor-in-chief ; Joseph E. Scherger, Nancy W. Dickey, co-editors.
    p. ; cm.
Rev. ed. of: Swanson's family practice review. 5th ed. c2005.
Includes bibliographical references and index.
ISBN 978-0-323-05554-3 (alk. paper)
1. Family medicine—Examinations, questions, etc. I. Swanson, Richard W. II. Tallia, Alfred F. III. Scherger, Joseph E. IV. Dickey, Nancy W. Swanson's family practice review. VI. Title: Family medicine review.
[DNLM: 1. Family Practice—Examination Questions. WB 18.2 S9718 2009]
RC58.S93 2009
616.0076—dc22   2008020397

Acquisitions Editor: Druanne Martin
Developmental Editor: Agnes H. Byrne
Design Direction: Steven Stave

Printed in China

Last digit is the print number: 9 8 7 6 5 4 3 2 1

To the lasting memory of

Dr. Richard Swanson

An extraordinary physician and educator

Suraj Achar, MD, FAAFP, CAQSM
Assistant Clinical Professor
Department of Family and Community Medicine
University of California, San Diego, School of
  Medicine
San Diego, California
*Preparticipation Evaluation; Exercise Prescription;
Concussions; Acceleration and Deceleration Neck Injuries;
Upper Extremity Injuries; Low Back Pain; Lower Extremity
Strains and Sprains; Fracture Management; Infectious Disease
and Sports; Female Athlete Triad*

Lani K. Ackerman, MD
Associate Professor
Department of Family and Community Medicine
Texas A&M Health Science Center College of
  Medicine
College Station, Texas
*Family-Centered Maternity Care; Routine Prenatal Care;
Immunization and Consumption of Over-the-Counter
Drugs during Pregnancy; Exercise and Pregnancy; Infant
Feeding; Immunizations; Diaper Rash and Other Infant
Dermatitis; Otitis Media; Childhood Asthma;
Physical Activity and Nutrition*

Ronelle Campbell, DO
Assistant Professor
Department of Internal Medicine
University of California, San Diego, School of
  Medicine
San Diego, California
Human Immunodeficiency Virus Infection

Jonathan P. Chan, MD
Associate Physician
Department of Family Medicine
Kaiser Permanente, San Diego
San Diego, California
*Concussions; Acceleration and Deceleration
Neck Injuries*

Robert P. Chen, MD, MBA
Assistant Professor
Department of Family Medicine
Robert Wood Johnson Medical School
University of Medicine and Dentistry of New Jersey
New Brunswick, New Jersey
Chronic Obstructive Pulmonary Disease; Seizures; Sleep Disorders

Suparna Chhibber, MD
Family Practice
Baytown, Texas
*Over-the-Counter Drugs; Common Cold; Allergic Rhinitis;
Viral Exanthems; Cardiac Murmurs; Vomiting and
Diarrhea; Recurrent Abdominal Pain*

Beth Choby, MD
Assistant Professor
Department of Family Medicine
San Jacinto Methodist Family Medicine Residency
Baytown, Texas
*Common Problems in Pregnancy; Thyroid Disease in Pregnancy;
Intrauterine Growth Restriction; Post-term Pregnancy; Labor;
Delivery Emergencies; Bronchiolitis and Pneumonia;
Mononucleosis; Adolescent Safety*

Arnold E. Cuenca, DO
Team Physician
Women's Basketball
San Diego State University
Family Medicine/Sports Medicine Physician
San Diego Sports Medicine and Family Health Center
San Diego, California
Low Back Pain; Lower Extremity Strains and Sprains

Nancy W. Dickey, MD
President
Texas A&M Health Science Center
College Station, Texas
*Physician–Patient Relationship; Palliative Care; Cultural
Competence; Adolescent Development*

Sharon McCoy George, MD, MPS
Associate Professor
Department of Family Medicine
University of California, Irvine, School of Medicine
Irvine, California
Fibromyalgia; Chronic Fatigue Syndrome; Cancer Pain Management

Isaac Goldberg, MD
University of Texas Medical School
Houston, Texas
Preconception Care; Gestational Diabetes and Shoulder Dystocia; Hypertension in Pregnancy; Postpartum Blues, Depression, and Psychoses; Colic; Fever; Failure to Thrive and Short Stature; Child Abuse; Croup and Epiglottitis

Jeffrey Hall, DO
Assistant Professor
Department of Family Medicine
Texas A&M University System Health
    Science Center,
Temple, Texas
Acute and Chronic Poisoning

Penelope Holland-Barkis, MD
Assistant Professor
Department of Family and Community Medicine
Texas A&M College of Medicine
Temple, Texas
How to Break Bad News

David Howarth, MD
Associate Professor
Department of Family Medicine
Director, Geriatric Services
Robert Wood Johnson Medical School
University of Medicine and Dentistry of
    New Jersey
New Brunswick, New Jersey
Functional Assessment of the Elderly; Polypharmacy and Drug Reactions in the Elderly; The Propensity and Consequences of Falls among the Elderly; Urinary Incontinence in the Elderly; Prostate Disease; Pressure Ulcers; Constipation in the Elderly; Pneumonia and Other Common Infectious Diseases of the Elderly; Polymyalgia Rheumatica and Temporal Arteritis; Hypertension Management in the Elderly; Cerebrovascular Accidents; Depression in the Elderly; Dementia and Delirium; Parkinson's Disease; Elder Abuse; Emergency Treatment of Abdominal Pain in the Elderly

Jeffrey P. Levine, MD, MPH
Associate Professor
Director of Women's Health Programs
Department of Family Medicine
Robert Wood Johnson Medical School
University of Medicine and Dentistry of New Jersey
New Brunswick, New Jersey
Osteoporosis; Breast Disease; Premenstrual Syndrome and Premenstrual Dysphoric Disorder; Postmenopausal Symptoms; Abnormal Uterine Bleeding; Infertility

Barbara J. McGarry, MD
Clinical Assistant Professor
Department of Family Medicine
Robert Wood Johnson Medical School
University of Medicine and Dentistry of New Jersey
New Brunswick, New Jersey
Irritable Bowel Syndrome; Headache

Julie Graves Moy, MD, MPH
Institute for Health Policy
University of Texas School of Public Health
Austin, Texas
Domestic Violence; Common Problems of the Newborn; Lymphoma and Leukemia; Sickle Cell Disease; The Limping Child; Foot and Leg Deformities; Cardiac Arrest; Advanced Trauma Life Support; Urticaria and Angioneurotic Edema; Heat and Cold Illness

Parita Patel, MD
Assistant Professor
Department of Family and Community Medicine
Texas A&M University System Health Science Center
Temple, Texas
Diabetic Ketoacidosis

Susan Pohl, MD
Assistant Professor
Department of Family Medicine
Texas A&M University System Health Science Center
Temple, Texas
Spontaneous Abortion

Terry Rascoe, MD
Assistant Professor
Department of Family and Community Medicine
Texas A&M University System Health Science Center
Temple, Texas
Integrative Medicine

Joshua J. Raymond, MD, MPH
Assistant Professor
Department of Family Medicine
Robert Wood Johnson Medical School
University of Medicine and Dentistry of New Jersey
New Brunswick, New Jersey
Geriatric Fellowship Director
Family Medicine Residency Program
Centrastate Medical Center
Freehold, New Jersey
Chronic Obstructive Pulmonary Disease; Seizures; Sleep Disorders

Alan H. Remde, MD, FAAFP, FABFP
Assistant Professor
Department of Family Medicine
Robert Wood Johnson Medical School
University of Medicine and Dentistry of New Jersey
New Brunswick, New Jersey
Assistant Director
Family Practice Residency at Capital Health Systems
Lawrenceville, New Jersey
Asthma; Diabetes Mellitus

R. Hal Ritter, Jr., PhD, LPC, LMFT
Associate Professor
Department of Family and Community Medicine
Texas A&M University System Health Science Center
Temple, Texas
Ethical Decision-Making Issues

Beatrix Roemheld-Hamm, MD, PhD
Associate Professor
Department of Family Medicine
Robert Wood Johnson Medical School
University of Medicine and Dentistry of New Jersey
New Brunswick, New Jersey
Irritable Bowel Syndrome; Headache

Joseph E. Scherger, MD, MPH
Clinical Professor
University of California, San Diego School of Medicine
Medical Director, AmeriChoice
San Diego, California
Acute ST Segment Elevation Myocardial Infarction; Acute Coronary Symptoms and Stable Angina Pectoris; Hyperlipoproteinemia; Congestive Heart Failure; Hypertension; Dysrhythmia; Multiple Sclerosis; Acne, Rosacea, and Other Common Dermatologic Conditions; Common Skin Cancers; Common Renal Diseases; Renal Stones; Urinary Tract Infections; Fluid and Electrolyte Abnormalities; Anemia; Certain Hematologic Conditions; Breast, Lung, and Brain Cancer; Developmental Disabilities

Martin C. Schulman, MD
Associate Clinical Professor
Department of Family and Community Medicine
University of California, San Diego
La Jolla, California
Immune-Mediated Inflammatory Disorders and Autoimmune Diseases; Rheumatoid Arthritis; Osteoarthritis; Acute Gout and Pseudogout; Travel Medicine

George Scott, MD
Manteca Medical Group
Manteca, California
High Altitude and Barotrauma

R. Christopher Searles, MD
Assistant Clinical Professor
Department of Family and Community Medicine and
    Department of Psychiatry
University of California, San Diego
Co-Director, UCSD Combined Family Medicine and
    Psychiatry Residency Training Program
San Diego, California
Depressive Disorders; Bipolar Disorder; Generalized Anxiety Disorder; Post-traumatic Stress Disorder; Obsessive–Compulsive Disorder; Attention-Deficit/Hyperactivity Disorder; Conduct Disorder and Oppositional Defiant Disorder; Diagnosis and Management of Schizophrenia; Drug Abuse; Eating Disorders; Somatoform Disorders; Sexual Dysfunction; Psychotherapy in Family Medicine

Alfred F. Tallia, MD, MPH
Professor and Chair
Department of Family Medicine
Robert Wood Johnson Medical School
University of Medicine and Dentistry of New Jersey
New Brunswick, New Jersey
Family Influence on Health and Disease; Clinical Decision Making; Consultation and Team Care; Managing Multiple Morbidities; Quality Improvement; Clinical Prevention; Tobacco Dependency; Alcohol; Diet, Exercise, and Obesity; Trends in Cancer Epidemiology; Cardiovascular Epidemiology; Bioterrorism; Influenza and Other Emerging Diseases; Deep Venous Thrombosis and Pulmonary Thromboembolism; The Diagnosis and Management of Pneumonia in the Adult; Esophageal Disorders; Peptic Ulcer Disease; Hepatitis and Cirrhosis; Pancreatitis; Pancreatic Carcinoma; Biliary Tract Disease; Inflammatory Bowel Disease; Colorectal Cancer and Other Colonic Disorders; Common Endocrine Diseases; Disorders of the Eye; Joint and Soft Tissue Injections

LCDR Tricia E. VanWagner, MD
U.S. Navy Sports Medicine Fellow
Department of Sports Medicine
Naval Hospital Camp Pendleton
Camp Pendleton, California
Upper Extremity Injuries; Fracture Management

Jason P. Womack, MD
Instructor
Department of Family Medicine
Robert Wood Johnson Medical School
University of Medicine and Dentistry
    of New Jersey
Piscataway, New Jersey
Acute Appendicitis; Thyroid; Ear, Nose, and Throat Problems

Justine P. Wu, MD, MPH
Clinical Assistant Professor
Department of Family Medicine
Robert Wood Johnson Medical School
University of Medicine and Dentistry of
    New Jersey
New Brunswick, New Jersey
Vulvovaginitis and Bacterial Vaginosis; Cervical Abnormalities; Dysmenorrhea; Ectopic Pregnancy; Contraception; Spontaneous and Elective Abortion; Sexually Transmitted Diseases

Maria Rosenthal-Dichter, MD, PhD
Assistant Professor
Department of Family Medicine
Robert Wood Johnson Medical School
University of Medicine and Dentistry of New Jersey
New Brunswick, New Jersey

Joseph E. Scherger, MD, MPH
Clinical Professor
University of California, San Diego School of Medicine
Medical Director, Graybill...
San Diego, California

Marilyn C. Schallnau, MD
Associate Clinical Professor
Department of Family and Community Medicine
University of California, San Diego
La Jolla, California

George Scott, MD
Midway Medical Group
Murrieta, California

R. Christopher Searles, MD
Assistant Clinical Professor
Department of Family and Community Medicine and
Department of Psychiatry
University of California, San Diego
Co-Director, UCSD Combined Family Medicine and
Psychiatry Residency Training Program
San Diego, California

LCDR Trisha L. VanWagner, MD
MC, Navy Sports Medicine Fellow
Department of...
Naval Hospital Camp Pendleton
Camp Pendleton, California

Jason P. Womack, MD
Instructor
Department of Family Medicine
Robert Wood Johnson Medical School
University of Medicine and Dentistry
of New Jersey
Piscataway, New Jersey

Justine P. Wu, MD, MPH
Clinical Assistant Professor
Department of Family Medicine
Robert Wood Johnson Medical School
University of Medicine and Dentistry of
New Jersey
New Brunswick, New Jersey

Swanson's Family Medicine Review has been a marvelous educational tool for several generations of clinicians. The product of the founding genius of Dr. Richard Swanson, who passed away in 1996, the text has been an effective tool not only for family physicians preparing for certification or recertification but also for clinicians simply desiring to hone their familiarity with the basic concepts pertinent to primary care.

The primary goals of the sixth edition are to update the content and retain the special essence that made previous editions such valued and popular educational instruments. Although the basic format has been retained, this edition is now arranged in a fashion designed to make it easier for readers to find their way through the content. The book is divided into 11 sections. Ten represent a clinical area tested by the American Board of Family Medicine (ABFM), while the 11th section is an illustrated review.

Each section contains chapters covering specific subjects relevant to that section. Each chapter presents clinical cases that simulate real clinical situations, providing the learner with a sense of reality designed to enhance retention of content. Each clinical case is followed by questions concerning diagnosis and management. The question section is followed by an answer section, which provides a detailed discussion relevant to each question. Finally, each chapter has a short summation of key learning points and selected readings and references, including Web sites. The overall process is designed to increase retention and to expand and refine the readers' knowledge of the diagnostic methods, therapeutics, and patient management techniques presented in each case.

Joining me in preparing this edition are two new distinguished family physician co-editors, Nancy W. Dickey, MD, President of the Texas A&M Health Science Center and Vice Chancellor for Health Affairs for the Texas A&M System, and Joseph E. Scherger, MD, MPH, Professor of Family and Preventive Medicine at University of California, San Diego and Founding Dean of the Florida State University College of Medicine. Together as a team, we have reviewed the chapters and case problems for relevance and have chosen areas of emphasis for, and organization of, the content. We selected the sixth edition's content to reflect the broad core of knowledge that the family physician should have, and we valued the input of other family medicine clinicians with special expertise in specific content areas.

We have recruited as chapter authors the finest practicing family medicine experts from academic centers across the United States, who have subsequently reaffirmed and updated chapter content on the basis of thorough needs analyses, including opinions of readers, participants, and faculty in live CME conferences, expert opinion, and other accepted methodologies. The editors and authors anticipate that the reader will both enjoy and profit from their work in preparing this volume. Happy studying and learning!

Alfred F. Tallia, MD, MPH
Editor-in-Chief

ACKNOWLEDGMENTS ■

As editor-in-chief, I am indebted to many individuals for their support and assistance in the preparation of the 6th edition of *Swanson's Family Medicine Review*. To begin, I wish to thank my two new co-editors, Nancy W. Dickey, MD, and Joseph E. Scherger, MD, MPH, for their hard work and understanding.

Collectively, we would like to thank my wife, Elizabeth; Dr. Scherger's wife, Carol; and Dr. Dickey's husband, Frank, and our entire families, as well as those of the authors, for their sacrifice of time and their understanding as we prepared this edition.

To Dr. Kenneth Ibsen, our trusted director of continuing education and one of our former co-editors, a true scholar and gentleman, our continuing thanks. And to Ms. Agnes Byrne and the staff at Elsevier, our thanks for their inspiration and support. Our thanks as well to our colleagues in the academic communities that we call home for their help and understanding of the demands that preparation of this edition required.

Alfred F. Tallia, MD, MPH
Editor-in-Chief

Blood thinner

Rivaroxaban
Xarelto
15mg

CONTENTS

This section briefly discusses the philosophy and techniques of passing board examinations or any other type of medical examination. Most examinations have moved to computer-based administration. Learn whether this applies to your examination, and if so, read and use the demonstrations provided either on the Internet or elsewhere.

First, realize that you are "playing a game." It is, of course, a very important game, but a game nevertheless. When answering each question you must ask yourself, "What is it that the examiner wants from this question?" Let us turn our attention to the most common type of question, the multiple-choice question.

What these tips provide the learner is a way to "outfox the fox." So, how do you outfox the fox? Following these rules will maximize the chances.

RULE 1: Allocate your time appropriately. At the beginning of the examination, divide the number of questions by the time allotted. Pace yourself accordingly, and check your progress every half hour.

RULE 2: If using a computer-administered examination, take time before the examination to become familiar with the mechanics of maneuvering through the examination program. Learn whether you can return to questions you weren't sure about, or whether this is not allowed.

RULE 3: Answer every question in order. On some computer-administered examinations you run the risk of not being able to return to an unanswered question. Although American Board of Family Medicine examinations allow you to return, not all examinations permit this. And some examinations use unfolding question sequences that do not let you return to a previous

question. On paper-administered examinations, you run the risk of mis-sequencing your answers and having all answers out of order.

RULE 4: Do not spend more than your allotted time on any one question. If you don't know the answer and you are not penalized for wrong answers, simply guess.

RULE 5: Even if you are penalized for wrong answers (most examinations no longer do this) and you can eliminate even one choice, answer the question. Percentages dictate that you will come out ahead in the end.

RULE 6: If there is a question in which one choice is significantly longer than the others and you do not know the answer, select the long choice.

RULE 7: If you are faced with an "all of the above" choice, realize that these are right far more often than they are wrong. Choose "all of the above" if you do not know the answer.

RULE 8: Become suspicious if you have more than three choices of the same letter in a row. Two of one choice in a row is common, three is less common, and four is almost unheard of. Something is probably wrong.

RULE 9: Answer choices tend to be very evenly distributed. In other words, the number of correct "a" choices is close to the number of correct "b" choices, and so on. However, there may be somewhat more "e" choices than any other, especially if there are a fair number of "all of the above" choices. If you have time, do a quick check to provide yourself with some reassurance.

RULE 10: Never, never change an answer once you have recorded it on the computer unless you have an extraordinary reason for doing so. Many people taking multiple-choice–question examinations, especially if they have time on their hands after completing the examination, start second-guessing themselves and thinking of all kinds of unusual exceptions. Resist this temptation.

RULE 11: Before you choose an answer, always, always read each and every choice. Do not get caught by seeing what you believe is the correct answer jump out at you. Read all of the choices.

RULE 12: Scan the lead-in to the answers and the answers first, then read the clinical case/vignette. This way you will know what is being tested and will better attend to the necessary facts. Read each question carefully. Be especially careful to read words such as *not*, *except*, and so on.

Success cannot be guaranteed with these or any other rules. I do, however, believe that these rules will help you achieve better results on your board examinations.

Alfred F. Tallia, MD, MPH
Editor-in-Chief

It has been estimated that it will take 89 hours to complete this activity. Accordingly, Kaplan Medical CME designates this educational activity for up to 89 hours in Category 1 credit toward the AMA Physician's Recognition Award. Each physician should claim only those hours of credit that he or she actually spent completing the educational activity. These credits will be available from January 1, 2009 to December 31, 2011.

TARGETED AUDIENCE

This activity is designed to meet the educational needs of family practice physicians preparing for certification, recertification, and/or review of contemporary recommended practice behaviors. However, experience with previous editions suggests that it will also meet the educational needs of physicians in other specialties as well as physician assistants and other health care professionals desiring an up-to-date review of the essentials of primary care.

LEARNING OBJECTIVES

Upon completion of all or selected parts of this activity, participants should have:

1. reinforced and/or expanded their pre-existing knowledge in a way that will help improve the quality of their patient care;
2. learned new information that will have updated their pre-existing knowledge concerning current diagnostic methodologies, medications, and treatments;
3. gained further knowledge concerning state-of-the-art diagnostic strategies, treatment protocols, and/or clinical management strategies;
4. gained further insight into sensitive and effective ways communicated with patients;

5. and, if applicable, enhanced their knowledge concerning topics relevant to their certification or recertification examinations.

DISCLOSURE POLICY

In order to ensure balance, independence, objectivity, and scientific rigor, the editors—as the faculty responsible for content—are expected to disclose to all potential CME activity participants any relationship they may have had with any pharmaceutical company, biomedical device manufacturer/distributor, or other commercial entity that may be construed as a real or apparent conflict of interest with respect to the subject matter presented in this CME activity. The intent of this policy is not to prevent faculty who have such relationships from contributing to the activity, but rather to openly identify such relationships to the participants so they may form their own judgments concerning potential bias. In addition, contributors should identify non-FDA approved use of products whenever possible. However, it remains the responsibility of the participants to identify such products before using them in their practice; the publisher, CME provider, or the contributors cannot be held liable for misuse of any such product.

Alfred F. Tallia MD, MPH	Has no conflict of interest regarding any product discussed in this enduring CME activity. No use of off-labeled products is anticipated.
Joseph E. Scherger, MD, MPH	Has no conflict of interest regarding any product discussed in this enduring CME activity. No use of off-labeled products is anticipated.

Nancy W. Dickey, MD	Has no conflict of interest regarding any product discussed in this enduring CME activity. Use of off-labeled products may occur.

PROCESS FOR OBTAINING CONTINUING MEDICAL EDUCATION CREDIT

In order to obtain CME credits, it is necessary to first register. After registration you will be sent a questionnaire asking a little about you, how many and what type of CME credits you earned, the approximate percent improvement in your ability to answer the multiple-choice questions, and other pertinent evaluation data. Once that form is filled out and returned with the appropriate fee, you will be sent a certificate for the credits earned.

REGISTRATION

For registration, we require your name, degree, address, telephone number, and a $25 fee. Although this registration fee is non-returnable, it will be applied to the overall fee.

Registration may be conducted by mail or FAX using the tear-out registration page. Payment should be made to Kaplan Medical CME. The method of payment may be by check, money order, or credit card (Visa, MasterCard, American Express, or Discover).

The address for registration is:

CME Administrative Secretary
c/o Kaplan Medical CME
700 South Flower Street
Suite 2900
Los Angeles, CA 90017
Phone: 1-800-533-8850, ext. 5720
FAX: 213-892-1367
E-mail: CME@kaplan.com

Further questions may be directed to the CME coordinator at 213-452-5720.

CREDIT AND FEE SCHEDULE

Physicians requesting continuing medical education credit may do so upon completion of each individual section or, alternatively, elect to request the credit after completing the full text and receive a 10% discount. The maximum number of credit hours* and the associated fee for each section is indicated below. (The fees shown are based on a charge of $7.50 per credit hour for individual sections.)

Section	Maximum Credit Hours*	Fee
1. Family, Community, and Population Health	7	$52.50
2. Communication	4	$30.00
3. Adult Medicine	27	$202.50
4. Women's Health	7	$52.50
5. Maternity Care	8	$60.00
6. Children and Adolescents	13	$97.50
7. Geriatric Medicine	7	$52.50
8. Behavioral Health	4	$30.00
9. Emergency Medicine	3	$22.50
10. Sports Medicine	7	$52.50
11. Illustrated Review	2	$15.00
Entire book (10% discount)	**89**	**$667.50 less 10% = $600**

*These hours represent the average number of hours reported by five different readers of the 4th edition, adjusted to account for the greater length of the 5th and 6th editions.

Registration Form for CME Credits

Swanson's Family Medicine Review, 6th Edition

Name _____ Degree _____

Address_____
                       Street   City   State   Zip

Day Phone _____ FAX _____

E-mail _____

A nonrefundable fee of $25 must be included with this registration form:

Method of Payment:

Credit Card:
Type of Card: Visa _____ MasterCard _____ Amer. Exp. _____ Discover _____

Credit Card Number _____ Expiration Date _____

Signature _____

Check _____ Money Order _____

Mail or FAX the completed form to:

CME Administrative Secretary
c/o Kaplan Medical CME
700 South Flower Street
Suite 2900
Los Angeles, CA 90017
Phone: 1-800-533-8850, ext. 5720
FAX: 213-892-1367
E-mail: CME@kaplan.com

FAMILY, COMMUNITY, AND POPULATION HEALTH

Family Influences on Health and Disease

CLINICAL CASE PROBLEM 1

A Calculated Risk

A 35-year-old African American male comes to your office for the first time requesting a health maintenance visit. He works as an accountant in a Fortune 500 company and is concerned about his risk for hypertension.

SELECT THE BEST ANSWER TO THE FOLLOWING QUESTIONS

1. Regarding his risk, you would ask him about which of the following:
   a. smoking history
   b. exercise type and frequency
   c. diet history
   d. family history
   e. alcohol intake
   f. all of the above
   g. none of the above

2. You discover that his father developed hypertension at age 25 and is still living at the age of 75. Which of the following is true about family and risk?
   a. family is one of the major influences on disease incidence and prevalence
   b. family risk is not modifiable
   c. family risk need not be ascertained because there is nothing you can do about it
   d. family risk of disease susceptibility is absolutely transmittable
   e. family risk is not ascertainable by current methods of genetic screening

CLINICAL CASE PROBLEM 2

All in the Family

Two 75-year-old patients are hospitalized after both had a stroke resulting in a left-sided hemiparesis. The size and location of the thrombotic events in these patients are almost identical, as is the initial degree of impairment. Treatment received is also the same. One patient lives alone and has a sibling living in a distant state. The other patient is part of an extended family with many social supports, including grandchildren who visit often while in the hospital.

3. What outcomes would you predict for these patients based on their family social circumstances?
   a. identical outcomes are likely given the identical lesions and initial impairments
   b. it is impossible to predict outcomes
   c. the patient with more family supports is likely to have a better outcome
   d. the patient with fewer family supports is at lesser risk of acute mortality
   e. outcomes achieved are independent of any family social factors

CLINICAL CASE PROBLEM 3

Risks of Omission and Commission

A 28-year-old female presents to your office for the first time for prenatal care. She is 14 weeks into her first pregnancy. She is HIV positive but not on any antiretroviral agents. She has a one-half pack per day tobacco smoking habit. She has been unable to stop despite multiple attempts at quitting, and she has a glass of wine with dinner each night. She works in sales at a local food bar. She has taken no medications during her pregnancy because she is afraid any and all pills may harm her baby. She asks you what she can do to give her child a better chance in life than she has had.

4. At this time, it is most appropriate to advise her of which of the following?
   a. perinatal transmission of the HIV virus poses the child's greatest risk
   b. smoking is by far the most hazardous factor in her prenatal history
   c. alcohol consumption during pregnancy is a major risk factor for fetal alcohol syndrome
   d. she must restart antiretroviral medications immediately or risk certain death
   e. none of the above

CLINICAL CASE PROBLEM 4

Unwanted Advice

A 25-year-old mother presents for the first time with her 2-week-old infant, her first child. Hovering in the background are the two grandmothers. The mother is visibly concerned that the baby is "only" at the same weight as he was at birth. One grandmother chimes in that she knew breast-feeding was a bad idea, and the other insists that it is time to introduce cereal to the baby's diet. They start arguing among themselves until you escort everyone except the mother and the infant from the examination room.

5. In addition to giving the mother accurate advice about breast-feeding and nutrition, which of the following is an appropriate intervention at this time?
   a. refocus the attention of the grandmothers to some other facet of the family experience
   b. establish and reinforce the competency of the mother in her breast-feeding
   c. use your expert authority as the physician to set family rules for decision making in the mother's favor
   d. acknowledge and reinforce the expert authority of the grandmothers
   e. a, b, and c are correct

6. Possible positive aspects of the previous family situation include which of the following?
   a. evidence of closeness and connectedness
   b. a lack of criticism and blame
   c. the absence of protectionism and rigidity
   d. all of the above
   e. none of the above

7. You handle the situation with skill and care, and the grandmothers leave feeling reassured of your careful attention to their first and only grandson, and they are impressed with his mother's newly identified and recognized competence. In future visits, anticipatory guidance in this family should likely take into consideration which of the following?
   a. family beliefs about child discipline
   b. family influences on exercise and diet
   c. family beliefs about health and illness
   d. none of the above
   e. a, b, and c

Answers

1. **f.** Family influences on health and disease are numerous and multifactorial. These influences can be expressed across the individual and family life cycles. One of the most pronounced family effects is on genetics and disease susceptibility. Although all the historical elements listed are important, the family history, often recorded in the medical record pictorially as a genogram, will provide a constant guide for the assessment of symptoms as they present across the individual life cycle.

2. **a.** Disease incidence and prevalence are directly related to the interplay of family genetics, behaviors, and the host environment. Physicians should attend to known cues regarding family historical factors that can often foreshadow overt disease in patients.

3. **c.** A large literature exists on the influence of family on survival and disease progression. Strong family supports are protective and promote healing in acute disease circumstances. Studies of disease outcomes in myocardial infarction and stroke reveal striking supportive effects of family supports even when other variables are controlled for.

4. **a.** Family influence on prenatal and perinatal disease transmission is another important influence of the family on health and disease. Sadly, mother-to-infant transmission of HIV infection is epidemic in many areas of the so-called Third World, developing countries, but family transmission still influences development of disease and illness in all areas of the world, even in developed countries.

5. **e.** How many of us have been confronted by the case illustrated? Most experienced family physicians will recognize the situation. Dealing with family members beyond the presumed present patient is a common

occurrence in family medicine. In fact, skillful use of family resources is a therapeutic advantage in the family physician's armamentarium if used carefully. The supportive closeness of this family must be counterbalanced by reinforcement of the competence of the mother in this often seen scenario. Although being careful not to alienate the grandparents is important, ultimately the mother's competence and skill must be reinforced, as well as her decision-making authority. Because the physician possesses all forms of social power (expert, legal, coercive, referent, and reward), this can readily be accomplished.

6. a. While answers b and c can be positive aspects of family, they are absent in this situation.

7. e. Understanding family influences on health and disease is essential for effective practice as a family physician. Understanding allows for not only appropriate interventions in acute disease but also anticipatory guidance in the prevention of morbidity and future illness, and the promotion of health and well-being. Family factors that have protective influence on health and illness include closeness and connectedness, well-developed problem-focused coping skills, clear organization and decision making, and direct communication. Family pathologies that can adversely influence health and illness include intrafamily hostility, criticism, and blame; perfectionism and rigidity; lack of extrafamily support systems; and the presence of chronic psychopathology.

Summary

The effects of family on health and disease are large and multifactorial, and they are expressed across the individual and family life cycles. Family physicians and other health care providers must be cognizant of these influences and help individuals and families navigate the positive and less positive effects. The potential effects of family on health and illness include the following:

1. Genetics and disease susceptibility

Family effects through genetics are particularly strong. Although they can be moderated by environment and behavior, the effects are with us for a lifetime. Certain diseases, such as Huntington's disease and Tay–Sachs disease, are directly related to our parents; others, such as hypertension and diabetes, are strongly mediated by family factors.

2. Prenatal and perinatal transmission of disease

Generations of families have experienced prenatal or perinatal transmission of diseases ranging from syphilis to human immunodeficiency virus. In many areas of the world, this family influence has charted the destiny of countless children.

3. Child rearing and nurturing

Belief systems ranging from when to have children to how children should be raised and whether and how much children should be held are all part of the family influences on having and raising children.

4. Nutrition and lifestyle

Family traditions and socioeconomics play an important role in access to adequate nutrition. Many lifestyle behaviors, such as smoking, diet, exercise, and alcohol consumption, are influenced by our parents and extended family and by their habits and beliefs.

5. Access to and quality of care

Again, family socioeconomics along with race and ethnicity are factors that influence the ability to access health care and successfully navigate complex health care systems.

6. Spread of infectious disease

Family living situations and contacts are major influences on the spread of many infectious diseases ranging from mycoplasm pneumonia to influenza. Many infectious illness are passed from one family member to others in a household, and families are important vectors in times of epidemics.

7. Outcomes in acute and chronic illness

Multiple studies have demonstrated different outcomes in acute and chronic illness based on the degree of social supports available in families. Similarly, family dysfunction can be a major contributor to illness and adverse health outcomes in many individuals.

Family factors that have protective influence on health and illness include closeness and connectedness, well-developed problem-focused coping skills, clear organization and decision making, and direct communication. Family pathologies that can adversely influence health and illness include intrafamily hostility, criticism, and blame; perfectionism and rigidity; lack of extrafamily support systems; and the presence of chronic psychopathology.

Family-level interventions used by family physicians to reduce risk factors and increase protective functioning of families include various psychoeducational and psychotherapeutic techniques to address and enhance family relationships.

Suggested Reading

Alvarez GF, Kirby AS: The perspective of families of the critically ill patient: Their needs. *Current Opin Crit Care* 12(6):614–618, 2006.

Berg CA, Upchurch R: A developmental-contextual model of couples coping with chronic illness across the adult life span. *Psychol Bull* 133(6):920–954, 2007.

Copello AG, Templeton L, Velleman R: Family interventions for drug and alcohol misuse: Is there a best practice? *Curr Opin Psychiatry* 19(3):271–276, 2006.

Ensenauer RE, Reinke SS, Ackerman MJ, et al: Primer on medical genomics. Part VIII: Essentials of medical genetics for the practicing physician. *Mayo Clinic Proc* 78(7):846–857, 2003.

Nickman SL, Rosenfeld AA, Fine P, et al: Children in adoptive families: Overview and update. *J Am Acad Child Adolesc Psychiatry* 44(10): 987–995, 2005.

CHAPTER

2   Clinical Decision Making

CLINICAL CASE PROBLEM 1

A Third-Year Medical Student Who Wants to Know How to Think

A third-year medical student asks you to teach her the secrets of clinical decision making, or how you think when you approach and treat a patient. You agree and take her to see a patient in the emergency department. After you talk with the patient, you ask the student to describe everything she has seen and heard. You carefully note she has missed approximately half of what happened in the conversation between you and the patient, and even more in the physical examination.

SELECT THE BEST ANSWER TO THE FOLLOWING QUESTIONS

1. This represents a problem with which step(s) of the clinical decision-making process?
   a. cue acquisition
   b. hypothesis formation
   c. the search process
   d. all of the above
   e. none of the above

2. The most common problem related to clinical decision making seen in practicing physicians is:
   a. not formulating enough hypotheses
   b. not formulating the correct hypotheses
   c. not attending to all the patient-relevant cues
   d. not knowing the prevalence of a condition
   e. not using time appropriately in treatment plans

3. The student returns with you to the office and sees a patient on her own initially to gather historical and physical examination data, which she then presents to you. After seeing the patient, she is absolutely convinced the patient has a particular diagnosis. You take her with you to see the patient, and you obtain more historical information and examine the patient. As you ask her questions about her reasoning, she proceeds to ignore a whole variety of things that do not support her original diagnostic hypothesis. She has made which of the following errors in clinical decision making?
   a. failure to acquire a cue
   b. failure to generate hypotheses
   c. premature closure
   d. all of the above
   e. none of the above

CLINICAL CASE PROBLEM 2

A 25-Year-Old Medical Student Who Is Having Anxiety Attacks Regarding His Upcoming Epidemiology Examination

A 25-year-old medical student comes to your office in a state of extreme anxiety manifested by palpitations and sweating throughout the previous week. He tells you he is scheduled to have a clinical epidemiology examination in 24 hours.

On physical examination, his blood pressure is 120/70 mmHg, pulse is 90 beats per minute and regular, and respirations are 24 per minute. His physical examination is normal. You order a thyroid-stimulating hormone test to exclude hyperthyroidism. You explain to him that given the low prevalence of thyroid disease in his age group and the higher prevalence of anxiety in his medical school population of students, the test's negative predictive value will be helpful. He looks confused and more anxious.

In an attempt to deal with his symptoms, you decide to spend some time tutoring the student regarding basic epidemiologic concepts. You

Table 2-1	Relationship Between Test A and Disease B	
	Disease B Present	Disease B Absent
Test A positive	30 ᵃ TP	50 FP
Test A negative	10 FN	80 TN

Table 2-2	Prevalence of Disease X in Certain Populations
Setting	Prevalence (Cases/100,000)
General population	50
Women, age ≥ 50 years old	500
Women, age ≥ 65 years old, with a suspicious finding on clinical examination	40,000

begin by explaining the basics of a 2 × 2 table that relates positive and negative test results to the presence or absence of disease in a specific population (Table 2-1).

Use the data from Table 2-1 for questions 4–9.

4. What is the sensitivity of test A for disease B?
   a. 25%
   b. 37.5%
   c. 75%
   d. 62.5%
   e. 11%

   Sens = $\frac{TP}{(TP+FN)}$

5. What is the specificity of test A for disease B?
   a. 25%
   b. 37.5%
   c. 75%
   d. 61.5%
   e. 11%

   Spec = $\frac{TN}{TN+FP}$

6. What is the positive predictive value (PPV) of test A in the diagnosis of disease B?
   a. 37.5%
   b. 25%
   c. 75%
   d. 61.5%
   e. 11%

   PPV = $\frac{TP}{TP+FP}$

7. What is the negative predictive value (NPV) of test A in the diagnosis of disease B?
   a. 37%
   b. 89%
   c. 25%
   d. 75%
   e. 61.5%

   NPV = $\frac{TN}{TN+FN}$

8. What is the likelihood ratio for test A in disease B?
   a. 0.39
   b. 1.95
   c. 3.80
   d. 0.79
   e. 1.51

9. What is the prevalence of disease A in this population?
   a. 15.5%
   b. 23.5%

   c. 40.0%
   d. 10.5%
   e. 18.4%

Consider the data in Table 2-2 illustrating the prevalence of disease X in various populations. Based on this information about disease prevalence and assuming the sensitivity of test A for disease X is 80% and the specificity of test A for disease X is 90%, answer questions 10–13.

10. What is the PPV of test A in the diagnosis of disease X in the general population?
    a. 0.4%
    b. 1.3%
    c. 5.4%
    d. 15.7%
    e. 39.6%

11. What is the PPV of test A in disease X in women age 50 or older?
    a. 0.4%
    b. 3.9%
    c. 10.7%
    d. 23.6%
    e. 52.7%

12. What is the PPV of test A in disease X in women older than 65 years of age with a suspicious finding on clinical examination?
    a. 0.4%
    b. 5.6%
    c. 34.7%
    d. 84.2%
    e. 93.0%

13. If the PPV of a test for a given disease in a given population is 4%, how many true positive test results are there in a sample of 100 positive test results?
    a. 4
    b. 10
    c. 40
    d. 96
    e. none of the above

Table 2-3	Sensitivity and Specificity of Blood Sugar Levels in the Diagnosis of Diabetes Mellitus		
Blood Sugar Levels 2 Hours after Eating		**Sensitivity**	**Specificity**
>140 mg/100 (7.8 mmol/L)		57%	99.4%

Table 2-4	Blood Pressure Readings versus Visit Number	
Visit Number	**Mean Diastolic Blood Pressure (mmHg)**	
1	99.2	
2	91.2	
3	90.7	

To answer question 14, consider the data in Table 2-3 regarding the sensitivity and specificity in the diagnosis of diabetes mellitus in the population.

14. Given that the data are correct, if the sensitivity of the test for a given blood sugar level was 38.6%, which of the following would be the most likely value for specificity?
    a. 99.2%
    b. 98.7%
    c. 92.4%
    d. 87.3%
    e. 100.0%

15. The validity of a test is best defined as which of the following?
    a. the reliability of the test
    b. the reproducibility of the test
    c. the variation in the test results
    d. the degree to which the results of a measurement correspond to the true state of the phenomenon
    e. the degree of biologic variation of the test

16. Which of the following terms is synonymous with the term reliability?
    a. reproducibility
    b. validity
    c. accuracy
    d. mean
    e. variation

17. Which of the following is not a measure of central tendency?
    a. mean
    b. median
    c. mode
    d. standard deviation
    e. none; all of the above are measures of central tendency Gaussian distribution

Consider the following experimental data: In a trial of the effect of reducing multiple risk factors on the subsequent incidence of coronary artery disease, high-risk patients were selected for study. Elevated blood pressure was one of the risk factors for people to be considered. People were screened for inclusion in the study on three consecutive visits. Blood

pressures at those visits, before any therapeutic interventions were undertaken, were as listed in Table 2-4. Use the data in Table 2-4 to answer question 18.

18. Which of the following statements regarding these data is true?
    a. these results are very strange; consider publication in any journal specializing in irreproducible results
    b. this is an example of regression to the mean
    c. this is an example of natural variation
    d. the most likely explanation is either inter-observer or intraobserver variation
    e. we likely are dealing with faulty equipment in this case; the most likely reason for this would be failure to calibrate all of the blood pressure cuffs

Consider the following experimental data: A population of heavy smokers (men smoking more than 50 cigarettes per day) are divided into two groups and followed for a period of 10 years.
Use the data from Table 2-5 to answer question 19.

19. Regarding these results, which of the following statements is true?
    a. these results prove that screening chest x-rays improve survival time in lung cancer
    b. these results prove that screening chest x-rays should be considered for all smokers
    c. these results are most likely an example of lead-time bias

Table 2-5	10-Year Mortality Data		
Group	**Description**	**Diagnosed with Lung Cancer**	**Average Survival Time from Diagnosis**
Group 1 (experimental group)	490 individuals with annual chest x-rays	37	14 mo
Group 2 (control group)	510 individuals with no annual chest x-ray	39	8 mo

d. these results are most likely an example of length-time bias

e. these results do not make any sense; the experiment should be repeated

20. Length-time bias with respect to cancer diagnosis is defined as which of the following?
    a. bias resulting from the detection of slow-growing tumors during screening programs more often than fast-growing tumors
    b. bias resulting from the length of time a cancer was growing before any symptoms occurred
    c. bias resulting from the length of time a cancer was growing before somebody started to ask some questions and perform some laboratory investigations
    d. bias resulting from the length of time between the latent and more rapid growth phases of any cancer
    e. none of the above

21. Concerning population and disease measurement, prevalence is defined as which of the following?
    a. the fraction (proportion) of a population having a clinical condition at a given point in time
    b. the fraction (proportion) of a population initially free of a disease but that develops the disease over a given period
    c. equivalent to incidence
    d. mathematically as $a + b/(a + b + c + d)$ in a 2×2 table relating sensitivity and specificity to PPV
    e. none of the above

22. Concerning population and disease measurement, incidence is defined as which of the following?
    a. the fraction (proportion) of a population having a clinical condition at a given point in time
    b. the fraction (proportion) of a population initially free of a disease but that develops the disease over a given period
    c. equivalent to prevalence
    d. of little use in epidemiology
    e. none of the above

23. Regarding clinical epidemiology in relation to the discipline of family medicine, which of the following statements is true?
    a. clinical epidemiology is higher mathematics that bears little relation to the world in general, much less the specialty of family medicine
    b. clinical epidemiology was invented to create anxiety and panic attacks that mimic hyperthyroidism in medical students and residents

c. clinical epidemiology is unlikely to contain any useful information for the average practicing family physician

d. clinical epidemiology is a passing fad; fortunately for all concerned, its time has passed

e. none of the above statements about clinical epidemiology are true

Answers

1. a. The clinical decision-making process in family medicine involves four iterative steps: cue acquisition, hypothesis formation, the search, and plan. Cues come in a variety of different forms, including traditional patient-specific historical, physical examination, and laboratory data cues. There are also sensory cues, such as what we see, smell, hear, and feel about a patient and his or her story that we attend to; contextual cues, such as physical location of the encounter; and temporal cues, such as frequency, repetitions, intensity, and persistence of symptoms or signs: These are all part of our clinical thinking. The major mistakes we make as clinicians in cue acquisition are either missing or ignoring a cue or cues. However, from research we know that not all cues are attended to by experienced clinicians to arrive at a correct diagnosis. Inexperienced clinicians such as medical students often fail to attend to key cues, and as a result they often fail to consider proper hypotheses about what is going on to explain the patient's chief complaint.

2. b. Hypotheses are explanatory models of what we believe is going on in a patient. Traditionally, they lead to or are diagnoses. Hypotheses are generated and rank ordered based on the cues acquired. Knowledge of mortality and morbidity linked to cues helps clinicians to generate and rank order hypotheses. Other factors that influence hypotheses formation include experience, curiosity, and novelty. A variety of hypotheses are possible and important to consider, but hypotheses can be broadly placed into biomedical and psychosocial categories. The average skilled clinician will actively consider an average of five active hypotheses at any one time. The major error in clinical decision making overall is failure to generate or consider the correct hypothesis.

3. c. The search process gathers more cues to test the hypotheses being considered, and it is based on the science of probability. Hypotheses are weighed based on the sensitivity, specificity, and predictive value of cues in support or refute of a hypothesis. The search process relies on knowledge of prevalence of conditions in different populations and knowledge of the value of the cue with respect to the hypothesis. The major error is making assumptions about the sensitivity, specificity, or predictive value of data and coming to premature closure about a hypothesis under consideration. The inexperienced or not very careful decision maker often tries to squeeze as many cues into the incorrect hypothesis and often ignores nonsupporting cues.

The plan can be diagnostic or therapeutic or both. The plan should be patient centered, and often it is negotiated with the patient. Diagnostic and therapeutic plans may involve use of time, laboratory studies, pharmaco- and/or behavioral therapy, and consultation to gather new cues, test hypotheses, or provide definitive care. Follow-up is essential, and it is a hallmark in the patient–doctor relationship that facilitates decision making in family medicine. The major error in plan formation is not listening and considering the patient's needs and desires. Patient nonadherence is often a direct result.

Table 2-6 illustrates the answers to questions 4–9.

4. c. Sensitivity is defined as the proportion of people with the disease who have a positive test result. A sensitive test rarely will miss patients who have the disease. In Table 2-6, sensitivity is defined as the number of true positives (TPs) divided by the number of true positives plus the number of false negatives (FNs). That is,

$$\text{Sensitivity} = \text{TP}/(\text{TP} + \text{FN})$$

$$\text{Sensitivity} = a/(a + c) = 30/40 = 75\%$$

A sensitive test (one that is usually positive in the presence of disease) should be selected when there is an important penalty for missing the disease. This would be the case if you had reason to suspect a serious but treatable condition—for example, obtaining a chest x-ray in a patient with suspected tuberculosis or Hodgkin's disease. In addition, sensitive tests are useful in the early stages of a diagnostic workup of disease, when several possibilities are being considered, to reduce the number of possibilities. Thus, in

Table 2-6	Disease X	
	Disease X Present	**Disease X Absent**
Test A positive	30 (*a*) TP	50 (*b*) FP
Test A negative	10 (*c*) FN	80 (*d*) TN

FN, false negative; FP, false positive; TN, true negative; TP, true positive.

situations such as this, diagnostic tests are used to rule out diseases.

5. d. Specificity is defined as the proportion of people without the disease who have a negative test result. A specific test rarely incorrectly classifies people without the disease as having the disease. In Table 2-6, specificity is defined as the number of true negatives (TNs) divided by the number of true negatives plus the number of false positives (FPs). That is,

$$\text{Specificity} = \text{TN}/(\text{TN} + \text{FP})$$

$$\text{Specificity} = d/(d + b) = 80/130 = 61.5\%$$

A specific test is useful to confirm, or rule in, a diagnosis that has been suggested by other tests or data. Thus, a specific test is rarely positive in the absence of disease—that is, it gives very few false positive test results. Tests with high specificity are needed when false positive results can harm the patient physically, emotionally, or financially. Thus, a specific test is most helpful when the test result is positive.

There is always a trade-off between sensitivity and specificity. In general, if a disease has a low prevalence, choose a more specific test; if a disease has a high prevalence, choose a more sensitive test.

6. a. Positive predictive value (PPV) is defined as the probability of disease in a patient with a positive (abnormal) test result. In Table 2-6, the PPV is as follows:

$$\text{PPV} = a/(a + b) = 30/80 = 37.5\%$$

7. b. Negative predictive value (NPV) is defined as the probability of not having the disease when the test result is negative. In Table 2-6, the NPV is as follows:

$$\text{NPV} = d/(c + d) = 80/90 = 89\%$$

8. b. The likelihood ratio of a positive test result is the probability of that test result in the presence of disease divided by the probability of the test result in the absence of disease. In Table 2-6, the likelihood ratio is as follows:

Likelihood ratio (+) test results $a/(a + c)$ divided by $b/(b + d) = 30/(30 + 10)$ divided by $50/(50 + 80)$ or 1.95

9. b. The prevalence of a disease in the population at risk is the fraction or proportion of a group with a clinical condition at a given point in time. Prevalence is measured by surveying a defined population containing people with and without the condition of interest (at a given point in time). Prevalence can be equated

Table 2-7 Calculations Involved in a General 2 × 2 Table

	TARGET DISORDER	
	Present	**Absent**
Test positive	Cell a = (sensitivity) $(a + c)$	Cell b = $(b + d) - d$
Test negative	Cell c = $(a + c) - a$	Cell d = (specificity) $(b + d)$
Column sums	$a + c$	Total − $(a + c)$
Total = $a + b + c + d$		

with pretest probability. In Table 2-6, prevalence is defined as follows:

$$Prevalence = (a + c)/(a + b + c + d)$$

that is, $(a + c)$ divided by $(a + b + c + d) = (30 + 10)/(30 + 10 + 50 + 80) = 23.5$

As prevalence decreases, PPV must decrease along with it and NPV must increase.

10. **a.** Answers 10 and 11 are explained in answer 12, including Table 2-7.

11. **b.** See answer 12.

12. **d.** The respective PPVs for test A in the diagnosis of disease X in the general population, women older than age 50 years, and women older than 65 years with a suspicious finding on clinical examination are 0.4%, 3.9%, and 84.2%, respectively.

To perform the calculations necessary to obtain these answers, the following steps are recommended:

Step 1: Identify the sensitivity and specificity of the sign, symptom, or diagnostic test that you plan to use. Many of these are published. If you are not certain, consider asking a consultant with expertise in the area.

Step 2: Using a 2 × 2 table, set your total equal to an even number (consider, for example, 1000 as a good choice). Therefore,

$$a + b + c + d = 1000$$

Step 3: Using whatever information you have about the patient before you apply this diagnostic test, estimate his or her pretest probability (prevalence) of the disease in question. Next, put appropriate column summation numbers at the bottom of the columns $(a + c)$ and $(b + d)$. The easiest way to do this is to express your pretest probability (or prevalence) as a decimal three places to the right. This result is $(a + c)$, and 1000 minus this result is $(b + d)$.

Step 4: Start to fill in the cells of the 2 × 2 table. Multiply sensitivity (expressed as a decimal) by $(a + c)$ and put the result in cell a. You can then calculate cell c by simple subtraction.

Step 5: Similarly, multiply specificity (expressed as a decimal) by $(b + d)$ and put the result in cell d. Calculate cell b by subtraction.

Step 6: You now can calculate PPVs and NPVs for the test with the prevalence (pretest probability) used.

For example, to calculate the PPV for test A in the diagnosis of disease in women older than 65 years of age with a suspicious finding on clinical examination, use the following equation:

$$Prevalence = 40,000 \, cases/100,000 = 400/1000$$

Setting the total number equal to 1000,

$$(a + c)/(a + b + c + d) = 400/1000$$

Therefore, $a + c = 400$ and $b + d = 600$.
Thus,

$$Cell \, a = sensitivity \times 400 = 0.8 \times 400 = 320$$

and

$$Cell \, c = 400 - 320 = 80$$

Similarly,

$$Cell \, d = specificity \times 600 = 0.9 \times 600 = 540$$

Therefore,

$$Cell \, b = 600 - 540 = 60$$

$$PPV = a/(a + b) = 320/(320 + 60) = 84.2\%$$

Similar calculations can be made for the general population (prevalence = 50/100,000) and for women older than age 50 years (prevalence = 500/100,000).

13. **a.** If the PPV of a test for a given disease is 4%, then only 4 of 100 positive test results will be TPs; the remainder will be FPs. Further testing (often invasive) and anxiety will be inflicted on the 96% of the population with a positive test result but without disease.

Thus, careful consideration should be given to the PPV of any test for any disease in a given population before ordering it.

14. **e.** Remember the inverse relationship between sensitivity and specificity: If the sensitivity decreases, the specificity increases, and if the sensitivity increases, the specificity decreases. The only value that is greater than the previous specificity of 99.4% is 100%; therefore, it is the most likely correct value of the values listed for the specificity of the test. The value in the table is actually the case at a cutoff blood sugar level of 180 mg/100 mL 2 hours after eating; if we use this value for the cutoff, there will be even more false negative results than at 140 mg/100 mL. That is, we will incorrectly label more individuals who actually have diabetes as being normal, whereas we will not label anyone who does not have diabetes as having diabetes.

15. d. Validity is the degree to which the results of a measurement of a test actually correspond to the true state of the phenomenon being measured.

16. a. Reliability is the extent to which repeated measurements of a relatively stable phenomenon fall closely to each other. Reproducibility and precision are other words for this characteristic.

17. d. A normal, or Gaussian, distribution is characterized by the following measures of central tendency: (1) a mean: the sum of values for observations divided by the number of observations; (2) a median: the value point where the number of observations above equals the number of observations below; and (3) a mode: the most frequently occurring value.

In the same normal, or Gaussian, distribution, expressions of dispersion are the following: (1) the range: from the lowest value to the highest value in a distribution; (2) the standard deviation: the absolute value of the average difference of individual values from the mean; and (3) the percentile: the proportion of all observations falling between specified values.

The most valuable measure of dispersion in a normal, or Gaussian, distribution is the standard deviation (SD). It is defined as follows:

$$SD = (\sqrt{\sum x} - x^2)/(n - 1)$$

In a normal, or Gaussian, distribution 68.26% of the values lie within ±1 SD from the mean, 95.44% of values lie within ±2 SD from the mean, and 99.72% of values lie within ±3 SD from the mean.

18. b. As can be seen in this trial, there was a progressive and substantial decrease in mean blood pressure between the first and third visits. The explanation for this is called regression to the mean. The following is the best explanation of regression to the mean.

Patients who are singled out from others because they have a laboratory test that is unusually high or low can be expected, on average, to be closer to the center of the distribution (normal or Gaussian) if the test is repeated. Moreover, subsequent values are likely to be more accurate estimates of the true value (validity), which could be obtained if the measurement were repeated for a particular patient many times.

19. c. This is an example of lead-time bias. Lead time is the period between the detection of a medical condition by screening and when it ordinarily would have been diagnosed as a result of symptoms.

For lung cancer, there is absolutely no evidence that chest x-rays have any influence on mortality. However, if, as in this case, the experimental group had chest x-rays done, their lung cancers would have been diagnosed at an earlier time and it would appear that they were longer survivors. The control group most likely would have had their lung cancers diagnosed when they developed symptoms. In fact, however, the survival time would have been exactly the same; the only difference would have been that men in the experimental group would have known that they had lung cancer for a longer period.

20. a. Length-time bias occurs because the proportion of slow-growing lesions diagnosed during a cancer screening program is greater than the proportion of those diagnosed during usual medical care. The effect of including a greater number of slow-growing cancers makes it seem that the screening and early treatment programs are more effective than they really are.

21. a. Prevalence is defined as the fraction (proportion) of a population with a clinical condition at a given point in time. Prevalence is measured by surveying a defined population in which some patients have and some patients do not have the condition of interest at a single point in time. It is not the same as incidence, and as previously discussed in relation to sensitivity, specificity, and PPV in a 2×2 table, it is defined in mathematic terms as $a + c/(a + b + c + d)$.

22. b. Incidence in relation to a population is defined as the fraction (proportion) initially free of a disease or condition that go on to develop it over a given period. Commonly, it is known as the number of new cases per population in a given time, often per year.

23. e. Clinical epidemiology is a specialty that will assume increasingly more importance in the specialty of family medicine. Clinical epidemiology allows us to understand disease, to understand laboratory testing, and to understand why we should do what we should do and why we should not do what we should not do. More important, as family physicians are called on by governments, patients, licensing bodies, and boards to justify clinical decisions and treatments, it will allow us to understand the difference between "defensive" medicine and defensible medicine (the latter being what we are trying to achieve) in the interest of optimizing the health care of patients.

Summary

1. The process of clinical decision making in family medicine is essentially a four-step iterative process: cue acquisition, hypothesis formation, the search, and plan.

2. Cues come in a variety of different forms, including traditional patient-specific historical, physical examination, and laboratory data cues, as well as sensory cues (e.g., what we see, smell, hear, and feel about a patient and their story) and contextual cues (e.g., physical location cues such as the emergency room, office, hospital, and home, and temporal cues such as frequency, repetitions, intensity, and persistence of symptoms or signs). The major mistakes we make as clinicians in cue acquisition are either missing or ignoring a cue or cues. However, we know that not all cues are attended to by experienced clinicians to arrive at a correct diagnosis.

3. Hypotheses are explanatory models of what we believe is going on in a patient. Traditionally, they lead to or are diagnoses. A variety of hypotheses are possible and important to consider, but hypotheses can be broadly classified into biomedical and psychosocial categories. Hypotheses are generated and rank ordered based on the cues acquired. Knowledge of mortality and morbidity linked to the cues acquired helps clinicians to generate and rank order hypotheses. Other factors that influence hypothesis formation include experience, curiosity, and novelty. The average skilled clinician will actively consider an average of five active hypotheses at any one time. The major error in clinical decision making with respect to hypothesis formation is failure to generate or consider the correct hypothesis.

4. The search process gathers more cues to test the hypotheses being considered and is based on the science of probability. Hypotheses are weighed based on the sensitivity, specificity, and predictive value of cues in support or refute of a hypothesis. The search process relies on knowledge of prevalence of conditions in different populations and knowledge of the value of the cue with respect to the hypothesis. The major error is making assumptions about the sensitivity, specificity, or predictive value of data and coming to premature closure about a hypothesis under consideration.

5. The plan can be diagnostic or therapeutic or both. It should be patient centered, often is negotiated with the patient, and can involve use of time, laboratory studies, pharmaco- and/or behavioral therapy, and consultation to gather new cues, test hypotheses, or provide definitive care. Follow-up is essential, and it is a hallmark in the patient–doctor relationship that facilitates decision making in family medicine. The major error in plan formation is not listening and considering the patient's needs and desires. Patient nonadherence is often a direct result.

6. The summary of calculations related to search process statistics is described by the following 2×2 table:

	Disease or Hypothesis Present	Disease or Hypothesis Absent
Test or cue positive	*a*	*b*
Test or cue negative	*c*	*d*

$$\text{Prevalence} = a + b + c + d$$
$$\text{Sensitivity} = a/(a + c)$$
$$\text{Specificity} = d(b + d)$$
$$\text{Positive predictive value} = a/(a + b)$$
$$\text{Negative predictive value} = d/(c + d)$$
$$\text{Likelihood ratio positive test results}$$
$$= a/(a + c) \div b/(b + d)$$

7. Remember the importance of sensitivity, specificity, and especially PPV; understand that the lower the prevalence (or likelihood) of a condition in the patient about to be tested, the lower the PPV of the test. In outpatient, low-prevalence situations, NPV is often more useful, if it is known.

8. Understand the importance of false negative results and especially false positive results in the laboratory tests that you order.

9. Be prepared to draw a 2×2 table and calculate the PPV of a test given the sensitivity, specificity, and prevalence of the condition in the population.

10. Misinterpretations of survival statistics in cancer are often caused by lead-time bias and length-time bias.

Suggested Reading

Greenberg RS: *Medical Epidemiology*, 4th ed. New York, McGraw-Hill, 2005.

Guyatt GH, Rennie D: *Users' Guides to the Medical Literature: A Manual for Evidence-Based Clinical Practice. JAMA* online, accessed January 6, 2008.

CHAPTER

3   Consultation and Team Care

CLINICAL CASE PROBLEM 1

Who Ya Gonna Call

You are a recently graduated family physician new to a community practice made up of two other family physicians, a family nurse practitioner, and a physician assistant. You see a 47-year-old patient for several visits and are concerned about whether he should undergo a cardiac catheterization because of a 2-year history of intermittent but stable chest pain and a strong family history of premature cardiac mortality.

SELECT THE BEST ANSWER TO THE FOLLOWING QUESTIONS

1. Which of the following is/are among the factors you will consider in choosing the consultant:
   a. the skill and reputation of the cardiologist
   b. the geographic convenience for the patient
   c. the experience of other practitioners in your practice with the subspecialist
   d. the skill of the consultant is the only important consideration
   e. a, b, and c are correct
   f. a and c are correct

2. After choosing the appropriate consultant, you dictate a letter. The content of the letter should include all of the following except:
   a. a brief history
   b. a brief physical examination
   c. a directive that catheterization be done as soon as possible
   d. the type of help you are asking for
   e. any supporting laboratory data

3. Your communication expectations of the consultant should reasonably include which of the following:
   a. clear response regarding the diagnosis and management plan
   b. justification for the course of action outlined
   c. communication regarding the patient via telephone or in writing or both
   d. a and b
   e. a, b, and c

4. Your patient sees the consultant and returns to see you 3 weeks later confused by what was told to him by the consultant. You call the consultant but are told by her receptionist that she is too busy right now to come to the phone. Options at this time include all of the following except:
   a. ask to speak directly to the physician later in the day when she is available
   b. ask the patient to return to the consultant for another visit to get a clearer understanding of the recommendations and plan
   c. not using this consultant again
   d. seeking the opinion of another consultant if communication does not improve
   e. asking the receptionist to fax the consultant's letter of consultation if there is one

5. You later learn from the patient that the consultant had referred the patient to another consultant without your knowledge. Circumstances and reasons why this is problematic for both you and the patient include which of the following:
   a. such behavior disrupts continuity of care
   b. it may result in unnecessary utilization of additional resources
   c. the problem may have been handled by you
   d. it may add unnecessary inconvenience and expense for the patient
   e. all of the above

CLINICAL CASE PROBLEM 2

Who's on First, What's on Second

You attend your first meeting of the practice clinicians and staff. The practice leader says she wants to improve teamwork in the office. She defines teamwork as people working together cooperatively and effectively. Knowing that you have just graduated from a residency program known for its team-based care, she asks your advice.

6. Factors that improve practice functioning and teamwork include all of the following except:
   a. building trusting relationships
   b. having a diversity of perspectives
   c. using mostly written communication
   d. encouraging varied interactions
   e. b and d

7. Techniques to build some of these factors include all of the following except:
   a. create opportunities for interprofessional education
   b. expand skills in feedback, negotiation, and conflict resolution
   c. have practice leaders model the desired behavior
   d. isolate and ignore behaviors that inhibit collaboration
   e. develop a routine for managing conflict

8. You decide it is time to implement an electronic medical record in your practice. Reasonable expectations of what a working system will bring to the practice include which of the following:
   a. communication is likely to improve
   b. office efficiency is likely to improve
   c. patient care is likely to improve
   d. billing is likely to improve
   e. none of the above

Answers

1. e. There are many factors to consider when choosing a consultant. Certainly the expertise and skill set of the consultant are important. Whether the consultant participates in the patient's health plan and whether the consultant is within a reasonable distance geographically are two other considerations. The family physician is also in a good position to match patient to consultant in terms of personality type. Prior experience with a consultant is a good guiding factor in considering subsequent use. Did the patients have a good experience? Did you have a good experience as the referring physician?

2. c. Good communication is essential to the patient–doctor relationship and also for the physician–consultant–patient triad. At a minimum, you should provide written communication that outlines a brief history, physical and laboratory findings, and a clear statement of the type of help you are seeking.

3. e. The consultant, at a minimum, should provide timely, clear written information about the help you are seeking, which may include a clear response regarding the help you were requesting, a diagnosis and recommended management plan, and justification for the course of action outlined. In urgent situations, communication by telephone or in person is appropriate, to be followed up by written communication.

4. b. What to do about a consultant who has not fulfilled expectations is a common problem. In this instance, 3 weeks is more than enough time to expect written communication regarding a consultation. Of course, direct communication is imperative, and you may have been the victim of an overly protective staff member. Or the physician may have been genuinely unable to come to the telephone. Requesting the physician notes or other information is perfectly reasonable, but in this case it should not substitute for a formal form of written communication. In any event, the patient should not bear the burden of the noncommunication. If communication difficulties become a pattern, using another consultant in the future is an option.

5. e. The ping-ponging of patients among consultants without the involvement and coordination of care by the primary care physician is one of the main contributing factors to poor quality and high costs of health care in the United States. Such behavior disrupts continuity of care, and it makes a joke of the idea of a medical home for patients. In addition to unnecessary inconvenience and expense for the patient, it may result in unnecessary utilization of additional resources for a problem that may have been handled by you in the first place, and in the worst-case scenario it may lead to iatrogenesis.

6. c. Teamwork can be defined as people working together cooperatively and effectively for some common purpose. Teamwork in family medicine offices is dependent on good work relationships among team members. Characteristics of work relationships associated with successful practices have been studied and include the following: high levels of trust among team members; the presence of respectful, mindful, and heedful interactions among all parties; a tolerance for the expression of a diversity of ideas; a mix of rich (face-to-face) and lean (written) communication; and the presence of both social and task-oriented interactions.

7. d. There are a number of ways to successfully build some of the work relationship characteristics listed in answer 6 that are associated with successful practices. These include creating opportunities for interprofessional education, such as noontime interdisciplinary seminars and lunches; holding training sessions to expand and model everyone's skills in feed-back, negotiation, and conflict resolution; engaging practice leaders to model desired behaviors; and developing a routine for identifying and managing conflict so that behaviors that inhibit collaboration are not ignored but surfaced and successfully addressed. Building successful work relationships is difficult work, but it is necessary for good patient care. If done correctly, it can enhance workplace productivity and contribute to growth and enjoyment of one's role as a team member in effective health care delivery.

8. e. Implementing an electronic medical record (EMR) is being promoted by many quality-oriented organizations as an important step toward safer and more effective health care for patients. Used properly under the correct conditions, it can add immensely to improvements in a practice's quality of care and efficiency. However, multiple studies have demonstrated that it is not the panacea many have proposed it to be. An EMR will not make a dysfunctional office functional. Paper systems perform just as effectively in some offices, and careful attention to the underlying work relationships is even more important to problem solving than implementing an EMR. Otherwise, what you will get is an office with the same old problems plus an EMR.

Summary

No physician is an island, and the arts of consultation and collaboration are essential for good patient care, particularly for patient safety. In many respects, consultation is about communication skills, and like every interprofessional encounter, communication is a two-way street.

Among the factors that should be considered in choosing a consultant are

- skill and reputation of the consultant
- convenience and "match" with the patient's need and personality
- prior experience with the consultant

The requestor of the consultation should provide the consultant with the following:

- brief history
- brief physical examination
- any supporting laboratory data
- clear communication about the type of help you are asking for

In return, it is reasonable to expect the following from consultants in an appropriate and reasonable time frame:

- clear response regarding the diagnosis and recommended management plan
- justification for the course of action outlined
- communication regarding the patient via telephone or in writing or both

- return of the patient to you for coordination of any additional care that is needed, unless you request otherwise

Similarly, teamwork in the office, hospital, or other settings requires relationship building among people caring for patients. Work relationships within primary care practices affect the functioning and quality of care delivered by practices.

- Characteristics of work relationships associated with successful practices include high levels of trust; the presence of respectful, mindful, and heedful interactions; a tolerance for diversity of ideas; a mix of rich (face-to-face) and lean (written) communication; and the presence of both social and task-oriented interactions.
- Enhanced work relationships invest all members in practice goals, empower everyone to share insights that improve information flow and decision making, and enable a process of continuous reflection and renewal that facilitates practice improvement.
- Techniques to build better work relationships include creating opportunities for interprofessional education; expanding everyone's skills in feedback, negotiation, and conflict resolution; modeling desired behavior (especially by leaders); and directly confronting behaviors that inhibit collaboration through the development of a routine for managing conflict.

Suggested Reading

Gerardi D, Fontaine DK: True collaboration: Envisioning new ways of working together. *AACN Advanced Crit Care* 18(1):10–14, 2007.

Kripalani S, LeFevre F, Phillips CO, et al: Deficits in communication and information transfer between hospital-based and primary care physicians: Implications for patient safety and continuity of care. *JAMA* 297(8):831–841, 2007.

Piterman L, Koritsas S: Part II. General practitioner–specialist referral process. *Internal Med J* 35(8):491–496, 2005.

Smith SM, Allwright S, O'Dowd T: Effectiveness of shared care across the primary–specialty care interface in chronic disease management. *Cochrane Database Syst Rev* 3:CD004910, 2004.

Tallia AF, Lanham HJ, McDaniel RR Jr, Crabtree BF: Seven characteristics of successful work relationships. *Fam Pract Manage* 13(1):47–50, 2006.

CHAPTER

4 Managing Multiple Morbidities

CLINICAL CASE PROBLEM

A Case of Discontinuitis Ma[...]

A new patient presents to yo[...] your community from a differ[...] year-old recently divorced m[...] a history of recent-onset dia[...] hypertension, moderate obe[...] She smokes half a pack of [...] gets insufficient exercise, tr[...] an erratic diet. She compla[...] are worsening with stress [...] intermittent fatigue with sn[...] somnolence, and hot flushes. [...] medications from six different doctors she has irregularly seen in her previous locale, but she has not been seen in follow-up by any of them for the past 4 months.

SELECT THE BEST ANSWER TO THE FOLLOWING QUESTIONS

1. Given her symptom complex, at this time she is likely to need the services of which of the following subspecialists:
   a. a cardiologist
   b. a psychiatrist
   c. a sleep specialist
   d. an endocrinologist
   e. none of the above

   On examination, vital signs are as follows: body mass index, 30; blood pressure, 150/85; pulse, 85/minute; and respirations, 18/minute. She appears well developed, overnourished, neat, and well spoken. There are boggy nasal passages, nicotine staining on her bucal

mucosa, clear lungs, and a normal sounding heart. Abdomen is obese, and skin is warm and dry. Extremities are without clubbing, cyanosis, or edema. Peripheral pulses are normal and symmetrical. Affect is appropriate, but mood [...]sed. *why no TSH?*

[...]tory data would you like to obtain at [...] blood count (CBC), comprehensive [...]c panel (CMP), lipid profile, and elec-[...]gram (ECG)
[...]MP, lipid profile, hemoglobin A1c, and
[...]CMP, lipid profile, hemoglobin A1c, [...]nd thyroid-stimulating hormone
[...]CMP, lipid profile, hemoglobin A1c, and [...]-ray
[...]w testing is necessary at this time; obtain [...]ords first

3. Results from the Medical Outcomes Study suggest which of the following is (are) true regarding systems of care for this patient:
   a. optimal clinical outcomes are best achieved when care is provided by a generalist
   b. optimal clinical outcomes are best achieved when care is provided by subspecialists
   c. Costs of care and resource utilization tend to be lower when care is provided by generalists
   d. Similar clinical outcomes are achieved when care is provided by either a generalist or subspecialists
   e. c and d are correct

4. This case points out that which of the following is (are) among the skills needed to manage patients with multiple morbidities:
   a. the capacity to thrive on managing complex medical problems
   b. the ability to integrate all of the medical and personal issues facing an individual
   c. the ability to break down medical terms and complex medical issues to make it easier for patients to understand

PRACTICE YOUR ENGLISH
MEET YOUR
CONVERSATION PARTNER

DATE: ✗ 24/ 1:30 - 2:30
        19/4 - 5

TIME: _____

TO CANCEL, CALL 703-689-2700

d. the capacity to know and understand peoples' limitations, problems, and personal beliefs when deciding on a treatment
e. all of the above

5. In addition to reviewing all her current medications, obtaining any previous medical records you can, and ordering some laboratory data, your next step in management should include which of the following:
a. assessing the patient's understanding of her health problems
b. getting a sense of the patient's priorities in dealing with her health problems
c. reordering all her medications and stressing the importance of compliance
d. identifying community resources that can be brought to bear in a treatment plan
e. a, b, and d

6. You decide to enter the patient in your office-based disease registry. Which of the following is (are) true regarding disease registries:
a. they are a useful way for tracking practice adoption of disease and patient-centered guidelines
b. they require the use of an electronic medical record
c. they can facilitate population-based interventions such as hemoglobin A1c tracking or influenza immunizations
d. a and c
e. they are primarily a research tool of little use clinically

7. Regarding adapting your practice to dealing with the complexities of patients with multiple morbidities, all of the following are true except:
a. as the population ages, the problem of multiple morbidities generally exacerbates
b. implementing a self-audit and feedback function in a practice is a valid way of assessing overall practice performance
c. using information from administrative data sets provides more than adequate understanding of practice performance in treating different conditions
d. enlisting all practice members in quality-focused initiatives builds practice capacity for dealing with patient complexity
e. understanding the epidemiology and interaction of multiple risk factors is increasingly important in patients with multiple morbidities

Answers

1. **e.** You are a long way from consulting or referring to anyone. You must first get a clearer understanding of this patient's problems and how they interrelate. As the family physician, you are in the best position to do so, and it is your responsibility to do so.

2. **b.** Normally, it would be best to get old records before obtaining laboratory tests, particularly if the situation is not urgent. However, in the case of the previously fractured care experienced by this patient and the time since the last visit to all the subspecialists, the likelihood of receiving timely information in a timely manner is limited. Therefore, obtaining baseline information in this patient's situation is most appropriate. Of the combinations listed, that of CBC, CMP, lipid profile, HgbA1c, and ECG is most reasonable to cover this patient's multiple morbidities listed in the history.

3. **e.** The Medical Outcomes Study is the classic well-designed comprehensive study that compared outcomes of care in generalists and subspecialists after controlling for patient mix. Reported in *The Journal of the American Medical Association* and other medical journals, the comprehensive study found no difference in medical outcomes between generalists and subspecialists for patients with diabetes and hypertension who were followed for 7 years. Outcomes included measures of physical and emotional (functional) health, mortality, and disease-specific physiologic markers. However, there were significant differences with regard to lower resource utilization and cost for patients of primary care physicians due to more judicious use of tests, procedures, drugs, office visits, and hospitalizations.

4. **e.** Multiple skills are needed to manage patients with multiple morbidities. These include the capacity to thrive on managing complex medical problems; the ability to integrate all of the medical and personal issues facing an individual and his or her family members; the ability to break down medical terms and complex medical issues to make it easier for patients to understand; the capacity to develop long-term healing relationships with patients; the capacity to know and understand peoples' limitations, problems, and personal beliefs when deciding on a treatment; the ability to provide care that includes long-term behavioral change interventions that lead to better health; the ability to empower patients with information and guidance that are needed to maintain health over time; and the ability to link patients to appropriate community resources and to mobilize and

facilitate proper use of and communication among those resources. The family physician, by virtue of his or her training, is uniquely positioned to deliver these skills to patients with multiple morbidities.

5. **e.** Without a clear knowledge of the patient's understanding of her medical conditions, or an assessment of the patient's priorities in dealing with her health problems, reordering all her medications is likely to be a wasted opportunity to identify and prioritize the patient's needs and conditions. Without this information, stressing the importance of compliance is a waste of time. This is also an opportunity to identify community resources that can be brought to bear in a treatment plan.

6. **d.** Disease registries are a useful way for tracking practice adoption of disease- and patient-centered guidelines. It is a common misunderstanding that in order to have a disease registry you need an electronic medical record. This is not the case. Registries can facilitate population-based interventions such as hemoglobin A1c tracking or influenza immunizations, as well as facilitate and track other patient-centered interventions. Although some have been used in practice-based research, their primary application is in clinical care.

7. **c.** As the population ages, the problem of multiple morbidities generally exacerbates. Many clinicians have implemented a self-audit and feedback function in their practice, and they have found these to be valid ways of assessing overall practice performance. The use of information from administrative data sets in an attempt to provide an understanding of practice performance in treating different conditions has been a common practice of insurance companies for many years. However, these databases have been fraught with poor quality of data and are generally inadequate to measure individual practice or provider performance. Combined with chart audit, they become more useful. Enlisting all practice members in quality-focused initiatives builds practice capacity for dealing with patient complexity. Understanding the epidemiology and interaction of multiple risk factors is increasingly important in patients with multiple morbidities.

Summary

Managing patients with multiple morbidities is one of the primary problems confronting the health care system in the 21st century. This problem is especially well suited for the skill set of primary care physicians. Complexities increase as problems multiply, and dealing with complexity is a particular skill set of the family physician. The specific skills needed to deal with patients with multiple morbidities include

- the capacity to thrive on managing complex medical problems
- the ability to integrate all of the medical and personal issues facing an individual and his or her family members
- the ability to break down medical terms and complex medical issues to make it easier for patients to understand
- the capacity to develop long-term healing relationships with patients

- the capacity to know and understand peoples' limitations, problems, and personal beliefs when deciding on a treatment
- the ability to provide care that includes long-term behavioral change interventions that lead to better health
- the ability to empower patients with information and guidance that are needed to maintain health over time
- the ability to link patients to appropriate community resources and to mobilize and facilitate proper use of and communication among those resources

Modifying the practice to equip all members to contribute to the problem of managing patients with multiple morbidities is important, as is developing systems and processes to monitor practice performance. Effective methodologies include the use of patient disease registries to monitor populations in need of particular care, and the use of audit and feedback to assess practice and physician performance with respect to particular conditions or groups of conditions.

Suggested Reading

Baicker K, Chandra A: Medicare spending, the physician workforce, and beneficiaries' quality of care. *Health Affairs*, April 7, 2004.

Greenfield S, Rogers W, Mangotich M, et al: Outcomes of patients with hypertension and non-insulin-dependent diabetes mellitus treated by different systems and specialties. Results from the Medical Outcomes Study. *JAMA* 274:1436–1444, 1995.

Shi L, Macinko J, Starfield B, et al: Primary care, social inequalities, and all-cause, heart disease, and cancer mortality in U.S. counties. *Am J Public Health* 95:674–680, 2005.

CHAPTER

5 Quality Improvement

CLINICAL CASE PROBLEM 1

Quality Matters

An official from one of the insurance companies you participate with sets up an appointment to discuss quality improvement measures you are thinking about implementing in your office. In preparation for the meeting, you review the literature on quality improvement.

SELECT THE BEST ANSWER TO THE FOLLOWING QUESTIONS

1. Among the many possible online Internet sources for information about quality improvement, you find which of the following to be most reliable?
   a. the American Academy of Family Physicians (www.aafp.org)
   b. the Agency for Healthcare Research and Quality (www.ahrq.gov)
   c. the National Committee for Quality Assurance (www.ncqa.org)
   d. all of the above
   e. none of the above

2. One of the products of the National Committee for Quality Assurance that you run across online is HEDIS. Which of the following is (are) true about HEDIS?
   a. HEDIS stands for Health Employer Data and Information Series
   b. HEDIS contains measures of health care effectiveness and patient satisfaction
   c. HEDIS measures are not concerned about cost, just quality
   d. HEDIS measures are designed to be primarily applicable to patients with Medicare insurance
   e. HEDIS measures are updated every 5 years

3. Examples of HEDIS effectiveness of care measures applicable to family medicine outpatient practice include which of the following?
   a. measures of childhood immunization status
   b. colorectal cancer screening rates
   c. measures of influenza vaccination rates
   d. measures of frequency of ongoing prenatal visits
   e. a, b, and c are correct
   f. a, b, c, and d are correct

CLINICAL CASE PROBLEM 2

Improving Practice Quality

After reviewing the literature and reflecting on what you have found, you decide that good doctors should actively learn from their practices. This means taking the time to reflect upon your patient care practices, assimilate new and existing scientific evidence into your care of patients, and always seek ways to improve patient care.

4. Among the following measures you consider taking in your office practice to improve quality, which has been shown to be most effective?
   a. systematic collection and analysis of information about the clinical care provided in the context of evidence-based guidelines
   b. systematic analysis of practice experience, including feedback from patients, families, and the community
   c. regularly engaging staff in learning activities to advance competence and performance
   d. Only c has been shown to be effective
   e. a, b, and c are effective

5. Which of the following is (are) an essential element(s) of high-performing family medicine practices?
   a. an electronic patient clinical information system
   b. open and direct communication among all members of the practice

c. a leader who tolerates little deviance of accepted thought from employees
d. a and b are correct
e. a and c are correct

CLINICAL CASE PROBLEM 3

Measuring Quality

You decide to implement performance measures in your practice based on evidence of effectiveness targeting several major diseases in your patient population. In this process, you rely on performance measures for ambulatory care derived from the National Quality Forum.

6. Which of the following is (are) a reasonable performance measure(s) to assess your practice's preventive care delivery?
   a. rates of fecal occult blood testing for the past year in eligible men and women age 50 years or older
   b. the percentage of women between age of onset of sexual activity and 65 years who have had one or more Pap tests in the past 2 years
   c. the percentage of patients who smoke who received advice to quit smoking in the past year
   d. a and c
   e. a, b, and c

7. Which of the following is not a reasonable performance measure to assess your practice's care of patients with coronary heart disease (CAD) or heart failure?
   a. percentage of patients with CAD who were prescribed a lipid-lowering therapy
   b. percentage of patients with heart failure and left ventricular systolic dysfunction who were prescribed an angiotensin converting enzyme inhibitor or receptor blocker
   c. percentage of patients with three or more major risk factors and without contraindications who are on aspirin therapy
   d. percentage of patients with atrial fibrillation who are on warfarin therapy
   e. percentage of patients with CAD who have had an exercise stress test in the past year

8. Which of the following is not a reasonable performance measure to assess your practice's care of patients with diabetes?
   a. percentage of patients with diabetes with one or more hemoglobin A1c tests conducted during the past year

b. percentage of patients with diabetes seen by a podiatrist during the past year
c. percentage of patients with diabetes who had their blood pressure documented in the past year to be less than 140/90 mmHg
d. percentage of patients who received a retinal or dilated eye exam by an eye care professional during the past year or during the prior 2 years if the patient is at low risk for retinopathy
e. percentage of patients with diabetes with most recent LDL cholesterol less than 100 mg/dL

Answers

1. **d.** There are many sources of reliable information on quality improvement measures and interventions on the Internet. For the family physician, reliable sources include the Web sites of the American Academy of Family Physicians (AAFP), the federal Agency for Healthcare Research and Quality (AHRQ), and the National Committee for Quality Assurance (NCQA). The AAFP Web site (www.aafp.org,) for example, contains links to practice management and clinical care and research information. The AHRQ Web site (www.ahrq.gov) contains links to evidence-based practice reports, clinical practice guidelines, and information on preventive services. The NCQA Web site (www.ncqa.org) contains information on a variety of accepted quality of care measures, including the widely used HEDIS measures.

2. **b.** HEDIS stands for Health Effectiveness Data and Information Set. It is a set of widely used measures for assessing health care quality produced by NCQA. Updated yearly and applicable to all health insurance plans, HEDIS contains measures that cover a variety of quality domains, including measures of effectiveness of care, access and availability of care, satisfaction with the experience of care, use of care, costs of care, and health plan description and stability.

3. **e.** Examples of effectiveness of care measures in HEDIS include measures of childhood immunization rates, colorectal cancer screening rates, and influenza vaccination rates for applicable populations. Measures of frequency of ongoing prenatal visits are examples of utilization measures. For a complete listing of the HEDIS measures, visit the NCQA Web site at www.ncqa.org

4. **e.** All measures described have been shown to improve the quality of care delivered by primary care practices. Systematic collection and analysis of information about the clinical care provided in the context of evidence-based guidelines leads to understanding where

changes can be made to improve care. Systematic analysis of the practice experience, including specific feedback from patients, their families, and members of the community through surveys, can provide useful information to improve access and the quality of the process of care. Regularly engaging staff in learning activities to advance competence and performance is also a successful method for improving patient care quality.

5. b. A large body of literature supports the finding that primary care practices are not just small businesses but complex organizations whose success is dependent on all members of the organization, including staff as well as the physicians. In addition, studies have demonstrated that the quality of work relationships among members of the practice is important for the successful functioning and delivery of patient care. Characteristics of work relationships associated with successful practices include high levels of trust; the presence of respectful, mindful, and heedful interactions; a tolerance for diversity of ideas; a mix of rich (e.g., face-to-face) and lean (e.g., manuals and memos)

communication; and the presence of both social and task-oriented interactions. Although electronic clinical information systems can be useful to practices in the care of patients, they are not essential. What is essential is a well-organized team with common goals that puts the patient first.

6. e. There are a host of reasonable measures one could use based on U.S. Preventive Services guidelines. Performance measurers should be chosen and tailored to the individual practice's patient populations.

7. e. Exercise stress testing is not recommended on an annual basis for all patients with CAD. All other measures are reasonable and built on evidence-based guidelines.

8. b. Although proper foot care is important for patients with diabetes, there is no evidence that an annual visit to the podiatrist reduces morbidity in diabetics. Other measures listed are reasonable and approved by various organizations based on effectiveness studies.

Summary

1. Poor quality care leads to sicker patients, more disabilities, higher costs, and lower confidence in the health care system. Overwhelming evidence exists that primary care reduces mortality and costs, and it improves overall quality of the health care of the nation. Family physicians are in key positions to serve patients as navigators through our often dysfunctional health care system by seeking and obtaining data about quality of care.
2. Being good doctors also means actively learning from our practices and continually seeking to improve care provided. This means taking the time to reflect on our patient care practices and assimilate new and existing scientific evidence into our care of patients.
3. Reliable sources of information about quality include Web sites of the American Academy of Family Physicians, the Agency for Healthcare Quality and Research, and the National Committee for Quality Assurance. Other organizations involved in quality include the Institute of Medicine, the Leapfrog Group, and the Joint Commission.
4. HEDIS is a widely used measurement for assessing health care quality. Produced by the National Committee for Quality Assurance, it is updated yearly and is applicable to all health insurance plans. HEDIS measures cover a variety of quality domains, including

measures of effectiveness of care, access and availability of care, satisfaction with the experience of care, use and costs of care, and health plan descriptions and measures of stability.
5. There are a host of reasonable, evidenced-based performance measures that physicians can implement in their practices. Systematic collection and analysis of information about the clinical care provided in the context of evidence-based guidelines leads to understanding where changes can be made to improve care. Systematic analysis of survey feedback from patients, their families, and members of the community can provide useful information to improve access and the process of care. Regularly engaging staff in learning activities to advance competence and performance is also a successful method for improving patient care quality.
6. Quality of work relationships among practice members is important to successful functioning and delivery of patient care. Characteristics of work relationships associated with successful practices include high levels of trust; the presence of respectful, mindful, and heedful interactions; a tolerance for diversity of ideas; a mix of rich (e.g., face-to-face) and lean (e.g., manuals and memos) communication; and the presence of both social and task-oriented interactions.

Suggested Reading

Tallia AF, Lanham HJ, McDaniel R, et al: Seven characteristics of successful work relationships in primary care practices. *Fam Pract Manage* 13(1):47–57, 2006.

CHAPTER

6 Clinical Prevention

CLINICAL CASE PROBLEM 1

A 51-Year-Old Male Who Presents for an "Executive" Examination

A 51-year-old male comes to your office requesting an "executive" examination. He has been in the habit of receiving a yearly "executive" examination at work but recently has changed jobs. His new employer does not offer these services. The patient had been told by a health professional at his previous job that "a complete physical, head to toe, with lots of tests is the best method of ensuring maintenance of good health." He recently heard a radio advertisement for a company that "specializes" in executive examinations but decided to see you instead.

SELECT THE BEST ANSWER TO THE FOLLOWING QUESTIONS

1. With regard to the relative effectiveness of yearly "executive" examinations, which of the following statements is most accurate?
   a. the efficacy of yearly executive examinations has been confirmed in randomized controlled clinical trials
   b. the effectiveness of yearly executive examinations has been confirmed by anecdotal evidence
   c. the efficacy of yearly executive examinations has been demonstrated in case–control trials
   d. the efficacy of yearly executive examinations has been confirmed in population cohort studies
   e. none of the above statements are true

2. Which of the following is a criterion (or criteria) for effective periodic health screening interventions?
   a. the condition tested must have a significant effect on quality of life
   b. the disease must have an asymptomatic phase during which detection and treatment significantly reduce morbidity and mortality
   c. acceptable treatment methods must be available
   d. tests must be available at a reasonable cost
   e. all of the above are true

3. Good reasons to consider recommending a health maintenance visit for an asymptomatic adult include which of the following?
   a. to learn the patient's wishes regarding his or her health care
   b. to perform or order preventive health service interventions
   c. to maximize your income
   d. a and b
   e. a, b, and c

4. Which of the following statements regarding a health maintenance visit is (are) true?
   a. the visit in itself may be therapeutic and provide the patient with reassurance
   b. the visit provides an opportunity to update information in the patient's "medical home"
   c. the visit may produce benefit to the patient through therapeutic touch
   d. the visit may help to develop or reinforce the patient–doctor relationship
   e. all of the above are true

CLINICAL CASE PROBLEM 2

A 52-Year-Old Male Technophile

A 52-year-old long-time "worried well" male patient of yours schedules an appointment to discuss a newspaper report of a new cancer screening test now being offered locally. He brings the article, which recommends a new imaging procedure to search for lung cancer in former smokers. Your patient is a former smoker, and he asks if he should have the test now available at the local imaging facility. The test costs $2000 and is not covered by insurance. Yet the article claims that the test picks up 80% of "even tiny lung cancers" not seen on other "screening" tests. He mentions that when he called the facility to ask the physician questions about the procedure, he was told "ask your family doctor."

5. Which of the following statements regarding health screening interventions is (are) true?
   a. health screening interventions such as mammography are a form of primary prevention
   b. interventions that target low-prevalence conditions are acceptable if costs are low
   c. if questions exist regarding an intervention's efficacy, it is better to err on the side of commission than omission
   d. many interventions fail to demonstrate a beneficial effect on mortality despite high sensitivity and specificity
   e. none of the above statements are true

6. The U.S. Preventive Services Task Force (USPSTF) is an excellent source of screening recommendations for which of the following reasons?
   a. the task force is made up of family physicians
   b. the task force uses an expert opinion approach for issuing recommendations
   c. the evidence for and against an intervention is weighed
   d. recommendations are fixed in stone and will stand up in court
   e. a and c are true

7. Which of the following statements is (are) true regarding false-positive findings of screening tests?
   a. false-positive findings can create needless patient anxiety
   b. false-positive findings often initiate an "intervention cascade"
   c. false-positive findings place a substantial burden on the entire health care system
   d. a and b
   e. a, b, and c

8. Which of the following statements is true regarding patient perceptions of yearly executive examinations and related laboratory tests?
   a. many patients believe that a routine executive, complete examination, along with a complete laboratory profile, will diagnose the majority of illnesses
   b. most patients understand the meaning of the term health maintenance examination
   c. most patients understand the importance of a focused, regional examination
   d. patients are generally sensitive to the costs of routine physical examinations and routine laboratory tests
   e. none of the above statements are true

CLINICAL CASE PROBLEM 3

A 35-Year-Old Female Who Presents for a Health Maintenance Examination

A 35-year-old female has come to your office for a health maintenance examination. The physician examines the skin in an effort to identify dysplastic nevi, other unusual nevi, or other skin lesions.

9. Which of the following statements is true?
   a. the examination for skin cancer in a health maintenance examination is highly sensitive and highly specific
   b. the examination for skin cancer in a health maintenance examination is highly sensitive but of low specificity
   c. the examination for skin cancer in a health maintenance examination is neither sensitive nor specific
   d. the examination for skin cancer in a health maintenance examination is highly specific but of lower sensitivity
   e. the examination for skin cancer is of variable sensitivity and specificity depending on the skill of the examiner

Answers

1. **e.** Efficacy studies answer the question, "Does it work?" Effectiveness studies answer the question, "Does it work in the real world?" Although the yearly examination, including executive examinations, had been a primary diagnostic tool throughout much of the 20th century, there is little, if any, evidence in the literature to support its efficacy or effectiveness as a screening tool. The yearly physical examination should not be confused with the health maintenance assessment, for which there is ample evidence supporting its efficacy. The health maintenance assessment is an assessment targeted at specific age and gender causes of morbidity and mortality. Recommendations for the periodic health maintenance examination are derived from epidemiologic data that assess population risk and intervention benefit. Specific evidence-based screening and counseling interventions are part of the health maintenance examination. The USPSTF is the preeminent body for the assessment and recommendation of interventions that are a part of the periodic health maintenance examination.

2. **e.** The criteria for effective periodic health screening are as follows: (1) The condition for which the physician is testing must have a significant effect on the quality of the patient's life; (2) acceptable treatment methods must be available for that particular condition; (3) the disease must have an asymptomatic phase during which detection and treatment significantly reduce morbidity and mortality; (4) treatment during the asymptomatic phase must yield a result superior to that obtained by delaying treatment until symptoms appear; (5) tests must be available at a reasonable cost; (6) tests must be acceptable to the patient; and (7) the prevalence of the condition must be sufficient to justify the cost of screening.

3. d. See answer 4.

4. e. Reasons to perform a periodic health maintenance examination in asymptomatic adults include the following: (1) to establish or reinforce a good patient–doctor relationship; (2) to provide opportunity to learn the patient's wishes and augment information in the medical record; (3) to reinforce the primary care office as the patient's medical home and best source for advice and guidance; (4) to provide the therapeutic benefit of touch; (5) to perform appropriate periodic health screening interventions; (6) to reinforce patient education, especially lifestyle and nutritional counseling; (7) to realistically reassure the patient (and the physician); (8) to establish and enhance the patient's self-management skills; (9) to determine if the patient is indeed asymptomatic; and (10) to avoid giving the patient the impression that he or she must have symptoms to be examined.

5. d. There has been an avalanche of health screening recommendations recently emanating from a variety of sources, some of which must be viewed as suspect due to the secondary benefits accrued by the recommenders. It is difficult to pick up a newspaper and not find a new test or procedure being touted as the next best thing since free air. How does the family physician help patients sort it all out? Health screening interventions, such as mammography and colonoscopy, are a form of secondary prevention, designed to catch a disease process early in its asymptomatic stage. Primary prevention interventions such as immunization prevent the disease from occurring. Tertiary prevention interventions favorably alter the course of an illness by preventing complications, an example of which is anticoagulation for stroke prevention in atrial fibrillation.

Answer 2 discussed the criteria for a good screening intervention. Interventions that target low-prevalence conditions are unacceptable even if costs are low because they are a waste of money and may have untoward effects such as false-positive test results that may lead to iatrogenesis. Thus, if questions exist regarding an intervention's efficacy, it is better to err on the side of not performing the test. Many interventions fail to

demonstrate a beneficial effect on mortality despite high sensitivity and specificity. This was found to be the case with certain very sensitive imaging procedures for lung cancer. The family physician should be the best source of information regarding screening interventions if the patient's interests are kept at the forefront. The USPSTF is the best source of evidenced-based recommendations to guide screening recommendations.

6. c. Although family physicians have led the way in the United States with the first scientific studies advocating targeted screening examinations based on the epidemiology of problems seen in patients at different ages and in different genders, the USPSTF is now multidisciplinary, adding to its strength and legitimacy as a body that issues recommendations based on the strength and weight of the evidence available. Recommendations for screening procedures are carefully weighed based on available evidence for or against a procedure. A five-category rating system informs both doctor and patient about the strength of a recommendation or whether insufficient evidence for or against a procedure exists. So-called "expert" opinion is not a factor in decisions, and recommendations have been known to change if the scientific evidence one way or another evolves. For these reasons, the task force's recommendations are considered the gold standard of periodic health screening interventions. Recommendations and the evidence supporting them are available for review at the Agency for Healthcare Research and Quality Web site (www.ahrq.gov).

7. e. The same excessive compulsiveness that serves as a survival skill in medical training is often dysfunctional in medical practice. False-positive findings are common in the face of low test sensitivity and specificity and low prevalence of the condition in the population tested. Even if a test has high sensitivity and specificity, the more tests or maneuvers that are performed on the same individual, the higher the likelihood of a false-positive result. Also, the likelihood that a positive test is true positive (positive predictive value) is directly related to the prevalence of the condition in the target population. Performing examinations in populations in which the condition has a low prevalence will thus generate a high false-positive rate. False-positive test results create needless anxiety in both patients and physicians. More important, such results often lead to an "intervention cascade," initiating further testing of greater invasiveness, which increases the potential for iatrogenic harm. A good example of this is the finding of a slightly enlarged ovary (you think) on pelvic bimanual examination, a situation in which a benign cause is much more likely than a malignant cause.

From this may result routine ultrasound, followed perhaps by laparoscopy to rule out a malignant tumor of very low prevalence. We all must ask ourselves before initiating any intervention, "What is the evidence that this action is likely to do the patient any good?"

8. **a.** Many patients believe that an executive complete examination, along with a large number of laboratory tests, will diagnose the majority of illnesses. This is obviously a mistaken impression. Sadly, some health professionals have taken financial advantage of this misconception, playing off patients' needs for reassurance. Conversely, most patients are unaware of the hazards of unnecessary interventions and testing, and many physicians do not take the time to educate their patients of the hazards. As in any intervention, patients should be informed of the rationale (evidence and expected outcomes), risks, benefits, and alternatives of laboratory testing.

Despite efforts aimed at increasing public awareness and understanding, many patients do not understand the concept of health maintenance visits or of focused examinations. In addition, many patients are still not very sensitive about costs of "routine" examinations and tests. Further patient education efforts are necessary to inform patients regarding these important issues.

9. **e.** The clinical examination of the skin can have significant variability in terms of sensitivity and specificity depending on variability of the examiner's expertise. Although studies have demonstrated the effectiveness of family physicians in skin cancer screening relative to other specialists, variability exists in this or any other procedure. The greater the training and expertise in skin lesion diagnosis and treatment, the higher the sensitivity and specificity of the examination. Another excellent example of this phenomenon is radiologists reading mammograms. The more training the radiologist has and the more mammograms the radiologist reads, the higher the sensitivity and specificity of mammograms. Most studies report test results obtained under optimal conditions. Similarly, adverse outcomes, such as perforation rates in colonoscopy, are often derived from ideal study conditions. An important question to ask on behalf of the patient is, Are study conditions likely to be seen in my practice environment? It may be that the 1/1000 to 1/3000 risk of major complications in colonoscopy reported in the literature is really 1/500 to 1/1000 in the community. The family physician's role is to be a patient advocate and a skeptic when it comes to everything "new" and "better." Demand to see the scientific evidence before recommending and subjecting patients to the latest intervention.

Summary

1. Efficacy studies answer the question about an intervention, "Does it work?" effectiveness studies answer the question, "Does it work in the real world?" Both are important to ask and answer when weighing patient interventions geared toward prevention.
2. There is little, if any, evidence that yearly executive physicals are efficacious or effective or address issues and conditions that are preventable. The health maintenance assessment, in contrast, is an assessment targeted at specific age and gender prevalent causes of morbidity and mortality. Recommendations for the periodic health maintenance examination are derived from epidemiologic data that assess population risk and intervention benefit. Specific evidence-based screening and counseling interventions are part of the health maintenance examination.
3. The USPSTF is the preeminent body for the assessment and recommendation of interventions that are a part of the periodic health maintenance examination. USPSTF recommendations are evidence based, and the evidence for or against a particular intervention is rated and weighed.
4. Health screening interventions, such as mammography and colonoscopy, are a form of secondary prevention, designed to catch a disease process early in its asymptomatic stage. Primary prevention interventions such as immunization prevent the disease from occurring. Tertiary prevention interventions favorably alter the course of an illness by preventing complications, an example of which is anticoagulation for stroke prevention in atrial fibrillation.
5. Criteria for effective periodic health screening interventions are as follows:
   a. the condition for which the physician is testing must have a significant effect on the quality of the patient's life;
   b. acceptable treatment methods must be available for that particular condition;
   c. the disease must have an asymptomatic phase during which detection and treatment significantly reduce morbidity and mortality;
   d. treatment during the asymptomatic phase must yield a result superior to that obtained by delaying treatment until symptoms appear;
   e. tests must be available at a reasonable cost;
   f. tests must be acceptable to the patient; and
   g. the prevalence of the condition must be sufficient to justify the cost of screening.

Suggested Reading

The following are some of the historical, classic articles that challenged the established practice of yearly complete physicals:

Breslow L, Somers AR: The lifetime health monitoring program. *N Engl J Med* 296(11):601–608, 1997.

Frame PS: A critical review of adult health maintenance. Part 1: Prevention of atherosclerotic disease. *J Fam Pract* 22(4):341–346, 1986.

Frame PS: A critical review of adult health maintenance. Part 2: Prevention of infectious diseases. *J Fam Pract* 22(5):417–422, 1986.

Frame PS: A critical review of adult health maintenance. Part 3: Prevention of cancer. *J Fam Pract* 22(6):511–520, 1986.

Frame PS: A critical review of adult health maintenance. Part 4: Prevention of metabolic, behavioral, and miscellaneous conditions. *J Fam Pract* 23(1):29–39, 1986.

The full scope of the USPSTF recommendations may be viewed at the Web site www.ahrq.gov, clicking on 'Preventive Services' under 'Clinical Information.' You can also register for periodic updates from the USPSTF via e-mail through this site.

CHAPTER

7 Tobacco Dependency

CLINICAL CASE PROBLEM 1

A 40-Year-Old Who Smokes Three Packs of Cigarettes a Day

A 40-year-old executive who smokes three packs of cigarettes a day comes to your office for his routine health maintenance assessment. He states that he would like to quit smoking but is having great difficulty. He has tried three times before, but he says, "Pressures at work mounted up and I just had to go back to smoking."

The patient has a history of mild hypertension. His blood cholesterol level is normal. He drinks 1 or 2 ounces of alcohol per week. His family history is significant for premature cardiovascular disease and death.

SELECT THE BEST ANSWER TO THE FOLLOWING QUESTIONS

1. Current evidence suggests that coronary artery disease (CAD) is strongly related to cigarette smoking. What percentage of deaths from CAD is thought to be directly related to cigarette smoking?
   a. 5%
   b. 10%
   c. 20%
   d. 25%
   e. 30% to 40%

2. Which of the following diseases has (have) been linked to cigarette smoking?
   a. carcinoma of the larynx
   b. hypertension
   c. abruptio placenta
   d. Alzheimer's disease
   e. all of the above

3. Which of the following statements with respect to passive smoking is false?
   a. spouses of patients who smoke are not at increased risk of developing carcinoma of the lung
   b. sidestream smoke contains more carbon monoxide than mainstream smoke
   c. infants of mothers who smoke absorb measurable amounts of their mothers' cigarette smoke
   d. children of parents who smoke have an increased prevalence of bronchitis, asthma, and pneumonia
   e. the most common symptom arising from passive smoking is eye irritation

4. Of the following factors listed, which is the most important factor in determining the success of a smoking cessation program in an individual?
   a. the desire of the patient to quit smoking
   b. a pharmacologic agent as a part of the smoking cessation program
   c. the inclusion of a behavior-modification component to the program
   d. physician advice to quit smoking
   e. repeated office visits

5. Which of the following agents is (are) now considered a first-line pharmacologic agent(s) that reliably increase(s) long-term smoking abstinence rates?
   a. bupropion SR
   b. nicotine gum
   c. nicotine inhalers or nasal sprays
   d. nicotine patch
   e. all of the above

6. Assuming patient interest in smoking cessation, which of the following smoking cessation methods results in the highest percentage of both short-term and long-term success?
   a. transdermal nicotine
   b. a patient education booklet
   c. physician counseling and advice

d. a contract for a "quit date"

e. a combination of all of the above

7. One of the best individual targeted smoking cessation programs is the widely recommended 5 A's approach (Ask, Advise, Assess, Assist, and Arrange) designed to help the smoker who is willing to quit. Which of the following is true about this approach?

   a. the approach includes implementation of an officewide system that ensures that, for every patient at every visit, tobacco-use status is queried and documented

   b. smokers should be approached intermittently and gently to avoid provoking anger

   c. smokers from households with other smokers present should be advised to change domiciles

   d. the approach fosters self-reliance without the support of any outside organizations or individuals

   e. the use of pharmacotherapy is reserved for counseling failures

8. What is the approximate percentage of patients who relapse following successful cessation of smoking?

   a. 10%

   b. 50%

   c. 75%

   d. 85%

   e. 99%

9. What is the most prevalent modifiable risk factor for increased morbidity and mortality in the United States?

   a. hypertension

   b. hyperlipidemia

   c. cigarette smoking

   d. occupational burnout

   e. alcohol consumption

   because of passive smoking?

10. Nicotine replacement is especially important in which group of patients who smoke cigarettes?

    a. those patients who smoke when work-related stressors become unmanageable

    b. those patients who smoke more than 20 cigarettes a day

    c. those patients who smoke within 30 minutes of awakening

    d. those patients who experience withdrawal symptoms

    e. all of the above

    f. b, c, and d

11. Which of the following statements regarding the economic burden of smoking is (are) true?

    a. the economic burden of smoking is placed not only on the individual but also on society

    b. in the United States the costs related to cigarette smoking exceed $50 billion annually

    c. smoking has a significant effect on work-related productivity

    d. it would cost an estimated $6.3 billion annually to provide 75% of smokers ages 18 years and older with the cessation interventions of their choice

    e. all of the above statements are true

Answers

1. **d.** Of deaths from CAD, 25% are directly attributable to smoking. The incidence of myocardial infarction and death from CAD is 70% higher in cigarette smokers than in nonsmokers. In the United States, 18% of all deaths are caused by cigarette smoking.

2. **e.** The health consequences of smoking are enormous. The major processes involved include active smoking, passive smoking, addiction, and accelerated aging. The following disease categories have been directly linked to smoking: cancer, respiratory diseases, and cardiovascular diseases. Pregnancy and infant health and other miscellaneous conditions also are affected by smoking.

   The actual diseases involved include the following:

   a. *Cancer*: (1) lung, (2) larynx, (3) mouth, (4) pharynx, (5) stomach, (6) liver, (7) pancreas, (8) bladder, (9) uterine cervix, (10) breast, and (11) brain

   b. *Respiratory diseases*: (1) emphysema, (2) chronic bronchitis, (3) asthma, (4) bacterial pneumonia, (5) tubercular pneumonia, and (6) asbestosis

   c. *Cardiovascular diseases*: (1) CAD, (2) hypertension, (3) aortic aneurysm, (4) arterial thrombosis, (5) stroke, and (6) carotid artery atherosclerosis

   d. *Pregnancy and infant health*: (1) intrauterine growth restriction, (2) spontaneous abortion, (3) fetal and neonatal death, (4) abruptio placenta, (5) bleeding in pregnancy not yet discovered, (6) placenta previa, (7) premature rupture of the membranes, (8) preterm labor, (9) preeclampsia, (10) sudden infant death syndrome, (11) congenital malformations, (12) low birth weight, (13) frequent respiratory and ear infections in children, and (14) higher incidence of mental retardation

   e. *Other miscellaneous conditions*: (1) peptic ulcer disease, (2) osteoporosis, (3) Alzheimer's disease, (4) wrinkling of the skin ("crow's feet" appearance on the face), and (5) impotence

   The mechanisms whereby the linkage between smoking and the aforementioned diseases occur are multifactorial. What is striking, however, is the number of medical disease categories that smoking affects and the number of diseases within each category that smoking affects.

3. a. Tobacco smoke in the environment is derived from either mainstream smoke (exhaled smoke) or sidestream smoke (smoke arising from the burning end of a cigarette). Exposure to sidestream smoking (also known as passive smoking) produces an increased prevalence of bronchiolitis, asthma, bronchitis, ear infections, and pneumonia in infants and children whose parents smoke.

The most common symptom arising from exposure to passive smoking is eye irritation. Other significant symptoms include headaches, nasal symptoms, and cough. Exposure to tobacco smoke also precipitates or aggravates allergies.

Spouses of patients who smoke are at increased risk of developing lung cancer and CAD. For lung cancer, the average relative risk is 1.34 compared to people not exposed to passive smoke. This risk, in comparison, is more than 100 times higher than the estimated effect of 20 years' exposure to asbestos while living or working in asbestos-containing buildings. It is estimated that of the 480,000 smoking-related deaths each year, 53,000 are associated with passive smoking.

4. a. The most important factor in determining the success of a smoking cessation program is the desire of the individual to quit. If the individual is not interested in quitting, the probability of success is very low. Physician advice to quit, behavior-modification aids, nicotine replacement, and repeated office visits are all important. However, without the will to quit, they will not be effective.

5. e. The first-line pharmacologic agents that may be considered for inclusion in a smoking cessation program are nicotine (delivered via inhalation, orally [via chewing gum], or transdermally) and bupropion (or bupropion SR, Zyban). The use of the antidepressant bupropion (Zyban) has proved to be effective in the treatment of cigarette smokers. The aim is to stop smoking within 1 or 2 weeks after starting the medication, with the duration of treatment between 7 and 12 weeks. This treatment modality helps address both the psychologic and the physiologic aspects of smoking addiction. It acts by boosting brain levels of dopamine and norepinephrine, thus mimicking the effects of nicotine.

Second-line agents proved effective include clonidine and nortriptyline. Clonidine has proven efficacy in the relief of symptoms of opiate and alcohol withdrawal. It has been shown to be superior to placebo in helping patients remain abstinent from smoking for periods up to 1 year. Mecamylamine is a nicotine receptor antagonist that is analogous to naloxone for the treatment of opiate abuse. Mecamylamine may be useful as a method of smoking cessation in the recalcitrant smoker. It has not been studied extensively in such a population. Propranolol has been shown to relieve some of the physiologic changes associated with alcohol withdrawal-induced anxiety, but it has been shown to be ineffective in smoking cessation and has no effect on reducing subjective satisfaction and extinction of smoking behavior.

Varenicline (Chantix), a selective nicotinic acetylcholine receptor agonist, may lessen craving and withdrawal while competitively blocking nicotine. Varenicline treatment seems to be as effective as sustained-release bupropion; it has not been compared with nicotine replacement therapy or with combination therapies.

6. e. A meta-analysis of controlled trials of smoking cessation compared the effectiveness of smoking cessation counseling, self-help booklets, nicotine replacement, and establishing a contract and setting a quitting date. The study found that each modality was effective, but no single modality worked significantly better than the others. When treatment modalities were combined, however, the following results were obtained: Two treatment modalities were more effective than one, three treatment modalities were more effective than two, and four treatment modalities were more effective than three.

7. a. The widely recommended 5 A's approach (Ask, Advise, Assess, Assist, and Arrange) is designed to be used with the smoker who is willing to quit. The following is taken from the Agency for Healthcare Research and Quality Web site (www.ahrq.gov).

Ask—Systematically identify all tobacco users at every visit. Implement an officewide system that ensures that, for every patient at every clinic visit, tobacco-use status is queried and documented. Expand the "vital signs" to include tobacco use, or use an alternative universal identification system such as chart stickers or an electronic medical record alert.

Advise—Strongly urge all tobacco users to quit. In a clear, strong, and personalized manner, urge every tobacco user to quit. *Clear*—"I think it is important for you to quit smoking now, and I can help you. Cutting down while you are ill is not enough." *Strong*—"As your clinician, I need you to know that quitting smoking is the most important thing you can do to protect your health now and in the future. The clinic staff and I will help you." *Personalized*—Tie tobacco use to current health/illness and/or its social and economic costs, motivation level/readiness to quit, and/or the impact of tobacco use on children and others in the household.

Assess—Determine willingness to make an attempt to quit. Ask every tobacco user if he or she is willing to make an attempt to quit at this time (e.g., within the next 30 days). Assess patient's willingness to quit. If the patient is willing to make an attempt to quit at this time, provide assistance. If the patient will participate in an intensive treatment, deliver such a treatment or refer to an intensive intervention. If the patient clearly states he or she is unwilling to make a quit attempt at this time, provide a motivational intervention. If the patient is a member of a special population (e.g., adolescent, pregnant smoker, and racial/ethnic minority), consider providing additional information.

Assist—Aid the patient in quitting.

- *Help the patient with a quit plan.* A patient's preparations for quitting include the following: *Setting a quit date*—ideally, the quit date should be within 2 weeks. *Telling* family, friends, and co-workers about quitting and request understanding and support. *Anticipating* challenges to the planned quit attempt, particularly during the critical first few weeks. These include nicotine withdrawal symptoms. *Removing* tobacco products from the patient's environment. Prior to quitting, the patient should avoid smoking in places where he or she spends a lot of time (e.g., work, home, and car).
- *Provide practical counseling* (problem solving/training). Assisting patients in quitting smoking can be done as part of a brief treatment or as part of an intensive treatment program. Evidence demonstrates that the more intense and longer lasting the intervention, the more likely the patient is to remain smoke-free; even an intervention lasting fewer than 3 minutes is effective.
- *Inform them that abstinence is essential.* "Not even a single puff after the quit date." Past quit experience (if any)—review past quit attempts, including identification of what helped during the quit attempt and what factors contributed to relapse. Anticipate triggers or challenges in upcoming attempt—discuss challenges/triggers and how patient will overcome them successfully. Limit alcohol use—because alcohol can cause relapse, the patient should consider limiting/abstaining from alcohol while quitting. Talk to other smokers in the household—quitting is more difficult when there is another smoker in the household. Patients should encourage housemates to quit with them or not smoke in their presence.
- *Provide intratreatment social support.* Provide a supportive clinical environment while encouraging the patient in his or her quit attempt. "My office staff and I are available to assist you."
- *Help the patient obtain social support outside of treatment.* Help the patient develop social support for his or her quit attempt in his or her environments outside of treatment. "Ask your spouse/partner, friends, and co-workers to support you in your quit attempt."
- *Recommend the use of approved pharmacotherapy*, except in special circumstances. Recommend the use of pharmacotherapies found to be effective. Explain how these medications increase smoking cessation success and reduce withdrawal symptoms. The first-line pharmacotherapy medications include bupropion SR, nicotine gum, nicotine inhaler, nicotine nasal spray, and nicotine patch.
- *Provide supplementary materials. Sources*—federal agencies, nonprofit agencies, or local/state health departments. *Type*—culturally/racially/educationally/age appropriate for the patient. *Location*—readily available at every clinician's workstation.

Arrange—Schedule follow-up contact. Schedule follow-up contact either in person or via telephone. *Timing*—follow-up contact should occur soon after the quit date, preferably during the first week. A second follow-up contact is recommended within the first month. Schedule further follow-up contacts as indicated. *Actions during follow-up contact*—congratulate success. If tobacco use has occurred, review circumstances and elicit recommitment to total abstinence. Remind patient that a lapse can be used as a learning experience. Identify problems already encountered and anticipate challenges in the immediate future. Assess pharmacotherapy use and problems. Consider use or referral to more intensive treatment.

8. **d.** Arranging follow-up appointments for the patient is extremely important. This, in effect, prepares the patient for the support and surveillance of the physician. At the follow-up visits there is an opportunity to review concerns, review continuing plans, and discuss relapses. This last issue is extremely important because lapses occur in 85% of those who quit. The reaction and counseling of the physician following a lapse are crucial and should be framed in the context of a positive learning experience. One of the key points that needs to be reinforced by the physician is that learning to live without cigarettes is like learning any new skill—you learn from mistakes until your action becomes a new habitual behavior. Most patients require a few trials before they quit completely.

9. **c.** Cigarette smoking continues to be the most prevalent modifiable risk factor for increased morbidity and mortality in the United States. Not only does the smoker incur medical risks attributable to cigarette smoking but also passive smokers and society bear the ill effects and the increased economic costs attributable to the smoker's habit.

10. **f.** Nicotine replacement is especially important for the following types of smokers: (1) smokers who smoke more than 20 cigarettes a day, (2) smokers who smoke within 30 minutes of waking up, and (3) smokers who experience withdrawal symptoms.

Smokers who smoke when exposed to extremely stressful work situations should be managed mainly by behavior-modification techniques, although bupropion may be a consideration for therapy.

11. **e.** The individual smoker and society in general incur enormous economic costs as a result of smoking. Here are some facts from the U.S. Public Health Service's *Treating Tobacco Use and Dependence Fact Sheet, 2000* (available at www.surgeongeneral.gov/tobacco/smokfact.htm). Surveys reveal that 25% of American adults smoke. More than 430,000 deaths in the United States each year are attributable to tobacco use, making tobacco use the number-one modifiable cause of death and disease in the United States. Smoking prevalence among adolescents increased dramatically since 1990—more than 3000 additional children and adolescents each day become regular users of tobacco. Medical care costs attributable to smoking (or smoking-related disease) have been estimated by the Centers for Disease Control and Prevention (CDC) to be more than $50 billion annually in the United States. In addition, lost earnings and loss of productivity total at least another $50 billion a year, according to the CDC.

It would cost an estimated $10 billion annually to provide 75% of smokers aged 18 years or older with the intervention—counseling, nicotine patches, nicotine replacement, or a combination—of their choice. This would be cost-effective in relation to other medical interventions such as mammography or blood pressure screening. Epidemiologic data suggest that more than 70% of the 50 million smokers in the United States today have made at least one prior quit attempt, and approximately 46% try to quit each year. Most smokers make several quit attempts before they successfully kick the habit. Only 21% of practicing physicians say that they have received adequate training to help their patients stop smoking.

Summary

1. Identify all patients in your practice who smoke. The major mistake is failing to screen all patients to identify smokers. Refamiliarize yourself with the 5 A's approach reviewed in answer 7.
2. Assess the patient's readiness to change. Present all the health consequences of smoking.
3. Present the health benefits of smoking cessation.
4. Assess and develop the desire to modify smoking behavior.
5. Develop and formalize a patient-centered plan for change.
6. Establish a quitting date, and have the patient sign a contract.
7. Use an alternate nicotine delivery system or bupropion as an adjunct to counseling.
8. Use behavior-modification techniques as part of counseling and advice. Have the patient keep a journal of at-risk times for smoking.
9. Consider using any and all available patient education booklets or Web sites from the American Lung Association (www.lungusa.org), the American Cancer Society (www.cancer.org), the American Academy of Family Physicians (www.aafp.org), the National Institutes of Health (www.nih.gov), or the Agency for Healthcare Research and Quality (www.ahrq.gov). Establish a quit date and a contract; advise and counsel the patient at regular intervals, and incorporate behavior-modification techniques; and try to enlist family and workplace supports.
10. Have the patient consider times at which he or she may relapse (which will happen in 85% of patients). Have a plan for relapse if it happens. Most important, be supportive, positive, and prepared to treat comorbidities.

Suggested Reading

Fiore MC, Jaén CR, Baker TB, et al: *Treating Tobacco Use and Dependence*. Rockville, MD: U.S. Department of Health and Human Services, Public Health Service, May 2008. Accessed at Agency for Healthcare Research and Quality, www.ahrq.gov.

Frishman WH, Mitta W, Kupersmith A, Ky T: Nicotine and non-nicotine smoking cessation pharmacotherapies. *Cardiol Rev* 14(2):57–73, 2006.

Nides M, Oncken C, Gonzales D, et al: Smoking cessation with varenicline, a selective alpha$_4$beta$_2$ nicotinic receptor partial agonist: Results from a 7-week, randomized, placebo- and bupropion-controlled trial with 1-year follow-up. *Arch Intern Med* 166:1561–1568, 2006.

Okuyemi KS, Nollen NL, Ahluwalia JS: Interventions to facilitate smoking cessation. *Am Fam Physician* 74(2):262–271, 2006.

Ranney L, Melvin C, Lux L, et al: Systematic review: Smoking cessation intervention strategies for adults and adults in special populations. *Ann Internal Med* 145(11):845–856, 2006.

CLINICAL CASE PROBLEM 1

*A 45-Year-Old Male with an
Enlarged Liver*

A 45-year-old executive comes to your office for his periodic health assessment. He tells you that he has been feeling "weak, tired, and just not myself lately." He also tells you that he has been so tired that he "has had to stay home from work for many days at a time." He is beginning to question his ability to function effectively as the chief executive officer of a transportation company. When you inquire about other symptoms, he tells you that he also has suffered from "profound headaches" and that his sex life with his wife is "the pits." On direct questioning, he tells you that the headaches "have been a problem for the past 6 months" and his "lack of interest in sex" has been a problem for approximately the same amount of time.

He has no serious past medical, surgical, or psychiatric illnesses. He tells you that he is taking no over-the-counter or prescription drugs.

The patient describes himself as a "social drinker," and his use of alcohol is "strictly to relax." He then states, "I hope you do not think that I'm an alcoholic, Doc!" There is no evidence of acute intoxication at this time.

He does state, on more persistent questioning, "Well, may be I am using more alcohol than I did a few years ago. Oh sometimes, I think it might be a good idea to cut down a bit. I do get annoyed with my wife who points out that I am drinking more than I used to. Sometimes I even feel guilty and wonder if that's affecting our sex life. There are mornings that I wake up with the shakes and having an 'eye opener' really helps."

His father died of complications of "yellow jaundice" at age 61. His mother died of complications of heart failure at age 69. He has three brothers and two sisters; all are well.

On physical examination, his blood pressure is 160/104 mmHg. His pulse is 96 and regular. Examination of the head and neck, respiratory system, and musculoskeletal system are normal. Examination of the cardiovascular system reveals a point of maximum impulse (PMI) in the fifth intercostal space on the anterior axillary line. He subsequently describes recent episodes of "waking up at night short of breath" and "shortness of breath on exertion." Examination of the gastrointestinal system reveals no tenderness or rebound tenderness. The liver edge is palpated approximately 5 cm below the right costal margin. Examination of the neurologic system reveals intermittent carpal spasms of both extremities. He has a fine tremor of his hands. He cannot perform serial 7s and has difficulty with recall of information on the mental status examination.

SELECT THE BEST ANSWER TO THE FOLLOWING QUESTIONS

1. With the history given, what is the best description of the most likely diagnosis in this patient?
   a. somatization disorder
   b. adjustment disorder with depressed and anxious mood
   c. major depressive disorder
   d. alcohol dependence
   e. alcohol abuse

2. Which of the following signs or symptoms further substantiate your diagnosis in this patient?
   a. the location of the PMI
   b. the patient's elevated blood pressure
   c. the abdominal signs on physical examination
   d. the hand tremors
   e. all of the above

3. What are signs and symptoms of acute alcohol intoxication?
   a. facial flushing
   b. slurred speech
   c. nystagmus
   d. ataxia
   e. all of the above

4. What is the most likely cause of the patient's liver edge palpated at 5 cm below the right costal margin?
   a. tricornute liver (congenital malformation)
   b. alcoholic hepatitis or cirrhosis
   c. congestive heart failure
   d. "the deep diaphragm pushing the liver down" syndrome
   e. hepatorenal syndrome

5. There is a high correlation between the disorder diagnosed in question 1 and which of the following syndromes?
   a. generalized anxiety disorder
   b. major depressive disorder

c. schizophrenia

d. opioid abuse

e. all of the above

f. b and d only

6. The patient's inability to perform serial 7s and information recall is most likely caused by which of the following?

a. Alzheimer's dementia

b. alcoholic dementia

c. alcoholic amnestic syndrome

d. all of the above are equally likely

e. b and c

7. At what amount of blood alcohol level is a driver determined to be "impaired" in most states?

a. 0.02% (20 mg/dL)

b. 0.05% (50 mg/dL)

c. 0.1% (100 mg/dL)

d. 0.5% (500 mg/dL)

e. 1.0% (1000 mg/dL)

8. Regarding risk factors for the condition diagnosed in question 1, which of the following statements most accurately reflects risk factor status and identification?

a. there are no risk factors for this disease; it just happens

b. there is no single factor that accounts for increased relative and absolute risk in first-degree relatives of patients with this disorder

c. genetic, familial, environmental, occupational, socioeconomic, cultural, personality, life stress, psychiatric comorbidity, biologic, social learning, and behavioral conditioning are all risk factors or risk environments for this disorder

d. there is a clear risk factor stratification for this disorder

e. b and c

9. Which organ systems can be affected by alcohol abuse?

a. cardiovascular system

b. endocrine system

c. pulmonary system

d. hematologic system

e. all of the above

10. Which drug(s) is (are) useful in the treatment of alcohol withdrawal?

a. benzodiazepine

b. clonidine

c. barbiturates

d. anticonvulsants

e. all of the above

11. How is alcohol withdrawal syndrome best defined?

a. a state in which a syndrome of drug-specific withdrawal signs and symptoms follows the reduction or cessation of drug use

b. a state in which the physiologic or behavioral effects of a constant dose of a psychoactive substance decrease over time

c. a pathologic state that follows cessation or reduction in the amount of drug used

d. a and b

e. all of the above

12. How is alcohol abuse syndrome best defined?

a. a maladaptive state leading to clinically significant impairment

b. a maladaptive state leading to clinically significant distress

c. a maladaptive state leading to significant impairment defined by laboratory value

d. either a or c

e. either a or b

13. Considering the patient described, which of the following diagnostic imaging procedures is (are) definitely indicated?

a. chest x-ray

b. cardiac echocardiogram

c. computed tomography (CT) scan of the head

d. abdominal ultrasound

e. all of the above

14. Which of the following is the most likely explanation for the tremors observed on physical examination?

a. delirium tremens (early)

b. alcohol withdrawal syndrome

c. thiamine deficiency

d. alcoholic encephalopathy (early)

e. Korsakoff's psychosis

15. A 26-year-old male comes to your office for a periodic health examination before he gets married. When you question him about his lifestyle and ask him about his alcohol intake, he replies that he is a "social drinker." Once that is established, what should you do?

a. congratulate him on avoiding problems with alcohol

b. accept "social drinking" at face value and move onto the next question

c. ask him whether he ever has a drink while alone

d. ask him to very specifically define social drinking

e. request an estimate of the number of drinks per week and a specification on the kind of alcoholic beverages consumed

CLINICAL CASE PROBLEM 2

A Patient with Short-Term Memory Deficits

A patient who you suspect of alcohol dependence demonstrates significant short-term memory deficits. He then tries to cover up those deficits by making up answers to questions.

16. Which of the following is the most likely diagnosis?
    a. Wernicke's encephalopathy
    b. alcohol-induced persisting amnestic disorder (Korsakoff's psychosis)
    c. alcohol-induced psychotic disorder with delusions
    d. alcohol-induced psychotic disorder with hallucinosis
    e. alcohol-induced persisting dementia

17. The feature described as "making up answers to questions" is known as which of the following?
    a. confabulation
    b. alcoholic lying
    c. alcoholic delirium
    d. alcoholic paranoia
    e. memory loss encephalopathy

18. What is the cause of the disorder described in this case?
    a. riboflavin deficiency
    b. thiamine deficiency
    c. zinc deficiency
    d. cerebral atrophy caused by alcohol abuse
    e. cerebellar atrophy caused by alcohol abuse

19. The word alcoholism means different things to different people. Of the following, which is the best definition of alcoholism?
    a. alcohol abuse and alcohol dependency
    b. alcohol abuse but not alcohol dependency
    c. alcohol abuse or alcohol dependency
    d. alcohol abuse and/or alcohol dependency
    e. none of the above represent an adequate definition of alcoholism

20. What is the percentage of the U.S. population who will suffer from alcohol abuse or dependence during the course of a lifetime?
    a. 5%
    b. 10%
    c. 14%
    d. 48%
    e. 75%

21. Which of the following behavioral interventions is (are) most effective in the long-term management of alcohol dependence?
    a. cognitive behavioral therapy
    b. social behavior and network therapy
    c. motivational enhancement therapy
    d. a and c
    e. no one therapy is superior to another

22. Which of the following pharmacotherapeutic–psychosocial approaches works best in the long-term treatment of alcohol dependence?
    a. naltrexone–cognitive behavioral therapy
    b. topiramate–social network therapy
    c. acamprosate–motivational enhancement therapy
    d. disulfiram–aversion therapy
    e. a and b

Clinical Case Management Problem

Part A: Provide a screening test for alcohol abuse that can be administered easily in the office setting.

Part B: List five objectives for short-term treatment of the patient and the patient's family in a case of alcohol dependence.

Answers

1. d. This patient has alcohol dependence, which is defined as at least three of the following occurring during a 12-month period: (1) tolerance (the need for increased amounts of a substance to achieve intoxication or another desired effect or markedly diminished effect with use of the same amount of the substance); (2) characteristic withdrawal symptoms or the use of alcohol (or a closely related substitute) to relieve or avoid withdrawal; (3) substance often taken in larger amounts over a longer period than the person intended; (4) persistent desire or one or more unsuccessful attempts to cut down or quit drinking; (5) a great deal of time spent in getting the alcohol, drinking it, or recovering from its effects; (6) important social, occupational, or recreational activities are given up or reduced because of the alcohol; and (7) continued alcohol use despite the knowledge of having a persistent or recurrent social, psychologic, or physical problem that is caused by, or exacerbated by, use of alcohol.

2. e. The physical signs and symptoms actually substantiate the diagnosis of alcohol dependence, not alcohol abuse. Alcohol dependence is defined as a maladaptive pattern of alcohol use with adverse clinical consequences. These physical symptoms include the following: (1) The location of the PMI in the fifth intercostal space suggests cardiomegaly, which could result from either alcoholic cardiomyopathy or hypertension (most likely also related to alcohol intake); (2) the obvious hepatomegaly suggests alcoholic hepatitis or cirrhosis of the liver; (3) the fine tremor suggests early alcoholic encephalopathy, which is substantiated by the cognitive dysfunction (lack of ability to perform serial 7s); and (4) the patient's hypertension suggests alcohol as a potential cause.

3. e. Acute alcohol intoxication is characterized by mood lability, poor judgment, ataxia, slurred speech, decreased concentration and memory, facial flushing, blood pressure elevation, enlarged pupils, and nystagmus. Increasing alcohol levels can result in depression of respiration and reflexes and a decrease in blood pressure and body temperature, potentially followed by stupor, coma, and death.

4. b. The most likely cause of the hepatomegaly is alcoholic hepatitis and possibly cirrhosis. Laboratory tests that may be abnormal in alcoholic liver disease include γ-glutamyltransferase (GGT), alkaline phosphatase aspartate aminotransferase (AST), and alanine aminotransferase (ALT). An ALT/AST ratio of more than 2 is especially suspicious.

Often, the mean corpuscular volume (MCV) is elevated in patients with chronic heavy alcohol consumption. Uric acid levels may be elevated; abnormalities in the lipid metabolism are often present.

5. e. The National Institute of Mental Health Epidemiologic Catchment Area Program found a very high correlation rate between alcoholism and (1) suicide, (2) homicide, (3) accidents, (4) anxiety disorders, (5) major depressive disorder, (6) schizophrenia, (7) narcotic drug abuse, (8) cocaine abuse, and (9) cigarette smoking.

6. e. Chronic alcohol use is associated with the cognitive and memory deficits of alcoholic dementia and the more restrictive memory deficits of alcohol amnestic disorder. Patients with alcohol-related amnestic syndrome have the most difficulty with short-term memory (remembering recent events). However, deficits may be noted in long-term memory as well.

7. b. Drivers are determined to be "impaired" at levels of 0.05% (50 mg/dL) in most states. They are considered to be "under the influence" at levels of 0.1% (100 mg/dL). Somebody who does not exhibit signs of intoxication at alcohol levels of 100 mg/dL or higher probably is alcohol dependent because alcohol tolerance is evident.

8. e. Factors that determine an individual's susceptibility to a substance use disorder are not well understood. Studies of populations at risk for developing substance abuse have identified many factors that foster the development and continuance of substance use. These include genetic, familial, environmental, occupational, socioeconomic, cultural, and personality factors; life stressors; psychiatric comorbidity; biologic and social learning factors; and behavioral conditioning. The concordance rate for alcoholism between fathers and sons and among identical twin pairs is very high. This suggests a strong genetic determination for this disease. Accordingly, family members of alcoholics, especially first-degree relatives, need to be screened and counseled for alcohol dependence/abuse.

9. e. Complications of the cardiovascular system include elevated blood pressures, as mentioned previously, which usually is reversible with abstinence; alcoholic cardiomyopathy; sinus tachycardia; and arrhythmias. Endocrine complications in men include low testosterone and increased estrogen levels, decreased libido, testicular atrophy, and impotence. Women experience menstrual irregularities and sexual dysfunction. Pulmonary complications include bacterial pneumonias and aspiration pneumonias (when vomiting occurs in intoxicated patients) and increased rates of tuberculosis. Very often, pulmonary complications from smoking are present because 80% to 90% of alcoholics are cigarette smokers. Gastrointestinal complications include gastroesophageal reflux disease and peptic ulcer disease, esophagitis and esophageal varices as a late complication, alcoholic hepatitis, cirrhosis, and pancreatitis. Except for esophageal varices and cirrhosis, these conditions are often reversible with alcohol abstinence. Neurologic complications include peripheral neuropathy of the lower extremities, Wernicke–Korsakoff syndrome, hepatic encephalopathy, and alcohol dementia. Hematologic complications include iron-deficiency anemia; macrocytosis; thrombocytopenia; and neutrophil, lymphocyte, and thrombocyte dysfunction.

10. e. The mainstay of therapy is long-acting benzodiazepines such as diazepam, chlordiazepoxide, and chlorazepate, given in decreasing doses. Clonidine is sometimes used to reduce noradrenergic symptoms. Antipsychotic agents such as haloperidol are useful in addition to benzodiazepines in patients with hallucinations and agitation. Barbiturates and anticonvulsants (carbamazepine and divalproex) sometimes are used as anticonvulsants.

11. a. Alcohol withdrawal syndrome is a substance-specific syndrome that develops following cessation or reduced intake of alcohol.

12. a. Alcohol abuse describes patterns of alcohol use that do not meet the criteria for alcohol dependence. Alcohol abuse is defined as a maladaptive pattern of substance use that causes clinically significant impairment. This may include impairments in social, family, or occupational functioning; the presence of psychologic or physical problems; or the use of alcohol while or before driving a motor vehicle or operating machinery. Alcohol abuse commonly progresses to alcohol dependence.

13. e. The imaging studies indicated in this patient include a chest x-ray, a CT of the head, an abdominal ultrasound, and an echocardiogram. An echocardiogram should be done to define the thickness of the left ventricular wall to determine whether left ventricular hypertrophy (LVH) is present, as indicated by the position of the PMI. In addition, an electrocardiogram will aid in the diagnosis of LVH and determine, among other things, the absence or presence of cardiac arrhythmias. A chest x-ray is justified on the basis of probable cardiac enlargement—that is, to measure the cardiac/thoracic ratio. A CT scan will rule out causes of cognitive disturbances that may be related to alcohol abuse, including intracranial bleeding. It may also detect causes of cognitive disturbances unrelated to alcohol. An abdominal ultrasound will determine the cause of the liver enlargement and help determine the spleen size.

14. d. The movement disorder that is demonstrated on physical examination suggests the early stages of liver failure and alcoholic (Wernicke's) encephalopathy. It may develop into asterixes (an arrhythmic flapping tremor of the fully extended hand), sometimes referred to as liver flap.

15. e. Social drinking is a term with little meaning. It is important to more precisely determine drinking patterns.

The first step is to determine whether a patient drinks. The second step is to determine how much alcohol a patient drinks. It helps to have the patient estimate the number of drinks per week because many drinkers have irregular patterns with heavier weekend use. Because alcoholism is a disease usually minimized, it is only when the need to drink starts to seriously interfere with social or occupational functioning or the patient is apprehended while driving under the influence of alcohol that the alcohol abuser will become

aware of having a "problem." If the family physician can express concern regarding the effect of the quantity of alcohol consumed on the patient's health, prior to there being dire consequences related to the drinking habit, treatment can be initiated at an earlier time and serious sequelae of the disease can be prevented.

A very useful instrument for screening for alcoholism in the primary care setting is the CAGE questionnaire. The CAGE questionnaire includes four questions:

1. Have you ever felt the need to *c*ut down on your drinking?
2. Have you ever felt *a*nnoyed by criticisms of your drinking?
3. Have you ever had *g*uilty feelings about drinking?
4. Have you ever taken a morning *e*ye-opener?

With the CAGE questionnaire, any more than one positive answer may suggest alcohol abuse.

Another reliable screening tool for heavy alcohol use is the Michigan Alcohol Screening Test (MAST). This 25-item scale identifies abnormal drinking through its social and behavioral consequences with a sensitivity of 90% to 98%. The Brief MAST, a shortened 10-item test, has been shown to have similar efficacy. These tests are less likely to be used in a primary care environment.

16. b. This patient has alcohol-induced persisting amnestic disorder, called Korsakoff's psychosis. Patients with alcohol-related amnestic disorder have the most difficulty with short-term memory (remembering recent events), although deficits in long-term memory may be noted as well.

17. a. Patients often try to conceal or compensate for their memory loss by confabulation (making up answers or talking around questions that require them to use their memory).

18. b. The cause of this particular disorder is a chronic deficiency in the vitamin thiamine. For this reason, whenever a patient is in a confused state that may be related to alcohol abuse, intravenous thiamine should be administered.

19. e. Alcoholism is defined as a repetitive but inconsistent and sometimes unpredictable loss of control of drinking that produces symptoms of serious dysfunction or disability.

20. c. In 1994, the National Comorbidity Survey found that 23% of the population in the United States reported alcohol abuse or dependence. Recent studies suggest that almost 14% of Americans have alcohol use-related problems in their lifetime, and almost 8% meet criteria for alcohol abuse, dependence, or both at any given time. Approximately 75% of the population drinks alcohol. Men are two to three times more likely than women to be problem drinkers, although women may hide their drinking more frequently. Excessive drinking causes serious digestive system disorders, such as ulcers, inflammation of the pancreas, gastritis, and cirrhosis of the liver, and leads to physical and nutritional neglect. Central and peripheral nervous system damage can result in blackouts, hallucinations, tremors, alcohol withdrawal syndrome, delirium tremens, and death.

When women drink even moderately during pregnancy, damage can occur to unborn children. This can include birth defects, mental retardation, learning problems, and fetal alcohol syndrome.

Heavy drinking also results in psychologic and interpersonal problems, including impaired thinking and judgment, and changes in mood and behavior. These consequences of drinking then lead to impaired social relationships, marital problems, and/or child abuse and scholastic, occupational, financial, and legal problems.

21. **e.** A large number of behavioral approaches have been tried, including the popular Alcoholics Anonymous 12-step program. However, in studies comparing the different psychosocial interventions, including cognitive behavioral therapy, social behavior and network therapy, and motivational enhancement therapy, no one method appears to be superior to another. The physician must individualize choice of therapy based on the long-term knowledge of the patient. Studies indicate that a combination of behavioral and pharmacotherapy may be best to treat long-term alcohol dependence.

22. **a.** Three medications—disulfiram, naltrexone, and acamprosate—are currently approved by the Food and Drug Administration for the treatment of alcohol dependence. Naltrexone is an opioid receptor antagonist whose efficacy in the treatment of alcohol dependence in conjunction with cognitive behavioral therapy has been demonstrated by several clinical trials. Its main drawback is the lack of a long-term dosing mode, which it is hoped will be addressed in the near future. Acamprosate, calcium acetyl homotaurinate, is thought to stabilize the chemical balance in the brain that would otherwise be disrupted by alcoholism, possibly by blocking glutaminergic N-methyl-D-aspartate receptors, while gamma-aminobutyric acid type A receptors are activated. A systematic review concluded that acamprosate is best for achieving abstinence, whereas naltrexone is better in conjunction with CBT for long-term control of drinking. Combining naltrexone and acamprosate showed no additional benefit. Alcohol is metabolized in the liver by the enzyme alcohol dehydrogenase to acetaldehyde, which is further broken down to acetic acid by the enzyme acetaldehyde dehydrogenase. Disulfiram blocks this last enzyme, causing buildup of acetaldehyde, which upon ingestion of alcohol results in severe hangover-like symptoms. It must be taken daily and is not used in many primary care settings because of multiple side effects and contraindications. It is contraindicated in patients who are taking metronidazole or have psychosis or cardiovascular disease. It is not recommended for patients with severe pulmonary disease, peripheral neuropathy, seizures, or cirrhosis with portal hypertension, chronic renal failure, diabetes, or those older than 60 years. A rare but potentially fatal adverse effect is hepatotoxicity. With the exception of topiramate, there are currently no new, effective medications for alcohol dependence. This medication has been used with some success; ongoing studies are in progress to determine the correct combinations with psychotherapy.

Solution to the Clinical Case Management Problem

Part A: A good primary care screening test for alcoholism is the CAGE questionnaire. The CAGE questionnaire was described in answer 15. Alternatives are the MAST (25 items) and the Brief MAST (10 items); however, these are not used as extensively in the family practice setting.

Part B: Five objectives for the short-term treatment of alcohol dependence in the patient and the patient's family are as follows: (1) relieving subjective symptoms of distress and discomfort caused by intoxication or withdrawal; (2) preventing or treating serious complications of intoxication, withdrawal, or dependence; (3) establishing sobriety; (4) preparing for and referral to long-term treatment or rehabilitation; and (5) engaging the family in the treatment process.

Summary

1. Prevalence

An estimated 5% to 7% of Americans have alcoholism in any given year, and 14% will have it sometime during their lifetime.

2. Economic costs

The direct economic costs of alcoholism in the United States are staggering. In 2005, total economic losses from lost productivity in the United States were more than $100 billion. This does not include indirect economic costs and noneconomic costs and losses.

3. Definitions

a. Alcoholism: a repetitive but inconsistent and sometimes unpredictable loss of control of drinking that produces symptoms of serious dysfunction or disability.

b. Alcohol dependence: a maladaptive pattern of alcohol use that includes any three of the following: (1) tolerance; (2) withdrawal; (3) increasing amounts of consumption; (4) desire or attempts to cut down or quit; (5) substantial time spent in "hiding the habit"; (6) important social, occupational, or recreational dysfunction; and (7) continued use of alcohol despite knowledge of having a persistent or recurrent social, psychological, or physical problem.

c. Alcohol abuse: a residual category that describes patterns of alcohol use that do not meet the criteria for alcohol dependence.

d. Alcohol intoxication: reversible, alcohol-specific physiologic and behavioral changes caused by recent exposure to alcohol.

e. Alcohol withdrawal: an alcohol-specific syndrome that develops following cessation or reduced intake of alcohol.

f. Alcohol-persisting disorder: an alcohol-specific syndrome that persists long after acute intoxication or withdrawal abates (e.g., memory impairments or dementia).

4. Systemic disease association

The following disease states are directly linked to the toxic effects of alcohol: (a) alcoholic cardiomyopathy; (b) systemic hypertension; (c) alcoholic hepatitis; (d) Laënnec's (alcoholic) cirrhosis; (e) esophageal varices, gastritis, ascites, and/or edema; f) peripheral neuropathy; and (g) alcoholic encephalopathy.

5. Neurologic syndromes

a. alcoholic dementia
b. alcoholic amnestic disorder
c. Korsakoff's psychosis
d. Wernicke's encephalopathy
e. alcoholic hallucinosis
f. alcoholic paranoia
g. alcohol delirium

6. Screening

a. CAGE questionnaire
b. MAST questionnaire
c. Brief MAST questionnaire

7. Laboratory testing

There are no diagnostic tests that are specific for alcohol dependence, but MCV, liver transaminases (ALT and AST), and GGT are the most common tests. The accuracy of a diagnosis of alcoholism increases when a number of tests are used together.

8. Treatment

a. General considerations: See the Solution to the Clinical Case Management Problem.

b. Long-term treatment must have the following characteristics to maximize its potential: (1) active involvement with comprehensive rehabilitation and recovery program; (2) a relapse-prevention program with individual and peer support components and pharmacologic components (see answer 22); and (3) inclusion of family and significant others in the recovery process.

c. Goals of long-term treatment are as follows: (1) to maintain sobriety; (2) to make significant changes in lifestyle, work, and friendships; (3) to treat underlying psychiatric illness (dual diagnosis); and (4) to maintain an ongoing involvement in Alcoholics Anonymous or similar groups for relapse prevention.

Suggested Reading

Assanangkornchai S, Srisurapanont M: The treatment of alcohol dependence. *Curr Opin Psychiatry* 20(3):222–227, 2007.

Ballesteros J, Duffy JC, Querejeta I, et al: Efficacy of brief interventions for hazardous drinkers in primary care: Systematic review and meta-analyses. *Alcoholism Clin Exp Res* 28(4):608–618, 2004.

Blondell RD: Ambulatory detoxification of patients with alcohol dependence. *Am Fam Physician* 71:495–502, 509–510, 2005.

Ritson B: Treatment for alcohol related problems. *BMJ* 330(7483): 139–141, 2005.

Weiss RD, Kueppenbender KD: Combining psychosocial treatment with pharmacotherapy for alcohol dependence. *J Clin Psychopharmacol* 26(Suppl 1):S37–S42, 2006.

Williams SH: Medications for treating alcohol dependence. *Am Fam Physician* 72:1775–1780, 2005.

Diet, Exercise, and Obesity

CLINICAL CASE PROBLEM 1

*A 45-Year-Old Male Weighing 320
Pounds and Complaining of Fatigue*

A 320-pound, 45-year-old male comes to your office saying he feels fatigued. He has been obese all his life. He tells you that his obesity has nothing to do with calorie intake and everything to do with his slow metabolic rate. He has been investigated extensively at many major centers specializing in "slow metabolic rates." The result of his encounters has been a conclusion that he is simply "eating too much" (with which he disagrees). He has heard from a friend that "you are different" and has come to you for "the truth."

On examination, his body mass index (BMI) is off the scale (46). He weighs 320 pounds and is 5 feet 10 inches tall. Although you cannot feel his point of maximal impulse (PMI), you believe it is in the region of the anterior axillary line, sixth intercostal space. S1 and S2 are distant, as are his breath sounds. His abdomen is obese with striae covering the abdomen. His liver and spleen can not be felt.

You refer him to your local dietician and promise that you will "investigate his slow metabolic rate" if he will agree to adhere to a diet. The dietician puts him on an 1800 kcal/day diet and calculates his ideal weight to be 170 pounds.

SELECT THE BEST ANSWER TO THE FOLLOWING QUESTIONS

1. Assuming that his total energy expenditure is 2300 kcal/day and he does, in fact, stick to his 1800 kcal/day diet, how long will it take for him to reach his ideal weight?
   a. 125 days
   b. 225 days
   c. 325 days
   d. 525 days
   e. 1050 days

2. How is obesity generally defined?
   a. an increase in the ponderal index of 20% above normal
   b. a decrease in the ponderal index of 30% below normal
   c. an increase in the BMI of 20% above normal

   d. a BMI of 30 kg/m² or greater
   e. none of the above

3. Which of the following statements is (are) true regarding obesity?
   a. obesity is associated with increased death rates from cancer
   b. obesity is associated with increased death rates from coronary artery disease
   c. obesity is associated with increased death rates from diabetes mellitus
   d. a and b are both true; c has not been proved
   e. a, b, and c are all true

4. What is the overall prevalence of obesity in the United States?
   a. 5%
   b. 10%
   c. 23%
   d. 34%
   e. 50%

5. Which of the following conditions is (are) most clearly linked with obesity?
   a. alveolar hypoventilation syndrome
   b. hypertension
   c. hyperlipidemia
   d. diabetes mellitus
   e. all of the above

6. The use of severe calorie-restricted diets (800 kcal/day) has been responsible for many deaths. What is the most common cause of death in these cases?
   a. sudden cardiac death, secondary to dysrhythmia
   b. congestive cardiac failure, secondary to anemia
   c. hepatic failure
   d. renal failure
   e. septicemia

7. What is the percentage of individuals in the United States who achieve recommended levels of weekly physical activity?
   a. 15%
   b. 21%
   c. 32%
   d. 48%
   e. none of the above

8. Which of the following statements is (are) true regarding the use of anorexic drugs?
   a. short-term studies demonstrate that weight loss is greater with these agents at 1 month than with placebo agents
   b. hypertension is a documented side effect of these agents

c. renal failure is a documented side effect of these agents
d. long-term studies suggest that these agents are not beneficial as part of a weight-loss program
e. all of the above

9. Which of the following is (are) advocated as part of a weight-loss program?
   a. a nutritionally balanced diet
   b. decreasing the percentage of calories derived from fat
   c. an exercise program
   d. caloric restriction to approximately 500 kcal/day less than maintenance
   e. all of the above

10. The practical management of weight loss by the family physician should involve which of the following?
    a. multiple office visits for 8 to 12 weeks
    b. changes to the act of eating
    c. keeping a daily food diary
    d. treatment of any comorbid depressive illness
    e. all of the above

11. Which one of the following statements concerning the use of pharmacotherapy in obese patients is true?
    a. orlistat is not indicated in obese patients
    b. sibutramine results in weight losses in excess of 10 kg at 12 months
    c. phenterimine is completely ineffective as a weight loss agent in obese patients
    d. gastric bypass surgery is relatively benign in its complication rate
    e. none of the above are true

Clinical Case Management Problem

The vast majority of patients with obesity have essential obesity (analogous to essential hypertension). There are, however, secondary causes. List the potential secondary causes of obesity.

Answers

1. **e.** One pound of fat is equal to 3500 kcal. Therefore, if his total energy expenditure is 2300 kcal/day and the patient is taking in only 1800 kcal/day (the recommended difference in a weight-loss program between energy expenditure and energy intake is

500 kcal), his energy deficit is 500 kcal/day. His excess weight above ideal body weight is 150 pounds. This 150 pounds is equal to 525,000 kcal. The corresponding time to lose this number of calories is 1050 days (2.87 years).

2. **d.** The National Institutes of Health defines obesity as a BMI of 30 kg/m^2 or more, and it defines overweight as a BMI of between 25 and 29.9 kg/m^2. BMI is calculated by multiplying the weight in pounds by 703, and dividing the product by the height in inches squared—i.e., BMI = (weight in pounds × 703) ÷ (height in inches)^2.

3. **e.** Obesity is a major public health issue. There is a certain stigmatization to the diagnosis of obesity not present in many other conditions. Some authorities suggest that we should label obesity as essential obesity in the same way that we label hypertension as essential hypertension. The comparison between hypertension and obesity does not end there. Obesity is a major risk factor for coronary artery disease and other cardiovascular conditions, including hypertension, congestive heart failure, cardiomyopathy, and angina pectoris.

Obesity is associated with an increased incidence of type 2, non-insulin-dependent diabetes mellitus, caused by an effective increase in insulin resistance, which, of course, is linked to increased mortality.

Obesity has been established indirectly as a risk factor for some cancers. For example, it appears from some studies that the high-fat diet usually associated with obesity is also associated with an increased risk of colon cancer.

The following have also been shown to be directly linked to obesity: (1) thromboembolic disease, (2) endometrial carcinoma, (3) restrictive lung disease, (4) Pickwickian syndrome, (5) gout, (6) degenerative arthritis, (7) gallstone formation and gallbladder disease, (8) infertility, (9) hyperlipoproteinemias, (10) hernias and esophageal reflux, (11) psychosocial disabilities, and (12) increased risk of obstetric and surgical morbidity.

4. **d.** The overall prevalence of obesity in the U.S. adult population is approximately 34% (BMI = 30), an astounding increase from approximately 15% in 1976. Results from the 2003–2004 National Health and Nutrition Examination Survey, using measured heights and weights, indicate that an estimated 17% of children and adolescents ages 2 to 19 years are overweight. Overweight increased from 7.2% to 13.9% among 2- to 5-year-olds and from 11% to 19% among 6- to 11-year-olds between 1988–1994 and 2003–2004. Among adolescents aged 12 to 19 years, overweight increased from 11% to 17% during the same period. In certain groups, such as the Pima Indians, the prevalence of obesity is 50%. A higher prevalence of obesity occurs in those individuals in the lowest socioeconomic groups; the prevalence does, in fact, decrease as socioeconomic status increases. Combining the categories of overweight (BMI 25–29.9) at 32% and obesity (BMI = 30) at 34%, fully 66% of the adult population in the United States is carrying excess weight.

5. e. Of the conditions already postulated as linked with obesity, the strongest associations are between obesity and hypertension and obesity and diabetes. It should be noted that the other conditions listed previously are also linked to obesity. Moreover, there is strong evidence that weight loss in an obese individual reduces blood pressure, hemoglobin A1c levels, and triglyceride, low-density lipoprotein and total cholesterol levels, and it increases high-density lipoprotein levels.

6. a. The most common cause of death reported among patients who are on severe calorie-restricted diets is sudden cardiac death as a result of ventricular arrhythmias or dysrhythmias.

7. d. Recommended weekly physical activity is defined as moderate-intensity activities (brisk walking, bicycling, vacuuming, gardening, or anything that causes small increases in breathing or heart rate) for at least 30 minutes per day, at least 5 days per week, or vigorous-intensity activities (running, aerobics, heavy yard work, or anything else that causes large increases in breathing or heart rate) for at least 20 minutes per day, at least 3 days per week, or both. This can often be accomplished through lifestyle activities (i.e., household, transportation, or leisure time activities), which means almost all patients should be able to incorporate recommended levels of physical activities in their lifestyle.

8. e. Although short-term weight loss is enhanced by these agents, long-term studies demonstrate that most patients suffer a rebound effect and actually may end up even heavier. In addition, hypertension, stroke, and renal failures have been documented in patients using anorexic drugs. These medications can be classified as catecholaminergic or serotonergic:

1. Catecholaminergic agents include amphetamines and appetite suppressants such as phentermine. Phenylpropanolamine was removed from the market in 2005 by the Food and Drug Administration.
2. The serotonergic agents fenfluramine and dexfenfluramine were withdrawn from the market in

1997, and although fluoxetine, sertraline, and other selective serotonin reuptake inhibitors are serotonergic and often used in obesity treatment, they are not approved for the treatment of obesity.

Newer medications, including sibutramine (Meridia) and orlistat (Xenical), may be useful adjuncts to low-calorie diets, physical activity, and behavior therapy in carefully selected patients.

Surgical intervention to treat obesity should be limited to those with a BMI of 40 or greater. More than 200,000 patients have undergone bariatric surgery.

9. e. A structured program is essential for successful long-term weight loss. Most successful weight-loss programs are multidisciplinary, concentrating on hypocaloric diets, behavior modification to change eating behaviors, aerobic and strengthening exercise, and social support. Also, concomitant depressive disorders, a frequent comorbidity, require attention for successful weight loss and maintenance.

The weight-loss program must contain three essential components: (1) a nutritionally balanced diet, (2) aerobic and strengthening exercise, and (3) a reduction in the percentage of calories derived from fat. It has been shown that reducing the percentage of calories derived from fat (compared to carbohydrates and proteins) by itself produces weight loss. Current recommendations suggest that the energy intake should be approximately 500 calories less than energy output in a weight-loss program. Low-carbohydrate diets, although effective in rapid short-term weight loss, have not been proven to be more effective long term than a balanced calorie-restricted diet. In addition, the long-term effects of carbohydrate-restricted diets are not known. Nevertheless, much attention is being focused on these diets, and these and other diets are a multimillion dollar per year industry. The importance in strength training is receiving new attention. Research has shown that larger muscle mass burns fat and calories more efficiently. Many weight-loss programs now emphasize a balance between aerobic activity and muscle strength training. There is good evidence that other benefits (e.g., improved proprioception and balance in the elderly) may derive from strength training. Newer research strongly implicates genetic influences in obesity. Some believe that the majority of obesity may be explained by genetic causes that influence behavior.

10. e. The practical management of weight loss in a patient by the patient's family physician should include the following: (1) making weekly office visits over a period of 8 to 12 weeks and gradual lengthening of time between visits after that, (2) modifying eating habits, (3) keeping a food diary, and (4) increasing aerobic and strength training exercise activity.

Home weighing is not recommended because of significant fluctuations in body weight as a result of body water. If it is necessary for the patient to weigh himself or herself at home, it should be done no more than once or twice every 2 weeks.

The modification of eating habits is an important and interesting component of the overall plan. First, patients must begin to regard eating as a conscious activity rather than something that happens while thinking of other things. Second, the suggestion of drinking two glasses of water just before the meal to decrease appetite has validity. Third, instructing the patient to eat more slowly and chew food more thoroughly also appears to be valid.

11. **e.** Sibutramine, orlistat, phentermine, diethylpropion, bupropion, fluoxetine, and topiramate all promote weight loss. All of these drugs have side effects. Sibutramine treatment results in a weight loss (compared to placebo) of 3.43 kg at 6 months and 4.45 kg at 12 months, and orlistat results in a mean weight loss of 2.51 kg at 6 months and 2.75 kg at 12 months. Subjects treated with phentermine lose on average 3.6 additional kilograms of weight at 6 months, whereas subjects treated with diethylpropion lose on average 3.0 additional kilograms of weight. Fluoxetine studies show a mean weight loss of 4.74 kg at 6 months and

3.05 kg at 12 months. Bupropion studies show weight loss of 2.8 kg at 6 to 12 months, and topiramate studies show 6.5% of pretreatment weight lost at 6 months. Surgical treatment is more effective than nonsurgical treatment for individuals with a BMI of 40 kg/m^2 or greater, but it is associated with a substantial number of complications and adverse events and a mortality rate of approximately 1%. Surgery results in a 20- to 30-kg weight loss, maintained up to 8 years and accompanied by significant improvements in several comorbidities. Bariatric surgical complication rates can be high, and they vary significantly by surgeon.

Sibutramine can substantially increase blood pressure and pulse in some patients; all patients treated with sibutramine should have regular monitoring of blood pressure and pulse. Frequently encountered side effects include dry mouth, paradoxically increased appetite, nausea, strange taste in the mouth, anorgasmia and delayed ejaculation, upset stomach, constipation, trouble sleeping, dizziness, drowsiness, menstrual cramps/pain, headache, flushing, or joint/muscle pain.

Orlistat side effects are primarily gastrointestinal. The stool may become oily or loose, and increased flatulence is also common. Bowel movements often can be frequent or urgent, and absorption of fat-soluble vitamins and other fat-soluble nutrients is inhibited. Patients should take a multivitamin tablet containing fat-soluble vitamins once a day, at least 2 hours before or after taking the drug.

Solution to the Clinical Case Management Problem

The most common causes of secondary obesity include the following:

1. Iatrogenic disease: drugs that produce either true weight gain (more fat) as a side effect or produce salt and water retention
2. Depression: many patients gain weight
3. Cushing's syndrome
4. Hypothyroidism

Remember, however, that less than 1% of patients who are obese have an identifiable secondary cause of obesity.

Summary

1. **Definition**
   a. BMI = 30 kg/m^2 or, alternatively
   b. 20% higher than suggested ideal body weight

2. **Prevalence**
   An epidemic of obesity exists in the United States. In 2006, 34% of adults in the United States were obese;

when combined with overweight (BMI 25–29.9) U.S. adults, more than 66% of adults carry excess weight and its health consequences. Children are of particular concern because obesity rates are increasing, portending increasing rates as adults with attendant morbidities. Already the rate of type 2 diabetes has increased significantly in children.

3. Significance

a. Obesity is now regarded as the most important public health problem in the United States. (Unfortunately, it often is ignored because of the social stigma attached to it.)

b. Even more important is the increase in prevalence of obesity in children and adolescents. More than 17% of the children in the United States are overweight.

4. Complications

This increase in obesity translates into increased prevalence of the following:

a. coronary artery disease
b. myocardial infarction (obese patients are 250% more likely to develop coronary artery disease than are nonobese patients)
c. cerebrovascular disease
d. left ventricular hypertrophy and congestive heart failure
e. hyperlipidemia
f. type 2 diabetes mellitus with macrovascular complications
g. osteoarthritis
h. cholelithiasis and cholecystitis
i. obstructive sleep apnea and Pickwickian syndrome
j. restrictive lung disease
k. cancer
l. gout

Because obesity is a major risk factor for type 2 diabetes, the complications associated with this disease can also largely be considered a consequence of diabetes. These include

a. diabetic nephropathy from chronic renal failure (diabetes mellitus type 2 is the most common cause of chronic renal failure in the United States because type 2 diabetes is 10 times more frequent than type 1 diabetes)
b. diabetic retinopathy
c. diabetic neuropathy
d. autonomic neuropathy
e. generalized atherosclerotic vascular disease

5. Treatment

a. Avoid all diet fads and diet "revolutions."
b. Avoid anorexic drugs.
c. Change the composition of the diet. Maintain carbohydrate and protein, and decrease fat. Avoid simple sugars.
d. Attend multiple office visits to establish a baseline and to motivate continual weight loss.
e. Decrease caloric intake to approximately 500 kcal/day less than energy expenditure. (This produces a weight loss of approximately 1 pound/week.)
f. Increase aerobic and strength-training exercise. (This is essential to long-term weight loss and maintenance.)
g. Receive positive reinforcement from a support group, the physician, family, and friends.
h. Treat comorbid conditions including depression.
i. Carefully select patients for use of any weight-loss pharmacotherapeutic agents or surgical procedures.

Suggested Reading

Agency for Healthcare Research and Quality: *Pharmacological and Surgical Treatment of Obesity*. Accessed from www.ahrq.gov.

Aggoun Y: Obesity, metabolic syndrome, and cardiovascular disease. *Pediatr Res* 61(6):653–659, 2007.

Floriani V, Kennedy C: Promotion of physical activity in primary care for obesity treatment/prevention in children. *Curr Opin Pediatr* 19(1):99–103, 2007.

Hennekens CH, Schneider WR, Barice EJ: Obesity in childhood: Introduction and general considerations. *Pediatr Res* 61(6):634–635, 2007.

Institute for Clinical Systems Improvement: *Prevention and Management of Obesity (Mature Adolescents and Adults)*. Bloomington, MN: Institute for Clinical Systems Improvement, 2006.

LaMonte MJ, Blair SN: Physical activity, cardiorespiratory fitness, and adiposity: Contributions to disease risk. *Curr Opin Clin Nutr Metab Care* 9(5):540–546, 2006.

Low AK, Bouldin MJ, Sumrall CD, et al: A clinician's approach to medical management of obesity. *Am J Med Sci* 331(4):175–182, 2006.

Malnick SD, Knobler H: The medical complications of obesity. *Q J Med* 99(9):565–579, 2006.

Melzer K, Kayser B, Pichard C: Physical activity: The health benefits outweigh the risks. *Curr Opin Clin Nutr Metab Care* 7(6):641–647, 2004.

Saper RB, Eisenberg DM, Phillips RS: Common dietary supplements for weight loss. *Am Fam Physician* 70:1731–1738, 2004.

Virji A, Murr MM: Caring for patients after bariatric surgery. *Am Fam Physician* 73:1403–1408, 2006.

10 Trends in Cancer Epidemiology

CLINICAL CASE PROBLEM 1

A 74-Year-Old Farmer with Abdominal Pain

A 74-year-old grain farmer comes to your office for assessment of abdominal pain of 6 months' duration. The pain is located in the central abdomen with radiation through to the back. It is a dull, constant pain with no significant aggravating or relieving factors. It is not affected in any way by food. It is rated by the patient as a 5/10 baseline with occasional increases to 7/10. It has been getting worse for the past 2 months.

On examination, vital signs are stable, but the sclerae are slightly icteric. The abdomen is scaphoid. The liver margin feels slightly irregular 2 cm below the right costal margin. No other masses are felt. Abdominal ultrasound reveals a solid mass lesion in the area of the head of the pancreas measuring 4 cm. There are also two or three nodular densities (1 cm each) in the liver.

SELECT THE BEST ANSWER TO THE FOLLOWING QUESTIONS

1. What is the most likely diagnosis in this patient?
   a. benign pseudocyst of the pancreas
   b. adenocarcinoma of the pancreas
   c. squamous cell carcinoma of the pancreas
   d. pancreatitis
   e. malignant pseudocyst of the pancreas

2. With regard to the diagnosis in this patient, which of the following statements is true?
   a. the incidence of this disease has remained constant during the past 10 years in the United States
   b. the death rate from this disease has decreased significantly during the past 10 years in the United States
   c. the survival rate from this disease has increased greatly during the past 10 years in the United States
   d. there are no accurate data on death rates from this disease in the United States for the past 10 years
   e. none of the above are true

3. With regard to cancer mortality in the United States, which of the following statements is true?
   a. during the past 20 years, the death rate from all cancers has decreased significantly in children
   b. during the past 20 years, the death rate from prostate cancer has increased by 20%
   c. during the past 20 years, there has been no significant change in the death rate from lung cancers
   d. during the past 20 years, the death rate from all cancers has increased by 20%
   e. during the past 20 years, the death rate from breast cancer has increased by 15%

4. Which of the following statements is true regarding the leading causes of cancer mortality in the United States?
   a. the leading causes of cancer death by site in men are lung, prostate, and colon
   b. the leading causes of cancer death by site in women are breast, lung, and uterine
   c. the most prevalent cancers in women are breast, uterine, and bladder
   d. the most prevalent cancers in men are lung, bladder, and colon
   e. African Americans have a lower death rate from cancers than white Americans

5. With respect to the statistics discussed in questions 3 and 4, which of the following statements is true?
   a. the number of cancer cases can be expected to increase because of the growth and aging of the population in coming decades
   b. a major cause of the recent decline in lung cancer mortality rates in women is an increase in smoking rates
   c. high colorectal cancer screening rates continue to counterbalance the effects of diet and lack of physical activity
   d. the epidemic of obesity is unlikely to have any effect on cancer incidence and mortality trends
   e. tobacco taxes have little effect on smoking initiation in adolescents

6. With respect to secondary prevention measures for cancer, which of the following is true?
   a. the use of screening tests for breast cancer is decreasing
   b. the use of screening tests for cervical cancer is decreasing
   c. screening rates of at-risk populations for colorectal cancer remain low

d. physician screening rates for tobacco use in patients are satisfactory
e. lung cancer screening tests have been shown to reduce mortality

7. What is the leading cause of cancer death in women in the United States today?
a. breast cancer
b. colon cancer
c. lung cancer
d. brain cancer
e. ovarian cancer

CLINICAL CASE PROBLEM 2

A 50-Year-Old Stockbroker Who Watches Television

A 50-year-old stockbroker with no first-degree relatives with cancer visits you for your recommendations on colon cancer screening. She has heard about colonoscopy from a celebrity on television but wants to know what the options are and what you think. She has heard of those stool tests, but thinks the idea sounds "icky." She asks you which test you are going to have when you turn 50 years old. You spend some time providing her with information regarding screening for colorectal cancer.

8. Which of the following facts regarding colon cancer screening is correct?
a. the U.S. Preventive Services Task Force (USPSTF) recommends only two screening methods: fecal occult blood testing and colonoscopy
b. patients should be informed that the risk of perforation or serious bleeding from colonoscopy is approximately 1 in 1000 procedures in the community
c. colonoscopy has been proved to reduce mortality in large-scale screening trials
d. colon preparation for colonoscopy involves the administration of two enemas before the procedure
e. fecal occult blood testing involves virtually no preparation on the part of the patient

Clinical Case Management Problem

Discuss the preventive measures your patients may undertake to lower their risk of cancer from all causes.

Answers

1. **b.** The most likely diagnosis in this patient is adenocarcinoma of the pancreas. With the clinical history of progressive pain, the finding of an irregular liver border (which suggests liver metastases), and the finding of a mass lesion on ultrasound, the diagnosis is almost certainly confirmed. None of the other choices are reasonable. Pseudocysts do not show solid mass lesions. Squamous cell carcinoma does not occur in the pancreas. The history, physical findings, and ultrasound findings are not compatible with a diagnosis of pancreatitis.

2. **a.** During the past 10 years, the incidence of carcinoma of the pancreas has not changed. Age-adjusted mortality from this cancer has also not changed in the past 10 years. Pancreatic cancer remains one of the most lethal forms of cancer, with a dismal 5-year survival rate of approximately 3%.

3. **a.** Death rates from cancer, all sites and types, increased through 1990, then stabilized until 1993, and fell from 1993 through 2004. Individuals 65 years old or older have experienced an increased mortality from cancer during the past 20 years. Between 1990 and 2004, lung and prostate cancer death rates deceased in men, as did breast and colon cancer deaths in women. Nevertheless, lung cancer mortality now surpasses breast cancer mortality in woman. However, during the past 20 years, the overall death rate in children from all cancers has decreased by 40% in the United States. This is despite an increase in incidence roughly equivalent to the decrease. Leukemia is the most common cancer among children ages 0 to 14 years, and it is responsible for approximately 30% of all cancers during childhood. Acute lymphocytic cancer is the most common form of leukemia in children, whereas cancer of the brain/other nervous system is the second most common.

4. **a.** In 2007, there were 559,650 cancer deaths in the United States, accounting for nearly one-fourth of deaths in the country, surpassed only by heart disease. In men, lung cancer is by far the most common fatal cancer, followed by prostate and colon and rectum cancer. In women, lung, breast, and colon and rectum cancer are the leading sites of cancer death. Overall, men experience cancer death rates that are higher than those of women in every racial and ethnic group. African American men and women have the highest rates of cancer mortality. Asian and Pacific Islander women have the lowest cancer death rates, at approximately half the rate for African American women. For many

sites, survival rates in African Americans are 10% to 15% lower than those in whites. African Americans are less likely to receive a cancer diagnosis at an early, localized stage, when treatment can improve chances of survival. Cancer prevalence rates (excluding skin cancers) by site in men are highest for prostate, lung, and colon; in women (again excluding skin cancers), it is breast, lung, and colon, respectively.

5. a. The rate of cancer incidence has declined since the early 1990s. Nevertheless, the huge demographic shift occurring in the U.S. population is likely to yield increased numbers of cancer prevalence for the foreseeable future. Age is a risk factor for the development of cancer, but it is not the only one. Because of reduced cigarette consumption, we are seeing a reduction in lung cancer death rates in men. Obesity is a risk factor for several cancers, including female breast (among postmenopausal women), colon, and prostate cancer. There is a definite cancer link to smoking, a possible link to dietary fat and physical inactivity, and a definite link to multiple environmental carcinogens, all of which may play a role in the changing cancer epidemiology. Despite the protestations of tobacco companies, tobacco taxes are extremely effective in curbing smoking initiation rates in children and adolescents.

6. c. Screening rates remain low in most populations despite evidence of effectiveness of many interventions. Whereas mammography and cervical cancer screening rates are increasing, colorectal cancer screening rates, although slowly increasing, still remain low, despite the fact that effective methodologies exist. Death rates from lung cancer, especially among women, have increased significantly during the past 20 years. Yet many clinicians fail to perform the basic screen of asking about tobacco use in their patients. Despite the proliferation of physician and health industry advertising to the contrary, no lung cancer screening methodology has been shown to reduce mortality.

7. c. Lung cancer is now the most common cause of cancer death in U.S. women. This primarily is associated with the significantly increased risk as a result of smoking, as previously discussed.

8. b. The USPSTF recommends only that screening take place, not the specific method, which should be the patient's choice after a coherent discussion of the options available with the clinician. Fecal occult blood testing, colonoscopy, and sigmoidoscopy are all acceptable screening methods. Patients should be informed of all the risks and benefits and alternatives available. That would include the risk of perforation or serious bleeding from colonoscopy, which is between 1 in 1000 and 1 in 3000 procedures, as reported in several series in the literature. As with any procedure, risks are reduced by using a colonoscopist who performs a large volume of procedures. Someday, clinician-specific outcome rates will be public knowledge, but until then, family physicians must act as information gatherers for their patients. Although colonoscopy has not been proved to reduce colorectal cancer mortality in large-scale screening trials, the presumption is that it will. Several trials are under way. Colon preparation for colonoscopy is extensive; it involves the administration of cathartics the night before the procedure and restricting oral intake, both of which are sometimes difficult for the elderly. Fecal occult blood testing involves careful attention to dietary intake and medications on the part of the patient to reduce false-positive and false-negatives results.

Solution to the Clinical Case Management Problem

The following are the most important preventive measures that your patients may undertake to lower their risk of cancer from all causes: (1) Discontinue cigarette, pipe, and cigar smoking or tobacco chewing; (2) decrease the amount of alcohol consumed; (3) decrease the amount of dietary fat, especially saturated fat; (4) maintain a normal weight (to be accomplished by a decrease in dietary fat, a decrease in overall caloric intake, and an exercise program); (5) decrease exposure to environmental carcinogens whenever possible (protect yourself when applying pesticides, herbicides, and related chemicals); (6) avoid sun exposure without a sunscreen with a sun protective factor of 15 or greater; and (7) follow the USPSTF recommendations concerning the periodic health examination.

Summary

1. Death rates from cancer among all ages, all sites and types, have declined from 1993 through 2004.
2. Cancer remains the second leading cause of death in the United States, responsible for one-fourth of deaths in the country.
3. In men, lung cancer is by far the most common fatal cancer, followed by prostate and colorectal cancer.
4. In women, lung, breast, and colon and rectum cancer are the leading sites of cancer death.
5. African Americans are less likely to receive a cancer diagnosis at an early, localized stage, when treatment can improve chances of survival.
6. Cancer prevalence rates (excluding skin cancers) by site in men are highest for prostate, lung, and colon; in women (again excluding skin cancers), it is breast, lung, and colon, respectively.
7. Screening rates remain low in most populations despite evidence of effectiveness of many screening interventions.

Suggested Reading

For more information, visit the following Web sites:

American Cancer Society: www.cancer.org
Centers for Disease Control and Prevention's Division of Cancer Prevention and Control: www.cdc.gov/cancer

National Cancer Institute: http://nci.nih.gov.
Surveillance, Epidemiology, and End Results home page of the National Cancer Institute: www.seer.cancer.gov

---

CHAPTER

11 Cardiovascular Epidemiology

CLINICAL CASE PROBLEM 1

A 52-Year-Old Male with Coronary Heart Disease Who Has Had Both a Coronary Artery Bypass Grafting Procedure and Percutaneous Transluminal Angioplasty Procedures Done

A 52-year-old male with a history of coronary artery disease treated by a coronary artery bypass grafting procedure following three percutaneous transluminal angioplasty procedures and who currently is undergoing "triple angina therapy" comes to your office for a discussion of his condition and of the implications of his condition for his children. He recently has read that family history is a strong risk factor for heart disease (HD).

SELECT THE BEST ANSWER TO THE FOLLOWING QUESTIONS

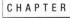

1. Since 1979, cardiovascular disease mortality in women in the United States has
   a. increased
   b. decreased by 30%
   c. stayed the same
   d. been exceeded by men
   e. decreased by more than 50%

2. Since 1979, cardiovascular disease mortality for men in the United States has
   a. increased by 50%
   b. decreased
   c. attained parity with women
   d. increased by 20%
   e. remained unchanged

3. Which of the following regarding stroke epidemiology is correct?
   a. 50% of stroke deaths occur outside of hospitals
   b. stroke is the second leading cause of death in the United States
   c. thrombotic strokes are more deadly than hemorrhagic or thromboembolic strokes
   d. age-adjusted death rates are lower in African Americans than in other groups
   e. Latinos have a higher age-adjusted death rate than other populations

4. What has been the major reason for the decline in the death rate from cardiovascular disease in the United States?
   a. new technology
   b. improved pharmacology
   c. better surgical techniques

d. risk factor reduction

e. nobody really knows for sure

5. The risk of developing cardiovascular disease in patients with hypertension compared with patients who do not have hypertension is
   a. three or four times as high for HD and seven times as high for stroke
   b. twice as high for HD and five times as high for stroke
   c. six times as high for HD and eight times as high for stroke
   d. the same for HD and twice as high for stroke
   e. the same for HD and the same for stroke

6. Regarding cigarette smoking and the risk of developing HD, which of the following statements is true?
   a. cigarette smokers have a 70% greater risk of developing HD than nonsmokers
   b. cigarette smokers have a 50% greater risk of developing HD than nonsmokers
   c. cigarette smokers have a 25% greater risk of developing HD than nonsmokers
   d. cigarette smokers have a 10% greater risk of developing HD than nonsmokers
   e. there is no difference in the risk of developing HD between smokers and nonsmokers

7. Regarding cigarette smoking, which of the following statements is true?
   a. the risk of HD is increased by up to 30% for those nonsmokers exposed to workplace or at-home environmental tobacco smoke
   b. smoking costs Americans approximately $20 billion in medical care per year
   c. after quitting, smokers' HD risk decreases by 50% after 10 years
   d. there is a direct correlation between smoking and education levels
   e. since 1969, the prevalence of smoking has increased by 20%

8. Regarding serum cholesterol and the incidence of HD, which of the following statements is true?
   a. for each 1% reduction in serum cholesterol there is a 6% reduction in the risk of heart disease death
   b. for each 1% reduction in serum cholesterol there is a 4% reduction in the risk of heart disease death
   c. for each 1% reduction in serum cholesterol there is a 2% reduction in the risk of heart disease death
   d. for each 1% reduction in serum cholesterol there is a 1% reduction in the risk of heart disease death

e. there is no established relationship between serum cholesterol and the risk of heart disease death

9. Regarding the risk of obesity in relation to cardiovascular disease, which of the following statements is (are) true?
   a. obesity is a risk factor for hypertension
   b. obesity is a risk factor for hypercholesterolemia
   c. obesity is a risk factor for diabetes
   d. obesity is an independent risk factor for HD
   e. all of the above statements are true

10. Body mass index (BMI) is defined as which of the following?
    a. the weight in pounds divided by the square of the height in meters
    b. the weight in kilograms divided by the square of the height in meters
    c. the square of the height in meters divided by the weight in pounds
    d. the square of the height in meters divided by the weight in kilograms
    e. none of the above

11. What is the definition of obesity?
    a. a weight 40% higher than normal weight for height
    b. a BMI of more than $25 \, kg/m^2$
    c. a weight 20% higher than normal weight for height
    d. a BMI of $30 \, kg/m^2$ or greater
    e. a weight 10% higher than normal weight for height

12. With respect to physical inactivity (sedentary lifestyle) and the risk of cardiovascular disease, which of the following statements is (are) true?
    a. sedentary lifestyle is an independent risk factor for cardiovascular disease
    b. sedentary lifestyle is associated with an increased death rate from cardiovascular disease
    c. sedentary lifestyle may be as strong a risk factor for cardiovascular disease as several other risk factors combined
    d. sedentary lifestyle is strongly correlated with obesity
    e. all of the above statements are true

13. What is the estimated percentage of Americans with hypertension whose blood pressure is under good control?
    a. 50%
    b. 75%
    c. 25%
    d. 10%
    e. 5%

14. With respect to primary prevention of hypertension, all except which of the following are proven to be effective?
    a. weight loss
    b. reduced dietary sodium intake
    c. moderation of alcohol intake
    d. increased physical activity
    e. calcium supplementation

15. Which of the following statements regarding the primary prevention of hypertension is true?
    a. the demonstrated reductions in blood pressure using lifestyle changes can be as large as those seen in pharmacotherapy
    b. lifestyle changes more effectively reduce blood pressure levels in males than in females
    c. blood pressure reductions as a result of lifestyle changes are sustained for an average of 6 to 12 months
    d. sodium added to processed food counts for an average of 20% of daily dietary sodium intake
    e. suburbanization of living patterns in the United States has no linkage to hypertension epidemiology

Answers

1. **a.** Since 1979, the cardiovascular disease mortality rate for women in the United States has increased. In 2004, cardiovascular disease claimed 459,000 lives. Since 1984, the number of cardiovascular disease deaths for females has exceeded that for males.

2. **b.** Since 1979, the cardiovascular disease mortality rate for men in the United States has decreased from 500,000 deaths per year to approximately 400,000.

3. **a.** Of stroke deaths, 50% occur outside of hospitals. Most patients do not make it to health care. That is why the first few hours, when thrombolytic therapy can be administered to nonhemorrhagic stroke victims, are so important. Stroke is the third leading cause of death in the United States, after heart disease and cancer; on average, every 3 minutes, someone dies of stroke. Thrombotic strokes are less deadly than hemorrhagic or thromboembolic strokes, but they are more common. Age-adjusted death rates from stroke are higher in African Americans than in other groups, and they are lower in Latinos.

4. **d.** The major reasons for the significant decrease in cardiovascular mortality in the United States are changes in lifestyle and risk factor reduction. Other contributing factors include new technology, improved pharmacology, better surgical techniques, and more effective medical management.

5. **a.** Americans with hypertension have three or four times the risk of developing HD and as much as seven times the risk of stroke as do those with normal blood pressure.

6. **a.** Cigarette smoking is a major risk factor for cardiovascular disease. Cigarette smokers are at increased risk for fatal and nonfatal myocardial infarctions and for sudden cardiac death. Smokers have a 70% greater HD prevalence rate, a twofold to fourfold greater incidence of acquiring HD, and a twofold to fourfold greater risk for sudden death than nonsmokers.

7. **a.** The risk of HD is increased by up to 30% for those nonsmokers exposed to workplace or at-home environmental tobacco smoke. Smoking costs Americans more than $200 billion in medical care per year and an estimated $400 billion in direct and indirect (e.g., time lost from work) costs per year. With numbers like these, which do not even begin to measure the human costs, it boggles the mind how politicians in the United States still can support tobacco farming subsidies year after year. After quitting, smokers' HD risk decreases by 50% after 1 year, making the rationale for quitting all the more potent. There is a relationship between smoking and education levels. They are inversely related: The higher the education levels, the lower the smoking rate. Tobacco sellers know this and target people of lower education levels with advertising. Since 1969, the prevalence of smoking in the United States has declined by 40% in people older than age 18 years.

8. **c.** Elevated serum cholesterol levels are associated with an increased risk of HD. Epidemiologic work in this area has suggested that for each 1% reduction in serum cholesterol, there is an associated 2% reduction in the risk of death from HD.

9. **e.** Being obese is a risk factor for hypertension, hypercholesterolemia, and diabetes mellitus. It is also an independent risk factor for HD. Being obese and being physically inactive increase all risks.

10. **b.** BMI is defined as the weight of a person in kilograms divided by the height of the person in meters squared. Tables are available that allow the calculation of BMI to be made easily in the office.

11. **d.** The definition of obesity is a BMI of 30 or greater.

12. e. Physical inactivity, or a sedentary lifestyle, is quickly becoming recognized as a powerful risk factor for cardiovascular disease. It is recognized as an independent risk factor for cardiovascular disease and cardiovascular death. There is extensive evidence that a vigorous exercise program, in fact, may counteract many other risk factors with regard to both the cardiovascular death rate and the cardiovascular disease prevalence rate. Physical inactivity is also associated with being obese, and these two risk factors are additive.

Weight-reduction programs are rarely successful in the absence of a reasonable exercise program. Most authorities suggest that to make a significant difference to the cardiovascular system, aerobic exercise must occur daily and last at least 30 minutes per session.

13. c. The percentage of Americans with hypertension whose blood pressure is under good control is estimated to be no more than 25%.

14. e. Weight loss, reduction of dietary sodium intake, moderation of alcohol intake, and increased physical activity are all (level of evidence A or B) effective in the prevention and control of hypertension. Calcium supplementation, although effective in some studies, has not been proved to be effective in large population studies or randomized controlled trials.

15. a. Multiple studies have demonstrated that reductions in blood pressure using lifestyle changes can be as large as those seen in pharmacotherapy. Yet most physicians largely continue to ignore this fact and fail to educate their patients about this or work with them to achieve success in lifestyle changes. Imagine the cost savings to us all if clinicians were as effective in helping to change people's behaviors as they are in prescribing pharmaceuticals. Blood pressure reductions as a result of lifestyle changes are equally effective in both male and female populations and in all ethnicities, races, and socioeconomic groups. Moreover, blood pressure reductions resulting from lifestyle changes are sustained well beyond 3 years in most studies. Sodium added to processed food counts for an astounding average of 70% of daily dietary sodium intake in the United States. This is why clinicians should encourage patients to pay careful attention to food labels. Dietary sodium reduction is linked directly to primary prevention of hypertension. Suburbanization of living patterns has also been linked to obesity epidemiology in the United States. Obesity is a risk factor in hypertension. With people becoming more dependent on the automobile even for basic activities of daily living such as eating lunch, physical activity levels have declined and obesity and hypertension have increased.

Summary

1. There has been a significant decrease in cardiovascular mortality rates in the United States during the past 15 years; however, the mortality rate among women is increasing.
2. The major reasons for the decrease in cardiovascular mortality rates in the United States are lifestyle modification and risk factor reduction.
3. Lifestyle modification, particularly weight loss and physical activity, are particularly important in efforts to further reduce cardiovascular mortality.
4. Hypertension, hypercholesterolemia, cigarette smoking, obesity, and physical inactivity are all independent risk factors for cardiovascular disease.
5. A vigorous exercise program may be enough to counteract several other cardiovascular risk factors and prevent cardiovascular morbidity and mortality.
6. Death rates from stroke are significantly higher in African Americans than in whites.
7. Cigarette smoking is estimated to account for 40% of deaths from HD in Americans younger than age 65 years.
8. The continuing education of the U.S. population with respect to what they can do for themselves to decrease risk of cardiovascular disease remains our number-one priority. Aggressive intervention with risk factors through lifestyle modification, education, and counseling will remain one of the greatest and most rewarding challenges for family physicians in this century.
9. The demonstrated reductions in blood pressure using lifestyle changes can be as large as those seen in pharmacotherapy. Clinicians need to educate their patients of this fact and learn effective means of helping to motivate patients to achieve these changes. Proven measures include restricting dietary sodium, increasing daily consumption of fruits and vegetables, increasing physical activity, losing weight, and eliminating tobacco use.

Suggested Reading

Ginsberg HN, Stalenhoef AF: The metabolic syndrome: Targeting dyslipidaemia to reduce coronary risk. *J Cardiovasc Risk* 10(2):121–128, 2004.

Hayes SN: Preventing cardiovascular disease in women. *Am Fam Physician*74:1331–1340, 1342, 2006.

Hooper L, Bartlett C, Davey Smith E, et al: Reduced dietary salt for prevention of cardiovascular disease. *Cochrane Database Syst Rev* (1):CD003656, 2003.

Mosca L, Banka CL, Benjamin EJ, et al: Evidence-based guidelines for cardiovascular disease prevention in women 2007 update. *Circulation* 115(11):1481–1501, 2007.

Oh RC, Lanier JB: Management of hypertriglyceridemia. *Am Fam Physician* 75:1365–1372, 2007.

Shaw K, Gennat H, O'Rourke P, Del Mar C: Exercise for overweight or obesity. *Cochrane Database Syst Rev* (4):CD003817, 2006.

Thom T, Haase N, Rosamond W, et al: Heart disease and stroke statistics—2006 update. *Circulation* 2006;113:e85–e151.

Wiysonge CS, Bradley H, Mayosi BM, et al: Beta-blockers for hypertension. *Cochrane Database Syst Rev* (1):CD002003, 2007.

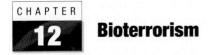

CHAPTER 12 · Bioterrorism

CLINICAL CASE PROBLEM 1

A Disturbing News Report

You are driving to your office after making hospital rounds and hear a news flash on the radio that several people in your community have come down with a mysterious respiratory illness that has caused three seemingly healthy middle-aged people to die suddenly and unexpectedly. The report says authorities have reason to suspect an act of bioterrorism. When you arrive at the office, your telephone lines are being flooded with incoming calls. Your receptionist says, "What's going on? Why is everyone panicked?"

SELECT THE BEST ANSWER TO THE FOLLOWING QUESTIONS

1. What is your best source of reliable information about the situation?
   a. local television news reports
   b. local health department
   c. police department
   d. Centers for Disease Control and Prevention (CDC) Web site
   e. local newspaper

2. You receive the necessary information from the appropriate source. The next day you speak by telephone to a patient at work who gives you a plausible exposure history and relates symptoms that are of concern to you. Your most appropriate next step for this patient is?
   a. send the patient home to await instructions
   b. send the patient to the hospital emergency department
   c. bring the patient into the office for an evaluation
   d. make a home visit to the patient
   e. none of the above

3. You make the correct choice in the next step for care for this patient. Whom should you immediately notify regarding the patient and your concerns?
   a. the local health department
   b. the hospital emergency department
   c. the local police
   d. no one because it would be a violation of the patient's privacy
   e. a, b, and c

4. The agents used in bioterrorism attacks are grouped into which of the following categories?
   a. biologic and radiologic
   b. biologic, radiologic, and chemical
   c. inhaled, topical, and ingested
   d. chemical and radiologic
   e. none of the above

5. Which of the following characteristics distinguish smallpox (variola) eruptions from those of chickenpox (varicella)?
   a. varicella eruptions are centripetal; variola are centrifugal
   b. variola eruptions break out all at once; varicella come in crops
   c. varicella eruptions are preceded by a highly febrile prodrome; variola are not
   d. variola eruptions are uncomfortable; varicella are not
   e. varicella eruptions progress slowly; variola eruptions progress to pustules in less than 12 hours

6. During which of the following times is the patient infected with variola not contagious?
   a. the incubation period
   b. the febrile prodrome
   c. during the initial rash on the tongue and in the mouth

d. during the pustular eruptions

e. after scab formation

7. Which of the following is true regarding smallpox?
   a. direct face-to-face contact is the most common means of smallpox spread
   b. smallpox can be spread through direct contact with infected bodily fluids or contaminated objects such as bedding or clothing
   c. smallpox can be spread through the air of enclosed buildings
   d. humans are the only natural hosts of variola
   e. all of the above

8. Which of the following is not true regarding plague?
   a. a swollen, tender lymph gland is the typical sign of the most common form of human plague
   b. signs of bubonic plague include a swollen gland with fever, chills, headache, and extreme exhaustion
   c. symptoms appear 12 to 16 days after being infected
   d. pneumonic plague causes high fever, chills, cough, difficulty breathing, and bloody sputum
   e. 14% of all plague cases in the United States are fatal

CLINICAL CASE PROBLEM 2

Show and Tell (and Pray It Never Happens)

As part of a bioterrorism preparedness program, you are asked to lecture to a group of your colleagues at the local hospital. Here are some of the questions you get. Choose the correct response.

9. What is (are) the appropriate choice(s) of antibiotic prophylaxis for a possible inhalation anthrax exposure?
   a. ciprofloxacin
   b. doxycycline
   c. amoxicillin
   d. clarithromycin
   e. a and b

10. Which of the following is (are) correct regarding inhalation anthrax?
    a. the average incubation period is 4 to 6 days
    b. the symptom complex includes fever, chills, sweats, fatigue, minimally productive cough, nausea or vomiting, and chest discomfort
    c. chest x-ray initially may show mediastinal widening, paratracheal/hilar fullness, and pleural effusions/infiltrates

d. pleural effusions are a common complication

e. all of the above

11. Chemical agents such as sarin typically work by causing neurotoxicity. Common routes of exposure to the agent sarin include which of the following?
    a. breathing contaminated air
    b. eating contaminated food
    c. drinking contaminated water or touching contaminated surfaces
    d. a, b, and c
    e. a and c

12. People exposed to chemical bioterrorism agents typically may experience which of the following symptoms within seconds to hours?
    a. runny nose, watery eyes, blurred vision, confusion, and headache
    b. drooling and excessive sweating
    c. cough, chest tightness, and rapid breathing
    d. nausea, vomiting, and diarrhea
    e. all of the above

13. Which of the following is (are) an effective antidote(s) to the common neurotoxic chemical agents?
    a. atropine
    b. succinylcholine
    c. ethanol
    d. 2-PAM (pralidoxime [2-pyrididine aldoxime])
    e. a and d

14. What are the short- and long-term effects of exposure to neurotoxic chemical agents?
    a. permanent neurologic impairment at any level of exposure
    b. mild or moderately exposed people usually recover completely
    c. even severely exposed people are likely to survive
    d. most neurologic impairments last 1 or 2 years
    e. even people who were mildly exposed are likely to die

15. Which of the following is true regarding the classic stages seen in acute radiation syndrome?
    a. in the prodromal stage, classic symptoms include nausea, vomiting, and possibly diarrhea (depending on dose) and occur from minutes to days following exposure
    b. the symptoms of the prodromal stage may last for up to several months
    c. in the latent stage, the patient feels weak and somnolent for a few weeks
    d. in the manifest illness stage, the symptoms are specific to the neurologic system and last several months

e. in the final stage, recovery or death, most patients who recover will be back to normal in a matter of days

Answers

1. **b.** Your local health department is your best source of information regarding any bioterrorist threats. Since the events in the United States of September and October 2001, a massive public health effort has been made to link local health departments to the state departments of health and the federal CDC. Although notification protocols should work from local to state to federal authorities, your local health department should have the most reliable information regarding events in your area.

2. **b.** The local hospital emergency department is the best place for an evaluation. Most local hospitals now have protocols in place for evaluation of patients with potential exposures or symptomology suggestive of an exposure. Clinicians should familiarize themselves with the protocols in place for their area hospitals.

3. **e.** The family physician's responsibility for appropriate notification is an important and crucial part of the response to a potential bioterrorist agent exposure. Clinicians are on the front lines of any community event and are advised by the CDC to notify the local health department (most county health departments in the United States have 24-hour access) and police department of any potential danger. In this case, in which a patient is being sent to the emergency department, the standard of care and public health is to notify the hospital at once. Early notification is critical to an early response, and it is a critical duty of all physicians.

4. **b.** The agents used in terrorism attacks are grouped into the following categories: biologic, radiologic, and chemical.

Bioterrorism agents are separated into three categories—A, B, or C—depending on how easily they can be spread and the severity of illness or death they cause. Category A agents are considered the highest risk and the highest priority. Category B agents are the second highest priority. Category C agents are the third highest priority and include emerging pathogens that could be engineered for mass spread in the future. Category A agents include organisms and toxins that pose the highest risk to the public and national security for the following reasons: (1) They can be easily spread or transmitted from person to person, (2) they result in high death rates and have the potential for major public health impact, (3) they could cause extreme concern and social disruption, and (4) they require special action for public health preparedness. Category A bioterrorism agents include smallpox, plague, and anthrax.

Examples of radiologic agents include traditional thermonuclear devices, so-called "dirty" bombs (small explosive devices containing radioactive materials), and radioactive waste in various delivery vehicles. Examples of chemical agents include the nerve agents sarin, VX, and mustard gases. Unfortunately, a veritable wealth of possible agents is at the disposal of determined terrorists. The clinician should become familiar with the more common agents and their effects. A good source of information is the CDC Web site (www.cdc.gov), which has multiple links to other reliable sites.

5. **b.** Smallpox (variola) is a serious, contagious infectious disease with an overall fatality rate of approximately 30% in unimmunized populations. There is no treatment for smallpox; the only prevention is vaccination. Naturally occurring smallpox was eliminated from the world in the late 1970s, after which routine vaccination was stopped. The eruptions of chickenpox (varicella) can be confused with smallpox (variola). Fortunately, there are ways to distinguish between the two. Varicella eruptions tend to be centrifugal, whereas variola are more centripetal. Variola eruptions, which typically begin on the tongue, break out all at once; varicella eruptions come in crops. Varicella eruptions are usually not proceeded by a febrile prodrome, whereas the highly febrile prodrome is characteristic of variola. Both variola and varicella eruptions are uncomfortable. Varicella eruptions progress rapidly, going from papules to vesicles sometimes in 24 hours; variola eruptions progress to pustules in several days. Pictures of each of these eruptions are available on the CDC Web site.

6. **a.** There is an incubation period of approximately 12 to 14 days during which time (and the only time) people are not contagious. The prodrome phase of 2 to 4 days consists of initial symptoms that include fever, malaise, head and body aches, and high fever of 101°F to 104°F. Rash begins as small red spots on the tongue, which develop into sores that break open. A rash will then appear on the face and spread to the arms, legs, and then to hands and feet. Within 24 hours, the rash spreads to all parts of the body. The rash then becomes raised bumps that are filled with a thick, opaque fluid and often have a depression in the center. These become pustules that crust over after 2 weeks.

7. e. Direct and prolonged face-to-face contact usually is required to spread smallpox. Smallpox also can be spread through direct contact with infected bodily fluids or contaminated objects (bedding or clothing) and rarely through the air in enclosed settings such as buildings and airplanes. Humans are the only natural hosts of variola.

8. c. A swollen, tender lymph gland is the typical sign of the most common form of human plague—bubonic plague. Signs of bubonic plague include a swollen gland with fever, chills, headache, and extreme exhaustion. Symptoms appear 2 to 6 days after being infected. In non-terror situations, the infection is spread most commonly by the bites of fleas from rodent carriers. Plague will spread through the bloodstream to the lungs causing pneumonic plague, which is characterized by high fever, chills, cough, difficulty breathing, and bloody sputum. Of all plague cases in the United States, 14% are fatal, but the illness is successfully treatable with antibiotics if caught early.

9. e. Ciprofloxacin and doxycycline are approved by the Food and Drug Administration for prophylaxis of inhalational *Bacillus anthracis* infection. Both have adverse effects in children. Amoxicillin is an option for children and pregnant or lactating women.

10. e. Inhalation anthrax incubation ranges from 1 to 3 days versus 2 to 8 days for flea-borne transmission. Typical symptoms include fever, chills, sweats, fatigue, minimally productive cough, nausea or vomiting, and chest discomfort. Sounds like influenza? This is the problem during winter months. Chest x-ray initially may show mediastinal widening, paratracheal fullness, hilar fullness, and pleural effusions or infiltrates or both. Pleural effusions are common complications. Patients can survive but require aggressive supportive care and multidrug antibiotic regimens.

11. d. Common routes of exposure to the agent sarin include breathing contaminated air, eating contaminated food, drinking contaminated water, or touching contaminated surfaces.

12. e. Patients may experience any or all of the following symptoms, often within seconds or minutes of exposure: runny nose, watery eyes, blurred vision, confusion, headache, drooling and excessive sweating, cough, chest tightness, rapid breathing, nausea, vomiting, and diarrhea. Rapid treatment is essential for survival.

13. e. Patients whose skin or clothing is contaminated with liquid nerve agent can contaminate rescuers by direct contact or through off-gassing vapor. Nerve agents are extremely toxic and can cause death within minutes to hours after exposure from respiratory failure. Atropine and pralidoxime (2-PAM Cl) are antidotes for nerve agent toxicity; however, pralidoxime must be administered within minutes to a few hours following exposure (depending on the specific agent) to be effective. Treatment consists of supportive measures and repeated administration of antidotes.

14. b. To quote from the CDC, "Mild or moderately exposed people usually recover completely. Severely exposed people are not likely to survive. Unlike some organophosphate pesticides, nerve agents have not been associated with neurological problems lasting more than 1 to 2 weeks after the exposure."

15. a. Acute radiation syndrome (ARS) is an acute illness caused by irradiation of the entire body by a high dose of ionizing radiation in a very short period (usually a matter of minutes). There are four stages of ARS:

- Prodromal stage: The classic symptoms for this stage are nausea, vomiting, and possibly diarrhea (depending on dose), which occur from minutes to days following exposure. The symptoms may last (episodically) for minutes up to several days.
- Latent stage: In this stage, the patient looks and feels generally healthy for a few hours or even up to a few weeks.
- Manifest illness stage: In this stage, the symptoms depend on the specific syndrome and last from hours up to several months.
- Recovery or death stage: Most patients who do not recover will die within several months of exposure. The recovery process lasts from several weeks up to 2 years.

There are three syndromes associated with the manifest illness stage: bone marrow syndrome, gastrointestinal syndrome, and cardiac syndrome (each named for the system affected). Individuals with the cardiac and gastrointestinal syndromes rarely survive. Treatment for acute radiation disease is supportive because the damage has been done; only the outcome is unknown.

Summary

Family physicians are likely to find themselves on the front line of response to bioterrorism. Each of us needs to became familiar with the local public health apparatus and establish lines of communication with authorities before such an event. The events of 2001 taught us that no locale is immune to the possibility of terror threats and actions. Agents used to create terror and injure the population can be biologic, chemical, and radiologic. Common agents of concern include smallpox, anthrax, plague, sarin, mustard gas, and a variety of radiologic weapons. A good source of information on this subject is the CDC. Please visit their Web site at www.cdc.gov.

Suggested Reading

The CDC Web site contains a wealth of up-to-date information. Please visit http://emergency.cdc.gov/agent.

CHAPTER

13 Influenza and Other Emerging Diseases

CLINICAL CASE PROBLEM 1

A 73-Year-Old Male with Fever, Headache, and Myalgias

You are called to see a 73-year-old boarding home resident with a 24-hour history of temperature of 103°F, headache, myalgias, cough, rhinorrhea, sore throat, and malaise. Seven other residents in the same boarding home have come down with similar symptoms. It is late winter, and there has been a significant outbreak of respiratory illness in the community. He has received no vaccinations in the previous 5 years. On examination, the patient appears acutely ill with fever, tachypnea, and tachycardia. The patient also has prominent pharyngeal erythema. There are a few expiratory rhonchi heard and intermittent bilateral rales in the lower lung fields.

SELECT THE BEST ANSWER TO THE FOLLOWING QUESTIONS

1. What is the most likely diagnosis in this patient?
   a. influenza A
   b. bronchiolitis
   c. bacterial pneumonia
   d. septicemia secondary to an unknown focus of infection
   e. peritonsillar abscess

2. Which of the following investigations may be indicated in this patient?
   a. complete blood cell count (CBC)
   b. blood cultures
   c. chest radiograph
   d. all of the above
   e. none of the above

3. Which of the following statements regarding the influenza virus(es) is (are) true?
   a. influenza epidemics occur annually and are of major public health importance worldwide
   b. influenza viruses are subclassified as influenza A, influenza B, and influenza C
   c. excess morbidity and mortality are reported consistently during influenza epidemics
   d. all of the above
   e. none of the above

4. Concerning the use of antibiotics in influenza infection in the elderly, which of the following statements most accurately describes a high practice standard?
   a. no elderly patients with influenza should receive prophylactic antibiotics
   b. all elderly patients with influenza should receive prophylactic antibiotics
   c. in most cases of uncomplicated influenza, the risk–benefit ratio favors withholding antibiotics
   d. basically, give the patient antibiotics if he or she asks for them; if the patient does not ask, do not give them
   e. nobody really knows for sure

5. What is the most common complication of the illness described in this patient?
   a. meningitis

b. pneumonia

c. serum sickness

d. agranulocytosis

e. brain abscess

6. Which of the following types of influenza is responsible for most of the world pandemics?

a. influenza A

b. influenza B

c. influenza C

d. influenza D

e. influenza E

7. Which of the following is the drug of choice for treating the symptoms of the patient described?

a. acetylsalicylic acid

b. acetaminophen

c. oseltamivir

d. meperidine

e. ibuprofen

8. What is the primary mode of transmission of the illness described?

a. via blood and blood products

b. oral–fecal contamination

c. sneezing and coughing

d. fomites

e. kissing

9. What is the most reliable method for preventing influenza?

a. gamma globulin

b. alpha-interferon

c. activated influenza vaccine

d. inactivated influenza vaccine

e. amantadine hydrochloride

10. Regarding influenza vaccine, which of the following statements is (are) true?

a. influenza vaccine is effective only against influenza A

b. the efficacy of influenza vaccine is approximately 95%

c. influenza vaccine should be administered every 2 years

d. the ideal time for administration of influenza vaccine is in the late spring

e. none of the above are true

11. Regarding influenza vaccination, which of the following statements is (are) true?

a. intramuscular (IM) influenza vaccination typically produces no adverse drug reactions

b. the recommended dosage of the IM influenza vaccine is 0.5 mL for adults

c. influenza vaccination reduces the severity of illness in vaccinated persons who become infected

d. b and c are true

e. a, b, and c are true

12. Which of the following statements regarding amantadine prophylaxis of influenza is (are) false?

a. amantadine prophylaxis is effective against both influenza A and influenza B

b. amantadine prophylaxis has been shown to reduce the duration of fever and other symptoms

c. amantadine has been shown to reduce the duration of viral shedding

d. amantadine prophylaxis is used in high-risk individuals in whom vaccine is contraindicated

e. all of the above statements are false

13. Which of the following groups should be considered for yearly vaccinations against influenza?

a. healthy adults older than age 65 years

b. children and adolescents receiving chronic aspirin therapy

c. health care workers

d. adults and children in chronic care facilities

e. all of the above

14. Which of the following is (are) a contraindication(s) to influenza vaccine?

a. history of asthma

b. allergy to hens' eggs

c. history of Ménière's disease

d. low-risk people who developed Guillain–Barré syndrome within 6 weeks of receiving a flu shot

e. b and d

CLINICAL CASE PROBLEM 2

Pandemic Pandemonium

A press report confirms that the avian influenza H5N1 virus, which has been widespread in bird populations in Asia, Africa, and Europe, is spreading among humans. Although nearly all human cases had been caused by direct contact with infected poultry, reports of human-to-human transmission have now been confirmed. There is widespread concern of an emerging global pandemic that may cause mortality in millions of cases.

15. Possible coordinated global responses to the threat may include which of the following actions?

a. taking measures to contain or delay the spread at the source, including restrictions on movement of people in and out of areas affected and mass immunizations and/or administration of stockpiled antiviral drugs

b. initiation of real-time monitoring methods to track the evolving pandemic

c. introduction of nonpharmaceutical interventions, including school closings, travel restrictions, and mass gathering bans

d. use of antiviral medications to protect priority groups such as first responders and health care workers

e. utilization of mass media to communicate risk and control measures

f. all of the above

Answers

1. **a.** This patient most likely has influenza A. Influenza A strains usually predominate in adults; influenza B strains tend to infect children. Bacterial pneumonia and a secondary septicemia may follow influenza, but at this time, with the history and physical examination reported, the most likely diagnosis is influenza. A very common symptom of influenza is a severe generalized or frontal headache, often accompanied by retro-orbital pain. Other early symptoms of influenza include diffuse myalgias, fever, and chills. Respiratory symptoms especially tend to follow the occurrence of the early symptoms. The term "flu" is used very loosely by both physicians and patients. Influenza consists of a set of symptoms that often can be used to differentiate it clinically from other viral infections. Nevertheless, because many viruses can cause symptoms like influenza, epidemiologic data are used in practice to help with diagnosis. Public health organizations gather viral cultures from sick individuals during times of high infection rates as a means to estimate influenza prevalence in the community. In children, the signs and symptoms of influenza are more subtle; they may appear simply as another upper respiratory tract infection or "cold."

2. **d.** At this time, it would be very reasonable to perform a CBC, blood cultures, and a chest radiograph (CXR). The CXR is indicated because rales are heard in the lung fields. A CBC and blood cultures, along with the CXR, will rule out a secondary bacterial pneumonia, most often caused by *Streptococcus pneumoniae* and the bacteremia that may accompany it.

3. **d.** Influenza epidemics occur annually and are of major public health importance worldwide. In the United States, annual epidemics of influenza occur during late fall and winter. Both morbidity and mortality are definitely associated with influenza epidemics. This is true especially of the very old and the very young. Those with chronic disease are at even greater risk.

Influenza is responsible for approximately 36,000 deaths annually and more than 200,000 hospitalizations during widespread outbreaks. Influenza viruses can cause disease in any age group, but rates of infection are highest among children. Serious illness and death are highest among the elderly, very young, and persons of any age who are immunocompromised or have serious underlying illnesses. There are two major influenza viruses that cause epidemic human disease, designated influenza A and influenza B. By far the most virulent and most significant is the influenza A virus. The epidemics are usually associated with an antigenic drift, which may be limited, or with an antigenic shift, which is more extensive and can be more serious. The antigenic drifts (a shift in the hemagglutinin and neuraminidase antigens) in most cases provide the next year's challenge for public health practitioners. The antigenic shifts are responsible for the major "pandemics" that have occurred with influenza. They are also responsible for the major epidemics. Influenza epidemics and influenza pandemics are almost always associated with influenza A.

4. **c.** In uncomplicated influenza viral infections, as in uncomplicated viral infections in general, there is no indication for the prescription of antibiotics. One could argue that those patients at high risk for the development of complications, such as those with chronic bronchitis, diabetes, renal failure, or other chronic diseases, may be treated prophylactically. However, no studies support the efficacy or effectiveness of such a course.

5. **b.** The most common complication of influenza is pneumonia. This pneumonia is initially a viral pneumonia but often develops, especially in susceptible elderly patients, into a bacterial pneumonia, with *Streptococcus pneumoniae* as the most common pathogen. Other pathogens include *Staphylococcus aureus* and *Haemophilus*. This is the reason for the recommendations of the U.S. Preventive Services Task Force on the periodic health examination with respect to influenza, namely (1) immunize all patients older than age 65 years annually with influenza vaccine, and (2) immunize all patients older than age 65 years and high risk with pneumococcal vaccine.

6. **a.** All of the world's pandemics are caused by major antigenic shifts associated with influenza A. Influenza B is not usually associated with epidemics or pandemics, but it can cause severe illness. Influenza C is a rare cause of illness, usually resulting in a mild

infection in adults; however, in infants and young children it can rarely cause more serious disease. There are no such things as influenza D and E.

7. **c.** Oseltamivir and zanamivir are antiviral medications effective in the treatment of all influenza variants. Thus, they are better choices than amantadine or rimantadine. Treatment should be started within 48 hours of onset of symptoms, and its use can shorten the duration and severity of symptoms. Antivirals can be used during the influenza season as an adjunct to late vaccination, as a supplement to preseason vaccination in people who are immunodeficient, and as chemoprophylaxis in the absence of vaccination. Antivirals can also be used to reduce the spread of the virus and to minimize disruption of patient care both in the community and in the institutional setting. See Table 13-1 from the CDC. Influenza vaccination, however, remains the preferred method of conferring protection.

8. **c.** The influenza virus is transmitted through respiratory secretions and thus is spread easily to susceptible persons. Sneezing, coughing, and close contact while talking are thought to be the major modes of transmission.

9. **d.** The most effective method for preventing influenza A is to immunize patients before the influenza season begins with inactivated (or killed) influenza vaccine. Influenza vaccine confers approximately 85% protection against the development of influenza and an even greater rate of protection against death from influenza.

10. **e.** Influenza vaccine is effective against both influenza A and influenza B, has an efficacy rate of approximately 85%, and should be administered yearly 1 or 2 months before the influenza season begins.

Table 13-1	**Recommended Daily Dosage of Influenza Antiviral Medications for Treatment and Chemoprophylaxis — United States**				
	AGE GROUP (YRS)				
Antiviral Agent	**1–6**	**7–9**	**10–12**	**13–64**	**≥65**
ZANAMIVIR*					
Treatment, influenza A and B	NA	10 mg (2 inhalations) twice daily	10 mg (2 inhalations) twice daily	10 mg (2 inhalations) twice daily	10 mg (2 inhalations) twice daily
	1–4	**5–9**			
Chemoprophylaxis, influenza A and B	NA	10 mg (2 inhalations) once daily	10 mg (2 inhalations) once daily	10 mg (2 inhalations) once daily	10 mg (2 inhalations) once daily
OSELTAMIVIR					
Treatment, influenza A and B†	Dose varies by child's weight§	Dose varies by child's weight§	Dose varies by child's weight§	75 mg twice daily	75 mg twice daily
Chemoprophylaxis, influenza A and B	Dose varies by child' weight‖	Dose varies by child's weight‖	Dose varies by child's weight‖	75 mg/day	75 mg/day

Note: Zanamivir is manufactured by GlaxoSmithKline (Relenza—inhaled powder). Zanamivir is approved for treatment of persons aged ≥7 years and approved for chemoprophylaxis of persons aged ≥5 years. Oseltamivir is manufactured by Roche Phamaceuticals (Tamiflu—tablet). Oseltamivir is approved for treatment or chemoprophylaxis of persons aged ≥1 year. No antiviral medications are approved for treatment or chemoprophylaxis of influenza among children aged <1 year. This information is based on data published by the Food and Drug Administration (available at http://www.fda.gov).

*Zanamivir is administered through oral inhalation by using a plastic device included in the medication pacakage. Patients will benefit from instruction and demonstration of the correct use of the device. Zanamivir is not recommended for those persons with underlying airway disease.

†A reduction in the dose of oseltamivir is recommended for persons with creatinine clearance <30 mL/min.

§The treatment dosing recommendation for children weighing ≤15 kg is 30 mg twice a day; for children weighing >15–23 kg. the dose is 45 mg twice a day; for children weighing >23–40 kg the dose is 60 mg twice a day; and for children weighing >40 kg, the dose is 75 mg twice a day.

‖The chemoprophylaxis dosing recommendation for children weighing ≤15 kg is 30 mg once a day; for children weighing >15–23 kg, the dose is 45 mg once a day; for children weighing >23–40 kg, the dose is 60 mg once a day; and for children weighing >40 kg, the dose is 75 mg once a day.

Reproduced from Advisory Committee on Immunization Practices: Prevention and control of influenza: Recommendations of the Advisory Committee on Immunization Practices (ACIP), 2007. *MMWR* 56:1–54, 2007.

11. d. Influenza vaccine typically produces some minor side effects, such as a sore arm, redness at the injection site, and low-grade fever. A history of anaphylactic hypersensitivity to eggs or egg products is a contraindication to receiving influenza vaccine. Details of vaccine dose are discussed in a later question, but the usual IM dose of whole virus vaccine for adults is 0.5 ml. An intranasal vaccine is now available and may supplant the injection in popularity, although it currently is a very expensive alternative. In those patients in whom immunization fails and in whom influenza does develop, influenza vaccine still reduces both the severity and the duration of symptoms.

12. a. Amantadine and its antiviral cousin rimantadine are effective only against influenza A. Antivirals reduce viral shedding and the duration and severity of influenza A symptoms (e.g., headache, fever, chills, myalgias, and cough) once the virus is established, and they may be used as treatment in high-risk patients in whom the influenza vaccine is contraindicated.

13. e. Individuals who should receive yearly influenza vaccine include the following:

- all persons aged 50 years or older. Although some people 50 to 64 years of age who do not have chronic (long-term) medical conditions may not be at high risk for serious complications, approximately 26% of people in this age group do have high-risk conditions. For this reason, beginning in 2000, yearly influenza vaccination was recommended for all people 50 years or older to increase the number of high-risk individuals immunized. An alternate strategy used in Europe and being considered in North America is to immunize all children. Either way, reducing the number of susceptible individuals should reduce the possibility of epidemic and spread.
- residents of nursing homes and other long-term care facilities that house persons of any age who have long-term illnesses
- adults and children 6 months of age or older who have chronic heart or lung conditions, including asthma

- adults and children 6 months of age or older who need regular medical care or had to be in a hospital because of metabolic diseases (e.g., diabetes), chronic kidney disease, or weakened immune system (including immune system problems caused by medicine or by infection with human immunodeficiency virus [HIV/AIDS])
- children and teenagers (aged 6 months to 18 years) who are undergoing long-term aspirin therapy and therefore could develop Reye syndrome after the flu
- women who will be more than 3 months pregnant during the flu season

Other folks in whom to consider immunization include the following: young, otherwise healthy children aged 6 to 23 months who are at increased risk for influenza-related hospitalization; doctors, nurses, and other employees in hospitals and doctors' offices, including emergency response workers; employees of nursing homes and long-term care facilities who have contact with patients or residents; employees of assisted living and other residences for people in high-risk groups; people who provide home care to those in high-risk groups; and household members (including children) of people in high-risk groups. The CDC recommends administration of the vaccine to anyone who wants to reduce their chances of getting the flu, particularly persons who provide essential community services (e.g., police officers and firefighters) and students or others in institutional settings (e.g., those who reside in dormitories).

14. e. People who should not get a flu shot include individuals with an allergy to hens' eggs, people with a history of a previous severe reaction to influenza vaccine, and people not at risk for complications of influenza who developed Guillain–Barré syndrome within 6 weeks after a flu shot. Asthma and other chronic illnesses are good reasons to get vaccinated.

15. f. All of the measures listed are possible global responses to emerging pandemics.

Summary

1. **Epidemiology**

   Influenza A is responsible for all major epidemics and pandemics of influenza. It is also the most virulent of the influenza types, which include A and B. Yearly outbreaks result mostly from antigenic drift in the H and N antigens. Influenza outbreaks begin in the late fall and can last until early into the new year.

2. **Signs and symptoms**

   Headache is a common symptom. Other symptoms include fever, chills, and myalgias, followed by the symptoms of cough and congestion.

3. Prevention

Influenza vaccine should be given to all high-risk groups discussed in this chapter. Ideally, immunization should take place in the fall, prior to the winter season. Vaccine efficacy averages approximately 85% and is effective for both influenza A and influenza B. Travelers to the tropics and winter-experiencing locales should also be immunized.

4. Antiviral medications

Antiviral medications may offer prophylaxis and treatment options, but they are still not a substitute for immunization. They may be used as an adjunct to vaccination in high-risk situations (especially chronic care facilities). When given early after onset of illness, they reduce the severity and duration of symptoms in persons who already have contracted the virus. As with all medications, they have potential side effects. Amantadine and rimantadine can cause central nervous system (CNS) side effects (e.g., nervousness, anxiety, difficulty concentrating, and light-headedness) and gastrointestinal side effects (e.g., nausea and loss of appetite). CNS side effects occur more often among persons taking amantadine than among persons taking rimantadine. Among some other persons with long-term illnesses, more serious side effects, such as delirium, hallucinations, agitation, and seizures, can occur. Side effects usually diminish and disappear after 1 week. Zanamivir is inhaled and can cause decreased respiratory function and bronchospasm, especially in those with asthma or other chronic lung disease. Therefore, zanamivir is generally not recommended for use in persons with underlying lung disease, such as asthma and chronic obstructive pulmonary disease. Other side effects reported by less than 5% of those who have used this drug are diarrhea, nausea, sinusitis, nasal infections, bronchitis, cough, headache, and dizziness. Oseltamivir can cause gastrointestinal side effects (i.e., nausea and vomiting), although these may be less severe if taken with food.

Please review answer 13 for a list of all those who should receive yearly influenza immunization.

Make sure you and your patients are immunized in a timely manner.

Suggested Reading

The Centers for Disease Control and Prevention Web site. Available at www.cdc.gov. (Web site has up-to-date recommendations and detailed information on immunization practices for influenza.)

Juckett G: Avian influenza: Preparing for a pandemic. *Am Fam Physician* 74:783–790, 2006.

Mandell LA, Wunderink RG, Aneveto A, et al: Infectious Diseases Society of America/American Thoracic Society consensus guidelines on the management of community-acquired pneumonia in adults. *Clin Infect Dis* 44(Suppl 2):S27–S72, 2007.

COMMUNICATION

Domestic Violence

CLINICAL CASE PROBLEM 1

A 25-Year-Old Female with Pelvic Pain, Low Back Pain, Insomnia, and Fatigue

A 25-year-old woman comes to the office for a new patient visit. Her complaints are 6 months of constant pelvic pain and low back pain, intermittent myalgias, insomnia for "many years," and feeling tired. When you ask about bruises of varying ages on arms, legs, and face, she notes that she is clumsy and bumps into things a lot. Her husband accompanies her to the visit and refuses to leave the exam room for the physical exam. On pelvic exam, purulent cervical discharge is noted, along with cervical motion tenderness. Her husband inquires as to why you are using so many tubes for lab specimens.

SELECT THE BEST ANSWERS TO THE FOLLOWING QUESTIONS

1. Which of the following should be considered to be part of the differential diagnosis in this patient?
   a. intimate partner violence (IPV)
   b. pelvic inflammatory disease
   c. pregnancy
   d. a bleeding disorder
   e. all of the above

2. What is the estimated lifetime prevalence of IPV in the United States?
   a. 1 in 100 women
   b. 1 in 50 women
   c. 1 in 25 women
   d. 1 in 10 women
   e. 1 in 3 or 4 women

3. Which of the following is not a characteristic of IPV?
   a. the association of violence with alcohol intake by the perpetrator
   b. violent behavior in the family of origin of both victim and batterer
   c. high risk of suicide attempt or gesture in the victim
   d. results in nearly 2 million injuries and 1300 deaths in the United States
   e. association of this disorder with poverty

4. Which of the following is not a common presenting symptom or complaint in a victim of IPV?
   a. back pain
   b. headache
   c. dyspareunia
   d. IPV itself
   e. abdominal pain

CLINICAL CASE PROBLEM 2

Clues to Domestic Violence

A 31-year-old African American woman with 6 years of education post high school presents at the emergency department with bruises, severe pain in the left forearm, and symptoms of depression. When the emergency department calls you regarding the patient's presence, you recall that she has had three appointments on your calendar but all three have been canceled at the last minute. Her husband is a laborer and often will not allow her to keep a physician's appointment unless he can accompany her. You indicate you will come in to see the patient.

5. Which of the following statements about screening by primary care physicians is true?
   a. only 15% of primary care physicians routinely screen their patients for IPV
   b. evidence is clear that routine screening of patients for IPV leads to improved health outcomes

c. screening tools such as HITS (Hurt, Insulted, Threatened, Screamed at), the Partner Abuse Interview, and the Women's Experience with Battering (WEB) scale have good internal consistency and have been validated against measurable health outcomes

d. clinicians should be alert to physical and behavioral signs and symptoms associated with abuse or neglect in all patients

e. evidence is clear that batterer intervention programs are effective in reducing rates of domestic violence

Following discussion and exam, you are convinced that this patient is a victim of IPV and recommend that she make a police report.

6. Which pair of IPV type/rate of report to police is correctly matched?
   a. IPV rape or sexual assault–20%
   b. physical assault–50%
   c. stalking–80%
   d. all of the above
   e. none of the above

7. With regard to IPV during pregnancy:
   a. 4% to 8% of pregnant women are abused at least once during pregnancy
   b. pregnant women who are being abused usually show no concern for the health of the unborn child
   c. sudden increase or decrease in frequency of office visits is not related to risk of being abused
   d. abusive partners accompany the patient to office visits rarely, if at all
   e. same-sex intimate partners are never involved in abuse of a pregnant woman

8. When women without symptoms are screened by clinicians for IPV
   a. the majority become angry or express being offended
   b. the risk of harm to the affected patient is increased when screening is done in the presence of the abusive partner
   c. few women believe that screening is of benefit or that it makes getting help easier
   d. posters, brochures, and other materials in an office with culturally sensitive information about IPV can lead to more victims providing information to clinicians when asked about IPV
   e. all of the above

9. Following discussion of involvement of the police, you discuss possible alternatives for the patient, including
   a. referral to a shelter since such referrals significantly reduce the likelihood of further physical injury
   b. confrontation of her husband and referral of him to counseling because evidence strongly supports such intervention
   c. allowing you to take photographs in case she later decides to press charges
   d. purchase of a gun to protect herself in case of another attack
   e. none of the above

Clinical Case Management Problem

Discuss the interventions and the order of those interventions that should take place for the victim, the victim's children, and the victim's mate in a situation similar to the one described in Clinical Case 2.

Answers

1. **e.** This patient has evidence of pelvic inflammatory disease (cervical discharge and cervical motion tenderness) and has multiple bruises of varying age. Although a bleeding disorder could be the cause of the bruises, she also has evidence of a sexually transmitted disease (STD), a partner who shows signs of mistrust of the physician, and bruises that could be associated with multiple injuries. She is of reproductive age and has evidence of STD, so pregnancy should also be considered. Patients who are victims of IPV often present to the physician not with this complaint but with complaints of fatigue, insomnia, or nonspecific complaints.

2. **e.** Approximately 32 million Americans were affected by IPV in 2000, with more than 1.5 million women and more than 800,000 men raped or physically assaulted by an intimate partner—approximately 47 assaults per 1000 women and 32 per 1000 men. The Centers for Disease Control and Prevention (CDC) reports that IPV results in nearly 2 million injuries and 1300 deaths per year in the United States. The U.S. Justice Department reports that IPV accounts for 20% of nonfatal violence against women, and that 85% of IPV victims are women. A 2002 study published in the *American Journal of Preventive Medicine* reported that

29% of women and 22% of men in the United States had experienced physical, sexual, or psychological IPV during their lifetime.

3. **a.** Even after leaving an abusive partner, women remain at risk; stalking is becoming increasingly prevalent, according to the U.S. Department of Justice. The *Journal of Trauma, Injury, Infection, and Critical Care* in 2004 reported the statistics in choice b, emphasizing the importance of suspicion for IPV when assessing injuries, as well as the need for primary care follow-up. Women who are victims of IPV are indeed more likely to be diagnosed with depression than the general population. The injury and death statistics in choice d were reported by the CDC and the risk data by the U.S. Department of Justice.

4. **d.** Although injury is a common presenting complaint in the emergency room, in the primary care setting physicians often hear complaints of somatic symptoms. When the patient is a victim of IPV, rarely is the IPV a presenting complaint.

5. **d.** The U.S. Preventive Services Task Force and the Canadian Task Force on Preventive Health Care both have promulgated statements addressing the lack of evidence that routine screening for IPV reduces harm, and they note that screening tools, although demonstrating good internal consistency, have not been validated against measurable health outcomes. However, this recommendation is noted to refer only to routine screening. When clinicians note evidence of IPV as part of the evaluation of a patient for other health complaints and findings, consideration of this violence should be part of a differential diagnosis.

Concerns that this screening causes any adverse effects have not been adequately examined. However, because improvements in health status cannot be demonstrated, justification for the cost, time, and materials involved is currently lacking. Half of women asked support routine screening. The U.S. Agency for Healthcare Research and Quality notes that only 6% of U.S. physicians ask patients about possible domestic violence, but 88% stated that they knew of female patients who were abused.

6. **a.** The U.S. Department of Justice in 2000 reported that 32 million Americans were affected by IPV, and that underreporting to law enforcement was a major issue. Approximately 20% of IPV rapes/sexual assaults are reported to police, but only 25% of physical assaults and 50% of stalkings are reported. These numbers are even lower with male victims.

7. **a.** The *Maternal and Child Health Journal* reported in 2000 that 4% to 8% of American pregnant women are abused at least once during the pregnancy. All other choices are false; female victims of IPV are characterized as being overly concerned and making frequent complaints about health issues. After abuse, they may withdraw from the health care system, change providers to avoid discussing the issue, or begin to seek care more frequently. Abusive partners can be male or female, and they often do not want the victim to seek medical attention without their presence. A sexual relationship is not necessary for IPV to occur.

8. **d.** The Institute for Clinical Systems Improvement discusses multiple strategies for improving the identification of and care for IPV victims in its 2006 statement. The office that provides information that can be viewed in private is a setting conductive to communication between doctor and patient about IPV. Screening in the presence of the abuser has not been shown to be harmful, but studies are not conclusive. Women who have been surveyed about IPV express support for routine screening and believe that screening makes it easier for victims to get help.

9. **c.** The evidence is insufficient to assure the patient that referral to a shelter or referral of her husband for counseling will reduce future violence. Clear documentation including photographs is important for a time when the patient may choose to press charges. Even if police are not notified of this instance, it provides evidence even after bruises have healed. Purchase of a gun is more likely to escalate the violence and potentially lead to a fatal wound for one of the partners.

Solution to the Clinical Case Management Problem

The interventions should include

Victim and Children

1. Establish the diagnosis using open-ended questions followed by more direct, closed-ended questions.
2. Explain the importance of the removal of the victim and her children to a safe environment, preferably a place that makes peer counseling and other therapy available.
3. Use supportive psychotherapy in the safe environment to reestablish the victim's self-esteem

and to reverse the ingrained feeling in the victim of learned helplessness.

Abuser

1. Referral for therapy, with some evidence supporting group psychotherapy, which facilitates sharing experiences with other abusers.
2. Treatment for substance abuse.
3. Treatment of any concurrent psychiatric problems.
4. Gradual, cautious reuniting with family.

Summary

1. **Definition and occurrence**
   a. IPV describes physical, sexual, or psychological harm by a current or former partner or spouse.
   b. IPV occurs among heterosexual or same-sex couples and does not require sexual intimacy.
   c. IPV occurs on a continuum, ranging from one hit that may or may not impact the victim to chronic, severe battering.
      i. Repeated abuse is also known as battering.
      ii. Most injuries are minor, such as scratches, bruises, and welts; more frequency leads to increased risk of bruises and knife wounds.
   d. Incidence
      i. Approximately 1.5 million women and more than 800,000 men are raped or physically assaulted by an intimate partner.
      ii. This translates into approximately 47 IPV assaults per 1000 women and 32 assaults per 1000 men.
      iii. 4% to 8% of pregnant women are abused at least once during pregnancy.

2. **Evaluation**
   a. There is insufficient evidence to recommend for or against routine screening of women for IPV.
      i. Evidence is lacking on whether interventions by clinicians reduce harm to women (recommendation at level I—insufficient evidence; U.S. Preventive Task Force).
      ii. There is insufficient evidence to recommend for or against counseling of abused women by primary care physicians; the same is true for referral to shelters.
   b. There is fair evidence to support referral of women who have spent at least one night in a shelter to a structured program of advocacy services.

   c. There is conflicting evidence regarding the effectiveness of batterer interventions in reducing rates of domestic violence. All clinicians should be alert to physical and behavioral signs and symptoms associated with abuse or neglect.
      i. One study found that only 6% of physicians ask their patients about possible domestic violence, but 88% admitted that they knew they had female patients who had been abused.
      ii. 48% of women support routine screening of all women, with 86% stating it would make it easier to get help.
      iii. Screening instruments: HITS (Hurt, Insulted, Threatened, Screamed at), the Partner Abuse Interview, and the Women's Experience with Battering (WEB) scale have good internal consistency, but none have been validated against measurable outcomes.
   d. Presenting physical symptoms: pelvic pain, headaches, back pain, fractures, low birth weight, STD, posttraumatic stress disorder symptoms (emotional detachment, sleep disturbance, flashbacks, depression, anxiety, and overuse of health services).
      i. Suspicious injuries/behavior: burns or bruises in unusual locations, central injuries (e.g., chest, breasts, abdomen, pelvis, and perineum), delay in seeking treatment, facial injuries (e.g., teeth, jaw, and ruptured eardrum), human bites, injuries at various stages of healing, injuries from weapons (old scars or new signs), pattern of injury not consistent with history, previous assault, and repeated visits for minor trauma.
   e. If abuse is suspected, clinicians should document history and physical findings, including photographs and drawings; provide treatment for injuries;

refer for counseling by a mental health professional; and provide telephone numbers of local crisis centers, shelters, and protective agencies (recommendations of the U.S. Preventive Task Force).

f. Domestic violence should be a consideration in all patient encounters and the interview should be conducted in private, with only the provider and the patient present. In certain situations, a trusted interpreter or language line service (not a friend or a family member) may be necessary.

3. Risk factors

a. Risk to be abused

    i. Females are more likely to be victims of IPV than are males.

    ii. American Indian/Alaskan native women and men, African American women, and Hispanic women are at highest risk.

    iii. Additional risk factors: young age, low income status, pregnancy, mental health problems, substance abuse by victim or perpetrator, separated or divorced status, history of child sexual and/or physical abuse, and those who are less educated or women more educated than their male partner (recommendation of the U.S. Preventive Task Force)

b. Increased risk to be perpetrator: low self-esteem, low income, low academic achievement, involvement in aggressive or delinquent behavior as a youth, heavy alcohol and drug use, depression, anger and hostility, personality disorders, prior history of being physically abusive, having few friends and being isolated from other people, unemployment, economic stress, emotional dependence and insecurity, belief in strict gender roles (e.g., male dominance and aggression in relationships), desire for power and control in relationships, being a victim of physical or psychological abuse (consistently one of the strongest predictors of perpetration)

Suggested Reading

Centers for Disease Control and Prevention: *CDC Fact Sheet: Intimate Partner Violence.* Available at www.cdc.gov./ncipc/dvp/ipv_factsheet.pdf.

Fox JA, Zawitz MW: Homicide trends in the United States. Washington, DC: U.S. Department of Justice, 2004. Available at www.ojp.usdoj.gov/bjs/homicide/homtrnd.htm.

Gazmararian JA, Petersen R, Spitz AM, et al: Violence and reproductive health: Current knowledge and future research directions. *Maternal Child Health J* 4(2):79–84, 2000.

Institute for Clinical Systems Improvement: *Domestic Violence.* Bloomington, MN: Institute for Clinical Systems Improvement, 2006.

Kass-Bartelmes BL: Women and domestic violence: Programs and tools that improve care for victims. *Res Action* 15:June 2004. Available at www.ahrq.gov/RESEARCH/domviolria/domviolria.htm.

Tjaden P, Thoennes N: Extent, nature, and consequences of intimate partner violence: Findings from the National Violence against Women Survey, Publication No. NCJ 181867. Washington, DC: U.S. Department of Justice, 2000.

U.S. Preventive Services Task Force: Screening for family and intimate partner violence: Recommendation statement. *Ann Intern Med* 140(5):382–386, 2004.

Wathen CN, MacMillan HL: Prevention of violence against women: Recommendation statement from the Canadian Task Force on Preventive Health Care. *Can Med Assoc J* 169(6):582–584, 2003.

How to Break Bad News

CLINICAL CASE PROBLEM 1

A 34-Year-Old Female Just Diagnosed with Metastatic Malignant Melanoma

You have just received the computed tomography (CT) scan report on a 34-year-old mother of three who had a malignant melanoma removed 3 years ago. Originally, it was a Clark's level I and the prognosis was excellent. The patient came to your office 1 week ago complaining of chest pain and abdominal pain. A CT scan of the chest and abdomen revealed metastatic lesions throughout the lungs and the abdomen. She is in your office, and you have to deliver the bad news of the significant spread of the cancer.

SELECT THE BEST ANSWER TO THE FOLLOWING QUESTIONS

1. Regarding the delivery of bad news to patients who are unaccompanied when they come to the office, which of the following statements is true?
   a. the fact that the patient is alone is irrelevant
   b. you have no right to interfere with her decision to come alone to the office
   c. you should go into the consultation room and explain that the situation is complex and it would be better if her husband or significant other were present when the test results were explained and treatment options were discussed
   d. patients do not remember much of anything after bad news is delivered, so it does not really matter whether someone else is present
   e. having a significant other present will only complicate an already difficult situation

2. Which of the following settings is not acceptable for the delivery of bad news?
   a. a physician's office
   b. a quiet room in a hospital setting
   c. the patient's home
   d. a private hospital room
   e. a multibed hospital room

3. The first step in breaking bad news is to
   a. deliver the news all in one blow and get it over with as quickly as is humanly possible
   b. fire a "warning shot" that some bad news is coming
   c. find out how much the patient knows
   d. find out how much the patient wants to know
   e. tell the patient not to worry

CLINICAL CASE PROBLEM 2

Communicating Bad News

A patient has had a breast biopsy for a suspicious lump seen on mammogram. The pathology report shows an adenocarcinoma. Arrangements for the patient to come to your office today, 3 days following surgery, were made when she left the surgicenter.

4. Which of the following were appropriate steps to have taken?
   a. discuss with the patient and her husband before the biopsy that you would like them to make arrangements for someone to drive her home if it is bad news
   b. suggest that she have someone accompany her to the follow-up so that there would be two sets of ears to hear the results and to recall the explanation and any plan for additional follow-up
   c. have your office call the husband when the report comes back positive for malignancy and demand that he accompany the wife to the follow-up visit
   d. check the next-of-kin listed on the hospital record and call that person to come to your office in case the patient chooses to come alone for the follow-up
   e. none of the above

5. Which of the following steps might be considered a communication aid and be helpful to the patient in the days following the diagnosis?
   a. an audiotape of the consultation discussion when you shared the results and plans
   b. a patient education hand-out that discussed the same material you discussed
   c. a follow-up letter after the consultation reiterating the information shared at the consultation
   d. a phone number of the last patient you treated who did well
   e. a, b, and c

6. Which of the following statements regarding finding out how much the patient wants to know is not true?
   a. every patient should be told everything about their condition
   b. some patients would rather not know all of the details of their disease

c. most patients initially do not know how much they want to be told

d. some patients want to know the whole truth right away

e. in some instances, patients should not be told the full extent of their condition

7. There are two languages that physicians use in talking to patients: English and "medispeak." Unfortunately, patients usually only understand English. Which of the following is an example of medispeak?
   a. lesion
   b. malignancy
   c. tumor
   d. cancer
   e. leukemia

8. Which of the following statements is false regarding the involvement of family physicians in the care of a patient with cancer?
   a. ideally, the family physician should be present when the patient is told of a bad diagnosis or prognosis
   b. the family physician and the primary consultant should be in contact and should be certain that the same message is delivered
   c. family physicians have a limited role to play once the patient is enrolled in a tertiary care cancer treatment center
   d. the family physician has a responsibility to follow up on the care of his or her patients regardless of whether he or she is actively involved in all aspects of care
   e. as cancer becomes a more chronic rather than fatal condition, much of the long-term care can be managed by the family physician

9. Which of the following is (are) true regarding the delivery of bad news to patients with a serious disease?
   a. check the patient's reaction to the situation frequently
   b. reinforce and clarify the information you are giving
   c. check the patient's understanding of the facts
   d. elicit the patient's concerns
   e. all of the above are true

10. In an interview in which news of a serious disease is presented, which of the following is the thing to do before the patient leaves the office?
    a. make sure the patient understands every word
    b. make sure the patient understands that you are doing everything you can
    c. make sure you leave the patient with a follow-up plan and provide the patient with some hope
    d. make sure the patient understands the dismal prognosis
    e. make sure that you have left no question unanswered

CLINICAL CASE PROBLEM 3

Life after the Bad News

A physician diagnosed with a terminal illness returns to his home university to continue the pursuit of his academic career to the best of his ability after having received bad news about his medical condition. He purposefully does not tell his colleagues the truth about his disease and continues to teach, write, receive grants, publish, and practice medicine. His condition deteriorates and he becomes increasing more physically disabled.

11. Which of the following scenarios is (are) most likely to occur?
    a. he is apt to receive more phone calls from concerned colleagues and more inquiries as to whether they can be of assistance to him
    b. when his colleagues see him in the hall, they will go out of their way to talk to him and offer any assistance they can
    c. once his colleagues are aware of the full extent of his illness, they will offer not only moral support but also support in terms of assistance in teaching, assistance in looking after his patients, and assistance in keeping his research programs viable
    d. all of the above are likely to occur
    e. none of the above are likely to occur

12. When Joanne, a 14-year-old, was diagnosed with leukemia, her mother asked you what Joanne should be told and by whom. You replied how?
    a. Joanne should be told she has mononucleosis and will feel very fatigued for a while but she will ultimately be cured
    b. Joanne should be told by the doctor that she has cancer and she may die from it, but if she survives the treatments she may also be cured of the disease
    c. Joanne and her parents should hear from the doctor together the diagnosis, including the name, a reasonable description of the treatment, and the hope for a cure as the outcome
    d. Joanne should be told she is too young to worry about a diagnosis and her parents and the doctor will take care of it

e. Joanne's parents should tell her whatever amount they are comfortable with and be the conduit for any questions that she might have about diagnosis or treatment

---

Clinical Case Management Problem

You are the physician caring for an 85-year-old woman who you have just diagnosed as having breast cancer. Before you have an opportunity to talk to the patient, her son and daughter come to your office to advise you that they do not wish you to tell their mother anything about her diagnosis. Describe how you would respond to the request.

Answers

1. c. You should go into the patient's room and explain that the situation is complex; it would be better if her husband or significant other were present when the test results were explained and treatment options were discussed. To have devastating news delivered to a patient in an unsupported environment is less than optimal. If a spouse, son, daughter, brother, sister, or other significant other cannot be present during the delivery of the news, it is useful to invite a social worker, psychologist, or member of the clergy to be present for patient support.

2. e. A multibed hospital room or an exposed area of an emergency room is not an acceptable location for the delivery of bad news. Patients in beds next to your patient obviously will be able to hear all or most of the conversation. Being in an exposed area would add to patients' feelings of vulnerability. Just pulling a hospital curtain is not an acceptable option.

When breaking bad news, attention to privacy, the physical environment, and the presence of a support person are important. Obviously, the other alternatives in the question are acceptable.

3. b. A "warning shot" prepares the patient psychologically to hear something negative.

4. b. You should encourage her to bring someone with her to the follow-up in order to increase the retention of diagnostic information as well as any further diagnostic or treatment steps that are necessary. It is inappropriate for your office to call someone to join the appointment without the patient's knowledge and consent. It can be as important to have someone

accompany a patient even when the diagnosis is not "bad news" because the stress of anticipating bad news can diminish the retention of information such as follow-up evaluations, medications, etc.

5. e. The National Breast Cancer Centre and National Cancer Control Initiative 2003 suggested that the patient's understanding, recall, satisfaction with care, or all three are increased with communication aids. These included provision of a tape of the consultation, sending a summary follow-up letter and/or having a support person present during the consultation or both. Giving one patient another's phone number without significant preplanning and permission would be inappropriate.

6. a. Most patients will want to be told the whole truth, but there are some exceptions. Every patient is different. The "whole truth" also does not have to be told all at once. Most patients initially are not even aware how much they want to be told. In some cultures, it may be inappropriate to convey medical facts directly to the patient. It is useful to encourage patients to ask questions and tailor your responses to meet their needs. Open-ended questions such as, "How much technical detail about your condition would you like me to share with you right now?" would be helpful.

7. a. Most health care professionals unconsciously use their own professional jargon. Using medispeak to explain something to a patient makes it less likely that the patient will be able to ask relevant questions. It also tends to isolate and alienate patients who find it unfamiliar. A comparison of English and medispeak is shown in Table 15-1.

8. c. Family physicians assume and maintain a coordinating role in the care of patients with cancer. Although at a certain time a patient may be receiving treatment in a tertiary care treatment center, the family physician must be seen as coordinating that care. Communication between the family physician, the family, and the specialist(s) involved should be maintained.

Table 15-1	Comparison of English and "Medispeak"
English	**Medispeak**
Leukemia	Blast cells
Multiple sclerosis	Demyelination
Cancer	Space-occupying lesion
The situation is serious	The prognosis is guarded

From Buckman R: *How to Break Bad News: A Guide for Health Care Professionals.* Toronto: University of Toronto Press, 1992.

Much of the long-term care can be managed by the family physician as cancer becomes a more chronic rather than fatal condition. The family physician's role can best be described in terms of the 5 Cs: continuous, comprehensive, compassionate, coordinated, and competent care.

9. **e.** While providing information to the patient, it is imperative that the physician keep the following principles in mind: (1) Provide the information in small chunks—after firing the "warning shot"; (2) use English, not medispeak; (3) check the patient's reaction in terms of both information processing and emotional state; (4) reinforce and clarify information you are giving; (5) elicit and address the patient's concerns; and (6) adjust your agenda to the patient's agenda.

10. **c.** Make sure before the patient leaves your office that you provide him or her with a follow-up plan. This will reinforce the belief that you are indeed in charge of his or her care and will ensure that the care plan is implemented. In addition, be sure to leave the patient with some hope for the future. That hope must be realistic hope, but hope nevertheless.

11. **e.** This case is a true story and was told eloquently by a physician named Rabin in the *New England Journal of Medicine* in 1982. The observations made of both the consultation with the neurologist and the reaction and treatment that the physician patient received when he returned to his home university have been summarized.

> My first reaction to the neurologist was one of deep disappointment from his impersonal manner. The neurologist exhibited no interest in me as a person and did not make even a perfunctory inquiry about my work. He gave me no guidelines about what I should do, either concretely in terms of daily activities or, what was more important, psychologically, to muster the emotional strength to cope with a progressive degenerative disease. The only thing my doctor did offer me was a pamphlet setting out in grim detail the future that I already knew about too well.

The reaction of colleagues to another problem is illustrated very well in the following description:

> By early 1980, however, the limp was worse, and I now held a cane in my right hand. The inquiries ceased and were replaced by a very obvious desire to avoid me. When I arrived at work in the morning I could see, from the corner of my eye, colleagues changing their pace or stopping in their tracks to spare themselves the embarrassment of bumping into me. As the cane became inadequate and was replaced by a walker, so my isolation from my colleagues intensified.

One has to ask why this happened. The author (Rabin D, 1982) suggests the following:

> Perhaps it is because we, as physicians, are the healers. We dispense treatment, counsel, and support; and we represent strength. The dichotomy of being both doctor and patient threatens the integrity of the club. To this guild of healers, becoming ill is tantamount to treachery. Furthermore, the sick physician makes us uncomfortable. He reminds us of our own vulnerability and mortality, and this is frightening for those of us who deal with disease every day while arming ourselves with an imaginary cloak of immunity against personal illness. This account is meant to draw attention to our frequent inability as physicians to deal with members of our profession who no longer fit the mold of complete healer.

The author also suggests some very simple steps that we can take to support our colleagues in time of illness, stress, trouble, or other difficulty. First, do not ignore ill colleagues. Greet them, inquire about their health, and visit them. Offer them support if they are physically handicapped. Second, be conscious of the physician patient's family and extend support to them. The spouse and children are suffering at least as much as the physician and need support, encouragement, and acknowledgment of their difficulties. Third, remember that the absence of a magic potion against the disease does not render you impotent. No one can assume the burden, but the patient knowing that he or she has not been forgotten does ease the pain.

This special type of communication and caring among physicians (or any other professional group) is essential as we enter an era of change unlike any other era health care has ever seen. Remember that the word doctor is translated from the Latin *doktor*, meaning teacher. As physicians we are all teachers, some in more diverse ways than others. Medical students, residents, patients, other health care professionals, and, most of all, students play the role at one time or another.

> When the student is ready, the teacher will appear.
> —Confucius

12. **c.** There is weak evidence that communicating information to young patients about the diagnosis and expected tests and interventions may help children and their families to better understand, prepare for, and cope with their illness; the medical or surgical procedures they may undergo; their discharge from hospital and return to school and community; any relapses that may occur; and, in some cases, their last weeks of life. Interventions that offer opportunities for children and adolescents with cancer to communicate their experience of their illness and treatment may be helpful to them.

Solution to the Clinical Case Management Problem

This is not an infrequent occurrence. In this situation, it is extremely important to remember who the patient is and what rights the patient has and does not have. Proceed in the following manner:

1. Assuming the mother is mentally competent, remember who the patient is: the mother, not the son or the daughter.
2. Invite the son and daughter to come in for a discussion with you. Start off by acknowledging that you understand how much they love their mother and obviously have her best interest in mind. Then, explain that as their mother's physician you have an ethical responsibility to talk to her about her disease. Offer to do it in such a way that allows their mother an opportunity to communicate how much information about the disease she wants. Ask the mother (in the presence of her son and daughter) how much detail she would like to hear about her condition and whether she wants to make her own decision or delegate this responsibility to her children.
3. In the unusual event that the son and daughter remain in disagreement about the process of information sharing and insist that their mother not be told about her condition, you might have to resort to including other parties such as a hospital ethics committee.

Summary

THE SEVEN-STEP PROTOCOL TO BREAKING BAD NEWS

1. Getting started:
   a. Get the physical setting right.
   b. Ensure family support at the time of breaking the news.
   c. Fire a warning shot.
2. Find out how much the patient already knows.
3. Find out how much the patient wants to know.
4. Decide on your objectives.
5. Share the information:
   a. Give the information in small chunks—start with the warning shot.
   b. Use English, not "medispeak."
   c. Reinforce and clarify the information frequently.
   d. Listen for the patient's concerns.
   e. Blend your agenda with the patient's agenda.
   f. Offer hope.
6. Respond to the patient's feelings.
7. Follow through with your planned objectives.

REMEMBER YOUR COLLEAGUES

Physicians and other health care providers as patients are just as vulnerable if not more vulnerable than patients who are not physicians and need our friendship, encouragement, help, and hope.

GUIDELINES AND SUGGESTIONS

1. Always leave the patient with realistic hope.
2. Realize that the patient will not absorb all the information on the first visit; schedule follow-up visits frequently. Give consideration to providing communication aids such as hand-outs, suggested questions, or even an audiotape of your conversation with the patient.
3. Facilitate and coordinate the patient's care from this point on.
4. Remember the 5 Cs of the family physician: continuous, comprehensive, compassionate, coordinated, and competent care.
5. Try to unlearn medispeak.

Suggested Reading

American Psychiatric Association: *Diagnostic and Statistical Manual of Mental Disorders IV-TR*, 4th ed. Washington, DC: American Psychiatric Association Press, 2000.

Buckman R: *How to Break Bad News: A Guide for Health Care Professionals.* Toronto: University of Toronto Press, 1992.

Lockhart K, Dosser I, Cruickshank S, Kennedy C: Methods of communicating a primary diagnosis of breast cancer to patients. *Cochrane Database Syst Rev* (3):CD006011, 2007.

Ptacek JT, Eberhardt TL: Breaking bad news: A review of the literature. *JAMA* 276(6):496–502, 1996.

Rabin D: Compounding the ordeal of ALS: Isolation from my fellow physicians. *N Engl J Med* 307(8):506–509, 1982.

Radziewicz R, Baile WF: Communication skills: Breaking bad news in the clinical setting. *Oncol Nurs Forum* 28(6):951–953, 2001.

Scott JT, Harmsen M, Prictor MJ, et al: Interventions for improving communication with children and adolescents about their cancer. *Cochrane Database Syst Rev* (3):CD002969, 2003.

16 Physician–Patient Relationship

CLINICAL CASE PROBLEM 1

"I Trust the Doctor, but…"

A 42-year-old male who has been your patient for 4 years comes to the office for a routine office visit. You have been treating chronic migraine headaches for the patient. He mentions that he would like to see a neurologist who he heard speak on the radio. Although you have done a complete evaluation of his headaches, he is concerned that he might have a brain tumor or other disease.

SELECT THE BEST ANSWER TO THE FOLLOWING QUESTIONS

1. Considering the situation, what should you do?
   a. explain to the patient that you have investigated the condition completely and that there is no need for a referral
   b. tell the patient that if that is the way he feels, he probably should find another family physician
   c. empathize with the patient regarding his symptoms and refer him to a neurologist of your choosing
   d. empathize with the patient regarding his symptoms and refer him to the neurologist he mentions
   e. tell the patient that you are deeply offended by his request; he has no right to question your competence

2. What is the primary purpose of consultation or referral to a specialist?
   a. to validate the findings of the family physician
   b. to ensure that the family physician has not missed anything
   c. to provide reassurance to the patient that the family physician is concerned about his or her welfare
   d. to improve the quality of health care by making available to patients and referring physicians the knowledge and skills of specialists or consultants at appropriate times
   e. to provide protection for the family physician against a malpractice suit

3. Trust in one's physician is described by patients as
   a. an inherent personality trait
   b. having no relationship to the institutions with which the physician is associated
   c. a learnable skill that can be improved
   d. separate from competence issues
   e. different than being a "good doctor""

CLINICAL CASE PROBLEM 2

You Can Be a Tool of Change

A 56-year-old female patient had been diagnosed with diabetes mellitus, insulin dependent, several years earlier. She had great difficulty maintaining her weight and medication schedule. She often denied that she needed to remain on the regimen recommended by her physician. Each visit, the physician would spend time discussing the importance of lifestyle and adherence to medication programs.

4. The patient's relatively long relationship with her physician is likely to
   a. enhance her ability and commitment to follow the treatment plan
   b. overburden the physician and encourage him to refer her elsewhere
   c. have no influence on the treatment process
   d. allow her to feel less guilt over her nonadherence to the plan
   e. enable her to set her own treatment regimen

5. Trust in one's physician contributes to
   a. discontinuity of care
   b. patient dissatisfaction
   c. elimination of need for second opinions
   d. improved treatment adherence
   e. more frequent office visits

6. "Trust" is defined as
   a. take the physician's word for recommended treatments
   b. expectation that physician will put the patient's interests first
   c. belief that the physician will not allow insurance incentives to influence him or her
   d. assumption that all consultants to whom the physician refers have the same perspective regarding patient care
   e. all of the above

CLINICAL CASE PROBLEM 3

"Do You E-mail?"

A couple and their two young children move to the West Coast due to job requirements. One of the first things that they must do is find acceptable primary care for the family. They have come to appreciate the flexibility of having a physician who is willing to use electronic communications. As they search for a physician or group that will support their needs, they outline the following concerns.

7. Access to "e-health" offers them
   a. convenience
   b. control
   c. choice
   d. a and b
   e. all of the above

8. The physician–patient relationship can be impacted by e-health options by
   a. causing greater distance because there is less face-to-face interaction
   b. improved sense of commitment because the physician can send reminders or quick, preprogrammed questions regarding how a patient is doing
   c. creating patient dissatisfaction because physicians answer e-mails at unacceptable times of the day
   d. reducing liability risk by keeping a copy of physician–patient interactions
   e. b and d

9. Soon after selecting a physician who is electronically savvy, one of the couple's children develops a significant asthma attack with very rapid breathing, wheezing, and some blue discoloration around his lips. They immediately e-mail the physician's office for instructions.
   a. this is unacceptable because e-mail should never be used for an emergency
   b. the physician's e-mail has a header that instructs that if the query is an emergency, the patient should call 911 and not use the e-mail contact
   c. the patient signed a release form when in the physician's office indicating that she understood the e-mail address was for making appointments, following up visits with brief questions, etc. and should not be used for emergent issues
   d. the couple take their child to the nearest emergency room and upon returning home use the physician's e-mail to provide his office with an update on the emergency room visit and request for a follow-up office visit
   e. all of the above

CLINICAL CASE PROBLEM 4

Communicating for Continuity

A 52-year-old white male presents at your office with prostate cancer. It has been previously treated with surgery and his primary care physician has been following his PSAs. He has moved across the country for job-related reasons and is seeking a new primary care physician.

10. Communication with cancer patients is particularly problematic because
    a. it is always bad news
    b. patients must process complex and, at times, controversial information
    c. all cancer patients maintain strong hope for a cure
    d. the physician–patient trust relationship has implications for the patient's adherence to follow-up and treatment
    e. b and d

11. Patient-centered clinicians use the following behavior(s):
    a. avoid eye contact because it threatens the patient
    b. frequent interruptions of the patient to seek clarification indicate concern and commitment to clarity
    c. calm listening with an absence of distracting movements such as fidgeting
    d. avoid repeatedly asking the patient to provide feedback or tell the physician that he or she understands because this insults the patient's intelligence
    e. lean back in the chair with arms and legs crossed to indicate that the clinician has all the time in the world

CLINICAL CASE PROBLEM 5

The Challenges of Nonorganic Disease

A 67-year-old female makes frequent visits to her primary care physician for complaints that frequently do not have identifiable organic causes. Her physician becomes frustrated by her demands for diagnoses, medication, and laboratory or imaging examinations to identify causation.

12. The appropriate steps for the primary physician are
    a. refer to an internist, who will be more able to assign diagnoses to her complaints
    b. avoid overuse of testing and reassure the patient that you will follow the symptoms

closely with her to determine the correct time for intervention

c. prescribe an anxiolytic medication to help the patient remain calm

d. order a comprehensive chemistry and hematologic evaluation followed by a positron emission tomography scan to rule out any pathology

e. none of the above

Answers

1. d. Unless there is a specific reason not to, you should refer the patient to the neurologist of his choice. Patients with chronic symptoms are difficult to manage. You may find that a second opinion not only validates your findings but also improves the relationship between you and the patient. He may in fact find the headache to be less of a problem. In this case, it would prove to be less of a problem for both you and him.

2. d. The primary purpose of consultation or referral is to improve the quality of health care by making available to patients and referring physicians the knowledge and skills of specialists or consultants at appropriate times.

There may be situations in complicated cases in which you wish to validate your findings or make sure that nothing has been overlooked. There also may be times when patients need additional reassurance.

To refer to specialists for the sole purpose of protecting yourself against malpractice (especially on a regular basis) is inappropriate.

3. c. Mechanic, as outlined in the Cochrane Review by McKinstry, notes that patients refer to learnable skills and not simply personality characteristics. Although competence is part of trust, it is not the full determinant of trust.

4. a. Evidence suggests that patients who have continuity with and trust in their physician are more likely to be adherent to the agreed upon treatment plan. The relationship serves as a positive reinforcement in care of chronic disease. Although progress may be slow, having a continuity relationship increases the likelihood of ultimate adherence to the regimen.

5. d. The Cochrane Review by McKinstry notes that trust can increase patient satisfaction, adherence to treatment, and improve continuity of care.

6. b. Although patients interpret trust as belief or confidence that the physician will provide reliable information and will act in the patients' interests, it does not mean that patients should not ask for further information or seek to confirm the reliable information that is provided. It creates an atmosphere in which patients can ask about influences on physician decision making, such as choice of inpatient facility or type of insurance incentives, but does not ensure that physicians would not be impacted by external incentives.

7. e. Convenience has never been more important with two parents working and an increased commitment to free time. Dealing electronically with appointments and answers to brief questions is more convenient than telephones and wait times. Having the ability to make their own appointments or request a refill at 2 AM allows them to have more control in the negotiation of receiving care. An increasing amount of disease management can be done online as well, allowing the patient with chronic disease to work with the physician to manage blood sugars or blood pressures without having to make frequent office visits.

8. e. The increased frequency of interactions allows patients to feel greater physician commitment even though the interactions are not face-to-face. The flexibility of sending both queries and answers at times that are convenient for patient and physician improves satisfaction. There is evidence that there is actually decreased liability because there is an easy record of the question and subsequent advice that may not exist for phone interactions.

9. e. E-mail offers a great deal of convenience to patients and physician offices. It is flexible with regard to the timing of queries and answers, allows detailed information to be attached to the answers, and allows a ready record of the interchange; however, it is not appropriate for emergency situations. It is imperative that physicians who provide e-mail interface for their patients take steps to ensure that at the time of an emergency, e-mail will not be used, although it does provide a way for timely update to a physician of other emergency interventions.

10. e. According to the National Cancer Institute at the National Institutes of Health, cancer patient communications are particularly problematic because the caregivers must help patients receive bad news, handle the emotional impact of a life-threatening illness, deal with uncertainty while maintaining hope, understand and remember complex information, communicate with multiple health professionals, and build trust that will sustain long-term clinical relationships. Many cancers are curable today, so not all news is bad; however, despite great progress in treating cancer, many patients have difficulty maintaining a positive, hopeful attitude.

11. **c.** Good patient-centered behavior includes maintenance of eye contact and seeking evidence of patient understanding by having them feedback what has been said. Listening without interruptions sends a message of interest and clarifying questions can come at the end. Crossed arms and legs often indicate a closed mind or barriers to a relationship. Calm listening without fidgeting sends the message that patients can take their time and tell their story.

12. **b.** Although avoiding overuse of prescriptions and/or testing can be very frustrating, the quality of the physician–patient relationship is particularly important when working with patients presenting with medically unexplained symptoms. While patients seek a diagnosis, prognosis, and some form of action, a longer running relationship is more likely to provide a context for reassurance and watchful waiting. If nonaction occurs in a setting without a relationship, the stage is set for patient dissatisfaction and overuse of medical services.

Summary

PRIMARY PHYSICIAN RELATIONSHIPS

1. Enhance patient adherence to treatment programs
2. Enhance patient satisfaction
3. Provide a trusting relationship in which to process complex, often controversial, information

WAYS CONSULTATIONS ENHANCE THE HEALTH CARE EXPERIENCE

1. By making available to patient and referring physician the knowledge and skills of experts in particular areas of concern
2. Best results occur with communication between referring physician and consultant before and following the consultation.
   a. This shows a team approach to caring for the patient.
   b. This maximizes use of available information and limits the likelihood of repeating evaluations unnecessarily.
3. As the arena of specialization based on site of care emerges (e.g., hospitalist), communication between physicians involved in the care of a patient becomes even more important to avoid loss of information and to identify and resolve conflicting recommendations or confirm agreements on interventions to be pursued.

ELECTRONIC COMMUNICATIONS

1. E-mail and Web sites offer an additional means of communicating complex information to patients.
2. E-mail offers a convenient way to conduct much of the business of care, including answering brief questions and tracking chronic disease measures.
   a. Care must be taken to ensure that patients understand that there are limitations to electronic communications and that in some instances an office visit or an emergency department evaluation will be required.

Effective Clinical Decisions—Shared Decision Making

Best course of action given current science
   Requires physicians to know and be able to fairly communicate best current evidence of risks and benefits of current options
Best course of action given health resources
   Requires physicians to be able to outline the costs/benefits of alternatives
Best course of action given clinical circumstances
Best course of action given patient preferences
   As clinical options multiply, need for patient guidance increases
   Patient values often drive decisions
Barriers to shared decision making
   Physician perception of time constraints
   Lack of applicability due to patient characteristics
   Lack of applicability due to clinical situation
Three most often reported facilitators of shared decision making
   Provider motivation
   Positive impact on the clinical process
   Positive impact on patient outcomes

Patient-Centered Care

Patient and Family Who Are	Clinicians/Physicians Who Are	Health Systems That Are
Informed	Patient centered	Accessible
Activated	Communicative	Responsive
Participatory	Responsive	Well-organized

Suggested Reading

Berry LL, Parish JT, Ogburn-Russell L, et al: Patients' commitment to their primary physician and why it matters. *Ann Fam Med* 6(1):6–13, 2008.

Epstein RM, Street RL: *Patient-Centered Communication in Cancer Care*. Bethesda, MD: U.S. Department of Health and Human Services, National Institutes of Health, National Cancer Institute, 2007.

Legare F, Ratte S, Kryworuchko J, et al: Interventions for improving the adoption of shared decision making by healthcare professionals. (Protocol) *Cochrane Database Syst Rev* (3):CD006732, 2007.

McKinstry B, Ashcroft RE, Freeman GK, Sheikh A: Interventions for improving patients' trust in doctors and groups of doctors. *Cochrane Database Syst Rev* (3):CD004134, 2006.

<table>
<tr><td>CHAPTER
17</td><td>**Palliative Care**</td></tr>
</table>

CLINICAL CASE PROBLEM 1

Depression Complicating Dementia

You are called to the home of a 75-year-old patient with progressive dementia. He has become increasingly depressed and agitated and now is unable to sleep at night. His family is concerned that he will wander away or perhaps set the house on fire. As you talk to the patient and review in your head the criteria for depression, you realize that this patient has an agitated depression.

SELECT THE BEST ANSWER TO THE FOLLOWING QUESTIONS

1. Which of the following may be indicated in the treatment of this patient's condition?
   a. a sedating tricyclic antidepressant in the evening
   b. an anxiolytic agent given on an as needed basis
   c. fluoxetine
   d. a and/or b
   e. all of the above

2. Which of the following statements is (are) true regarding use of palliative care and dementia patients?
   a. more than 32% of dementia patients are referred for palliative care
   b. since dementia patients have flawed memory, they do not suffer psychological distress and palliative care is unnecessary
   c. estimating survival of end-stage dementia patients complicates referral to palliative care/hospice care
   d. dementia patients rarely have pain, so they rarely need palliative care
   e. all of the above

3. Referral for palliative care of patients who have life-threatening, nonmalignant care is compromised by which of the following:
   a. disagreements between physicians regarding appropriateness and timing of referral
   b. difficulty predicting actual anticipated time of death
   c. concern that expansion of palliative care to this group might lead to a shortage of expertise available for patients with malignant disease
   d. overly optimistic estimates of survival leading to failure to refer patients in a timely manner
   e. all of the above

4. Barriers to timely referral to hospice/palliative care include which of the following:
   a. association of hospice with death
   b. physician reluctance to make referrals
   c. physician lack of awareness of available resources
   d. misperception of hospice as a place rather than a service
   e. all of the above

CLINICAL CASE PROBLEM 2

A 51-Year-Old Female with Severe Nausea, Vomiting, and Anorexia in Severe, Advanced Ovarian Cancer

A 51-year-old female patient with advanced ovarian cancer has terminal disease. She is constantly nauseated, vomiting, and anorexic. You are called to see her at home. In addition to the symptoms mentioned, the patient complains of a "sore abdomen," and she is having significant difficulty breathing. She also has a "sore mouth."

The patient has gone through chemotherapy with cisplatinum. This therapy ended 8 months ago. Her ovarian cancer was first discovered 12 months ago. Since that time, her condition has deteriorated to the point where she has lost 40 pounds and is feeling "weaker and weaker" every day.

On examination, the patient's breathing is labored. Her respiratory rate is 28 beats/minute. The breath sounds heard in both lungs are normal. Her mouth is dry, and there are whitish lesions that rub off with a tongue depressor. She looks significantly cachectic. Her abdomen is significantly enlarged. There is a level of shifting dullness, and there is a large abdominal mass that is approximately 8 × 35 cm.

5. What is (are) the drug(s) of choice for the management of cancer-associated cachexia and anorexia?
a. prednisone
b. prochlorperazine
c. megestrol acetate
d. cyproheptadine
e. a or c

6. The nausea and vomiting that this patient has developed may be treated with various measures or drugs. Which of the following could be recommended as first-line agents for this patient's nausea and vomiting?
a. prochlorperazine
b. dimenhydrinate
c. metoclopramide
d. all of the above
e. none of the above

7. The drug that you selected for the treatment of the nausea and vomiting unfortunately was not effective. What would you do at this time?
a. forget drugs and use a nasogastric (NG) tube
b. combine two or three of the previously mentioned drugs
c. forget treatment and attempt hydration with intravenous (IV) fluids
d. select ondansetron as an antiemetic
e. b or d

8. Based on the history of her "sore mouth" and white lesions that scrape off with a tongue depressor, what would you recommend treatment with?
a. ketoconazole
b. penicillin
c. amphotericin B
d. chloramphenicol
e. methotrexate

9. The patient described undergoes palliative radiotherapy for severe bone pain that develops 1 month after the problems described. Following this, significant diarrhea develops. Which of the following agents may be helpful in the treatment of this problem?

a. diphenoxylate hydrochloride
b. loperamide
c. codeine
d. all of the above
e. none of the above

10. What is the most prevalent symptom in patients with cancer?
a. anorexia
b. asthenia
c. pain
d. nausea
e. constipation

11. What is the most frequent cause of chronic nausea and vomiting in advanced cancer?
a. bowel obstruction
b. raised intracranial pressure
c. narcotic bowel syndrome
d. hypercalcemia
e. autonomic failure

12. The patient described becomes increasingly short of breath. You suspect a pleural effusion. A chest x-ray confirms the diagnosis of a left pleural effusion. Which of the following is the treatment of first choice for the treatment of this complication?
a. a thoracocentesis
b. home oxygen
c. a hospital bed that is elevated at the head
d. decreased fluid intake
e. prochlorperazine

13. Which of the following treatments may also be useful in treating this symptom?
a. palliative radiotherapy
b. prednisone
c. morphine sulfate
d. dexamethasone
e. all of the above

Answers

1. **d.** An agitated depression is best treated by a combination of a sedating tricyclic antidepressant and/or an anxiolytic agent given as needed. In this case, fluoxetine may actually make the situation worse. Although fluoxetine and other selective serotonin reuptake inhibitors represent very important advances in the treatment of depressive disorders, fluoxetine has the potential to make an agitated depression worse. In this case, it is safer to stick to the older, proven reliable tricyclic antidepressants (TCAs), especially a TCA with sedating properties.

2. **c.** Less than 2% of dementia patients are referred for palliative care. Studies examining distress have found significant measures of distress as well as a correlation between distress and duration of life in dementia patients. Referral for palliative care should be for relief of symptoms, not just pain relief. Dementia patients often have distress if not somatic pain. However, due to definitions of who can be referred for hospice care, it is very difficult to predict the timing of the last 6 months of a dementia patient's life, thereby complicating the referral process.

3. **e.** Often, physicians disagree about the timing and appropriateness of referral for palliative/hospice care. United States regulations requiring referral for the last 6 months of life are difficult in that many nonmalignant life-threatening diseases seem to have a waxing and waning course with a slow downhill course. There is concern that since nonmalignant causes outnumber malignant causes of death, if regular use were made of palliative care specialists, there would not be adequate numbers to treat those in need. Often, physicians are overly optimistic and tell patients they have much more time than they actually have and referral is made too late to receive the greatest benefit from the specialized services.

4. **e.** A number of barriers exist to full and effective use of hospice. Some of the barriers are family and patient based and some are health care provider based. Families often do not want to have the conversation about hospice or change to palliative rather than curative care because they believe death is imminent. Physicians often do not want to make a referral until patients and family are ready, and they often lack knowledge of available resources. Many want to go home and have a misperception of hospice as a place rather than a set of services.

5. **e.** Prednisone (a corticosteroid) and megestrol acetate (a progestational agent) are the pharmacologic treatments of choice in patients with advanced cancer who have significant anorexia.

In patients with anorexia, oral nutrition should be the first priority, with particular attention being paid to the timing of meals in relation to medical and nursing procedures and to the administration of drugs. Selected patients in whom oral nutrition or hydration is not possible may benefit from enteral nutrition or hypodermoclysis. Parenteral nutrition has shown no significant benefit in terms of improving survival or comfort, and its routine use is not indicated in palliative care.

Megestrol acetate in a dosage of 460 mg/day is rapidly becoming the pharmacologic agent of choice in the treatment of anorexia. An alternative to progestational agents is prednisone. Prednisone may be given in doses of approximately 10 to 15 mg/day. This may

be increased if necessary. Dronabinol has also been effective in weight gain for younger adults with specific conditions, such as AIDS and cancer.

With anorexia, particular attention must be paid to the mouth to prevent candidiasis and other problems.

Other potential choices for the pharmacologic treatment of anorexia include cyproheptadine, hydrazine sulfate, and cannabinoids.

6. **d.** The nonpharmacologic treatment of nausea and vomiting should include (1) attempting to find the cause; (2) the avoidance of a supine position to prevent the dangers of aspiration of vomit; (3) a general assessment of the environment of the patient and how it could be improved; (4) attention to body odors; (5) small, frequent meals (that the patient likes; not a bland diet); and (6) attractive food presentation.

Antiemetics can be divided into several classes: (1) anticholinergics such as hyoscine and atropine; (2) phenothiazines such as prochlorperazine and chlorpromazine; (3) butyrophenones such as haloperidol and droperidol; (4) antihistamines such as cyclizine and promethazine; (5) gastrokinetic agents such as domperidone and metoclopramide; (6) 5-HT$_3$ receptor antagonists such as ondansetron; (7) corticosteroids such as prednisone and dexamethasone; and (8) miscellaneous agents such as ibuprofen, tricyclic antidepressants, benzodiazepines, and nabilone.

There are some specific indications for certain antinauseants, such as the treatment of a partial bowel obstruction with a gastrokinetic agent, cyclizine for vestibular-associated emesis, and ondansetron for chemotherapy-induced emesis. In most cases, however, an antinauseant from any of the classes can be tried for any cancer-associated nausea.

Three general rules should be followed when prescribing antinauseants in cancer and palliative care management: (1) Before prescribing an antinauseant on a long-term basis, conduct a vigorous search for the underlying cause; (2) if you are using combination antinauseant therapy, do not combine antinauseants from the same class of drugs; and (3) if you are using combination antinauseant therapy, remember that antinauseants that work on the same neurotransmitter (dopamine, muscarinic/cholinergic, and histamine) tend to be less effective when combined than antinauseants that work on different receptors.

Although a discussion of the receptors involved in each antinauseant is too detailed for this book, the following approach to treating the nausea and vomiting associated with cancer and palliative care is suggested:

1. Always consider nonpharmacologic therapy first—small, frequent meals with appropriate food

presentation and consisting of foods that the patient likes.

2. Begin with prochlorperazine, dimenhydrinate, or metoclopramide.
3. Combine any two of the previously mentioned drugs or all three for resistant nausea.
4. Consider adding a corticosteroid such as prednisone or dexamethasone to the treatment regimen.
5. Consider ondansetron for chemotherapy-induced nausea and vomiting.
6. If emesis continues despite the previous treatment suggestions, try the rectal, subcutaneous, or suppository route.

7. **e.** As mentioned, a combination of two or three of the antinauseants discussed in the choices in question 2 would be appropriate. It is surprising that a few significant problems with extrapyramidal side effects occur with combination therapy.

Ondansetron is a 5-HT receptor antagonist. However, it is very expensive, and this certainly should be considered when selecting between this and a combination of older agents.

Try to avoid an NG tube in patients undergoing palliative care whenever possible. NG tubes are uncomfortable and thus tend to have a negative, rather than a positive, impact on symptom control in patients with cancer.

8. **a.** White lesions that scrape off with a tongue depressor are almost certainly oral thrush. Oral thrush is extremely common in patients undergoing palliative care, even with good mouth care. Treatment with clotrimazole troches or fluconazole is recommended.

9. **d.** The diarrhea in this case is likely the effect of the radiotherapy on the bowel. Diphenoxylate, loperamide, and codeine are all good treatment choices. In most patients, the diarrhea will settle down 1 or 2 weeks after the completion of the course of radiotherapy.

10. **b.** Asthenia (fatigue) is the most prevalent symptom in patients with advanced cancer. The prevalence of symptoms in patients with advanced cancer is as follows: (1) asthenia, 90%; (2) anorexia, 85%; (3) pain, 76%; (4) nausea, 68%; (5) constipation, 65%; (6) sedation, 60%; (7) confusion, 60%; and (8) dyspnea, 12%.

11. **a.** Although autonomic failure, hypercalcemia, narcotic bowel syndrome, and raised intracranial pressure can cause nausea and vomiting, the most frequent cause is bowel obstruction from pressure of an intraabdominal tumor on the bowel, involvement of the bowel in the tumor process, associated gastric stasis, or other causes.

12. **a.** A large pleural effusion initially should be treated by thoracentesis. If it recurs at infrequent intervals, this technique can be used repeatedly and with a sclerosing agent, such as infused talc. This can reduce the reoccurrence of a malignant effusion but often is irritating to the patient.

13. **e.** However, if pleural effusion recurs frequently, you may decide to use other symptom-relieving measures, including elevating the head of the bed, providing oxygen, breathing fresh air, decreasing fluid intake, prescribing prednisone or dexamethasone, prescribing morphine, and conducting palliative radiotherapy.

Summary

MANAGEMENT OF LATE STAGES OF LIFE-THREATENING DISEASES

1. Discussions with the patient (occasionally with family, either with patient's consent or in case of incompetent patient) regarding the prognosis, what is known about the timeline, and types of decisions that need to be made
   a. This would include the possibility of using palliative care or hospice teams at some point.
   b. This should include discussion of living wills, durable powers of attorney for health, or other means of communicating desires about end-of-life care.
   c. Discussions should occur about the importance of communicating symptoms, desires, etc. in order to provide the highest quality of life possible.
   d. As the end of life nears, it is appropriate to discuss how to handle possibly terminal symptoms, including respiratory distress, bradycardia, and recalcitrant pain. This discussion should include whether the patient or family desires transfer to the hospital or wants to die at home.

MANAGEMENT OF PHYSICAL SYMPTOMS

1. Nausea and vomiting
   a. Eat small, frequent meals.
   b. Avoid bland foods. Give the patient what he or she wants to eat.
   c. Take antiemetics: prochlorperazine, dimenhydrinate, metoclopramide, prednisone, hycosin/atropine, and ondansetron.
   d. Consider combination of antiemetics if one is not sufficient.
   e. If vomiting continues, consider suppository or subcutaneous route.
2. Constipation
   a. Attempt to find the cause—do not automatically assume it is from taking narcotics.
   b. Lactulose appears to be the agent of choice for the treatment of constipation in palliative care. A combination of a stool softener and a peristaltic stimulant is a good alternative.
3. Anorexia
   a. Eat small, frequent meals.
   b. Avoid blended, pulverized foods; give the patient what he or she wants to eat.
   c. Megestrol acetate is the most effective agent for treating anorexia and cachexia in patients who are terminally ill. Prednisone is a good alternative.
4. Dry mouth/oral thrush
   a. Mouth care is very important.
   b. Avoid drying agents such as lemon-glycerine swabs.
   c. Hydrogen peroxide at one-fourth strength, lemon drops, pineapple chunks, and tart juices are helpful.
   d. Look for oral thrush every day; treat with clotrimazole troches. If treatment is resistant, prescribe Diflucan.
5. Dehydration: Dehydration is usually not symptomatic; that is, it usually does not have to be treated. Always base your decision to use fluids on whether you think it will make the patient feel better and improve the patient's quality of life. Remember, the most common complication of treating patients receiving palliative care with IV fluids is iatrogenic pulmonary edema.
6. Diarrhea
   a. Try to identify the cause.
   b. Diphenoxylate, loperamide, and codeine are equally effective.
7. Dyspnea and pleural effusion: Open windows, supplementary oxygen, semi-Fowler's position, bronchodilators, prednisone, narcotic analgesics, anxiolytics, diuretics, and palliative radiotherapy may all be of help with recurrent pleural effusions. Treat first occurrence with thoracocentesis. How often you repeat this procedure depends on the patient's comfort level and how quickly the fluid reaccumulates.
8. Partial bowel obstruction
   a. Restrict fluids.
   b. Antiemetics: Consider prokinetic agents such as metoclopramide first.
   c. Corticosteroids: Prednisone.
   d. Narcotic analgesics.
   e. Try to avoid the use of a NG tube, if possible.
9. Malignant ascites
   a. Paracentesis is often effective: How often you perform this procedure is again dependent on the reaccumulation of fluid.
   b. Spironolactone alone or with thiazide and/or loop diuretics may be helpful.
10. Cerebral edema: Dexamethasone with an H_2 receptor antagonist is both diagnostic and therapeutic.
11. Fungating growths
    a. Frequent dressing changes; normal saline or hydrogen peroxide
    b. Yogurt or buttermilk dressings
    c. Charcoal briquettes around the house
    d. Fresh air
12. Depression and anxiety
    a. Remember bio-psycho-social-spiritual model of pain and symptom control.
    b. Psychotherapy: "Be there, be sensitive, be silent."
    c. Antidepressant medication
    d. Anxiolytics (sublingual especially effective)
13. Hypercalcemia
    a. Most common serious metabolic abnormality in palliative care.
    b. Think about the diagnosis: Otherwise, you will not make it.
    c. Fluids will treat hypercalcemia effectively in most cases.

Suggested Reading

Aminoff BZ, Adunsky A: Their last 6 months: Suffering and survival of end-stage dementia patients. *Age Ageing* 35(6):597–601, 2006.

Feeg VD, Elebiary H: Exploratory study on end-of-life issues: Barriers to palliative care and advance directives. *Am J Hospice Palliative Med* 22(2):119–124, 2005.

National Cancer Institute. Pain (PDQ), 1999. Available at www.cancer.gov/cancertopics/pdf/supportivecare/pain/HealthProfessional.

Stevens LM: JAMA patient page: Palliative care. *JAMA* 296(11):1323, 2006.

Rakel RE, Bope ET (eds): *Conn's Current Therapy 2003: Pain Management.* Philadelphia: Saunders, pp 1–10, 2002.

CHAPTER

18 Ethical Decision-Making Issues

CLINICAL CASE PROBLEM 1

Withholding Information from an Aging Patient

An 89-year-old woman lives with her daughter and family. At times, the living arrangement has been difficult. Recently, the daughter was concerned because her mom was not eating. You have been the primary care physician for the mother and the family for approximately 10 years. The concerned daughter brings her mom to see you. After seeing you, the mother is hospitalized. In the hospital, the mother is started on IV fluids and nutrition. Even though she complains about the hospitalization, the mother is basically compliant with treatment. The physician orders several tests, and the results are not good. The daughter is concerned that her mother will not be able to emotionally manage the difficult report, which includes an intestinal malignancy and the recommendation of intestinal surgery. With or without surgery, life expectancy is probably only a matter of 6 to 8 months. The mother is asking about the test results, but the daughter says, "Doctor, don't tell my mother what is going on. She has a hard enough time with things as it is."

SELECT THE BEST ANSWER TO THE FOLLOWING QUESTIONS

1. Who is the decision maker for mother?
   a. mom: "What do the tests show?"
   b. daughter: "Don't tell mom."
   c. doctor: "I know what is best."
   d. call risk management
   e. nursing staff: They are with the mother all the time

2. What ethical principles are most relevant to this case?
   a. justice and fidelity
   b. beneficence and noncompliance
   c. autonomy and beneficence
   d. nonmaleficence and justice
   e. all of the above

In determining whether someone has the capacity for medical decision making, the physician often says, "The patient is oriented ×3."

3. What does this mean?
   a. place, employment, time
   b. place, time, person
   c. time, place, decision
   d. family, age, place
   e. family, person, time

CLINICAL CASE PROBLEM 2

Decision Making and the Confused Patient

Assume the previous case as it is presented but with the following difference: As a physician, you have determined that the mother is somewhat confused by the environment and what is going on. The daughter agrees with you, and she says she just wants her mom to be comfortable. The mother still asks to know what the test results show, and the daughter says not to tell the mother the bad news.

4. Who is the decision maker for mom?
   a. mom: "What do the tests show?"
   b. daughter: "Don't tell mom."
   c. doctor: "I know what is best."
   d. call risk management
   e. refer the decision to another physician

CLINICAL CASE PROBLEM 3

When Siblings Disagree

Continue to assume the original case but with the following difference: Rather than being confused, the mother is delirious and in and out of conscious awareness.

Since you have treated the mother and family for 10 years, you have in the mother's medical record three documents. First, there is a do not resuscitate order in the event that the situation becomes critical. Second, there is an advance directive that states that the mother does not want anything "heroic" for her care. She wants only to be comfortable. Third, there is a Power of Attorney for Health Care Decisions that the mother has executed naming the daughter as surrogate in case of her incapacity. There is a brother present who insists that the mother be told everything. He says, "She always taught us to tell the truth. Lying is just plain wrong, and she would never agree to that."

5. Who it the decision maker for mom?
   a. mom: "What do the tests show?"
   b. daughter: "Don't tell mom."
   c. doctor: "I know what is best."
   d. call risk management
   e. refer the decision to another physician

6. Which is true about a Durable Power of Attorney for Health Care?
   a. it allows the surrogate to make medical decisions about what the surrogate thinks is best in this situation
   b. it can be overruled by the attending physician
   c. it mandates that the surrogate make decisions for the patient based on what the patient would decide if he or she had the capacity for decision making
   d. it is a democratic process, and family members, by majority vote, can overrule the decisions of the appointed surrogate
   e. Because the Power of Attorney is a voluntary process, the immediate next of kin always has veto authority over any medical decision that is made

CLINICAL CASE PROBLEM 4

When Technology and Religion Conflict

A 16-year-old boy is brought to the emergency department with a lacerated leg from a lawnmower accident. The father tied a tourniquet around the leg, but the boy has lost a lot of blood. On entering the emergency department, the parents identify themselves as Jehovah's Witnesses and say they do not want the boy to receive any blood. However, they do want the boy's life to be saved. The doctors assess the situation and quickly tell the parents that the boy needs blood immediately or he will die. The boy, who is conscious, says, "Give me the blood. I do not want to die. It's a stupid rule any way." The parents overrule the boy and say it is not his decision.

7. It is a life or death decision. What do you do?
   a. tell the parents that they are wrong and that you know what is best for the boy

   b. inform the parents that in your opinion, the Jehovah's Witnesses are incorrect in their views of not accepting blood
   c. view the decision as a medical emergency, give the boy blood, and then address the difficult issues with the parents at a later time
   d. knowing he will die, you refuse to give the boy blood, realizing that to do so against the parents' instructions will be battery against a minor child
   e. tell the parents to take the boy to another hospital

CLINICAL CASE PROBLEM 5

Unmarried, Pregnant, 18-Year-Old Female

You work in an area with a large adolescent population. An 18-year-old woman comes to you because she has had sexual intercourse for the first time, and she has missed her last period. She is very distraught and concerned that she may be pregnant. You are emotionally touched by her story. In addition, you are an advocate for unwed mothers to complete their pregnancy. When the pregnancy test comes back, it is positive. When you inform the young woman of the test results, she immediately says she wants an abortion. Through further conversation, you learn that the father of the baby does not know about the pregnancy, and she has no intention of telling him. She says it was all a mistake, and she does not want to ever see him again. She insists on an abortion. However, because of your pro-life views, you personally and morally oppose abortion.

8. What should you do?
   a. explain to the patient your opposition to abortion and that you will not help in doing what you believe is morally wrong
   b. inform the patient that all you can do is help her through her pregnancy, and she can either keep the child or put the child up for adoption
   c. tell her to find another doctor who is pro-choice
   d. discuss her health options with her, namely carry the baby to term and keep it, carry the baby to term and place it for adoption, or have a therapeutic abortion. You also strongly advise her to seek professional counseling during this time
   e. none of the above

9. The 2002 law that states that any fetus born alive must receive appropriate care is called what?
   a. No Child Left Behind Act
   b. Born Alive Infants Protection Act
   c. Fetal Birth Viability Act
   d. Full-Term Birth Act
   e. none of the above

10. The right to life movement is actively involved in:
    a. the beginning of life
    b. the end of life
    c. health care for the disabled
    d. health care in decisions of futility
    e. all of the above

CLINICAL ETHICS AND CASE ANALYSIS

11. In the case analysis method of ethical decision making, which of the following categories must be considered?
    a. indications for medical intervention
    b. patient preferences
    c. quality of life
    d. contextual features
    e. all of the above

12. In the case analysis method of ethical decision making, the category "Indications for medical intervention" includes which of the following ethical principles?
    a. beneficence
    b. nonmaleficence
    c. clinical judgment
    d. a and b
    e. a and c

13. In the case analysis method of ethical decision making, the category "Patient preferences" includes which of the following?
    a. paternalism
    b. informed consent
    c. medical capacity
    d. all of the above
    e. none of the above

14. The clinical case method for deciding "quality of life" includes which of the following?
    a. physician-assisted suicide
    b. palliative care
    c. euthanasia
    d. life support
    e. all of the above

Clinical Case Management Problem

A 17-year-old male is involved in a motorcycle/automobile crash and is brought to the emergency room with multiple trauma including coma. He is stabilized and sent to the intensive care unit. Over the course of the next several hours, he is placed on a respirator and administered IV fluids, intracranial pressure monitoring, and multiple medications. His heart and kidneys appear to be functioning well. However, at 48 hours postadmission he is found to have no electrical activity on an electroencephalogram (EEG). His parents are adamant that everything continue to be done, citing a case recently reported in the newspaper about a man who awoke from a long coma and returned to work and family. His driver's license indicates that he is willing to be an organ donor.

Using the clinical case management system, outline the steps that might be taken in providing care for this young man and his family.

Answers

1. **a.** As a patient, the mother is inquiring about the test results, and she has a right to know the information. Even though the mother is very ill, the fact that the daughter is concerned about her mother's reaction is not sufficient reason to withhold the information. If there are other complicating factors, they are not presented in this case. There is no purpose in seeking a consult from risk management. The daughter's comments are not hostile or argumentative, and the mother is clear in her thinking and in her desire to know the results. The nursing staff does provide regular care of the patient, but they are not the decision makers for treatment decisions.

2. **c.** Autonomy is a significant principle with regard to respect of persons. It assumes the individual has the right to determine what happens to him or her. In this case, the mother has a right to know, she is inquiring about the test results, and her agreement is essential for further treatment or refusal of treatment. In addition, truth telling is often understood as beneficence, doing good, whereas lying, or withholding truth, may be viewed as harmful. Answers a and d are not correct because justice does not play a significant part in the situation in terms of fairness or allocation of resources.

Answer b is incorrect because noncompliance is a behavior and not an ethical principle.

3. **b.** Place, time, person, often referred to as "time, place, person." The determination of one's capacity for medical decision making is always an issue when ethical decisions are being made, including procedures about one's body. Time is the most sensitive indicator of confusion because time changes constantly. Place changes are next in sensitivity. Person, or identity, is permanently embedded information and does not change. Someone who is identity confused may be seriously impaired.

In this case, the daughter can be reassured that you know and have treated her and her family, including her mother, and that knowing her mother as you do, you believe the mother when she says she wants to know the test results. You can also assure the daughter that you will proceed in a sensitive way with giving the information to her mother. You can offer to sit down with the three of them in a quiet way with minimal distractions, and you will begin by asking her mother what it is that she wants to know and how much information she wants. In addition, you will give the mother plenty of time to think about the conversation and ask questions. It is hoped that the daughter will find this collegial approach acceptable.

4. **a.** The mother is still the decision maker. Confusion does not necessarily mean incapacity for all decisions. The physician will be very sensitive about the situation of telling the mother the difficult information, and the mother may or may not fully understand. It may take several different conversations for the information to become clear, and even then, the mother may complain that she has not been told anything. However, by having the daughter present for each conversation, the daughter knows what has been said.

The physician needs to also be aware that there may be other family members involved in this case. If so, they should be invited into the conversation. We assume the mother is a widow, so her husband is not available. However, he could be living in a nursing home while his wife lives with her daughter. Also, there may be other siblings, even in another city or state. Some sensitivity to, and awareness of, these other family members is necessary for managing the total situation.

Consultation with the ethics committee may become necessary if the family cannot agree on a course of care.

5. **b.** With a Power of Attorney for Health Care Decisions, the daughter is the surrogate decision maker, and she has the right to manage the information about her mother who is delirious and mentally incapacitated. This document also simplifies the situation in case there are other family members who desire to be involved in the decision making. However, because some surgery is indicated to relieve the intestinal blockage, the mother is still going to have to be informed, probably in a similar manner as previously recommended, and given time to comprehend what is going to happen. The daughter will have to decide if some surgery, or no surgery, is what her mother needs in order to be comfortable. If she decides not to have surgery, then limiting the information given to the mother is more acceptable. However, the physician must realize that a decision to withhold information is a medical decision.

6. **c.** The Power of Attorney for Medical Decisions is a legal document that cannot be overruled by other interested parties, including physicians. The purpose of the document is for the surrogate to exercise "substituted judgment," which means that the surrogate is to represent, as accurately as possible, what the patient would decide if the patient were capable of medical decision making. It is not designed for the surrogate to do whatever he or she thinks is "best," and it is not what the surrogate thinks the patient needs. Rather, it is what the patient would decide if the patient had the capacity to make the decision. For this reason, it is very important for physicians to know who has power of attorney. In addition, discussing the question, "Who do you want to be medical decision maker for you in case of your incapacity?" with a continuity patient is an important part of continuity of patient care.

7. **c.** Answers a and b are incorrect because they have a similar logic. Patients have rights that are to be respected by physicians. Similarly, getting into an argument about one's personal opinions on another's religion is counterproductive to respecting the patient or the parents. Answers d and e also have similar logic. The physician does not refuse care in an emergency, or send the patient somewhere else, knowing death is imminent.

Although answer c is correct, it has several dimensions. Generally, the courts do allow a "mature minor" to make medical decisions, including decisions that may be in opposition to those of the parents, when it is a life or death decision. The age of a mature minor is generally 16 or 17 years. Courts generally support the minor's decision if the benefit or risk that the mature minor is choosing is greater than 50%. In other words, if the mature minor, in opposition to parents, wants to choose a benefit that is greater than 50%, or refuse a risk that is greater than 50%, then the courts will, generally, accept the decision of a mature minor. In the current case, clearly there is a benefit to receiving blood.

In a ruling by a Massachusetts court in 1944 (*Prince v Massachusetts*), the court ruled against the parents of a Jehovah's Witnesses child: "Parents may be free to become martyrs themselves, but it does not follow that they are free … to make martyrs of their (minor) children."

The physician will not commit battery against the boy if the boy is transfused. However, in the eyes of the parents, even though their son is alive, the physician may have condemned the boy to an eternity in hell for giving him blood. The decision is further complicated by the disagreement between the boy and his parents regarding the teachings of their religion on blood transfusion.

In working with Jehovah's Witnesses patients, it is very important to ask the patient about blood preferences. There is great variability in Witness beliefs about blood. It is also very important to be confidential in these conversations so that church elders will not know if a member makes a decision against the church.

Generally, whole blood products are not acceptable—red cells, white cells, plasma, and platelets. However, some Witness groups do allow individual choice for blood divided into fractions. Autotransfusion of predeposited blood is not acceptable. Intraoperative collection and hemodilution are objectionable to many, but others will accept intraoperative salvage where the extracorporeal circulation is not interrupted.

8. d. Someone who is pregnant is considered an adult for the purposes of health care decisions. In this case, she is 18 years old, a legal adult, and also pregnant. However, the physician has personal moral values that contradict what the patient wants. Nevertheless, the physician is obligated to provide her with quality health care, including all of the options for decision making regarding the pregnancy. Patients often make personal life and death decisions that are contrary to what is medically or morally acceptable according to some value system. The physician must maintain a therapeutic doctor–patient relationship with the patient while respecting the patient's autonomy for decision making.

9. b. The Born Alive Infants Protection Act states that any fetus born that is alive must receive appropriate care. This law does prohibit no care, in which case death occurs by a form of exposure and neglect. However, it does permit comfort care for extreme situations in which circumstances are extraordinary. No Child Left Behind is an educational act, and there is no Fetal Birth Viability Act or Full-Term Birth Act.

10. e. The right to life movement is actively involved in various legislative processes, including the writing of laws governing life and death issues. The movement's concerns are that in life and death decisions, the value of life may be diminished and viewed as disposable or inconvenient. Some will also view these decisions as "playing God."

11. e. See answer 13.

12. d. See answer 13.

13. e. Albert Jonsen et al have written about the clinical case method for ethical decision making in medical ethics. In this work, the authors list a four-category approach—sometimes referred to as the "four box method"—for understanding the ethical decision and its context. First, the situation is clarified for the *medical indications*. What is the problem, diagnosis, and prognosis? The ethical principles of beneficence and nonmaleficence are relevant here. Beneficence is doing good for the patient, and nonmaleficence is at least doing no harm to the patient. What is a good medical outcome, and what must be avoided? In question 12, clinical judgment is not an ethical principle, but it is certainly required for good decision making.

Second, *patient preferences* are addressed. Is the patient mentally capable of medical decision making? Assuming the patient is fully informed, what are the patient's preferences for the situation? Respect for patient autonomy is a key ethical factor. Paternalism is a behavior, not an ethical principle. Medical capacity and informed consent are both necessary but are not ethical principles.

Third, what are the *quality of life* issues? What are the prospects of returning to a normal life? Are there plans for stopping treatment and only providing palliative care? Key ethical principles include beneficence, nonmaleficence, and respect for autonomy. Autonomy is respect for the patient, realizing the patient has the final say about what happens to his or her body.

Finally, what are the *contextual factors* for the ethical analysis? Are there family issues or provider issues that influence treatment? Are there financial issues or religious and cultural issues that influence the decision? The principle of justice—that is, loyalty and fairness—is relevant. Justice means giving a patient the best care within the confines and limits of the contextual situation, regardless of the patient's background.

14. **e.** Quality of life is a subjective standard that is based on the individual's satisfaction with one's physical, mental, and social condition. Any pain management or end of life consideration raises a question of what quality the patient may experience. The subjective standard of quality of life has great variability from person to person. However, the subjective evaluation of one's quality of life is not to be confused with the general moral principle of "sanctity of life." Sanctity of life tends to place more restrictive limits on all end of life decisions based on a higher objective value for life than limits that are based on a standard of subjective quality.

Quality of life can be a very difficult decision. Who determines when a life has, or does not have, quality? What are the standards for quality? What is the quality of life for a child born with severe disabilities and extreme mental challenges? Does the moral concept of "all life is sacred"—sanctity of life—demand that extraordinary and artificial means be used to keep the newborn alive, or is the potential for any quality of life so compromised that ordinary comfort care should be provided, in which case natural death is certain?

Solution to the Clinical Case Management Problem

Medical intervention: Indications for medical intervention include the need to stabilize the patient until adequate time has passed to assess neurological function. The clinical status is very disturbing to family, but the patient is unaware. Life support is necessary until adequate data can be compiled for decision making.

Conclusions regarding indication for treatment: It was reasonable to intervene and stabilize until data were collected. However, it is illogical to continue to provide support in light of brain death.

Patient preferences: Although this patient is a minor, he apparently gave some thought to what he would do/like to do in the case of catastrophe. Because he is incapable of decision making, his written preference can at best help to reassure parents through their decision making.

Quality of life: Issues include the parents' perception that the monitoring devices indicate life while sophisticated testing reveals that the patient's brain has ceased to function.

Conclusion: A discussion(s) must occur with the family including the legal status, the opportunity for a short time to come to acceptance of the status (although this would ideally have been done in the 48 hours leading up to the first EEG and during the interval before a confirmatory test), the steps to be taken in disconnecting the technical support, and the opportunity to fulfill their son's desire to be an organ donor.

Contextual features: The main contextual feature is the need for the parents to understand the difference between a person being sustained on life support even with little chance of recovery and brain death when the state has determined that the person is already dead and continuation of mechanical support is not an option.

During the time the patient is in the intensive care unit, his family must be kept up to date on the condition of the patient and the implications. Prognosis and meaning of technical issues such as "brain death" should be included in the discussion, with the realization that it takes time to internalize such issues for a grieving family.

Legally, once the patient has been diagnosed as brain dead, he is dead and it is no longer an issue of continuing life support. This is not an issue of medical futility but a legal definition of death. However, helping the family to understand the issues can occasionally take some time and should include counseling support from ministers, chaplaincy, health care providers, and family support systems.

Once the family has been fully informed, time with the patient before disconnecting support equipment might be helpful in their grieving.

Summary

1. Ethical decision making can be based on a case analysis method.
2. Case analysis considers four categories: indications for medical intervention, patient preferences, quality of life, and contextual (or societal) features.
3. The most common disagreements involve indications for intervention; patient preferences; and quality of life disagreement between individual patients' values or autonomy, indications or lack of same for treatment, and one or another of various societal pressures.
4. Golden Rule 1 of medical ethics: *Primum non nocere*—first, do no harm (nonmaleficence).
5. Golden Rule 2 of medical ethics: Consider first the welfare of the patient (beneficence).
6. Medical futility: A treatment that has no or an extremely remote chance of doing any good should not be undertaken. For purposes of security, that should mean zero chance (as with CPR in a patient with terminal cancer with Cheyne–Stokes respiration).
7. There is absolutely no substitute for good doctor–patient communication and good interprofessional health care communication in biomedical ethics.

Suggested Reading

Beauchamp TL, Childress JF: *Principles of Biomedical Ethics*, 5th ed. Oxford: Oxford University Press, 2001.

Jonsen AR, Siegler M, Winslade WJ: *Clinical Ethics: A Practical Approach to Ethical Decisions in Clinical Medicine*, 6th ed. New York: McGraw-Hill, 2006.

Lo B: *Resolving Ethical Dilemmas: A Guide for Clinicians*, 3rd ed. Philadelphia: Lippincott Williams & Wilkins, 2005.

Pence GE: *Classic Cases in Medical Ethics: Accounts of Cases that Have Shaped Medical Ethics, with Philosophical, Legal, and Historical Backgrounds*, 4th ed. New York: McGraw-Hill, 2004.

Pence GE (ed): *Classic Works in Medical Ethics: Core Philosophical Writings*. New York: McGraw-Hill 1998.

Integrative Medicine

CLINICAL CASE PROBLEM 1

"Are Those All *the Medications You Take?"*

A 35-year-old white female schoolteacher presents to your office to establish care. She completes a medical history survey that states she has fibromyalgia and hypoglycemia. The only medication listed on her form is an oral contraceptive agent, but when interviewed she adds that she also takes multiple dietary supplements. She requests that you perform a general well woman exam and renew her birth control pills.

SELECT THE BEST ANSWER TO THE FOLLOWING QUESTIONS

1. Which of the following aspects of this case does not match the typical user of complementary and alternative medicine (CAM) therapies?
   a. a higher percentage of users are female
   b. after prayer, use of "natural products" is the most common form of CAM therapy
   c. the majority of users have at least some college education
   d. despite the use of CAM, the majority of users continue to see conventional practitioners
   e. the majority of CAM users inform their doctor

2. Which of the following statements is true regarding CAM in general?
   a. CAM therapies are rarely covered by health insurance
   b. usage of CAM peaked in the 1990s and has steadily declined
   c. the U.S. government funds several hundred million dollars of CAM-related research annually
   d. the majority of U.S. medical schools do not have curriculum regarding CAM
   e. most CAM users turn to these therapies due to their dissatisfaction with conventional biomedical care

3. In this case, which of the following options would be the least appropriate?
   a. ask the patient to provide you with a complete list of her supplements
   b. obtain additional information regarding her diagnoses of fibromyalgia and hypoglycemia
   c. inquire into other CAM therapies that the patient may be utilizing

d. when dictating this encounter, simply state that she is taking dietary supplements since it is not necessary to list each one in the record

e. perform a complete exam that is appropriate for her age and medical condition

4. Which of the following is not true regarding dietary supplements?

   a. the Food and Drug Administration (FDA) does not regulate these products

   b. they are not considered drugs, and therefore do not have to prove their efficacy or safety

   c. supplements are not allowed to make any claims of curing or mitigating disease

   d. they must state on their labels "this statement has not been evaluated by the Food and Drug Administration"

   e. the most common reason people take these products is a belief that doing so promotes good health

5. Which of the following is not true regarding herbal products?

   a. St. John's Wort has been shown in studies to be effective in the treatment of mild to moderately severe depression

   b. St. John's Wort has been shown to elevate the levels of some drugs, such as cyclosporine and digoxin, due to inhibition of the cytochrome P450 (CYP3A4) pathway in the liver

   c. some herbal products have been found to have contaminants such as heavy metals or prescription drugs

   d. ginkgo biloba, commonly taken for dementia-related concerns, can interfere with platelet function

   e. studies have shown that some herbal products may not contain the dosage that is stated on the package label

6. Match the following supplements with the condition most associated with its usage:

   a. saw palmetto   A. respiratory infections
   b. milk thistle   B. menopausal symptoms
   c. black cohosh   C. prostate enlargement
   d. echinacea   D. anxiety
   e. kava kava   E. liver disease

7. In the current case, which would be the least appropriate option?

   a. ask the patient to describe the reason why she is taking each of the herbals

   b. discuss any potential harm, such as drug–herb interactions, that may occur with the specific supplements being used

c. try to convince the patient to stop taking all of the supplements since they do not have the same level of evidence as drugs

d. provide the patient with a list of reliable resources for CAM therapies, including appropriate web sites

e. invite the patient to be an active participant in decisions regarding her health care, such as treatment options and any laboratory testing

8. During the office visit, the patient states that she is interested in a "holistic" approach to her health care. Which of the following would be your least appropriate response?

   a. respectfully explain that you are a family physician and holistic care is not part of your scope of practice

   b. discuss the use of low-impact cardiovascular exercise for the treatment of her fibromyalgia

   c. explain the importance of small, frequent, nutritious meals to help alleviate her hypoglycemic reactions

   d. discuss the benefits of relaxation techniques, such as meditation and guided imagery, to reduce pain

   e. offer to set up appropriate referrals as needed and help coordinate her care

CLINICAL CASE PROBLEM 2

When Traditional Medicine Fails…

Mr. Smith is a 72-year-old male who has been in your practice for several years. He has a history of prostate cancer that was successfully treated with radical prostatectomy 2 years ago. His only other known medical problems are hyperlipidemia and moderate osteoarthritis, which tends to limit his daily activities. He has tried several nonsteroidal anti-inflammatory agents but did not tolerate them for various reasons. He presents to your office for a routine follow-up visit, but his main objective is to ask your opinion regarding several CAM therapies that he is considering.

9. Regarding CAM in general, which of the following is true?

   a. patients diagnosed with cancer rarely use CAM therapies due to the serious nature of this diagnosis

   b. CAM treatments have not been shown to be effective in reducing pain

   c. patients using prescription drugs rarely use dietary supplements

d. when taken according to the package label by relatively healthy adults, dietary supplements tend to have fewer side effects than do prescription drugs

e. most CAM users are older, retired individuals

10. Which of the following would be the least appropriate advice to offer this patient?

a. it is best to use either conventional treatments alone or only CAM therapies due to the potential for significant adverse interaction between them

b. some studies have demonstrated benefit with the use of glucosamine products for the treatment and prevention of osteoarthritis of the knee

c. there are data to support the use of acupuncture to treat knee arthritis

d. lifestyle modifications, such as maintaining ideal body weight, can have a positive effect on arthritis

e. tai chi, an oriental movement therapy, has been shown to have a favorable impact on strength and balance in elderly patients

11. Regarding acupuncture in the United States, which of the following is not true?

a. the majority of acupuncture is provided by licensed practitioners

b. it can only legally be administered by a person specifically licensed in acupuncture

c. the National Institutes of Health (NIH) has stated that there is evidence to support the use of acupuncture for certain conditions, such as nausea and postoperative pain

d. pregnancy is a relative contraindication to the use of acupuncture

e. increased pain, bruising, fainting, and pneumothorax are all possible adverse effects of acupuncture

12. Regarding manual therapies, which of the following is not true?

a. back and neck pain, along with headaches, are common reasons people seek manual therapy, such as osteopathic manipulative treatment

b. chiropractic care has been demonstrated to provide a higher degree of patient satisfaction than typical conventional care for the treatment of acute low back pain

c. the majority of acute low back pain episodes resolve within 6 months regardless of the therapy used

d. the risk of a serious adverse effect, such as stroke or spinal cord damage, from manipulation is approximately 1 case per 1000 manipulations

e. osteoporosis, pathologic fractures, and significant rheumatoid arthritis are contraindications to thrusting-type therapies

13. Since your patient in this case has been treated for prostate cancer, he is naturally concerned about other forms of malignancy. He is wondering if he should start a special "detoxification" diet that has been recommended by his granddaughter. Which of the following is the most appropriate response?

a. inform him that his body naturally detoxifies itself daily and this regimen is a waste of time and money

b. tell the patient that you are unfamiliar with the treatment so there is not much you can do to help him

c. inform him that diet has no impact on one's risk of cancer

d. offer to review the information that he has brought to the visit and set up a follow-up appointment to discuss this

e. set up a referral for him to see a gastroenterologist to discuss "detoxification diets"

14. Which of the following statements is not true?

a. patients wanting "holistic" cancer therapy typically must go to Mexico since these services are not available at reputable centers in the United States

b. mind–body therapies, such as hypnosis, have been shown to reduce the need for narcotics in some cancer patients

c. support groups are often helpful when a patient is facing a serious medical problem such as cancer

d. acupuncture can be used as a complementary therapy to help palliate the nausea associated with chemotherapy

e. guided imagery has been shown to have a positive effect in some cancer patients

15. Regarding hyperlipidemia, match the following treatments with the best corresponding statement:

a. fish oil	A. contains statin-like properties
b. garlic	B. often derived from sugarcane
c. red yeast rice	C. high dosages can lower triglycerides
d. walnuts	D. common herbal with some evidence of very mild lipid lowering
e. policosanol	E. daily small amount may have a beneficial effect

16. Which of the following statements pertaining to cardiovascular health is true?
 a. chelation therapy has been demonstrated in large randomized controlled trials to have a positive effect on coronary artery disease
 b. fish oil has been shown to reduce the risk of fatal arrhythmias in postinfarction patients
 c. the American Heart Association diet has been proven more effective at preventing coronary events than the Mediterranean diet
 d. although herbals may have significant drug–herb interactions, no negative effects have been shown between herbals and aspirin therapy
 e. diets with less than 10% of the total calories from fat are the most effective at preventing further coronary events and are the easiest to adhere to

---

Clinical Case Management Problem

A 55-year-old, moderately obese attorney presented last week to your office to establish care. At that visit, he proudly told you that he does not take any prescription drugs due to their toxic side effects. He also asserted that doctors are too quick to prescribe pills due to the influence of the pharmaceutical industry. You obtained some basic health screening tests that day which included a fasting lipid panel and glucose. The lab demonstrates that his triglycerides and low-density lipoprotein cholesterol are markedly elevated and his fasting glucose was 200. Explain how you would approach this patient when he returns to discuss his results.

Answers

1. e. CAM has been defined as a group of diverse medical and health care systems, practices, and products that are not currently considered to be part of conventional medicine. The term "integrative medicine" has been used to describe the combination of evidenced-based CAM modalities with conventional medicine. Despite the relatively common usage of these therapies, often estimated to be between 35% and 65%, the majority of users do not disclose this use to their medical doctor. The most common reasons given are "it wasn't important for the doctor to know" and "the doctor never asked."

2. c. The National Center for Complementary and Alternative Medicine, which is part of NIH, was established in 1998. It, along with other NIH centers, funded approximately $300 million in CAM research in 2005.

CAM use continues to be common in the United States. Although much of it remains an out-of-pocket expense, treatments such as chiropractic and osteopathic manipulation are frequently covered by insurers.

According to the latest surveys, the majority of U.S. medical schools offer curriculum covering CAM.

The majority of CAM users continue to see conventional medical doctors but use complementary therapies due to a belief that these other treatments are "more congruous with their personal values, beliefs, and philosophical orientation toward health and life."

3. d. "Dietary supplements" is a term given to a broad range of products that include vitamins, minerals, herbals, and amino acids. Since many drug–supplement interactions have been documented, it is best to have a complete listing of these products in the patient's health care record.

4. a. In 1994, the Dietary Supplement Health and Education Act was passed by Congress. Since that time, the FDA has regulated supplements as food products and not as drugs. If the ingredients in a supplement were sold in the United States prior this act, then safety data are not required. Also, no efficacy studies are needed as long as the product does not claim to treat, cure, or mitigate any disease. The most common reason vitamins and herbals are taken is a belief that they promote good health.

5. b. St. John's Wort has been shown in several studies to induce the CYP 450 system, which may lead to subtherapeutic levels of some drugs, such as cyclosporine, digoxin, and oral contraceptives.

6. a. saw palmetto — C. prostate enlargement
b. milk thistle — E. liver disease
c. black cohosh — B. menopausal symptoms
d. echinacea — A. respiratory infections
e. kava kava — D. anxiety

7. c. Although dietary supplements do not usually have the same level of evidence as prescription drugs, favorable data do exist for many products. Whenever possible, it is best to honor a patient's preferences regarding therapeutic options, including use of CAM, if there are no significant contraindications.

8. a. Treating the "whole person" has always been a basic tenet of family medicine. However, time pressures and other demands on us as physicians can easily hinder the delivery of holistic, patient-centered care.

9. d. Although supplements can occasionally have adverse side effects, most are well tolerated when taken as directed on the label.

Patients diagnosed with cancer or HIV represent some of the highest users of CAM therapies.

Many modalities, such as hypnosis and acupuncture, have been shown to reduce pain.

With the exception of prayers for healing, CAM use tends to decline after age 60 years.

10. a. Most patients use complementary therapies along with conventional treatments. As long as each treatment is noted and evaluated within the context of benefit versus risk for the patient, the chance of adverse reactions should be minimized.

Published studies demonstrate favorable outcomes for glucosamine, acupuncture, and tai chi for the conditions listed.

11. b. Acupuncture is an ancient healing art that, in the United States, utilizes sterile needles that are inserted into specific points in order to treat, mitigate, or prevent disease. The majority of states have licensing requirements for acupuncturists that typically include completion of an accredited school, passing a national standardized test, and maintenance of continuing education hours. However, other practitioners who have their own licensing boards, such as physicians and chiropractors, may also perform acupuncture in many states.

12. d. The risk of a serious complication from manipulative therapy is estimated to be between 1 in several hundred thousand to 1 in 1 million.

Although most acute low back pain does resolve within 6 months regardless of the therapy used, chiropractic has been associated with higher patient satisfaction levels according to a study published in the *New England Journal of Medicine* (October 5, 1995).

13. d. Summarily dismissing his concerns and questions, especially those validated by friends or relatives,

can easily undermine your relationship with this patient. If unfamiliar with the therapy in question, offer to spend some time researching this for the patient. Patients are usually much more receptive to hearing that a particular treatment has no documented benefit once they know you have actually evaluated it in an objective manner.

In this case, unless the gastroenterologist has a particular interest in CAM therapies, it is unlikely that he or she will be any more capable than you with regard to answering his questions.

14. a. Many medical centers that treat patients with cancer now offer complementary therapies. These offerings may include mind–body techniques, acupuncture, and nutritional support, along with conventional therapies to patients that are interested in those options.

15. a. fish oil — C. high doses can lower triglycerides

b. garlic — D. common herbal with some evidence of very mild lipid lowering

c. red yeast rice — A. contains statin-like properties

d. walnuts — E. daily small amounts may have beneficial effect

e. policosanol — B. often derived from sugarcane

16. b. Omega-3 fatty acids, found in the oil of many coldwater fish, have been shown to have several positive effects on cardiovascular health, including a reduction in triglycerides, fatal arrhythmias, and ischemic strokes.

Chelation therapy, the use of EDTA to remove cholesterol plaque, has not been demonstrated in any large randomized study to have a positive effect on coronary disease. The Mediterranean diet consists of lean meats, nuts, fresh fruits/vegetables, moderate amounts of fat from olives and fish, along with some wine. This diet has been shown in some studies to have a more favorable effect on cardiovascular disease than the American Heart Association diet. Diets with moderate fat levels, such as this, are typically easier to commit to than ultra-low-fat diets, such as the Ornish diet.

Solution to the Clinical Case Management Problem

The practice of medicine should always take into account the best available scientific evidence, patient preferences, and your own experience. If a patient is strongly opposed to a certain therapy, other sensible options often still exist. The ability and willingness to provide your patients with reasonable therapeutic modalities that include more than pharmaceuticals and surgery is at the heart of integrative medicine. In this particular case, aggressive lifestyle interventions, such as diet modification and weight loss, can have a significant positive effect on the patient's health. Specific short-term goals (e.g., 8- to 10-pound weight loss and improvement in glucose and lipids during the next 2 months) should be mutually agreed upon up front. If the patient is unable to achieve these goals in the specified time frame, then he or she will often be more receptive to discussing other therapies. Ultimately, however, you must decide whether or not you are willing to accept the patient's terms and preferences, and then communicate your intentions clearly to the patient.

Summary

CAM is defined by the NIH as "a group of diverse medical and health care systems, practices, and products that are not presently considered to be part of conventional medicine." Conventional medicine, also referred to as Western medicine, is typically what is practiced by medical and osteopathic doctors, along with other allied health professionals, such as psychologists and registered nurses. A distinction is sometimes made regarding those practices that are used instead of conventional medicine, termed *alternative therapies*, versus those practices used in addition to conventional medicine, termed *complementary therapies*. Integrative medicine often refers to blending of one or more CAM therapies into conventional medicine.

The NIH further defines CAM practices into four broad areas of study; mind–body medicine, biologically based practices, manipulative and body-based practices, and energy medicine. Examples of each of these include hypnosis, herbal products, massage, and qi gong, respectively. Another category—termed "whole medical systems"—represents therapies like traditional Chinese medicine, which utilizes practices from the other four general categories.

A sizable body of research data already exists regarding CAM practices. However, high-quality randomized control trials are often lacking, inconclusive, or have demonstrated negative results. The National Center for Complementary and Alternative Medicine, a component of the NIH, was established to facilitate and partially fund additional high-quality research in this area.

While rigorous scientific data is not always available to support many forms of CAM therapies, a large number of Americans routinely utilize them for both minor and serious health concerns. A majority of these people will continue to seek conventional medical care. While some practices, such as mind–body therapy, are unlikely to conflict with Western medical treatments, other remedies, such as certain herbal products, may have significant adverse reactions. It is therefore important for medical and osteopathic physicians to become familiar with these practices in order to best advise their patients and provide safe and effective care.

Suggested Readings

Barnes P, Powell-Griner E, McFann K, Nahin R: *CDC Advance Data Report #343. Complementary and Alternative Medicine Use among Adults: United States, 2002.* Bethesda, MD: National Institutes of Health, National Center for Complementary and Alternative Medicine, May 27, 2004. Available at www.cdc.gov/nchs/data/ad/ad343.pdf.

Eisenberg DM, Davis RB, Ettner SL, et al: Trends in alternative medicine use in the United States, 1990–1997: Results of a follow-up national survey. *JAMA* 280(18):1569–1575, 1998.

National Center for Complementary and Alternative Medicine: http://nccam.nih.gov.

Office of Dietary Supplements: http://ods.od.nih.gov.

20 Cultural Competence

Battering Is Battering—Or Is It?

A 27-year-old African American female comes to the office to seek care for a badly sprained wrist. When asked about the mechanism of injury, she indicated she had fallen. However, when questioned further she admitted that she was the victim of spousal abuse. She indicated that she did not call the police because she was afraid they would not arrest her husband.

SELECT THE BEST ANSWER TO THE FOLLOWING QUESTIONS

1. She did not want to go to a shelter. Her reasons for not choosing to go to the shelter likely included
   a. there were unlikely to be any persons of color working at the shelter
   b. she had been there before and knew they were not sensitive to food preferences and personal hygiene needs
   c. professional staff are perceived to be judgmental about individuals who have been "helpless"
   d. African American women have a distinct mistrust of standardized social service agencies
   e. all of the above

2. She indicated she was not willing to report the abusive situation because
   a. the legal system is often unresponsive to the needs of African American women
   b. police are more likely to arrest the abuser in an African American home
   c. often, the abuse decreases in frequency after a visit by police
   d. none of the above
   e. all of the above

"So You Think You Understand Me?"

A third-year medical student is about to participate in her first clinical rotation. She will be doing family medicine in a clinic located in an area of the city with a very diverse population. She is excited and knows she will do very well because she has done a great deal to prepare for this type of rotation.

3. Which of the following will most enhance her care of a diverse panel of patients?
   a. a working knowledge of Spanish so she can talk with her patients
   b. having passed a course that taught her the meaning and content of cultural sensitivity
   c. developing an understanding of any given culture requires asking questions about knowledge, values, and philosophy of the patient's culture and the impact of those in the treatment plan
   d. having spent a summer in a Honduran village, she has acquired an understanding of different cultures
   e. she has no biases about skin color, religious belief, or country of origin, so she will have no difficulty providing quality care

4. As the student begins to see patients in the clinic, she might encounter cultural differences, such as
   a. being noncompliant with meds because the color of the pill is believed to be unlucky
   b. refusing treatments because of religious beliefs about surgery or transfusions
   c. refusing examination because of cultural prohibitions on exposure of the body
   d. none of the above
   e. all of the above

5. As the rotation progresses, the student is struck by the frequency with which African American women seem to have breast cancer. When she studies the available data, she finds that African American women continue to have higher rates of mortality from breast cancer than Caucasian women. She believes it is because
   a. many African American women have not received regular mammograms
   b. African American women do not breast-feed, so they are at higher risk
   c. African American women have larger breasts and are unable to palpate the mass until it is relatively larger
   d. African American women are fearful of exposure to the radiation of mammograms, so early detection is unlikely
   e. African American women have a genetic predisposition to breast cancer

6. As the student begins to see patients with a translator for languages she does not speak, she finds that often a short question by her ends with a lengthy exchange between the translator and the patient. Which of the following describes why this phenomenon occurs?

a. this always means that the translator is adding his or her biases to the medical information
b. this often means that the translator is trying to ensure the patient understands the question or the information being provided
c. this cannot be tolerated because it is impossible to trust the communication that is occurring
d. it is important to talk to the translator to ascertain what is being said beyond the question or information provided by the physician or student
e. b and d

Answers

1. e. Studies show that lack of sensitivity to the cultures of individuals who might use the resources makes the resource less acceptable. Studies have shown that African American women perceive that there are too few women of color working in therapeutic areas and admissions. Often, food and hygiene products are not welcoming and comforting. It is often perceived that African American women are being judged for being in need of the shelter; furthermore, they perceive the same judgment is not transferred to other ethnicities. Thus, the caregiver needs to try to find shelters, consultants, and other sources of aid that are sensitive to the needs and cultural issues of the African American woman.

2. a. Police are actually less likely to arrest an abuser in an African American home, and the abuse is more likely to increase if the police are called but the abuser is not removed. Perceptions are reported that the legal system seems to expect more violence in the African American community and thus is more tolerant than they would be of a similar complaint in another home. Thus, if the caregiver is not sensitive to the concerns, abuse may escalate without social intervention.

3. c. Even if one is knowledgeable about one culture different from one's own, that does not translate to knowledge or understanding of other cultures.

Understanding the vast impact of culture on one's health choices best influences a health provider by teaching him or her to ask questions and seek to understand values and philosophies that might impact a patient's health decisions. One of the major problems in treating someone with a different language is being less than fluent in a language. Even with interpreters, a major problem is that errors are made due to minor mistranslations. A course in cultural sensitivity should teach one to ask questions; it is unlikely to teach one to be sensitive. Believing that one has no biases is likely to increase the impact on decision making because the provider is less likely to heighten his or her sensitivity to any unacknowledged biases.

4. e. As described in Fadiman's book, *The Spirit Catches You and You Fall Down*, patients' beliefs can have a significant impact on their decision making. Her patient's family refused medications due to pill color (unlucky) and refused spinal taps and surgery secondary to religious beliefs. In other cultures, female patients still point to dolls to describe sites of pain or dysfunction because they are prohibited from disrobing for male physicians.

5. a. Many African American women do not have access to or are not referred for regular mammograms, and this is believed to account for later diagnosis and subsequent higher mortality. However, many physicians and other providers "blame" other cultural and lifestyle reasons for the disparate numbers.

6. e. Learning to work with a translator means developing confidence in the process and the need for the translator to ensure that the patient understands the question or the information being provided. It is important for providers to talk with translators even after patients have left to understand the complexity of the process. Because languages are not translated word for word, sometimes a translation takes longer than the original question. However, it is important to ensure that the translator is not inserting his or her own biases.

Summary

Cultural competence is the integration and transformation of knowledge about individuals and groups of people into specific standards, policies, practices, and attitudes used in appropriate cultural settings to increase the quality of services, thereby producing better outcomes.

The fundamental value of racial/ethnic concordance is improved communication.
1. The ability of health care providers to understand and respond sensitively and effectively to the cultural and linguistic needs of patients.

a. Research suggests that patients in racially concordant relationships are more likely to use needed services and less likely to postpone seeking care. Often, the difference is not language but, rather, the milieu in which the conversation and interpretation occur. At times, the interpreter may have to serve as a cultural bridge between patient and caregiver. They may both speak the same language but come from such varied perspectives that meanings are not clear and misunderstandings occur.

2. The U.S. population is increasing in diversity, so cultural sensitivity is increasing in importance.

a. Evidence suggests that language of the interview is a significant contributor to the outcome of the interaction.

b. Medical interpreters are a primary addition to the scope of services as our communities become more culturally and racially diverse. Their role is to convert one language into another without changing the original meaning because shared meaning is critical. Medical interaction with individuals whose primary language is different from that of the caregiver often leads to medical mistakes with frequent incorrect translation of words, clinical misdiagnosis, adverse drug reactions, and problems understanding drug labels. At least one survey suggests that many health providers do not know how to work with interpreters. In 2001, 14 standards were created related to culturally and linguistically appropriate services in health care. The standards cover three broad areas of requirements in health care for racial or ethnic minorities: culturally competent care, language access services, and organizational support for these initiatives.

Suggested Reading

Brown TT, Scheffler RM, Tom SE, Schulman KA: Does the market value racial and ethnic concordance in physician–patient relationships? (Quality and satisfaction). *Health Services Res* 42(12):706–727, 2007.

Carillo-Zuniga G, Dadig B, Guion KW, Rice VI: Awareness of the national standards for culturally and linguistically appropriate services at an academic health center. *Health Care Manager* 27(1): 45–53, 2008.

Fadiman, A: *The Spirit Catches You and You Fall Down*. New York: Farrar, Straus, and Giroux, 2002.

Gillum TL: Community response and needs of African-American female survivors of domestic violence. *J Interpersonal Violence* 23(1):39–57, 2008.

Tanabe MKG: Cultural competence in the training of geriatric medicine fellows. *Educational Gerontol* 33:421–428, 2007.

U.S. Department of Health and Human Services, Office of Minority Health: A physician's practical guide to culturally competent care. Available at https://cccm.thinkculturalhealth.org/GUIs/GUI_About thissite.asp.

ADULT MEDICINE

Acute ST Segment Elevation Myocardial Infarction

CLINICAL CASE PROBLEM 1

A 60-Year-Old Male with Acute Chest Pain

A 60-year-old farmer is brought to the local emergency department with his wife by the county sheriff. Apparently he developed a "twinge of chest pain" while shoveling grain 3 hours ago. He insisted on staying home until "he collapsed on the floor." Even then, he wanted to stay home and rest, but his wife insisted on calling 911. The call was answered by the sheriff's department, and a county sheriff rushed him and his wife to the emergency room (ER) at the nearest hospital in the rural area in which he resides. At his admission, he states that the pain is "almost gone"—"what a fuss about nothing." On taking a history, he tells the admitting physician that he smokes two packs of cigarettes daily, that he drinks a "goodly amount of beer," and that he had been told that his serum cholesterol level is good; the doctor even told him his was one of the best values he had ever seen for a man his size and age. On further questioning, he admits to a dull, aching, viselike pain around his chest, with radiation to the left shoulder. He also discloses that when the pain was at its worst he experienced nausea and vomiting, but he adds that because he is already doing better it must have been something he ate. His wife adds that she has never seen him in so much pain, but he is a "stubborn old goat."

He still insists that it is just a little stomach trouble, but on physical examination he is sweating and diaphoretic. He has vomited twice since coming to the ER. His blood pressure is 160/100 mmHg, and his pulse is 120 and irregular. His abdomen is obese, and you believe you can detect an enlarged aorta by deep palpation.

His electrocardiogram (ECG) results reveal significant Q waves in V1 to V4, with significant ST segment elevation in the same leads. There are reciprocal ST changes (ST segment depression) in the inferior leads (II, III, and avF).

SELECT THE BEST ANSWER TO THE FOLLOWING QUESTIONS

1. The most likely diagnosis in this patient is
   a. acute inferior wall myocardial infarction (MI)
   b. acute anterior wall MI
   c. acute myocardial ischemia
   d. acute pericarditis
   e. musculoskeletal chest wall pain

2. Given the history, physical examination, and ECG, your first priority is to
   a. call the ambulance for immediate transport to another hospital that "knows how to treat this thing"
   b. admit the patient for observation
   c. administer streptokinase or tissue plasminogen activator (t-PA) intravenously (IV)
   d. administer heparin IV
   e. none of the above

3. The nearest big city hospital is a 6-hour drive. Given your attention to your first priority, you would now
   a. call the ambulance for immediate transport to another hospital that "knows how to look after this thing"
   b. admit the patient to the coronary care unit for observation
   c. administer streptokinase or alteplase IV immediately
   d. administer heparin IV immediately
   e. none of the above

4. Which of the following criteria should be met before a patient is given thrombolytic therapy

following the history, physical examination, and ECG previously described?

a. typical chest pain suggestive of a MI
b. ECG changes confirming MI
c. the absence of other diseases that would explain the symptoms
d. all of the above
e. none of the above

5. The most correct statement regarding thrombolytic therapy in acute myocardial infarction (AMI) is
a. patients younger than age 65 years benefit more than elderly victims of MI
b. no benefits have been realized when therapy has been instituted after 6 hours of onset of chest pain
c. thrombolytic therapy has improved the prognosis of patients with prior coronary artery bypass grafting (CABG)
d. patients with non-Q MI have benefited as well as patients who sustain Q-wave MIs with thrombolytic therapy
e. A 50% reduction in mortality has been realized when therapy is administered within 3 hours of onset of chest pain

6. Which of the following statements regarding the use of heparin in patients with AMI is (are) true?
a. heparin therapy is used almost routinely with thrombolytic therapy during the acute phase of MI treatment, provided certain criteria are met
b. heparin is recommended whenever there is echocardiographic evidence of left ventricular thrombi
c. heparin should be administered (unless contraindicated) to all patients with acute anterior wall MI
d. heparin is contraindicated in patients with uncontrolled hypertension
e. all of the above

7. Which of the following is (are) a contraindication(s) to the use of thrombolytic therapy in patients with AMI?
a. active gastrointestinal bleeding
b. recent surgery (2 weeks postoperative)
c. history of cerebrovascular accident
d. suspected aortic dissection
e. all of the above

8. Which of the following statements regarding patients admitted to the coronary care unit following presumed MI is (are) true?
a. patients with suspected MIs should have the left ventricular ejection fraction measured before leaving the hospital

b. patients should have an exercise tolerance test on the fourth or fifth hospital day
c. patients should have an exercise stress test performed 4 to 6 weeks after hospitalization
d. a and c
e. none of the above

9. Which of the following is (are) a significant feature(s) of the pathophysiology of MI?
a. endothelial cell wall damage
b. coronary atherosclerosis
c. thromboxane A_2 production
d. all of the above
e. a and b

10. Which of the following is (are) true concerning aspirin in the treatment of AMI?
a. aspirin may serve as a substitute for streptokinase or t-PA
b. aspirin may serve as a substitute for heparin
c. aspirin may serve as a substitute for beta blockade
d. all of the above
e. none of the above

11. Which of the following statements regarding thrombolytic therapy is false?
a. thrombolytic therapy limits myocardial necrosis
b. thrombolytic therapy preserves left ventricular function
c. thrombolytic therapy reduces mortality
d. all of the above statements are false
e. none of the above statements are false

12. Which of the following is true regarding primary angioplasty in the treatment of acute ST segment elevated MI?
a. primary angioplasty is not a substitute for thrombolytic therapy
b. its universal adoption is likely to be limited by geography
c. it can be performed in hospitals that do not perform CABG surgery
d. stent placement worsens outcomes
e. operator variables are insignificant

13. Which of the following statements concerning dysrhythmias and dysrhythmic drugs in patients who have sustained an MI is (are) true?
a. premature ventricular contractions are common and should be treated with lidocaine
b. sustained runs of ventricular tachycardia frequently progress to ventricular fibrillation (VF)
c. prophylactic lidocaine is recommended to prevent dysrhythmias in all patients who have sustained an MI

d. none of the above

e. all of the above

14. One of the major patient concerns following an MI is the risk of a second or subsequent attack. In which of the following circumstances is the risk of reinfarction and/or mortality following MI significantly increased?

a. left ventricular ejection fraction, 40%

b. exercise-induced ischemia

c. non-Q-wave infarction (subendocardial infarction)

d. a and b

e. all of the above

15. Which of the following medications have been shown to be of benefit in some patients who have had an MI?

a. beta blockers

b. calcium channel blockers

c. aspirin

d. a and c

e. all of the above

16. Which of the following statements concerning rehabilitation of the patient after an MI is (are) true?

a. sexual intercourse should not resume for at least 3 months

b. patients who have sustained an MI should not work for at least 4 months

c. patients who have sustained an MI gradually may increase activity over 6 to 8 weeks

d. no significant psychologic distress regarding the MI has been shown to occur in the patient's spouse or significant other

e. all of the above

17. The best single confirmatory investigation for AMI is

a. the ECG

b. the height of ST segment elevation in the affected area (in millimeters) plus the depth of ST segment depression in the reciprocally affected leads (in millimeters)

c. the creatine kinase isoenzyme MB fraction

d. the presence of dysfunctional heart muscle as demonstrated by echocardiography

e. cardiac troponin levels

18. Sudden death as a result of MI is almost always the result of

a. third-degree heart block resulting from infarction of the atrioventricular node

b. ventricular tachycardia

c. ventricular fibrillation

d. ventricular standstill

e. none of the above

19. Which of the following statements regarding shock and its treatment in AMI is (are) true?

a. the patient with AMI may develop shock secondary to hypovolemic hypotension

b. the patient with AMI may develop shock secondary to persistent hypotension and a poor cardiac index

c. both forms of shock respond well to treatment with intravenous fluids (Ringer's lactate or normal saline solution)

d. a and b

e. all of the above

20. Coronary reperfusion with thrombolytic agents has been shown to be of benefit when commenced within which of the following maximum number of hours from the onset of pain?

a. 4

b. 6

c. 12

d. 24

e. 48

21. In this clinical case, there is a key finding on physical examination of the patient's abdomen that should be further assessed by

a. an abdominal ultrasound

b. an intravenous pyelogram

c. a digital subtraction angiogram

d. a computed tomography (CT) scan

e. a magnetic resonance imaging (MRI) scan

Answers

1. **b.** This patient most likely has suffered an anterior wall MI. The history suggests that he is at high risk for an infarct, and the Q waves and ST segment elevations in V1 to V4 and ST segment elevation in the anterior chest leads plus reciprocal changes in the inferior wall confirm the diagnosis. An acute inferior wall MI would have ST segment elevation and possibly Q waves in the inferior leads. Acute pericarditis would have ST segment elevation in all leads. Musculoskeletal chest wall pain does not produce the abnormalities in the ECG that are seen in this patient.

2. **e.** The history, physical examination, and ECG clearly point to an acute anterior wall MI. First, ascertain that the patient's airway is patent (without obstruction, vomit, or any blockage) and administer 100% oxygen.

3. **c.** Administer fibrinolytic agents such as streptokinase or alteplase (t-PA). The recombinant t-PA alteplase, a fibrin-specific agent, and streptokinase, a nonspecific agent, have been used most extensively. The recommended dose of streptokinase in AMI is 1.5 million U IV over 30 to 60 minutes. The regimen for the administration of alteplase is 15 mg IV bolus, then 0.75 mg/kg over 30 minutes (maximum 50 mg), and then 0.5 mg/kg for a 60-minute period (maximum 35 mg).

Newer recombinant DNA fibrinolytic-specific agents are reteplase and tenecteplase. Reteplase is given via a 10 + 10 MU double bolus administered 30 minutes apart. For tenecteplase, the dose is 0.5 mg/kg single bolus (maximum 50 mg). The advantages of the recombinant DNA sources, alteplase, reteplase, and tenecteplase, are high clot selectivity and few allergic reactions. Because of ease of administration, tenecteplase is often favored as an agent.

4. **d.** Thrombolytic therapy should be administered only when the following criteria are met: (1) typical chest pain suggestive of an MI, (2) ECG changes confirming MI, and (3) the "absence" of other diseases that would explain the symptoms.

Age older than 70 years was formerly a criterion for exclusion of patients for thrombolytic therapy; this is no longer the case. Contraindications to thrombolytic therapy include (1) active internal bleeding, (2) suspected aortic dissection, (3) prolonged or traumatic cardiopulmonary resuscitation, (4) recent head trauma or known intracranial neoplasm, (5) hemorrhagic retinopathy, (6) pregnancy, (7) history of recent (6 months or less) stroke or cerebral neoplasm, and (8) trauma or surgery within the past 2 weeks.

5. **e.** Although the benefits of thrombolytic therapy are greatest within the first 1 to 3 hours, a 10% mortality benefit can be achieved up to 12 hours after the onset of pain. Older patients, who have a higher complication rate, actually benefit more from thrombolytic therapy because they have a higher pretreatment hospital mortality rate. Treatment should be considered for patients as old as 80 years—or even older if the benefit-to-risk ratio seems favorable.

Patients with non-Q-wave infarcts have not benefited from thrombolytic therapy, nor have patients with prior CABG.

6. **e.** The role of concomitant heparin in the initial treatment of AMI has become increasingly clear over time. Studies have shown that early, effective anticoagulation with heparin maintains t-PA-induced coronary artery patency more effectively than aspirin alone. Subgroup analyses have shown that patients receiving therapeutic heparin, as measured by the activated partial thromboplastin time, have an extremely high patency approaching 95% following t-PA administration. Current guidelines call for the use of either unfractionated heparin or low-molecular-weight heparin for increased safety and ease of use.

Heparin therapy, however, has not been found to outweigh the harms in patients receiving streptokinase, except in cases of anterior wall MI, or in patients with complications prone to thromboembolism such as atrial fibrillation or congestive heart failure.

The two most important indications for concomitant use of heparin are acute anterior wall MI and echocardiographic evidence of left ventricular thrombi.

7. **e.** The major contraindications to adjunctive heparin therapy in MI are history of major surgery with time from discharge of less than 14 days, history of cardiovascular accidents, suspected aortic dissection, and acute gastrointestinal hemorrhage.

8. **d.** Before leaving the hospital, the patient should have his left ventricular ejection fraction measured, and an exercise stress tolerance test should be performed after 4 to 6 weeks.

9. **d.** The pathophysiology of AMI centers around the formation and rupture of a vulnerable atherosclerotic plaque. The progression of atherosclerosis is as follows: (1) Superficial atherosclerotic fatty streaks form in the coronary arteries even in children; (2) the fatty streaks progress to elevated fibrous plaques by the third and fourth decades of life; and (3) these fibrous plaques progress to complex, eccentric, ulcerated, and hemorrhagic plaques by the fifth and sixth decades, culminating in plaque rupture or intraplaque hemorrhage and formation of a clot leading to coronary artery occlusion.

The fragile endothelium is damaged by hypertension, elevated low-density lipoprotein cholesterol, diabetes, smoking, and other factors. Simple denudation exposes the vascular collagen, which triggers circulating platelet adhesion and aggregation and a cascade of growth-factor release including thromboxane A_2, prostacyclin, and platelet-derived growth factor. Smooth muscle cell and monocyte proliferation, along with lipid accumulation under the influence of growth factors, leads to severe atherosclerosis. For reasons that are not entirely clear, some atherosclerotic lesions, particularly those near vessel branch points and possibly triggered by viral infection or other causes of inflammation, become vulnerable and rupture, leading to the AMI syndrome.

10. **e.** Acetylsalicylic acid (aspirin) is the only adjunctive agent that has been shown unequivocally to reduce mortality alone or in conjunction with thrombolytic agents in patients with AMI. The ISIS-II study showed that acetylsalicylic acid (ASA) reduced mortality by 25%. However, when ASA was added to streptokinase, the effect was synergistic, and mortality from MI was reduced by 42%.

Thus, aspirin has been shown to reduce rethrombosis and recurrent MI. However, it is not a substitute for anything; it should be used along with other acute agents in the treatment of MI.

11. **e.** Thrombolytic therapy and interventional angioplasty are the cornerstones of treatment of acute ST segment elevated MI. Thrombolytic therapy is an established, effective therapy that limits myocardial necrosis, preserves left ventricular function, and reduces mortality.

12. **b.** Primary angioplasty with stenting is becoming the intervention of choice for acute ST segment elevated MI in many hospitals. Primary angioplasty with stenting is safe and confers advantages over balloon angioplasty alone. The addition of glycoprotein IIb/IIIa inhibitor abciximab treatment improves flow characteristics, prevents distal thromboembolization, and reduces the need for repeat angioplasty. A strategy of primary stenting in association with abciximab is the current gold standard of care for patients with AMI. The use of medication-eluding stents is promising and may surpass results of primary angioplasty with stenting plus glycoprotein inhibitors. However, primary angioplasty has the following limitations: Outcomes vary according to the skills of interventionist, and the procedure is effective only for patients presenting early (less than 12 hours after AMI). Complications are more common than with elective angioplasty, as are ventricular arrhythmias, although the latter are generally treatable. Right coronary artery procedures have high complication rates of sinus arrest, atrioventricular block, idioventricular rhythm, and severe hypotension. Surgical backup is required because up to 5% of patients require bypass surgery. Primary angioplasty, although an effective procedural intervention, requires facilities and experienced staff, and many adults with AMI in the United States and Canada are out of timely reach of such facilities and personnel.

13. **d.** Premature ventricular contractions (PVCs) occur frequently following AMI but do not require treatment. Couplets, triplets, multifocal PVCs, and short runs of nonsustained ventricular tachycardia are treated effectively with intravenous lidocaine. However, although they are treated with intravenous lidocaine, no survival advantage has been shown with lidocaine in this setting.

Most clinicians do not treat these nonmalignant ventricular dysrhythmias because they rarely progress to life-threatening situations; if they do, they can be treated effectively with cardioversion or defibrillation.

Lidocaine is not recommended in the routine prophylaxis of AMI. In addition, long-term prophylaxis with oral antiarrhythmics, such as flecainide and encainide, following AMI has been shown to drastically increase mortality.

14. **e.** The risk of subsequent infarction and/or mortality following discharge from the hospital following an MI is increased in patients with (1) postinfarction angina pectoris, (2) non-Q-wave infarction, (3) congestive cardiac failure, (4) left ventricular ejection fraction less than 40%, (5) exercise-induced ischemia diagnosed by ECG or by scintigraphy, and (6) ventricular ectopy (frequency > 10 PVCs/minute).

15. **e.** Beta blockers, aspirin, and coumadin have improved the prognosis in some patients following an MI. Beta blockers appear to reduce the risk of sudden death in patients who are at increased risk. Antiplatelet agents, particularly aspirin, have been shown to be of benefit in patients who have had an MI. Aspirin reduces both rethrombosis and recurrent MI. Coumadin has been shown to decrease the risk of thromboembolic events in high-risk patients after infarction. Other antiarrhythmics have not been shown to be as effective as beta blockers as prophylactic agents.

16. **c.** Patients who have suffered an MI should increase activity levels gradually over a period of 6 to 8 weeks. Patients can return to work by approximately 8 weeks. Patients who have suffered an uncomplicated MI may be safely started in an activity program by 3 or 4 weeks postinfarct. Sexual intercourse can resume within 4 to 6 weeks of the infarction. There does not seem to be any logical reason for the patient to wait 3 months to resume intercourse. The following is a good rule to follow in this case: "If the patient can climb the stairs to the bedroom, the rest is probably okay too."

In many patients, the psychologic impact of an MI outweighs the physical impact. Also, in a significant percentage of families, the spouse is affected as much as, if not more than, the patient. One of the most common errors in cardiac rehabilitation is not to involve the spouse or significant other at every stage of the program.

17. **e.** The best confirmatory test of the choices offered for the diagnosis of AMI is cardiac troponins. Cardiac troponins I and T are the preferred markers because they are more specific and reliable than creatine kinase or its isoenzyme creatine kinase MB. Elevation of the ST segment can result from either injury or infarction. It is neither sensitive nor specific enough for the diagnosis of infarction in the absence of Q waves. For the diagnosis of AMI, the ECG is sensitive (70% to 90% with more than 1 mm of elevation in two contiguous leads); unfortunately, it is less specific. The presence of dysfunctional heart muscle on echocardiography means that there is likely to be a lowering of both the ejection fraction and the cardiac index; it says nothing about whether an MI has occurred or anything regarding the age of same.

18. c. Sudden death as a result of AMI is almost always the result of VF induced by the electrical instability of the ischemic/infarction zone. VF is most common either at the immediate onset of coronary occlusion or at the time of coronary reperfusion (reperfusion arrhythmia).

19. d. Shock in the presence of an AMI can be of two pathophysiologic varieties. Either there is hypovolemia and associated hypotension (hypovolemic shock), or there is persistent hypotension and a poor cardiac index in the presence of adequate left ventricular filling pressures.

Hypovolemic shock is best treated with volume replacement using either Ringer's lactate or normal saline solution. Care must be taken to avoid "volume overloading," which may produce pulmonary edema and congestive cardiac failure.

Cardiogenic shock generally is associated with severe left ventricular dysfunction and occurs with large infarcts that produce damage to more than 40% of the left ventricle. Treatment is urgent, and mortality is high. The treatments of choice include the following: (1) intraaortic balloon pump placement to increase coronary flow and decrease afterload; (2) coronary reperfusion with percutaneous transluminal balloon angioplasty (the mainstay of treatment); and (3) pharmacologic agents, including morphine, dopamine, and dobutamine.

20. c. One clinical trial has shown unequivocally that there is a significant survival advantage to patients with AMI, even when thrombolytic agents are given up to 12 hours after the onset of the chest pain.

21. a. The finding on physical examination of the abdomen of "an enlarged aorta" should be further assessed by an abdominal ultrasound study. The patient probably has an aortic aneurysm. Although this finding could also be assessed by CT or MRI, an abdominal ultrasound is considerably less expensive and just as sensitive.

Summary

1. Signs and symptoms

Acute ST segment elevation MI occurs when a thrombus forms on a ruptured atheromatous plaque and thereby occludes a coronary artery. The pain of MI, unlike angina pectoris, usually occurs at rest. The pain is similar to angina in location and radiation but is more severe and builds up rapidly. Usually it is described as retrosternal tightness or as a squeezing sensation or sometimes as a dull ache. Radiation to the left shoulder is common. Other common symptoms include sweating, weakness, dizziness, nausea, vomiting, and abdominal discomfort. Abdominal discomfort is especially common in inferior wall MIs.

2. ECG changes

The classical evolution of changes is from peaked (hyperacute) T waves to ST segment elevation, Q-wave development, and then T-wave inversion. This sequence may occur over a few hours or may take several days. (Note: If ECG changes are not present, do not assume an MI has not occurred. If signs and symptoms suggest MI, it is an MI until proved otherwise.)

3. Confirmatory evidence

Evidence of infarction is confirmed by elevation of the cardiac troponins or creatine kinase MB fraction. Cardiac troponin I and T are the preferred markers because they are more specific and reliable than creatine kinase or its isoenzyme creatine kinase MB.

4. Other diagnostic procedures

Scintigraphic studies including technetium-99 and thallium-201 imaging and radionuclide angiography, as well as echocardiography, may help document the extent of the damage but are not performed until after treatment.

5. Treatment of acute MI

a. Supplementary oxygen
b. Morphine sulfate for pain relief
c. Coronary reperfusion

There are currently two means of reopening a blocked coronary artery in acute MI: thrombolytic therapy and primary angioplasty. Both are effective in reducing mortality but have limitations.

Thrombolysis, the most common form of treatment, is contraindicated in 20% of patients primarily because of bleeding risk. The recanalization rate is up to 55% with streptokinase and up to 60% with alteplase. There is a 5% to 15% risk of early or late reocclusion and a 1% or 2% risk of intracranial hemorrhage with an attendant 40% mortality. Nevertheless, thrombolytic therapy is readily available and widely used. Indications for thrombolysis in acute MI are as follows: clinical history and presentation strongly suggestive of MI within 6 hours plus one or more of a 1- to 2-mm ST elevation in two or more contiguous limb leads, new left bundle branch block, or 2-mm ST depression in V1 to V4 suggestive of true posterior MI. Patients presenting with the previous symptoms within 7 to 12 hours of onset with persisting chest pain and ST segment elevation are also candidates. Patients younger than 75 years presenting within 6 hours of anterior wall MI should be considered for recombinant t-PA. Absolute contraindications to thrombolysis include the following: aortic dissection, history of cerebral hemorrhage, cerebral aneurysm, arteriovenous malformation or intracranial neoplasm, recent (within past 6 months) thromboembolic stroke, or active internal bleeding. Patients previously treated with streptokinase should receive a recombinant t-PA (e.g., reteplase).

Primary angioplasty with stenting is becoming the intervention of choice for acute ST segment elevated MI in many hospitals. Primary angioplasty with stenting is safe and confers advantages over balloon angioplasty alone. In early trials, the addition of glycoprotein IIb/IIIa inhibitor abciximab treatment was shown to improve flow characteristics, prevent distal thromboembolization, and reduce the need for repeat angioplasty. A strategy of primary stenting in association with abciximab is the current gold standard of care for patients with AMI. The use of medication-eluding stents is promising and may surpass results of primary angioplasty with stenting plus glycoprotein inhibitors.

However, primary angioplasty has the following limitations: Outcomes vary according to skills of interventionist, and the procedure is effective only for patients presenting early (less than 12 hours after AMI). Complications are more common than with elective angioplasty, as are ventricular arrhythmias, although the latter are generally treatable. Right coronary artery procedures have high complication rates of sinus arrest, atrioventricular block, idioventricular rhythm, and severe hypotension. Surgical backup is required because up to 5% of patients require bypass surgery. Primary angioplasty, although an effective procedural intervention, requires facilities and experienced staff, and many adults with AMI in the United States and Canada are out of timely reach of such facilities and personnel.

d. Aspirin one stat, 160 mg/day: Concurrent use of aspirin with a thrombolytic drug reduces mortality far more than either drug alone. In the ISIS-2 trial, aspirin with streptokinase reduced mortality by 42% without any increased incidence of stroke or major bleeding.

e. Heparin therapy for patients receiving streptokinase: Heparin is used only for those at high risk of thromboembolism, such as those with large infarctions, atrial fibrillation, or congestive heart failure. For patients receiving fibrin-specific agents (alteplase and tenecteplase), heparin should be administered to reduce the risk of late reocclusion.

f. Beta blockade limits the extent of infarction

g. Nitroglycerin for pain control

h. Warfarin: again used as was heparin, for those at high risk for thromboembolism

i. Consider magnesium sulfate as analgesic/anxiolytic

j. Note: Lidocaine prophylaxis is not indicated for the prevention of dysrhythmias

6. Post-MI

a. Submaximal stress ECG test and echocardiogram

b. Discharge medications: aspirin; beta blocker, and possibly angiotensin-converting enzyme inhibitor if there was a large infarct or thrombolytic therapy was administered; consider statin or another cholesterol lowering agent unless contraindicated. If aspirin is not tolerated, clopidogrel is an as effective, although expensive, antiplatelet alternative. Clopidogrel plus aspirin may be used and offers some additional benefit according to a Cochrane review.

c. Exercise program within 3 or 4 weeks

d. Return to work within 8 weeks

e. Sexual intercourse within 4 weeks

f. Involvement of the spouse or significant other is critical

Suggested Reading

Antman EM, Morrow DA, McCabe CH, et al: Enoxaparin versus unfractionated heparin with fibrinolysis for ST-elevation myocardial infarction. *N Engl J Med* 354(14):1477–1488, 2006.

Cannon CP, Turpie AG: Unstable angina and non-ST-elevation myocardial infarction: Initial antithrombotic therapy and early invasive strategy. *Circulation* 107(21):2640–2645, 2003.

Grech ED, Ramsdale DR: Acute coronary syndrome: ST segment elevation myocardial infarction. *BMJ* 326(7403):1379–1381, 2003.

Keller T, Squizzato A, Middeldorp S: Clopidogrel plus aspirin versus aspirin alone for preventing cardiovascular disease. *Cochrane Database Syst Rev* (3):CD005158, 2007.

Mukherjee D, Eagle KA: The use of antithrombotics for acute coronary syndromes in the emergency department: Considerations and impact. *Prog Cardiovasc Dis* 50:167–180, 2007.

Natarajan MK, Yusuf S: Primary angioplasty for ST-segment elevation myocardial infarction: Ready for prime time? *Can Med Assoc J* 169(1):32–35, 2003.

CLINICAL CASE PROBLEM 1

A 55-Year-Old Male with Chest Pain

A 55-year-old male presents for the first time to your office for assessment of left-sided shoulder pain. The pain comes on after any strenuous activity, including walking. The pain is described as follows:

Quality: dull, aching
Quantity: 8/10 when doing any activity—otherwise he is asymptomatic
Location: mainly retrosternal
Radiation: appears to be radiating to the left shoulder area
Chronology: began approximately 8 months ago and has been getting worse ever since
Continuous/intermittent: intermittent
Aggravating factors: exercise of any kind
Relieving factors: rest
Associated manifestations: occasional nausea
Pain history: no previous pain before 8 months ago; no other significant history of pain syndromes
Quality of life: definitely affecting quality of life by limiting activity

The patient tells you that the pain seems somehow worse today. For the first time, it did not go away after he stopped walking. The patient's blood pressure is 130/90 mmHg; his pulse is 72 beats/minute and regular. His heart sounds are normal. There are no extra sounds and no murmurs.

SELECT THE BEST ANSWER TO THE FOLLOWING QUESTIONS

1. Which of the following statements regarding this patient's chest pain is (are) false?
   a. the patient may have suffered a myocardial infarction
   b. the patient's chest pain may be the result of angina pectoris
   c. the patient's chest pain may be the result of esophageal motor disorder
   d. the administration of sublingual nitroglycerin is a very sensitive test to distinguish angina pectoris from esophageal causes

   e. the patient should be admitted to the coronary care unit until the origin of the pain is firmly established

2. The patient is admitted to a chest pain unit and monitored. Which of the following investigations is not indicated at this time as part of this initial inpatient evaluation?
   a. an exercise tolerance test
   b. coronary angiography
   c. a serum thyroid-stimulating hormone (TSH) level
   d. a complete blood count (CBC)
   e. a fasting blood sugar

   His pain remits with aspirin and intravenous nitroglycerin. His cardiac troponin levels and electrocardiogram (ECG) are normal. The patient does well and has an exercise tolerance test. This test reveals a 2.5-mm ST segment depression at 5 METS (metabolic equivalents of oxygen consumption) of activity as the patient achieved 50% of his age-predicted maximum heart rate.

3. Which of the following statements regarding this test result is (are) true?
   a. result indicates probable coronary artery disease (CAD)
   b. coronary angiography is indicated
   c. his inability to achieve maximum heart rate predicts CAD
   d. a and b
   e. all of the above statements are true

4. In addition to aspirin, which of the following medications is indicated as a first-line therapy for the treatment of this patient?
   a. diltiazem
   b. atenolol
   c. isosorbide dinitrate
   d. prazosin
   e. hydrochlorthiazide

CLINICAL CASE PROBLEM 2

A 67-Year-Old Male with a History of Angina Pectoris

A 67-year-old male with a history of angina pectoris is brought to the emergency room (ER) by his wife. For the past 3 days, he has been having increasing chest pain. The retrosternal chest pain has been occurring intermittently while at rest during the day, while in bed at night, and while walking (he is able to walk only very slowly because of pain). The pain has been getting progressively persistent and worse during the past 8 hours. On physical examination, his blood pressure is 120/70 mmHg. His pulse is 96 beats/minute and regular. The rest of his examination is unchanged from previous visits to the office. His ECG shows ST segment depression of 1.5 mm in leads V5 and V6. There is also flattening of the T waves seen across the precordial leads.

5. Which of the following statements regarding this patient is (are) true?
   a. this patient has unstable angina
   b. intravenous nitroglycerin and morphine may be used for pain relief
   c. the patient should be started on heparin and clopidogrel
   d. this patient should already be taking daily aspirin
   e. all of the above are true

CLINICAL CASE PROBLEM 3

A 50-Year-Old Female with a Sharp Retrosternal Chest Pain

A 50-year-old female presents to the ER with a sharp retrosternal chest pain that awoke her. This is the fourth episode in as many nights, but she is sure that she is not having a heart attack because she saw her physician only 3 weeks ago. At that time, he gave her a "clean bill of health." She was told that her ECG, blood pressure, and cholesterol were completely normal. She is a nonsmoker and has no family history of CAD.

On physical examination, her blood pressure is 100/70 mmHg. Her pulse is 96 beats/minute and regular, and the remainder of the cardiovascular and respiratory examination is normal.

Her ECG reveals a significant ST segment elevation in the anterior limb leads. Within 1 hour, the ST segment has returned to normal. Cardiac troponin levels are normal.

6. Which of the following statements regarding this patient is (are) true?
   a. this patient probably has Prinzmetal's angina
   b. calcium channel blockers are the treatment of choice for this type of angina

c. beta blockers are advised for this type of angina
   d. a, b, and c
   e. a and b

7. Which of the following statements regarding percutaneous coronary angioplasty (PTCA) and mortality from CAD is (are) true?
   a. PTCA reduces overall mortality
   b. PTCA improves morbidity from CAD
   c. PTCA usually includes intracoronary stent placement
   d. optimal lesions for angioplasty are proximal in location, noneccentric, and located at branch (bifurcation) points in the vessel
   e. b and c

8. In which of the following patients would PTCA most likely be used?
   a. a 55-year-old male smoker with left main stem disease
   b. a diabetic patient with four-vessel disease
   c. an elderly patient with a ventricular aneurysm
   d. an obese patient with distal left anterior descending artery disease
   e. any of the above are good indications for PTCA

9. Which of the following is least likely to be used as a combination therapy in patients with angina pectoris?
   a. nitroglycerin–atenolol–nifedipine
   b. nitroglycerin–enalapril–nifedipine
   c. nitroglycerin–propranolol–verapamil
   d. nitroglycerin–metoprolol–diltiazem
   e. nitroglycerin–atenolol–nifedipine

10. Which of the following complications is seen with ticlopidine?
    a. thrombocytopenia
    b. ventricular arrhythmias
    c. atrial arrhythmias
    d. syncope
    e. b and d

11. Coronary artery bypass surgery (CABG) may be indicated as the treatment of choice for angina pectoris with which of the following patients with angina?
    a. a patient with triple-vessel disease
    b. a patient with one-vessel disease
    c. a patient with two-vessel disease
    d. CABG may be first-line therapy in any of the above
    e. b or c

CLINICAL CASE PROBLEM 4

A 65-Year-Old Male with Angina and Hypertension

A 65-year-old male presents to your office with a history strongly suggestive of angina pectoris. He also has a long history of hypertension.

On physical examination, his blood pressure is 170/100 mmHg. Exercise tolerance testing reveals a 2.5-mm Hg ST segment depression in the lateral leads. A 2D/M mode echocardiogram reveals apical akinesis and an estimated ejection fraction of 50%.

12. Which of the following medications would you consider as the agent of first choice in the treatment of this patient?
    a. hydrochlorothiazide
    b. nifedipine
    c. clonidine
    d. atenolol
    e. prazosin

13. Which of the following investigations should be performed on a patient with possible angina pectoris?
    a. CBC
    b. chest x-ray
    c. fasting lipid profile
    d. thyroid function testing
    e. all of the above

14. The pathophysiology of angina pectoris is best explained by which of the following?
    a. significantly increased peripheral vascular resistance
    b. a balance between oxygen supply and oxygen demand
    c. an imbalance of oxygen supply and oxygen demand plus or minus coronary artery spasm
    d. significant peripheral venous and arterial vasoconstriction
    e. none of the above

15. Which of the following criteria indicate a diagnosis of unstable angina pectoris?
    a. new-onset angina (2 months) that is either severe or frequent (three episodes/day) or both
    b. patients with accelerating angina
    c. patients with angina at rest
    d. b and c
    e. all of the above

Clinical Case Management Problem

Briefly describe the phenomenon of asymptomatic coronary artery ischemia.

Answers

1. **d.** Acute chest pain is a very common and often difficult diagnostic problem. Angina pectoris is the pain of myocardial ischemia associated with acute coronary syndromes and chronic stable angina. Acute coronary syndromes include ST segment elevated myocardial infarction (discussed in Chapter 21), non-ST segment elevation myocardial infarction, and unstable angina. The distinction between unstable angina and non-ST segment myocardial infarction is the presence of elevated markers of myocardial necrosis (troponins) in infarction. The distinction between unstable angina and chronic stable angina is made on the basis of history and/or progressive ECG changes. Myocardial infarction must be assumed until proven otherwise in patients with any significant risk factors. Of course, not all angina pectoris is the result of CAD, although this is the first hypothesis to entertain and test. Noncardiac causes of ischemia include anemia and hyperthyroidism. Other causes of chest pain are musculoskeletal disorders, gastroesophageal reflux disease, and pulmonary lesions. Pain from esophageal motor disorder is often confused with pain from myocardial ischemia. This differential is often exceedingly difficult. Often, quality of pain, quantity of pain, radiation of pain, and some aggravating factors are the same in both conditions. Although many physicians believe that relief with nitroglycerin is specific for myocardial ischemia and myocardial infarction, this is not the case. Sublingual nitroglycerin will relieve pain from esophageal motor disorder; it will also relieve pain from myocardial ischemia and myocardial injury.

2. **b.** We are not yet far enough down the diagnostic pathway of angina pectoris to justify the invasive procedure of coronary angiography. Normal cardiac troponin levels essentially rule out myocardial infarction. However, the origin of this patient's chest pain is still unclear and must be pursued in a systematic manner. At this time, the following are diagnostic considerations: myocardial ischemia secondary to CAD or other causes, esophageal motor or reflux disorder, and musculoskeletal chest wall pain. Because this patient has other significant risk factors, such as age and male gender, he should be assumed to have a cardiovascular cause for his pain until

proved otherwise. Thus, all testable risk factors should be measured, and the presence of underlying causes of angina should be ascertained. To rule out the possibilities of diabetes, anemia, and thyroid disease as underlying causes for his angina, a fasting blood sugar, CBC, and TSH level should be performed. Chest radiograph and pulse oximetry should be performed to evaluate for intrapulmonary causes of hypoxemia. A treadmill exercise stress test should be performed because this patient has a relatively high pretest probability of having CAD (Bayes' theorem).

3. **d.** The 2.5-mm ST segment depression quite likely represents severe coronary ischemia from CAD. Although we are not told the results of blood pressure monitoring during this patient's exercise tolerance test, if he had experienced a "hypotensive response," this would be another indication of severe ischemia. Failure to achieve his targeted maximum heart rate in and of itself does not predict CAD. However, taken together with the other information provided—ST segment depression at less than 6 METS and at less than 70% of his predicted maximal heart rate—it indicates a high probability of myocardial ischemia. With this information, coronary angiography should now be performed.

4. **b.** Medications used for treating angina pectoris of CAD include several classes of drugs: (1) antiplatelets/anticoagulants, (2) beta blockers, (3) lipid-lowering agents (3-hydroxy-3-methylglutaryl coenzyme A [HMG-CoA] reductase inhibitors), (4) nitrates, and (5) calcium channel blockers.

The underlying cause of angina of myocardial origin is the mismatch between oxygen supply and demand. There may be many causes of this mismatch, many of which are correctable by treating the underlying condition (e.g., anemia and hyperthyroidism). Certainly the major cause to rule out or diagnose and treat is CAD. Narrowing or obstruction of the coronary arteries leads to ischemia. In the acute coronary syndromes of unstable angina and non-ST segment elevation myocardial infarction, there is generally a platelet-rich, partially occlusive thrombus present. Microthrombi can embolize and obstruct flow downstream. In the acute coronary syndrome of ST segment elevation (or Q-wave) myocardial infarction discussed in Chapter 10, a fibrin-rich, more stable occlusive thrombus is the cause of symptoms. In the past decade, much progress has been made in the development and use of several categories of medications used for the treatment of angina of CAD. Drugs listed here are the standard classes of agents used and are designed in large part to target the aforementioned pathophysiology.

Antiplatelet/anticoagulant treatment: Aspirin is the most widely used antiplatelet drug and is effective at doses from 75 to 300 mg daily. This is the agent of choice in CAD angina. Other antiplatelet agents include dipyridamole and ticlopidine. Ticlopidine is effective, but it is associated with the side effects of neutropenia and thrombocytopenia. Clopidogrel is another effective agent, and it can be used if aspirin is contraindicated or not tolerated. Newer agents include the glycoprotein IIb/IIIa antagonists, which have been used primarily in conjunction with thrombolysis in acute myocardial infarction. They are expensive, and their role is imprecisely defined in different forms of angina. Anticoagulations with low-molecular-weight heparin (LMWH) or standard heparin followed by warfarin have been tried in various forms of angina and are effective in reducing morbidity primarily in persons at high risk for embolization. Warfarin should be continued for 2 or 3 months, except in atrial fibrillation, when it should be maintained indefinitely. If the patient is taking warfarin, aspirin may be taken concomitantly, but there is a higher risk of bleeding.

Use of beta blockers is a standard therapy for the prevention of second myocardial infarction, the reduction of myocardial ischemia, and mortality reduction in the perioperative period in individuals with underlying angina. These drugs are still underutilized despite multiple guidelines and studies of effectiveness.

Good evidence exists indicating that lipid-lowering HMG coenzyme reductase inhibitors (statins) stabilize plaques of CAD and may reduce myocardial events. They are also effective in reducing low-density lipoprotein cholesterol, a potent risk factor in CAD.

Nitrates are the old war horses of pain relief, for which they are effective but do little for long-term mortality reduction. Still, they are widely used.

A calcium channel blocker (diltiazem) is used particularly for coronary artery spasm. These agents are applied in a cascade to the spectrum of disease ranging from chronic stable angina to the acute coronary syndromes. At a minimum, all patients with chronic stable angina and no contraindications should be on aspirin, beta blockers, and statins. Long-acting nitrates, calcium channel blockers, and additional antiplatelet/anticoagulant therapy may also be considered. In acute coronary syndromes, hospitalized patients at lower risk for CAD are treated with aspirin, clopidogrel, and either heparin or LMWH until the diagnosis is clear. For acute coronary syndrome hospitalized patients with intermittent or worsening symptoms but no ST segment changes, with positive or negative troponins, treatment includes the use of those medications for low-risk patients plus glycoprotein IIb/IIIa inhibition and early invasive intervention by cardiac catheterization.

5. e. The history given by this patient is one of unstable angina pectoris. Unstable angina pectoris is the term used to describe accelerating or "crescendo" angina in a patient who has previously had stable angina. Unstable angina can be diagnosed when the angina is new in onset, occurs with less exertion or at rest, lasts longer, or is less responsive to medication. Aspirin is the first treatment that should be given. For pain relief, nitrates or morphine may be used. In addition, a beta blocker, if not already in use, plus clopidogrel, standard heparin or LMWH, and a glycoprotein IIb/IIIa inhibitor should be started until the coronary arteries' anatomy is defined via catheterization. Nitrates are often used for the initial presentation of unstable angina. Nonparental therapy with sublingual or oral nitrates or nitroglycerin ointment may be sufficient, although IV is an option. Despite the ECG showing only 1.5 mm of ST segment depression and no acute changes indicative of myocardial infarction, the patient should be hospitalized and placed in the coronary care unit. Serial ECGs and serial cardiac troponins or other markers of myocardial damage should be performed.

6. d. Prinzmetal's angina (coronary artery vasospasm) is angina that occurs in the absence of precipitating factors. Its symptoms most commonly occur in the early morning, often awakening the patient from sleep. It is usually associated with ST segment elevation rather than ST segment depression. Coronary angiography should be performed to rule out coexisting fixed stenotic lesions. Calcium channel blockers are probably the drugs of choice for Prinzmetal's angina. Nitrates are also effective. Beta blockers are not indicated in patients who have vasospasm without fixed, stenotic lesions.

7. e. Although overall mortality reduction from PTCA compared with medical treatment has not been shown, the procedure reduces symptoms and, in some instances, medication use. The use of new medication eluting stents inserted as part of the procedure may change mortality outcomes. Primary complications are restenosis requiring repeat procedure; arrhythmias, particularly with right coronary artery procedures; and artery rupture, necessitating surgery.

8. d. PTCA as a treatment for dilating stenotic coronary arterial lesions was introduced in 1977. Today, successful dilatation rates per stenosis exceed 90%, complication rates have fallen to 4%, and procedure-related myocardial infarction and death remain uncommon. PTCA most often involves stent placement to maintain vessel patency. In many centers, PTCA is the most commonly used invasive therapy for CAD. Significant restenosis used to occur within the first year in up to 40% of lesions, resulting in both symptomatic recurrence and high reintervention rates. Various strategies—from the use of intravascular medication eluting stents to concomitant treatment with glycoprotein IIb/IIIa inhibitors—have demonstrated improvement in rates of acute closure and restenosis. In retrospective studies comparing the long-term results of PTCA and CABG, angina recurrence and event-free survival rates are better in the CABG for diabetics with multivessel disease and patients with main stem and proximal left anterior descending artery lesions. Hence, answers a and b are incorrect. Although older patients benefit from PTCA because it is better tolerated than surgery, a major ventricular aneurysm would be a contradiction. In summary, at this time the success rates of PTCA are under intensive scrutiny. Older studies comparing mortality and morbidity of PTCA with those of medical therapy and CABG surgery may not apply to current use of PTCA with drug eluting stents. Operator skill is another unknown with major effects on outcomes. The family physician must stay tuned to ongoing developments in this field and seek to know the local interventionists' rates of successful outcomes to better advise and manage the patient.

9. b. Of the combinations listed, the least likely combination of drugs to treat angina pectoris is nitroglycerine–enalapril–nifedipine. Enalapril is an ACE inhibitor. Unless the patient also has congestive heart failure, ACE inhibitors are generally not used as medical therapy for angina pectoris.

10. a. Ticlopidine is an effective antiplatelet agent. Patients must be monitored for the possibility of thrombocytopenia and neutropenia.

11. d. CABG may be the treatment of choice in any of the choices listed, although it is specifically indicated on the basis of better mortality outcomes for individuals with left main stem disease and diabetics with multiple vessel disease.

12. d. A patient with both angina pectoris and hypertension should be treated with a cardioselective beta blocker. Hydrochlorothiazide, although effective in hypertension, will not reduce mortality as effectively as a beta blocker. The calcium channel blocker verapamil would be a reasonable treatment option only in addition to the beta blocker.

13. **e.** Patients suspected of having angina pectoris need (1) a CBC, (2) a fasting lipid profile, (3) a chest x-ray, (4) an ECG, and (5) thyroid function testing. Moreover, renal function should be evaluated, and electrolyte and blood glucose measurements should be made. Testing for hyperhomocystinemia may also be warranted. If the patient appears to have significant chronic obstructive pulmonary disease, then pulse oximetry and spirometry may also be helpful.

14. **e.** The basic pathophysiology in patients with angina pectoris due to myocardial ischemia is an imbalance between oxygen supply and demand due to narrowing of the coronary arteries.

15. **e.** Unstable angina pectoris is characterized by new-onset angina (>2 months) that is severe and/or frequent (>3 episodes/day), patients with accelerating angina, or patients with angina at rest.

Solution to the Clinical Case Management Problem

Obstructive CAD, acute myocardial infarction, and transient myocardial ischemia are frequently asymptomatic. The majority of patients with typical chronic angina pectoris are found to have objective evidence of myocardial ischemia (ST segment depression). However, many of these same patients and some other patients who are always asymptomatic are at high risk for coronary events. Longitudinal studies have demonstrated an increased incidence of coronary events including sudden death and myocardial infarction in asymptomatic patients with positive exercise tests for ischemia. In addition, patients with asymptomatic ischemia following a myocardial infarction are at far greater risk for a secondary coronary event than symptomatic patients. Patients who are found to have asymptomatic ischemia should be evaluated by stress thallium ECG. The management of asymptomatic ischemia must be individualized and depends on many factors, including the patient's age, occupation, and general medical condition. However, patients with severe asymptomatic ischemia on noninvasive testing should have aggressive risk factor modification and, at a minimum, should be placed on aspirin, beta blockers, and possibly statins. Strong consideration should be given to referral for coronary arteriography.

Summary

DEFINITION

Angina pectoris simply means chest pain. Angina pectoris is often the pain of myocardial ischemia associated with acute coronary syndromes and chronic stable angina. Acute coronary syndromes include ST segment elevated myocardial infarction (discussed in Chapter 21), non-ST segment elevation myocardial infarction, and unstable angina. The distinction between unstable angina and non-ST segment myocardial infarction is the presence of elevated markers of myocardial necrosis (troponins and others) in infarction. The distinction between unstable angina and chronic stable angina is made on the basis of history and/or progressive ECG changes. In all of the previous instances, angina implies an imbalance between myocardial requirements for oxygen and the amount of oxygen delivered through the coronary arteries. This can occur via a mechanism of increased demand, diminished or extinguished delivery, or both. Acute coronary syndromes of unstable angina and non-ST segment elevation myocardial infarction have a much worse prognosis than chronic stable angina, with a 30-day mortality of between 10% and 20% despite treatment. These patients may also have higher long-term risk of death than patients with ST segment elevation myocardial infarction. Of course, not all angina pectoris is due to CAD, although this is the first hypothesis to entertain and test. Noncardiac causes of ischemia—such as anemia, hyperthyroidism—as well as nonischemic conditions—such as musculoskeletal disorders, gastrointestinal conditions (e.g., gastroesophageal reflux disease), pulmonary lesions, and others—must be considered. In the end, however, myocardial ischemia from CAD must be examined and ruled out by the clinician because the consequences of missing this diagnosis can be fatal.

SYMPTOMS

Patients with angina pectoris from underlying CAD frequently describe the discomfort as either an anterior chest "tightness" or "pain." Other descriptions include anterior chest "burning," "pressing," "choking," "aching," "gas," and "indigestion." These symptoms are typically located in the retrosternal area or the left chest. Usually, radiation to the left shoulder, left arm, or jaw occurs. Typical angina is aggravated by exercise and relieved by rest. Although there is no universally accepted definition of unstable angina, it has three main presentations: angina at rest, new-onset angina, and increasing angina.

SIGNS

Physical examination is often normal, although hypertension is sometimes present.

RISK STRATIFICATION

Patients with chronic stable angina symptoms are at lower risk than those with unstable angina and generally can be monitored and treated as outpatients. Patients with angina at rest, new-onset angina, or increasing angina should be risk stratified through ECG testing and measurement of cardiac troponins, preferably in a chest pain unit or hospital emergency department. Patients should have serial ECGs performed and cardiac biomarkers drawn; if these are negative, early stress testing should be performed to evaluate for coronary disease. Patients with persistent or worsening symptoms, or positive cardiac troponins, despite normal ECGs, should be managed in a hospital cardiac unit as described later.

INITIAL LABORATORY EVALUATION

CBC, urinalysis, electrolytes, blood glucose, blood lipids, uric acid, renal and thyroid function tests, chest radiographs, ECG, and cardiac troponins are basic. Stress ECG testing with thallium is generally indicated in non-acute coronary syndrome initial evaluations. Radionuclide scintigraphy, echocardiography, and coronary angiography may follow.

TREATMENT

Underlying, reversible noncardiac causes of angina should be treated as appropriate. In general, three forms of treatment exist for angina of CAD: medical therapy, percutaneous revascularization, and coronary artery bypass grafting. Older clinical trials of medical therapy must be interpreted with caution because many were completed before more recent antiplatelet, antifibrin, and cholesterol-lowering agents were available. Patients with chronic stable angina have an approximately 2% average annual mortality, which is only twice that of age-matched controls, a key factor to bear in mind when considering revascularization interventions. Higher risk patients, however, often stand to benefit the most from revascularization procedures.

Higher risk patients include those with poor exercise capacity and easily provoked ischemia, recent-onset angina, previous myocardial infarction, impaired left ventricular function, underlying diabetes, more than one stenosed artery, and those with disease that affects the left main stem or proximal left anterior descending artery.

1. For chronic stable angina
   a. Acute attacks
      i. Mild: sublingual nitroglycerin or nitroglycerin spray
      ii. Severe: hospitalization and evaluation
   b. Long-term prophylaxis and treatment: risk factor reduction and aspirin, HMG coenzyme reductase inhibitors (statins), and beta blockers with or without long-acting nitroglycerin, or long-acting calcium channel blockers. Addition of clopidogrel and LMWH may be considered.
   c. Intervention/surgery
      i. Percutaneous transluminal angioplasty has not demonstrated reduction in overall mortality compared to medical treatment, and patients undergo more procedures and have greater complications. However, patients do experience greater symptom relief and require fewer medications. Trials with newer medication eluting stents may change these outcomes.
      ii. Coronary artery bypass surgery has less mortality compared with medical treatment for patients with severe left main stem coronary disease, three-vessel disease, two-vessel disease with a severely affected proximal left anterior descending artery, or diabetics with multivessel disease. For lower risk patients, surgery provides symptom relief and improves exercise tolerance when medical treatment fails. Comparisons of PTCA with surgery suffer from the fact that most trials predate the more recent introduction of PTCA interventions that include medication eluting stents. In older trials examining single-vessel disease, mortality is similar between surgery and PTCA, but rates of infarction, persistent symptoms, and repeat revascularization are higher in PTCA. In multivessel disease, mortality is similar, but PTCA is necessarily reserved for vessels with suitable, less tortuous, anatomy, making comparisons with surgery difficult.

2. For acute coronary syndromes
   a. Low-risk patients: Treat with aspirin, clopidogrel, and either heparin or LMWH. Consider early invasive intervention.
   b. For patients with intermittent or worsening symptoms but no ST segment changes, with positive

or negative troponins, treat with the medications for low-risk patients in (a) plus glycoprotein IIb/IIIa inhibition and early invasive intervention by cardiac catheterization.

c. For treatment of ST segment elevation MI, see Chapter 10.

d. Prinzmetal's angina is an angina variant caused by coronary artery spasm with or without fixed stenotic lesions. It is more common in women than in men. ST segment elevation is more common than ST segment depression. Calcium channel blockers are the treatment of choice.

Suggested Reading

Cannon CP, Turpie AG: Unstable angina and non-ST-elevation myocardial infarction: Initial antithrombotic therapy and early invasive strategy. *Circulation* 107(21):2640–2645, 2003.

Gibbons RJ, et al: American College of Cardiology. American Heart Association clinical practice guidelines. Part I: Where do they come from? *Circulation* 107(23):2979–2986, 2003.

Grech ED, Ramsdale DR: Acute coronary syndrome: Unstable angina and non-ST segment elevation myocardial infarction. *BMJ* 326(7401):1259–1261, 2003.

Mukherjee D, Eagle KA: The use of antithrombotics for acute coronary syndromes in the emergency department: Considerations and impact. *Prog Cardiovasc Dis* 50:167–180, 2007.

O'Toole L, Grech ED: Chronic stable angina: Treatment options. *BMJ* 326(7400):1185–1188, 2003.

Snow V, Barry P, Fihn SD, et al: Evaluation of primary care patients with chronic stable angina: Guidelines from the American College of Physicians. *Ann Intern Med* 141:57–64, 2004.

Hyperlipoproteinemia

CLINICAL CASE PROBLEM 1

A 51-Year-Old Male with High Blood Cholesterol

A 51-year-old male comes to your office for his "yearly workup." He is a typical type A personality: hard driving and "married to my job and proud of it." He is, however, married to his wife as well, as he points out in retrospect. He has had previous problems with "high blood cholesterol" and wishes to have his cholesterol checked today.

On examination, his blood pressure is 170/100 mmHg. His pulse is 84 beats/minute and regular. His body mass index is 31. His abdomen is obese.

His family history is significant for hypertension in both parents. His uncle sustained a myocardial infarction (MI) at the age of 51 years, and his older brother had "heart problems" at age 53 years. His total cholesterol in your office (nonfasting) is 328 mg/dL.

You ask the patient to return in 1 week for a fasting sample. The results are as follows: total cholesterol (TC), 288 mg/dL; triglycerides, 262 mg/dL; high-density lipoprotein (HDL), 37 mg/dL; and low-density lipoprotein (LDL), 199 mg/dL.

SELECT THE BEST ANSWER TO THE FOLLOWING QUESTIONS

1. Regarding this patient's lipid profile, which of the following statements is (are) true?
   a. this is a normal profile given his age and family history
   b. determination of his smoking status must be made prior to any recommendations
   c. intense dietary therapy and drug therapy should be considered immediately
   d. although this is an abnormal profile, in the absence of known coronary disease, careful observation of the cholesterol is all that is required at this time
   e. treatment decisions should be based on apoprotein levels

2. Which of the following, according to the National Cholesterol Education Program (NCEP), defines high blood cholesterol?
   a. TC > 180 mg/dL; LDL > 100 mg/dL
   b. TC > 200 mg/dL; LDL > 130 mg/dL
   c. TC > 240 mg/dL; LDL > 160 mg/dL
   d. TC > 250 mg/dL; LDL > 180 mg/dL
   e. TC > 270 mg/dL; LDL > 200 mg/dL

3. What is the single most important risk factor for coronary artery disease (CAD)?
   a. an elevated HDL level
   b. an elevated triglyceride level
   c. an elevated LDL level

d. a depressed HDL level

e. an elevated total blood cholesterol

4. The NCEP defines all of the following conditions as major risk factors for CAD except

a. smoking

b. obesity

c. low HDL cholesterol

d. hypertension

e. age older than 45 years in males

5. All of the following conditions are at high risk for CAD except

a. peripheral arterial disease

b. diabetes mellitus

c. abdominal aortic aneurysm

d. symptomatic carotid artery disease

e. chronic kidney disease

6. An elevated triglyceride level is associated most closely with which of the following?

a. impaired glycemic control

b. hyperthyroidism

c. weight loss

d. low serum very low-density lipoprotein (VLDL) cholesterol

e. elevated total serum cholesterol level

7. At what level of LDL cholesterol is treatment definitely indicated?

a. above 160 mg/dL

b. above 150 mg/dL

c. above 130 mg/dL

d. above 125 mg/dL

e. above 120 mg/dL

8. Which of the following is the treatment of choice for hypercholesterolemia?

a. gemfibrozil

b. colestipol

c. nicotinic acid

d. simvastatin

e. none of the above

9. What is the drug class of choice for the management of mild to moderate elevations of plasma LDL?

a. the fibric acid derivatives

b. the nicotinic acid derivatives

c. the 3-hydroxy-3-methylglutaryl coenzyme A (HMG-CoA) reductase inhibitors

d. the bile acid sequestrants

e. any of the above

10. Recommendations for lifestyle modification to reduce CAD risk include

a. regular aerobic exercise

b. plant stanol ester use

c. low-dose aspirin therapy

d. a and c

e. all of the above

11. Which of the following nutritional supplements helps decrease the risk of CAD?

a. vitamin E

b. dietary fiber

c. hormone replacement therapy

d. aspirin

e. a and d

12. Which of the following is (are) an independent risk factor(s) for CAD?

a. increased LDL concentration

b. decreased HDL concentration

c. increased total cholesterol concentration

d. increased triglyceride concentration

e. all of the above

13. Which of the following antihypertensive drugs do not have an adverse effect on plasma lipids?

a. hydrochlorothiazide

b. fosinopril

c. atenolol

d. nifedipine

e. b and d

14. The American Heart Association's (AHA) Step 1 diet allows how much total cholesterol in the daily intake?

a. 500 mg

b. 400 mg

c. 350 mg

d. 300 mg

e. 200 mg

15. Which of the following statements is (are) true regarding fish oil supplements?

a. fish oils have been shown to lower plasma triglyceride levels

b. fish oils inhibit platelet aggregation

c. fish oils have been shown to increase HDL levels

d. fish oils may decrease blood pressure and blood viscosity

e. all of the above are true

16. What is the drug of choice for the treatment of hypertriglyceridemia?

a. nicotinic acid

b. gemfibrozil

c. lovastatin

d. a and b

e. all of the above

17. Secondary causes of hyperlipidemia include all of the following except
    a. hypothyroidism
    b. cirrhosis
    c. systemic lupus erythematosus
    d. nephrotic syndrome
    e. pregnancy

18. All of the following statements regarding abnormal lipid diagnosis and management are true except
    a. if HDL cholesterol is greater than 60 mg/dL, then one risk factor may be subtracted from the CAD risk factor total
    b. the U.S. Preventive Services Task Force (USPSTF) recommends that cholesterol screening begin at age 18
    c. statin medications are best given in the evenings
    d. start a statin medication in a patient with diabetes mellitus with an LDL cholesterol of 100 mg/dL
    e. LDL cholesterol can be calculated as total cholesterol – (triglycerides/5 + HDL cholesterol)

Clinical Case Management Problem

List the risk factors shown to increase the risk of CAD in the population.

Answers

1. **c.** Given this patient's age and risk factors, it was appropriate to proceed directly to a full (fasting) lipid profile. Normal serum cholesterol is defined as a value less than 200 mg/dL. Any level above 200 mg/dL is considered high unless the HDL cholesterol is high enough to give a normal ratio of TC/HDL.

The question of which patients should be screened for hypercholesterolemia continues to be debated. The third USPSTF report recommends the following: (1) All men aged 35 years or older and all women aged 45 years or older should be screened routinely for lipid disorders (this extends the recommendations of the second USPSTF, which recommended that adults not be screened until age 65 years); (2) younger adults—men aged 20 to 35 years and women aged 20 to 45 years—should be screened if they have other risk factors for heart disease (these risk factors include tobacco use, diabetes, a family history of heart disease

or high cholesterol, or high blood pressure. This recommendation expands on the recommendations of the second USPSTF, which focused on screening middle-aged men and women); and (3) clinicians should measure HDL in addition to measuring TC or LDL. The USPSTF found insufficient evidence to recommend for or against measuring triglycerides. In addition, the current recommendation is to screen with a nonfasting sample.

2. **b.** The National Institutes of Health Adult Treatment Guidelines III (2004) defines high blood cholesterol as equal to or greater than the following: (1) TC, 200 mg/dL; and (2) LDL, 130 mg/dL.

3. **c.** The most important risk factor for CAD is an elevated LDL. The second most important risk factor is depressed HDL.

4. **b.** The five major risk factors for CAD are (1) having hypertension, (2) smoking, (3) having diabetes, (4) being older than age 45 years in males and older than age 55 years in females, and (5) having a family history of MI in a first-degree relative (male relative younger than age 55 years or a female relative younger than age 65 years). Obesity is not a specific risk factor but is strongly associated with the conditions that are major risk factors.

5. **e.** The following conditions are considered CAD risk factor equivalents: peripheral arterial disease, diabetes mellitus, abdominal aortic aneurysm, and symptomatic carotid artery disease.

6. **a.** An elevated triglyceride level, defined as 250 mg/dL or greater, is often observed in people with diabetes with poor glucose control. Weight loss and a low-carbohydrate and low-fat diet are recommended for lifestyle treatment of hypertriglyceridemia. An elevated triglyceride level is associated most closely with an elevated VLDL. TC may be elevated with high triglycerides but can also be in the normal range.

7. **c.** An LDL level is considered elevated when it is higher than 130 mg/dL.

8. **e.** The treatment of choice for hypercholesterolemia is diet therapy. The AHA has produced Step 1 and Step 2 diets. The Step 1 diet includes less than 30% of total calories from fat, less than 10% of calories from saturated fat, and less than 300 mg/day of cholesterol. The Step 2 diet includes less than 30% of total daily calories as fat, less than 7% of calories

from saturated fat, and less than 200 mg/day of cholesterol.

Management of hypercholesterolemia with drugs is indicated only after dietary treatment over a reasonable amount of time has failed to reduce the cholesterol level to a sufficiently low level, although there is a newfound sense of more aggressive treatment, even for primary prevention, as the result of studies such as the Air Force/Texas Coronary Atherosclerosis Prevention Study. The current recommendations that diet therapy be continued for 6 months before drug therapy is started are often supplanted because this study and others have shown conclusively that aggressive treatment of even low-risk middle-aged adults with statin therapy can reduce cardiac morbidity and mortality.

9. **c.** The drug class of choice for mild to moderate LDL elevation is one of the HMG-CoA reductase inhibitors on the market. These include lovastatin (Mevacor), pravastatin (Pravachol), simvastatin (Zocor), atorvastatin (Lipitor), and rosuvastatin (Crestor). All patients who are started on HMG-CoA inhibitors should have not only the plasma lipids but also the liver function tests at baseline and then after 12 weeks. If no further dose changes are made, then liver function tests may be evaluated every 6 months and then yearly when stable. There is a low risk of myositis; therefore, creatinine kinase levels should be measured if patients report leg pain or muscle cramps. In patients with mild to moderate isolated LDL elevation (type IIA), plasma lipids may be normalized with 10 to 20 mg once daily of any of these agents. Patients with higher LDL levels may require higher doses of single-agent therapy or, alternately, multidrug therapy. With such therapy, LDL cholesterol may be lowered up to 40%, and triglyceride levels may be lowered 10% to 15%. There appears to be little change in the HDL level. All the previously mentioned drugs have been known to produce hepatic and skeletal muscle toxicity, insomnia, and weight gain. These side effects, however, are relatively uncommon, dose related, and occur much more frequently in patients who are undergoing multidrug therapy.

The drug of second choice for type IIA hyperlipoproteinemia is niacin. The total daily dose (500-mg tablets) is up to 3 g. All patients taking niacin require monitoring of liver function tests and creatine phosphokinase monthly for 3 months, then every 3 months for 6 months, and every 4 to 6 months thereafter. Niacin may decrease plasma LDL by up to 35% and may decrease triglyceride levels by up to 75%; at the same time, it may increase HDL by up to 100%. In addition, the apolipoprotein A level is

decreased by up to 50%. Unfortunately, niacin has a considerable number of significant side effects, including (1) induction of gastric irritation and gastritis; (2) activation of long-dormant peptic ulcers; (3) elevation of plasma uric acid levels, precipitating an attack of gout; (4) elevation of blood glucose levels; (5) exacerbation of diabetes; and, most commonly, (6) cutaneous flushing, dry and even scaly skin, and, in rare instances, acanthosis nigricans.

Some of these nuance side effects can be ameliorated by coadministering aspirin and/or prescribing the long-acting formulation of niacin. Fortunately, all side effects disappear when the drug is discontinued.

Resins, including cholestyramine (Questran) and colestipol (Colestid), are the drugs of third choice for patients with type IIA hyperlipoproteinemia. The dose ranges are 4 to 8 g once or twice daily for cholestyramine and 5 to 10 g once or twice daily for colestipol.

Their advantages include an almost complete lack of absorption and potential for systemic toxicity that goes with it. Their disadvantages include an unpleasant grittiness and multiple gastrointestinal side effects, including abdominal bloating, abdominal pain, sometimes severe constipation, and gastrointestinal bleeding. Because resins may decrease the absorption of other drugs, they and other drugs should be taken 2 hours apart.

10. **e.** Healthy lifestyle choices that reduce the risk of coronary events include diet, aerobic exercise, weight management, smoking cessation, multivitamin supplements with folic acid, aspirin therapy, and plant stanol ester nutritional supplements. The Food and Drug Administration permits food labels to indicate that daily use of plant stanol esters will help reduce LDL levels. These esters are produced by the esterification of the plant steroid stanol with canola oil, and they act by blocking the intestinal absorption of cholesterol. This reduces the serum LDL but not serum HDL.

11. **d.** Vitamin E, although popular as an antioxidant, has not been shown to favorably or unfavorably alter the course of CAD. Dietary fiber also has no beneficial effect on heart disease, but it does show favorable effect on colorectal disease. Hormone replacement therapy was shown to increase the risk of CAD by the Women's Health Initiative. However, primary and secondary prevention trials have shown that aspirin decreases CAD risk.

12. **e.** Risk factors for CAD include (1) increased LDL concentration (most important lipid risk factor),

(2) decreased HDL (second most important risk factor), (3) increased TC, and (4) increased triglyceride concentration.

13. e. Nifedipine, a calcium channel blocker, and fosinopril, an angiotensin converting enzyme inhibitor, are the only drugs listed that do not have an adverse effect on plasma lipids. (Angiotensin receptor blockers are also neutral with respect to plasma lipids, and alpha blockers appear to have a beneficial effect on HDL levels.) The beta blocker listed, metoprolol, and hydrochlorothiazide adversely affect plasma lipids.

14. d. As mentioned previously, the treatment of first choice for hyperlipidemia is diet. The AHA's Step 1 diet and Step 2 diet are listed in the table.

AHA Step 1 and 2 Diets		
	Step 1	Step 2
Cholesterol	300 mg	200 mg
Total fat	30% of calories	30% of calories
Saturated fat	10% of calories	7% of calories

15. e. Fish and fish oil supplements may reduce plasma lipid levels (especially triglycerides), inhibit platelet aggregation, decrease blood pressure and viscosity, and increase HDL cholesterol. The active ingredients are the long-chain omega-3 fatty acids, eicosapentaenoic acid and docosahexaenoic acid. Well-controlled long-term studies conducted by the Brigham and Women's Hospital and the Harvard Public School of Health and released in 2002 showed an 81% decrease in sudden cardiac-related death risk in men and a 34% decrease in women who consumed fish on a regular basis. Female nurses who consumed fish at least once a week also were found to have a 25% decline in nonfatal heart attacks and a significant decline in deaths in general. The authors believed that both fish and fish oil supplements had a positive effect. However, the beneficial use of fish oil supplements for general use remains more controversial, perhaps because it may not generally be appreciated that efficient absorption requires the presence of other nutrients, particularly additional lipid. In addition, these polyunsaturated fatty acids readily autooxidize.

The essential C-18 omega-3 fatty acid, linolenic acid (also known as alpha-linolenic acid), can be converted to the 20-carbon eicosapentaenoic acid, which in turn is converted to the 22-carbon docosahexaenoic acid and as a consequence can substitute for fish oils. The typical U.S. diet, however, tends to limit this conversion because the linoleic/linolenic acid ratio in the diet is too high. This conversion may also be inhibited by other fatty acids; trans fatty acids in particular have been implicated. Unfortunately, the distribution of alpha-linolenic acid is limited. Studies suggest the optimal linoleic/linolenic acid ratio is between 5 and 10 to 1. The oils obtained from flaxseed, walnuts, rapeseed (canola), safflower, soybean, and wheat germ are the only natural substances with these fatty acids in this optimal range. The best way to ensure the oils are not partially oxidized is to consume them in the foods from which they are derived.

16. b. The drug of choice for most cases of hypertriglyceridemia is gemfibrozil or another fibric acid derivative. Hypertriglyceridemia may be associated with type 2a, type 2b, type 3, or type 4 hyperlipoproteinemia. The usual dose of gemfibrozil is 0.6 g twice a day. Gemfibrozil will decrease hypertriglyceridemia by 40% to 80% and will increase HDL by 10% to 40%.

Until very recently, combining a reductase inhibitor with gemfibrozil was not recommended. This combination still should be used with caution but may be tolerated if a low dose of one drug is given 12 hours apart from a low dose of the other (e.g., pravastatin 10 to 20 mg in the morning with gemfibrozil 600 mg in the evening).

17. b. Hypothyroidism, lupus, pregnancy, oral contraceptive use, and nephritic syndrome are associated with elevations of cholesterol. Cirrhosis is usually associated with a decrease in cholesterol.

18. b. The USPSTF recommends general screening at age 35 years for males and age 45 years for females and targeted screening in adults age 20 to 45 years. If HDL cholesterol is greater than 60 mg/dL, then one risk factor may be subtracted from the CAD risk factor total.

Start a statin medication in a patient with diabetes mellitus with a LDL cholesterol of 100 mg/dL or greater. The Heart Protection Study suggests that statins may even be beneficial in people with diabetes who have LDL values of less than 100 mg/dL. LDL cholesterol can be calculated as total cholesterol − (triglycerides/5 + HDL cholesterol). (Statin medications are best given in the evening.)

Solution to the Clinical Case Management Problem

The risk factors for CAD in the population are as follows: (1) family history of CAD, (2) male sex, (3) hypertension, (4) hypercholesterolemia, (5) high LDL levels, (6) low HDL levels, (7) hypertriglyceridemia, (8) high VLDL levels, (9) cigarette smoking, (10) high alcohol intake (via its effect on hypertension), (11) lack of aerobic exercise, (12) obesity, (13) type 1 diabetes, (14) type 2 diabetes, (15) postmenopausal women, and (16) hyperhomocystinemia.

Summary

1. Screening

The third USPSTF report recommends the following: (1) All men aged 35 years or older and all women aged 45 years or older should be screened routinely for lipid disorders; (2) younger adults—men aged 20–35 years and women aged 20–45 years—should be screened if they have other risk factors for heart disease (including tobacco use, diabetes, a family history of heart disease or high cholesterol, or high blood pressure); and (3) clinicians should measure HDL in addition to measuring TC or LDL. The USPSTF found insufficient evidence to recommend for or against measuring triglycerides. The current recommendation is to screen with a nonfasting sample, and all patients should receive periodic counseling regarding dietary intake of fat (especially saturated fat) and cholesterol.

2. Recommended cholesterol values (ATP III Guidelines, 2004)

a. TC: normal, equal to or less than 5.2 mmol/L (200 mg/dL); borderline, 5.2 to 6.2 mmol/L (200 to 240 mg/dL); elevated, equal to or greater than 6.2 mmol/L (240 mg/dL)

b. LDL cholesterol: ideal, equal to or less than 3.4 mmol/L (13,000 mg/dL); borderline, 3.4 to 4.1 mmol/L (13,000 to 15,929 mg/dL); elevated, equal to or greater than 4.1 mmol/L (15,930 mg/dL)

c. HDL cholesterol: ideal, equal to or greater than 40 mg/day in men and postmenopausal women, and equal to or greater than 50 mg/day in premenopausal women.

d. VLDL cholesterol (triglycerides): ideal, equal to or less than 1.4 mmol/L (125 mg/dL); borderline, 1.4 to 2.8 mmol/L (125 to 250 mg/dL); elevated, equal to or greater than 2.8 mmol/L (250 mg/dL)

3. Dietary treatment of hypercholesterolemia

Treat hypercholesterolemia if LDL cholesterol is greater than 130 mg/dL or greater than 100 mg/dL with two or more risk factors. Dietary management is the treatment of first choice.

a. Begin with the Step 1 diet of the AHA: no more than 300 mg cholesterol, no more than 30% total fat, and no more than 10% saturated fat.

b. Continue for at least 6 months. If cholesterol levels do not normalize, consider AHA Step 2 diet: no more than 200 mg cholesterol, no more than 30% total fat, and no more than 7% saturated fat.

4. Drug treatments for hypercholesterolemia

Drugs should be used if dietary treatment is insufficient or if multiple risk factors are present.

a. Drugs of first choice are HMG Co-A reductase inhibitors. The Scandinavian Simvastatin Survival Study showed that cholesterol-lowering drugs reduce deaths from CAD and sudden cardiac death. In this study, the HMG-CoA reductase inhibitor simvastatin substantially improved survival, reducing the overall risk of death by 30% and the risk of coronary death by 42%. This adds even more credibility to the recommendation that HMG-CoA reductase inhibitors be considered the drugs of first choice for the treatment of hyperlipidemia.

b. Drug of second choice: niacin

c. Drug of third choice: bile acid sequestrants

5. Hypertriglyceridemia

Hypertriglyceridemia has been established as an independent risk factor for CAD. Always search for a secondary cause of hypertriglyceridemia, such as the presence of diabetes mellitus, alcohol use, or oral contraceptive use.

Treatments for hypertriglyceridemia include the AHA Step 1 and Step 2 diets, and the drug of choice for drug treatment of hyperlipoproteinemia primarily resulting from elevated triglycerides is gemfibrozil.

Suggested Reading

Agency for Healthcare Research and Quality: *Screening Adults for Lipid Disorders. What's New from the USPSTP*, AHRQ Publication No. APPIP 01-0011. Rockville, MD: Agency for Healthcare Research and Quality, 2001.

Expert Panel on Detection, Evaluation, and Treatment of High Blood Cholesterol in Adults (Adult Treatment Panel III), National Heart, Lung, and Blood Institute: *ATP III Update 2004*. Bethesda, MD: National Heart, Lung, and Blood Institute. Available at www.nhlbi.nih.gov

Hu FB, et al: Fish and omega-3 fatty acid intake and risk of coronary heart attack in women. *JAMA* 287:1818–1821, 2002.

Institute for Clinical Systems Improvement: *Lipid Management in Adults*. Bloomington, MN: Institute for Clinical Systems Improvement, 2007. Available at www.icsi.org.

CHAPTER

24 Congestive Heart Failure

CLINICAL CASE PROBLEM 1

A 78-Year-Old Female with Shortness of Breath

A 78-year-old female comes to the emergency department with a 6-month history of fatigue and shortness of breath, aggravated especially when performing any exertional activity including those associated with activities of daily living. She has found that occasionally she has to get up at night and open the window to get air. There has been a weight gain of 15 pounds during the 6 months, and there has been gradual swelling of her ankles and legs. Her history reveals no previous myocardial infarction, but it does reveal the presence of type 2 diabetes for 15 years, severe hypertension for 30 years, and obesity for 8 years. Although the shortness of breath has been a significant problem for only 6 months, she does mention having "some breathing problems" intermittently for at least 4 years, and she has been treated for intermittent atrial fibrillation and moderate chronic obstructive pulmonary disease. She is taking glyburide, hydrochlorothiazide, diltiazem, coumadin, ipratropium, and captopril.

On physical examination, the patient's blood pressure is 140/90 mmHg. The respiratory rate is 28 breaths/minute, and the pulse is 98 beats/minute and regular; she is afebrile. Head, ears, eyes, nose, and throat are unremarkable; there is no elevated jugular venous distention (JVD). Both S1 and S2 are normal, but a fourth heart sound is present; there are no murmurs. Chest examination reveals bibasilar rales in both lung bases. Abdominal examination is benign; the hepatojugular reflex is negative. Extremities reveal bilateral 3+ pitting edema to both knees. Pulse oximetry shows an O_2 saturation of 90% on room air. Electrocardiogram (ECG) reveals normal sinus rhythm, no acute changes, and left ventricular (LV) hypertrophy. You suspect a form of heart failure and order a chest radiograph.

SELECT THE BEST ANSWER TO THE FOLLOWING QUESTIONS

1. Your working hypothesis, based on the history and physical examination, is that the patient has which of the following?
   a. diastolic heart failure
   b. systolic heart failure
   c. biventricular heart failure
   d. cor pulmonale
   e. heart failure secondary to pulmonary fibrosis

2. Based on the type of failure this patient has, what is most likely to be found on chest radiograph?
   a. normal chest
   b. congestion and cardiomegaly
   c. pulmonary edema
   d. congestion with or without cardiomegaly
   e. cardiomegaly

3. The chest x-ray is consistent with the history and physical examination and your diagnosis of diastolic failure. The patient is admitted for therapy. You order an echocardiogram. Again, based on the type of failure this patient has, what is this likely to show?
   a. normal LV cavity size
   b. an ejection fraction of more than 40%
   c. a dilated left ventricle
   d. an ejection size of less than 40%
   e. a and b

4. The targeted range of the diastolic blood pressure in this patient should be
   a. <90 mmHg
   b. <80 mmHg
   c. between 80 and 90 mmHg
   d. it does not matter
   e. >90 mmHg to maintain perfusion

CLINICAL CASE PROBLEM 2

A 62-Year-Old Male with Exertional Dyspnea, Orthopnea, and Wheezing

A 62-year-old male, with a long history of smoking two packs of cigarettes a day, presents to your office with a history of worsening shortness of breath with exertion for the past 3 weeks. He also relates recent onset of fatigue, two-pillow orthopnea, and scattered wheezes when climbing a flight of stairs. Five years ago, he had an anterior wall myocardial infarction but had been doing well until his recent symptoms. He has no other medical problems. He takes a baby aspirin and atenolol daily.

On examination, his vital signs were as follows: pulse 100 beats/minute and regular, respiration 24 breaths/minute, blood pressure 129/89, afebrile. Weight has increased by 10 pounds since the last visit 6 months ago. There is JVD at 30 degrees elevation, rales a third of the way up in both lung fields, moderate hepatic congestion, and a positive hepatojugular reflux. Heart examination reveals an S4 but no murmurs. There is also 1+ pitting edema in both legs to his midcalves. You perform an ECG, which shows sinus rhythm and no acute changes but poor R-wave progression in the anterior leads. Chest radiograph reveals cardiomegaly and pulmonary vascular congestion.

5. Which of the following medications is (are) appropriate for acute management?
   a. furosemide
   b. captopril
   c. diltiazem
   d. labetalol
   e. a, b, and c

6. The nonpharmacologic treatments(s) of choice for this condition may include which of the following?
   a. salt restriction
   b. fat restriction
   c. water restriction
   d. none of the above
   e. a, b, and c

The patient described here is treated with the appropriate medication and improves. He returns in 2 weeks with dyspnea and fatigue, although it is not as severe as before. Vital signs are normal. At this time, the JVD has resolved and the hepatojugular reflex is absent. The cardiac examination is unchanged. There is trace pitting edema in his ankles bilaterally. He has lost 10 pounds. Results of an echocardiogram are pending.

7. At this time, which of the following is (are) appropriate medication(s) to consider instituting?
   a. an angiotensin-converting enzyme (ACE) inhibitor or adrenogenic receptor binder (ARB)
   b. a second beta blocker
   c. a calcium channel blocker
   d. digitalis
   e. a and d

8. Which of the following pathophysiologic mechanisms may underlie heart failure in this patient and should be searched for as part of a comprehensive evaluation?
   a. LV chamber remodeling
   b. coronary artery disease
   c. valvular heart disease
   d. abnormal excitation–contraction coupling
   e. all of the above

9. What is (are) the current indication(s) for the use of digitalis in this condition?
   a. a dilated left ventricle
   b. an S3 or S4 gallop
   c. decreased ejection fraction
   d. atrial fibrillation with a rapid ventricular rate
   e. c and d

10. Which of the following is (are) correct about the effects of digitalis on patients with this condition?
    a. digoxin reduces long-term mortality
    b. digoxin decreases rates of worsening of heart failure
    c. lower digoxin maintenance doses may be as effective as higher doses
    d. digoxin use reduces hospitalizations
    e. b, c, and d

11. In evaluating a patient for systolic dysfunction, the most important characteristic found on echocardiogram is
    a. myocardial hypertrophy
    b. valvular heart disease
    c. cor pulmonale
    d. low ejection fraction
    e. wall motion abnormalities

12. Which of the following correctly defines the American Heart Association (AHA) stages of heart failure?
    a. stage A are asymptomatic patients at high risk but with no identifiable structural abnormalities

b. stage B are asymptomatic patients with identifiable structural abnormalities

c. stage C are symptomatic patients with structural abnormalities

d. stage D are end-stage patients refractory to standard therapy

e. all of the above

13. All but which of the following has been shown to reduce hospitalizations and mortality in selective patients with congestive heart failure (CHF)?

a. beta blockers

b. spironolactone

c. ACE inhibitors

d. biventricular pacing

e. calcium channel blockers

Clinical Case Management Problem

A major error in treating heart failure is assuming that all patients who appear to be in heart failure need furosemide. When given furosemide, some patients actually get worse. Provide an example of a practical situation in which this could occur.

Answers

1. a. This patient has a classic history for diastolic heart failure. An estimated 20% to 40% of patients with CHF have preserved or normal systolic function. In these patients, contraction is normal, but diastole (relaxation phase) is abnormal. During exertion, normal filling during diastole does not occur, and cardiac output is impaired. Therefore, dyspnea is particularly profound during exertion. Dyspnea is the most common sign of both systolic and diastolic CHF. Initially, the dyspnea is present only with moderate amounts of exertion, but as the severity of the heart failure increases, the shortness of breath may occur with only minimal exertion or even at rest. Other common symptoms of heart failure are fatigue and lethargy.

Patients with diastolic cardiac failure are, like the patient presented, frequently elderly and female, with a history of hypertension, diabetes, and obesity. Atrial fibrillation, if present, is usually paroxysmal, and a fourth heart sound (S4 gallop) is often present. In systolic heart failure, which can occur in all ages and more often in males, atrial fibrillation tends to be persistent, a third heart sound is present (S3 gallop), and there is often a history of previous myocardial infarction.

In both forms of failure, lying flat is often followed by increasing shortness of breath. Paroxysms of nocturnal dyspnea (PND) are suggestive of heart failure. On careful questioning, the patient describes the bouts as marked breathlessness—a "suffocating feeling"—and these symptoms are often accompanied by significant anxiety. The patient has to sit upright or even stand up to breathe and may have the urge to rush to an open window to relieve the "suffocating feeling." Extra pillows are needed to reduce the number and severity of attacks. Some patients even have to resort to sleeping upright in a chair at all times.

2. d. Patients with diastolic failure will present with congestion with or without cardiomegaly on chest radiograph. Do not be fooled into thinking that the absence of cardiomegaly rules out failure. In systolic failure, in contrast, cardiomegaly almost always is present. Heart failure also can be distinguished by which ventricle is failing the most. Whereas LV cardiac failure is manifested by symptoms such as shortness of breath, right ventricular cardiac failure is manifested by signs such as enlargement of the liver, a positive hepatojugular reflex, and an elevated jugular venous pressure. In severe cases of elevated right-sided atrial pressure, splanchnic engorgement may accompany anorexia, nausea, vomiting, ascites, and eventually cachexia. In most instances of chronic failure, however, both ventricles are usually involved, making the distinction less useful.

3. e. The cardinal features of diastolic heart failure are the presence on echocardiogram of a normal LV ejection fraction and a usually normal LV cavity size. Concentric LV hypertrophy is usually present as well. In systolic heart failure, LV ejection fraction is usually less than 40% and the ventricular cavity is dilated.

4. b. This patient has diabetes and, as a result, evidence-based guidelines suggest targeting diastolic blood pressure to be less than 80 mmHg to reduce mortality and morbidity.

5. a. The most appropriate acute pharmacotherapeutic intervention is the administration of diuretics, particularly loop diuretics, preferably intravenously. Careful attention should be given to the patient's urine output and weight as a measure of successful diuresis. Reasonable investigations in acute failure include the following: 12-lead ECG; chest radiograph; blood chemistries including blood urea nitrogen (BUN), creatinine, glucose, and electrolytes; complete blood count (CBC); thyroid-stimulating hormone (TSH); liver function tests and lipids; urinalysis for protein and sugar; and echocardiography. Diuresis should be accomplished with careful attention to electrolytes, especially potassium, with adequate replenishment of depleted salts. Oxygen should be administered to correct any hypoxia.

6. e. Nonpharmacologic therapy for CHF involves the following in order of importance: (1) bed rest, (2) salt restriction (2 or 3 g sodium/day), (3) fluid restriction (related to sodium restriction), and (4) fat restriction (as a reasonable approach to a healthy lifestyle using the AHA Step 1 diet, which is 300 mg cholesterol, 30% total calories from fat, and 10% of calories from saturated fat).

7. a. Two drugs have been proven to be particularly useful in the treatment of chronic heart failure: ACE inhibitors and beta blockers, the latter of which this patient is already taking. ACE inhibitor drugs such as captopril, enalapril, or lisinopril have been shown to reduce both morbidity and mortality in patients with severe systolic heart failure. Little outcome difference exists between those taking higher or lower doses, so the latter is preferred to reduce potential side effects. For patients who cannot tolerate ACE inhibitors, ARBs are a reasonable alternative, although no studies have produced evidence that they should be used as a first-line agent in chronic CHF. This may be more of an issue of the dosages used in trials, and a head-to-head study of an ACE inhibitor with or without ARB suggests the ARB agent may be as effective as an ACE alone, but the two together confer no additive advantage. Whether this is true for the entire class of ARBs remains to be determined. Beta blockers, when used with caution and introduced carefully, also have had a positive effect on mortality and morbidity in multiple studies and are thought to work primarily by countering the harmful effects of the sympathetic nervous system. Initiation often may exacerbate symptoms, so patients must be monitored carefully and titrated slowly. Because the echocardiogram results are pending, it is uncertain whether digoxin is appropriate in this patient. Calcium channel blockers have not demonstrated the effectiveness of ACE inhibitors or beta blockers.

8. e. CHF is a syndrome in which a large number of pathophysiologic mechanisms may underlie the symptoms and signs of heart failure. Some of these include structural abnormalities of the myocardium, LV chamber, and coronary arteries and functional abnormalities of the valves and electrical systems. In this patient, a comprehensive evaluation would include a search for evidence of LV chamber remodeling, coronary artery disease, valvular heart disease, abnormal excitation–contraction coupling, and arrhythmias. Coexisting noncardiac diseases also should be identified and treated. That would include search for and control of tobacco addiction, alcohol abuse, diabetes, hypertension, obesity, anemia, sleep apnea, and renal disease.

9. e. The use of digitalis (in the form of digoxin) has come full circle. This drug, isolated from the foxglove plant, used to be the mainstay of treatment for CHF. For various reasons, it then fell into disfavor, to the point where it was virtually never used. The completion of the circle has resulted in digoxin once again being used extensively. Its primary indications are in cases of CHF with a reduced ejection fraction and atrial fibrillation with a rapid ventricular rate. Physicians should be aware of drug interactions that may increase digoxin levels. These include use of digoxin with verapamil, quinidine, procainamide, nifedipine, or amiodarone. Physicians should also be aware of electrolyte abnormalities (hypokalemia and hypomagnesemia) induced by diuretics and overdosing in the elderly, who may have decreased renal clearance.

10. e. True statements about the use and effects of digoxin include the following: Digoxin decreases rates of worsening of heart failure, lower digoxin maintenance doses may be as effective as higher doses, and digoxin use in appropriate patients reduces the rate of hospitalizations in CHF. Elderly patients and those with renal insufficiency are also more prone to the toxic effects of the drug. Remember that the primary indications for its use are those patients with CHF and both a low ejection fraction and atrial fibrillation with rapid ventricular rate.

11. d. In evaluating patients for systolic dysfunction, the most important characteristic found on echocardiogram is the ejection fraction, which is usually less than 40% in systolic heart failure. Although myocardial hypertrophy, valvular heart disease, and wall motion abnormalities may be found, it is the ejection fraction that defines systolic dysfunction.

12. e. The AHA has developed a classification system that defines the different stages of heart failure, thereby emphasizing the preventive, albeit usually progressive, nature of the condition. People with stage A heart failure are asymptomatic patients at high risk but with no identifiable structural abnormalities. People with stage B heart failure are asymptomatic patients with identifiable structural abnormalities. Stage C is symptomatic patients with structural abnormalities; stage D is end-stage patients refractory to standard therapy. People with stage A disease should have risk factor reduction, such as treatment of hypertension, dyslipidemia, or diabetes, and patient and family education. Stage B patients should be treated with ACE inhibitors or ARBs (all patients) and beta blockers (in selected individuals). Stage C patients should all be taking ACE inhibitors and beta blockers; should be treated with dietary sodium restriction, diuretics, and digoxin (selectively, if indicated); may be candidates for cardiac resynchronization if bundle block is present; may be revascularized or have correction of valvular heart disease (if present); and may be treated with an aldosterone antagonist. Stage D refractory disease may be treated with all of the previously mentioned methods as appropriate plus the use of inotropics, transplantation, ventricular assistive devices, or hospice.

13. **e.** Calcium channel blockers are the exception in this list of interventions that have been found to be effective in reducing hospitalizations and mortality.

Solution to the Clinical Case Management Problem

A practical example of a patient becoming worse after being given furosemide is the following:

A 55-year-old male with uremia and a history of CHF manifests an increasing shortness of breath and increasing edema of the extremities. You naturally assume that his CHF is worsening, and you administer furosemide. He deteriorates rapidly. The cause: uremic pericarditis. What appeared to be CHF was not. The lesson to be learned is as follows: Make sure the patient has CHF before you treat the CHF.

Summary

CHF is a syndrome in which a large number of pathophysiologic mechanisms may underlie the symptoms and signs of heart failure. Some of these include structural abnormalities of the myocardium, LV chamber, and coronary arteries and functional abnormalities of the valves and electrical systems. A comprehensive evaluation includes a search for evidence of diminished pump function, LV chamber remodeling, coronary artery disease, valvular heart disease, abnormal excitation–contraction coupling, and arrhythmias. Coexisting noncardiac diseases should also be identified and treated. That would include a search for and control of tobacco addiction, alcohol abuse, diabetes, hypertension, obesity, anemia, sleep apnea, and renal disease.

The AHA has developed a classification system that defines the different stages of heart failure, thereby emphasizing the preventive, albeit usually progressive, nature of the condition. People with stage A heart failure are asymptomatic patients at high risk but with no identifiable structural abnormalities. People with stage B heart failure are asymptomatic patients with identifiable structural abnormalities. Patients in stage C are symptomatic with structural abnormalities, and stage D consists of end-stage patients refractory to standard therapy.

Dyspnea is the most common symptom of both systolic and diastolic CHF. Other common symptoms of heart failure are fatigue, lethargy, and PND. An estimated 20% to 40% of patients have diastolic heart failure with preserved or normal systolic function. In these patients, contraction is normal, but diastole (relaxation phase) is abnormal. During exertion, normal filling during diastole does not occur, and cardiac output is impaired. Therefore, dyspnea is particularly profound during exertion, and as the severity of the heart failure increases, the shortness of breath may occur with only minimal exertion or even at rest. In systolic heart failure, the more common form of heart failure, systolic function is impaired and the cardiac systolic ejection fraction is diminished (<40%) as measured by echocardiogram.

Patients with diastolic cardiac failure are frequently elderly and female, with a history of hypertension, diabetes, and obesity. Atrial fibrillation, if present, is usually paroxysmal, and a fourth heart sound (S4 gallop) is often present. In systolic heart failure, which can occur in all ages and more often in males, atrial fibrillation tends to be persistent, a third heart sound is present (S3 gallop), and there is often a history of previous myocardial infarction. Classic signs of both types of failure include tachypnea, tachycardia, JVD, rales, hepatojugular reflux, hepatosplenomegaly, cephalization and congestion on chest radiograph with or without cardiomegaly, and diminished oxygen saturation on pulse oximetry.

Reasonable investigations in acute failure include the following: 12-lead ECG; chest radiograph; blood chemistries including BUN, creatinine, glucose, and electrolytes; CBC; TSH; liver function tests and lipids; urinalysis for protein and sugar; echocardiography; and pulse oximetry.

Patients with stage A disease should have risk factor reduction, such as treatment of hypertension, dyslipidemia, or diabetes, and patient and family education. Stage B patients should be treated with ACE inhibitors or ARBs (all patients) and beta blockers (in selected individuals). Stage C patients are symptomatic, and, in addition to oxygen, the most appropriate acute pharmacotherapeutic intervention is the administration of diuretics, particularly loop diuretics, preferably intravenously. Careful attention should be given to the patient's urine output and weight as a measure of successful diuresis. In addition, all stage C patients should be taking ACE inhibitors and beta blockers and should be treated with dietary sodium restriction. Other therapies include the use of chronic diuretics, digoxin (selectively, if indicated), aldosterone antagonists, cardiac resynchronization if bundle block is present, and revascularization and/or correction of valvular heart disease (if present). Stage D refractory disease may be treated with all of the previously mentioned methods as appropriate plus the use of inotropics, transplantation, ventricular assistive devices, or hospice.

Suggested Reading

Cowie MR, Zaphiriou A: Management of chronic heart failure. *BMJ* 325(7361):422–425, 2002.

Hunt SA, Abraham WT, Chin MH, et al: ACC/AHA 2005 guideline update for the diagnosis and management of chronic heart failure in the adult. *Circulation* 112:e154–e235, 2005.

Jessup M, Brozena S: Medical progress: Heart failure. *N Engl J Med* 348(20):2007–2018, 2003.

O'Connor CM: The new heart failure guidelines: Strategies for implementation. *Am Heart J* 153(4 Suppl):2–5, 2007.

CHAPTER

25 Hypertension

CLINICAL CASE PROBLEM 1

An Obese 47-Year-Old Male with Hypertension

A 47-year-old male presents to your office for a yearly checkup. He is 5 foot 10 inches tall, weighs 250 pounds, smokes two packs of cigarettes a day, and "slams down" 12 ounces of whiskey a day. He is a truck driver and is on the road a lot. He frequently eats at "fast-food joints."

On physical examination, you find his blood pressure to be 180/105 mmHg. His point of maximum impulse is detected in the sixth intercostal space in the anterior axillary line. His funduscopic examination is normal. He has no carotid bruits.

SELECT THE BEST ANSWER TO THE FOLLOWING QUESTIONS

1. Which of the following statements about this patient's blood pressure is (are) false?
   a. a single blood pressure reading of diastolic 105 mmHg is satisfactory for a diagnosis of hypertension
   b. this patient's alcohol intake may be a significant contributing factor to his elevated blood pressure
   c. the patient should have his blood pressure rechecked after a period of rest in the office
   d. the patient should return for reassessment of his blood pressure in 1 week
   e. the patient's cigarette smoking may be a significant contributing factor to his elevated blood pressure

2. Which of the following blood pressure values meets the definition of prehypertension in the report on *Prevention, Detection, Evaluation and Treatment of Hypertension* of the Joint National Committee on Detection, Evaluation, and Treatment of High Blood Pressure (JNC) 7?
   a. 122/82 mmHg
   b. 140/90 mmHg
   c. 118/78 mmHg
   d. 135/85 mmHg
   e. a and d

3. The minimum goal in hypertension therapy is to reduce his blood pressure to a level less than which of the following?
   a. 150/90 mmHg
   b. 140/90 mmHg
   c. 130/90 mmHg
   d. 120/80 mmHg
   e. 110/70 mmHg

4. A week later, the patient returns to your office with blood pressure measurements taken by his company's nurse. They are as follows: 148/95, 144/92, and 150/90 mmHg. At this time, you would prescribe
   a. a thiazide diuretic
   b. a beta blocker
   c. a calcium channel blocker
   d. an angiotensin-converting enzyme (ACE) inhibitor
   e. none of the above

5. What is the first-line pharmacologic therapy now recommended for most patients with hypertension?
   a. a beta blocker
   b. a thiazide diuretic
   c. a calcium channel blocker
   d. an ACE inhibitor
   e. any of the above

6. Which of the following statements is false?
   a. in chronic congestive heart failure, ACE inhibitors, beta blockers, and aldosterone inhibitors have been shown to decrease morbidity and mortality
   b. recurrent strokes are decreased by a combination of ACE inhibitors and thiazide diuretics
   c. calcium channel blockers are beneficial in reducing cardiovascular disease and stroke in patients with diabetes mellitus
   d. hypertension in older individuals is best treated with calcium channel blockers
   e. ACE inhibitors should be avoided in women of childbearing age or pregnant women

7. Which statement(s) is (are) true regarding the use of antihypertensive drugs with other comorbidities?
   a. thiazide diuretics are useful in slowing demineralization in osteoporosis
   b. beta blockers are useful in prophylactic treatment of migraine headache
   c. beta blockers are useful in the comanagement of Raynaud's phenomenon
   d. a and b
   e. all of the above

8. The initial diagnostic workup of a patient with hypertension should include which of the following?
   a. electrolytes
   b. blood urea nitrogen (BUN), creatinine
   c. electrocardiogram (ECG)
   d. 24-hour urine for vanillylmandelic acid (VMA) and metanephrines
   e. a, b, and c
   f. all of the above

9. Based on the patient's history and physical examination, which of the following statements concerning his hypertensive complications is most likely true?
   a. this patient is unlikely to have any hypertensive complications
   b. this patient likely has hypertensive retinopathy
   c. this patient likely has cardiac hypertrophy
   d. this patient likely has hypertensive renal failure
   e. none of the above are true

10. Which of the following statements accurately applies to mild hypertension?
    a. the term is no longer considered appropriate in defining hypertension
    b. mild hypertension describes a systolic level of 140 to 159 mmHg
    c. mild hypertension describes a diastolic level of 90 to 104 mmHg
    d. b and c
    e. none of the above

11. Which of the following statements regarding the treatment of hypertensive emergencies and urgencies is false?
    a. patients with marked blood pressure elevations and acute target organ damage require hospitalization
    b. patients with marked blood pressure elevations without target organ damage should receive immediate combination oral hypertensive therapy
    c. the oral medication of choice for hypertensive urgencies is sublingual nifedipine
    d. all of the above
    e. none of the above

CLINICAL CASE PROBLEM 2

A 50-Year-Old Male with Resistant Hypertension

A 50-year-old male is being treated for hypertension with a low-salt diet, hydrochlorothiazide 25 mg/day, and propranolol 120 mg twice daily. His blood pressure is currently 180/100 mmHg.

12. Which of the following would be a reasonable third-line agent for the treatment of this patient's blood pressure?
    a. atenolol
    b. metoprolol
    c. labetalol
    d. furosemide
    e. enalapril

13. What is the most common side effect of ACE inhibitors?
a. cough
b. constipation
c. headache
d. skin rash
e. depression

14. What is the recommended starting dose for hydrochlorothiazide (HCTZ)?
a. 25 mg
b. 50 mg
c. 75 mg
d. 100 mg
e. none of the above

15. Which one of the following prescribing considerations concerning HCTZ is true?
a. it can be used without concern in patients taking digoxin
b. it is safe for use in patients with uric acid metabolism disorders
c. it can cause hyperkalemia
d. it can be associated with osteoporosis development
e. its use should be avoided in patients allergic to sulfonamides

16. Based on the history and physical examination of the patient described in Clinical Case Problem 1, which of the following additional investigations should be undertaken?
a. digital subtraction angiography
b. intravenous pyelogram (IVP)
c. echocardiogram
d. retinal ultrasound
e. renal ultrasound

17. Which medication would be the least optimal in a patient with asthma?
a. hydrochlorothiazide
b. propranolol
c. lisinopril
d. nifedipine
e. prazosin

18. Which antihypertensive medication is best avoided in chronic kidney disease?
a. lisinopril
b. furosemide
c. amlodipine
d. triamterene
e. atenolol

19. Which medication is contraindicated in gout?
a. atenolol

b. hydrochlorothiazide
c. lisinopril
d. nifedipine
e. prazosin

20. The 47-year old male patient described in Clinical Case Problem 1 is admitted to the hospital a few months later for an acute myocardial infarction. He has disregarded your previously prescribed therapies. What medications would you now prescribe for his blood pressures that average 160/90 mmHg?
a. metoprolol
b. amlodipine
c. lisinopril
d. a and c
e. a, b, and c

CLINICAL CASE PROBLEM 3

A 49-Year-Old Obese Postmenopausal Woman with Type 2 Diabetes Mellitus

The next day, the wife of the patient described in Clinical Case Problem 2, a teacher, sees you in your office. She is a 49-year-old postmenopausal obese woman with type 2 diabetes mellitus. She brings in a list of blood pressures taken by the school nurse during the past 3 months. The blood pressure readings average 136/86 mmHg.

21. Your approach to this clinical case problem could include:
a. recommend lifestyle changes and a return visit in 3 months
b. prescribe lisinopril, when her blood pressure is unchanged in 3 months
c. prescribe metoprolol, when her blood pressure is unchanged in 3 months
d. a and b
e. a and c

Clinical Case Management Problem

Specify the recommended and contraindicated antihypertensive drugs for the following patients:

Patient 1: A young patient with hyperdynamic circulation
Patient 2: An elderly patient with no particular chronic diseases other than hypertension

Answers

1. a. Hypertension should not be diagnosed until a sustained, repetitive elevation of blood pressure has been documented. For diagnosis, at least three readings averaging greater than 140 mmHg systolic or 90 mmHg diastolic must be documented, preferably by the same observer using the same technique. The classification is based on two or more properly measured seated blood pressure readings on two or more office visits. Alcohol abuse is a significant cause of hypertension. Any patient with hypertension should be questioned regarding alcohol intake. Although a low dose of alcohol has been shown to be cardioprotective, "low" must be carefully defined. An absolute maximum of two drinks per day may be cardioprotective; any more than that may be harmful and, indeed, an additional risk factor for coronary artery disease.

The patient described in this clinical case problem should have his blood pressure taken again after 5 minutes of controlled rest. If his arm circumference is greater than 33 cm, obtain his blood pressure reading with the obese blood pressure cuff. Also instruct this patient to abstain from caffeine and cigarette smoking for at least 2 hours before his pressure is checked on his next visit.

A patient whose blood pressure returns to normal after a period of rest is known as a "labile hypertensive." Of patients who are labile hypertensive, approximately 50% go on to develop sustained hypertension.

2. e. JNC 7 describes prehypertension as a 120 to 139 mmHg systolic and 80 to 89 mmHg diastolic blood pressure reading. Those with blood pressures in the 130/80 to 139/89 mmHg range are at twice the risk to develop hypertension as those with lower values. Treatment is to prescribe lifestyle modifications. It has been well established that home blood pressure readings (if done correctly and taken with a blood pressure recording device that has been calibrated against a mercury manometer) are more accurate and a more significant predictor of cardiovascular morbidity and mortality than office blood pressure readings.

The patient should not be started on antihypertensive medication at this time. First, the diagnosis must be established. Second, before considering antihypertensive medication you must consider nonpharmacologic therapy and attempt to lower his or her blood pressure without drugs.

3. b. The minimum goal in antihypertensive therapy is to reduce the blood pressure to a level of 140 mmHg systolic and 90 mmHg diastolic. Ideally, the blood pressure should be less than 120/80 mmHg.

4. e. The first step in treating this patient's blood pressure is to use nonpharmacologic therapy. There is no doubt that nonpharmacologic therapy has a major role to play in the management of hypertension. Nonpharmacologic therapies that have been shown to make a difference and should be prescribed for this patient include (1) weight reduction, (2) alcohol elimination (for a person such as this, who "slams down" 12 ounces of whiskey per day, your best bet would be to attempt to eliminate the "slamming" completely), (3) cigarette smoking cessation, (4) aerobic exercise 4 hours per week or 1200 kcal (however, this patient should first be given an exercise tolerance test), (5) salt intake reduction, and (6) fat intake reduction.

The fat-reduction program should follow the American Heart Association's Step 1 diet formula (decreasing the fat content of the diet without changing the total caloric intake will automatically begin the weight-reduction process) or the National Heart, Lung, and Blood Institute's DASH diet (a combination diet rich in fruits, vegetables, and low-fat dairy foods and low in saturated and total fat), which has been shown to lower blood pressure.

You need to decide which of these therapies to begin with; obviously, attempting to alter everything at once will not work. An alcohol rehabilitation program or a smoking cessation program would be an excellent first choice.

5. b. The JNC 7 recommends thiazide diuretics for most patients and specific drugs for compelling indications. For instance, in diabetes mellitus type 1, with proteinuria, an ACE inhibitor is recommended. In heart failure, ACE inhibitors and diuretics and aldosterone antagonists are recommended. In isolated systolic hypertension of older individuals, diuretics are preferred, and long-acting dihydropyridine calcium antagonists are also acceptable. In the face of myocardial infarction, beta blockers and ACE inhibitors are recommended. In chronic kidney disease, ACE inhibitors and antitension II receptor blockers (ARBs) have shown favorable effects on the progression of diabetic and nondiabetic renal disease. Recurrent stroke rates are lowered by a combination of ACE inhibitors and thiazide diuretics. The most recent studies discourage the use of beta blockers as first-line therapy for hypertension unless there are specific indications.

6. d. In chronic congestive heart failure, ACE inhibitors, beta blockers, and aldosterone inhibitors have been shown to decrease morbidity and mortality. Recurrent strokes are decreased by a combination of ACE inhibitors and thiazide diuretics. Calcium channel blockers are beneficial in reducing cardiovascular disease and stroke in patients with diabetes mellitus. Hypertension in older individuals is best treated with diuretics. ACE inhibitors should be avoided in women of childbearing age or pregnant women because they are teratogenic.

7. d. Thiazides are useful in the treatment of osteoporosis because they slow the demineralization process. Beta blockers are useful in migraine headache prophylaxis but are contraindicated in Raynaud's phenomenon.

8. e. The basic (and cost-effective) hypertensive workup includes (1) complete urinalysis, (2) hemoglobin and hematocrit, (3) BUN and creatinine, (4) serum calcium and potassium, (5) fasting lipid profile, (6) plasma glucose, and (7) ECG.

Other tests, including renal ultrasound, IVP, or 24-hour urine for VMA and metanephrines, are indicated only in special circumstances. A patient that is, for example, 55 years old and develops hypertension for the first time should be suspected of having a secondary cause. (As a general rule, if essential hypertension is going to develop, it will develop before the age of 50 years). In a 50-year-old patient, the most common secondary cause of hypertension is renal artery stenosis. This would call for investigation with magnetic resonance angiography of the renal arteries or Doppler

flow analysis of the renal arteries. Another secondary cause is pheochromocytoma (hypertension, sweating, and palpitations).

9. c. This patient probably has cardiac hypertrophy. This is suspected from the physical examination of the heart, when the point of maximal impulse is found in the sixth intercostal space–anterior axillary line. The normal apical impulse is located at or medial to the midclavicular line in the fourth or fifth intercostal space. The physical examination described provided no evidence concerning retinopathy or nephropathy.

10. a. The term mild hypertension is no longer considered appropriate in defining hypertension because it may very well give some a false sense of security ("I've been told I have hypertension, but I've also been told it is mild; therefore, I really don't have to worry about it"). See the following table for the newer JNC 7 classification.

Classification of Blood Pressure for Adults		
Classification	**Systolic mmHg**	**Diastolic mmHg**
Normal	<120	<80
Prehypertension	130–139	80–89
Hypertension		
Stage 1	140–159	90–99
Stage 2	≥160	≥100

11. d. Hypertensive emergencies and hypertensive urgencies are defined as follows: A hypertensive emergency is a clinical situation in which blood pressure must be lowered immediately and carefully to prevent or limit target organ damage. Examples of hypertensive emergencies are malignant hypertension, acute myocardial ischemic syndromes, acute pulmonary edema, acute renal insufficiency, acute intracranial events, postoperative bleeding, eclampsia, and pheochromocytoma. Generally, a 25% reduction in the initial blood pressure values is required to prevent further complications.

A hypertensive urgency is a clinical situation in which blood pressure should be lowered within 24 to 48 hours. Examples of hypertensive urgencies are accelerated hypertension, marked hypertension associated with congestive cardiac failure, stable angina pectoris, transient cerebral ischemic attacks, and perioperative hypertension. Previously used sublingual nifedipine was found in studies to cause acute coronary events and ischemic strokes when used in hypertensive emergencies.

Hypertensive emergency/urgency drug selection must be made on a pathophysiologic basis.

A summary of current recommendations follows:

1. Central nervous system disorder
   a. Drug of choice: sodium nitroprusside
   b. Alternative: labetalol
2. Intracranial hemorrhage
   a. Drug of choice: sodium nitroprusside
   b. Alternative: labetalol
3. Acute left ventricular failure
   a. Drug of choice: enalaprilat
   b. Contraindicated: labetalol
4. Acute coronary ischemia
   a. Drug of choice: nitroglycerin
   b. Alternatives: labetalol and sodium nitroprusside
5. Unstable angina
   a. Drug of choice: nitroglycerin
   b. Alternative: labetalol
6. Aortic dissection
   a. Drug of choice: esmolol hydrochloride
   b. Alternatives: sodium nitroprusside and propranolol
   c. Contraindicated: hydralazine
7. Eclampsia
   a. Drug of choice: $MgSO_4$ (magnesium sulfate)
   b. Alternative: hydralazine
8. Pheochromocytoma
   a. Drug of choice: phentolamine
   b. Contraindicated: beta-adrenoreceptor blockers

12. e. This patient is currently on a thiazide diuretic and a beta blocker. Therefore, the most reasonable alternative as a third-line agent would be either an ACE inhibitor or a calcium channel blocker.

Atenolol and metoprolol are also beta blockers and thus would not be reasonable choices.

Labetalol is a combination alpha–beta blocker and thus would also be a poor choice.

Furosemide is a loop diuretic and would not be a reasonable choice for the management of this patient's hypertension.

Enalapril is an ACE inhibitor and would be an excellent choice for a third-line agent.

13. a. The most common side effect of ACE inhibitors is cough. The mechanism of the cough appears to be bradykinin induced. It does not appear to be truly allergic in nature. Approximately 15% of patients taking chronic ACE inhibitors develop a chronic cough. ARBs do not have this side effect.

14. a. The starting dose of a hydrochlorothiazide is 25 mg. A low dose (25 mg) has been shown in many studies to be just as efficacious as a higher dose (50, 75, or 100 mg). The only difference between the low dose and the higher doses is the greatly increased incidence of side effects with the higher doses. The same principle, with dose adjusted for molecular weight difference, holds true for other thiazides.

15. e. Thiazide diuretics may produce any of six metabolic side effects: hyperglycemia, hyperuricemia, hyperlipidemia, hypomagnesemia, hyponatremia, and hypokalemia. Some patients who are allergic to sulfonamides are also allergic to HCTZ. Because HCTZ can cause hypokalemia, concurrent digoxin use must be monitored. Thiazide diuretics slow the demineralization process in bone.

16. c. The patient's point of maximum impulse is in the sixth intercostal space in the anterior axillary line. This suggests left ventricular hypertrophy secondary to hypertension (and perhaps also as a result of the obesity). An echocardiogram is indicated to evaluate the thickness of the left ventricle.

17. b. In a patient with asthma, a nonselective beta blocker should be avoided because it may lead to bronchoconstriction and wheezing.

18. d. Triamterene possibly would lead to hyperkalemia, which is problematic in chronic kidney disease. ACE inhibitors and ARB medications provide a favorable prognosis for kidney disease until hyperkalemia develops. To manage fluid balance in kidney disease, a loop diuretic is often needed, particularly in combination with an ACE or ARB medication.

19. b. HCTZ is contraindicated in gout because it may raise uric acid levels.

20. d. Administration of beta blockers and ACE inhibitors is associated with a favorable outcome in cases of myocardial infarction.

21. d. Lifestyle changes are the cornerstone of hypertension and diabetes mellitus management. Prevention of nephropathy is a compelling indication to prescribe an ACE inhibitor in a patient with diabetes. Beta blockers have not shown as compelling an indication with respect to prevention of diabetic nephropathy.

Solution to the Clinical Case Management Problem

Patient 1: A young patient with hyperdynamic circulation
Recommended drugs: beta blockers
Contraindicated drugs: none

Patient 2: An elderly patient with no particular chronic diseases other than hypertension
Such a person is liable to suffer from isolated systolic hypertension resulting from increased vascular stiffness (decreased compliance).
Recommended drugs: First-line agents: diuretics, with reduced drug dose; second-line agents: ACE inhibitors and long-acting calcium channel blockers
Contraindicated drugs: none

Patient 3: An African American patient
Recommended drugs: thiazide diuretics are preferred for initial therapy, calcium channel antagonists also are effective
Contraindicated drugs: none, but in the absence of concomitant thiazide therapy the effect of ACE inhibitors or beta blockers is blunted

Patient 4: A patient with gout
Recommended drugs: any drug but diuretics
Contraindicated drugs: diuretics

Patient 5: A patient with ischemic heart disease
Recommended drugs: beta blockers, calcium channel blockers
Contraindicated drugs: none

Patient 6: A patient with asthma
Recommended drugs: calcium channel blockers
Contraindicated drugs: beta blockers

Patient 7: A patient with peripheral vascular disease
Recommended drugs: calcium channel blockers or other vasodilators
Contraindicated drugs: beta blockers

Patient 8: A patient with non-insulin-dependent diabetes
Recommended drugs: ACE inhibitors
Contraindicated drugs: none, although diuretics may increase blood sugar levels

Patient 9: A patient with insulin-dependent diabetes
Recommended drugs: ACE inhibitors
Contraindicated drugs: beta blockers

Patient 10: A patient with hypercholesterolemia
Recommended drugs: ACE inhibitors, calcium channel blockers, alpha blockers, beta blockers with intracarotid sodium amytal (ISA)
Contraindicated drugs: high-dose beta blockers without ISA, high-dose diuretics

Patient 11: A patient with congestive heart failure
Recommended drugs: ACE inhibitors, diuretics
Contraindicated drugs: none, although beta blockers should be used with caution

Patient 12: A pregnant patient
Recommended drugs: alpha methyldopa, hydralazine
Contraindicated drugs: diuretics, ACE inhibitors

Summary

1. Diagnosis

Blood pressure measurement in three readings, separated by a time of at least 1 week. Each of the three readings should be taken after at least 5 minutes of controlled rest and after having not consumed caffeine or smoked during the past hour. Hypertension is diagnosed if the average systolic pressure is at least 140 mmHg and/or the average diastolic pressure is at least 90 mmHg. A single reading of a diastolic pressure of 110 mmHg is also probably sufficient for the diagnosis of hypertension.

2. Evaluation

History, physical examination, and laboratory evaluation should include the evaluation of other risk factors, including family history of hypertension and other cardiovascular disease, the presence of diabetes mellitus,

obesity, alcohol intake, hyperlipidemia, smoking, exercise pattern, and stress.

Search for evidence of end-organ damage: cardiac hypertrophy (may need echocardiogram), funduscope, and renal function.

Laboratory evaluation should include complete blood count, urinalysis, electrolytes, BUN, creatinine, calcium, cholesterol, glucose, and ECG.

3. Classification

Staging system outlined in answer 10. Stages have replaced mild, moderate, and severe hypertension.

4. Treatment

Nonpharmacologic treatment: Treatment with medication includes weight reduction, increase in aerobic exercise, restriction of sodium, restriction of saturated fat (DASH diet), discontinued smoking, and decreased stress.

Pharmacologic treatment: JNC 7 recommends use of thiazide diuretics in most patients. Optimal formulation should be effective for 24 hours, requiring only a once-daily dose, if possible. Long-acting formulations are preferred over short-acting agents because adherence to therapy is better, control is consistent and persistent, cost may be lower, and nighttime protection from sudden increases in blood pressure is present. Combinations of low doses of two agents from different classes are recommended and practically inevitable in stage 2 hypertension. JNC 7 also recommends specific medications when compelling indications exist.

Suggested Reading

Chobanian AV, Bakris GL, Black HR, et al: The seventh report of the Joint National Committee on Prevention, Detection, Evaluation, and Treatment of High Blood Pressure: The JNC 7 report. *JAMA* 289(19):2560–2572, 2003.

Godlee F (ed): *Clinical Evidence, Cardiovascular Concerns.* London: BMJ Books, 2003.

Hall WD: A rational approach for the treatment of hypertension in special populations. *Am Fam Phys* 60:156–162, 1999.

Institute for Clinical Systems Improvement: *Hypertension Diagnosis and Treatment.* Bloomington, MN: Institute for Clinical Systems Improvement, 2006.

Rosendorff C, Black HR, Cannon CP, et al: Treatment of hypertension in the prevention and management of ischemic heart disease: A scientific statement from the American Heart Association Council for High Blood Pressure Research and the Councils on Clinical Cardiology and Epidemiology and Prevention. *Circulation* 115:2761–2788, 2007.

CHAPTER

26   Dysrhythmia

CLINICAL CASE PROBLEM 1

A 37-Year-Old Male with "Skipping Heart Beats"

A 37-year-old male comes to your office for assessment of "skipping heartbeats." These skipped beats have been a concern for the past 8 months. The patient reports no other symptoms accompanying these skipped beats. Specifically, he reports no increased sweating, no palpitations, no weight loss, no chest pain, no pleuritic pain, and no anxiety.

On physical examination, his blood pressure is 100/70 mmHg. On auscultation of his heart, you observe that S1 and S2 are normal—there are no extra sounds or murmurs. You hear approximately five premature beats per minute.

SELECT THE BEST ANSWER TO THE FOLLOWING QUESTIONS

1. What is the most commonly encountered "premature contraction"?
   a. a ventricular premature beat
   b. an atrial premature beat
   c. atrial flutter
   d. atrial fibrillation
   e. none of the above

2. Most atrial premature beats discovered on clinical examination are
   a. associated with chronic obstructive pulmonary disease (COPD)
   b. completely benign
   c. associated with valvular heart disease
   d. associated with an increase in cardiovascular mortality
   e. none of the above

3. Most ventricular premature beats discovered on clinical examination are
   a. associated with COPD
   b. completely benign
   c. associated with valvular heart disease
   d. associated with an increase in cardiovascular mortality
   e. none of the above

CLINICAL CASE PROBLEM 2

A 51-Year-Old Male with Acute Chest Pain

A 51-year-old male presents to the emergency room (ER) with an acute episode of chest pain. He has a history of atrial fibrillation. On examination, his blood pressure is 80/60 mmHg and his ventricular rate is approximately 160 beats/minute. He is in acute distress. His respiratory rate is 32 breaths/minute. His electrocardiogram (ECG) shows atrial fibrillation with a rapid ventricular response.

4. What should your first step in management be?
a. digitalize the patient
b. give the patient intravenous (IV) verapamil
c. give the patient IV adenosine
d. start synchronized cardioversion
e. start rapid IV hydration

CLINICAL CASE PROBLEM 3

A 44-Year-Old White Male with Palpitations

A 44-year-old white male comes to your ER saying he has palpitations. He denies chest pain or shortness of breath. There is no history of known heart disease or cardiac risk factors except for mild obesity. He does admit to drinking heavily the night before at an office retirement party.

On physical examination, his blood pressure is 120/80 mmHg and his ventricular rate is 160 beats/minute. His ECG confirms atrial fibrillation with a rapid ventricular response.

5. What should you do at this time?
a. digitalize the patient
b. treat the patient with IV verapamil
c. treat the patient with IV procainamide
d. cardiovert the patient
e. have him perform a Valsalva maneuver by rebreathing into a paper bag

6. What is the recommended treatment for paroxysmal supraventricular tachycardia (PSVT) with hemodynamic compromise?
a. synchronized cardioversion
b. direct-current countershock
c. IV adenosine
d. IV verapamil
e. IV digoxin

7. Patients with chronic atrial fibrillation are at increased risk for which of the following conditions?
a. acute myocardial infarction (MI)
b. ventricular tachycardia
c. sudden cardiac death
d. cerebrovascular accident
e. ventricular fibrillation

8. What is the drug of choice for prevention of the complication described in question 7?

a. prophylactic streptokinase
b. prophylactic warfarin
c. prophylactic heparin
d. prophylactic lidocaine
e. no drug is recommended

9. Which of the following statements regarding the medical treatment of atrial premature beats with antiarrhythmic drugs is true?
a. the benefit outweighs the risk
b. the risk outweighs the benefit
c. the risk and the benefit are equal
d. the risk and benefit depend on the patient
e. nobody really knows for sure

10. Which of the following statements regarding the medical treatment of ventricular premature beats with antiarrhythmic drugs is true?
a. the benefit outweighs the risk
b. the risk outweighs the benefit
c. the risk and the benefit are equal
d. the risk and benefit depend on the patient
e. nobody really knows for sure

Answers

1. b. Atrial premature beats are the most common premature beats encountered in the adult population. They are almost always asymptomatic and are often discovered incidentally during a medical examination. Patients with atrial premature beats often complain of "palpitations" or "a feeling of skipped heartbeats" during periods of emotional stress or during periods of quiet, such as while resting in bed. Atrial premature beats may be associated with tachycardias that, particularly if nonsustained (less than 30 seconds), may not be perceived by the patient.

2. b. Atrial premature beats require no treatment except reassurance of the patient. Reassurance is particularly important because the more convinced the patient is that something is seriously wrong, the more atrial premature beats he or she will sustain.

There are obviously other causes of palpitations that must be considered, such as thyrotoxicosis, panic disorder, and pheochromocytoma. However, benign premature atrial contractions are much more common than premature atrial contractions as a result of thyrotoxicosis, panic disorder, or pheochromocytoma.

3. b. Most ventricular premature contractions, as with atrial premature contractions, turn out to be completely benign. As with atrial premature contractions, most patients simply need reassurance. Also as with atrial premature contractions, most ventricular premature contractions are asymptomatic and are often discovered during a medical examination. Occasionally, premature ventricular contractions (PVCs) (unlike premature atrial contractions [PACs]) may be symptoms of more serious underlying heart disease. With runs of ventricular premature beats (ventricular tachycardia), the patient may develop angina, dyspnea, dizziness, syncope, and even cardiac arrest.

If there is a serious question about the number of ventricular premature beats per minute, a 24-hour Holter monitor is an excellent way to measure. The risk of prescribing a patient a prophylactic antiarrhythmic drug for ventricular ectopy outweighs the benefit.

4. d. This patient presents with what appears to be an acute attack of atrial fibrillation with rapid ventricular response. This is an unstable tachycardia. The treatment of choice for this patient is synchronized cardioversion at 100 J of energy. Advanced cardiac life support (ACLS) protocol recommends cardioversion energies of (1) 100 J, (2) 200 J, (3) 300 J, and (4) 360 J in that order and in succession if the previous energy level was not successful.

5. b. In this case, the patient has the same condition, atrial fibrillation. However, in this case he is hemodynamically stable instead of hemodynamically unstable. Therefore, a less dramatic intervention than cardioversion can be attempted at this time. The scenario of atrial fibrillation following alcohol ingestion ("holiday heart syndrome") is seen frequently during holidays and weekends. Generally, the acute cardiac rhythm disturbance occurs in the background of heavy chronic alcohol consumption. Occasionally, the arrhythmia may be induced acutely without chronic abuse, especially after a period of prolonged sleeplessness.

ACLS protocol suggests that for rate control in this situation, both beta blockers and calcium channel blockers are appropriate.

6. a. Unstable PSVT is treated with immediate cardioversion.

A patient who presents with stable PSVT first should be treated with vagal maneuvers and adenosine. Vagal maneuvers have therapeutic and diagnostic value. These maneuvers can help differentiate PSVT from other rhythms such as atrial flutter. Carotid sinus massage, Valsalva maneuver, and the placement of a cold ice pack on the skin are examples of vagal maneuvers. Pressing on the eyeballs is not a recommended vagal maneuver.

7. d. These patients are at increased risk for sudden stroke.

8. b. Anticoagulation therapy is underused for patients with chronic atrial fibrillation. Because these patients are at risk for embolic cerebrovascular accidents, it is recommended they start taking warfarin prophylaxis, provided there is no contraindication. All of the trials to date have shown that chronic warfarin therapy maintained with an international normalized ratio (INR) of 2 to 3 significantly reduces the incidence of strokes in patients with chronic atrial fibrillation (whether persistent or intermittent). In high-risk patients, warfarin is approximately twice as effective as aspirin in reducing risk of stroke. Younger patients (<65 years old) with no risk factors (previous stroke or transient ischemic attack, hypertension current or in the past, diabetes, or congestive heart failure) may be treated with aspirin alone.

9. b. The risk outweighs the benefit; see answer 10.

10. b. In patients with either PACs or PVCs, it is obvious that unless the circumstances are unusual and have been documented electrophysiologically, the risk of treatment with antiarrhythmic drugs outweighs the benefit. A number of trials have confirmed this.

Summary

1. Atrial premature beats: These are benign and extremely common; reassurance is the only treatment recommended.
2. Ventricular premature beats: The vast majority are benign, they are extremely common, and reassurance is the only treatment recommended after a complete cardiovascular status is determined for the patient.

    According to the Cardiac Arrhythmia Suppression Trial, with ventricular ectopy, even in patients at high risk (i.e., following an MI), the risk of treating this dysrhythmia is greater than the risk of doing nothing.
3. Treatment for PSVT when the patient is stable consists of vagal maneuvers and adenosine.
4. Treatment for atrial fibrillation is:
    a. If hemodynamically unstable: synchronized cardioversion: 100 J–200 J–300 J–360 J
    b. If hemodynamically stable: calcium channel blockers or beta blockers
    c. Prophylaxis against embolic cerebrovascular accidents with warfarin is recommended. The INR should be maintained between 2 and 3. If warfarin is contraindicated, or in younger patients with no risk factors, aspirin therapy is effective.

Suggested Reading

American Heart Association: American Heart Association guidelines for cardiopulmonary resuscitation and emergency cardiovascular care. *Circulation* 112(Suppl 1):IV1–IV203, 2005.

Fuster V, Ryden LE, Cannom DS, et al: ACC/AHA/ESC 2006 guidelines for the management of patients with atrial fibrillation. *Circulation* 114:e257–e354, 2006.

CHAPTER

27 Deep Venous Thrombosis and Pulmonary Thromboembolism

CLINICAL CASE PROBLEM 1

A 65-Year-Old Female with Cyanosis, Shortness of Breath, and Substernal Chest Pain

A 65-year-old female is admitted to the emergency room with a 3-hour history of cyanosis, shortness of breath, and substernal chest pain. She had been discharged 5 days earlier after having a total hip replacement for severe osteoarthritis. The hip surgery was uneventful.

On physical examination, the patient is in obvious acute respiratory distress. Her respiratory rate is 40 breaths/minute and her breathing is labored. Her blood pressure is 100/70 mmHg. Cyanosis is present. There appear to be decreased breath sounds in the lower lobe of the right lung, as well as adventitious breath sounds in all lobes.

SELECT THE BEST ANSWER TO THE FOLLOWING QUESTIONS

1. Based on the information provided, what is the most likely diagnosis in this patient?
   a. fat embolus
   b. acute myocardial infarction
   c. dissecting aortic aneurysm
   d. acute pulmonary embolism
   e. cholesterol emboli syndrome

2. Which of the following findings if present in the history and physical exam increases the likelihood of a patient having a pulmonary embolism?
   a. heart rate > 100 beats/minute
   b. hemoptysis
   c. surgery within the previous 4 weeks
   d. previous deep venous thrombosis
   e. all of the above

3. Which of the following statements is true concerning examination of a patient with suspected deep venous thrombosis (DVT)?
   a. clinical examination is diagnostic in every case
   b. clinical examination is, in most cases, diagnostic
   c. clinical examination is of some value but has low sensitivity and low specificity
   d. clinical examination is of no value
   e. nobody really knows for sure

4. Which of the following blood gas combinations occur most commonly in the condition described in this clinical case?
   a. decreased Po_2 and decreased Pco_2
   b. decreased Po_2 and increased Pco_2
   c. increased Po_2 and increased Pco_2
   d. increased Po_2 and decreased Pco_2
   e. none of the above

5. What is the most common cause of morbidity and mortality among hospitalized immobile patients?
   a. myocardial infarction
   b. cerebrovascular accident
   c. deep venous thrombosis/pulmonary embolism
   d. nosocomial infection
   e. none of the above

6. Which of the following best describes D-dimer screening for suspected venous thromboembolism (VTE)?
   a. high sensitivity, low specificity
   b. low sensitivity, high specificity
   c. high sensitivity, high specificity
   d. low sensitivity, low specificity
   e. none of the above

7. Which of the following is correct regarding treatment of patients with VTE?
   a. low-molecular-weight heparin (LMWH) is as effective as unfractionated heparin (UFH)
   b. warfarin therapy should be started after a minimum of 2 days of heparin
   c. LMWH is safe to use in patients with a history of heparin-induced thrombocytopenia
   d. early ambulation and use of graded compression stockings increases risk of pulmonary embolism (PE) in DVT
   e. none of the above

CLINICAL CASE PROBLEM 2

A 35-Year-Old Female Who Has Recently Returned from a Trip Overseas

A 35-year-old recently pregnant female, now on oral contraceptives, presents to the office with 1 week of unilateral painful right leg swelling. There is no history of trauma, but 12 days ago the patient returned from overseas via a 12-hour airplane ride. On physical examination, her right calf is 5 cm greater in circumference than her left, and there is tenderness when you squeeze the gastrocnemius muscle.

8. Which of the following is (are) a risk factor(s) for the condition described here?
   a. prolonged immobilization
   b. long leg fractures
   c. pregnancy
   d. malignancy
   e. all of the above

9. Which of the following statements about treatment modalities for venous thromboembolism disease is correct?
   a. LMWH increases the partial thromboplastin time (PTT) to the same degree as UFH
   b. protamine reverses the anticoagulant activity of UFH but not LMWH
   c. in hemodynamically stable patients, thrombolytic therapy has been shown to reduce mortality and the risk of recurrent PE
   d. leafy green vegetables can potentiate the anticoagulant effect of warfarin
   e. inferior vena cava (IVC) filters are indicated in patients with VTE and a contraindication to anticoagulation

10. Which of the following statements regarding DVT prophylaxis is correct?
    a. patients undergoing hip replacement surgery should receive either LMWH or warfarin
    b. low-dose subcutaneous heparin has been shown to be as effective as LMWH in patients undergoing knee replacement surgery
    c. intermittent pneumatic compression of the legs should not be used in combination with LMWH or coumadin
    d. intermittent pneumatic compression of the legs decreases endogenous fibrinolytic activity
    e. warfarin therapy should be continued a minimum of 12 months after uncomplicated DVT to prevent recurrence

Answers

1. **d.** VTE is a disease entity comprising PE and DVT. This patient most likely has a PE. Hip surgery is a common predisposing factor for PE. Symptoms of PE are often subtle. It is often impossible to distinguish PE from myocardial infarction on the basis of symptoms alone. Chest pain, dyspnea, anxiety, hyperventilation, and syncope are common to both conditions. Signs of PE include adventitious breath sounds, fever, and cyanosis. Pulmonary embolism is suggested by the triad of cough, hemoptysis, and pleuritic chest pain.

Pulmonary embolism may lead to acute cor pulmonale. This complication produces (1) distended neck veins, (2) tachycardia, (3) an accentuated and split pneumonic heart sound, (4) Kussmaul's sign (distention of the jugular veins on inspiration), and (5) pulsus paradoxus (exaggerated decrease in blood pressure on inspiration). Systemic hypotension and shock suggest massive PE. Massive PE should also be considered in the following circumstances: hemodynamic instability, severe hypoxemia or respiratory distress, a massively abnormal perfusion defect in a V/Q scan, right heart strain or failure, elevated pulmonary artery pressure, and severe occlusion seen on computed tomography (CT) angiogram. Massive PE should be treated with thrombolytics.

In the postoperative setting, fat and cholesterol emboli syndromes always need to be considered. A hallmark of both of these disorders is the presence of purpura. Fat embolism typically occurs on the upper body 2 or 3 days after a major injury. Through the use of special fixatives, the emboli can be demonstrated in biopsy specimens of the petechiae. Cholesterol emboli are usually seen on the lower extremities of patients with atherosclerotic vascular disease. They often follow anticoagulant therapy or an invasive vascular procedure such as an arteriogram. Associated findings include livedo reticularis, gangrene, cyanosis, subcutaneous nodules, and ischemic ulcerations.

2. **e.** When evaluating a patient for a possible embolism, risk factors that increase the probability of the diagnosis include having (1) signs and symptoms of DVT, (2) a heart rate greater than 100 beats/minute, (3) immobilization or surgery in the past 4 weeks, (4) a history of DVT or PE, (5) hemoptysis, or (6) cancer (receiving treatment or palliative care or received treatment within the past 6 months).

3. **c.** The clinical diagnosis of DVT is difficult and unreliable. DVT is frequently present in the absence of

clinical signs (e.g., pain, heat, or swelling) and is absent in approximately 75% of patients in whom clinical signs or symptoms of PE suggest its presence. The Wells criteria for DVT risk assessment include active cancer/treatment, immobilization/paralysis, recent major surgery/bedridden 3 or more days, localized tenderness along deep vein, entire leg swelling, calf swelling greater than 3 cm compared with other leg, pitting edema in symptomatic leg, collateral superficial veins, and history of previous DVT. In the absence of a likely alternative diagnosis, a patient having three or more of the previous criteria suggests a high probability of DVT.

4. a. Massive embolism is commonly associated with arterial hypoxemia, hypocapnia, and respiratory alkalosis. In addition, the difference between the alveolar Po_2 and the arterial Po_2 ($PAo_2 - Pao_2$) may be widened due to the increase in alveolar dead space. However, a normal alveolar–arterial gradient does not exclude the diagnosis.

5. c. The most common cause of morbidity and mortality among hospitalized immobile patients is DVT and PE. This is directly related to the immobile state. In the United States, the incidence of fatal plus nonfatal PE exceeds 500,000 annually. This overall incidence is verified by autopsy statistics. Evidence of recent or old embolism is detected in 25% to 30% of routine autopsies.

6. a. D-Dimer testing (a measurement of the degradation products of cross-linked fibrin circulating in plasma) is a highly sensitive but nonspecific screening test for suspected VTE. It is most useful to help rule out VTE. If the D-dimer test is negative, VTE is highly unlikely. D-Dimer is elevated in almost all patients with an embolism but is also elevated with advancing age, pregnancy, trauma, cancer, inflammatory conditions, and during the postoperative period.

7. a. LMWH is as effective as UFH and is preferred initial therapy in DVT. LMWH is administered on a weight-determined dosing schedule. Many cases of uncomplicated DVT can be treated out of the hospital with LMWH, which requires no frequent blood monitoring of coagulation values. Use of LMWH may be limited in the face of renal insufficiency.

Heparin therapy should be started as soon as VTE disease is suspected, as long as there are no contraindications. Absolute contraindications include active hemorrhage or recent intracranial bleeding. Relative contraindications include recent or impending surgery, active peptic ulcer disease with bleeding, liver disease, recent major trauma, severe anemia, and renal disease.

Warfarin therapy in VTE disease should be started immediately with either LMWH or UFH. Heparin therapy should be continued for at least 5 days after the initiation of warfarin therapy and until the international normalized ratio is above 2 for two consecutive days. Early ambulation and the use of graded compression stockings reduce the duration of pain and swelling in DVT and are not associated with any increased incidence of PE.

Heparin-induced thrombocytopenia (HIT), a complication that occurs in approximately 3% of patients treated with UFH and 1% or 2% of patients treated with LMWH, is an immune-mediated reaction. HIT requires cessation of heparin therapy and the use of alternative anticoagulants.

The value of PTT in monitoring the safety and efficacy of UFH administration remains controversial. With respect to safety, the risk of hemorrhage (the principal complication of heparin therapy) is not clearly related to coagulation test alterations; rather, it appears to be related to factors such as the coexistence of other diseases associated with bleeding risk (gastric or duodenal ulcer, coagulopathies, or uremia) and advanced age. Likewise, achievement of the desired effect of UFH (cessation of thrombus growth *in vivo*) has not been related consistently to coagulation tests. Current recommendations suggest keeping the PTT measured just prior to the next intermittent dose at or above 1.5 times the control and at 1.5 to 2.5 times the control with the continuous infusion regime.

8. e. The risk of DVT and PE is increased by (1) immobility (both posttraumatic and postoperative), (2) long leg fractures, (3) a prior history of DVT, (4) oral contraceptive or estrogen use, (5) cerebrovascular accident (CVA) or a history of CVA, (6) pregnancy, (7) malignancy, (8) autoimmune disease, (9) nephrotic syndrome, (10) polycythemia, (11) inflammatory bowel disease, (12) congestive heart failure, or (13) obesity.

9. e. IVC filters are indicated in patients with VTE and a contraindication to anticoagulation. The filters are also indicated when there is a recurrence of VTE despite anticoagulation. LMWH does not increase the PTT. Protamine reverses the anticoagulant activity of UFH and LMWH. Thrombolytic therapy has not been shown to decrease mortality or risk of recurrent PE in hemodynamically stable patients. If there is no contraindication, thrombolytic therapy is indicated in patients with PE and circulatory shock. Leafy green vegetables, along with medications such as rifampin, griseofulvin, sucralfate, and barbiturates, can reduce the anticoagulant effect of warfarin.

10. **a.** Patients undergoing hip or knee replacement surgery should receive prophylaxis with LMWH or warfarin. Low-dose subcutaneous heparin has not been shown to be as effective as LMWH for DVT prophylaxis in patients undergoing knee replacement surgery. There can be additional benefit when intermittent pneumatic compression of the legs is used in combination with other preventive strategies. In addition to improving blood flow, intermittent pneumatic compression of the legs also increases endogenous fibrinolytic activity. The duration of warfarin therapy should be individualized based on risk of VTE recurrence and risk of potential complications of treatment. In uncomplicated, first-instance DVT, in the absence of risk factors outlined previously, warfarin therapy may be safely discontinued after a minimum of 3 months.

Summary

Wells criteria for DVT risk assessment include active cancer/treatment, immobilization/paralysis, recent major surgery/bedridden 3 or more days, localized tenderness along deep vein, entire leg swelling, calf swelling greater than 3 cm compared with other leg, pitting edema in symptomatic leg, collateral superficial veins, and history of previous DVT. In the absence of a likely alternative diagnosis, the presence of three or more of the previous criteria suggests a high probability of DVT.

1. Diagnosis

Most patients who develop DVT and subsequent PE have previously described risk factors. However, remember that DVT is often clinically silent, and the clinical diagnosis can be notoriously inaccurate. PE is often heralded by the abrupt onset of dyspnea, chest pain, apprehension, hemoptysis, or syncope. When massive PE is present, the signs of acute cor pulmonale are evident. With PE, rhonchi or wheezing are frequently heard in the chest.

2. Laboratory diagnosis

The current investigational modalities for DVT and PE include

a. D-Dimer testing: This is a valuable test that, if negative (negative predictive value), helps to rule out DVT and PE. A patient with low clinical pretest probability combined with a negative D-dimer can be considered to have DVT ruled out. As already discussed, D-dimer levels are elevated in many different circumstances. Higher negative predictive values are required to rule out PE given the consequences of a missed diagnosis.

b. Duplex ultrasonography with compression: This is a good initial screening tool for DVT in moderate to high-risk patients, and if negative, a D-dimer should also be ordered. Results need to be interpreted with caution in PE: Ultrasonography is negative in up to 50% of patients with proven PE; also, up to 20% of patients without an embolism will have positive ultrasonographic findings.

c. Venography: Ascending contrast venography is the gold standard for the diagnosis of DVT. However, it has many drawbacks, including cost, availability, and discomfort. Serial ultrasonography is an acceptable alternative in situations in which there is a high likelihood of DVT with an initial negative duplex ultrasound. In many institutions, contrast CT venography has shown good results and is a good alternative.

d. The chest x-ray and electrocardiogram (ECG): The chest x-ray in PE may show a parenchymal infiltrate and evidence of a pleural effusion if pulmonary infarction has occurred; ECG findings are used to help eliminate acute myocardial infarction as an alternative diagnosis.

e. Arterial blood gases: Low Po_2, low Pco_2, and respiratory alkalosis are seen in PE. Blood gas results are most useful when used in conjunction with other information.

f. The ventilation/perfusion scan: A valuable test for PE when the results are definitive. A normal or low-probability scan is very good for ruling out a PE, and a high-probability scan is strongly associated with a PE. The problem is that many patients without a PE will have abnormal findings on V/Q scanning, and many patients with a PE will not have findings that indicate a high probability.

g. CT pulmonary angiography: In many centers, this is the preferred test for diagnosing PE. It allows direct visualization of emboli and detection of parenchymal abnormalities. In studies, the sensitivity of CT angiography scanning for diagnosis of PE has ranged from 85% to 100% depending on a number of variables, including location of emboli and differences in technology. CT angiography has mostly replaced invasive pulmonary angiography as the gold standard for the diagnosis of PE in the presence of an equivocal V/Q scan.

3. Treatment
a. Supplemental oxygen for PE
b. Heparin: UFH or LMWH
c. Warfarin
d. IVC filter: indicated for patients with VTE who have a contraindication to anticoagulation, for patients with recurrence of PE despite anticoagulation therapy, or for some patients at high risk for initial or recurrent PE.
e. Thrombolytic therapy: reserved for patients with massive PE and cardiovascular compromise. Many centers now perform direct injection of thrombolytics.
f. Direct thrombin inhibitors: indicated for patients with VTE and heparin-induced thrombocytopenia. Lepirudin and argatroban are Food and Drug Administration-approved direct thrombin inhibitors.

Suggested Reading

Chunilal SD, Eikelboom JW, Attia J, et al: Does this patient have pulmonary embolism? *JAMA* 290(21):2849–2858, 2003.

Fancher TL, White RH, Kravitz RL: Combined use of rapid D-dimer testing and estimation of clinical probability in diagnosis of deep vein thrombosis: Systematic review. *BMJ* 329(7470):821, 2004.

Institute for Clinical Systems Improvement: *Venous Thromboembolism.* Bloomington, MN: Institute for Clinical Systems Improvement, 2006. Available at www.guidelines.gov.

Quiroz R, Kucher N, Zou KH, et al: Clinical validity of a negative computed tomography scan in patients with suspected pulmonary embolism: A systematic review. *JAMA* 293(16):2012–2017, 2005.

Roy PM, Colombet I, Durieux P, et al: Systematic review and meta-analysis of strategies for the diagnosis of suspected pulmonary embolism. *BMJ* 331(7511):259, 2005.

Stein PD, Hull RD, Patel KC, et al: D-dimer for the exclusion of acute venous thrombosis and pulmonary embolism: A systematic review. *Ann Intern Med* 140(8):589–602, 2004.

Wells PS, Owen C, Doucette S, et al: Does this patient have deep vein thrombosis? *JAMA* 295(2):199–207, 2006.

CHAPTER
28 Chronic Obstructive Pulmonary Disease

CLINICAL CASE PROBLEM 1

A 55-Year-Old Male with a Chronic Cough

A 55-year-old male presents to your office for assessment of a chronic cough. He complains of "coughing for the last 10 years." The cough has become more bothersome lately. The cough is productive of sputum that is usually mucoid; occasionally it becomes purulent.

He has a 35-year history of smoking two packs of cigarettes a day (a history of 70 pack years). He quit smoking approximately 2 years ago.

On physical examination, his blood pressure is 160/85 mmHg. His pulse is 96 beats/minute and regular. He has a body mass index of 34. He weighs 280 pounds. He wheezes while he talks. On auscultation, adventitious breath sounds are heard in all lobes. His chest x-ray reveals significant bronchial wall thickening. There are increased markings at both lung bases.

SELECT THE BEST ANSWER TO THE FOLLOWING QUESTIONS

1. What is the most likely diagnosis in this patient?
   a. smoker's cough
   b. subacute bronchitis
   c. emphysema
   d. chronic bronchitis
   e. allergic bronchitis

2. What is the most likely cause of this condition?
   a. right-sided heart failure
   b. cor pulmonale
   c. cigarette smoking
   d. obstructive sleep apnea
   e. hypercarbia

3. Which of the following statements regarding this condition is (are) true?
   a. the disease develops in 10% to 15% of cigarette smokers
   b. cigarette smokers in whom this disease develops usually report the onset of cough with expectoration 10 to 12 years after smoking began
   c. dyspnea is noted initially only on extreme exertion; as the condition progresses, it becomes more severe and occurs with mild activity

d. pneumonia, pulmonary hypertension, cor pulmonale, and chronic respiratory failure characterize the late stages of the disease

e. all of the above are true

4. Which of the following regarding the patient is (are) true?
   a. this patient is a "pink puffer"
   b. this patient's blood gases likely will show a decreased P_{CO_2}
   c. this patient's chest x-ray will demonstrate normal to increased lung markings
   d. this patient's disease is a disease of the terminal bronchi
   e. all of the above are true

5. Which of the following pulmonary function results is not associated with the condition described here?
   a. reduced FEV_1 (forced expiratory volume)
   b. reduced FEV_1/FVC (forced vital capacity)
   c. reduced FEF_{25-75} (forced expiratory flow)
   d. decreased residual volume
   e. none of the above are associated with this disease state

6. Regarding the pathophysiology of chronic bronchitis, which of the following statements is (are) false?
   a. most histologic studies in patients with chronic bronchitis have shown an increase in the size of mucus-secreting glands as measured by the Reid index (a ratio of gland to bronchial wall thickness)
   b. smooth muscle hyperplasia occurs in patients with chronic bronchitis
   c. chronic bronchitis is characterized by chronic, excessive secretion of mucus
   d. in chronic bronchitis, there is a clear relationship between smooth muscle hyperplasia and bronchodilator responsiveness or methacholine sensitivity
   e. none of the above are false

7. Which of the following is (are) an established risk factor(s) for chronic obstructive pulmonary disease (COPD)?
   a. smoking
   b. atopy
   c. elevated levels of immunoglobulin E (IgE)
   d. bronchial hyperresponsiveness
   e. all of the above

8. Which of the following is (are) accurate regarding the role of bacteria in chronic bronchitis?
   a. the delay in mucociliary clearance allows inhaled bacteria to colonize the normally sterile airways

and to multiply, leading to further infectious exacerbations
   b. *Haemophilus influenzae, Streptococcus pneumoniae,* and *Moraxella catarrhalis* account for 75% of all exacerbations of chronic bronchitis
   c. bacteria may act synergistically with tobacco smoke to impede mucociliary clearance and allow organisms to colonize the airways further
   d. nicotine stimulates the growth of *H. influenzae*
   e. a, b, and c
   f. all of the above are true

9. Which of the following is least likely to be considered in the diagnosis of chronic bronchitis?
   a. asthma
   b. pneumothorax
   c. chronic angiotensin-converting enzyme (ACE) inhibitor therapy
   d. Gastroesophageal reflux disease
   e. postnasal drip from sinusitis

10. Which of the following statements regarding smoking cessation is true?
    a. cessation of smoking dramatically increases symptoms in patients with established COPD
    b. cessation is difficult with a high relapse rate
    c. stopping cold turkey is most successful
    d. relapse should be considered a failure on the part of the patient and clinician
    e. none of the above

11. Which medications are most effective in long-term management of COPD?
    a. beta agonists
    b. anticholinergic drugs
    c. methylxanthines
    d. inhaled glucocorticoids
    e. oral glucocorticoids

12. Which of the following drugs is (are) recommended as symptomatic management for a patient with chronic bronchitis?
    a. tiotropium
    b. salmeterol
    c. fluticasone
    d. b and c
    e. all of the above

13. Long-term home oxygen therapy is indicated in which of the patients with chronic bronchitis?
    a. all patients who have established chronic bronchitis and who have met the criteria of symptoms for at least 5 years
    b. all patients who have a resting P_{aO_2} of 55 mmHg or less

c. all patients who have a resting Pao_2 of 60 mmHg or less with evidence of chronic tissue hypoxia as demonstrated by cor pulmonale or polycythemia

d. b and c

e. all of the above

CLINICAL CASE PROBLEM 2

A Patient Whose Symptoms Are Exacerbated by Second-Hand Smoke

The patient described in Clinical Case Problem 1 is stabilized with long-term therapy. Unfortunately, during the winter holiday, he travels to his son's home in a distant state and finds himself in an environment in which six packs of cigarettes a day are being smoked by his son and his son's wife (four packs for the son and two packs for his wife). There is a layer of definite haze that hangs approximately 1 foot below all the ceilings in the house. As he sits in the house 1 day (unable to go outside or walk any distance at all because of significantly increased shortness of breath since arriving), he counts the number of ashtrays; there are 21. His son, through the haze of smoke, finally notices that his dad is out of breath and his lips appear very blue. He takes him to the nearest emergency room (ER).

The ER doctor diagnoses his condition as an acute exacerbation of chronic bronchitis. His major symptoms at this time include dyspnea, increased sputum production, and purulence. The patient's Pao_2 when measured in the ER is 44 mmHg.

14. Which of the following should be instituted as therapy for this condition?

a. low-flow oxygen

b. intravenous corticosteroids

c. oral ciprofloxacin

d. a and b only

e. all of the above

15. Which of the following organisms that have been implicated in the pathogenesis of acute exacerbations of chronic bronchitis has (have) exhibited resistance *in vivo* to ampicillin?

a. *Haemophilus influenzae*

b. *Streptococcus pneumoniae*

c. *Moraxella catarrhalis*

d. a and b only

e. all of the above

CLINICAL CASE PROBLEM 3

An 82-Year-Old Female with Shortness of Breath Recently Admitted to a Nursing Home

An 82-year-old female with dementia is admitted to your nursing home service after a recent hip fracture due to her severe osteoporosis and kyphosis. There is no documentation of COPD in her transfer records. A nurse pages you regarding this patient and reports increased shortness of breath. The nurse also informs you that the patient is a retired millworker and has a 20 pack-year smoking history with multiple hospitalizations for "respiratory problems." However, secondary to her dementia, the patient is unable to report a history of "emphysema." Although the patient was transferred that day, the full history and physical were not completed yet. The nurse reports a temperature of 97.3°F, respiratory rate of 24 breaths/minute, heart rate 96 beats/minute, blood pressure 110/66 mmHg, and diminished breath sounds through all fields with occasional wheezes. She has an involved family and the nurse gives you the daughter's telephone number.

You call and speak with the daughter who has power of attorney. She reports a long history of COPD with one prior episode of respiratory failure that required intubation and mechanical breathing. After the hospitalization for respiratory failure, her memory worsened and overall the daughter believes her mother is "failing." The daughter reports a 30-pound weight loss during the past year and notes increased frailty; she now weighs 114 pounds. The daughter starts crying on the phone and asks you to do "what you think is best." Before the daughter hangs up, however, you are able to confirm that the patient has do-not-resuscitate (DNR) and do-not-hospitalize directives.

16. Which is the least likely cause of this shortness of breath?

a. asthma exacerbation

b. congestive heart failure (CHF) exacerbation

c. COPD exacerbation

d. aspiration pneumonia

e. pulmonary embolism

17. Which is the least helpful test in the management of this case?

a. chest x-ray

b. complete blood count
c. alpha-antitrypsin deficiency
d. electrocardiogram
e. lower extremity ultrasound

18. What risk factors does this woman have for COPD?
    a. smoking history
    b. occupational exposure to respiratory irritants
    c. recurrent respiratory-related hospitalizations
    d. the presence of comorbidities: severe osteoporosis with kyphosis
    e. All of the above

19. What would be the most worrisome symptom of an acute COPD exacerbation in this woman?
    a. increased shortness of breath
    b. change in sputum production
    c. change in mental status
    d. fever
    e. chest tightness

20. What is the least realistic goal of treating this patient?
    a. improve shortness of breath
    b. improve endurance
    c. prevent additional lung damage
    d. optimize current lung function
    e. reversal of lung damage

21. A care plan would include all of the following except
    a. maximizing exercise tolerance
    b. patient education
    c. control of cough and secretions
    d. relief of anxiety and depression
    e. avoiding unnecessary, disabling, or expensive therapy

22. Which is the most appropriate nutritional recommendation for this patient?
    a. consuming infrequent large meals
    b. drinking fluids during meals
    c. consuming very hot or extremely cold foods
    d. minimizing foods that require excessive chewing
    e. consuming foods that will cause gas and bloating

23. Palliative therapy for this patient would include all of the following except
    a. hospitalization
    b. oxygen
    c. opiates
    d. benzodiazepines
    e. fluids

Clinical Case Management Problem

Describe the difference between the two major types of COPD in terms of (1) the part of the airway affected, (2) the color of lips in severely affected individual, (3) the definition of both types, (4) the pathophysiology, and (5) the causes.

Answers

1. **d.** This patient has chronic bronchitis. Chronic bronchitis is defined as cough and sputum production on most days for at least 3 months of the year for at least 2 years. Chronic bronchitis and emphysema are the two underlying conditions in COPD.

Emphysema is a destructive process involving the lung parenchyma. It is defined as abnormal permanent enlargement of air spaces distal to the terminal bronchioles accompanied by destruction of alveolar walls.

Acute bronchitis is an inflammation of the bronchi caused by an infectious agent or acute exposure to a nonspecific irritant. Acute bronchitis most often is caused by a viral infection. Acute bronchitis may occur as a complication of chronic bronchitis.

2. **c.** Chronic bronchitis most commonly is caused by cigarette smoking. Right-sided heart failure and cor pulmonale may result from chronic bronchitis and/or emphysema. Obstructive sleep apnea is often a complication of COPD. Hypercarbia (increased Pco_2 level) is a valuable prognostic sign in chronic bronchitis and allows the prediction (along with decreased Po_2) of when certain therapies, especially home oxygen, should be used.

3. **e.** Chronic bronchitis usually develops in cigarette smokers approximately 10 to 12 years after smoking initiation. Patients with chronic bronchitis have an increased susceptibility to recurrent respiratory tract infections. COPD develops in 10% to 15% of patients who are cigarette smokers. In these patients, airflow obstruction worsens over time if cigarette smoking is continued.

Dyspnea initially is noted only on extreme exertion, but as the COPD progresses, it becomes more severe and occurs with mild activity. In severe disease, dyspnea may occur at rest.

Complications of COPD include pneumonia, pulmonary hypertension, cor pulmonale, and chronic respiratory failure.

4. **c.** Patients with COPD can be classified into two basic types: type A COPD patients, or "pink puffers," and type B COPD patients, or "blue bloaters." The patient described in this question is a typical blue bloater who typically has the following characteristics: (1) is stocky or obese, (2) has cough and sputum production, (3) has normal or increased lung markings, (4) has a markedly reduced P_{O_2} and an elevated P_{CO_2}, and (5) often develops pulmonary hypertension and/or cor pulmonale. Blue bloaters have chronic bronchitis. Type A COPD pink puffers typically have the following characteristics: (1) are thin, (2) have dyspnea, (3) have hyperinflated lungs on chest x-ray, and (4) have a slightly decreased P_{O_2} and a normal or slightly decreased P_{CO_2}. Pink puffers have emphysema.

5. **d.** Chronic bronchitis is characterized by several abnormalities observed on pulmonary function testing. Abnormalities noted most frequently include (1) an increased (not decreased) residual volume, (2) a decrease in FEV_1 (the forced vital capacity in 1 second), (3) a decrease in FEV_1/FVC, and (4) a decrease in FEF_{25-75}.
COPD is divided into the following stages:

Stage 0 (at risk): FEV is normal, FEV_1/FVC is normal

Stage I (mild COPD): FEV > 80%, FEV_1/FVC < 70% predicted

Stage II (moderate COPD): FEV_1 50% to 80%, FEV_1/FVC < 70%

Stage IIa (moderate COPD): FEV_1 30% to 50%, FEV_1/FVC < 70%

Stage III (severe COPD): FEV_1 < 30%, FEV_1/FVC < 70%

6. **d.** Most mucus is secreted by subepithelial glands in the large airways. It follows that chronic bronchitis, a disorder characterized by chronic, excessive secretion of mucus, is a disease of the large airways. Most histologic studies of chronic bronchitis have shown an increase in the size of the mucus-secreting glands as measured by the Reid index (a ratio of gland to bronchial wall thickness), although no clear-cut relation between this index and the degree of airflow obstruction has been established. Patients with chronic bronchitis also have smooth muscle hyperplasia; however, unlike the situation for asthma, there is no clear-cut relationship between their responsiveness or methacholine sensitivity. Bronchial hyperresponsiveness, which is present in at least 50% of patients with COPD, may lead to dyspnea and hypoxemia.

7. **e.** It is commonly thought that cigarette smoking is the only risk factor for COPD. In fact, a number of other risk factors are implicated: (1) exposure to tobacco smoke; (2) domestic and occupational pollutants and recurrent respiratory tract infections, particularly in infancy; (3) atopy, which is characterized by eosinophilia or an increased level of serum IgE; (4) the presence of bronchial hyperresponsiveness; (5) a family history of COPD; and (6) certain protease deficiencies, such as α_1-antitrypsin deficiency, which may also be responsible for a positive family history.

8. **f.** Cigarette smoking, as the most common cause of chronic bronchitis, leads to loss of ciliated epithelium and more viscous secretions, compromising the local defenses of the respiratory tract. The delay in mucociliary clearance allows inhaled bacteria to colonize the normally sterile airways and to multiply, leading to further infectious exacerbations. *Haemophilus influenzae* is present in the sputum of approximately 60% of patients with stable chronic bronchitis. *Haemophilus influenza*, *S. pneumonia*, and *M. catarrhalis* account for 75% of all exacerbations of chronic bronchitis and 85% to 95% of bacterial exacerbations. *Haemophilus influenzae* may act synergistically with tobacco smoke to impede mucociliary clearance and allow further multiplication and colonization of the airway. By-products of *H. influenzae* metabolism have been shown to cause further impairment of ciliated cells *in vitro*, stimulate mucus production, and secrete IgA protease that may further impair host defenses. In addition, nicotine has been shown to stimulate the growth of this organism, and *H. influenzae* has been shown to engender an immune reaction in the airways.

9. **b.** The diagnosis of chronic bronchitis rests on clinical criteria that have already been described. There are no characteristic physical findings and no specific radiographic changes or laboratory features diagnostic of this disease.
The differential diagnosis of chronic cough, however, must be considered. This includes (1) asthma, (2) postnasal drip, (3) gastroesophageal reflux, (4) foreign body aspiration, (5) congestive heart failure, (6) bronchiectasis, and (7) chronic ACE inhibitor therapy (15% of patients taking ACE inhibitors develop a chronic cough).

10. **b.** Tobacco dependence is a chronic disease. Relapse is common and reflects the nature of dependence: It should not be regarded as a failure on the part of either the clinician or the patient. The average smoker makes three or four attempts to quit before success. Frequent physician counseling and reinforcement makes the attempts more successful. In addition to referrals to formal smoking cessation programs, consider nicotine replacement. Numerous studies indicate that nicotine replacement in any form (gum, lozenge, or transdermal patch) increases long-term cessation.

11. **b.** Three types of bronchodilator are in common clinical use: beta agonist, anticholinergic drugs, and methylxanthines. Despite differences in their site of action, the most important consequence of action is smooth muscle relaxation. Tiotropium improves health status and reduces exacerbations compared to ipratropium. Theophylline is a weak bronchodilator with some anti-inflammatory properties. Long-acting beta agonists improve health to a greater extent than short-acting beta agonists.

12. **d.** Combining medications of different classes is a convenient way of delivering treatment and obtaining better results. Combining long-acting inhaled beta agonists and inhaled corticosteroids shows improvement in pulmonary function and a reduction in symptoms. The TORCH study, published in the *New England Journal of Medicine* in February 2007, found significant advantages for health status, frequency of exacerbations, use of oral steroids, and protection against decline in lung function. *In vitro* and *in vivo* evidence suggests that a mechanistic interaction at the molecular level between inhaled corticosteroids and beta agonists may explain the improved efficacy of therapy with combination therapy compared with either medication alone.

13. **d.** Symptomatic therapy for patients with chronic bronchitis includes the use of (1) inhaled bronchodilators, (2) oral bronchodilators, (3) inhaled corticosteroids, (4) oral corticosteroids, (5) inhaled anticholinergics, (6) home oxygen therapy, and (7) rehabilitation programs.

The use of inhaled bronchodilators by patients with airflow obstruction may increase flow rates and reduce dyspnea. Inhaled anticholinergic agents appear to produce greater bronchodilatation than inhaled β_2 agonists in COPD, with fewer side effects. This may be related to increased cholinergic tone in the airways as the degree of obstruction progresses. Combination therapy with agents from both groups may have an additive effect in some patients. Patients who demonstrate symptomatic or physiologic improvement, or both, with these medications should be maintained on the inhaled drugs indefinitely. In patients who remain symptomatic while taking inhaled bronchodilators, a trial of an oral theophylline medication is warranted. These medications are weaker bronchodilators than inhaled anticholinergics or beta agonist drugs but may have additional beneficial effects in chronic bronchitis by increasing respiratory muscle strength and endurance, improving mucociliary clearance, and increasing central respiratory drive, all of which may lead to a symptomatic improvement in patients with the disease.

The benefits of home oxygen therapy have been clearly demonstrated in major clinical trials. To be considered candidates for treatment, patients must (1) be in a stable clinical state, (2) have a resting Pao$_2$ of 55 mmHg or less, or (3) have a Pao$_2$ of 60 mmHg with evidence of chronic tissue hypoxia as demonstrated by cor pulmonale or polycythemia. In properly selected patients, the use of home oxygen for more than 18 hours a day may increase the life span of patients with COPD by 6 or 7 years. Oxygen is also indicated in patients with signs and symptoms of cor pulmonale or pulmonary hypertension or with desaturation during sleep.

14. **e.** Treatment of an acute exacerbation of chronic bronchitis provides symptomatic relief and prevents any transient decline in pulmonary function. Low-flow oxygen should be instituted if hypoxemia is present (as in this case). The goal of oxygen therapy in this case is to get the Pao$_2$ higher than 60 mmHg. In addition, oral or intravenous corticosteroids should be given because they have been shown to hasten the resolution of patients in the acute exacerbation phase of chronic bronchitis.

Patients with all three of the following "acute exacerbative symptoms" have been shown to benefit from antibiotic therapy: (1) increasing dyspnea, (2) increased sputum production, and (3) purulence of sputum. In patients with fewer than the three symptoms, the situation is less clear.

15. **e.** Antibiotic choices obviously should be based on both host and pathogen factors. The latter relate to resistance problems. The three most common isolates associated with acute exacerbations of chronic bronchitis are *H. influenzae*, *S. pneumoniae*, and *M. catarrhalis*.

All have exhibited resistance *in vivo* to ampicillin and other first-line agents. Nevertheless, most U.S. and international guidelines recommend initial treatment of acute exacerbations of chronic bronchitis with amoxicillin or tetracycline derivatives. Other potential first-line agents include trimethoprim–sulfamethoxazole and cefaclor. In the most complicated cases of acute exacerbation of chronic bronchitis, most guidelines recommend quinolones, macrolides, and a second- or third-generation cephalosporin as the initial agent.

16. **a.** Shortness of breath is a common issue among newly admitted residents of nursing homes. Frequently, the information/history of COPD is not communicated to the long-term care facility. Symptoms of CHF, asthma, or pulmonary embolism are similar in the frail elderly. The patient recently had hip surgery; therefore, she is at an increased risk for pulmonary embolism. The patient has a history of dementia; with her recent surgery, this predisposes her to dysphagia and aspiration. Asthma can present later in life but is unlikely.

17. **c.** A physical examination is rarely diagnostic in mild COPD. The following tests are recommended to develop a differential diagnosis: (1) chest x-ray, (2) complete blood count, (3) chemistry profile, (4) electrocardiogram, and (5) lower extremity ultrasound (which will help in the evaluation of a pulmonary embolism). Testing for α-antitrypsin deficiency is limited to younger patients with COPD.

18. **e.** Few symptoms and physical signs clearly differentiate COPD from other respiratory conditions, such as asthma and CHF. It is important that the history of a new patient with known or suspected COPD includes (1) exposure to smoking, (2) exposure to occupational irritants, (3) history of exacerbations or previous hospitalizations for respiratory disorders, and (4) the presence of comorbidities that may contribute to restriction of activity.

19. **c.** Patients with COPD need frequent assessments. A history of prior exacerbations as well as knowledge of precipitating events is helpful in the evaluation of the patient's stability. Increased shortness of breath with or without wheezing, change in sputum production, chest tightness, and fever may signal an acute exacerbation. A change in mental status is particularly worrisome and warrants urgent medical evaluation. This may represent hypoxia and respiratory decompensation.

20. **e.** COPD is a chronic disorder that is only partially reversible. Complete resolution of symptoms and reversal of damage is not a realistic goal. It is most important to focus on improving quality of life and preventing lung damage rather than "curing" the damage already suffered.

21. **b.** When designing a care plan, it is important to take into account the patient's comorbidities, prognosis, life expectancy, and individual preference. Education would be appropriate for patients without dementia, but in this situation, the patient would not retain information.

22. **d.** It is important to maintain food nutrition and healthy body weight. Ventilatory muscles have enhanced energy requirements as COPD progresses. Patients with chronic shortness of breath may not eat; it is important to consume foods that are easy to eat. Patients should have a healthy diet, and underweight patients should eat nutritionally dense foods.

23. **a.** If a patient is DNR, care should be palliative. Treatment of end-stage COPD may include fluids, oxygen, opiates, and benzodiazepines. End-of-life care must balance the adverse effects of respiratory depression and decreased mental alertness against the symptomatic relief they offer patients.

Solution to the Clinical Case Management Problem

1. The two forms of COPD are chronic bronchitis and emphysema.
   a. Chronic bronchitis affects the large airways of the lung.
   b. Emphysema affects the terminal bronchi.
2. The color of lips in severely affected individuals is:
   a. Blue; the "blue bloater" equals chronic bronchitis.
   b. Pink; the "pink puffer" equals emphysema.
3. Definitions
   a. Chronic bronchitis: Excessive cough, productive of sputum on most days for at least 3 months a year during at least 2 consecutive years.
   b. Emphysema: Defined histologically by abnormal permanent enlargement, without obvious fibrosis, of the airspaces distal to the terminal bronchi, accompanied by destruction of their walls.
4. Pathophysiology
   a. Chronic bronchitis
      i. chronic, excessive secretion of mucus
      ii. increase in the size of the mucus-secreting cells
      iii. smooth muscle hyperplasia
      iv. bronchial airway hyperresponsiveness
   b. Emphysema
      i. distal airspace enlargement
      ii. no significant fibrosis
      iii. loss of alveolar attachments
      iv. decrease in elastic recoil
      v. increase in lung compliance
      vi. hyperinflation
      vii. ventilation–perfusion mismatching
5. Causes
   Most cases of both chronic bronchitis and emphysema are the result of cigarette smoking; α_1-antitrypsin deficiency is a factor in some cases of emphysema.

Summary

1. Definitions
See Solution to the Clinical Case Management Problem.

2. Pathophysiology
See Solution to the Clinical Case Management Problem.

3. Differentiation of disease entities in COPD
See Solution to the Clinical Case Management Problem.

4. Signs and symptoms
a. Symptoms: dyspnea, cough, sputum production, and sputum purulence. When cor pulmonale and right-sided heart failure are present, there is extremity swelling.
b. Signs: increased respiratory rate, respiratory distress, cyanosis, barrel chest, distant heart sounds, and increased jugular venous pressure.
c. Three most important signs/symptoms indicating deterioration are (i) increasing dyspnea, (ii) increased sputum volume, and (iii) increased purulence.

5. Pulmonary function test abnormalities
a. Decreased FEV_1
b. Decreased ratio of FEV_1/FVC
c. Decreased FEF_{25-75}
d. Increased residual volume
e. Normal to increased functional residual capacity
f. Decreased diffusion capacity

6. Pathologic organisms associated with infection in COPD
a. *Haemophilus influenzae*
b. *Streptococcus pneumoniae*
c. *Moraxella catarrhalis*

7. Treatment
a. Bronchodilators
   i. The best single agent for long-term treatment in chronic bronchitis is an inhaled anticholinergic ipratropium (Atrovent) or tiotropium bromide (Spiriva).
   ii. Beta agonists should be combined with (i) above.
b. Corticosteroids: Routine use of inhaled corticosteroids cannot be recommended in chronic care. Corticosteroids (both inhaled and intravenous/oral) are most helpful in acute exacerbations. Macrolides in atypical cases are expected.
c. Antibiotics: Routine prophylactic use of antibiotics cannot be recommended. They are most useful in acute exacerbations if all three of the following are present: (i) increasing dyspnea, (ii) increasing sputum production, and (iii) increasing sputum purulence.

   Antibiotics of choice include ampicillin, trimethoprim–sulfamethoxazole, amoxicillin, doxycycline, and cefaclor. Floxin is effective for severe exacerbations, and macrolides should be used if atypical organisms are suspected. Note: Resistance is constantly increasing and recommendations may rapidly change.
d. Home oxygen: Home oxygen is indicated if Pao_2 is 55 mmHg or less at rest or if Pao_2 is 60 mmHg with evidence of chronic tissue hypoxia as demonstrated by cor pulmonale or polycythemia.
e. Diuretics: Use of diuretics is indicated only for treatment of cor pulmonale and right-sided heart failure.
f. Smoking cessation: At any time in the course of COPD, smoking cessation can be and is of benefit. Do not accept "I've smoked too long and I am too old to quit."
g. Counseling/support groups: Group therapy with other patients with COPD often helps the patient come to terms with the disease.

Suggested Reading

American Academy of Family Practice: COPD: Putting guidelines into practice (Web program). Available at www.aafp.org/online/en/home/cme/selfstudy/cases/copd.html.

American Medical Directors Association: *COPD Management in the Long-Term Care Setting: Clinical Practice Guidelines.* Columbia, MD: American Medical Directors Association, 2003.

Aull L: Pharmacologic management of chronic obstructive pulmonary disease in the elderly. *Ann Long-Term Care* 14(12):27–35, 2006.

Celli BR, MacNee W, committee members: Standards for the diagnosis and treatment of patients with COPD: A summary of the ATS/ERS position paper. *Eur Respir J,* 23:932–946, 2004.

Hanania N, Darken P, Horstman D, et al: The efficacy and safety of fluticasone propionate 250 mcg/salmeterol 50 mcg combined in the diskus inhaler for the treatment of COPD. *Chest* 124:834–843, 2003.

Rabe KF: Treating COPD—The TORCH trial, P values and the Dodo. *N Engl J Med* 356:8, 2007.

CLINICAL CASE PROBLEM 1

A 22-Year-Old Male with a Chronic Cough

A 22-year-old male presents to your office for assessment of a chronic cough. He has just moved to your city and will be attending the university there. He has moved into an apartment in the basement of a house.

As soon as he moved in, he began to notice a chronic, nonproductive cough associated with shortness of breath. He has never had these symptoms before, and he has no known allergies. When he leaves for school for the day, the symptoms disappear. The symptoms are definitely worse at night.

His landlady has three cats. He did not think he was allergic to cats, but now he thinks that might be the problem.

On examination, his respiratory rate is 16 breaths/minutes and regular. He is in no distress at the present time. There are a few expiratory rhonchi heard in all lobes. His blood pressure is 120/70 mmHg, and his pulse is 72 beats/minute and regular.

SELECT THE BEST ANSWER TO THE FOLLOWING QUESTIONS

1. What is the most likely diagnosis in this patient?
   a. paroxysmal nocturnal cough syndrome
   b. hyporesponsive airways disease
   c. cough variant asthma
   d. allergic bronchitis
   e. none of the above

2. For children, which of the following statements is (are) true?
   a. it is sometimes difficult to differentiate asthma from bronchiolitis
   b. some children with an episode of bronchiolitis do not develop asthma
   c. the relationships among bronchiolitis, ongoing bronchial hyperactivity, and asthma are unclear, although many children with bronchiolitis develop asthma
   d. a, b, and c
   e. none of the above

3. Which of the following is (are) included in the working definition of asthma?
   a. reversible airway obstruction
   b. bronchial airway inflammation
   c. bronchial airway hyper-responsiveness to a variety of stimuli
   d. expiratory rhonchi
   e. a, b, and c
   f. all of the above

4. Which of the following statements on incidence and mortality regarding asthma is (are) false?
   a. the mortality from asthma is decreasing (presumably because of improved therapies)
   b. the number of cases of asthma from various causes continues to increase at a rapid rate
   c. asthma mortality tends to be higher in inner cities in minorities
   d. all of the above statements are false
   e. none of the above statements are false

5. Asthma, on a pathophysiologic basis, is primarily:
   a. a bronchoconstricting process
   b. an allergenic stimulus process
   c. an inflammatory process
   d. a bronchial hyper-reactivity process
   e. an immunoglobulin E-mediated antigen–antibody reaction

6. Following antigenic stimulation of the bronchial airway, which cell is most responsible for the beginning of the airway's response?
   a. the basophil
   b. the mast cell
   c. the eosinophil
   d. the bronchial epithelial cell
   e. the bronchial mucus-producing goblet cells

7. What is (are) the substance(s) released by the cell that is most responsible for the beginning of the airway's response?
   a. histamine
   b. proteolytic enzymes
   c. heparin
   d. chemotactic factors
   e. all of the above

8. The parameter most useful in evaluating a patient with asthma is
   a. peak flow
   b. peak inspiratory flow rate
   c. the forced expiratory volume in 1 second (FEV_1)
   d. none of the above
   e. all of the above

9. The main classification classes for asthma as provided by the American Academy of Allergy, Asthma, and Immunology include
   a. severe persistent
   b. moderate persistent
   c. mild persistent
   d. mild intermittent
   e. all of the above

10. The reversible airflow obstruction seen in asthma results from which of the following?
    a. bronchoconstriction
    b. mucus plug formation
    c. edema
    d. a and b
    e. all of the above

11. Which of the following is (are) a clinical hallmark(s) of asthma?
    a. cough
    b. nocturnal dyspnea
    c. wheezing
    d. shortness of breath
    e. a, c, and d

12. Which of the following is (are) associated with an increase in asthma incidence?
    a. migration from a rural to urban environment
    b. migration from more developed countries to Indonesia, Greece, or India
    c. migration from a Third World country to a Westernized country
    d. migration to from temperate to more tropical countries
    e. a and c

CLINICAL CASE PROBLEM 2

A 24-Year-Old Runner with Wheezing and Shortness of Breath

A 24-year-old, otherwise healthy, woman cross-country runner reports wheezing and shortness of breath only when exercising, especially in the cold air. These symptoms are getting worse.

13. True statements regarding exercise-induced bronchospasm (EIB) include all of the following except
    a. most patients with EIB already have clinically recognized asthma
    b. EIB can occur in exercisers with no history or other symptoms of asthma
    c. during the past few decades, the prevalence of EIB has increased in elite athletes

d. EIB is found especially in those who engage in endurance sports
e. EIB is accurately diagnosed by the characteristic history

14. Which of the following is the agent of choice for the treatment of acute symptoms in these circumstances?
    a. inhaled β_2-agonists
    b. oral aminophylline
    c. inhaled anticholinergics
    d. inhaled sodium cromoglycate
    e. oral corticosteroids

15. What is the mechanism of action of the agent of choice in question 14?
    a. mast cell stabilizer
    b. inhibitor of early phase reaction
    c. inhibitor of late-phase reaction
    d. bronchodilator
    e. none of the above

16. What is (are) the best medication(s) to give immediately before exercise to prevent an EIB attack?
    a. β_2-agonist such as albuterol or a mast cell stabilizer such as cromolyn or nedocromil inhaler
    b. inhaled epinephrine
    c. an inhaled anticholinergic such as Atrovent
    d. inhaled steroid
    e. a and b

17. Nonpharmacologic means of reducing EIB include all of the following except
    a. a high-salt diet may decrease EIB by improving vascular volume
    b. nose breathing
    c. warming up for a 5-kilometer run by doing short sprints 20 minutes beforehand
    d. avoid exercising in cold, dry air
    e. a and c are both false

18. For a patient with EIB who has frequent symptoms despite nonpharmacologic treatment modalities and a β_2-agonist for acute symptoms, choose the list of long-term medications for better control in the correct order of efficacy (most effective to least effective):
    a. salmeterol inhaled (Serevent) > inhaled corticosteroid > montelukast (Singulair) > theophylline
    b. cromolyn inhaled (Intal) > montelukast (Singulair) > theophylline > salmeterol inhaled (Serevent)
    c. tiotropium inhaled (Spiriva) > cromolyn inhaled (Intal) > montelukast (Singulair) > theophylline

d. inhaled corticosteroid > montelukast (Singulair) > salmeterol inhaled (Serevent) > theophylline

e. salmeterol inhaled (Serevent) > cromolyn inhaled (Intal) > montelukast (Singulair) > theophylline

19. Vocal cord dysfunction (VCD) can masquerade as EIB or asthma. Characteristics of VCD include all of the following except
    a. hallmark symptoms include a sense of throat closing or choking with severe shortness of breath
    b. it is usually found in highly competitive adolescent and young adult men
    c. a bronchial provocation challenge test often needs to be done to exclude other entities such as EIB
    d. directly witnessing an attack during exercise is often key in making a diagnosis
    e. it usually occurs in 20- to 40-year-old women, often with a history of a psychological disorder

20. What are the chief characteristics of exercise-induced hyperventilation?
    a. excess CO_2 buildup during exercise leading to compensatory deep rapid breathing
    b. loss of control of breathing, often during intense exercise, resulting in rapid shallow breaths
    c. a method of banking oxygen just prior to intense exercise that may be mistaken for EIB
    d. a recurrent syndrome triggered by even mild exercise in patients with panic disorder
    e. none of the above

CLINICAL CASE PROBLEM 3

A 30-Year-Old New Patient with Chronic Asthma

Mr. Smith is a 30-year-old accountant who has noticed that his asthma, which he has had since he was a young child, has gotten worse. He has recently moved from a rural area to the urban area where you practice.

21. Which of the following stepped care classifications used to guide pharmacotherapy in asthma requires environmental control as the necessary first step for his treatment?
    a. mild intermittent asthma
    b. mild persistent asthma
    c. moderate persistent asthma
    d. severe persistent asthma
    e. all of the above

22. All the following are characteristics of mild persistent asthma except

a. symptoms occurring more than twice a week but less than once a day
b. exacerbations that affect activity
c. peak expiratory flow (PEF) greater than 80% of personal best
d. PEF variability of 20% to 30%
e. nocturnal symptoms two or three times per week

23. Which of the following most accurately describes the preferred pharmacologic treatment of moderate persistent asthma in adults?
    a. inhaled sodium cromoglycate alone
    b. inhaled β_2-agonists alone
    c. inhaled corticosteroids alone
    d. daily inhaled corticosteroids plus long-acting inhaled β_2-agonists, if needed
    e. inhaled sodium cromoglycate continually plus intermittent inhaled β_2-agonists

24. All the following are characteristics of severe persistent asthma except
    a. continual symptoms
    b. frequent exacerbations that may last days
    c. infrequent nighttime symptoms
    d. PEF rates less than 60% of personal best
    e. PEF variability of more than 30%

25. Pharmacotherapy of severe persistent asthma includes
    a. high-dose steroids via mask
    b. long-acting bronchodilator
    c. sustained-released theophylline
    d. quick relief with an inhaled β_2-agonist as needed
    e. all of the above

26. In a patient whose PEF rate is less than 50% of personal best, suggesting a severe exacerbation, the initial home treatment includes which of the following?
    a. an inhaled short-acting β_2-agonist administered three times via metered-dosed inhaler or one time via nebulizer
    b. inhaled cromolyn, three times via metered-dosed inhaler or one time via nebulizer
    c. an inhaled corticosteroid, administered three times via metered-dosed inhaler or one time via nebulizer
    d. subcutaneous self-administered epinephrine
    e. none of the above

27. Which of the following pulmonary function tests is the most useful for diagnosis of asthma?
    a. decreased forced vital capacity (FVC)
    b. increased residual volume
    c. a ratio of FEV_1/FVC of 75%
    d. increased functional residual capacity
    e. increased total lung capacity

28. Which of the following pulmonary function tests is most easily performed at home?
   a. FEV_1/FVC ratio
   b. FCV
   c. midexpiratory flow rate
   d. PEF rate
   e. residual volume

29. Which of the following is the most common abnormality observed on the chest x-ray of a patient with asthma?
   a. hyperinflation
   b. increased bronchial markings
   c. atelectasis
   d. flattening of the diaphragm
   e. all of the above are equally common

30. What is the most common abnormality seen on physical examination of a patient with asthma?
   a. increased respiratory rate
   b. inspiratory rales
   c. inspiratory rhonchi
   d. expiratory rales
   e. expiratory wheezes

31. Environmental control as a part of the therapeutic intervention involves a search for and elimination of which of the following agents from the patient's environment?
   a. air pollution
   b. pollens, molds, mites, cockroaches, and pets
   c. tobacco smoke, wood stoves, and fumes
   d. workplace exposures
   e. sulfates, aspirin, other nonsteroidal anti-inflammatory drugs, and other potential offending drugs
   f. all of the above

32. Pure cough variant asthma has which of the following characteristics?
   a. patients often have to go from doctor to doctor until someone makes the diagnosis
   b. patients are treated in the same manner as non-cough variant asthma
   c. cough variant asthma is very uncommon
   d. a and b
   e. all of the above

33. A patient who presents to the emergency room in acute respiratory distress resulting from a severe attack of asthma should be treated with all of the following except
   a. warm, humidified, high-flow-rate oxygen
   b. constant bedside monitoring
   c. intravenous corticosteroids
   d. intravenous fluids
   e. intravenous antibiotics

34. Which of the following statements regarding childhood asthma is (are) false?
   a. there is a very significant hereditary component to the probability of a child acquiring asthma
   b. asthma in children is often associated with parental smoking
   c. asthmatic children are often allergic to aspirin (acetylsalicylic acid)
   d. inhaled corticosteroids, administered properly, do not pose a major risk or hazard to childhood growth
   e. many children who are asthmatic go on to outgrow it completely

35. Which of the following viral agents has been implicated as a cause of asthma?
   a. respiratory syncytial virus
   b. parainfluenza virus
   c. adenovirus
   d. rhinovirus
   e. influenza virus

36. Long-acting β_2-agonists such as salmeterol
   a. improve peak flow levels and symptoms in asthma patients not adequately controlled on inhaled corticosteroids alone
   b. are appropriately used as rescue inhalers
   c. are associated with increased asthma-related hospitalization and death
   d. help decrease bronchial inflammation
   e. a and c

Clinical Case Management Problem

Jill is a 25-year-old with newly diagnosed moderate persistent asthma who has been found on allergy testing to be severely allergic to dust mites and mold and moderately allergic to cats and tree pollens common to her area. She recently moved into a townhouse with wood floors on the first and second floors but wall-to-wall carpeting in her bedroom. There are many throw rugs throughout the house. She has approximately 10 houseplants. There is an unfinished basement that periodically has minor flooding during heavy rainstorms. She has a cat that likes to sleep on her bed during the day. Heating is via a heat pump with electric heating backup that is distributed through forced hot air vents. She does not have much furniture for her new home but plans to make some major purchases within the near future.

How would you advise Jill on environmental controls to help her asthma?

Answers

1. c. This patient has cough variant asthma. Physicians should be aware that cough variant asthma is particularly common in children but can occur, as in this case, in adults as well. The diagnosis is often missed because in many cases there is no wheezing.

2. d. First, it is sometimes difficult to differentiate on the basis of symptoms, signs, and laboratory findings between asthma and bronchiolitis. Second, some children with an episode of bronchiolitis do not develop asthma. Third, the relationship between bronchiolitis and asthma is unclear. There is good evidence that bronchiolitis may be a risk factor for asthma and may predispose to asthma.

3. e. The current working definition of asthma is as follows: (1) a lung disease with airway obstruction that is usually reversible, (2) a lung disease that is characterized by airway inflammation, and (3) a lung disease that is characterized by increased bronchial hyperresponsiveness to various stimuli.

4. a. The morbidity and mortality from asthma are increasing, not decreasing. Asthma is often referred to as an obstructive lung disease manifested by recurring wheezing. The obstruction is secondary to inflammation, mucosal edema, mucous hypersecretion, and smooth muscle contraction.

Asthma affects more than 17 million Americans each year. Despite efforts to provide better diagnostics, prevention, and treatment, the prevalence of and mortality from asthma continue to increase.

5. c. Our understanding of the pathophysiology of asthma has undergone considerable change in the past few years. This has had a substantial impact on treatment. Asthma is now recognized as an inflammatory disorder. Although bronchoconstriction and bronchial hyper-reactivity are characteristics of asthma, the basic underlying pathophysiologic process is inflammation in the bronchial wall.

6. b. For further comment, see answer 11.

7. e. For further comment, see answer 11.

8. c. The FEV_1 is the most useful parameter in evaluating patients with asthma. The rate in disciplined patients is helpful in following lung function, especially when exposed to various allergens. For further comment, see answer 11.

9. e. These characteristic classes are important to identify because they lead to a stepwise approach to the identification and treatment of asthma. For further comment, see answer 11.

10. e. For further comment, see answer 11.

11. e. The diagnosis of asthma is often made on the basis of a typical history of abrupt dyspnea, with a dry, nonproductive cough and wheezing.

Questions 6 through 11 describe the pathophysiology of asthma. The events are as follows:

Event 1: Beginning of the response of the bronchial wall to the particular antigenic stimulation.

Event 2: Antigenic stimulation leads to mast cell degranulation.

Event 3: Mast cell degranulation leads to the following:
- Immediate release of preformed mediators from granules.
- Release of secondary mediators, including (i) histamine, (ii) chemotactic factors, (iii) proteolytic enzymes, and (iv) heparin.

Event 4: The release of these mediators leads to significant smooth muscle bronchoconstriction.

Event 5: The initial bronchial constriction leads to recruitment of other inflammatory cells, including neutrophils, eosinophils, and mononuclear cells.

Event 6: The recruitment of these "secondary mediator cells" has demonstrated the release of cytokines, vasoactive factors, and arachidonic acid metabolites.

Event 7: Activation of epithelial and endothelial cells occurs, enhancing inflammatory responses.

Event 8: Release of interleukins 3 to 6, tumor necrosis factor, and interferon-gamma has been demonstrated in the inflammatory response.

The importance of these series of events is as follows:

- The early phase reaction of asthma is mediated by the "primary mediators": neutrophils, eosinophils, and mononuclear cells.
- The late-phase reaction of asthma is mediated by the "secondary mediators": cytokines, vasoactive factors, and arachidonic acid metabolites.
  Important summary points include the following:
- Asthma is a chronic inflammatory disorder of the lower airways characterized by episodes of acute symptomatic exacerbations overlaying chronic inflammation. Inflammation results in the following:
  - Increased bronchial hyperresponsiveness to stimuli
  - Reversible airflow obstruction by bronchoconstriction, mucus plug formation, and edema
- Atopy is a predisposing factor in many patients.

12. **e.** Asthma incidence increases with migration from rural or Third World countries to Westernized or urban environments. The cause of this is unknown, and it may include exposure to multiple antigens, pollution, the effects of a stressful lifestyle, and alterations in diet.

13. **e.** EIB occurs commonly in known asthmatics (up to 80%), but it can occur in isolation with no other asthma symptoms. Endurance sports especially increase the volume of air contaminated with allergens and pollutants that are believed to injure the airways and trigger EIB. Up to one fifth of recent Olympic team members in endurance sports have been diagnosed with EIB—more than twice that reported in the 1970s. Diagnosis based only on a history of exercise-induced respiratory symptoms has been shown to be quite inaccurate. The differential diagnosis of EIB includes VCD, exercise-induced hyperventilation, and poor fitness, as well as cardiac causes. If symptoms do not improve with standard treatment, assessment of FEV_1 via spirometry with a bronchial provocation test may be indicated. Nose breathing or the wearing of masks may help EIB. Warming up with brief sprints of submaximal workouts may markedly reduce bronchospasm during exercise performed soon thereafter, perhaps by inducing a refractory period, as well as improving blood flow and hydration of the bronchial tubes.

Pharmacologic preexercise treatment of EIB includes mast cell stabilizers such as cromolyn or nedocromil and β_2-agonists. Short-acting β_2-agonists such as albuterol are the treatment of choice for acute EIB symptoms. Inhaled corticosteroids and leukotriene inhibitors help reduce EIB if long-term maintenance treatment is needed.

14. **a.** The agent of choice for acute symptoms due to exercise-induced or cold air-induced asthma is a short-acting β_2-agonist, such as albuterol. See answer 13.

15. **d.** Albuterol works as a bronchodilator. See answer 13.

16. **a.** β_2-Agonists such as albuterol or mast cell stabilizers such as cromolyn are the best preexercise treatments for EIB. Inhaled albuterol should be taken 15 to 30 minutes prior to exercise. Cromolyn inhaler should be taken 10 to 60 minutes prior to exercise. Cromolyn lasts approximately 2 hours, whereas nedocromil lasts up to 4 hours. Both have minimal side effects. See answer 13.

17. **a.** Warming up, such as by doing sprints, helps improve blood flow and hydration of the bronchial tubes and induce a refractory period that may reduce EIB. Breathing through the nose ("nature's humidifier") or wearing a mask if practical may also help. Increased sodium has not been shown to help and may actually worsen bronchial hypersensitivity. See answer 13.

18. **d.** Inhaled corticosteroids are generally the treatment of choice for long-term management of difficult to treat EIB, just as they are for asthma in general. Leukotriene inhibitors are effective but less efficacious. Long-term β_2-agonists such as salmeterol may work but reduce acute bronchoprotection. Theophylline has very limited use in EIB. Tiotropium is indicated for chronic obstructive pulmonary disease, not EIB. See answer 13.

19. **b.** VCD is characterized by abnormal closing of the vocal cords during exercise leading to a sense of throat tightness, choking, and dyspnea with inspiratory stridor. These symptoms resolve within minutes of stopping exercise. It is thought to be largely psychogenic and occurs mainly in 20- to 40-year-old women who are anxious or depressed or have a history of other psychiatric disorders. Bronchial provocation tests are often needed to rule out other entities. Direct witnessing of an attack, in which the exerciser chokes, leans forward, and complains of a strangling sensation in the throat, can help make the diagnosis.

20. **b.** Exercise-induced hyperventilation is a relatively common disorder in athletes in which they lose control of their breathing and breath high in the chest with rapid shallow breathes rather than using the abdominal muscles. It can coexist with EIB. Patients will complain of throat tightness and shortness of breath. Laryngoscopy is required to rule out VCD, and a bronchial provocation test may be required to rule out or clarify if there is also EIB. It is important to suspect in the exerciser who is not responding to the usual treatment of EIB. Treatment consists of abdominal breath training exercises, often with the assistance of a psychologist.

21. **e.** All of the above.

22. **e.** The characteristics of mild persistent asthma include symptoms twice a week but less than once a day. Exacerbations may affect activity. Nighttime symptoms occur more than twice per month, FEV_1 or PEF is 80% or more, and PEF variation is 20% to 30%.

23. **d.** The pharmacotherapy for moderate persistent asthma in adults and children 5 years of age or older includes the use of a daily medium-dose inhaled corticosteroid and the addition, if needed, of a long-acting inhaled β_2-agonist or sustained-released theophylline.

24. c. Infrequent nighttime symptoms is incorrect. Nighttime symptoms occur frequently.

25. e. The treatment for severe persistent asthma includes the following: (1) anti-inflammatory treatment with an inhaled corticosteroid, (2) long-acting bronchodilators with inhaled β_2-agonists, (3) sustained-released theophylline or long-acting β_2-agonist tablets, and (4) corticosteroid tablets or syrup (2 mg/kg/day, with no more than 60 mg/day). Short-acting inhaled β_2-agonists can be used as needed to control symptoms.

26. a. A PEF less than 50% of personal best suggests a severe exacerbation. Initial treatment should include an inhaled short-acting β_2-agonist administered three times via metered-dosed inhaler or one time via nebulizer. If the PEF rate remains less than 50% of personal best or wheezing and shortness of breath persist, the patient should repeat the β_2-agonist and proceed to the nearest emergency room.

27. c. Remember, however, that FEV_1 is most sensitive in evaluating patients with asthma.

28. d. The PEF rate is a useful tool for clinician assessment and patient self-assessment of their asthma. It is also useful to monitor and change therapy and to diagnose exacerbations. Patients should establish their personal best PEF rate. PEF requires maximal effort and therefore is not useful if the patient does not cooperate. This is established after therapy extinguishes symptoms. For 2 or 3 weeks, the patient records daily his or her PEF rate in the early afternoon with the same meter. An average is obtained. The PEF rate should be recalculated every 6 months to account for growth in children or disease progression.

29. b. Increased bronchial markings is the most common abnormality observed on the chest x-ray in a patient with asthma.

30. a. The following is an overview of the clinical findings and their importance in asthma.

Physical examination signs and symptoms: (1) increased respiratory rate; (2) use of accessory muscles of respiration (intercostals, sternocleidomastoid, and scalene muscles); (3) dyspnea and anxiety; (4) the most characteristic lung finding on auscultation is expiratory rhonchi (wheezes), which are high-pitched sounds that occur when air has to travel through a constricted or inflamed passageway; (5) nasal flaring; (6) cyanosis in severe cases (lips); and (7) paroxysmal cough.

Chest x-ray findings: (1) The most characteristic chest x-ray abnormality in asthma is the presence of increased bronchial wall markings (This is most prominent when viewed from the end-on position. This finding results from the increase in the thickness of the bronchial wall and changes in the epithelium, which are associated with inflammation. These changes are translated into increased radio-opacity.); and (2) there is also flattening of the diaphragm in some cases as a result of chronic inflammation and use of the accessory muscles of respiration.

The most useful pulmonary function tests: (1) PEF rate (discussed previously); (2) FEV_1/FVC in percentage (normal 80%) (This measures the amount of air volume that can be expressed in 1 second over the total amount of lung air volume that can be expressed. It is by far the most important test done in a spirometry laboratory for the diagnosis and management of asthma.); (3) MEF_{25-75} in percentage (normal 75%). (This is the maximum expiratory flow that occurs between 25% and 75% of the vital capacity.)

31. f. All of the above.

32. d. The following features of cough variant asthma should be borne in mind: First, cough variant asthma is very common. At least 33% of children with asthma will have only the cough, no wheezing. Second, adults, as with the patient described, may also develop cough variant asthma.

33. e. An acute, severe asthmatic attack is an emergency. The basic elements of treatment are as follows: (1) give inhaled β_2-agonist via nebulizer; (2) ensure the patient is sitting up; (3) immediately give the patient warm, humidified 100% oxygen via a Venturi mask; (4) start two intravenous lines; (5) begin an intravenous corticosteroid immediately; (6) obtain blood gases and electrolytes analyses; (7) monitor vital signs continuously (with an electrocardiogram hooked into the main computer at the nurses' desk); and (8) once the patient is stable, transfer him or her to an observation unit ward if this has been a severe attack and you have had trouble controlling it—do not discharge the patient.

34. e. First, there is a very significant heredity component to asthma. If one parent has it, the child may have up to a 25% risk. If two parents have it, the child's risk may be up to 50%. Second, there is a very strong association between parental smoking and asthma in children. Third, many children who have asthma are allergic to aspirin and other nonsteroidal anti-inflammatory drugs.

Remember that asthma, nasal polyps, and aspirin allergy constitute a recognized triad.

Finally, patients do not "outgrow" asthma. Children who have asthma may experience less severe attacks as adults, or they may never experience problems. However, they have not outgrown it—they still have a tendency for chronic inflammation in the bronchial tubes.

35. a. There appears to be a very strong association between respiratory syncytial virus (the main virus causing bronchiolitis) and asthma. Although it is difficult to state that the relationship is cause and effect, there is sufficient evidence to suggest that it might be. More research in this area may help resolve this issue.

36. e. Long-acting β-agonists appear to be a double-edged sword: They improve asthma control but lead to worse outcome when exacerbations do occur, probably because tolerance develops. Thus, they are associated with increased rates of hospitalization and death from asthma, which has led the Food and Drug Administration to issue a boxed warning limiting their use to second-line when low- or medium-dose inhaled corticosteroids are insufficient for adequate asthma control. They should never be used as rescue inhalers—such inappropriate use has led to a number of deaths. They do not decrease bronchial inflammation.

Solution to the Clinical Case Management Problem

Environmental control is considered a central part of asthma management. It is recommended by all major medical associations involved in asthma care and should be done with all levels of severity of asthma. It is based on the inherent logic that if a patient is allergic to an allergen, minimizing exposure to that allergen should help. An environmental survey is done first; then, based on the specific allergy, testing is done to document clinical suspicion of specific allergies. The National Environmental Education Foundation is a good resource for implementing environmental controls.

Although there is a fair amount of evidence indicating that various control methods reduce the allergen in question, there is much less evidence that this translates into better asthma control, mainly because few rigorous studies have been done. Despite their widespread recommendation, certain specific environmental controls have not been shown to be beneficial. For example, Gotzsche and others found no evidence that commonly prescribed methods of house dust mite control led to any improvement in asthma in a major Cochrane meta-analysis. Whether this is because environmental control of these specific allergens simply does not work, current methods of doing so are insufficient, or the effects of control on asthma take longer than the length of most studies to manifest is an open question.

Commonly accepted environmental controls that (might) help include the following (controls especially helpful for Jill's situation are italicized):

1. *Minimize indoor air pollution* (which is often worse than outdoor air pollution) by
   a. Having a rigorous no smoking rule for the household.
   b. Keeping the house clean. Use only vacuum cleaners that are equipped with a HEPA/micro filter system.
   c. Ensuring adequate ventilation. *Put filters on vents bringing air into rooms.*
   d. Venting to the outside any particle-producing appliance, such as a range or wood stove.
   e. Minimizing use of strong chemicals, odors, and dusts, including insect sprays, hair sprays, cleaning products, paint fumes, sawdust, and air fresheners. Ensure adequate ventilation if they must be used in the house.
2. Minimize exposure to outdoor pollution
   a. Stay inside or limit vigorous exercise when the air quality index is poor.
   b. *Filter air coming into the house with a HEPA filter.*
   c. Consider moving to a low-pollution area if effects on quality of life are major.
   d. Do not exercise vigorously next to busy roads.
3. If one did want to reduce dust mites
   a. *Encase especially pillows* but also mattresses and box springs in allergen impermeable covers.
   b. Wash bedding weekly in hot water (130°F or higher). This entails buying special blankets that can tolerate this washing.
   c. *Minimize "dust collectors"* (e.g., plush fabric upholstery, draperies, and stuffed toys). *Use wipeable surface furniture and blinds instead.*

d. Avoid excess humidity, which favors dust mite growth.

e. *Avoid wall-to-wall carpet. Periodically put throw rugs upside down in the sun to kill dust mites.*

f. Vacuum with a micro filter/HEPA filter-equipped vacuum cleaner when the asthmatic person is not around, or use a mask.

g. Damp mop or use dust magnet, special rags to clean dust.

4. Eliminate mold and mildew

a. Repair leaky faucets and pipes.

b. Properly seal tiles in wet areas such as shower stalls to avoid mildew growth.

c. Clean shower curtains regularly.

d. Control relative humidity to less than 50%. Use a dehumidifier if necessary.

e. Vent moisture-producing appliances such as dryers to the outside.

f. Ensure adequate ventilation in damp areas. Install exhaust fans if necessary.

g. *Seal leaky basements. Provide a sump pump for backup.*

h. Avoid working with decaying leaves, mulch, or similar materials, or wear a mask.

i. *Avoid standing water in saucers or waterlogged houseplants.*

j. Mold can be cleaned with a 10% chlorine bleach solution. (Never mix with other types of cleaning solutions because this may produce toxic fumes.)

k. HEPA filters, either central or stand-alone portable units, are effective at cleaning any airborne allergen.

5. Cockroaches

a. Keep eating areas clean.

b. Store garbage in closed containers.

c. Seal crevices where cockroaches enter. Boric acid powder in crevices will discourage cockroaches.

d. If you must use pest management services, choose a company that specializes in integrated pest management, which uses the least toxic options possible.

e. Do not use strong pesticides yourself, especially the spray type, inside the house.

6. Avoid animal dander

a. Cats are one of the most allergenic of animals. Avoid them if possible, or give them to another home. If you insist on keeping a cat, do not let it sleep in the bedroom or on the laundry. Try washing the cat regularly (twice a week) with an allergen removal wash.

b. If the family wants a pet, get one that does not have fur or feathers. If one must have a dog, choose one that has hair instead of fur, such as a poodle.

Summary

1. All that wheezes is not asthma, and all asthma does not wheeze.

2. A moderately severe to severe attack of asthma is an emergency. Do not discharge the patient unless you are very sure that the asthma attack is resolved completely.

3. Asthma is an inflammatory disease.

4. The prevalence of and mortality from asthma are increasing.

5. There is effective prophylaxis for exercise-induced asthma.

6. Cough variant asthma is very common but often misdiagnosed.

7. There is nothing wrong with a short course (several days) of oral steroids (prednisone 20 to 60 mg/day) for a severe case of asthma. It works, and it will keep the patient out of the hospital and out of danger.

8. Suggest peak flow meters to all of your patients with asthma for home monitoring.

9. Suggest use of a spacer with all metered-dosed inhalers—they improve efficiency of medication delivery.

10. Stepped care provides a rational rubric for pharmacotherapy.

11. Education and good environmental control of allergens and triggers are key to good management of asthma.

STEP CARE FOR ASTHMA

The following information is from the National Asthma Education and Prevention Program Expert Panel Report.

Quick Relief: All Patients

- Short-acting bronchodilator: Two to four puffs of short-acting inhaled β₂-agonists as needed for symptoms.
- Intensity of treatment will depend on severity of exacerbation—up to three treatments at 20-minute intervals or a single nebulizer treatment as needed. A course of systemic corticosteroids may be needed.
- Use of short-acting β₂-agonists more than two times per week in intermittent asthma (daily, or increasing use in persistent asthma) may indicate the need to initiate (increase) long-term control therapy.

Notes on the Stepwise Approach

The stepwise approach is meant to assist, not replace, the clinical decision making required to meet individual patient needs.

- Classify severity: Assign patient to most severe step in which any feature occurs (PEF is percentage of personal best; FEV1 is percentage predicted) (Table 29-1).

- Gain control as quickly as possible (consider a short course of systemic corticosteroids), then step down to the least medication necessary to maintain control.
- Minimize use of short-acting inhaled β2-agonists. Overreliance on short-acting inhaled β2-agonists (e.g., use of short-acting inhaled β2-agonists every day, increasing use or lack of expected effect, or use of approximately one canister a month even if not using it every day) indicates inadequate control of asthma and the need to initiate or intensify long-term-control therapy.
- Provide education on self-management and controlling environmental factors that make asthma worse (e.g., allergens and irritants).
- Refer to an asthma specialist if there are difficulties controlling asthma or if step 4 care is required. Referral may be considered if step 3 care is required.

Table 29-1 Stepwise Approach for Managing Asthma in Adults and Children Older Than 5 Years of Age: Treatment

	CLINICAL FEATURES BEFORE TREATMENT OR ADEQUATE CONTROL		Daily Medications Required to Maintain Long-Term Control
	Symptoms, Day/Night	PEF or FEV₁ PEF Variability	
Step 4: Severe persistent	Continual/frequent	≤60%; >30%	Preferred treatment High-dose inhaled corticosteroids *and* Long-acting inhaled β₂-agonists *and, if needed* Corticosteroid tablets or syrup long term (2 mg/kg/day, generally do not exceed 60 mg/day). (Make repeat attempts to reduce systemic corticosteroids and maintain control with high-dose inhaled corticosteroids.)
Step 3: Moderate persistent	Daily >1 night/wk	>60% to <80%; >30%	Preferred treatment Low to medium-dose inhaled corticosteroids and long-acting inhaled β₂-agonists Alternative treatment Increase inhaled corticosteroids within medium-dose range *or* Low- to medium-dose inhaled corticosteroids and either leukotriene modifier or theophylline *If needed (particularly in patients with recurring severe exacerbations):* Preferred treatment Increase inhaled corticosteroids within medium-dose range and add long-acting inhaled β₂-agonists Alternative treatment Increase inhaled corticosteroids within medium-dose range and add either a leukotriene modifier or theophylline

(Continued)

Table 29-1	Stepwise Approach for Managing Asthma in Adults and Children Older Than 5 Years of Age: Treatment—cont'd		
	CLINICAL FEATURES BEFORE TREATMENT OR ADEQUATE CONTROL		
	Symptoms, Day/Night	**PEF or FEV₁ PEF Variability**	**Daily Medications Required to Maintain Long-Term Control**
Step 2: Mild persistent	>2/wk, but <1×/day >2 nights/mo	≥80%; 20–30%	Preferred treatment: Low-dose inhaled corticosteroids Alternative treatment Cromolyn, leukotriene modifier, nedocromil, *or* sustained-release theophylline to serum concentration of 5–15 µm/mL
Step 1: Mild intermittent	≤2 days/wk ≤2 nights/mo	≥80%; <20%	No daily medication needed Severe exacerbations may occur, separated by long periods of normal lung function and no symptoms. A course of systemic corticosteroids is recommended.

Step down: Review treatment every 1–6 months; a gradual stepwise reduction in treatment may be possible.

Step up: If control is not maintained, consider step up. First, review patient medication technique, adherence, and environmental control.

Suggested Reading

Boushey HA, Corry, DB, Fahy, JV, et al: *Murray & Nadel's Textbook of Respiratory Medicine*, 4th ed. Philadelphia: Saunders, 2005.

Gotzsche PC, Johansen HK, Schmidt LM, Burr ML: House dust mite control measures for asthma. *Cochrane Database Syst Rev* 4:CD001187, 2004.

Holzer K: Respiratory symptoms during exercise. In Bruckner P, ed., *Clinical Sports Medicine*, 3rd ed. Sidney: McGraw–Hill, 2007.

Mark JD: Asthma. In Rakel D, ed., *Integrative Medicine*, 2nd ed. Philadelphia: Saunders, 2007, pp. 347–358.

National Asthma Education and Prevention Program Expert Panel Report: Guidelines for the diagnosis and management of asthma update on selected topics—2002. *J Allergy Clin Immunol* 110(5 pt 2):S141–S219, 2002.

National Environmental Education Foundation, www.neefusa.org.

Salpeter SR, Buckley NS, Ormiston TM, Salpeter EF: Meta-analysis: Effect of long-acting β-agonists on severe asthma exacerbations and asthma-related deaths. *Ann Intern Med* 144:904–912, 2006.

Sonia AB, Vollmer WM, Wilson SR, Frazier EA, Hayward AD: A randomized clinical trial of peak flow versus symptom monitoring in older adults with asthma. *Am J Respir Crit Care Med* 174: 1077–1087, 2006.

CHAPTER

30   The Diagnosis and Management of Pneumonia in the Adult

CLINICAL CASE PROBLEM 1

A 24-Year-Old University Student with a Dry, Hacking Cough

A 24-year-old university student presents to the student health service with a 3-day history of a dry, hacking cough that was initially nonproductive but has become productive of scant, white sputum. The patient also complains of malaise, headache, and fever, as well as muscle aches and pains. The patient had no other upper respiratory tract symptoms before this illness began (no rhinorrhea, sore throat, or conjunctivitis).

The patient has had no episodes like this in the past; however, her roommate developed the same symptoms 2 days ago.

On examination, the patient has a temperature of 39°C (102.2°F). You hear a few scattered rales in the left lung base but find no other abnormalities.

SELECT THE BEST ANSWER TO THE FOLLOWING QUESTIONS

1. Which of the following is the most cost-effective strategy at the present time?
   a. order no laboratory tests or imaging investigations; assume that it is viral and will clear up on its own
   b. order no laboratory tests or imaging investigations; treat with ampicillin just to be on the safe side

c. order the complete work-up: every possible test; no matter what the patient has, you will not be the one to get sued

d. on the basis of your clinical findings, order a chest x-ray

e. forget the tests; just treat her with "big-gun" therapy

2. What is the most likely diagnosis in this patient?
   a. viral pneumonia
   b. *Mycoplasma pneumoniae* pneumonia
   c. *Streptococcus pneumoniae* pneumonia
   d. *Klebsiella pneumoniae* pneumonia
   e. no pneumonia of any kind, a case of simple acute bronchitis

3. If you ordered a chest x-ray, what would be the most likely finding?
   a. nothing: clear and normal
   b. left lower-lobe pneumonia
   c. patchy bilateral lower-lobe infiltrates
   d. right middle-lobe infiltrates
   e. bilateral upper-lobe infiltrates

4. What is the treatment of choice for this patient?
   a. symptomatic treatment only
   b. ribavirin for respiratory syncytial virus
   c. clarithromycin
   d. ampicillin
   e. penicillin G

CLINICAL CASE PROBLEM 2

A Very Sick 55-Year-Old Woman

A 55-year-old woman, previously healthy and recovering from an episode of bronchitis, suddenly develops a "shaking chill," followed by the onset of a high fever of 40°C (104°F); pleuritic chest pain, and cough productive of purulent, rust-colored sputum.

On examination, the patient appears ill. Her respiratory rate is 40 breaths/minute, and bronchial breath sounds are heard in the left lower lobe. Chest x-ray reveals consolidation present in the left lower lobe.

5. On the basis of the history, the physical examination, and the chest x-ray findings, what is the most likely laboratory finding if sputum is obtained?
   a. gram-negative bacillus
   b. gram-negative cocci
   c. gram-positive bacillus
   d. gram-positive cocci (lancet-shaped)
   e. mixed flora

6. What is the most likely organism responsible for this patient's illness?
   a. *S. pneumoniae*
   b. *K. pneumoniae*
   c. *M. pneumoniae*
   d. influenza A
   e. *Haemophilus influenzae*

7. What is the initial treatment for this patient?
   a. ceftriaxone
   b. ciprofloxacin
   c. gentamicin
   d. macrolide
   e. a and d

CLINICAL CASE PROBLEM 3

A 35-Year-Old Renal Transplant Patient with Fever, Dyspnea, and 2 Days of Diarrhea

A 35-year-old man with chronic renal failure presented 4 days ago with fever, dyspnea, and 2 days of diarrhea. He had a renal transplant 6 months ago and is being treated with corticosteroids and cyclosporine. The chest x-ray showed an area of consolidation in the right middle lobe and a diffuse interstitial infiltrate. He has failed to respond to ceftriaxone and has a continued fever and cough. Today he is lethargic and confused.

8. What is the most likely organism causing his pneumonia?
   a. *Pneumocystis carinii*
   b. *Legionella pneumoniae*
   c. *Mycobacterium tuberculosis*
   d. *Mycobacterium avium intracellulare*
   e. *Cytomegalovirus*

9. What is the drug of first choice for this patient?
   a. macrolide
   b. cephalosporin
   c. quinolone
   d. tetracycline
   e. a and c

CLINICAL CASE PROBLEM 4

A 75-Year-Old Alcoholic Patient with Fever, Shortness of Breath, Chest Pain, and Cough Productive of Purulent Sputum and Blood

A 75-year-old alcoholic patient, with a history of congestive heart failure and suffering from fever, shortness of breath, chest pain, and cough productive of purulent sputum and blood, is admitted to hospital. On physical examination, the patient has a temperature of 39°C (102.2°F), a respiratory rate of 28 breaths/minute, and bronchial breath sounds in the right upper lobe.

A chest x-ray confirms the diagnosis of right upper-lobe pneumonia, with a small cavitary lesion.

10. What is the most likely organism responsible for this patient's illness?
a. *S. pneumoniae*
b. *K. pneumoniae*
c. *M. pneumoniae*
d. influenza A
e. *H. influenzae*

11. What is (are) the treatment(s) of choice for this patient?
a. erythromycin
b. ceftriaxone plus azithromycin
c. penicillin G
d. ampicillin
e. ampicillin plus gentamicin

CLINICAL CASE PROBLEM 5

A 55-Year-Old Male Smoker with COPD, High Fever, Chills, Cough, and Shortness of Breath

A 55-year-old male with a 60 pack-year history of smoking and documented chronic obstructive pulmonary disease (COPD) presents with a high fever, chills, a productive cough (yellowish-green sputum), and shortness of breath.

Examination yields decreased breath sounds in the right middle lobe and right lower lobe. You suspect a pneumonia.

A chest x-ray confirms right middle-lobe and right lower-lobe pneumonia. A Gram stain reveals gram-negative rods in abundance.

12. Based on his 60 pack-year history of smoking, the Gram stain result, and his history of chronic bronchitis, what is the most likely organism in this patient?
a. *Moraxella catarrhalis*
b. *M. pneumoniae*
c. *H. influenzae*
d. a or b
e. a or c

13. What is (are) the treatment(s) of choice for this patient?
a. erythromycin
b. cefuroxime plus azithromycin
c. penicillin G
d. ampicillin
e. ampicillin plus gentamicin

14. An elderly patient in a long-term care facility develops influenza A pneumonia in spite of both vaccination and amantadine prophylaxis. What is the organism most likely to complicate influenza pneumonia?
a. *S. pneumoniae*
b. *H. influenzae*
c. *Chlamydia trachomatis*
d. *Chlamydia pneumoniae*
e. *M. pneumoniae*

15. Which of the following is the most common cause of community-acquired pneumonia?
a. *M. pneumoniae*
b. *H. influenzae*
c. *S. pneumoniae*
d. *Staphylococcus aureus*
e. *Varicella* pneumonia

16. What is the most common cause of nosocomial pneumonia?
a. *M. pneumoniae*
b. aerobic gram-negative bacteria
c. *S. pneumoniae*
d. *H. influenza*
e. viral pneumonia

Clinical Case Management Problem

Discuss the characteristics of a sputum specimen satisfactory for Gram stain and for culture.

Answers

1. **d.** Certainly the most reasonable course of action following the history and physical examination is to perform a chest x-ray.

2. **b.** This patient most likely has a *Mycoplasma* pneumonia. *M. pneumoniae* is a common respiratory tract pathogen in young adults. The most common respiratory symptom is a dry, hacking, usually nonproductive cough. Systemic symptoms include malaise, headache, and fever. Rash, serous otitis media, and joint symptoms occasionally accompany the respiratory symptoms.

3. **c.** Physical findings are usually either minimal or unremarkable. Auscultation of the chest usually reveals only scattered rhonchi or fine, localized rales. Conversely, the chest x-ray often reveals fine or patchy lower-lobe or perihilar infiltrates. The white blood cell count is often elevated (10,000 to 15,000/mm³). Cold agglutinins are nonspecific and found in only 30% to 50% of cases. The diagnosis can be confirmed by acute and convalescent *Mycoplasma* complement fixation or enzyme immunoassay titers.

Clinically and radiographically, pneumonia caused by adenovirus is often difficult to differentiate from *Mycoplasma* pneumonia. The clinical picture does not fit that of *S. pneumoniae*, and the patient has no risk factors that should produce *K. pneumoniae*.

Mycoplasma pneumonia is the favored diagnosis over viral pneumonia (adenovirus) because of age, the absence of other upper respiratory tract symptoms, the prevalence of *Mycoplasma* pneumonia in students of colleges and universities, and the disparity of findings on auscultation relative to the findings on chest x-ray.

4. **c.** The treatment of choice is a macrolide antibiotic such as azithromycin or clarithromycin, or tetracycline for 10 days.

5. **d.**

6. **a.** This patient has a classic history of pneumococcal pneumonia. *S. pneumoniae* (pneumococcus) is the most common cause of bacterial pneumonia in the adult population.

Pneumococcal pneumonia often presents with a "shaking rigor" (as in this patient), followed by fever, pleuritic chest pain, and cough with purulent or rust-colored sputum. Viral upper or lower respiratory tract infections can precede pneumococcal pneumonia.

Elderly or debilitated patients can have an atypical presentation. Fever can be low grade, behavior disturbances might seem more significant than respiratory symptoms, and cough might not be prominent. Patients appear acutely ill, frequently having dyspnea, with minimal execution and chest splinting. Signs of consolidation are frequently present.

An elevated white blood cell count with left shift is common. Chest x-ray usually shows disease confined to one lobe (frequently a lower lobe), but several lobes can be involved, with either consolidation or bronchopneumonia. Gram stain of the sputum shows polymorphonuclear leukocytes and lancet-shaped gram-positive diplococci.

Sputum cultures should be obtained, but because up to 40% of patients with bacteremic pneumococcal pneumonia have negative sputum cultures, blood cultures should be obtained in these patients.

7. **e.** With the patient's clinical picture including a respiratory rate of 40 breaths/minute and chest splinting, hospitalization with intravenous therapy is indicated. Initial empiric treatment prior to the availability of organism susceptibility for a hospitalized patient with presumed streptococcal pneumonia would include a β-lactam plus a macrolide antibiotic such as azithromycin (Zithromax) or clarithromycin (Biaxin). An alternative is a respiratory quinolone as monotherapy (e.g., gatifloxacin [Tequin], levofloxacin [Levaquin], or moxifloxacin [Avelor]); however, beware of resistance. Because it is impossible to exclude *Legionella* given these clinical findings, a macrolide should be added to the β-lactam. Erythromycin has little coverage for *H. influenza* and should not be used. Treatment is ultimately guided by culture and susceptibilities.

8. **b.** The combination of pneumonia plus failure to respond to standard antibiotics such as ceftriaxone in an immunocompromised host points to the diagnosis of *Legionella*. The patient should be hospitalized for monitoring.

9. **a.** Newer macrolides and quinolones are considered the agents of choice. From the macrolide class, azithromycin is the most active against *Legionella*. Alternatives include the fluoroquinolones, moxifloxacin, gatifloxacin, and levofloxacin. A response is usually seen in 3 to 5 days. Note that interactions between some of the fluoroquinolones and immunosuppressive agents used in renal transplantation warrant careful monitoring of patients. Consultation with a transplant center team is a good idea.

10. **b.** Although the most likely cause of pneumonia in an elderly, debilitated person remains *S. pneumoniae*, the gram-negative organism *K. pneumoniae* is commonly found in alcoholic patients. *K. pneumoniae* is frequently seen in nosocomial pneumonias. The chest x-ray results described point to this latter organism.

Although the presentation in *Klebsiella* pneumonia can be similar to pneumococcal pneumonia, the upper lobes are more frequently involved than the lower lobes. Sudden onset is common, and pleuritic chest pain and hemoptysis are common features. Sputum is thick and often bloody. Because this is a necrotizing pneumonia, cavitary lesions can be found, which do not occur with *S. pneumoniae*. Other important causes of pneumonia in elderly patients include other gram-negative organisms, such as *Escherichia coli* and *H. influenzae*, and gram-positive organisms, such as *S. pneumoniae* and *S. aureus*.

11. **b.** The treatment of first choice for this patient is the cephalosporin cefuroxime (or ceftriaxone) plus azithromycin. This drug combination is effective against all the pathogens listed. An alternative is to use one of the quinolones (e.g., levofloxacin) alone.

12. e. In a patient with a pneumonia complicating chronic bronchitis, likely organisms include *H. influenzae* and *M. catarrhalis*.

13. b. The treatment of choice is the same as for the patient in Clinical Case Problem 4: a cephalosporin (e.g., cefuroxime or ceftriaxone) plus a macrolide (e.g., azithromycin [Zithromax] or clarithromycin [Biaxin]).

14. a. The most likely organism to complicate influenza pneumonia is *S. pneumoniae*.

15. c. The most common cause of community-acquired pneumonia is *S. pneumoniae*.

16. b. The most common cause of nosocomial pneumonia is aerobic gram-negative bacteria, although recent studies have shown that *S. aureus* now occurs with almost equal frequency.

Solution to the Clinical Case Management Problem

Sputum cytology is essential to make an accurate diagnosis of pneumonia. Saliva or nasopharyngeal secretions are of little value in determining the etiology of pneumonia, because colonization with gram-negative bacilli and other organisms is common.

If more than 25 squamous epithelial cells are seen per low-power magnification (LPM) field, the specimen is considered inadequate for culture. The ideal sputum specimen contains fewer than 10 squamous epithelial cells per LPM field and many polymorphonuclear leukocytes.

Summary

1. **Community-acquired pneumonia**

   The most common bacterial cause in all age groups is *S. pneumoniae*. Another common cause is *C. pneumoniae*, which causes approximately 15% of all pneumonias. Certain risk factors (i.e., age, underlying illness) can suggest other possible causes.

2. **Young adults**

   M. pneumoniae is a common causative agent, and *Mycoplasma* pneumonia is common among young adults. *Mycoplasma* pneumonia can often be differentiated from other pneumonias by the signs and symptoms elicited on history and physical examination and the findings on chest x-ray. Diagnostic clues to *M. pneumoniae* are a harsh, nonproductive, constant cough with little evidence of the shaking chills and high fever seen in streptococcal pneumonia. The major differential diagnosis is adenoviral pneumonia.

3. **Middle-aged adults with COPD**

   H. influenzae: *H. influenzae* pneumonia is a common pneumonia complicating COPD. Another common cause is *M. catarrhalis*, which is seen primarily in patients with underlying cardiopulmonary disease.

4. **Immunocompromised patients or those with COPD who fail to respond to conventional therapy**

   Suspect *Legionella* pneumonia: The signs and symptoms of *Legionella* pneumonia include malaise, headache, myalgia, weakness, and fever. Following these symptoms are intermittent rigors for 24 hours. There is also a nonproductive or minimally productive cough, and scant hemoptysis and pleuritic chest pain are common.

5. **Elderly patients with immune compromise secondary to alcohol**

   Suspect *K. pneumoniae*: *Klebsiella* pneumonia has much the same signs and symptoms as other bacterial pneumonias (see the following section).

6. **Bacterial versus viral pneumonia**

   a. Bacterial pneumonia: fever, chills (sudden onset of shaking chills in pneumococcal pneumonia), pleuritic chest pain, productive cough, purulent sputum, tachycardia, tachypnea, bronchial breath sounds.

   b. Viral pneumonia: gradual onset, general malaise, headache, prominent cough (often nonproductive), sometimes few abnormalities on examination of the lung (auscultation). The chest x-ray findings are more prominent.

c. *Mycoplasma* pneumonia: As in viral pneumonia, except cough can be almost constant, harsh, nonproductive, and irritative.

7. Treatment

Note guidelines do change. Although the following empiric treatment recommendations are up to date as of printing, please consult www.guidelines.gov for the latest recommendations. For uncomplicated patients with community-acquired pneumonia who do not require hospital admission, the treatment of choice is either a macrolide (erythromycin, azithromycin, or clarithromycin) or doxycycline. If there has been recent antibiotic use, choose one of the fluoroquinolones (e.g., levofloxacin) or an advanced macrolide (azithromycin, clarithromycin) plus high-dose amoxicillin clavulanate.

For patients with comorbidities (e.g., diabetes, COPD, cancer, congestive heart or renal failure) who do not require hospital treatment, the treatment of choice is an advanced macrolide or a fluoroquinolone. If there has been recent antibiotic use, a fluoroquinolone alone or an advanced macrolide plus a beta-lactam antibiotic is indicated.

For patients who require hospital admission, the treatment of choice is either a β-lactam cephalosporin (e.g., cefuroxime or ceftriaxone) plus a macrolide (erythromycin or azithromycin), or one of the quinolones (levofloxacin) alone. For seriously compromised hospitalized patients in whom *Pseudomonas* is not a consideration, add clindamycin to a fluoroquinolone. Imipenem or piperacillin can be added to ciprofloxacin if *Pseudomonas* is an issue. In-hospital treatment should always be guided by culture and sensitivities when possible. Consultation with an infectious disease subspecialist should be considered, because guidelines change and local resistance is always a problem.

8. Prevention

a. Pneumococcal vaccine: All patients at high risk.
b. Influenza vaccine (annually): All patients and health care workers at high risk.

Suggested Reading

Bjerre LM, Verheij TJ, Kochen MM: Antibiotics for community-acquired pneumonia in adult outpatients. *Cochrane Database Syst Rev* (2):CD002109, 2004.

Brunton S, Carmichael B, Fitzgerald M, et al: Community-acquired bacterial respiratory tract infections. *J Fam Pract* 54(3):255–262, 2005.

Brunton S: Treating community-acquired bacterial respiratory tract infections: Update on etiology, diagnosis, and antimicrobial therapy. *J Fam Pract* 54(4):357–364, 2005.

Community-Acquired Pneumonia in Adults. Bloomington, MN: Institute for Clinical Systems Improvement (ICSI), 2006. Available at www.guidelines.gov.

Morris CG, Safranek S, Neher J: Clinical inquiries: Is sputum evaluation useful for patients with community-acquired pneumonia? *J Fam Pract* 54(3):279–281, 2005.

CHAPTER

31 Esophageal Disorders

CLINICAL CASE PROBLEM 1

A 33-Year-Old Male with Substernal and Retrosternal Pain and Hypertension

A 33-year-old overweight male comes to the emergency room in an agitated state complaining of substernal and retrosternal pain radiating to his neck, accompanied by a congested feeling in his chest. He states that this pain started upon arising that morning and he is convinced he is having a heart attack.

On physical examination, his blood pressure is 210/95 mmHg and his pulse is 106 beats/minute and regular. His heart sounds and electrocardiogram (ECG) pattern are normal. His lungs are clear. His abdomen is soft; no masses and no tenderness are felt. He was given nitroglycerine tablets and his blood pressure quickly decreased.

As his blood pressure subsided and after he was told his ECG pattern was normal, he calmed down and remembered a history of intermittent upper abdominal chest pain that was quickly relieved with antacids. A burning sensation was not predominant, but he said that on some occasions it left a feeling of pins and needles in the throat. These pains had no relationship to exercise or exertion but were exacerbated by eating and relived by antacids. Furthermore, he states he had been agitated and slept poorly the previous night because he had been informed the day before that he will be laid off from work at the end of the month. In an attempt to console himself, before going to bed the previous night he polished off a pound of chocolates washed down with a bottle of red wine. He also smoked a pack of cigarettes in a few hours rather that his usual rate of a pack a day.

SELECT THE BEST ANSWER TO THE FOLLOWING QUESTIONS

1. Which of the following must be considered in the differential diagnosis of this patient's problem?
   a. acid reflux disease
   b. myocardial ischemia
   c. peptic ulcer disease
   d. panic disorder
   e. a and d only
   f. all of the above

2. Given the history and physical examination, which of the following conditions is (are) most likely responsible for the symptoms noted?
   a. acid reflux disease
   b. myocardial ischemia
   c. peptic ulcer disease
   d. panic disorder
   e. a and d

3. What is the major pathophysiologic mechanism underlying the chronic symptoms described in this case?
   a. transient relaxation of the lower esophageal sphincter (LES)
   b. decreased resting pressure of the LES
   c. achalasia
   d. excess production of hydrogen ions (H^+) in the stomach
   e. esophageal spasm

4. Which of the following is not an acceptable treatment for gastroesophageal reflux disease (GERD)?
   a. antacids and over-the-counter histamine 2 (H_2) antagonists
   b. certain lifestyle changes
   c. prescription-strength H_2 antagonists
   d. pro-kinetic agents
   e. proton pump inhibitors (PPIs)

5. Which of the following is not associated with severe chronic GERD?
   a. difficulty in swallowing
   b. esophageal cancer
   c. Barrett's esophagus
   d. esophageal varices
   e. esophagitis

CLINICAL CASE PROBLEM 2

A 68-Year-Old Male Who Finds Swallowing Difficult

A 68-year-old male presents to your office with a complaint about an apparent lump in his throat and difficulty in swallowing. He finds that solid foods and pills tend to stick in his throat, sometimes causing him to choke. He also has some trouble swallowing liquids. He has smoked a pack or two of cigarettes per day since he was 14 years old and admits to liking a few shots of whiskey on an almost daily basis.

Vital signs are normal. No abnormalities are discerned upon physical examination.

6. Which of the following is the least likely cause of his dysphagia?
   a. achalasia
   b. diffuse esophageal spasm
   c. a lower esophageal ring (Schatzki ring)
   d. pharyngeal paralysis
   e. an esophageal stricture

7. Which of the following is (are) not true concerning malignant dysphagia?
   a. a risk factor for squamous cell cancer is Barrett's esophagus
   b. most esophageal cancers occur in the more distal parts of the esophagus
   c. malignant dysphagia can usually be distinguished from other dysphagias by the rapid progression of symptoms
   d. due to more sophisticated modes of diagnosis and treatment developed within the past 5 years, the overall 5-year survival rate is 50%
   e. a and d are false statements
   f. b and c are false statements

Answers

1. **f.** All choices should be considered.

2. **e.** It is most important to rule out myocardial ischemia with further testing including blood analysis of cardiac enzymes and/or troponins and, perhaps, hospitalization and an exercise stress test. However, the most likely cause of the symptoms described is GERD complicated by anxiety brought about by job-related stress coupled with his fresh chest pain. When he awoke, his underlying anxiety was increased due to chest pain. This raised his blood pressure, inducing a feeling of heaviness in his chest, further raising his anxiety level to

that of panic, which in turn further increased his blood pressure. The nitroglycerine helped break this vicious cycle, allowing him to calm down, think more rationally, and remember past symptoms, which included a history of probable GERD. Although a final diagnosis cannot be made on the basis of the described symptoms alone, the absence of abnormal cardiac exam findings and the normal ECG point away from heart problems. Moreover, a number of factors point toward GERD being an underlying cause, including (1) the relatively high prevalence of GERD in the population (in one study, 25% to 40% of adults were found to be affected at least monthly and 7% to 10% daily), (2) his history of acid reflux symptoms relived by antacids, and (3) his indulgence in "comfort eating" of GERD-inducing foods the previous night. In addition, the stress of being laid off and a night of poor sleep made conditions ripe for onset of his symptoms.

Although GERD usually manifests as heartburn, a sizable minority report chest pain with minimal or no burning sensation, making diagnosis more difficult. Others report hoarseness or even shortness of breath as the presenting symptom. Peptic ulcer can produce aching discomfort in the upper abdomen or lower chest and thus must be included in the differential. However, it rarely is described as retrosternal pain radiating to the neck; moreover, eating generally relieves, not worsens, symptoms.

3. **a.** The most common cause of acid reflux is a transient relaxation of the LES. However, permanent relaxation and increased abdominal pressure that overcomes the LES may also be causative factors. Transient relaxation may be caused by foods (chocolates, coffee and other sources of caffeine, alcohol, fatty meals, and peppermint/spearmint) or by drugs (beta blockers, nitrates, calcium channel blockers, and anticholinergics) and by smoking (nicotine).

In addition to relaxation of the LES, other potential precipitants are poor esophageal motility and delayed gastric emptying. Hiatal hernias are also found in high frequency in patients with symptoms of GERD. Achalasia is characterized by dysphagia, not by acid regurgitation. Although excess gastric acid may exacerbate symptoms, GERD can occur with normal acid secretion. Esophageal spasm can cause acid reflux, but it is a relatively rare condition and not a major mechanism.

Although some of the symptoms described were due to anxiety, it was described as an acute attack, not a chronic condition.

4. **d.** The prokinetic motility agents metoclopramide (Reglan) and cisapride (Propulsid) were once marketed as the drugs of choice to prevent GERD relapse. However, in July 2000, Jansen voluntarily withdrew cisapride from the market because of concern about possible adverse side effects, and in March 2003 the Food and Drug Administration required metoclopramide to carry warnings concerning neuroleptic malignant syndrome as a possible adverse reaction and suggested limiting its use. Antacids and/or over-the-counter H_2 antagonists coupled with certain lifestyle changes comprise the most conservative line of treatment.

The following lifestyle changes were found to be effective in an evidence-based review: weight loss and elevation of the head of the bed by approximately 6 inches. Commonsense measures include avoid lying down after meals, avoid late night meals or midnight snacks, and avoid tight-fitting clothes. Interestingly, commonly made recommendations such as the avoidance of dietary irritants (e.g., fat, chocolate, caffeine, spearmint/peppermint, and alcohol), drugs that lower LES pressure (e.g., calcium channel blockers, beta blockers, and theophyline), and discontinuation of tobacco use had little effect on outcome. Nevertheless, if the patient encounters a pattern of known precipitants such as use of anti-inflammatory drugs, certainly recommend avoidance of the irritant.

Should symptoms persist despite lifestyle changes, a PPI can be added to increase the pH of the material being regurgitated. Many patients have tried H_2 receptor blockers before seeing the physician. H_2 receptor blockers are available mostly without prescription: cimetidine (Tagamet), ranitidine (Zantac), nizatidine (Axid), and famotidine (Pepcid). The PPIs include omeprazole (Prilosec), lansoprazole (Prevacid), rabeprazole (Aciphex), esomeprozole (Nexium), and pantoprazole (Protonix). PPIs are more effective than H_2-receptor antagonists but cost more, even though they only need to be taken once a day. Although PPIs effectively reduce symptoms, they do so by reducing the gastric acidity, which may in the long term lead to other problems, such as reducing the ability to absorb vitamin B_{12} and/or protection against ingested pathogens. Also, PPIs interfere with the bioavailability of many other drugs dependent on low gastric pH for absorption, such as digoxin and ketoconazole.

As in the case described, anxiety can provoke additional symptoms and can also exacerbate the gastric reflux systems. Supportive counseling and possibly the temporary addition of an anxiolytic can also be considered.

Patients should be evaluated every 8 to 12 weeks, and if symptoms are alleviated the dosage of the drug used may be decreased with the aim of titrating to the lowest possible dose and, ideally, eventual discontinuation. Should a relapse occur, treatment can be started again.

If patients do not have an adequate response to therapy, or for patients 50 years old or older, endoscopy should be considered because of the higher incidence of gastric malignancies and peptic ulcer disease.

5. **d.** Esophageal varices are a by-product of portal hypertension, not esophageal reflux disease.

The potential pathological sequence of events associated with chromic GERD is as follows: (1) The acid irritates the esophageal lining, causing inflammation and esophagitis; (2) the esophagitis can lead to ulcer and stricture formation, causing difficulty in swallowing; (3) chronic inflammation may also induce metaplasia and transformation of the cells lining the esophageal lumen, causing Barrett's esophagus; and (4) Barrett's esophageal cells can transform into malignant cells. Only approximately 5% of people with GERD develop Barrett's esophagus, but once diagnosed, there is at least a 30-fold greater chance of developing a malignancy.

6. **d.** All listed choices are potential causes of dysphagia. An additional cause for consideration in this case is malignant dysphasia. Although not listed in this question, it is critical to always first rule out malignancy as a potential cause of even mild dysphagia because failure to diagnose and start treatment of esophageal cancer in a timely manner is almost a certain death sentence. Moreover, the patient described in Clinical Case Problem 2 has several risk factors for esophageal cancer, including his age, sex, and smoking and drinking habits. (See answer 7 for further discussion.)

However, among the five conditions listed, pharyngeal paralysis is the least likely cause of dysphagia in the case described. This condition is produced by weakness and incoordination of the muscles in the pharynx that propel food into the esophagus. Both liquids and solids are difficult to swallow, and aspiration into the windpipe and regurgitation into the nose commonly occurs. It is a result of faulty transmission of nerve impulses to the pharyngeal muscles generally caused by an associated neuromuscular disease, such as myasthenia gravis, amyotrophic lateral sclerosis, or stroke. No such neurological condition was described.

Achalasia, meaning failure to relax, is a rare disorder with an incidence in the United States of approximately 1 per 100,000. It is caused by incoordination of the esophageal peristaltic muscles and the failure of the LES to relax due to a lack of inhibitory input from nonadrenergic, noncholinergic, ganglionic cells. As a consequence, food cannot pass into the stomach. The cause is not known, and swallowing of liquids and solids is affected. The most effective treatment is endoscopical dilation, including injection of botulism toxin into the LES to block acetylcholine release, with the aim of restoring the balance between excitatory and inhibitory stimulation. A less effective but less abrasive treatment worth trying as the first line of treatment, particularly for elderly or other more fragile patients, is the use of medications that relax the LES. Calcium channel blockers or nitrates are the drugs of choice. However, such treatment is successful in only approximately 10% of the cases. If all else fails, the patient can be advised to hold his or her arms straight up in the air. This has been alleged to facilitate swallowing.

Diffuse esophageal spasm is characterized by multiple high-pressure, poorly coordinated esophageal contractions that usually occur after a swallow. The cause is unknown, and symptoms mimic GERD. However, if the cause is spasm, the symptoms will continue intermittently over a period of years and may become progressively worse. Esophageal dilation may provide relief. If not, surgery may be necessary.

A Schatzki ring is a diaphragm-like mucosal ring that forms at the esophagogastric junction (the B ring). If the lumen of this ring becomes too small, symptoms occur. The cause is not clear, but such rings are usually found in older individuals and have been observed in 6% to 15% of patients undergoing a barium swallow; however, only 0.5% of those being examined have significant symptoms. Symptoms correlate with the size of the lumen of the ring: A lumen greater than 20 mm in diameter provides few, if any, symptoms; if it is less than 13 mm in diameter, chronic and more severe symptoms occur. Most patients have an intermittent, nonprogressive dysphagia for solid foods that occurs while consuming a heavy meal with meat that was "wolfed down"; hence the pseudonym the "steakhouse syndrome." Sometimes the meal is regurgitated, relieving the block, and eating can be resumed. Patients with a Schatzki ring are also at risk for GERD. A diagnosis is confirmed by radiographic barium swallow or endoscopic means, and if symptoms are sufficiently troublesome, the treatment of choice is rupture of the ring by dilatation.

An esophageal stricture is a narrowing of the lumen of the esophagus preventing the passage of foods. Typically, it is at the distal end of the tube and is the result of scarring after chronic exposure to gastric juice due to GERD. Scaring and consequently stricture formation can also occur in response to other types of trauma, including swallowing caustic solutions, chronic swallowing of pills without water, or residual scarring after surgery. Usual treatment is dilatation.

7. **e.** Prior to 1970 in the United States, and still in many areas of the world, squamous cell carcinoma accounted for 90% to 95% of the cases of esophageal cancer. However, since that time, the relative incidence of adenocarcinoma has increased markedly in the United States and by the early 1990s it accounted for approximately 50% of all cases. Currently, the proportion of adenocarcinomas is probably even higher.

In the United States, the incidence of all types of esophageal cancer is 3 to 6 cases per 100,000; it is more prevalent in males (male:female ratio is 7:1) and in African American males than in white males. It is generally diagnosed in the sixth or seventh decade.

Nonkeratinizing stratified epithelial squamous cells line the esophagus. Irritations of these cells and/or exposure to carcinogens cause a malignant transformation inducing a squamous cell carcinoma. Tobacco use and excess alcohol consumption account for most squamous cell cases and are the major modifiable risk factors in the United States. Other potential factors include nitrosamines and other nitrosyl compounds commonly found in smoked or pickled foods. In some environments, there are nitrosyl compounds in the water and certain mineral deficiencies lead to the accumulation of these compounds in ceratin food plants. Both events have been suggested to cause squamous cell carcinoma. It has also been reported that chronic ingestion of very hot liquids, very spicy foods, or other irritants promotes squamous cell tumors. Long-standing cases of achalasia or strictures as well as radiation and a host of other relatively uncommon factors have also been reported to induce squamous cell carcinomas, but squamous cell cancer does not arise from Barrett's esophagus. A diet rich in fruits and vegetable seems to protect against this malignancy.

In contrast to the multiple causes of the squamous cell malignancies, adenocarcinomas arise from a well-characterized sequence. In response to chronic exposure to acid reflux, the normal stratified epithelium first becomes inflamed, and then metaplasia occurs and these columnar epithelia cells are transformed into a specialized glandular epithelium called Barrett's epithelium. The Barrett epithelial cells can then undergo a progressive dysplasia from low to high grade and ultimately to adenocarcinoma. Most adenocarcinomas occur in the more distal parts of the esophagus because this area is more likely to be exposed to regurgitated acid.

Because very early symptoms are only a very mild dysphagia, early cancers tend to be ignored. Unfortunately, both squamous cell and adenocarcinomas are very aggressive, and by the time the tumors have grown large enough to obscure the lumen and produce severe symptoms, they also are likely to have grown through the esophageal wall and have invaded other tissues. The fact that the esophageal wall is thin, composed of only two tissue layers, facilitates this escape. Because of this tendency to overlook early symptoms, many patients have a stage IV cancer at the time of diagnosis with a 5-year survival rate of only 5%; the overall 5-year survival rate at all stages is 20% to 25% and is the same for both squamous cell and adenocarcinoma.

Summary

ACID REFLUX DISEASE (GERD)

The most common cause is a transient relaxation of the LES. Permanent LES relaxation, increased abdominal pressure, and strictures are less common causes. Diagnosis can usually be made by a detailed history, confirmed if desired by a therapeutic challenge with an antacid (if symptoms immediately improve the diagnosis is probable). In cases in which symptoms persist despite treatment, or risk factors such as smoking or alcohol use are present, endoscopy should be pursued. Most important, Barrett's esophagus or adenocarcinoma can be ruled in or out by endoscopy.

The first line of treatment should be lifestyle changes (see A4) supplemented with over-the-counter antacids. Over-the-counter calcium carbonate antacids generally are effective, inexpensive, and also increase the daily intake of calcium. If acid reflux continues, a PPI should be prescribed; PPIs are more effective than H_2 blockers, but H_2 blockers are less expensive and generally available without a prescription.

Potential long-term consequences include esophagitis, strictures, Barrett's esophagitis, and adenocarcinoma.

DYSPHAGIA

1. Archetypal esophageal-based causes
   a. Achalasia is characterized by the loss of peristalsis and constriction of the LES. Achalasia is diagnosed by esophageal manometry (to measure intraluminal pressure, pH, and transit time) and pneumatic dilatation of the esophagus. It is treated by endoscopic dilatation with injection of botulism toxin or by LES relaxants (calcium channel blockers or nitrates).
   b. Esophageal spasm is characterized by an increased percentage of uncoordinated peristolic waves with some preserved peristalsis. It is diagnosed by esophageal manometry, and it is treated with bougienage or calcium channel blockers or nitrates. Anxiolytics may also be prescribed to reduce anxiety induced by the spasms.
   c. Esophageal stricture is a narrowing in one or more parts of the esophagus, most often caused by chronic gastric reflux but very serious cases are caused by ingestion of toxic liquids or solids. The latter most commonly occurs in children, and all

family physicians have an obligation to inform parents about the danger of having easy access to corrosive substances. It is diagnosed by history and confirmed by barium swallow or endoscopy. The treatment of choice is progressive dilatation.

d. Esophageal ring (Schatzki ring) is a narrowing of the diameter of the esophageal lumen at the point of the ring, which is generally at the level of the LES. The degree of blockage is correlated with the diameter of the retained opening. As a rule, symptoms are intermittent and are associated with swallowing solid foods without chewing them sufficiently; the larger chunks tend to get caught in the narrowed passageway. The diagnosis can be confirmed by barium swallow or endoscopy. The first line of treatment is behavioral modification—learning to eat more slowly. If symptoms are severe and/or occur often, treatment is dilatation and fracture of the ring.

e. Acute foreign body obstruction is a commonly experienced phenomenon—"food is felt to be going down the wrong pipe." Usually, the offending particle is coughed up. However, occasionally a particle remains lodged. If this occurs high in the esophagus or in the lower pharynx, it may block the air passage, resulting in an inability to breathe or talk. The affected individual will turn blue and pass out within a matter of minutes; the "Heimlich maneuver" is a practical and effect way to quickly dislodge the offending object. More often, the foreign body is lodged more deeply in the esophagus, where it can best be removed by a fiberoptic endoscope. Small children are prone to put all sorts of foreign objects into their mouths. If one of these is swallowed, it too may become stuck in the esophagus. Although the basic principles remain the same, the swallowed object is more likely to be a hard, often sharp, object with the potential of perforating the esophagus or other parts of the gastrointestinal tract.

f. Almost all esophageal malignancies are either squamous cell or adenocarcinomas. Adenocarcinoma of the esophagus occurs as a secondary response to Barrett's esophagus and recently has become the most common esophageal cancer in the United States. Squamous cell carcinoma was the most common form in the United States and still is in many areas of the world. It arises in response to many carcinogenic factors, the most modifiable ones being smoking and excess alcohol consumption. Diagnosis of either type is confirmed by endoscopy with biopsy. Unfortunately, this is rarely done until dysphagia has become marked and weight loss has started; by that time, prognosis has become poor. Regrettably, endoscopy cannot be conducted on every patient with heartburn, but ongoing research is trying to develop newer diagnostic methods able to screen for early esophageal cancer in a practical way. However, treatment modalities have become more aggressive in recent years. Surgical resection is the procedure of choice supported by chemo- and radiotherapy. Although the 5-year survival rate is still miserable, it has improved significantly during the past two decades.

2. Miscellaneous causes of dysphagia

a. Systemic sclerosis is characterized by progressive muscle atrophy and fibrosis, leading to loss of peristalsis as well as reduction of sphincter pressure. This may lead to substantial GERD and its complications. Treatment is similar to that for GERD.

b. Candidal esophagitis associated with the acquired immunodeficiency syndrome (AIDS)

c. AIDS

d. Herpes simplex esophagitis

e. Cerebrovascular accidents and neurologic disorders such as acute lateral sclerosis

f. Pharyngeal paralysis and pharyngeal diverticula: Although these are not esophageal problems, they should be considered in a differential diagnosis of dysphagia.

Suggested Reading

Blot WJ, McLauglin JK: The changing epidemiology of esophageal cancer. *Semin Oncol* 26(5 Suppl 15):2–8, 1999.

Chawla S, Seth D, Mahajan P, Kamat D: Gastroesophageal reflux disorder: A review for primary care providers. *Clin Pediatr* 45(1):7–13, 2006.

Heath EI, Limburg PJ, Hawk ET, Forastiere AA: Adenoma of the esophagus, risk factors and prevention. *Oncology* 4:507–514, 518–520, 2000.

Kaltenbach T, Crockett S, Gerson LB: Are lifestyle measures effective in patients with gastroesophageal reflux disease? An evidence-based approach. *Arch Intern Med* 166(9):965–971, 2006.

Kirby TJ, Rice TW: The epidemiology of esophageal cancer. The changing face of a disease. *Chest Surg Clin North Am* 4(2):217–225, 1994.

Lagergren J, Bergström R, Lindgren A, Nyrén O: Symptomatic gastropharyngeal reflux as a risk factor for esophageal adenocarcinoma. *N Engl J Med* 340(11):825–831, 1999.

Liker H, Hungin P, Wiklund I: Managing gastroesophageal reflux disease in primary care: The patient perspective. *J Am Board Fam Pract* 18(5):393–400, 2005 .

Patti MG, Way LW: Evaluation and treatment of primary esophageal motility disorders. *West J Med* 166(4):263–269, 1997.

Scott M, Gelhot AR: Gastroesophageal reflux disease: Diagnosis and management. *Am Fam Physician* 59:1170–1177, 1999.

Spechler SJ: American Gastroenterological Association medical position statement on the treatment of patients with dysphagia caused by benign disorders of the distal esophagus. *Gastroenterology* 117(1):229–233, 1999.

Van Pinxteren B, Numans ME, Bonis PA, Lau J: Short-term treatment with proton pump inhibitors, H2-receptor antagonists and prokinetics for gastro-oesophageal reflux disease-like symptoms and endoscopy negative reflux disease. *Cochrane Database Syst Rev* (4):CD002095, 2004.

Wildi SM, Tutuian R, Castell DO: Rapid food intake induces gastroesophageal reflux. Your mother was right. *Gastroenterology* 124:A72, 2003.

32 Peptic Ulcer Disease

CLINICAL CASE PROBLEM 1

A 58-Year-Old Male with Epigastric Pain

A 58-year-old male with a 4-month history of epigastric pain presents to your office. The pain is described as dull and achy and is intermittent. There is no radiation of the pain. Exacerbating factors include coffee intake. Infrequently, he is awakened at night from the pain. Temporary alleviating factors include eating a meal or taking nonprescription H_2-antagonists. The baseline intensity of the pain is approximately a 6 out of 10, but it can fluctuate in intensity to an 8 out of 10. The pain has not changed since it began 4 months ago. No weight loss, vomiting, melena, or hematochezia have been noted, but nausea does occur at times. The patient denies any dramatic increase in his usually stressful career, and he describes his position as a "high-powered executive." He admits that he is a "workaholic." He has no prior history of chronic abdominal pain, and he takes no regular prescription medications or nonprescription analgesics.

On exam, the patient has some epigastric tenderness with no rebound or guarding. The remainder of the exam is unremarkable.

SELECT THE BEST ANSWER TO THE FOLLOWING QUESTIONS

1. What is the most likely diagnosis in this patient?
   a. gastric carcinoma
   b. gastric ulcer
   c. duodenal ulcer
   d. cholecystitis/cholelithiasis
   e. irritable bowel syndrome

2. Which of the following statements regarding the patient described is (are) false?
   a. upper endoscopy with biopsy for *Helicobacter pylori* is indicated
   b. cigarette smoking may aggravate the condition
   c. drinking alcohol aggravates the condition
   d. this patient should be treated with a bland diet
   e. this condition may be aggravated or caused by the ingestion of certain medications

3. Which of the following is most sensitive and specific for detection of *Helicobacter* infections?
   a. serology for IgG against *H. pylori*
   b. urea breath test
   c. *Helicobacter pylori* stool antigen
   d. endoscopic biopsy with histologic examination
   e. none of the above are particularly sensitive

4. The patient is found to be *H. pylori* positive and placed on a combination of lansoprazole, clarithromycin, and amoxicillin for 14 days for his condition. His symptoms improve rapidly, and he is essentially pain free in 2 weeks. Which of the following statements is (are) true about this treatment?
   a. amoxicillin was prescribed because of a high probability of sepsis in his condition
   b. a combination of omeprazole, clarithromycin, and amoxicillin for 14 days would probably be equally effective
   c. a combination of bismuth, metronidazole, and an H_2-blocker for 14 days would probably be equally effective
   d. a combination of clarithromycin, amoxicillin, and lansoprazole for 7 days would be less effective
   e. none of the above

5. What is the mode of action of omeprazole?
   a. an H_1-receptor antagonist
   b. an H_2-receptor antagonist
   c. a proton pump inhibitor (PPI)
   d. a cytoprotective agent
   e. an anticholinergic agent

6. The condition described should respond to treatment with complete healing within a maximum of how many weeks?
   a. 1 or 2 weeks
   b. 3 to 6 weeks
   c. 8 to 12 weeks
   d. 16 to 20 weeks
   e. 26 to 52 weeks

7. Which of the following drugs is classified as a cytoprotective agent?
   a. metoclopramide
   b. misoprostol
   c. bismuth subsalicylate
   d. ondansetron
   e. nizatidine

8. Which of the following statements regarding the role of drugs in the condition described is false?
   a. cyclooxygenase type 2 (COX-2) inhibitors do not cause this condition

b. the use of dexamethasone is a risk factor for this condition

c. aspirin may precipitate this condition

d. some nonsteroidal anti-inflammatory drugs (NSAIDs) seem more likely to precipitate this condition than others

e. the incidence of this condition in patients taking indomethacin or other NSAIDs is increased

9. Which of the following statements regarding *H. pylori* is true?

a. chronic infection is uncommon in most areas of the world

b. organisms are found in human feces but not saliva

c. income and socioeconomic factors do not influence prevalence

d. approximately 10% of adults with dyspepsia recolonized

e. prevalence of infection is higher in Hispanics and African Americans

10. Which of the following statements regarding the diagnosis and treatment of gastric ulcers is false?

a. the pain of gastric ulcers, in contrast with duodenal ulcers, is sometimes aggravated rather than relieved by food

b. gastric ulcers do not present with bleeding or perforation as the initial presentation

c. endoscopy should follow the identification of a gastric ulcer on a gastrointestinal (GI) series

d. the healing rate and the time to heal for gastric ulcers are generally longer than those for duodenal ulcers

e. anorexia, nausea, and vomiting are more common in patients with gastric ulcer than duodenal ulcer

11. Advantages of PPIs over H_2-blockers include all of the following except

a. superior acid suppression

b. faster healing rates

c. safe for use in hepatically impaired patients

d. faster symptom relief

e. lower and less frequent dosing requirement

12. Endoscopy is indicated for all of the following except

a. a 57-year-old male with new dyspepsia and weight loss

b. a 35-year-old female with epigastric pain that is worse with eating and associated with anorexia and early satiety

c. a 40-year-old female with a duodenal ulcer seen on upper GI series

d. a 45-year-old male with *H. pylori* peptic ulcer disease (PUD) with persistent symptoms after 3 weeks of acid suppression therapy

e. a 47-year-old male with history of PUD with recurrence of symptoms soon after completion of treatment

13. Which of the following types of *H. pylori* testing is not useful for confirming eradication?

a. stool antigen test

b. urea breath test

c. enzyme-linked immunosorbent assay (ELISA) serology

d. culture

e. Steiner's stain of gastric biopsy specimen

14. In the United States, the most common cause of the condition described here is

a. alcohol

b. aspirin

c. Zollinger–Ellison syndrome

d. *H. pylori*

e. idiopathic

Clinical Case Management Problem

Discuss the pathophysiology of NSAID and *H. pylori*-induced peptic ulcers.

Answers

1. c. This patient has a duodenal ulcer. Duodenal ulcer pain is characterized by a deep, aching, recurrent pain located in the midepigastrium. It is often relieved by food or antacids and aggravated by aspirin, coffee, or other irritants. Nocturnal pain is common, and it may awaken the patient at night.

Anorexia, weight loss, and vomiting are infrequently associated symptoms of duodenal ulcer. The occurrence of these symptoms should lead one to suspect a gastric ulcer, which may be worse with food and is a risk for developing gastric carcinoma.

2. d. Upper endoscopy with a culture and biopsy for *H. pylori* is indicated given this patient's age and persistent symptoms. It is reasonable and safe, however, to treat many patients with typical duodenal ulcer symptoms with no alarm signs without endoscopy. Patients should be tested for *H. pylori* and treated if positive. Alarm signs include age older than 55 years, rectal bleeding or melena, weight loss, anorexia/early satiety, anemia, dysphagia, jaundice, family history of gastric cancer, and previous history of gastric cancer or complicated ulcer disease. If the symptoms improve with a PPI and *H. pylori* eradication treatment, then no investigation is needed. If they do not, investigation with endoscopy should proceed.

Cigarette smoking has been shown to aggravate peptic ulcer disease and delay healing of peptic ulcers. Patients who smoke also have an increased probability of recurrence. Aspirin and other NSAIDs may aggravate or produce a peptic ulcer. Alcohol is a strong stimulant of acid secretion. Bland diets or other special diets are of no use in PUD.

3. d. Endoscopy with biopsy and histologic examination has a sensitivity of more than 95% and 100% specificity. Not everyone can or needs to have endoscopy, however, and other noninvasive tests have excellent sensitivity and specificity. In the office setting, stool for *H. pylori* antigen has a sensitivity of 93% and a specificity of 98%, and it is a good tool for the identification of infection in symptomatic outpatients. The urea breath test has a sensitivity of 95% and a specificity of 98%, but it requires special equipment not often found in family medicine offices. The serum IgG antibody test is 85% sensitive and 78% specific, but it is not useful for assessing eradication because it remains positive for quite some time after treatment.

4. b. Initial studies identified *H. pylori* in 95% of duodenal ulcers and 80% of gastric ulcers, but recent studies have shown that the prevalence of *H. pylori* has decreased to 60% to 75% due to eradication treatment. With PPIs alone, 75% of patients who are *H. pylori* positive will have an endoscopically documented recurrence within 1 year. With the successful eradication of *H. pylori*, the recurrence rate is less than 10% within 1 year. Increasingly, however, the problem of resistance is being seen. The eradication of *H. pylori* is quite difficult and multiple drugs are required. Current regimens include triple and quadruple therapies for varying durations. Single and dual drug combination therapies are not recommended because of unacceptably low cure rates. The use of amoxicillin in the treatment of PUD has nothing to do with sepsis. The 14-day combinations of omeprazole or lansoprazole plus amoxicillin and clarithromycin have an approximately 85% to 90% eradication rate. Smaller studies examining a 7-day combination of clarithromycin, amoxicillin, and lansoprazole have found eradication rates similar to those of longer therapies with better compliance and reduced cost. One study that examined bismuth subsalicilate combined with amoxicillin, metronidazole, and lansoprazole for 1 day found a 95% eradication rate. Recurrence is problematic, and it usually requires higher and longer dosing of different agents.

5. c. Omeprazole binds to the proton pump of the parietal cell, inhibiting secretion of hydrogen ions into the gastric lumen. In doses of 20 to 40 mg/day, it inhibits more than 90% of total 24-hour gastric acid secretion, which is a significant improvement compared to the 50% to 80% inhibition achieved with an H_2-blocker. This greater inhibition of gastric acid secretion results in greater pain relief and a decrease in healing time for the peptic ulcer.

6. b. A duodenal ulcer, treated appropriately, should respond to treatment and heal completely within 3 to 6 weeks. *H. pylori* treatment should last 10 to 14 days. A course of acid suppression therapy following eradication treatment is no longer thought to be needed.

7. b. Misoprostol is a prostaglandin analogue and is a cytoprotective agent to gastrointestinal mucosa. It is approved for the prevention of NSAID-induced ulcers in persons at high risk; however, PPIs are better at preventing duodenal ulcers and as good as misoprostol in preventing gastric ulcers. Metoclopramide is a prokinetic and may be useful as an adjunct therapy for GERD; however, the Food and Drug Administration required labels to carry warnings concerning the neuroleptic malignant syndrome as a possible adverse reaction. Bismuth is an agent available as part of the combination therapies used for *H. pylori* eradication. Ondansetron is a 5-HT_3 antagonist that is used to prevent nausea and vomiting in chemotherapy patients. Nizatidine is an H_2-receptor antagonist. H_2 receptor antagonists inhibit the action of histamine at the histamine H_2-receptor of the parietal cell, decreasing both basal and food-stimulated acid secretion. All H_2-receptor antagonists are equally efficacious. The treatment of choice for peptic ulcer disease not associated with *H. pylori* is a PPI.

8. a. COX-2-specific NSAIDs still have a risk of causing PUD but perhaps at a reduced rate than typical NSAIDs. They are used with caution because of their increased risk of fatal cardiovascular events. NSAIDs including indomethacin are well-known to be causative agents in both gastritis and PUD. There is a 10% to 20% prevalence of gastric ulcers and a 25% prevalence of duodenal ulcers in chronic NSAID users.

Dexamethasone (a potent corticosteroid) is extensively used in palliative care to reduce cerebral edema and inhibit centrally mediated nausea and/or vomiting. However, it is a potent stimulator of gastric acid secretion and must be used with an H_2-receptor antagonist or a PPI to prevent gastritis or peptic ulcer formation.

Aspirin is one of the most ulcerogenic NSAIDs. The risk appears to be dose related and is present even at doses of 325 mg every other day. Risk of PUD with NSAID use increases with age, prior GI disease, steroid use, anticoagulant use, female sex, and increased dose.

9. e. Infection with *H. pylori* can be lifelong. In most of the developing world, the prevalence of infection is 80% to 90% of the population. In the United States, approximately 30% of those with dyspepsia are colonized with *H. pylori*. Transmission is through oral–oral and fecal–oral routes, and organisms can be found in infected individuals' feces and saliva. The prevalence of infection in African Americans, Asian Americans, and Hispanics is on average one-third higher than in white Americans. Persons with lower income and socioeconomic status seem to be at risk for higher prevalence.

10. b. NSAID-induced gastric ulcers can be asymptomatic, and initial presentation can be perforation or bleeding. A gastric ulcer identified endoscopically must be followed by another endoscopy to confirm that healing has occurred. The pain of gastric ulcer disease is aggravated rather than relieved by food. Anorexia, nausea, and vomiting are more common in patients with gastric ulcers than in patients with duodenal ulcers. Also, the healing rate for gastric ulcers generally is slower than for duodenal ulcers.

11. c. Several of the PPIs, namely lansoprazole and rabeprazole, need to be used with caution in patients

with hepatic impairment. PPIs do provide better acid suppression, healing rates, and symptom relief than the H₂ blockers. The dose and frequency of dosing are also less for PPIs.

12. c. It is acceptable to empirically treat a patient with documented duodenal or suspected duodenal ulcer who has no alarm signs, as reviewed in answer 2.

13. c. ELISA serology testing, although very convenient and commonly used, is not reliable to determine successful eradication of *H. pylori*. Antibody titers are slow to decline and can therefore lead to many false positives even after successful treatment. Serology testing is appropriate for patients never treated for the organism in the past. Steiner's stain of gastric biopsy and culture require invasive endoscopy but are sensitive and specific for detecting persistence of *H. pylori* after treatment. Stool antigen and urea breath tests are also accurate tests to check for persistence of infection. Stool tests are more convenient since they are office based compared to the urea breath test, which requires special equipment not usually available in the office.

14. d. *H. pylori* continues to be the number one cause of PUD, followed by NSAIDs. Zollinger–Ellison syndrome is not common but causes multiple duodenal and gastric ulcers. Idiopathic ulcers are on the increase as *H. pylori* prevalence declines.

Solution to the Clinical Case Management Problem

NSAIDs can cause acute mucosal injury with submucosal hemorrhages and erosions with gross bleeding as a topical effect, and chronic use leads to ulceration from systemic effect by inhibiting prostaglandins that protect against injury in the GI tract.

H. pylori infection causes gastric inflammation. Infected persons have increased gastric acid

secretion, and in patients with ulcers this may be sixfold higher than in normal individuals. There are also interactions between NSAIDs and *H. pylori*. NSAID users are more prone to developing an ulcer if they are *H. pylori* positive; in fact, they have a twofold higher risk of having a bleeding peptic ulcer with concomitant *H. pylori* infection.

Summary

SYMPTOMS AND SIGNS

Approximately 40% of the population experiences symptoms referable to the upper GI tract every 6 months, and the two most common symptoms are epigastric pain and heartburn, frequently coexisting. When to obtain endoscopy is an ongoing controversy. Dyspepsia under the age of 55 years in the absence of warning signs (weight loss, persistent symptoms despite treatment, and blood in the stool) is often functional, and most guidelines do not call for endoscopy. Persistent symptoms, however, suggest the presence of PUD. PUD occurs in the stomach and duodenum, and although discernment between the two loci on the basis of symptoms is poor, there are some overall principles. First, duodenal ulcer tends to produce midepigastric pain sometimes radiating to the back and often relieved by ingestion of food or antacids. Second, gastric ulcer tends to produce midepigastric pain relieved by antacids but often aggravated by food. Nocturnal pain is often present. Third, nausea and vomiting are frequently associated with PUD. Anorexia and weight loss in the presence of PUD symptoms should be investigated by endoscopy.

Epigastric tenderness, although frequently present, is of little help in discerning upper GI pathology (sensitivity, 64%; specificity, 30%). A palpable epigastric mass or a supraclavicular lymph node (Virchow's node) should raise concern for a gastric malignancy.

1. Etiology

The two most common causes of PUD are use of NSAIDs and infection with *H. pylori*.

2. Differential diagnosis

Cholecystitis; pancreatitis; appendicitis; carcinoma of the esophagus, stomach, or pancreas; ischemic bowel disease in the elderly; inflammatory bowel disease

3. Investigations

a. *Helicobacter pylori* testing can be done noninvasively and treatment provided if positive.

b. Upper endoscopy is used for direct visualization, culture, and biopsy of the esophagogastroduodenal mucosa. There are no reliable clinical guidelines to assist in the decision of when to use endoscopy. In general, age older than 55 years and/or symptoms unresponsive to therapy warrant consideration for endoscopy. Examining stool for blood and a complete blood count may be indicated if there are signs or symptoms suggestive of blood loss.

4. Treatment

a. NSAID-associated peptic ulcer: Stop the NSAID and begin a PPI (e.g., omeprazole); 2-week courses are effective in many patients.

b. *H. pylori*-associated peptic ulcer: See treatment protocols in answer 4; beware of resistance, which is an increasing problem.

Suggested Reading

Ables AZ, Simon I, Melton ER: Update on *Helicobacter pylori* treatment. *Am Fam Physician* 75(3):351–358, 2007.

Delaney B, Ford AC, Forman D, et al: Initial management strategies for dyspepsia. *Cochrane Database Syst Rev* (4):CD001961, 2005.

Ford AC, Delaney BC, Forman D, Moayyedi P: Eradication therapy for peptic ulcer disease in *Helicobacter pylori* positive patients. *Cochrane Database Syst Rev* (2):CD003840, 2006.

Gisbert JP, Khorrami S, Carballo F, et al: *H. pylori* eradication therapy vs. antisecretory non-eradication therapy (with or without long-term maintenance antisecretory therapy) for the prevention of recurrent bleeding from peptic ulcer. *Cochrane Database Syst Rev* (2):CD004062, 2004.

Huang JQ, Zheng GF, Hunt RH, et al: Do patients with non-ulcer dyspepsia respond differently to Helicobacter pylori eradication treatments from those with peptic ulcer disease? A systematic review. *World J Gastroenterol* 11(18):2726–2732, 2005.

Louw JA: Peptic ulcer disease. *Curr Opin Gastroenterol* 22(6):607–611, 2006.

Moayyedi P, Soo S, Deeks J, et al: Eradication of Helicobacter pylori for non-ulcer dyspepsia. *Cochrane Database Syst Rev* (2):CD002096, 2006.

Moayyedi P, Talley NJ, Fennerty MB, Vakil N: Can the clinical history distinguish between organic and functional dyspepsia? *JAMA* 295(13):1566–1576, 2006.

Hepatitis and Cirrhosis

CLINICAL CASE PROBLEM 1

A 50-Year-Old Male with Ascites

A 50-year-old male is brought into your office by his wife. His wife states that for the past several months he has experienced extreme weakness and fatigue. In addition, he has gained 20 pounds in the past 3 weeks. She states that during the past few weeks, the patient has eaten virtually nothing. When you question the patient, he states that his wife is overreacting. The patient's wife is extremely concerned about his alcohol intake. When you question the patient, he states that he is a social drinker. When you pursue this line of questioning further and ask him what he means by being a social drinker, you find out that he drinks a few drinks before and after most meals plus a few drinks before he goes to bed.

You decide to pursue the question of drinking even further. When you ask him what he drinks, he says vodka. When you ask him if he drinks two 26-ounce bottles a day, he says, "Heck, no! I would never put away more than a bottle a day."

On physical examination, you find a middle-aged gentleman looking much older than his age. He has a ruddy complexion and scleral icterus. The patient has a significantly enlarged abdominal girth. There is a level of shifting dullness present. The patient's liver edge is felt 6 cm below the right costal margin. It has a nodular edge. In addition, spider nevi are present over the upper part of the patient's body. Palmar erythema is noted.

SELECT THE BEST ANSWER TO THE FOLLOWING QUESTIONS

1. Which of the following statements regarding this patient's condition is (are) false?
   a. the most likely diagnosis is cirrhosis of the liver
   b. this condition probably is associated with alcohol abuse
   c. jaundice is a rare sign in the disorder described
   d. approximately 30% of patients with a history of alcohol abuse will develop alcoholic hepatitis
   e. approximately 50% of patients with this condition (in an advanced stage) will die within 2 years

2. Which of the following statements regarding alcoholic hepatitis is (are) false?
   a. alcoholic cirrhosis develops in approximately 90% of patients with alcoholic hepatitis
   b. serum bilirubin often may be 10 to 20 times what is normal in this condition
   c. serum alanine aminotransferase (ALT) is almost always lower than serum aspartate aminotransferase (AST; formally SGOT)
   b. hepatomegaly is seen in 80% to 90% of patients with alcoholic hepatitis
   e. a mortality rate of 10% to 15% is seen in acute alcoholic hepatitis

3. What is the most common cause of cirrhosis in the United States?
   a. hepatitis A
   b. hepatitis B
   c. hepatitis C
   d. alcoholism
   e. cytomegalovirus hepatitis

4. The ascites associated with cirrhosis generally should be treated by which of the following?
   a. sodium restriction
   b. water restriction
   c. spironolactone
   d. a and c
   e. a, b, and c

5. Clinical manifestations of cirrhosis include which of the following?
   a. fatigue
   b. jaundice
   c. splenomegaly
   d. hypoalbuminemia
   e. all of the above

6. The pathophysiology of alcoholic cirrhosis includes all of the following except
   a. macronodular and micronodular fibrosis
   b. nodular regeneration
   c. decreased portal vein pressure
   d. increase in hepatic size followed by a decrease
   e. development of ascites and esophageal varices

7. Which of the following is (are) appropriate treatment for cirrhosis of the liver?
   a. cessation of alcohol use
   b. beta blockers
   c. maintenance of proper nutrition
   d. liver transplantation
   e. all of the above

CLINICAL CASE PROBLEM 2

A Nauseated 25-Year-Old Schoolteacher with Icterus and Right Upper Quadrant Pain

A 25-year-old schoolteacher presents with nausea, vomiting, anorexia, aversion to her usual one pack a day tobacco habit, and right upper quadrant abdominal pain. She has been sick for the past 3 days. On questioning, she does complain of passing dark-colored urine for the past 2 days. She has just returned from a 2-week trip to Mexico. Her boyfriend, who was on vacation with her, is not sick. She has had no exposure to blood products, has no history of intravenous drug use, and has no significant risk factors for sexually transmitted disease. On examination, she looks acutely ill. Her pulse is 100 beats/minute, blood pressure 110/70 mmHg, respirations 18, and temperature 101°F. Her sclera are icteric, and her liver edge is tender.

8. What is the most likely diagnosis in this patient?
a. hepatitis A
b. hepatitis B
c. hepatitis C
d. atypical infectious mononucleosis
e. none of the above

9. Which of the following tests is the most sensitive in confirming the diagnosis suspected in this patient?
a. complete blood count with differential
b. anti-hepatitis A virus (HAV)-immunoglobulin M (IgM)
c. HAV core antigen
d. anti-hepatitis B core antigen
e. anti-hepatitis C virus

10. Initial screening for hepatitis B should include which of the following?
a. hepatitis B surface antibody (anti-HBsAg) and hepatitis B core antibody (anti-HBc)
b. hepatitis B early antigen (HBeAg) and anti-HBe
c. HBsAg and anti-HBsAg
d. HBsAg and anti-HBc
e. anti-HBe and anti-HBc

11. Which of the following laboratory tests is (are) usually abnormal in a patient with acute viral hepatitis?
a. serum AST
b. serum bilirubin
c. serum ALT
d. serum alkaline phosphatase
e. all of the above

12. Indications for the use of hepatitis B vaccine include which of the following?
a. health care personnel
b. patients undergoing hemodialysis
c. all children
d. all previously unvaccinated adults
e. all of the above

13. Which of the following types of viral hepatitis is (are) associated with the development of chronic active hepatitis?
a. hepatitis B
b. hepatitis C
c. hepatitis A
d. a and b only
e. all of the above

14. Which of the following is (are) a complication(s) of alcoholic cirrhosis?
a. hypersplenism
b. hepatic encephalopathy
c. congestive gastropathy
d. spontaneous bacterial peritonitis
e. all of the above

Clinical Case Management Problem

Describe the relationship between cirrhosis of the liver and right-sided heart failure.

Answers

1. c. This patient has alcoholic hepatitis with cirrhosis of the liver. Alcohol abuse is thought to be related to one in five hospitalizations in the United States. Many cases of cirrhosis of the liver are directly attributable to alcohol abuse, although infectious agents, particularly hepatitis C, are an emerging cause. Cirrhosis is an irreversible inflammatory disease that disrupts liver structure and function. Alcoholic hepatitis is seen in approximately 30% of heavy drinkers. Men with alcoholic hepatitis usually consume at least 70 g of alcohol daily and have done so an average of 10 years. In women, a lower threshold of 20 to 40 g for the same period is average for the development of hepatitis. Cirrhosis is the disorganization of hepatic tissues caused by diffuse fibrosis and nodular regeneration. Nodules of regenerated tissue form between fibrous bands, giving the liver a cobbled appearance.

Symptoms of early alcoholic liver disease include weakness, fatigue, and weight loss. In advanced disease, the patient develops anorexia, nausea and vomiting, swelling of the abdomen and the lower extremities, and central nervous system symptoms related to the cirrhotic liver disease. Other symptoms that may occur include loss of libido in both sexes, gynecomastia in men, and menstrual irregularities in women.

The liver of patients with alcoholic hepatitis and cirrhosis is usually enlarged, palpable, and firm. In advanced cirrhosis, the liver may actually shrink. Dermatologic manifestations include spider nevi, palmar erythema, telangiectases on exposed areas, and occasional evidence of vitamin deficiencies. Although jaundice is rarely an initial sign, it usually develops later. Other later developing signs include ascites, lower extremity edema, pleural effusion, purpuric lesions, asterixis, tremor, delirium, coma, fever, splenomegaly, and superficial venous dilatation on the abdomen and thorax. There appears to be a genetic predisposition to the development of these complications. Of patients with advanced cirrhosis, 50% will be dead in a period of 2 years; 65% will be dead in 5 years. Hematemesis, jaundice, and ascites are unfavorable signs.

2. **a.** The first clinical stage of alcoholic liver disease is termed alcoholic hepatitis. Alcoholic hepatitis is a precursor of cirrhosis that is characterized by inflammation, degeneration, and necrosis of hepatocytes and infiltration of polymorphonuclear leukocytes and lymphocytes.

During the past 10 years in the United States, deaths from alcohol-related liver disease have increased. The incidence is greatest in middle-aged males, and mortality from cirrhosis is higher in blacks than in whites. Although alcoholic cirrhosis is a prevalent type of cirrhosis, only approximately 15% of alcoholics actually develop the disease. There appears to be a genetic predisposition to its development. The amount and duration of alcohol consumption are directly correlated with the extent of damage to the liver.

The symptoms of alcoholic hepatitis include anorexia, nausea, vomiting, weight loss, emesis, fever, and generalized abdominal pain. Hepatomegaly is found in 80% to 90% of these patients. Other signs include jaundice, ascites, splenomegaly, and spider angiomas.

Laboratory abnormalities in alcoholic hepatitis include hyperbilirubinemia and elevated serum transaminase. The ratio of serum AST/ALT is often 2:1 or greater. This can help differentiate alcoholic hepatitis from viral hepatitis. Other laboratory abnormalities include elevated alkaline phosphatase, hypoalbuminemia, and a prolonged prothrombin time.

The prognosis of alcoholic hepatitis is variable; many patients develop only a mild illness. However, there is a 10% to 15% mortality rate from the acute event.

The treatment of alcoholic hepatitis involves cessation of alcohol consumption, increased caloric and protein intake, and vitamin supplementation (especially thiamine).

Alcoholic cirrhosis develops in approximately 50% of patients surviving alcoholic hepatitis. In the other 50%, various degrees of hepatic fibrosis develop.

3. **c.** The most common cause of cirrhosis in the United States is now hepatitis C, surpassing alcohol-induced cirrhosis. Hepatitis C virus (HCV) is also the most common cause of hepatocellular carcinoma. More than 4 million Americans are infected with HCV, and the yearly incidence is 35,000. Patients with HCV go on to develop chronic active hepatitis in more than 50% of cases and subsequent cirrhosis in approximately 20% to 40% of cases. HCV is also the leading cause of liver transplantation. Hepatitis A does not progress to chronic active hepatitis. Hepatitis B progresses to chronic active hepatitis and subsequently to cirrhosis in up to 10% to 15% of cases. Cytomegalovirus infection does not produce cirrhosis.

4. **d.** The treatment of ascites and the edema associated with ascites includes the following: (1) sodium restriction to 800 mg of Na^+/day (or 2 g of NaCl); (2) spironolactone (Aldactone) 25 to 100 mg four times per day (effective in 40% to 75% of cases); (3) paracentesis; (4) combination diuretic therapy with furosemide in those patients who do not respond, with either spironolactone plus hydrochlorothiazide or spironolactone plus furosemide; and (5) paracentesis with albumin (or dextran) infusion in refractory cases. There must be complete abstention from alcohol. Fluid restriction is unnecessary unless serum sodium is less than 120 to 125 mEq/L.

The 1-year survival rate of patients with cirrhosis with ascites is 50%, compared with 90% in patients with uncomplicated cirrhosis. Formation of ascites results from a combination of portal hypertension, hypoalbuminemia, lymphatic leakage, and sodium retention. The management of ascites in patients with cirrhosis is complicated. Diagnostic paracentesis should be performed in any patient with cirrhosis who undergoes clinical deterioration. Defined indications for the treatment of ascites include significant patient discomfort, respiratory compromise, a large umbilical hernia, and recurrent bacterial peritonitis.

Sodium restriction is considered the cornerstone of therapy for ascites. Patients with cirrhosis require significant curtailment of sodium intake (800 mg/day) to obtain clinical benefit. Approximately 10% to 20% of patients who maintain a strict low-salt diet achieve complete resolution of ascites without additional therapy.

However, hyponatremia may accompany sodium restriction, and severe hyponatremia (serum Na less than 125 mEq) is a reason to begin fluid restriction as well. The vast majority of patients will also require diuretics.

Spironolactone (Aldactone), an aldosterone antagonist, is the first-line diuretic of choice in the treatment of cirrhotic ascites. It is effective in controlling up to 50% of patients with cirrhosis. Other potassium-sparing diuretics may be substituted for spironolactone, including triamterene and amiloride. The addition of loop diuretics (e.g., furosemide) is sometimes needed to achieve maximum benefit. Alternatives to furosemide include bumetanide and torsemide. Watch for hypokalemia with diuretics. Up to 90% of patients with cirrhosis and ascites will respond to diuretics and salt restriction. For those who do not, periodic paracentesis with albumin replacement is an alternative, as are portocaval shunts and transjugular intrahepatic portosystemic shunts, the latter for those requiring frequent large-volume paracentesis.

5. e. The clinical manifestations of cirrhosis were discussed previously. Another common finding in cirrhosis is hypoalbuminemia due to poor hepatic synthetic function.

6. c. Cirrhosis is an irreversible inflammatory condition of disordered and disrupted liver structure and function. Cirrhosis results from the disorganization of hepatic tissues caused by diffuse fibrosis and nodular regeneration. Micronodular and macronodular fibrosis occurs. Nodules of regenerated tissue form between the fibrous bands, giving the liver a cobbled appearance. The liver is initially larger than normal in size and then usually becomes smaller than normal in the later stages. The changes in the liver result in increased portal vein pressure, which leads to the formation of ascites and to esophageal varices.

7. e. In uncomplicated cirrhosis, treatment includes cessation of alcohol use, maintenance of proper nutrition, and use of beta blockers to reduce portal hypertension. Patients with uncomplicated cirrhosis may have a relatively benign course of illness for many years. Once the patient has an episode of decompensation, such as fluid retention, variceal bleeding, encephalopathy, spontaneous bacterial peritonitis, or hepatorenal syndrome, mortality is high without transplantation.

8. a. This patient most likely has hepatitis A. Hepatitis A occurs either spontaneously or in epidemics. Transmission is via the oral–fecal route. The presenting signs and symptoms of hepatitis A include (1) general malaise and fatigue; (2) general myalgias; (3) arthralgias; (4) abdominal pain; (5) nausea and vomiting; (6) severe anorexia, out of proportion to the degree of illness; and (7) aversion to smoking (if the patient smokes). Hepatitis B and hepatitis C are unlikely in this case because risk factors are absent. Although infectious mononucleosis may involve the liver and present with some of the same signs and symptoms, hepatitis A is much more likely, given the history of travel to an endemic area.

9. b. Acute infection with hepatitis A is confirmed by the demonstration of IgM antibodies to HAV (IgM-anti-HAV). These antibodies persist for approximately 12 weeks after appearance. IgG antibodies to HAV follow and simply indicate exposure at some time in the past. HAV core antigen is incorrect because hepatitis A does not possess a recognizable core antigen; the tests using core antigen apply to hepatitis B only, and antibodies to HB core antigen have nothing to do with hepatitis A. Choice e, anti-hepatitis C virus, is incorrect because it does not give any information about hepatitis A infection.

10. d. There are so many antigens and antibodies associated with hepatitis virology that it is difficult to determine what is what. However, it can be simplified considerably. Initial screening for hepatitis B should include HBsAg and anti-HBc (HBcAb, the antibody to the core antigen). These two tests will identify most cases of acute hepatitis B. There is a period between the clearance of HBsAg and the appearance of anti-HBs (HBsAb) that lasts for 4 to 6 weeks. During this time, the only marker for hepatitis B that can detect the infection with any certainty is anti-HBc (HBcAb). If acute hepatitis B is suggested from the initial screening, then further laboratory tests should be ordered. These include the following:

1. HBeAg: The e antigen indicates the presence of a highly infectious or contagious state or a chronic infection.
2. anti-HBe (HBeAb, the antibody to the previously listed antigen): The presence of this antibody indicates low infectivity and predicts the later seroconversion or resolution of hepatitis B.
3. anti-HBs (HBsAb, the antibody to the surface antigen): The presence of this antibody indicates past hepatitis B infection and current immunity.

11. e. In acute viral hepatitis, the serum transaminases (serum AST and serum ALT) are markedly elevated, along with serum bilirubin and serum alkaline phosphatase.

12. **e.** Hepatitis B vaccine should be offered to all people not previously immunized and is particularly important for those at high risk and those with continued exposure to hepatitis B infection. Those at high risk for acquiring hepatitis B include the following: (1) all health care personnel, (2) patients undergoing hemodialysis, (3) patients requiring frequent blood transfusions, (4) employees and residents of institutions for people with developmental disabilities, (5) men who have sex with men and all of their contacts, (6) intravenous drug users, (7) sexual contacts of chronic HBsAg carriers, and (8) children born to mothers who have chronic hepatitis B. The Centers for Disease Control and Prevention (CDC) recommends all children be immunized with hepatitis B vaccine.

13. **d.** Chronic active hepatitis (which may lead to cirrhosis of the liver, liver failure, and hepatocellular carcinoma) is associated with hepatitis B, hepatitis C, and hepatitis D (delta virus hepatitis, which occurs only in patients who are also chronically infected with hepatitis B). Chronic active hepatitis is not associated with hepatitis A or hepatitis E.

14. **e.** Complications of cirrhosis include the following: (1) portal hypertension, leading to esophageal varices, congestive gastropathy, and hypersplenism; (2) hepatic encephalopathy; (3) ascites, leading to spontaneous bacterial peritonitis and umbilical hernia (spontaneous rupture); (4) hepatorenal syndrome; (5) coagulation abnormalities; (6) hepatocellular carcinoma; (7) pulmonary dysfunction; (8) hepatic osteodystrophy; (9) cholelithiasis; (10) pericardial effusion; and (11) impaired reticuloendothelial system function.

Solution to the Clinical Case Management Problem

Briefly, the relationship between cirrhosis of the liver and right-sided heart failure is that micronodular fibrosis, macronodular fibrosis, and nodular regeneration eventually lead to portal hypertension with all of its complications, one of which can be right-sided heart failure.

Summary

INFECTIOUS FORMS OF HEPATITIS

1. Hepatitis A
   a. The etiologic agent is an RNA hepatovirus.
   b. Sporadic or epidemic infections are spread by the fecal–oral route.
   c. The primary symptoms are anorexia, nausea, vomiting, malaise, and aversion to smoking.
   d. The clinical signs are fever, enlarged tender liver, and jaundice.
   e. The relevant laboratory findings are normal to low white blood cell count and abnormal ALT, AST, bilirubin, and alkaline phosphatase values.
   f. Diagnostic clues include elevated transaminase levels and the presence of serum IgM-anti-HAV.

   The only treatment required is symptomatic, namely rest; it is rarely fulminating and does not become chronic.

   Prevention is meticulous hand washing because the oral–fecal route is the main route of spread. Although important for all, it is essential for food handlers. Hepatitis A vaccine is now available for patients at risk.

2. Hepatitis B
   a. The etiologic agent is a DNA hepadnavirus.
   b. It is usually transmitted sexually or by blood or blood products and is particularly common in intravenous drug users and in patients with acquired immune deficiency syndrome (AIDS).
   c. Up to 30% of infected individuals may be carriers.
   d. It is diagnosed by finding an elevation of liver transaminases and HBsAg and anti-HBc in the serum.

   The treatment is symptomatic unless it becomes fulminating—as it will in 0.1% to 1% of cases—or chronic—as it will in 1% to 10% of infected adults and 90% of neonates. The recommended treatment of symptoms is with interferon, which has a 40% success rate.

   Hepatitis B hyperimmunoglobulin is used to prevent symptoms after known or suspected exposure and prevention is obtained via hepatitis B vaccine, the administration of which is now recommended for all children and adults by the CDC.

3. Hepatitis C
   a. The etiologic agent is a single-stranded virus belonging to the Flaviviridae family.
   b. There are more than 100 strains belonging to six major "genotypes."
   c. The disease is usually transmitted by blood or blood products, and sexual transmission is also possible.
   d. The development of a screening test in 1990 virtually eliminated spread via transfusions, and it is thought that sharing of contaminated needles is the main route of transfer.

The disease course is quite variable. Approximately 15% to 25% of infected individuals recover spontaneously. The remaining individuals become chronically infected, of whom approximately 20% will develop cirrhosis and another 1% to 5% will develop hepatocellular cancer.

Hepatitis C is the most common chronic bloodborne infection in the United States, with an incidence of approximately 35,000 cases per year. Approximately 4 million people in the United States are infected, and as the population ages hepatitis C–related deaths—currently approximately 8000 to 10,000 per year—will increase. Currently, it is the most common cause of cirrhosis and liver transplantation.

Treatment of hepatitis C is symptomatic and depends on liver biopsy staging and viral genotyping. As mentioned previously, it often progresses to become a chronic disease, which can be treated with pegylated interferon and ribavirin. Factors associated with successful treatment include genotypes other than 1, lower baseline levels, less fibrosis on biopsy, and lower body surface area and weight. Major side effects of treatment include flulike symptoms, neuropsychiatric symptoms, and cytopenias. Sustained responses (the absence of viral HCV-RNA in serum) of 55% in carefully selected individuals are typical.

4. Delta hepatitis (hepatitis D)
   Delta hepatitis is found only in association with chronic hepatitis B. This combination is particularly likely to lead to chronic active hepatitis and its complications, including cirrhosis, liver cell failure, and hepatocellular carcinoma.

5. Hepatitis E
   This is an enterically transmitted form of hepatitis. Like hepatitis A, it never leads to chronic infection.

ALCOHOLIC HEPATITIS

The signs and symptoms of alcoholic hepatitis closely resemble the symptoms of viral hepatitis. In alcoholic hepatitis, the ratio of AST to ALT is usually 2:1.

Patients who develop alcoholic hepatitis are at high risk for developing cirrhosis of the liver. The symptoms and signs of cirrhosis are weakness, fatigue, weight loss, anorexia, hepatomegaly, spider nevi, palmar erythema, asterixis, tremor, and ascites. Patients with cirrhosis often develop portal hypertension with its complications and hepatic encephalopathy.

The treatment is supportive. The use of glucocorticoids in acute alcoholic hepatitis is controversial. Colchicine may slow disease progression. Complete abstinence from alcohol is important. Treatments for ascites include sodium restriction, diuretics (especially spironolactone) with or without thiazides or loop diuretics, paracentesis, and shunts.

Cirrhotic liver complications include upper gastrointestinal bleeding from varices, hemorrhagic gastritis, or gastroduodenal ulcers; liver failure; hepatic encephalopathy; hepatorenal syndrome; and hepatocellular carcinoma.

Suggested Reading

Flamm SL: Chronic hepatitis C virus infection. *JAMA* 289(18): 2413–2417, 2003.

Heidelbaugh JJ, Bruderly M: Cirrhosis and chronic liver failure: Part 1. Diagnosis and evaluation. *Am Fam Physician* 74:756–762, 781, 2006.

Heidelbaugh JJ, Sherbondy MA: Cirrhosis and chronic liver failure: Part 2. Complication and treatment. *Am Fam Physician* 74:767–776, 781, 2006.

Iredale JP: Cirrhosis: New research provides a basis for rational and targeted treatments. *BMJ* 327(7407):143–147, 2003.

Lin KW, Kirchner JT: Hepatitis B. *Am Fam Physician* 69:75–82, 86, 2004.

Madhotra R, Gilmore IT: Recent developments in the treatment of alcoholic hepatitis. *QJM* 96(6):391–400, 2003.

Marsano LS: Hepatitis. *Prim Care* 30(1):81–107, 2003.

Russo MW, Fried MW: Side effects of therapy for chronic hepatitis C. *Gastroenterology* 124(6):1711–1719, 2003.

Ryder SD, Beckingham IJ: ABC of diseases of liver, pancreas, and biliary system: Acute hepatitis. *BMJ* 322(7279):151–153, 2001.

Schiff ER: Update in hepatology. *Ann Intern Med* 132(6):460–466, 2000.

CLINICAL CASE PROBLEM 1

50-Year-Old Male with a History of Severe Abdominal Pain

A 50-year-old male with a 20-year history of heavy drinking comes to your emergency room with his wife complaining of severe abdominal pain. The pain began 4 days ago and has been getting progressively worse. The pain has been so severe that the patient has been crying at night. Despite this severe pain, the patient managed to make it to his local bar last evening and straggled home at 3 AM. He has also been nauseous and vomited a few times yesterday. The pain is described as constant, sometimes burning in nature, and seems to go to the back. The patient has not eaten for the past 4 days.

On examination, you observe a stoic, overweight male who looks much older than his stated age; he looks pale and slightly diaphoretic. As you examine him, you clearly smell alcohol on his breath. The patient's blood pressure is 90/70 mmHg, respirations are 20 breaths/minute, and pulse is 100 beats/minute. Examination of his heart and lungs is normal except for mild tachycardia. He has a marked tenderness in the epigastric region along with guarding. The bowel sounds are slightly diminished. There is also a sensation of fullness present in the epigastric area. No other abnormalities are present.

SELECT THE BEST ANSWER TO THE FOLLOWING QUESTIONS

1. The differential diagnosis at this point would be
   a. acute gastritis
   b. acute pancreatitis
   c. perforated peptic ulcer
   d. acute cholecystitis
   e. all of the above

2. All of the following tests should be ordered next except
   a. complete blood count with differential
   b. serum amylase and lipase level
   c. computed tomography (CT) scan of the abdomen with contrast
   d. comprehensive metabolic panel
   e. arterial blood gases

3. Which of the radiological imaging techniques is the most sensitive in diagnosing acute pancreatitis and pancreatic pseudocyst?
   a. transabdominal ultrasonography
   b. contrast-enhanced CT of the abdomen
   c. magnetic resonance cholangiopancreatography
   d. plain x-ray (abdominal series)
   e. endoscopic ultrasonography

4. Patients with acute pancreatitis sometimes present with bruising around the umbilicus and flank area. This is due to
   a. trauma to the abdomen
   b. ruptured spleen
   c. retroperitoneal bleeding
   d. superior mesenteric artery erosion
   e. disseminated intravascular coagulation

5. Fullness in the epigastric region and a palpable mass in this patient are most likely due to
   a. a pancreatic pseudocyst formation
   b. a palpable gallbladder
   c. an enlarged spleen
   d. an enlarged liver
   e. abdominal wall hematoma

6. What is (are) the essential diagnostic feature(s) of the condition of the patient described here?
   a. abrupt onset of epigastric pain with radiation to the back
   b. nausea and vomiting
   c. elevated serum amylase
   d. all of the above
   e. none of the above

7. The treatment of this condition must include all of the following except
   a. eliminate oral intake for the first 48 hours
   b. aggressive fluid replacement
   c. calcium replacement
   d. pain control
   e. intravenous H_2-receptor blockers

8. Which of the following statements about the disease discussed is (are) true?
   a. many cases of this disease are associated with gallstones
   b. strong evidence suggests a link between this disease and alcohol
   c. the chronic condition of this disease is more likely to be associated with alcohol abuse rather than biliary tract disease

d. all of the above statements are true

e. none of the above statements are true

9. In approximately two-thirds of patients with this disease, a plain film of the abdomen is abnormal. Which of the following abnormalities is this plain film most likely to show?
   a. a "sentinel loop"
   b. the "colon cutoff sign"
   c. air under the diaphragm
   d. distention in both the small bowel and the large bowel
   e. feces throughout the colon

10. Complications of the condition described here include all of the following except
    a. ascites
    b. pleural effusion and acute respiratory distress syndrome (ARDS)
    c. pancreatic necrosis
    d. pseudocyst formation
    e. membranous enterocolitis

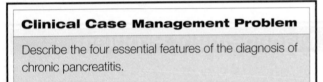

Clinical Case Management Problem

Describe the four essential features of the diagnosis of chronic pancreatitis.

Answers

1. e. All of the mentioned conditions can present with an acute abdomen and the signs and symptoms demonstrated by this patient. At this early stage, all these conditions should be considered as differential diagnoses.

2. c. The initial laboratory evaluation should include a complete blood count with differential, amylase and lipase level, metabolic panel (blood urea nitrogen, creatinine, glucose, and calcium levels), and liver function tests and arterial blood gases. Results from these tests should be used to guide further evaluation. CT scan of the abdomen would help in diagnosing pancreatitis and pseudocyst formation but should be done after the initial laboratory investigations and stabilization of the patient.

3. b. Contrast-enhanced CT has become the standard imaging technique for detection of acute pancreatitis and pseudocyst formation. Not only does it help in diagnosis but also some studies have shown that a CT severity index is helpful in predicting the severity of acute pancreatitis compared with the Ranson's criteria and the APACHE II scale. Transabdominal ultrasonography is a better tool for diagnosis of cholelithiasis. Bowel gas can often limit the accuracy of pancreatic imaging by ultrasonography. Plain x-ray of the abdomen can demonstrate the sentinel loop in two-thirds of patients but is not sensitive or specific enough for diagnosis. Magnetic resonance cholangiopancreatography can be used as a noninvasive test to determine which patients will need endoscopic retrograde cholangiopancreatography (ERCP). It is no more sensitive than a CT scan in determining the severity of acute pancreatitis, and it is much more expensive and not always available.

4. c. Ecchymosis in the periumbilical area (Cullen's sign) and in the flank area (Grey–Turner's sign) is caused by retroperitoneal bleeding. Ruptured spleen is not associated with acute pancreatitis. Superior mesentric artery occlusion does not present with bruising in the abdominal wall. Disseminated intravascular coagulation presents with generalized bleeding.

5. a. The palpable mass in this patient is most likely due to pancreatic pseudocyst formation. A palpable gallbladder is seen in obstruction at the ampulla or sphincter of Oddi. These patients are jaundiced and do not present with such acute symptoms and pain. An enlarged spleen is unlikely in this patient given the clinical history, as is an enlarged liver. This patient did not give a history of trauma to suggest an abdominal wall hematoma.

6. d. The essential diagnostic features of acute pancreatitis include abrupt onset of epigastric pain with radiation to the back and lower lumbar spine, nausea and vomiting, and elevated serum amylase and lipase. Acute pancreatitis is usually caused by gallstones or alcoholism. The essential diagnostic features of pancreatic pseudocyst include an epigastric mass and pain, mild fever and leukocytosis, persistent serum amylase or serum lipase elevation, and demonstration of pseudocyst by CT scan.

7. e. The essentials of treatment of severe acute pancreatitis include (1) keeping the patient NPO for the first 48 hours and gastric suction via nasogastric tube if severe gastric distension is present; (2) fluid replacement to replace sequestered fluid in the retroperitoneal space; (3) replacement of calcium and magnesium and other electrolytes (in severe attacks of pancreatitis, both hypocalcemia and hypomagnesemia may occur and need to be treated); (4) oxygen therapy (severe hypoxemia develops in 30% of patients; the onset is often insidious and can result in adult respiratory distress syndrome); (5) adequate pain relief; (6) nutrition—enteral nutrition when the patient can tolerate PO intake; and (7) antibiotics if pancreatic necrosis and infection are present. Although the use of H₂-receptor blockers, anticholinergic drugs, and glucagon is reasonably common, their efficacy has not been demonstrated.

8. d. Gallstone disease and alcohol abuse are each responsible for approximately 40% of cases of acute pancreatitis. Other causes include hyperparathyroidism, hypertriglyceridemia, familial pancreatitis, postoperative (iatrogenic) pancreatitis, protein deficiency, use of certain drugs, obstruction of the pancreatic duct, and trauma.

Chronic pancreatitis is much more likely to be associated with alcoholism than with biliary tract disease. In fact, a patient with alcoholism who presents with one attack of acute pancreatitis is very likely to have subsequent attacks and chronic disease.

9. a. In approximately two-thirds of cases, a plain film of the abdomen is abnormal. The most frequent finding is isolated dilatation of a segment of gut (the sentinel loop) consisting of jejunum, transverse colon, or duodenum adjacent to the pancreas.

Gas distending the right colon that abruptly stops in the mid or left transverse colon is called the colon cutoff sign. This is caused by colonic spasm adjacent to the pancreatic inflammation but is not as common as the sentinel loop.

Air under the diaphragm is suggestive of a perforated peptic ulcer.

A completely distended small and large bowel suggests a distal bowel obstruction.

Constipation is not associated with acute pancreatitis.

10. e. In addition to chronic pancreatitis and pancreatic pseudocyst formation, acute pancreatitis may also lead to necrotic pancreatitis, pancreatic abscess (which is fatal if not treated surgically), ascites, pleural effusion, and ARDS. Membranous enterocolitis is not a complication of acute pancreatitis.

Solution to the Clinical Case Management Problem

The four essential features of chronic pancreatitis are as follows: (1) persistent or recurrent abdominal pain in almost all cases; (2) pancreatic calcification on x-ray in 50% of cases; (3) pancreatic insufficiency in 30% of cases, which may lead to either steatorrhea (loss of exocrine function) or diabetes mellitus (loss of endocrine function); and (4) it is most often caused by alcoholism.

Summary

1. Acute pancreatitis is usually caused by either alcohol abuse or biliary tract disease (40% biliary tract–gallstone associated; 40% alcohol intake). Other causes include hypertriglyceridemia, medications such as antiretroviral therapy, hypercalcemia and hyperparathyroidism, pancreatic or ampullary tumors, iatrogenic causes (e.g., operative trauma during ERCP), and autoimmune diseases.

2. Essential features of diagnosis are a history of alcohol abuse, abrupt onset of epigastric pain radiating through to the back, nausea and vomiting, and elevated serum amylase and serum lipase levels.

3. Laboratory investigations include complete blood count with differential, serum amylase and urine amylase, serum lipase, serum glucose, serum lactate dehydrogenase, serum bilirubin, serum aspartate aminotransferase/alanine aminotransferase, serum calcium, serum magnesium, electrolytes, serum triglycerides, and arterial blood gases. Radiological imaging includes plain film of abdomen, abdominal ultrasound, and contrast-enhanced CT scan of the abdomen. CT scan of the abdomen is the most sensitive imaging modality to diagnose the severity of acute pancreatitis and pseudocyst formation.

4. Clinical criteria to determine the severity of acute pancreatitis
   a. Ranson's criteria initially present
      i. age > 55 years
      ii. white blood cell count > 16,000/mm³
      iii. blood glucose > 200 mg%
      iv. serum lactate dehydrogenase > 350 IU/L
      v. aspartate aminotransferase (serum glutamate oxaloacetate transaminase) > 250 IU/L
   Criteria developing within 48 hours of admission
      i. hematocrit decreases more than 10%

    ii. blood urea nitrogen increases more than 5 mg/dL
   iii. serum Ca: 8 mg/dL or less
   iv. arterial Po$_2$ < 60 mmHg
    v. base deficit > 4 mew/L
   vi. estimated fluid sequestration = 600 mL (volume requirement)

  Morbidity and mortality rates correlate with number of criteria present
    i. 0 to 2 criteria, 1% mortality
   ii. 3 or 4 criteria, 15% mortality
  iii. 5 or 6 criteria, 40% mortality
   iv. 7 or 8 criteria, 50% or greater mortality

  b. CT severity index

    A is normal pancreas: 0 points

    B is edematous pancreas: 1 point

    C is B plus mild extrapancreatic changes: 2 points

    D is severe extrapancreatic changes plus one fluid collection: 3 points

    E is multiple or excessive fluid collections: 4 points

    A CT severity index score of 5 or more was associated with mortality 15 times higher than those with a score less than 5.

  c. APACHE II scoring system: Acute Physiology and Chronic Health Evaluation includes the following factors: age, rectal temperature, mean arterial pressure, heart rate, Pao$_2$, arterial pH, serum potassium, serum sodium, serum creatinine, hematocrit, white blood cell count, Glasgow Coma Scale scores, and chronic health status. APACHE II scores of 8 or more at 24 hours are associated with the need for the intensive care unit, secondary pancreatic infection, pancreatic necrosis, mortality, and increased hospital stay.

5. Essentials of management include NPO and nasogastric suction in severe cases with gastric distension, strict intake/output measurement (a measure of fluid sequestration), fluid replacement of sequestered fluid, replacement of calcium and magnesium if low, oxygen, pain control, and enteral nutrition as soon as tolerated.

6. Resolution within 1 week in most cases.

7. Complications include pseudocyst formation, abscess formation, hemorrhage, ascites, pleural effusion, and chronic pancreatitis.

8. Chronic pancreatitis is almost always associated with alcohol-induced problems; complications of chronic pancreatitis include malabsorption (steatorrhea), diabetes mellitus, and chronic pain.

Suggested Reading

Beckingham IJ, Bornman PC: ABC of diseases of liver, pancreas, and biliary system. Acute pancreatitis. *BMJ* 322(7286):595–598, 2001.

Carroll JK, Herrick B: Acute pancreatitis: Diagnosis, prognosis, and treatment. *Am Fam Physician* 75:1513–1521, 2007.

Munoz A, Katerndahl DA: Diagnosis and management of acute pancreatitis. *Am Fam Physician* 62:164–174, 2000.

Vlodov J, Tenner SM: Acute and chronic pancreatitis. *Prim Care* 28(3):607–628, 2001.

Yousaf M, McCallion K, Diamond T, et al: Management of severe acute pancreatitis. *Br J Surg* 90(4):407–420, 2003.

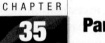

CHAPTER

35 **Pancreatic Carcinoma**

CLINICAL CASE PROBLEM 1

A 62-Year-Old Male with Abdominal Pain

A 62-year-old male comes to your office for a third opinion. He has seen two other physicians during the past 3 months regarding an abdominal pain that is, according to the patient, "getting worse and worse." It is unrelated in any way to food intake except that the patient has become significantly anorexic since developing the pain. The first physician told him that he had irritable bowel syndrome; the second physician told him that the pain was a psychoneurotic pain: "Basically, sir, that means it is all in your head." The patient tells you that he was very disappointed with the two physicians, especially because the first one had been his family doctor for more than 15 years.

You decide to spend your time today on a very focused history. The most important information you gather is (1) the patient has lost 20 pounds in 3 months; (2) the pain is constant; (3) the patient has never had abdominal pain before; (4) the patient's mood has definitely changed during this period (in fact, the first symptom was depression, even before the pain started); and (5) the pain is central abdominal, radiating through to the back, dull and aching in character, and described as a 7/10 in terms of severity.

On examination, the patient looks "unwell." You cannot describe it any more clearly than that. He just looks unwell. There is no clinical evidence of anemia, jaundice, or cyanosis. Examination of the abdomen reveals some tenderness in the midabdominal region. The liver edge is felt 2 cm below the left costal margin.

SELECT THE BEST ANSWER TO THE FOLLOWING QUESTIONS

1. The differential diagnosis in this patient would include all except which of the following?
   a. inflammatory bowel disease
   b. carcinoma of the stomach
   c. carcinoma of the pancreas
   d. irritable bowel syndrome
   e. none of the above can be excluded

2. If you could order only one investigation at this time, which one of the following would you order?
   a. a magnetic resonance imaging scan of the abdomen
   b. gastroscopy
   c. a dual-phase helical computed tomography (CT) scan of the abdomen
   d. a colonoscopy
   e. serum amylase or serum lipase

3. The appropriate investigation is ordered. What is the sensitivity of this investigation in the disorder described?
   a. 70%
   b. 80%
   c. 90%
   d. 95%
   e. 100%

4. Which of the following statements regarding the relationship between this patient's depressive symptoms and his abdominal symptoms is correct?
   a. the abdominal symptoms are unrelated to the depression
   b. the abdominal symptoms are indirectly related to the depression
   c. the abdominal symptoms are directly related to the depression
   d. the abdominal symptoms and the depressive symptoms usually do not coexist in this disorder
   e. nobody really knows for sure

5. The patient had planned a vacation for the week after the investigation was performed. You persuaded him to return to your office when he returns from his vacation in 6 weeks for further evaluation. You encourage him to take his vacation because of your suspicions regarding his disease. Before he leaves for his vacation, however, you must provide the patient with one other treatment. What is the single most important treatment to be undertaken at this time?
   a. begin the patient on an anti-inflammatory medication
   b. begin the patient on an oral corticosteroid
   c. begin the patient on an antidepressant
   d. begin the patient on an oral chemotherapeutic agent
   e. none of the above

6. Cancer pain is an extremely important medical problem. Which of the following statements regarding the management of cancer pain in the United States is true?
   a. cancer pain is extremely well managed by most U.S. physicians
   b. the overtreatment of cancer pain is much more of a problem than the undertreatment of cancer pain in the United States
   c. the undertreatment of cancer pain is much more of a problem than the overtreatment of cancer pain in the United States
   d. most Americans with cancer pain die in very good control; few have cancer pain that is not well controlled
   e. none of the above statements are true

7. The patient returns to your office in 6 weeks following an overseas tour. Because of your therapy, he was able to enjoy most of his holiday. Three days ago, his pain began to become acutely worse. The patient now appears jaundiced. He has lost another 15 pounds, and there is a palpable mass in the periumbilical region. The investigation performed earlier is repeated, and a mass measuring 6 cm × 5 cm is now seen in the appropriate region. At this time, what should you do?
   a. explore with a surgeon the possibility of a Whipple's procedure
   b. begin aggressive radiotherapy and chemotherapy
   c. begin high-dose prednisone to increase his weight
   d. explore with a surgeon the possibility of the total removal of the organ in question
   e. none of the above

8. What is the most clearly established risk factor for the disease described?
   a. alcohol consumption
   b. cigarette smoking
   c. high fat intake
   d. environmental toxins
   e. previous exposure to radiation

9. With respect to the molecular biology of this disease, which of the following statements is true?
   a. no tumor markers have been established for this disease
   b. the CA-19-9 and 72-4 serum markers may help to confirm the diagnosis in symptomatic patients
   c. the CA-19-9 serum antigen has a sensitivity of 90% in patients with this disease
   d. the CA-19-9 serum antigen has a specificity of 90% in patients with this disease
   e. the CA-19-9 and 72-4 serum markers are good screening tests for this disease

10. A patient with this disease will demonstrate which of the following physical findings?
    a. decreased pain when assuming the supine position
    b. increased pain when assuming the supine position
    c. decreased pain with flexion of the spine
    d. increased pain with flexion of the spine
    e. b and c
    f. a and d

Clinical Case Management Problem

Discuss the impact of this disease on the U.S. population under the following headings: (1) this disease's place as a killer of Americans (among all cancers), (2) risk factors, (3) symptoms and signs, (4) treatment, and (5) prognosis.

Answers

1. d. From the history and the physical examination, you determine that the patient has a serious disease. The severity, constant nature of the pain, and physical findings make irritable bowel syndrome implausible. In forming a differential diagnosis, you should consider diagnostic possibilities in the following categories: (1) infectious/inflammatory, (2) neoplastic or not, (3) circulatory, or (4) traumatic.

From the history alone, the following are diagnostic possibilities:

A. Infectious/inflammatory: (1) inflammatory bowel disease, Crohn's disease, or ulcerative colitis; (2) pancreatitis; or (3) cholecystitis
B. Neoplastic: (1) carcinoma of the stomach (linitis plastica); (2) carcinoma of the head of the pancreas; or (3) carcinoma of the colon
C. Circulatory: (1) aortic aneurysm (leaking) or (2) mesenteric ischemia
D. Traumatic: pancreatic pseudocyst

2. c. Obviously, before you decide on which investigation to order, you have to make a commitment to your primary diagnosis. The most likely diagnosis is adenocarcinoma of the pancreas. The reasons are as follows: (1) The abdominal pain is constant and unrelated to food, (2) the patient has experienced a 20-pound weight loss, and (3) the patient is depressed.

Therefore, the investigation of choice is a dual-phase helical CT scan of the abdomen. No other test provides such high sensitivity and specificity.

3. d. The sensitivity of the CT scan in the diagnosis of adenocarcinoma of the pancreas is between 95% and 98%—that is, only 1 of every 20 patients with adenocarcinoma will have false-negative CT scan results.

4. c. There is a significant correlation between carcinoma of the pancreas and depression. In many cases, as in this Clinical Case Problem, the depression actually precedes the abdominal pain.

5. e. Although it is reasonable to start the patient on an antidepressant, it is the second most important treatment. The most important treatment is to start the patient on an adequate pain relief program. It would seem that, because of the severity of the pain, an oral narcotic analgesic would be the drug of first choice. You suggest that while he is on vacation he telephone on a regular basis so you can advise medication changes.

6. c. Cancer pain is an enormous medical problem in the United States and Canada. It is likely to become an even more serious problem in the future as the population ages. It is estimated that approximately 50% of patients in North America with cancer die in moderately severe to severe pain. The reason appears to be multifactorial and related to inadequate education in medical school, residency, and continuing medical education; reluctance to use narcotic analgesics when they need to be used; and fear of licensure difficulties if "too many narcotics" are prescribed.

7. e. You should (1) break the news to the patient with his spouse or significant other present, if possible; (2) discuss with the patient his treatment options, including palliative radiotherapy, palliative chemotherapy, and palliative radiotherapy and chemotherapy; (3) suggest an aggressive pain control program, consider a celiac plexus block, changing narcotic analgesics, and continuing to increase his dosage of narcotics; and (4) in terms of symptoms, maintain control of nausea or vomiting, maintain control of constipation, and consider an appetite stimulant (Megace).

8. b. The most likely established risk factor for adenocarcinoma of the pancreas is cigarette smoking. There is some controversy regarding alcohol intake, but most authorities consider it a significant risk factor as well.

9. b. There is no effective screening test for this disease. However, the tumor antigens CA 19-9 and 72-4 are present in many patients with pancreatic carcinoma. These serum markers have a sensitivity of 50% to 75% and a specificity of less than 83%, making them inadequate tools for screening. However, in symptomatic patients, they may help with the diagnosis if the CT imaging test is equivocal, and they may provide some prognostic information.

10. e. One of the most important tests in the physical examination of a patient suspected of having a malignancy is known as a provocative maneuver. A provocative maneuver attempts to reproduce the pain (gently). An example of a provocative maneuver for somatic pain caused by bony metastatic disease is to put pressure on the bone in question. The provocative maneuver for a patient with a tumor that is retroperitoneal is to have the patient lie flat or lie with a pillow or other object underneath the small of his or her back. This will reproduce the pain. The same patient will obtain relief from his or her pain when leaning forward.

Solution to the Clinical Case Management Problem

Adenocarcinoma of the Pancreas

1. Mortality from adenocarcinoma: Approximately 31,000 new cases of adenocarcinoma of the pancreas occur each year, and there are an equivalent number of deaths each year. Adenocarcinoma of the pancreas is the fourth leading cause of death due to cancer.

2. Risk factors for adenocarcinoma of the pancreas: Women account for 57% of new cases—a number that is rising. Approximately 10% of patients have a familiar history. Cigarette smoking in all cases is clearly the number one risk factor. Other implicated factors include diabetes and obesity. High intake of fruits and vegetables and exercise appear to have protective effects.

3. Symptoms and signs
   a. Abdominal symptoms and signs: (i) central abdominal pain radiating through to the back; dull, aching, and steady in character; most commonly described as a "deep" pain; (ii) weight loss; (iii) hepatomegaly (50% of patients); (iv) palpable abdominal mass (indicates inoperability); (v) a palpable nontender gallbladder in a jaundiced patient suggests neoplastic obstruction of the common bile duct (Courvoisier's law).
   b. Nonabdominal symptoms and signs: Painless jaundice from obstruction of the common bile duct is a common sign seen in 80% of patients

with cancer in the head of the pancreas. Approximately two-thirds of pancreatic cancers occur in the pancreatic head. Depression as a result of the patient's general medical condition is often the initial symptom appearing before any of the abdominal symptoms or painless jaundice.

4. Treatments
   a. Surgical: Carcinoma of the head of the pancreas is resectable in only 20% of patients (Whipple's procedure).
   b. Chemotherapy/radiotherapy: More than half of patients with pancreatic carcinoma have metastases at the time of diagnosis. Palliative chemotherapy or radiotherapy can be offered; currently, several clinical trials have shown some promise of reducing mortality.
   c. Pain control: Pain control appears to be the most important part of therapy (celiac plexus block and/or narcotic analgesics).
   d. Symptom control: Control nausea and vomiting with combination antiemetics, and control constipation with lactulose or stool softener and a peristaltic stimulant.

5. Prognosis: The prognosis for adenocarcinoma of the pancreas is dismal. The 5-year survival rate is approximately 4%. However, moderately encouraging results have been obtained with the use of gemcitabine and other adjuvant, x-ray, and molecular biologic therapies.

Suggested Reading

Freelove R, Walling AD: Pancreatic cancer: Diagnosis and management. *Am Fam Physician* 73:485–492, 2006.

CLINICAL CASE PROBLEM 1

33-Year-Old Female with Right Upper Quadrant Abdominal Pain

A 33-year-old female comes to the emergency room with a 12-hour history of right upper quadrant (RUQ) abdominal pain. The pain is severe now but waxes and wanes and is associated with nausea and some episodes of vomiting. The pain sometimes radiates through to the back. She feels warm but has not checked her temperature. There is no diarrhea. Her last bowel movement was 1 day ago and was normal. The patient has no similar history in the past.

On examination, the patient is an obese young female in some discomfort. Her vital signs reveal a temperature of 100 °F and pulse of 102 beats/minute. Her blood pressure is 130/70 mmHg and her respirations are 18 breaths/minute. There is no scleral icterus. The chest is clear, and the cardiovascular exam is normal. Abdominal examination reveals marked upper abdominal tenderness with guarding, especially in the right upper quadrant. On palpation of the right upper quadrant of the abdomen when the patient is asked to take a deep breath, there is a marked increase in pain. The bowel sounds are present but seem slightly sluggish. The patient has no drug allergies and is not taking any medications at the present time.

SELECT THE BEST ANSWER TO THE FOLLOWING QUESTIONS

1. What is the most likely diagnosis in this patient?
   a. acute cholecystitis
   b. biliary colic
   c. acute gastroenteritis
   d. ileocecal appendicitis
   e. Crohn's disease

2. Given this patient's signs and symptoms, which of the following investigative procedures will you order next to help with the diagnosis?
   a. computed tomography (CT) scan of the abdomen
   b. a hydroxy iminodiacetic acid (HIDA) scan
   c. an abdominal ultrasound
   d. magnetic resonance imaging (MRI) of the abdomen
   e. plain x-ray of the abdomen

3. What is (are) the treatment(s) of choice for the patient at this time?
   a. intravenous fluids
   b. parenteral antibiotics
   c. adequate pain control
   d. laparoscopic cholecystectomy within 24 to 48 hours
   e. all of the above

4. Complications of gallstones include all of the following except
   a. acute cholecystitis
   b. hydrops of the gallbladder
   c. gastric outlet obstruction
   d. hepatic vein thrombosis
   e. acute biliary pancreatitis

5. Regarding the definite procedure to correct this condition, which of the following statements is true?
   a. a definite surgical procedure should not be contemplated at this time; if required, it should be performed several months later
   b. a definitive surgical procedure should not be contemplated at this time; if symptoms continue to recur, you can reconsider
   c. a definitive surgical procedure should be performed at this time
   d. a definitive surgical procedure is contraindicated given the signs and symptoms with which this patient presents
   e. a definitive surgical procedure should not be considered until all other methods of treatment have failed

6. Which of the following statements about gallbladder disease in the United States is (are) true?
   a. more than 20 million Americans have gallstones
   b. more than 300,000 cholecystectomies are performed annually
   c. most gallstones are composed predominantly of cholesterol
   d. diabetics have an increased prevalence of gallstones
   e. all of the above statements are true

7. Regarding the use of nonsurgical therapy in gallstone disease, which of the following statements is true?

a. oral dissolution therapy is an excellent option for most patients
b. few, if any, gallstones that are dissolved with oral dissolution therapy recur
c. the preferred agent for oral dissolution therapy is ursodiol
d. oral dissolution therapy should not be combined with extracorporeal shock wave lithotripsy (ESWL)
e. oral dissolution therapy works best in patients with large gallstones

8. Which of the following statements regarding the treatment of asymptomatic gallstones is most accurate?
   a. asymptomatic gallstones should be treated with oral dissolution therapy
   b. asymptomatic gallstones should not be treated
   c. treatment of asymptomatic gallstones depends on the presence or absence of comorbid conditions
   d. asymptomatic gallstones should be treated with laparoscopic cholecystectomy, whereas symptomatic gallstones should be treated with open cholecystectomy
   e. for asymptomatic gallstones, the treatment of choice is ESWL

9. What is the most common complication during laparoscopic cholecystectomy?
   a. excessive bleeding
   b. small bowel perforation
   c. injury to the biliary tract system
   d. inability to remove the gallbladder through the laparoscope
   e. liver laceration

10. Which of the following statements is (are) true regarding laparoscopic cholecystectomy?
    a. laparoscopic cholecystectomy provides a safe and effective treatment for most patients with symptomatic gallstones; it is the treatment of choice
    b. laparoscopic cholecystectomy provides distinct advantages over open cholecystectomy
    c. laparoscopic cholecystectomy can be performed at a treatment cost equal to or slightly less than that for open cholecystectomy
    d. during laparoscopic cholecystectomy, when the anatomy is obscured because of excessive bleeding or other problems, the operation should be converted promptly to open cholecystectomy
    e. all of the above statements are true

Clinical Case Management Problem

The two most common diagnostic conditions associated with gallbladder disease are biliary colic and acute cholecystitis. Describe the differences in presentation and pathophysiology between biliary colic and acute cholecystitis.

Answers

1. **a.** The persistent nature of the pain in acute cholecystitis is a major clinical symptom that differentiates it from bilary colic. In addition, there is RUQ abdominal tenderness, voluntary guarding, and a positive Murphy's sign. The pain is sometimes referred to the right scapula, and the gallbladder may be palpable. Moreover, mild jaundice may occur.

Acute cholecystitis is manifested pathologically by gallbladder distention (hydrops), serosal edema, and infection secondary to obstruction of the cystic duct. Although the other choices can sometimes can present atypically with RUQ pain, the probability is low.

2. **c.** The diagnostic procedure of choice in this patient is an abdominal ultrasound. Gallstones will be demonstrated in approximately 95% of cases, and the specificity of the procedure is very high. Ultrasound should be done after 8 hours of fasting because gallstones are visualized better in a distended, bile-filled gallbladder. Ultrasound findings that suggest acute cholecystitis are pericholecystic fluid, gallbladder thickening, and sonographic Murphy's sign. A CT scan or MRI is more sensitive in diagnosing choledocholithiasis; however, they are expensive and offer no more sensitivity in the diagnosis of gallstones or acute cholecystitis. The HIDA scan is expensive and reserved for cases in which the ultrasound or CT scan is nondiagnostic but there is a high suspicion of cholecystitis.

3. **e.** In a patient with acute cholecystitis, intravenous fluids should be given to correct dehydration and possible electrolyte imbalance, and a nasogastric tube may be inserted if the patient has protracted vomiting. For acute cholecystitis, appropriate parenteral antibiotics should be given. Most physicians agree that early laparoscopic cholecystectomy within 24 to 48 hours is indicated once the diagnosis of acute cholecystitis is made. Advantages of laparoscopic over open cholecystectomy are a reduction in postoperative pain, a short hospital stay, and a more rapid return to work and other activities.

4. **d.** Acute cholecystitis is the most common complication of gallstones after biliary colic. Approximately 90% of cases of acute cholecystitis are associated with cholelithiasis. In the event of delayed diagnosis, the cystic duct remains obstructed and the lumen may become distended, causing hydrops of the gallbladder. Although rare, a large gallstone may sometimes erode through the wall into an adjacent viscus, usually the duodenum. The stone may become obstructed in the terminal ileum, causing small bowel obstruction, or in the duodenal bulb and pylorus, causing gastric outlet obstruction (Bouveret's syndrome). There is no known relationship between gallstones and hepatic vein thrombosis. A gallstone that migrates into the common bile duct may obstruct the duct and cause acute biliary pancreatitis and acute cholangitis.

5. **c.** In years past, acute cholecystitis was managed either aggressively or conservatively. Because the disease resolves spontaneously in approximately 60% of cases, the conservative approach was to manage the patient expectantly, with a plan to perform elective cholecystectomy after recovery, reserving early surgery for those patients with severe or worsening disease.

Currently, the preferred treatment plan is to perform laparoscopic cholecystectomy in all patients following an episode of acute cholecystitis unless there are specific contraindications to performing the operation. The most common contraindication is severe concomitant disease, which makes the patient a poor surgical risk. The reasoning for this approach is as follows: (1) The incidence of technical complications is no greater with early surgery; (2) early surgery reduces the total duration of illness by approximately 30 days, the length of hospitalization by 5 to 7 days, and direct medical costs by several thousands of dollars; and (3) in the absence of surgery, recurrent episodes are not uncommon, which may increase morbidity. In addition, the following factors affect the decision as to when to operate: (1) the diagnostic certainty; (2) the general health of the patient; and (3) signs of local complications of acute cholecystitis, such as gangrene or empyema.

6. **e.** More than 20 million Americans have cholelithiasis; approximately 300,000 operations are performed annually for the disease. Cholecystectomy is the most commonly performed abdominal surgery in medicine. The incidence of cholelithiasis increases with age. Most gallstones (70% to 95%) are composed predominantly of cholesterol. The remainder is pigment stones. The composition of the gallstone affects neither the symptoms associated with biliary colic nor the symptoms associated with acute cholecystitis. People with diabetes have an increased prevalence of gallstones. These patients have a propensity for obesity and hypertriglyceridemia. Therefore, it has been difficult to prove diabetes as an independent risk factor.

7. **c.** Oral dissolution therapy with bile acids was first introduced in the early 1970s. The first agent available was chenodiol, which has been replaced by ursodiol. Oral dissolution therapy is indicated only in a small minority of patients because there is a 50% recurrence rate. The most effective use of bile acids occurs with small gallstones (5 mm in diameter or less), which are floating, cholesterol in nature, and within a functioning gallbladder. This represents approximately 15% of patients. Patients must be treated between 6 and 12 months, and monitoring is necessary with ultrasound until dissolution is achieved. In such patients, 60% to 90% of gallstones will dissolve. Unfortunately, at least half of these stones recur within 5 years. Dissolution rates are higher and recurrence rates are lower in patients with single stones, in nonobese individuals, and in young patients. Unfortunately, many patients suffer distressing side effects from this treatment, such as nausea. Indications for bile acid therapy are limited to patients with a comorbid condition that precludes safe operation and patients who choose to avoid operation. ESWL is not commonly used by itself; it is used with oral dissolution therapy. This technique may be successful in up to 95% of patients with a functioning gallbladder and solitary noncalcified stones 20 mm in diameter or less. Recurrence is infrequent following therapy with ESWL for a single small stone, but it is more common in patients with multiple stones. Again, the gallbladder remains and the probability of further stone formation is high.

8. **b.** Current opinion suggests that asymptomatic gallstones should not be treated. The vast majority of gallstones remain silent throughout life. Only 1% to 4% per year of asymptomatic patients will develop symptoms or complications of gallstone disease. Existing data suggest that 10% of patients will develop symptoms within the first 5 years following diagnosis and approximately 20% within 10 years. Almost all patients will experience symptoms for a time period before they develop a complication. Therefore, with few exceptions, prophylactic treatment of asymptomatic patients cannot be justified.

9. **c.** All of the complications listed are possible, but the most common complication of laparoscopic cholecystectomy is bile duct injury. The frequency of bile duct injury is dependent on the skills of the surgeon and has been decreasing consistently as more experience with this procedure has been gained.

10. e. Laparoscopic cholecystectomy provides a safe and effective treatment for most patients with symptomatic gallstones. It is currently the treatment of choice for most patients, providing distinct advantages over open cholecystectomy. It decreases pain and disability without increasing mortality or overall morbidity. Although the rate of common bile duct injury is slightly increased, this rate is still sufficiently low to justify the use of this procedure.

Laparoscopic cholecystectomy can be performed at a treatment cost that is equal to or slightly less than that of open cholecystectomy and will result in substantial cost savings to the patient and society because of reduced loss of time from work.

The outcome of laparoscopic cholecystectomy is influenced greatly by the training, experience, skill, and judgment of the surgeon performing the procedure. Multiple studies have found that improved outcome is directly related to volume of procedures performed. Therefore, choosing a surgeon is often the critical decision a family physician can make that influences a patient's outcome. During laparoscopic cholecystectomy, when anatomy is obscured, excessive bleeding occurs, or other problems arise, the operation should be converted promptly to open cholecystectomy. Conversion in these circumstances reflects sound surgical judgment and should not be considered a complication of laparoscopic cholecystectomy.

Solution to the Clinical Case Management Problem

Biliary colic results from transient obstruction of the cystic duct with a gallstone. The pain associated with biliary colic usually begins abruptly after a meal and subsides gradually, lasting from a few minutes to several hours. It is located in the upper right quadrant and may or may not be associated with abdominal tenderness. There is no associated inflammation of the gallbladder with biliary colic because of the transient nature of the condition.

Acute cholecystitis, however, is associated pathophysiologically with inflammation of the gallbladder wall, with secondary infection in the gallbladder caused by blockage of the cystic duct. The first symptom is abdominal pain in the RUQ, with referral of the pain to right scapula and along the costal margin to the back. The pain persists and becomes associated with abdominal tenderness and guarding in the RUQ. There is nausea, vomiting, and a positive Murphy's sign (arrest of inspiration with palpation in the RUQ). The pain does not resolve spontaneously. There may be fever.

Summary

ACUTE CHOLECYSTITIS

1. Symptoms and signs: (a) acute RUQ pain, (b) mild fever and leukocytosis, (c) nausea and vomiting, (d) tenderness and guarding in the RUQ with or without a palpable gallbladder, and (e) gallstones on ultrasound scan
2. Treatment: (a) hospital admission, (b) parenteral fluids, (c) analgesics, (d) intravenous antibiotics, and (e) laparoscopic cholecystectomy as soon as possible

BILIARY COLIC

1. Symptoms and signs: (a) recurrent abdominal pain (usually RUQ), (b) dyspepsia, and (c) gallstones on ultrasound

2. Treatment: laparoscopic cholecystectomy when recurrent episodes occur. Oral dissolution therapy and extracorporeal shock wave lithotripsy may be considered in patients who are high risk for surgery.
   a. Choledocholithiasis/cholangitis: Choledocholithiasis occurs in 15% of patients with gallstones. Preoperative endoscopic retrograde cholangiography with sphincterotomy or intraoperative common duct exploration are options in concert with cholecystectomy.
      Choledocholithiasis is the major cause of cholangitis. Symptoms of cholangitis include biliary colic, jaundice, fever, and chills. Treatment of cholangitis

includes intravenous antibiotics, cholecystectomy, and intervention to the common duct.

b. Laparoscopic cholecystectomy: Laparoscopic cholecystectomy is the treatment of choice for the vast majority of patients with biliary tract disease. It is a much more conservative operation, causes much less postoperative pain, and is associated with a much earlier return to work. Choice of surgeon is key, with higher quality outcomes associated higher volume of cases performed.

c. Asymptomatic gallstones: Asymptomatic gallstones should be left where they are; do not create a problem where one does not exist.

Suggested Reading

Ahmed A, Ramsey C, Cheung RC, Reeffe EB: Management of gallstones and their complications. *Am Fam Physician* 61:1673–1680, 2000.

Indar AA, Beckingham IJ: Acute cholecystitis. *BMJ* 325(7365):639–643, 2002.

Langham MR Jr, Mekeel KL: Hepatobiliary disorders. *Surg Clin North Am* 86(2):455–467, x–xi, 2006.

Trowbridge RL, Rutkowski NK, Shojania KG: Does this patient have acute cholecystitis? *JAMA* 289(1):80–86, 2003.

CHAPTER 37
Inflammatory Bowel Disease

CLINICAL CASE PROBLEM 1

A 32-Year-Old Female with Fever, Weight Loss, and Chronic Diarrhea

A 32-year-old female comes to your office with a 6-month history of loose bowel movements, approximately eight per day. Blood has been present in many of them. She has lost 30 pounds. For the past 6 weeks, she has had an intermittent fever. She has had no previous gastrointestinal (GI) problems, and there is no family history of GI problems.

On examination, the patient looks ill. Her blood pressure is 130/70 mmHg. Her pulse is 108 beats/minute and regular. There is generalized abdominal tenderness with no rebound. A sigmoidoscopy reveals a friable rectal mucosa with multiple bleeding points.

SELECT THE BEST ANSWER TO THE FOLLOWING QUESTIONS

1. What is the most likely diagnosis in this patient?
   a. irritable bowel syndrome
   b. Crohn's disease
   c. ulcerative colitis
   d. Crohn's colitis
   e. bacterial dysentery

2. At this time, which of the following represent(s) the investigation(s) of choice?
   a. colonoscopy
   b. barium enema
   c. upper GI series and follow-through
   d. a and c
   e. a, b, and c

3. Which of the following may be indicated in the management of the acute phase of the condition described?
   a. steroid enemas
   b. oral corticosteroids
   c. parenteral corticosteroids
   d. a and b
   e. a, b, and c

4. Which of the following statements regarding the use of sulfasalazine in the condition described is (are) false?
   a. sulfasalazine is structurally related to both aspirin and sulfa drugs
   b. sulfasalazine is effective in maintaining remission in this condition and in the acute treatment of mild disease
   c. sulfasalazine may impair folic acid metabolism
   d. all of the above are false

5. Which of the following completions regarding the long-term prognosis of the patient described in the case history is false? Following an initial attack
   a. 66% of patients go into remission with medical therapy
   b. 80% of treatment-compliant patients maintain remission for many years

c. 10% of patients continue to have active disease until surgical intervention is undertaken

d. 5% of patients die within a year

e. none of the above are false

6. Which of the following complications occur in the disease described?
   a. toxic megacolon and strictures
   b. colonic cancer
   c. iritis
   d. a and b
   e. a, b, and c

CLINICAL CASE PROBLEM 2

A 25-Year-Old Male Presents with an 18-Month History of Chronic Abdominal Pain

A 25-year-old male presents with an 18-month history of chronic abdominal pain. The patient has seen several physicians and has been diagnosed as having "nervous stomach," irritable bowel syndrome, and "depression." Associated with this abdominal pain for the past 3 months have been nonbloody diarrhea, anorexia, and a weight loss of 20 pounds. He has developed a painful area around the anus.

On examination, the patient has diffuse abdominal tenderness. He looks thin and unwell. He has a tender, erythematous area in the right perirectal area.

7. What is the most likely diagnosis?
   a. irritable bowel syndrome
   b. Crohn's disease
   c. ulcerative colitis
   d. bacterial dysentery
   e. amebiasis

8. Pathologically, what is the difference between the patient in this case and the patient described in Clinical Case Problem 1?
   a. inflammation in this case involves all layers of the bowel; the former involves only the mucosa
   b. inflammation in the former case involves all layers of the bowel; the latter involves only the mucosa
   c. inflammation in the former case involves the first two layers of the bowel (mucosa and submucosa); the latter involves only the mucosa

d. inflammation in this case involves the first two layers of the bowel (mucosa and submucosa); the former involves only the mucosa

e. the two diseases are essentially identical on a pathophysiologic basis

9. Which of the following investigations is the most sensitive test for confirming the diagnosis in this patient?
   a. sigmoidoscopy
   b. colonoscopy
   c. barium enema
   d. computed tomography (CT) scan of the abdomen
   e. magnetic resonance imaging (MRI) scan of the abdomen

10. Which of the following drugs is (are) appropriate initial therapy in the acute phase of the condition described in Clinical Case Problem 2?
    a. budesonide
    b. sulfasalazine
    c. metronidazole
    d. 6-mercaptopurine
    e. all of the above

11. Metronidazole is effective in which of the following subtypes of Crohn's disease?
    a. mild Crohn's disease
    b. perianal disease
    c. Crohn's disease of the small bowel
    d. a and b
    e. a, b, and c

12. Which of the following is (are) not associated with Crohn's disease?
    a. skip lesions on x-ray
    b. thumbprinting on x-ray
    c. anti-*Saccharomyces cerevisiae* antibodies
    d. perinuclear-staining anti-neutrophil cytoplasmic antibodies
    e. a and c

13. Which of the following statements regarding complications of the condition described in Clinical Case Problem 2 is false?
    a. rectal fissures, rectocutaneous fistulas, and perirectal abscesses are common complications of this condition
    b. arthritis sometimes is seen as a complication of this condition
    c. erythema nodosum and pyoderma gangrenosum sometimes are found with this condition
    d. patients with this condition are not at increased risk of colorectal cancer
    e. none of the above statements are false

*A Thin, Anemic-Appearing,
31-Year-Old Female*

A 31-year-old female comes to your office with a 6-month history of GI problems including abdominal distention, excessive flatus, foul-smelling stools, weight loss, and nonspecific complaints of weakness and fatigue. The patient describes the symptoms as being especially severe after the intake of cereal grains and bread of any kind. The patient has not traveled to any specific area in the recent past. She has not left the country.

She is thin and looks anemic. Vital signs are normal. The patient is in no acute distress, but her abdomen reveals active bowel sounds, mild distention, and diffuse discomfort to palpation.

14. On the basis of this information, what is the most likely diagnosis in this patient?
    a. lactase deficiency
    b. acute pancreatitis
    c. celiac sprue
    d. tropical sprue
    e. bacterial overgrowth syndrome

15. What is the pathophysiology of this disease?
    a. an immunologic disorder of the small bowel mucosa
    b. a disaccharide deficiency of the small intestinal mucosa
    c. a deficiency of pancreatic exocrine
    d. secondary contamination of the small intestine by coliform bacteria
    e. none of the above

*A 15-Year-Old Female Who can no
Longer Drink Milk*

A 15-year-old female presents to your office with a 1-month history of abdominal cramping, abdominal bloating, and increased flatulence following the ingestion of milk or milk products. The patient drank three glasses of milk 2 hours ago.

On examination, the abdomen is tympanic and appears to be slightly distended. No other abnormalities are found on examination.

16. What is the most likely diagnosis in this patient?
    a. tropical sprue
    b. celiac sprue

    c. lactase deficiency
    d. regional enteritis
    e. chronic pancreatitis

Clinical Case Management Problem

Discuss the relationship between inflammatory bowel disease (ulcerative colitis and Crohn's disease) and the risk of acquiring carcinoma of the colon.

Answers

1. **c.** This patient almost certainly has ulcerative colitis. Ulcerative colitis usually presents with (1) abdominal pain, (2) diarrhea, (3) passage of blood via the rectum, (4) tenesmus, (5) fever, (6) chills, (7) malaise and fatigue, and (8) weight loss. Sigmoidoscopy usually reveals friability (with easy bleeding) and granularity. Crohn's disease (regional enteritis) is usually not associated with rectal bleeding, although it may be. Crohn's disease is discussed in a subsequent question. Bacterial dysentery would not be as long-lasting as this illness. Irritable bowel syndrome is a diagnosis of exclusion and does not present with systemic symptoms.

2. **a.** Barium enema or colonoscopy may be performed in this patient. However, colonoscopy is preferable to barium enema because it identifies the extent of disease and at the same time allows biopsies to be taken. Again, friability is the hallmark finding, as is involvement of the rectum. Radiographic findings in ulcerative colitis include the following: (1) continuous involvement of the colon, (2) superficial ulcerations, and (3) "backwash ileitis"

Although the rectum and the distal colon are the most common sites of involvement, patients with more severe disease may have involvement of the entire colon. A GI series and follow-through would not add any useful information to the investigation of a patient strongly suspected of having ulcerative colitis.

3 **e.** Therapy of ulcerative colitis depends on the site and severity of the disease. Corticosteroids remain the cornerstone of management of patients with severe acute ulcerative colitis. They are not, however, efficacious in the maintenance of remission. Patients with severe, acute disease are usually severely ill and require hospitalization and close monitoring for the potential development of toxic megacolon and silent perforation. Current treatments for mild and moderate, severe, refractory, and remission states of illness are listed as follows for distal (rectal) and extensive (entire colon) forms of the disease.

Distal Disease

1. Mild to moderate
   a. Oral or rectal aminosalicylates, known as 5-ASAs (Sulfasalazine, mesalamine, or olsalazine remain the initial therapy of choice in the treatment of patients with mild to moderate acute disease and in the maintenance of remission. Sulfasalazine is structurally related both to aspirin and to sulfa drugs. It inhibits folic acid, and patients taking it thus need a supplement of at least 1 mg of folic acid per day.)
   b. Rectal corticosteroids (given as a retention enema, hydrocortisone 100 mg once or twice per day)
2. Severe
   a. Oral or parenteral corticosteroids (They usually are given as prednisone in the range of 20 to 60 mg/day as a single oral dose for 2 to 4 weeks or methylprednisolone intravenously. When the relief of symptoms has been attained, the dose can be tapered gradually.)
   b. Rectal corticosteroids
3. Refractory
   a. Oral or intravenous (IV) corticosteroids, plus
   b. Oral azathioprine, mercaptopurine (the purine analogues, azathioprine [Imuran] and 6-mercaptopurine, have corticosteroid-sparing effects and are useful in the induction and maintenance of remission), or infliximab (e.g., Remicade)—an anti-tumor necrosis factor monoclonal antibody
   c. If refractory to medical therapy, surgical management indicated
4. Remission
   a. Oral or rectal aminosalicylates
   b. Oral azathioprine or mercaptopurine

Extensive Disease

1. Mild to moderate: oral aminosalicylates
2. Severe
   a. Oral or parenteral corticosteroids
   b. Intravenous cyclosporine (an immunosuppressant that works by inhibiting the production of cytokine by helper T cells)
3. Refractory
   a. Oral or IV corticosteroids, plus
   b. Oral azathioprine or mercaptopurine, infliximab (e.g., Remicade)—an anti-tumor necrosis factor monoclonal antibody
   c. If refractory to medical management, surgical management indicated

4. Remission
   a. Oral aminosalicylates
   b. Oral azathioprine or mercaptopurine

4. d. Sulfasalazine, like the other aminosalicylates, has a proven efficacy in the management of patients with ulcerative colitis. It is the therapy of choice in the treatment of patients with mild to moderately severe active disease. It is the treatment of choice for the maintenance of remission in patients with established ulcerative colitis.

5. e. All of the statements are true. Following an initial attack of ulcerative colitis, 66% of patients go into remission with medical treatment. Of treatment-compliant patients, 80% maintain remission, 10% have continually active disease, and 5% die within 1 year of the initial attack. Of all patients with ulcerative colitis of any severity, 25% of patients will undergo total proctocolectomy within 5 years of the first attack. The risk of colonic cancer increases with time. By 15 years after initial diagnosis, patients with colonic disease are at a risk significant enough to consider prophylactic colectomy.

6. e. Complications of ulcerative colitis include the following: (1) toxic megacolon, (2) perforation, (3) colorectal carcinoma, (4) colonic stricture, and (5) hemorrhage.

Extracolonic complications include the following: (1) skin disease (erythema nodosum and pyoderma gangrenosum), (2) aphthous ulcers, (3) iritis, (4) arthritis, and (5) hepatic disease.

7. b. This patient has Crohn's disease (regional enteritis).

8. a. Pathologically, Crohn's disease involves an inflammation of all layers of the bowel, in contradistinction to ulcerative colitis, which involves just the mucosa.

Associated anorectal complications include the following: (1) fistulas, (2) fissures, and (3) perirectal abscesses.

The peak incidence of Crohn's disease is at 30 years of age; most cases occur between the ages of 20 and 40 years. Crohn's disease may follow an indolent course resulting in diagnostic delay. The signs and symptoms include the following: (1) mild chronic abdominal pain, (2) mild nonbloody diarrhea, (3) anorexia, (4) weight loss, and (5) fatigue.

Pain is often confined to the lower abdomen and is "aching" or "cramping." A misdiagnosis of irritable bowel syndrome is often made.

9. b. In most cases, no one test is sufficient for diagnosis, but endoscopy does allow for biopsy of abnormal tissue and pathologic confirmation of the disease. Colonoscopy is more sensitive than sigmoidoscopy, but it will not show the transmural involvement. Sigmoidoscopy alone will miss Crohn's disease in 30% to 50% of patients. Barium air-contrast enema and upper GI series with small bowel follow-through are also valuable diagnostic procedures in the evaluation for diagnosis of Crohn's disease in this patient. Crohn's disease often presents as segmental involvement of two or more colonic areas; between these areas the colon is normal. The transmural involvement is often suggested by radiologic features including the protrusion of a defect into the lumen (thumbprinting). CT scanning and MRI scanning are often performed in Crohn's disease, but they can miss many subtle lesions. Gadolinium-enhanced MRI with oral dilute barium sulfate and rectal water depicts intestinal and extraintestinal changes of Crohn's disease and shows promise as a diagnostic aide.

10. e. The drug of choice for the treatment of patients with Crohn's disease varies according to the severity of illness. Mild to moderate disease is often treated with a combination of oral aminosalicylates, oral antibiotics (metronidazole and ciprofloxacin), and oral corticosteroids (budesonide). Oral azathioprine or mercaptopurine have also been used. In severe disease, oral or systemic corticosteroids are used with subcutaneous or IV methotrexate and the anti-tumor necrosis factor infliximab, a monoclonal antibody. The latter drug has been particularly useful in refractory disease. As in ulcerative colitis, steroid dosage should be tapered after a few weeks of therapy. Maintenance of remission has been a challenge in Crohn's disease. The 5-aminosalicylates have been, at best, variable in effectiveness. Azathioprine and mercaptopurine have been used extensively with satisfactory results, although the long-term use of immunosuppressants is always a concern. The use of probiotics seems effective in subgroups of patients with Crohn's disease, and antibiotics, especially metronidazole, have been useful in all forms of disease and particularly for patients with perianal fistulas. Attention to maintenance of proper nutrition is a constant task in all inflammatory bowel diseases.

11. d. Metronidazole is effective in the management of Crohn's colitis and Crohn's perianal disease. It is not, however, effective in the treatment of Crohn's disease of the small bowel.

12. d. Radiographic manifestations of Crohn's disease include skip lesions on x-ray (normal and abnormal alternating sections of bowel) and thumbprinting (characteristic defect protruding into the lumen).

Anti-*Saccharomyces cerevisiae* antibodies are seen in more than 50% of patients with Crohn's disease and only occasionally in patients with ulcerative colitis. Perinuclear-staining anti-neutrophil cytoplasmic antibodies are seen in more than 70% of patients with ulcerative colitis and only occasionally in patients with Crohn's disease.

13. d. Rectal fissures, rectocutaneous fistulas, or perirectal abscesses occur in up to 50% of patients with Crohn's disease at some time during their illness. Extracolonic manifestations of Crohn's disease occur in 10% of patients with the disease. These include arthritis (which in fact may precede the GI symptoms), iritis, erythema nodosum, pyoderma gangrenosum, and aphthous ulcers. The risk of colorectal cancer is less in patients with Crohn's disease than in patients with ulcerative colitis. Patients who have had the disease for more than 15 years, however, are still at increased risk for this malignancy.

14. c. This patient most likely has celiac sprue (gluten enteropathy).

15. a. Gluten enteropathy is an immunologic disorder of the small bowel observed in both children and adults. Exposure of the small intestine to antigenic components of certain cereal grains in susceptible people causes subtotal or total villous atrophy with reactive crypt hyperplasia.

Common GI complaints include the following: (1) abdominal distention; (2) excessive flatus; (3) large, bulky, foul-smelling stools; and (4) weight loss.

Other nonspecific complaints that commonly occur are weakness or fatigue. Patients may present with anemia from either an iron-deficiency anemia or a megaloblastic anemia (folic acid deficiency). Other patients suffer from deficiency of a fat-soluble vitamin or vitamin B_{12}.

Therapy consists of a gluten-free diet (avoiding any products containing wheat, rye, barley, or oats). Cereals such as corn, rice, buckwheat, sorghum, and millet are not pathogenic and may be substituted. Clinical improvement is generally seen after several days on a gluten-free diet. Restoration of normal histologic architecture takes weeks to months.

16. c. This patient has a lactase deficiency in the small intestine. Thus, symptoms characteristic of malabsorption (bloating, diarrhea, crampy abdominal pain, and foul-smelling stools) occur when milk or milk products are ingested. The treatment of choice for these patients is replacement of the deficient enzyme with an enzyme supplement such as Lactaid tablets and/or replacement of lactose-rich dairy products with low-lactose products, such as yogurt, lactose-reduced milk, and most hard (fermented) cheeses.

Solution to the Clinical Case Management Problem

Inflammatory bowel disease, which includes ulcerative colitis and Crohn's disease, is directly related to the risk of acquiring carcinoma of the colon. The risk is related to the following:

1. Which disease: Ulcerative colitis has a greater risk than Crohn's disease, but both have increased risk.
2. Severity of the disease: The more severe the disease, the greater the risk of carcinoma of the colon.
3. The length of time with the disease: The longer the patient has had the disease, the greater the risk.

4. The site of the disease: The risk of cancer of the colon is much higher in patients who have ulcerative colitis compared to ulcerative proctitis.

Patients with ulcerative proctitis, ulcerative colitis, and Crohn's colitis should be screened by endoscopy (colonoscopy) every 1 or 2 years depending on the factors listed. For ulcerative colitis, the screening process may indicate the appropriate time for a prophylactic hemicolectomy (average 15 years since disease onset).

Summary

Studies suggest that chronic inflammation in inflammatory bowel disease may be due to cellular immune responses to a certain bacteria residing in the luminal wall. Disease susceptibility is determined genetically, and the immune responses and inflammation are triggered by environmental stimuli.

ULCERATIVE COLITIS

1. Pathophysiology involves the mucosa only.
2. Local symptoms include the following: (a) diarrhea (bloody), (b) mucus from the rectum, (c) tenesmus, (d) constipation (may alternate with diarrhea), and (e) abdominal pain. Complications such as toxic megacolon and perforation are uncommon.
3. Systemic symptoms include fever, chills, anorexia, weight loss, malaise, fatigue, erythema nodosum, pyoderma gangrenosum, aphthous ulcers, iritis, arthritis, and hepatic disease.
4. Investigations include sigmoidoscopy, colonoscopy, and air-contrast barium enema. If there is danger of perforation (megacolon), barium enema is contraindicated. Perinuclear-staining anti-neutrophil cytoplasmic antibodies are seen in more than 70% of patients with ulcerative colitis.
5. Therapy of ulcerative colitis depends on the site and severity of the disease. See answer 3.

CROHN'S DISEASE

1. Pathophysiology involves all layers of the bowel wall.
2. Local symptoms include abdominal pain, nonbloody diarrhea, and mucus from the rectum.
3. Systemic symptoms include fever, chills, anorexia, malaise, fatigue, weight loss, erythema nodosum, pyoderma gangrenosum, aphthous ulcers, arthritis, and iritis.
4. Other features include rectal fistulas, rectal fissures, and perirectal abscesses.
5. Investigations include endoscopy and biopsy, barium enema, and GI series and follow-through; anti-*Saccharomyces cerevisiae* antibodies are seen in more than 50% of patients with Crohn's disease.
6. The drug of choice for the treatment of patients with Crohn's disease varies according to the severity of illness. See answer 10.

OTHER DISEASES THAT MAY RESEMBLE INFLAMMATORY BOWEL DISEASE

1. Celiac sprue
   a. Pathophysiology is gluten-sensitive enteropathy. It is an immunologic reaction of the small bowel wall that causes villous atrophy and crypt hyperplasia.
   b. Symptoms include bloating; diarrhea; foul-smelling stools; and weight loss, especially after eating gluten-containing products (breads, pasta, etc.).
   c. Treatment involves elimination of gluten from the diet.
2. Lactase deficiency
   a. Pathophysiology is deficiency of the disaccharide enzyme lactase.
   b. Symptoms include crampy abdominal pain, bloating, foul-smelling stools, and diarrhea after the ingestion of milk or dairy products.
   c. Treatment involves replacement enzymes, such as lactase supplements, before ingesting milk and milk products.

Suggested Reading

De La Rue SA, Bickston SJ: Evidence-based medications for the treatment of the inflammatory bowel diseases. *Curr Opin Gastroenterol* 22(4):365–369, 2006.

Grover P, Kamat D: Management of inflammatory bowel disease. *Clin Pediatr* 46(4):359–364, 2007.

Hanauer SB: Inflammatory bowel disease: Epidemiology, pathogenesis, and therapeutic opportunities. *Inflammatory Bowel Dis* 12(Suppl 1): S3–S9, 2006.

Kucharzik T, Maaser C, Lugering A, et al: Recent understanding of IBD pathogenesis: Implications for future therapies. *Inflammatory Bowel Dis* 12(11):1068–1083, 2006.

Langan RC, Gotsch PB, Krafczyk MA, Skillinge DD: Ulcerative colitis: Diagnosis and treatment. *Am Fam Phys* 76:1323–1331, 2007.

Razack R, Seidner DL: Nutrition in inflammatory bowel disease. *Curr Opin Gastroenterol* 23(4):400–405, 2007.

CHAPTER

38 Irritable Bowel Syndrome

CLINICAL CASE PROBLEM 1

A 40-Year-Old Female with Chronic Constipation and Abdominal Pain

A 40-year-old female comes to your office with a several-year history of lower abdominal pain associated with constipation (one hard bowel movement every 3 days) and the passage of mucus per rectum on a regular basis. She states that her abdominal pain feels better after she has a bowel movement. She has never passed blood per rectum. She describes no fever, chills, weight loss or gain, jaundice, or any other symptoms. There is no relationship between the abdominal pain and specific food intake.

On physical examination, the abdomen is scaphoid, and no hepatosplenomegaly or masses are palpated. There is a very mild generalized abdominal tenderness, but it does not localize.

SELECT THE BEST ANSWER TO THE FOLLOWING QUESTIONS

1. What is the most likely diagnosis in this patient?
   a. hypothyroidism
   b. Crohn's disease
   c. ulcerative colitis
   d. lactose intolerance
   e. Irritable bowel syndrome

2. Which of the following statements regarding the condition described is (are) false?
   a. the typical location of the abdominal pain is the lower abdomen
   b. intermittent diarrhea can be seen in this condition
   c. there is often a perception of incomplete emptying of the rectum
   d. bowel movements are often irregular
   e. very severe abdominal tenderness is a hallmark of the disease

3. Which treatment would be least helpful for this patient?
   a. methylcellulose (Citrucel)
   b. psyllium fiber supplements
   c. Alosetron (Lotronex)
   d. peppermint oil capsules
   e. guar gum

4. Which of the following would be most unlikely in a patient with the condition described?
   a. family history of this condition
   b. increased pain at times of stress
   c. pain on awakening from sleep
   d. abdominal bloating
   e. increased passage of flatus

5. Which of the following tests is not indicated for this patient?
   a. a complete blood count
   b. liver function tests
   c. electrolytes
   d. abdominal ultrasound
   e. thyroid function studies

CLINICAL CASE PROBLEM 2

A 34-Year-Old Female with Crampy Abdominal Pain

A 34-year-old female presents with a long history of crampy abdominal pain that is relieved by defecation. She normally has three to five loose but formed stools per day. When she is stressed, she has increased abdominal pain, flatus, and bowel movements. She was recently promoted at work and is excited about her job but is intimidated by her new boss. For the past 3 days, she has called in sick for work and is at your office requesting a note for work. She denies fever, nausea, vomiting, bloody stool, and weight loss. She does not drink alcohol or caffeine, and she does not smoke cigarettes. Her family history is significant for her mother having a "sensitive stomach."

6. What treatment would be least helpful in this patient?
   a. desipramine
   b. alosetron
   c. fiber supplements
   d. loperamide
   e. hyoscyamine

7. Which of the following conditions (symptoms) is not associated with the condition?
   a. fibromyalgia
   b. cholelithiasis
   c. interstitial cystitis
   d. depression
   e. migraine headaches

8. What specialized testing is indicated in the described patient?
   a. anti-gliadin antibody
   b. stool culture
   c. computed tomography (CT) of abdomen and pelvis
   d. urea breath test
   e. anti-mitochondrial antibody

9. Which of the following is the most important component of management of the condition described?
   a. single-agent pharmacologic therapy
   b. multiple-agent pharmacologic therapy
   c. a therapeutic physician–patient relationship
   d. a focused diet
   e. intensive psychotherapy

10. Which of the following medications should not be used in the treatment of the condition described?
    a. psyllium
    b. loperamide
    c. cholestyramine
    d. codeine phosphate
    e. amitriptyline

Clinical Case Management Problem

Discuss "red flag" signs that indicate an alternate diagnosis and warrant additional testing.

Answers

1. e. The most likely diagnosis is irritable bowel syndrome (IBS). The current diagnostic criteria for IBS (Rome II criteria, 1999) include abdominal pain or discomfort present for at least 12 weeks (not necessarily consecutive) in the past year that cannot be explained by structural or biochemical abnormalities and two of the following three features: (1) pain relieved with defecation, (2) onset associated with a change in the frequency of bowel movements (diarrhea or constipation), and/or (3) onset associated with a change in the form of the stool (loose, watery, or pelletlike). Supportive symptoms are either fewer than three stools per week or more than three stools per day. In addition, the stools are described as hard or lumpy.

Hypothyroidism is associated with constipation, but fatigue and weight gain would be part of the patient's presentation.

Crohn's disease is unlikely in the absence of systemic symptoms, including nonbloody diarrhea, anorexia, weight loss, fever, and fatigue.

Ulcerative colitis is unlikely in the absence of weight loss and the passage of bright red blood per rectum.

Lactose intolerance is linked specifically to the intake of milk and milk products.

2. e. The perception of incomplete emptying of the rectum, irregular bowel action, and the relief of the abdominal pain with defecation are common in IBS. Both diarrhea and constipation are seen in IBS. Abdominal pain is confined to the lower abdomen, usually in the area of the sigmoid colon. Although abdominal tenderness may be present, it is usually not severe and is not a hallmark of the disease.

3. c. Alosetron (Lotronex) is used in special cases of women with severe diarrhea-predominant IBS. It can only be prescribed by providers who have enrolled in a special prescribing program. It is associated with severe constipation and ischemic bowel disease. Tegaserod (Zelnorm), until recently used for women with constipation-predominant IBS, was withdrawn from the market in March 2007 due to a higher than expected risk for heart attack, stroke, and chest pain. Fiber, such as psyllium and methylcellulose, has been found to be helpful in constipation-predominant IBS, but it may exacerbate diarrhea-predominant IBS. Peppermint oil enteric coated capsules have been found to be helpful in adults and children with IBS. Guar gum was shown to be as effective as fiber supplementation in controlled studies.

4. c. IBS is a functional condition. Pain on awakening from sleep is suggestive of an organic etiology.

In addition, pain that interferes with normal sleep patterns, diarrhea that awakens the patient from sleep, visible or occult blood in the stool, weight loss, and fever also suggest organic disease. IBS is seen with increased frequency in first-degree relatives. Stress, caffeine, and various foods can exacerbate symptoms of IBS but do not cause IBS.

5. **d.** A physical exam, complete blood count, metabolic profile, and stool for occult blood testing are indicated. Thyroid function studies are also reasonable to rule out hypothyroidism. An abdominal ultrasound is not indicated for the diagnosis of this condition.

6. **c.** For diarrhea-predominant IBS, fiber supplementation can exacerbate symptoms. Alosetron is indicated in select cases of women with diarrhea-predominant IBS, although its use is restricted in the United States. Tricyclic antidepressants, anticholinergics, and antidiarrheal medications such as norpramin, hyoscyamine, and loperamide can be helpful in diarrhea-predominant IBS.

7. **b.** Patients with IBS have a higher incidence of functional disorders, such as fibromyalgia, interstitial cystitis, and migraine headaches. Conditions that are more common in patients with IBS include fatigue and depression. Cholelithiasis is not associated with IBS.

8. **a.** Anti-gliadin antibody testing is recommended in diarrhea-predominant IBS presentations to rule out celiac sprue. Stool cultures are not indicated without recent onset or other accompanying constitutional symptoms. A CT scan of the abdomen and pelvis is not indicated. Urease breath testing is used for the diagnosis of *Helicobacter pylori* infection; anti-mitochondrial antibodies are useful to diagnose primary biliary cirrhosis.

9. **c.** The most important component of treatment in IBS is establishing a therapeutic, communicative, and trusting physician–patient relationship and educating the patient regarding the benign nature of the condition and favorable long-term prognosis.

The important components of the physician–patient relationship that should be emphasized include a nonjudgmental attitude, concern regarding the patient's understanding of the illness, expectations and consistent limits, and involvement of the patient in treatment decisions. Because of the long-term nature of IBS, primary management by a family physician is essential. Although consultants may be needed in some cases for both patient and family physician reassurance, this should be the exception rather than the rule.

Pharmacologic, behavioral, and dietary approaches play an important but subordinate role in the treatment of this disorder.

10. **d.** Treatment of IBS includes the following:

1. Eliminating certain foods, including gas-forming foods such as legumes, caffeine, alcohol, fatty foods, and products containing sorbitol. Patients should keep a diary to identify foods that exacerbate symptoms.
2. Supplementing with high-fiber foods such as bran.
3. Engaging in supportive therapy, relaxation exercises, hypnosis, cognitive behavioral therapy, and psychodynamic interpersonal psychotherapy.

Other agents used in the treatment of IBS include the following:

1. Psyllium (another bulking agent)
2. Antispasmodic or anticholinergic agents
3. Antidiarrheal agents such as diphenoxylate, loperamide, or cholestyramine in cases in which diarrhea is the predominant symptom
4. Tricyclic antidepressants such as amitriptyline or desipramine
5. Osmotic laxatives such as milk of magnesia when constipation is the predominant symptom. Fiber supplements and a high-fiber diet are also important in treating constipation-predominant IBS. Alosetron, a 5-HT$_3$ receptor antagonist, is used short term in women whose primary bowel symptom is diarrhea.
6. Complementary and alternative treatments that have evidence favoring their use include peppermint oil enteric coated capsules, Chinese herbal supplements, and the probiotic *Bifidobacterium infantis*.

Codeine phosphate or other narcotic agents are contraindicated in the treatment of IBS.

In the management of a patient with IBS, consider doing and not doing the following:

You Should
1. Do a complete history including a psychosocial history, a family history, and a marital history.
2. Attempt to ascertain the patient's understanding and concerns about the condition.
3. Establish a strong, trusting family physician–patient relationship. This forms the basis for the therapy (supportive psychotherapy) that follows.
4. Have the patient ask all of his or her questions in an unhurried atmosphere.
5. Perform a complete physical examination to rule out other conditions and to reassure the patient that you are truly interested in the problem.

You Should Not

1. Repeat investigations or order other, more costly investigations unless red flags are present.
2. Criticize your colleagues for failure to completely investigate this problem until a cause was found; this is not appropriate.
3. Promise what you cannot deliver, which is a cure for IBS. Instead, you will provide the empathic sup-

port necessary to help the patient understand and deal with the condition.
4. Rely on a polypharmacy approach to achieve better results. Use the suggested drugs with prudence and caution.
5. Use narcotic analgesics as a treatment for IBS.

Solution to the Clinical Case Management Problem

The presence of red flags in a patient's history, physical exam, or initial laboratory workup makes an alternate, more serious diagnosis more likely and warrants additional investigations. These red flags include a family history of colon cancer or irritable bowel disease, an onset of symptoms after age 50 years, recent antibiotic use, weight loss, nocturnal symptoms, fever, persistent severe diarrhea or constipation, rectal bleeding, the presence of anemia or occult blood in the stool, or a palpable rectal mass on exam.

Summary

1. IBS is extremely common; prevalence estimates suggest that 15% of the population has symptoms compatible with this diagnosis.
2. IBS is the most common condition that gastroenterologists see in referral or consultation practice.
3. Consider IBS as a diagnosis of inclusion rather than exclusion. Base your diagnosis on the positive criteria discussed previously.
4. Consider the minimal investigations that have been suggested as sufficient; do not overinvestigate.
5. After establishing a strong physician–patient relationship, consider dietary manipulation as primary therapy.
6. Antispasmodics, anticholinergics, tricyclic antidepressants, antidiarrheal agents, and osmotic laxatives and 5-HT$_3$ receptor agonist agents are drugs that can be used for the treatment of IBS. Use caution combining them.
7. Reassurance regarding the benign nature of the condition and the provision of hope for control of the symptoms are likely the most important therapy for this condition (supportive psychotherapy).
8. Other behavioral approaches include cognitive–behavioral therapy, hypnosis, and stress management/relaxation therapy.

Suggested Reading

Hadley SK, Gaarder SM: Treatment of irritable bowel syndrome. *Am Fam Physician* 72(12):2501–2506, 2005.
Liu JP, Yang M, Liu YX, et al: Herbal medicines for treatment of irritable bowel syndrome. *Cochrane Database Syst Rev* (1):CD004116, 2006.
Podovei M and Kuo B: Irritable bowel syndrome: A practical review. *South Med J* 99(11):1235–1244, 1284, 2006.
Quartero AO, Meineche-Schmidt V, Muris J, et al: Bulking agents, antispasmodic and antidepressant medication for the treatment of irritable bowel syndrome. *Cochrane Database Syst Rev* (2):CD003460, 2005.

CLINICAL CASE PROBLEM 1

*A 29-Year-Old Female with Nausea,
Vomiting, and Central Abdominal Pain*

A 29-year-old female comes to your office with a
1-day history of nausea, mild vomiting, and vague
central abdominal pain. The pain has begun to
move down and to the right. She also describes
mild dysuria. Anorexia began 24 hours ago, and the
patient has "felt warm." Her last menstrual period
was 2 weeks ago.

Her past health has been excellent. She has no
drug allergies and is not taking any medications.
On physical examination, she appears ill. Her
temperature is 38.1°C. She has tenderness in both
the right lower quadrant and the left lower quadrant,
but tenderness is greatest in the right lower
quadrant. Rebound tenderness is present. The rectal
examination discloses tenderness on the right side.
There is no costovertebral angle tenderness.

SELECT THE BEST ANSWER TO THE FOLLOWING QUESTIONS

1. What is the most likely diagnosis in this patient?
   a. pelvic inflammatory disease (PID)
   b. ovarian torsion
   c. acute appendicitis
   d. acute cholecystitis
   e. acute pyelonephritis

2. At this time, what would be the most reasonable
   course of action?
   a. advise the patient to go home and return for
      follow-up in 24 hours
   b. hospitalize the patient for observation, evalua-
      tion, and possible operation
   c. begin outpatient oral antibiotic therapy and see
      the patient in 48 hours
   d. advise the patient to go home and call you if no
      improvement occurs within the next 72 hours
   e. none of the above

3. Which of the following laboratory markers would
   be most helpful in supporting the diagnosis?
   a. amylase
   b. white blood cell (WBC) count

   c. C-reactive protein
   d. urinalysis
   e. pregnancy test

4. A consultant sees your patient and makes an
   appropriate suggestion. Which of the following is
   the suggestion likely to be?
   a. perform an abdominal laparoscopy or laparotomy
   b. begin intensive triple-drug intravenous antibiotics
   c. continue the period of observation
   d. perform further diagnostic tests
   e. order another consult

5. Which of the following is not a clear complication
   of the original condition and definitive therapy?
   a. wound infection
   b. intra-abdominal abscess formation
   c. portal pyelophlebitis
   d. bowel obstruction
   e. infertility

6. In which of the following groups are the signs and
   symptoms of the condition described likely not to
   be classic?
   a. infants
   b. young adult males
   c. the elderly
   d. a and c
   e. b and c

7. In which of the following age groups is the diagnosis of the condition described here most likely to
   be confused with another serious intra-abdominal
   inflammatory condition?
   a. infants
   b. young children
   c. young adult males
   d. young adult females
   e. elderly males and females

8. Regarding the pathophysiology of the described
   condition, which of the following is not a usual
   component of the pathologic process?
   a. obstruction of the organ accounting for early
      symptoms and signs
   b. hypoperistalsis leading to abdominal cramping
   c. rapid invasion of the wall of the organ by bac-
      teria leading to inflammation
   d. spreading of the inflammation to involve the
      whole wall of the organ
   e. gangrene and perforation of the organ

9. Mortality is highest in which of the following
   groups?
   a. infants

b. young adults with rupture of the organ
c. children with rupture of the organ
d. elderly with rupture of the organ
e. pregnant women

10. All of the following statements about the management of this condition when rupture occurs are true except
a. more aggressive fluid resuscitation is usually necessary
b. intravenous antibiotics should be given for 7 to 10 days or until the patient is afebrile
c. insertion of a percutaneous drain prior to surgery is recommended
d. open laparotomy or laparoscopy can be performed
e. expect a prolonged recovery with longer duration of fever and elevated WBC count

11. The radiographic test with the highest sensitivity in diagnosing this condition is
a. ultrasonography
b. barium enema
c. abdominal x-ray
d. computed tomography (CT) with intravenous and oral contrast
e. nuclear medicine WBC-labeled scan

CLINICAL CASE PROBLEM 2

A 3-Year-Old Male with 4 Days of Abdominal Pain

A 3-year-old boy is brought into your office by his parents after 4 days of abdominal pain. His parents state that it appeared their son had some pain in his abdomen and assumed he had a simple "stomach virus" with some associated vomiting and malaise. They decided to bring him to the office since he was not completely better. They noted he "felt warm" during the past few days and had not been eating much. Per the parents, the pain seems to be improved today but he is still not himself. On examination, the temperature is 38°C and the pulse is 105 beats/minute. The boy appears ill but is not lethargic or in any distress. Abdominal exam reveals tenderness in the RLQ with deep palpation. The abdomen is otherwise soft and there is no guarding or rebound tenderness. You suspect the patient has appendicitis.

12. You call the local radiologist and she is able to see your patient right now. What imaging modality is most appropriate in this setting to confirm you suspicions?

a. CT scan with rectal contrast
b. CT scan with oral contrast
c. CT without contrast
d. ultrasound
e. magnetic resonance imaging

13. All of the following may be positive physical exam signs in acute appendicitis except
a. Rovsing's sign
b. pain at McBurney's point
c. McMurphy's sign
d. psoas sign
e. obturator sign

14. Which statement is true regarding imaging modalities in appendicitis?
a. oral contrast has no role when CT is performed for appendicitis
b. rectal contrast has no role when CT is performed for appendicitis
c. ultrasound is sensitive for visualizing a normal appendix to rule out appendicitis
d. intravenous contrast is useful in diagnosis of acute appendicitis
e. plain radiographs should be performed prior to other radiologic studies

15. Which of the following is not consistent with acute appendicitis on ultrasound?
a. the appendix is greater than 4 mm on ultrasound
b. the appendix is noncompressible
c. periappendiceal fluid
d. brightly echogenic periappendiceal fat
e. the presence of appendicolith

16. You perform the appropriate imaging modality and a filled RLQ mass is identified. Which of the following is the most appropriate treatment at this time?
a. appendectomy alone
b. appendectomy with intravenous antibiotics
c. percutaneous drainage alone
d. percutaneous drainage with intravenous antibiotics
e. intravenous antibiotics alone

Clinical Case Management Problem

Discuss the management of the condition described in Clinical Case Problem 2, ruptured appendicitis, when it presents with abscess formation.

Answers

1. **c.** The most likely diagnosis in this patient is acute appendicitis.

The typical history of acute appendicitis is vague central abdominal discomfort followed by anorexia, nausea, and some vomiting. The pain, which is continuous but often not severe, usually moves into the right lower quadrant. The pain is aggravated by movement, walking, or coughing.

In patients with retrocecal appendicitis (which this description fits), there may be dysuria and hematuria with rectal tenderness because of the proximity of the appendix to the ureter and bladder. With perforation there is generalized abdominal tenderness and rebound tenderness. Retrocecal appendicitis often produces poorly localized epigastric pain and only mild nausea and vomiting. Thus, retrocecal appendicitis can be significantly more difficult to diagnose than classic appendicitis. Peritonitis can develop very rapidly. Temperature elevation is usually mild in appendicitis.

The most important differential diagnosis in this case is acute pelvic inflammatory disease. This is often very difficult to differentiate from appendicitis in a woman of childbearing age. The constellation of signs and symptoms, however, favors appendicitis. Acute cholecystitis, acute pyelonephritis, and acute PID are discussed in separate problems.

2. **b.** This patient has an acute abdomen and therefore should be hospitalized for further evaluation and possible operation. With an acute abdomen, definitive treatment should not be delayed.

A WBC count is often elevated. In acute appendicitis, the average leukocyte count is 15,000/mm^3, and 80% of patients have a leukocyte count greater than 11,000/mm^3. The differential count will often show a left shift. A leukocytosis can be helpful in supporting a diagnosis of appendicitis but does not differentiate it from other intra-abdominal processes.

A urinalysis and a serum pregnancy test are all laboratory investigations that should be performed in this patient, but their value is to rule out other diagnoses. Urinalysis may be misleading because 50% of these studies may display hematuria or pyuria due to urinary tract irritation from the inflamed appendix.

Oral antibiotics are not a recommended treatment for appendicitis.

3. **b.** See answer 2.

4. **a.** The most appropriate action at this time would be an abdominal laparoscopy or laparotomy to confirm the diagnosis and treat the condition. The laparoscope is now being used for the removal of appendices by most surgeons. Advantages of laparoscopy include the ability to examine the entire abdomen without the need for extending the operative incision. In addition, there are significantly fewer infectious wound complications. Once the decision to operate has been made, the patient may receive a dose of prophylactic antibiotics, but this is not often extended postoperatively in a case of nonperforated appendix.

5. **e.** The risk of infertility in women who have had appendicitis is not clear. One large study found no increased risk of infertility in women with nonperforated disease but a severalfold increase in infertility in women with perforated appendicitis. Another study showed no increased risk.

Clear complications of appendectomy include the following:

1. Wound infection: For patients with an acute, nonperforated appendix, rates of wound infection are less than 5%. This statistic is thought to be even less in those who undergo laparoscopic removal. If a superficial wound infection is suspected, treatment consists of opening the wound followed by sterile dressing changes.
2. Intraabdominal abscess: Risk of this complication is less than 1% in those with uncomplicated appendicitis, but it increases substantially in those with appendicitis complicated by perforation. Treatment of intraabdominal abscess is discussed later.
3. Portal pyelophlebitis: This is an uncommon but serious complication of appendicitis. It is a septic thrombophlebitis of the portal vein that can lead to hepatic abscesses and considerable mortality. Diverticulitis is the most common etiology, but it can be caused by appendicitis. Treatment consists of controlling the cause of infection and long-term IV antibiotics.
4. Bowel obstruction: Bowel obstruction is a complication of any laparotomy. The incidence after appendicitis is approximately 1%, with the majority occurring within the first 6 months post-op.

6. **d.** Infants, young children, and elderly patients may all present with atypical symptoms, making the diagnosis of appendicitis difficult. In infants and young children, the presenting symptoms may be nonspecific and include only lethargy and irritability, especially in the early stages. They may also have difficulty communicating their symptoms. In elderly patients, the same situation applies. Moreover, in elderly patients, the probability of rupture increases. This may be due to atypical presentations and minimally abnormal lab results.

7. d. This question is meant to demonstrate the importance of distinguishing acute appendicitis from acute PID and its complications, such as tuboovarian abscess.

Young women with right-sided ovarian disease are particularly difficult to differentiate from young women with acute appendicitis. One clue may lie in the point of maximal tenderness. In appendicitis, the point of maximal tenderness is McBurney's point (two-thirds of the distance from the umbilicus to the anterior superior iliac spine). In right-sided ovarian disease, the point of maximal tenderness is 2 or 3 cm below this point.

8. b. The small size of the appendix accounts for its ability to produce symptoms quickly. The pathologic process can be divided into stages:

Stage 1 involves the obstruction of the appendix by a fecalith, a mucous plug, a foreign body, a parasite, lymphoid hyperplasia, or a tumor. This obstruction and hyperperistalsis (not hypoperistalsis) is associated with the early signs of periumbilical cramping and vomiting as a result of distension of the appendix.

Stage 2 involves an increase in intraluminal pressure over venous pressure, causing ischemia and ulceration. Next, there is rapid invasion of the wall of the organ by bacteria, with secondary inflammation.

Stage 3 involves spreading of the infection/inflammation to involve the entire wall of the organ and neighboring peritoneum, leading to a change in character of the pain to constant and localized. Continued swelling and hypoxia leads to gangrene and eventual perforation. This leads to signs and symptoms of peritonitis.

Stage 4 is the last stage and involves perforation of the appendix. All four stages may develop within a very short period (24 to 48 hours).

9. d. Elderly patients with rupture have the highest mortality rates. Overall mortality from appendicitis is less than 1% since the era of antibiotics; however, mortality rates increase to 3% in the general population with rupture. Although rupture in infants and the elderly is common, elderly patients have a much higher mortality rate (up to 15%). Pregnant women do not have high rates of mortality but are much more likely (two or three times more likely) to perforate, in which case maternal death is rare but fetal abortion reaches a rate of 20%.

10. c. Percutaneous drainage is indicated only with late perforated appendix that has resulted in abscess formation at the time of diagnosis. Morbidity increases from 0.1% to almost 4% with perforation (and is much higher in the elderly), and perforation always results in a prolonged recovery compared to nonperforated appendicitis. Surgery in the scenario of perforated appendicitis is an option, but some studies have shown less postoperative complications if an interval appendectomy is performed after a course of IV antibiotics. Once appendicitis has been diagnosed, antibiotics are indicated. For uncomplicated appendicitis, one preoperative prophylactic dose of broad-spectrum antibiotic such as cefotetan or cefoxitin should be administered. For ruptured appendicitis, a broad-spectrum antibiotic should be continued for 7 to 10 days or until the patient is afebrile and has a normal WBC count. Before surgery, fluid resuscitation is always necessary, but with perforation the patient usually will be even more volume depleted and will need much more aggressive fluid replacement.

11. d. The sensitivity of CT is 94%. The sensitivity of ultrasonography is 83% to 88% and is very operator dependent. Barium enema is 80% to 90% sensitive but is no longer recommended because up to 40% of studies can be equivocal secondary to only partial filling of the appendix. Abdominal radiographs are not routinely recommended because of very low sensitivity and specificity. Nuclear medicine scans are 87% to 93% sensitive but are time-consuming and do not distinguish appendicitis from other inflammatory conditions in the right lower quadrant. Note that although imaging can be very helpful, the diagnosis of appendicitis is primarily made by history and physical, and imaging study results can be equivocal.

12. d. CT scanning is the most sensitive radiologic study to diagnose appendicitis, but evaluation in children presents a few challenges. In addition to cost and potential side effects of contrast media, there is a relative high amount of radiation that may increase the risk of cancer throughout a child's lifetime. Some studies have shown this to be significantly greater than the risk conferred to adults. Young children may not be able to cooperate for CT scanning and may require sedation, which poses its own risks. The American College of Radiology advocates the use of ultrasound over CT in children in most cases. CT can be used if sonographic findings are uncertain.

13. c. McMurphy's sign is a clinical exam finding in acute cholecystitis. Rovsing's sign is pain referred to the right lower quadrant when the left lower quadrant is palpated. Psoas sign is worsened pain with active flexion and extension of the hip and is thought to be due to irritation of the psoas muscle by an inflamed adjacent appendix. Obturator sign is pain elicited when the hip is flexed and externally rotated. Pain at McBurney's point represents the anatomic location of the inflamed appendix at 2 cm away from the anterior superior iliac spine toward the umbilicus.

14. **d.** Contrast agents are all helpful in the diagnosis of acute appendicitis. Rectal contrast, although invasive, provides a rapid and accurate way to determine the patency of the appendix. Lack of contrast filling the appendix is suggestive of appendicitis. Oral contrast serves the same purpose, but it takes at least 1 hour before the contrast reaches the cecum, delaying diagnosis. Intravenous contrast is helpful in enhancing the surrounding fat, which may help provide other radiologic signs suggesting acute appendicitis. CT scans may be performed without oral or IV contrast, but this decreases the likelihood of finding an alternative diagnosis when appendicitis is not present. Contrast medium is not required but can be a useful adjunct in the diagnosis of appendicitis. Ultrasound has a good positive likelihood ratio but a poor negative likelihood ratio. It is a very good test to diagnose appendicitis when it is present, but it is not helpful in ruling out appendicitis because a normal appendix is very difficult to identify sonographically. Plain radiographs are insensitive and nonspecific. Studies show that 82% of plain radiographs are negative or misleading in children with appendicitis.

15. **a.** The most useful sonographic sign in appendicitis is an appendix greater than 6 mm in diameter (not 4 mm). Other signs that support the diagnosis of appendicitis are the presence of an appendicolith, brightly echogenic periappendiceal fat suggesting inflammation, and periappendiceal fluid suggesting perforation. A noncompressible appendix is also suggestive of appendicitis.

16. **d.** Treatment of RLQ mass in the setting of appendicitis requires different treatment than simple appendicitis. Early operation on such a mass results in a high incidence of postoperative complications, including peritonitis and wound infection. The primary treatment goal should be percutaneous drainage of the mass with concomitant IV antibiotics. After a prolonged course of antibiotics, interval appendectomy can be performed.

Solution to the Clinical Case Management Problem

Of patients with appendicitis, 2% present with a right lower quadrant mass, which can be an abscess or phlegmon. Currently, the preferred management of these patients includes ultrasound or CT-guided percutaneous drainage and intravenous antibiotics. Elective appendectomy can then be pursued after 6 weeks. This approach is favored over immediate surgery for appendiceal abscess, which can lead to the dissemination of a local infection and result in fistulas and the need for more extensive surgeries such as cecectomy or right hemicolectomy with subsequent longer hospitalization.

Summary

Acute appendicitis is the "great imitator." If you do not think of appendicitis, you will not make the diagnosis. Maintain a high index of suspicion, especially in the young and in the elderly.

1. Classic symptoms of appendicitis: periumbilical abdominal pain, initially vague, but later localizes to the right lower quadrant (McBurney's point); anorexia; low-grade fever; and leukocytosis.
2. Diagnosis can be difficult, particularly in young women, in whom other diagnoses such as PID, tuboovarian abscess, and ovarian torsion may present similarly.
3. Anatomical variations such as retrocecal or retroileal appendicitis: poorly localized abdominal pain, mild nausea and vomiting, mild diarrhea, urinary frequency, and hematuria.
4. Diagnostic tests: WBC, urinalysis, and diagnostic imaging if the diagnosis is in question.
5. CT scan is the most useful imaging technique in most settings. Ultrasound should be considered in certain cases, including children and pregnancy.
6. Definitive therapy: laparoscopic appendectomy or laparotomy with open removal. (Laparoscopic appendectomy is now performed more commonly.

The procedure is associated with fewer postoperative complications.)
7. Complications: wound infection, intra-abdominal abscess, bowel obstruction, and portal pyelophlebitis.
8. Patients who present with RLQ mass associated with presumed appendicitis should be treated with percutaneous drainage and IV antibiotics because complications of surgery are increased in this scenario. Interval appendectomy may be performed at a later date.

Suggested Reading

Kwok M, Kim M, Gorelick M: Evidence-based approach to the diagnosis of appendicitis in children. *Pediatr Emergency Care* 20(10):690–698, 2004.

Lally K, Cox C, Andrassy R: Appendix. In *Sabiston Textbook of Surgery: The Biological Basis of Modern Surgical Practice*, 17th ed. Philadelphia: Saunders, 2004.

Rybkin A, Thoeni R: Current concepts in imaging of appendicitis. *Radiol Clin North Am* 45:411–422, 2007.

Sarosi J, George A, Richard H: Appendicitis. In *Sleisenger & Fordtran's Gastrointestinal and Liver Disease*, 8th ed. Philadelphia: Saunders, 2006.

Wolfe JM, Henneman PL: Acute appendicitis. In Marx J, ed., *Rosen's Emergency Medicine: Concepts and Clinical Practice*, 6th ed. St. Louis: Mosby, 2006.

CHAPTER

40 Colorectal Cancer and Other Colonic Disorders

CLINICAL CASE PROBLEM 1

A 48-Year-Old Male with Weakness, Fatigue, and Lower Right-Sided Abdominal Fullness

A 48-year-old male comes to your office with a vague lower right-sided abdominal fullness (not pain). He describes to you a general feeling of "not feeling well," fatigue, and a somewhat tender area "down near my appendix." He states, "I have no energy. I'm tired all the time." He also suspects that his skin changed color, first to a pale color and then to a slightly yellow color.

On direct questioning, he admits to anorexia, weight loss of 30 pounds in 6 months, nausea most of the time, vomiting twice, some diarrhea that seems to be mucus, and blood in the stool almost every day for the past 3 months. When you ask him what he makes of all this, he tells you, "Maybe a very bad flu."

On examination, the patient looks very pale. Examination of the abdomen reveals abdominal distention. You record the abdominal girth as a baseline. There is a sensation of "fullness" in the right lower quadrant of the abdomen. This area is also dull to percussion and is slightly tender. There is definite percussion of tympani on both sides of the area of dullness. The liver span is approximately 20 cm. The sclerae are yellow.

SELECT THE BEST ANSWER TO THE FOLLOWING QUESTIONS

1. At this time, what would you do?
   a. tell the patient to relax and recheck with your office in 6 months
   b. diagnose irritable bowel syndrome and start the patient on dietary therapy
   c. tell that patient that he probably is going through a viral illness; relax and come back in 2 months if the symptoms have not improved
   d. order a complete workup on the patient
   e. none of the above

2. What is the definitive diagnostic procedure of choice in this patient?
   a. complete blood count (CBC)
   b. fecal occult blood samples
   c. air-contrast barium enema
   d. colonoscopy
   e. three views of the abdomen

3. What is the most likely diagnosis in this patient?
   a. irritable bowel syndrome
   b. lactose intolerance
   c. adenocarcinoma of the pancreas
   d. adenocarcinoma of the colon
   e. ruptured appendix

4. Having made a correct diagnosis from question 3, what is the definitive treatment of choice?
   a. total colectomy
   b. surgical removal of the mass
   c. removal of the appendix
   d. abdominoperineal resection of the rectum

e. neodymium:yttrium-aluminum garnet (Nd:YAG) laser photocoagulation of the identified lesion

5. Carcinoma of the colon most commonly originates in which of the following?
   a. an adenomatous polyp
   b. an inflammatory polyp
   c. a hyperplastic polyp
   d. a benign lymphoid polyp
   e. a leiomyoma

6. Adenomatous polyps are found in approximately what percentage of asymptomatic patients who undergo screening?
   a. 5%
   b. 10%
   c. 15%
   d. 20%
   e. 25%

7. A barium enema is performed on a patient with a suspected carcinoma of the descending colon following an unsuccessful colonoscopy. What is the best radiologic description that fits the probable diagnosis in this patient?
   a. a "strawberry cutout" lesion
   b. an "orange dimpled" lesion
   c. an "apple core" lesion
   d. a "cabbage fulgurating" lesion
   e. a "banana peel" lesion

8. Colorectal polyps are thought to be the origin of most colorectal cancers. Which of the following statements regarding colorectal polyps is false?
   a. the larger the colorectal polyps, the greater the chance of malignancy
   b. hyperplastic polyps have the highest malignant potential of all colorectal polyps
   c. adenomatous polyps increase in incidence with each decade after the age of 30 years
   d. routine removal of adenomas from the colon reduces the incidence of subsequent adenocarcinoma
   e. villous adenomas carry the highest malignant potential of all adenomas

9. Which of the following statements best describes the current evidence for fecal occult blood screening as a measure to reduce the morbidity and mortality from colorectal cancer?
   a. there is good evidence to include fecal occult blood testing in screening asymptomatic patients older than age 50 years for colorectal carcinoma
   b. there is fair evidence to include fecal occult blood testing in screening asymptomatic patients older than age 50 years for colorectal carcinoma

c. there is insufficient evidence to include or exclude fecal occult blood testing as an effective screening test for colorectal cancer in asymptomatic patients older than age 50 years
   d. none of the above

10. Which of the following statements regarding carcinoembryonic antigen (CEA) and colorectal cancer is true?
    a. CEA is a cost-effective screening test for colorectal cancer
    b. elevated preoperative CEA levels correlate well with postoperative recurrence rate in colorectal cancer
    c. CEA is a sensitive test for colorectal cancer
    d. CEA is a specific test for colorectal cancer
    e. CEA has no value in predicting recurrence in colorectal cancer

---

CLINICAL CASE PROBLEM 2

A 78-Year-Old Male with Acute and Severe Abdominal Pain

A 78-year-old male comes to your office with acute and severe abdominal pain, left lower quadrant tenderness, a left lower quadrant mass, and a temperature of 39°C. The patient has had no significant illnesses in the past. He is very healthy. He sees his physician once a year and has had a normal heart, normal blood pressure, and normal "everything else," as he says, for many years.

On examination, the patient's temperature is 39.5°C. His pulse is 102 beats/minute and regular. His blood pressure is 210/105 mmHg. There is significant tenderness in the left lower quadrant. Rebound tenderness is not present. There is a definite sensation of a mass present.

11. What is the most likely diagnosis in this patient?
    a. adenocarcinoma of the colon
    b. diverticulitis
    c. diverticulosis
    d. colorectal carcinoma
    e. atypical appendicitis

12. What is the treatment of choice for this patient?
    a. primary resection of the diseased segment with anastomosis
    b. primary resection of the diseased segment without anastomosis
    c. colectomy
    d. abdominal perineal resection
    e. none of the above

13. Which of the following is (are) a component(s) of the acute treatment of this patient's condition?
    a. intravenous (IV) fluids
    b. IV (broad-spectrum) antibiotics
    c. nasogastric (NG) suction, if abdominal distention or vomiting are present
    d. all of the above
    e. a and c

14. Which of the following investigations is contraindicated at this time in this patient?
    a. computed tomography (CT) scan of the abdomen and pelvis
    b. magnetic resonance imaging scan of the abdomen and pelvis
    c. three views of the abdomen
    d. air-contrast barium enema
    e. none of the above are contraindicated

15. Which of the following statements regarding this patient's blood pressure elevation is true?
    a. this patient most likely has essential hypertension
    b. this patient's abdominal pain is most likely related to his hypertension
    c. this elevation of blood pressure could be caused by the pain he is experiencing
    d. this patient's physician (the one he has been seeing every year) obviously has made a very serious mistake in labeling this patient as normotensive
    e. none of the above statements are true

16. What is the analgesic of choice for control of pain in this patient?
    a. morphine
    b. hydromorphone
    c. methadone
    d. pentazocine
    e. codeine

17. Which of the following organism(s) is (are) most likely involved in the condition described?
    a. *Escherichia coli*
    b. *Bacteroides fragilis*
    c. *Streptococcus pneumoniae*
    d. a and b
    e. all of the above

CLINICAL CASE PROBLEM 3

A 35-Year-Old Male with Rectal Bleeding and Mucoid Discharge from the Rectum

A 35-year-old male comes to your office with rectal bleeding, mucoid discharge from the rectum, and

protrusion of certain structures through the anal canal. On proctoscopic examination, large internal hemorrhoids are seen.

18. What is the best next step in the management of this patient?
    a. proceed with definitive treatment
    b. proceed with further investigations
    c. prescribe a hemorrhoidal cream
    d. do nothing; ask the patient to return in 6 months for review
    e. none of the above

19. What is the treatment of choice for this patient?
    a. a hemorrhoidal cream
    b. a hemorrhoidal ointment
    c. hemorrhoidectomy
    d. injection of phenol into the hemorrhoidal tissue
    e. rubber band ligation of the internal hemorrhoids

20. Which of the following statements regarding angiodysplasia is (are) true?
    a. angiodysplasia is an acquired condition most often affecting individuals older than age 60 years
    b. angiodysplasia is a focal submucosal vascular ectasis that has the propensity to bleed profusely
    c. most angiodysplastic lesions are located in the cecum and proximal ascending colon
    d. multiple lesions occur in 25% of cases
    e. all of the above statements are true

Clinical Case Management Problem

The fourth edition of this book stated, "Regarding colorectal cancer, there appears to be almost universal support for the following: (1) decreasing the amount of fat in the diet, especially saturated fat (this also will lead to decreased body mass index or total body weight); (2) increasing the amount of fiber in the diet; (3) increasing the intake of cruciferous vegetables and fiber; (4) decreasing alcohol intake; and (5) decreasing the intake of salted, smoked, and nitrate-based foods." In which way has this belief been altered by recent evidence-based randomized clinical trials?

Answers

1. **e.** None of the answers are appropriate or sufficiently focused.

2. **d.** The colonoscopy will allow for a tissue biopsy and diagnosis as well.

3. **d.** In this patient, the problem list at this point is as follows: (1) a middle-aged male with nonspecific feelings of "ill health;" (2) there is a right lower quadrant mass on physical examination, raising suspicion of carcinoma; (3) the liver is enlarged, possibly indicating metastases; (4) the pale appearance suggests anemia; (5) icterus suggests elevated conjugated hyperbilirubinemia; and (6) the clinically apparent abdominal distention indicates possible ascites.

With this constellation of symptoms and signs, the working diagnosis is adenocarcinoma of the colon, possibly the cecum, with liver metastases.

The investigations that must be performed at this time include the following:

1. Laboratory: (a) CBC, (b) serum bilirubin, (c) liver enzymes (aspartate aminotransferase, alanine aminotransferase, and γ-glucuronosyltransferase), (d) alkaline phosphatase, (e) serum calcium, (f) serum electrolytes, and (g) CEA.
2. Radiology: (a) chest x-ray and (b) CT scan of the abdomen with contrast.
3. The diagnostic procedure of choice in this patient is a total colonoscopy to confirm a mass lesion, to determine the location of that lesion, and to obtain a biopsy of the lesion if possible.
4. For colon carcinoma, the essentials of diagnosis are as follows:
   a. Right colon: (i) an unexplained weakness or anemia, (ii) occult blood in the feces and diarrhea with mucus, (iii) dyspeptic symptoms, (iv) persistent right abdominal discomfort, (v) palpable abdominal mass, (vi) characteristic x-ray findings, and (vii) characteristic colonoscopic findings
   b. Left colon: (i) change in bowel habits with thin stools, (ii) gross blood in the stool, (iii) obstructive symptoms, (iv) characteristic x-ray findings, and (v) characteristic colonoscopic or sigmoidoscopic findings
   c. Rectum: (i) rectal bleeding, (ii) alteration in bowel habits, (iii) sensation of incomplete evacuation, (iv) intrarectal palpable tumor, and (v) sigmoidoscopic findings

4. **b.** The definitive surgical treatment of choice in this patient (if feasible) is resection of the colonic mass. The preliminary location of the lesion based on physical examination is in the area of the cecum. If this proves to be correct, the colonic resection will involve the removal of the area from the vermiform appendix to the junction of the ascending and transverse colons. With the presence of liver metastasis, this procedure is palliative.

5. **a.** The vast majority of colonic adenocarcinomas evolve from adenomas. Adenomas are a premalignant lesion, and in the large bowel the sequence is adenoma, dysplasia in the adenomas, and adenocarcinoma.

6. **e.** Both adenomas and the subsequent evolved adenocarcinomas increase in incidence with age, and the distribution of adenomas and cancer in the bowel is similar. Overall, adenomatous polyps are found in approximately 25% of asymptomatic patients who undergo screening colonoscopy. The age-related prevalence of adenomatous polyps is 30% at age 50 years, 40% at age 60 years, 50% at age 70 years, and 55% at age 80 years. The mean age of patients with adenomas is 55 years, which is approximately 5 to 10 years earlier than the mean age for patients with adenocarcinoma of the colon. Approximately 50% of polyps occur in the sigmoid colon or in the rectum and thus can be revealed by sigmoidoscopy. Approximately 50% of patients with adenomas have more than one adenoma, and 15% have more than two adenomas. There is an interesting correlation between patients with breast cancer and adenomatous polyps in the colon and rectum. Patients with breast cancer have an increased risk of adenomatous polyps.

The malignant potential of the adenoma depends on the growth pattern, the size of the polyp, and the degree of atypia or dysplasia. Adenocarcinoma of the colon is found in approximately 1% of adenomas less than 1 cm in diameter, in approximately 10% of adenomas between 1 cm and 2 cm in diameter, and in approximately 45% of adenomas with a diameter greater than 2 cm.

The potential for cancerous transformations increases with increasing degrees of dysplasia.

Sessile lesions are more apt to be malignant than pedunculated ones. The time it takes an adenoma to proceed through the process to frank adenocarcinoma is believed to be between 10 and 15 years.

The following is a summary of the types of adenomas and their malignant potential: (1) villous adenoma, 40% become malignant; (2) tubulovillous adenoma, 22% become malignant; and (3) tubular adenoma, 5% become malignant.

7. **c.** This patient most likely suffers from a constricting carcinoma of the descending colon. A barium enema (preferably an air-contrast barium enema) of a constricting carcinoma of the descending colon presents what is best described as an "apple core" lesion. On the barium enema, you will note the loss of mucosal patterns, the "hooks" at the margins of the lesion, the relatively short length of the lesion, and the abrupt ending of the lesion.

8. b. Hyperplastic polyps are designated as "unclassified" but are totally benign. The highest malignant potential is carried by villous adenomas.

9. a. The current U.S. Preventive Services Task Force recommends colorectal cancer screening for all people aged 50 years or older. Screening reduces mortality. Acceptable screening methods include annual fecal occult blood testing, colonoscopy, and contrast barium enema. Colonoscopy provides an alternative that will find abnormalities throughout the colon and allows removal of polyps at the same time; however, the major complication rate of 1 in 1000 procedures and the difficult preparation make many patients concerned about the process. Flexible sigmoidoscopy also provides a clear picture but only of the distal third of the colon. So-called virtual colonoscopy done via a CT scan cannot replace colonoscopy at this time.

10. b. CEA is a glycoprotein found in the cell membranes of a number of tissues, a number of body fluids, and a number of secretions including urine and feces. It is also found in malignancies of the colon and rectum. Because some of the CEA antigen enters the bloodstream, it can be detected by the use of a radioimmunoassay technique of serum.

Elevated CEA is not specifically associated with colorectal cancer; abnormally high levels of CEA are also found in patients with other gastrointestinal (GI) malignancies and non-GI malignancies. CEA levels are elevated in 70% of patients with an adenocarcinoma of the large bowel, but less than 50% of patients with localized disease are CEA positive. Thus, because of these difficulties with sensitivity and specificity, CEA does not serve as a useful screening procedure, nor is it an accurate diagnostic test for colorectal cancer at a curable stage. However, elevated preoperative CEA levels correlate with postoperative recurrence rate, and failure of CEA to fall to normal levels after resection implies a poor prognosis. CEA is helpful in detecting recurrence after curative surgical resection; if high CEA levels return to normal after operation and then increase progressively during the follow-up period, recurrence of cancer is likely.

11. b. This patient has diverticulitis, an infection and inflammation of one or more diverticula that, in its noninflammatory state, is known as diverticulosis. In the United States and Canada, approximately 50% of patients have diverticula, 10% by age 40 years and 65% by age 80 years. The prevalence of diverticula varies widely throughout the world.

Cultural factors, especially diet, play an important causative role. Among dietary factors, the most important one is the fiber content of ingested food.

The essentials of diagnosis of diverticulitis are as follows: (1) acute abdominal pain (usually left lower), (2) left lower quadrant tenderness with or without a mass in the same area, and (3) fever with leukocytosis.

The imaging findings are as follows:

1. Plain films: If inflammation is localized—ileus, partial colonic obstruction, small bowel obstruction, or left lower quadrant mass.
2. CT scans: No perforation—effacement of pericolic fat with or without abscess or fistulas.
3. Barium enema: Contraindicated during an acute attack of diverticulitis; the risk of perforation and barium escape into the peritoneal cavity is high.

12. e. The treatment of choice for diverticulitis is expectant unless surgical treatment is necessary because of rupture and subsequent peritonitis or multiple recurrences.

The natural history of diverticulitis follows: (1) 10% to 20% of patients with diverticulosis develop diverticulitis; (2) approximately 75% of complications of diverticular disease develop in patients with no prior colonic symptoms; and (3) approximately 25% of patients hospitalized with acute diverticulitis require surgical treatment. In the past few decades, the operative mortality of primary resection has decreased from 25% to less than 5%.

13. d. Treatment includes (1) nothing by mouth, (2) IV fluids with potassium, (3) NG suction if abdominal distension or vomiting is present, and (4) IV antibiotics.

14. d. See answer 11.

15. c. The elevation of blood pressure in this patient is almost certainly directly associated with the pain that he is experiencing. Acute and chronic pain (but especially acute pain) increases the release of the "pressor hormones" such as norepinephrine. This produces vasoconstriction that ultimately results in elevated blood pressure. The patient thus experiences a vicious pain cycle that is circular in dimension: more pain, pressor hormone release, elevated blood pressure, increase in pressor hormone release, more pain, and so on.

16. a. Morphine will readily relieve the pain, decrease anxiety, and lower the elevated blood pressure.

17. **d.** The most common organisms involved in the development of diverticulitis are *E. coli* and *B. fragilis*.

18. **a.** The next step in the management of this patient is to proceed with definitive treatment.

19. **e.** This patient has internal hemorrhoids. The treatment of choice for the protruding internal hemorrhoids that this patient has is rubber band ligation. Rubber band ligation is especially useful in situations in which the hemorrhoids are enlarged or prolapsing.

To accomplish this procedure, the anoscope is used and the redundant mucosa above the hemorrhoid is grasped with forceps and advanced through the barrel of a special ligator. The rubber band is then placed snugly around the mucosa and the hemorrhoidal plexus. Ischemic necrosis occurs over several days, with eventual slough, fibrosis, and fixation of the tissues. One hemorrhoidal complex at a time is treated, with repeat ligations performed at 2- and 4-week intervals as needed.

The major, but uncommon, complication of this procedure is pain severe enough to require removal of the band. To avoid this, the band must be placed high and well above the junction of the mucocutaneous region (dentate line). In this location, the innervation is autonomic, not somatic. If pain begins and does not resolve, infection should be suspected and investigated immediately. At the time the dead tissue falls off, there may be significant bleeding; the patient should be aware of this.

20. **e.** Angiodysplasia is an acquired colonic condition that mainly affects elderly individuals. Pathophysiologically, angiodysplasia can be described as a focal submucosal vascular ectasis that has a high probability of producing significant bleeding. The vast majority of angiodysplastic lesions occur in the cecum and in the proximal ascending colon. In at least 25% of patients, multiple lesions are present.

The primary symptom is bright red rectal bleeding that can be extensive and that may require transfusion.

Diagnosis is made by colonoscopy. The diagnosis is made when two of the following three features are present: (1) an early filling vein (within 4 or 5 seconds after injection), (2) a vascular tuft, and (3) a delayed-emptying vein.

If searched for carefully, as many as 25% of individuals older than age 60 years have angiodysplasia. In many cases, expectant management or colonoscopic cauterization is all that is needed. If surgery is required, the operative procedure of choice appears to be hemicolectomy.

Solution to the Clinical Case Management Problem

Evidence-based, randomized clinical studies have found no evidence that consumption of fat, fiber, or vegetables decreases the reoccurrence of colorectal cancer. However, other well-controlled epidemiologic studies still support obesity and physical inactivity as primary risk factors. Possible effects of alcohol and smoked foods are yet to be investigated. Common sense would argue for commonly underadhered to nutritional recommendations: Eat real (nonprocessed), fresh food; mostly plants, and not too much.

Summary

COLORECTAL CANCER

1. Incidence: In the United States, cancer of the colon and rectum ranks second after cancer of the lung in incidence and death rates. Approximately 6% of Americans will develop colorectal cancer in their lifetime, and the 5-year survival rate is 62.1%.
2. Age and sex
   a. Age: The incidence of carcinoma of the colon increases with age, starting slowly at age 40 years and then doubling for each decade thereafter.
   b. Sex: Carcinoma of the colon, particularly the right colon, is more common in women, and carcinoma of the rectum is more common in men.
3. Genetic predisposition: Genetic predisposition to cancer of the large bowel is well recognized. Relatively rare cases are inherited in a Mendelian fashion, namely familial adenomatous polyposis and hereditary nonpolyposis colorectal cancer. However, a familial tendency also exists among the general population; by the age of 79 years, a person with no affected relative has a

4% chance of developing colorectal cancer. With one first-degree relative, there is a 9% chance; with more than one first-degree relative, there is a 16% chance; and with a first-degree relative who developed cancer before the age of 45 years, there is a 15% chance.

4. Risk factors for carcinoma of the colon include (a) ulcerative colitis, (b) Crohn's disease, (c) exposure to radiation, (d) colorectal polyps, (e) cigarette smoking, and (f) high-fat diets.

5. Essentials of diagnosis: See answer 3.

6. Distribution of cancer of the colon and rectum: (a) rectum, 30% of all colorectal cancers; (b) sigmoid, 20% of all colorectal cancers; (c) descending colon, 15% of all colorectal cancers; (d) transverse colon, 10% of all colorectal cancers; and (e) ascending colon, 25% of all colorectal cancers.

7. Pathophysiology: The vast majority of colorectal cancers originate in colonic polyps. Tubular adenomas (tubulovillous adenoma) and villous adenomas are both premalignant.

8. Treatment of colorectal cancer
   a. Basic treatment for cancer of the colon consists of wide surgical resection of the lesion and its regional lymphatic drainage after preparation of the bowel.
   b. Basic treatment for cancer of the rectum consists of abdominoperineal resection of the rectum or a low anterior resection of the rectum.
   c. Adjuvant therapy includes radiotherapy and combination chemotherapy.

9. Prevention
   a. Aspirin in high doses.
   b. Increased physical activity and weight loss.

POLYPS OF THE COLON AND RECTUM

1. Prevalence: Adenomatous polyps are found in approximately 25% of asymptomatic adults who undergo screening colonoscopy. The prevalence of adenomatous polyps is 30% at age 50 years, 40% at age 60 years, 50% at age 70 years, and 55% at age 80 years.

2. Malignant potential: Adenomas are a premalignant lesion, and most authorities believe that the majority of adenocarcinomas of the large bowel evolve from adenomas (adenoma-to-carcinoma sequence). The mean age of patients with polyps is 5 to 10 years younger than the mean age of patients with colorectal cancer.

3. Benign polyps include hematomas, inflammatory polyps, and hyperplastic polyps.

4. Essentials of diagnosis: The essentials of diagnosis of polyps of the colon and rectum include the passage of blood per rectum and sigmoidoscopic, colonoscopic, or radiologic discovery of polyps.

5. Treatment: Adenomatous polyps should be removed by methods that include electrocautery, Nd:YAG laser therapy, and laparotomy if removal through the colonoscope is unsuccessful.

6. Prevention: Eating a high-fiber diet will help prevent colonic disease.

DIVERTICULOSIS AND DIVERTICULITIS

1. Prevalence: Approximately 50% of individuals in the United States develop colonic diverticula. Diverticular disease is much more common in the United States than in Japan or other Eastern countries.

2. Symptomatic versus asymptomatic: Diverticulosis probably remains asymptomatic in 80% of individuals.

3. Essentials of diagnosis of diverticulitis are as follows: (a) acute abdominal pain, (b) left lower quadrant tenderness with or without a mass, (c) fever and leukocytosis, and (d) characteristic radiologic signs showing diverticula.

4. Treatment
   a. Conservative: Some patients can be treated at home with oral antibiotics and analgesics.
   b. In-hospital treatment consists of NPO; insertion of an NG tube; and administration of IV fluids, antibiotics, and pentazocine for analgesia.
   c. Surgical: Surgical treatment is necessary when there is a diverticula rupture or when abscess and peritonitis ensue. Approximately 25% of hospitalized patients need surgery.

5. The "DO NOT" of diverticulitis: DO NOT do a barium enema in the acute phase (potential rupture and peritonitis).

6. Organisms associated with diverticulitis include *E. coli* and *B. fragilis*.

7. Prevention: Eating a high-fiber diet will help prevent colonic disease.

OTHER CONDITIONS OF NOTE

1. Internal hemorrhoids with prolapse: Treatment consists of rubber band ligation.

2. Angiodysplasia: Consider angiodysplasia as another cause of rectal bleeding in elderly patients.

Suggested Reading

Bingham SA, Day NE, Luben R, et al: Dietary fibre in food and protection against colorectal cancer in the European Prospective Investigation into Cancer and Nutrition (EPIC): An observational study. *Lancet* 361:1496–1501, 2003.

Collins JF, Lieberman DA, Durbin TE, Weiss DG: Accuracy of screening for fecal occult blood on a single stool sample obtained by digital rectal examination: A comparison with recommended sampling practice. *Ann Intern Med* 142:81–85, 2005.

Dube C, Rostom A, Lewin G, et al; U.S. Preventive Services Task Force: The use of aspirin for primary prevention of colorectal cancer: A systematic review prepared for the U.S. Preventive Services Task Force. *Ann Intern Med* 146(5):365–375, 2007.

Levin B, Brooks D, Smith RA, Stone A: Emerging technologies in screening for colorectal cancer: CT colonography, immunochemical fecal occult blood tests, and stool screening using molecular markers. *CA Cancer J Clin* 53:44–55, 2003.

Lin OS, Kozarek RA, Schembre DB, et al: Screening colonoscopy in very elderly patients: Prevalence of neoplasia and estimated impact on life expectancy. *JAMA* 295:2357–2365, 2006.

Nadel MR, Shapiro JA, Klabunde CN, : A national survey of primary care physicians' methods for screening for fecal occult blood. *Ann Intern Med* 142:86–94, 2005.

Pignone M, Rich M, Teutsch SM, et al: Screening for colorectal cancer in adults at average risk: A summary of the evidence for the U.S. Preventive Services Task Force. *Ann Intern Med* 137(2):132–141, 2002.

Pignone M, Saha S, Hoerger T, et al: Cost-effectiveness analyses of colorectal cancer screening: A systematic review for the U.S. Preventive Services Task Force. *Ann Intern Med* 137(2):96–104, 2002.

Schatzkin A, Lanza E, Corle D, et al: Lack of effect of a low-fat, high-fiber diet on the reoccurrence of colorectal adenomas. *N Engl J Med* 342:1149–1155, 2000.

Walsh JM, Terdiman JP: Colorectal cancer screening: Scientific review. *JAMA* 289(10):1288–1296, 2003.

Wender RC: Barriers to screening for colorectal cancer. *Gastrointest Endosc Clin North Am* 12:145–170, 2002.

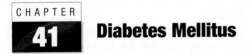

CHAPTER 41 Diabetes Mellitus

CLINICAL CASE PROBLEM 1

An 18-Year-Old Female with Weight Loss and Feeling Poorly

Jackie is an 18-year-old female with no previous chronic medical problems who comes to your office with a chief complaint of "feeling rotten." She tells you that she has lost 15 pounds in the past 2 months and has had increasing thirst and urination. The patient has been feeling fatigued and nauseous, which has gotten especially worse in the past 2 days after she "caught a cold" that had been going around her family members.

On examination, the patient is well below the 5th percentile for weight. She looks thin and pale, and seems a little sluggish, but answers questions appropriately. Her nose is slightly congested, but otherwise her mucous membranes are dry. Her temperature is 99°F, blood pressure is 95/70 mmHg, and her pulse is 110 beats/minute. Respirations are deep at a rate of 30 breaths/minute and her breath smells "fruity." She has a few anterior cervical and axillary nodes, each measuring 1 cm. Lungs are clear to auscultation. Her abdomen is slightly tender. No other abnormalities are found.

SELECT THE BEST ANSWER TO THE FOLLOWING QUESTIONS

1. The most likely diagnosis is?
   a. diabetes insipidus
   b. early diabetic ketoacidosis
   c. type 2 diabetes mellitus (DM) under poor glycemic control
   d. alcohol abuse
   e. mild type 1 DM

2. What is the most appropriate course of action?
   a. advise Jackie to begin psychotherapy for an eating disorder with comorbid alcohol abuse and monitor her weight carefully during the next several months
   b. treat Jackie's cold symptomatically; have her increase fluids such as juice and soups; order some basic labs, such as basic metabolic panel, glycosylated hemoglobin (HgbA$_{1c}$), complete blood count (CBC), and urinalysis (U/A); see her in 1 week for follow-up and to discuss the results; and tell her to call if she is feeling worse
   c. check an office finger-stick glucose level and a urine dipstick, and if your suspicions are confirmed, admit Jackie to the hospital for stabilization and management with possible consultation with an endocrinologist
   d. treat her in the office with 1 L of intravenous (IV) normal saline to correct her dehydration, and then send her home with a prescription for an anti-nausea agent. Tell her to continue to push fluids; order a CBC, chemistry screen, and U/A; and see her back in 3 days for follow-up and to discuss the results. She is to call if she is feeling worse
   e. start the patient on desmopressin (DDAVP), order some basic labs, have the patient push fluids, and refer her to an endocrinologist

She follows your advice and is subsequently seen in the emergency department. Laboratory data include serum glucose greater than 600, ketones in the urine at 4+, and a serum Na of 128.

3. Initial treatments should include
   a. IV bicarbonate should be routinely used to correct the likely acidosis
   b. high-volume IV isotonic or half-normal saline fluids and IV regular insulin via IV pump
   c. subcutaneous insulin every 4 to 6 hours in a sliding scale, with labs every 12 hours until the situation is stabilized

d. give D5NS IV fluid until the Jackie can re-establish adequate oral intake

e. avoid adding potassium to the IV (unless the patient is frankly hypokalemic) since these patients tend to have excess potassium levels

4. To minimize risk of cerebral edema, lowering of blood glucose level should be done no faster than what rate per hour in a patient with severe hyperglycemia?
   a. 10 mg/dL
   b. 20 mg/dL
   c. 30 mg/dL
   d. 80 mg/dL
   e. 200 mg/dL

5. Principles regarding evaluating possible triggers that worsen the underlying condition include
   a. cocaine abuse can trigger this condition
   b. infection rarely triggers acute worsening of control of this condition
   c. it is clinically useful to repeat a chest x-ray in 24 to 48 hours, even if the initial one was negative, if one suspects pneumonia
   d. a and c
   e. because of changes induced by the underlying disease, it is not useful to get a urinalysis and culture when searching for a trigger for this condition

6. All of the following are true regarding type 1 DM except
   a. it is associated with other autoimmune disorders
   b. age of onset is usually before 30 years
   c. islet cell antibodies are found in approximately 90% of cases
   d. suboptimal vitamin D nutrition is associated with increased incidence
   e. there is approximately a 90% concordance in monozygotic twins for this type of DM

7. The Diabetes Control and Complications and other landmark trials clearly demonstrated which one of the following?
   a. myocardial infarction and stroke were markedly improved in patients with tight glycemic control
   b. once-daily combined insulin or oral medications were adequate for tight glycemic control in most patients
   c. primary care physicians can easily accomplish tight glycemic control in their type 1 diabetic patients

   d. tight glycemic control tends to lead to better weight control
   e. intensive glycemic control of type 1 DM decreases microvascular complications

8. True statements regarding macrovascular complications in type 1 or type 2 DM include all of the following except
   a. low-density lipoprotein (LDL) should be kept at least <2.6 mmol/L (100 mg/dL), and likely <70 mg/dL, if the patient has confirmed vascular disease
   b. blood pressure goal is <130/80 mmHg
   c. treatment with insulin or sulfonylureas has clearly been shown to worsen macrovascular disease via worsening hyperinsulinemia
   d. strict blood pressure control is more beneficial than tight glycemic control in reducing macrovascular complications
   e. virtually all type 2 diabetics older than age 40 years who do not have a contraindication to them should be on statins

9. True statements regarding diabetic ketoacidosis (DKA) management include
   a. serum sodium level – (serum chloride + Bicarbonate) is usually elevated
   b. DKA only occurs in type 1 DM
   c. in a patient with a serum potassium level of 4.5 mEq/L (mmol/L), there is likely total body potassium depletion that needs replacement
   d. a and c
   e. DKA usually develops over a period of 1 or 2 weeks

10. Regarding fluid and electrolyte management in DKA, all of the following are true except
    a. fluid deficits are often on the order of 6 to 8 L
    b. the initial fluid replacement should generally be normal (0.9%) saline unless there is severe hypernatremia
    c. in the otherwise healthy adult with DKA, a reasonable rate of infusion generally needed for the first 3 hours of treating full DKA is 150 mL/hour
    d. potassium level should be monitored frequently (every hour at first and then every 2 to 4 hours) during the initial treatment phase of DKA
    e. in a patient with acute DKA but otherwise normal organ function, 20 to 40 mEq KCl/L can be added to the IV fluid if the serum potassium is 4 or 5 mEq/L

A 35-Year-Old Male Who Comes in for a Routine Periodic Health Exam

Mr. Couchpo is a 35-year-old male who comes to your office for a routine health exam. He works as a computer programmer, is recently married, and came in because "he wants to make sure he is healthy." The following are other key elements of the history and physical:

Feels fine, except occasionally a little "sluggish" after a long day at the office.

No past medical history.

Family history: His mother and an older brother both have type 2 DM, both with onset in their 40's, and his father has had hypertension since his 30's. His father developed coronary artery disease in his 50's.

Patient states that his diet is "regular."

Exercise: He used to play varsity soccer in college. Now he plays golf occasionally on a weekend in the warmer months when he can get away from his job. He likes to walk when he can, but he feels that he "doesn't have the time."

Stress level: "High"—many deadlines and long hours at work; commutes into the city by train.

Physical exam: height, 5 feet, 10 inches; weight, 195 pounds; body mass index, 28; waist circumference, 43 inches. Blood pressure, 135/88 mmHg; pulse 76 beats/minute. Physical exam is otherwise unremarkable.

Screening labs: fasting blood glucose, 115; C-reactive protein, 4.3 mg/L; total cholesterol = 230; high-density lipoprotein (HDL) = 35; LDL = 125; and triglycerides = 180.

11. Correct statements about this symptom complex include all of the following except
    a. this syndrome affects approximately one-fifth of U.S. adults and is increasing in prevalence
    b. the elevated C-reactive protein is an added risk factor that the patient will progress to frank type 2 DM and coronary artery disease
    c. body mass index is a better predictor of risk for progression to related chronic diseases than is waist circumference
    d. lifestyle issues superimposed on a genetic distribution are the main cause
    e. other associated disorders of this syndrome include chronic kidney disease and fatty liver

A 3-day dietary diary for this patient is summarized as follows:

Breakfast: usually a mug of coffee and a Danish or bagel

Midmorning: often snacks or treats or pastries brought in by colleagues

Lunch: has a 1-hour lunch break during the workday and usually goes out to a local diner and has a sandwich such as ham and cheese on rye or a burger, with a soft drink or coffee

Dinner: starch such as mashed potatoes with butter or french fries, a serving of green beans or other vegetable, and an 8- to 10-ounce piece of chicken or steak

Use this diet diary to answer questions 12 through 17.

12. Choose the best answer regarding this patient's carbohydrate sources:
    a. the patient tends to eat high glycemic index (GI) and load foods with a low nutrient/calorie ratio that will likely worsen his overweight, C-reactive protein, dyslipidemia, and vascular disease risk
    b. most whole wheat commercial breads have a low GI
    c. avoiding commercial flour products, such as by switching to sprouted grain flourless breads, and substituting nonwhite starchy vegetables, such a squash or yams, would much improve the quality of his carbohydrate intake
    d. a and c
    e. carrots have a high glycemic load and should be avoided by those with metabolic syndrome or diabetes

13. Choose the best answer regarding this patient's caloric intake:
    a. total caloric balance is more important than whether the calories come from fat, carbohydrate, or protein in determining body weight
    b. the caloric (energy) density of foods has not been demonstrated to be important for weight control
    c. a redistribution of calories, with more at breakfast and less at dinner, would likely benefit the patient, such as by decreasing midmorning snacking
    d. a and c
    e. adequate fiber in the diet to improve caloric balance is 10 to 15 g/day

14. Choose the best answer regarding the fat sources:
    a. different types of fats are basically equal in their affect on health—it is the total fat that counts

b. the patient needs to increase polyunsaturated seed oils, such as corn, sunflower, or safflower oil

c. substituting stick margarine containing partially hydrogenated corn or soybean oil for the butter he currently uses would be a good first step in improving the quality of fats in his diet

d. the balance between omega-3 and -6 fatty acids is likely distorted, with excess saturated and trans-fatty acid intake

e. flax and walnut oils would be excellent cooking/sauteing oils

15. Choose the best answer regarding the protein sources in his diet:

a. total protein is likely excessive and may, over time, lead to impaired renal function

b. substituting a protein powder diet drink for a meal would be an effective way to help him lose weight and build muscle

c. emphasizing plant sources of protein such as those made from legumes would improve multiple aspects of his diet

d. a and c

e. a high-protein, low-carbohydrate diet (with protein >2 g/kg body weight/day and total carbohydrates <130 g/day), when combined with regular vigorous aerobic and muscle strengthening exercises, is an excellent strategy for the patient with glucose intolerance or DM

16. Choose the best answer regarding this patient's vegetable and fruit intake:

a. adding iceberg lettuce and a slice of tomato to his sandwich, switching from soft drinks to fruit juice, and snacking on dried fruit rather than pastries would be a major step in improving his vegetable and fruit intake

b. recommending a standard daily multivitamin/multimineral supplement would be the best strategy—it has all the necessary nutrients found in fruit and vegetables and would be easier for the patient to implement

c. although fruit and vegetable intake is slightly low, there is no credible evidence that increasing them leads to better health outcomes

d. the patient needs to gradually increase his intake to three to five servings of vegetables, ideally with at least one a dark leafy green, and two or three servings of whole fruit per day

e. recommending a nutraceutical food bar with extra antioxidants and vitamins is a more practical way to help this patient attain the equivalent nutrition found in fruit and vegetables

17. Choose the best answer regarding how this patient might handle sweets and sugar intake:

a. it is critical to ban sugar from the diet of patients with DM and metabolic syndrome since they are a main cause of these disorders and are empty calories that deplete the body of necessary nutrients

b. because recent studies do not show worsening of glycemic control from sugar, there is no reason to limit these in patients with metabolic syndrome or DM

c. establishing a reasonable quota and teaching the patient to mindfully and slowly savor sweets and treats can naturally limit them so that they do not derail the patient's treatment when done in the context of a balanced whole foods diet

d. switching from table sugar (sucrose) to high-fructose corn syrup sweeteners has been shown to decrease sweet craving and associated over-eating and to lower triglyceride levels

e. whole fruit in general should be avoided in patients with metabolic syndrome and DM since the high fructose content has been shown to bypass normal satiety mechanisms and worsen glycemic control

18. Regarding this patient's exercise habits, assuming he has been medically cleared and can safely exercise, the best advice would be:

a. encourage the patient to exercise vigorously each weekend by jogging or swimming

b. get a stationary bike and try to do 30 minutes of biking and 30 minutes of calisthenics each evening

c. do not emphasize the need for exercise—although often recommended, there is little evidence that regular exercise improves health outcomes

d. assuming a suitable area to do so is available, encourage him to "brown bag" a lunch and then go for a 30- to 45-minute walk for the remainder of his lunchtime during the workweek. On weekends, after 2 or 3 months of reconditioning, take up a sport or activity that he finds fun and meaningful, such as amateur soccer

e. direct the patient to join a semiprofessional traveling soccer league since he already has skills in soccer from his college years, and people tend to continue activities they are good at

19. Which of the following statements regarding type 2 DM is false?
   a. impaired glucose tolerance is defined by a fasting blood sugar range of 100 to 125 mg/dL
   b. elevated fasting blood sugar provides the first evidence of loss of glucose control
   c. lifestyle changes of increased physical activity and improved nutrition can decrease the risk of developing DM by 50% or more
   d. metformin may be effective in decreasing the risk of developing diabetes
   e. lifestyle changes are more effective than treatment with metformin

20. Choose the best answer regarding the endocannabinoid system:
   a. a collection of weight-loss medicines that work at the level of the hypothalamic–pituitary–adrenal axis
   b. a newly discovered and conceptualized endocrine system involved in stress recovery, homeostasis, and energy balance including food intake
   c. a new weight-loss system using plant-derived medicines
   d. a new approach to treating metabolic syndrome and early DM using a complex herbal system that is unproven clinically but is very popular
   e. a weight-loss system that utilizes modulation of endogenous cannabinoid receptors

CLINICAL CASE PROBLEM 3

A 45-Year-Old African American Woman with Type 2 DM Diagnosed 6 Months Ago

Mrs. Jones is a 45-year-old asymptomatic obese African American female who comes to your office for the first time for follow-up of her DM. She has transferred to you from her primary care physician out of state and was diagnosed with type 2 DM 6 months ago. She states her previous physician started her on glyburide 5 mg daily before breakfast, told her to "cut out sugar and heavy foods," and advised her to try to walk for 20 minutes three times a week. She is on no other prescription medications, but she does take over-the-counter ibuprofen, a few pills a day, for knee osteoarthritis. She also takes chromium piccolinate 200 μg/day and α-lipoic acid 600 mg/day because she heard from a friend at church that it helps diabetes. He also gave her a 2000-calorie American Diabetes Association (ADA) diet leaflet to follow. She has run out of test strips, but the last time she checked her fasting blood sugar 2 months ago, it was 160, which is approximately average for her. She brings the results of his office records and most recent labs from 6 months ago, which show the following:

Past medical history: positive for mild hypertension (range, 130/85 mmHg to 140/90 at various office visits), hyperlipidemia (fasting total cholesterol = 230, LDL = 125, HDL = 38, triglycerides = 180), obesity (weight, 190 pounds; height, 5 feet, 8 inches), mild osteoarthritis of knees

No known drug allergies

Health insurance: Has a basic plan that covers visits but no prescription plan

Family history: Positive for DM in her mother and older sister, hypertension (HTN) and coronary artery disease in her mother, father, older sister and younger brother

Social history: Negative for smoking, alcohol, or illicit drug abuse. Married with three adult children. Works as a cashier at a local supermarket. Recreation: Likes to socialize and dance

Labs (from 6 months ago): basic metabolic profile: blood urea nitrogen/creatinine ratio, 15/1.1; estimated glomerular filtration rate, 67 mL/minute/1.73 m²; electrolytes normal; albumin, 3.5; CBC, within normal limits; HgbA$_{1c}$, 8.2%

Her exam is consistent with the history and laboratory findings.

21. Choose the best answer regarding Mrs. Jones's overall health status:
   a. her diabetes, HTN, weight, and lipids are inadequately controlled, and she would benefit from a multidisciplinary approach to resolution of these issues
   b. her diabetes, weight, and lipids need better control, but HTN is adequately controlled for her age
   c. Mrs. Jones, as an African American, statistically has a poorer prognosis for her diabetes
   d. instructing her to continue to follow her 2000-calorie ADA diet brochure will likely resolve her medical problems
   e. a and c

22. Initial management at your first visit should include all of the following except
   a. refill her medications and glucometer supplies
   b. order an HgbA$_{1c}$, chemistry screen, urine dip and microalbumin/creatinine ratio, and fasting lipid panel

c. start her on regular insulin three times daily before meals

d. give her diet and blood sugar diaries to return within 1 or 2 weeks

e. referral to an ophthalmologist

23. When Mrs. Jones returns for her next visit, her HgbA$_{1c}$ is 8.8%. What lifestyle changes would you suggest next?

a. encourage her to continue her walks, perhaps increasing these to four times a week if she is comfortable with this

b. have her start jogging for 45 minutes, 5 days a week to maximize weight loss and metabolic control

c. review her diet and blood sugar diary and arrange for her to receive ongoing dietary instruction, with a goal of losing 1 pound per week during the next 3 months

d. a and c

e. since she seemed to have failed to lose weight on the 2000-calorie ADA diet, give her an 1800-calorie ADA diet brochure to follow instead

24. Mrs. Jones does lose 10 pounds during several months of coaching, but her repeat HgbA$_{1c}$ is 7.5%. If you wanted to add a second medication to her glyburide, what would you choose?

a. add metformin to her regimen, starting at 1 g twice daily

b. add pioglitazone (Actos)

c. add metformin, but start at 500 mg or 850 mg daily

d. add regular insulin given three times daily before meals

e. add nateglinide (Starlix) three times daily before meals

25. Which of the following statements regarding type 2 DM is true?

a. most patients present to their physicians with symptoms directly related to their diabetes

b. most patients are essentially asymptomatic at diagnosis (apart from being obese)

c. most patients can control the DM by diet and exercise

d. most patients will not manifest complications

e. most patients are younger than age 40 years

26. Choose the best answer regarding the patient's use of chromium for DM:

a. it appears to facilitate uptake of glucose into cells

b. chromium natural sources include brewer's yeast and whole grains, but supplementation is likely required to achieve a clinically significant effect.

c. there is level B (moderate) scientific evidence of efficacy in at least some subpopulations of diabetics, although some high-quality studies show no benefit

d. a, b, and c

e. there is no credible scientific evidence that chromium supplements improve type 2 DM control

27. Choose the best answer regarding the patient's use of α-lipoic acid:

a. adding a teaspoon of this low pH supplement to each meal of the day lowers the glycemic load of the meal, but it can lead to hypoglycemia if medications are not adjusted

b. this supplement is a "fat burner" that is popular for weight loss

c. this potent antioxidant enhances glucose uptake, helps prevent glycosylation, and appears to help diabetic neuropathy in some studies, although it can induce thiamine deficiency if this vitamin is not supplemented

d. this supplement has been shown in multicenter trials to reduce macular degeneration

e. α-lipoic acid is a fad supplement with no credible scientific basis to support its use in diabetics

28. What is the best way to manage Mrs. Jones's hyperlipidemia?

a. prescribe a fibric acid derivative such as gemfibrizol

b. assuming she has no contraindications, place her on a "statin" while continuing diet and exercise efforts

c. prudent diet and exercise will likely be sufficient, providing she can lower her LDL to less than 130 mg/dL and raise her HDL to, more than 35 mg/dL within 6 months.

d. better glycemic control will likely improve her lipid profile sufficiently

e. adding a 500-mg fish oil capsule daily will likely normalize her triglycerides

29. Initial steps in helping Mrs. Jones manage her mild knee osteoarthritis include all of the following except

a. tell her to try to limit her ibuprofen use to when she has flare-ups of her arthritis

b. add glucosamine sulfate

c. even modest weight loss may improve her symptoms

d. a regular program of knee muscle strengthening will likely help her symptoms

e. place her on a stronger dose of nonsteroidal antiinflammatory drugs (NSAIDs) such as

Naprosyn 500 mg once or twice a day for better control of her symptoms

30. All of the following are true regarding sulfonylureas except
    a. they are contraindicated in a patient with sulfa allergy
    b. they tend to cause weight gain
    c. most are metabolized by the liver to substances that are cleared by the kidney; thus, they are generally not used in significant liver or kidney disease
    d. their efficacy tends to wear out after approximately 5 years of treatment
    e. they help improve insulin sensitivity

31. Situations in which it would be advisable to hold or not use metformin include
    a. anytime blood sugar is greater than 250 mg/dL; in patients who are on sulfonylureas, any radio contrast dye and history of lactic acidosis
    b. iodinated radio contrast dye, hypoxia, acidosis from any reason, major surgery, serious kidney or liver disease, and anyone who is seriously ill or not taking anything by mouth
    c. history of lactic acidosis, major surgery, kidney disease, dehydration, and iodinated contrast dye, and in patients on thiazolidinediones
    d. history of lactic acidosis, radio contrast dye, major surgery, and kidney disease, and anyone more than 50 years old
    e. metformin is safe in most clinical situations, which is one of its chief advantages

32. Choose the best answer regarding thiazolidinediones such as pioglitazone (Actos) and rosiglitazone (Avandia):
    a. they should be avoided in patients with severe classes of congestive heart failure because of their tendency toward fluid retention
    b. by improving insulin sensitivity, they lead to weight loss
    c. they should never be combined with sulfonylureas because of serious drug interactions
    d. they are insulin secretagogues
    e. one of their main advantages is that liver function tests do not have to be monitored

CLINICAL CASE PROBLEM 4

A 64-Year-Old Male with Burning Feet

A 64-year-old male with type 2 DM is complaining of a burning sensation in his feet at night. On physical examination, you note decreased sensations in his toes and calluses on his lateral fifth digits.

33. Appropriate care of this patient's neuropathy includes
    a. referral to podiatry
    b. checking a B_{12} level, especially if the patient is on metformin
    c. improved glycemic control
    d. a and c
    e. a, b, and c

34. Which one of the following statements is true regarding diabetic nephropathy in the United States?
    a. the prevalence of diabetic nephropathy is contributed to mainly by people with type 1 DM
    b. the prevalence of diabetic nephropathy is contributed to mainly by people with type 2 DM
    c. the ratio of people with type 2 DM to people with type 1 DM in the United States is 10 to 1
    d. the ratio of people with type 1 DM to people with type 2 DM in the United States is 2 to 1
    e. a and d
    f. b and c

35. Credible ways to prevent or improve eye complications of DM include all of the following except
    a. annual ophthalmologic visits for a dilated exam
    b. supplementing with lutein at a preventative dose of 6 mg/day
    c. eating a daily serving of dark leafy green vegetables such as kale or spinach
    d. tight glycemic and blood pressure control
    e. vitamin A 20,000 units daily

36. Credible ways to reduce vascular complications in diabetics include all of the following except
    a. place the patient on a dihydropyridine calcium channel blocker
    b. adjust intake ratio of omega-3/omega-6 fatty acid to approximately 1 to 2
    c. add a HMG CoA reductase inhibitor ("statin") to virtually all diabetics older than 40 years of age even if their LDL is already in the general population normal range
    d. increase vegetable servings to three to five per day and whole fruit to two or three per day and ensure regular aerobic exercise appropriate for the patient's level of fitness
    e. start aspirin 81 mg/day

37. All of the following are true regarding depression and DM except
  a. depression is more common in diabetics, especially in those with comorbid conditions
  b. primary care physicians successfully diagnose most depression in diabetics
  c. depressed diabetic patients take less care of themselves
  d. collaborative care models improve care of depressed diabetic patients
  e. depression is associated with increased risk of coronary heart disease in diabetic women

38. Choose the best answer regarding sexual dysfunction in diabetics:
  a. loss of vaginal lubrication, dyspareunia, and decreased libido may be signs of autonomic neuropathy in women
  b. patients generally volunteer to discuss sexual concerns with their doctor
  c. erectile dysfunction may be one of the earliest signs of diabetic neuropathy
  d. a and c
  e. sexual function is not affected in diabetics any more than in the general population

39. Medications that can predispose to type 2 DM include
  a. beta blockers, atypical antipsychotics, protease inhibitors, high-dose thiazides or niacin, and corticosteroids
  b. beta blockers, angiotensin-converting enzyme (ACE) inhibitors, moderate-dose inhaled corticosteroids, and glucosamine sulfate
  c. hydrocortisone 1% topical cream, oral contraceptives, raloxifene, and glucosamine sulfate
  d. protease inhibitors, hydrochlorothiazide 25 mg daily, and calcium channel blockers
  e. corticosteroids, beta blockers, ACE inhibitors, albuterol, and fluconazole

CLINICAL CASE PROBLEM 5

A 27-Year-Old Patient with Type 1 DM with Protein in Her Urine

A 27-year-old patient with type 1 DM presents to your office for her regular 3-month checkup. Her urine microalbumin is in the 80s on three spot samples. A 24-hour urine test produces a protein reading of 150 mg.

40. What should your next management step be?
  a. do nothing—this is microalbuminuria

  b. do nothing—this is still considered normal
  c. start the patient on an ACE inhibitor
  d. change the patient's diet—decrease protein by 10% a day
  e. refer the patient to a diabetologist

41. Which one of the following statements regarding dietary recommendation for type 1 DM is false?
  a. make an effort to distribute carbohydrate intake evenly throughout the day
  b. eating a high-fiber diet improves glycemic control, allowing the patient to consume more carbohydrate
  c. total fat intake should be limited to reduce total caloric consumption
  d. a prudent diabetic diet limits high-sugar foods
  e. high-protein diets should be avoided in patients with long-standing DM

42. Which statement is false regarding insulin therapy in DM?
  a. human insulin is the only available insulin in the United States
  b. average insulin doses are 0.6 to 0.8 units/kg of body weight per day
  c. glargine insulin (Lantus) should be given within 30 minutes of starting a meal
  d. insulin can be coadministered with oral sulfonylureas
  e. in long-time type 2 DM, insulin can be added at bedtime to improve control

43. A newly diagnosed patient with type 1 DM is started on a total insulin dose of 18 units. Which of the following is likely to be the correct morning/evening: regular/intermediate insulin dose?
  a. morning: total 12 units: regular 6 units, intermediate 6 units
     evening: total 6 units: regular 3 units, intermediate 3 units
  b. morning: total 9 units: regular 6 units, intermediate 3 units
     evening: total 9 units: regular 6 units, intermediate 6 units
  c. morning: total 12 units: regular 4 units, intermediate 8 units
     evening: total 6 units: regular 2 units, intermediate 4 units
  d. morning: total 6 units: regular 4 units, intermediate 2 units
     evening: total 12 units: regular 4 units, intermediate 8 units

e. morning: total 6 units: regular 3 units, intermediate 3 units
   evening: total 12 units: regular 8 units, intermediate 4 units

44. What is the most likely explanation for the "abnormal gas in the stomach" seen in upright abdominal radiographs of many patients with DM?
    a. gastroparesis as a result of diabetic autonomic neuropathy
    b. gastroparesis as a result of sympathetic dysfunction
    c. associated with diabetic ketoacidosis
    d. associated with hyperosmolar coma
    e. none of the above

45. Choose the best answer regarding inhaled insulin (Exubera):
    a. it is indicated only in type 1 DM
    b. it can be used in both pediatric and adult diabetics
    c. it can be used in smokers
    d. it is indicated only in adults free of lung disease
    e. it cannot be used with sulfonylureas or metformin

46. Choose the best answer regarding glycemic control in hospitalized patients:
    a. intensive glycemic control that maintains blood sugar in the range of 80 to 110 mg/dL in critically ill patients has been shown to improve outcomes
    b. maintaining blood sugar less than <200 mg/dL in critically ill patients is adequate to optimize outcomes
    c. glycemic goals for general medical and surgical hospital patients should be as follows: preprandial blood sugar levels <110 mg/dL and maximum blood sugar levels <180 mg/dL
    d. a and c
    e. tight glycemic control should be avoided in hospital patients because of the serious risk of hypoglycemia

47. Choose the best answer regarding consultations in the care of diabetic patients:
    a. because primary care physicians have a large breadth of skills, they generally do not need consultations in routine cases of DM
    b. the primary care physician functions best as part of a collaborative multidisciplinary team to take optimal care of diabetic patients
    c. most primary care physicians maintain adequate glycemic control of their hospitalized patients

d. most primary care physicians have enough skills and time to adequately counsel diabetics on proper diet and exercise by themselves
e. the patient should be encouraged to take on the role of "recipient of care" from the entire diabetes team

Clinical Case Management Problem

A patient who has transferred to your care for his type 2 DM and obesity has been struggling to adhere to a sensible diet. He comes to your office for a follow-up appointment and wants to know the value of incorporating the concept of glycemic index (GI)/load into his eating habits. What should your response be? How do you explain what the GI is? Is there any value to the GI concept? What can you tell your patient about the GI that may help him develop better eating habits?

Answers

1. b. Her fruity breath is from ketosis, which can very rarely occur in poorly controlled type 2 DM but is much more likely to be type 1 DM in this age group and clinical presentation.

2. c. DKA should always be handled in a hospitalized setting, usually an intensive care unit, and often with an endocrinologist's consultation, if appropriate.

3. b. Patients with DKA are always dehydrated and need large-volume IV fluid resuscitation, usually isotonic fluids such as normal saline. If corrected serum sodium level is high, this can be reduced to half-normal saline. Insulin should always be administered via an IV pump to guard against accidental overdose. Bicarbonate should not be used routinely to correct acidosis—the acidosis will correct itself with fluid and insulin. Bicarbonate is used only in extreme acidosis. Subcutaneous insulin is inappropriate in the setting of DKA. Virtually all DKA patients are total body potassium depleted, even if their serum potassium level is normal (acidosis raises serum potassium).

4. d. Lowering blood glucose too fast is believed to predispose to cerebral edema, although this is not completely proven.

5. d. Cocaine may induce hyperglycemia as well as interfere with self-care. Patients with DKA are dehydrated, so an admission chest x-ray may be falsely negative but later pick up a pneumonia once the patient is hydrated.

6. **e.** Type 1 DM has a less strong genetic component than type 2 DM. Identical twins have a 30% to 70% concordance rate for type 1 DM, not 90%. Type 1 DM is associated with other autoimmune disorders such as Hashimoto's hypothyroidism, and onset is usually in late childhood or adolescence. Islet cell antibodies are found in the majority of newly diagnosed type 1 DM but disappear once the β cells are "burnt out." A cohort study in Finland found an 80% decreased incidence of type 1 DM in children supplemented with high-dose vitamin D, strongly suggesting that suboptimal vitamin D levels are a risk factor in the genetically susceptible.

7. **e.** Intensive glycemic control decreases microvascular complications such as retinopathy, nephropathy, and neuropathy. It may also decrease macrovascular complications such as myocardial infarction and stroke, but this is not clear. The goal is as tight glycemic control as possible while avoiding hypoglycemia. This is difficult even for a multidisciplinary team, requiring multiple tests and medicine doses per day. Tight glycemic control tends to induce weight gain.

8. **c.** Goals to reduce macrovascular complications include improving the lipid profile in the following order of priority: LDL <100 mg/dL (<70 mg/dL if confirmed atherosclerotic vascular disease), HDL >40 mg/dL in men and >50 mg/dL in women, and triglycerides <150 mg/dL.

Blood pressure <130/80 mmHg (note: this is lower than the general hypertensive population goal of <140/90 mmHg). The effects of various medications used for tight glycemic control on macrovascular disease are unclear, but a major study did not show increased risk from sulfonylureas or insulin. Unlike glycemic control, strict blood pressure control has been clearly demonstrated to lower both micro- and macrovascular complications. Statins have been shown to lower cardiovascular risk even in diabetics with "normal" lipid profile; therefore, they should likely be used in virtually all DM patients older than 40 years of age whenever there is no contraindication.

9. **d.** Anion gap is elevated in DKA, and total body potassium is almost always depleted, even if serum potassium is normal. The acidosis of DKA, which generally develops over a period of 24 hours, drives potassium out of cells and into the extracellular space, raising serum potassium. DKA can occur in type 2

DM, especially in African Americans and Hispanics, although it is much less common.

10. **c.** DKA requires large volumes of fluid resuscitation, generally normal saline at 5 to 10 mL/kg/hour or 2 or 3 L during the first few hours. Electrolytes need to be monitored closely and corrected as needed.

11. **c.** This patient has "metabolic syndrome," an insulin resistance/excess inflammation syndrome. Twenty percent of U.S. adults are affected, mainly because of poor lifestyle choices (sedentary or poor diet with associated overweight) superimposed on a genetic predisposition. Also called "cardiometabolic risk" or "syndrome X," it is a precursor of type 2 DM as well as a risk factor for atherosclerotic vascular disease, hypercoagulable state, HTN, fatty liver, chronic kidney disease, gout, impotence, female sexual dysfunction, gallstones, kidney stones, polycystic ovarian syndrome, and likely some cancers. Elevated markers of inflammation such as C-reactive protein are predictors of increased risk of progressing to type 2 DM. Increased waist circumference reflects visceral fat/central obesity, which is a stronger predictor of chronic disease risk than body mass index.

12. **d.** High GI foods (i.e., carbohydrates that quickly raise blood sugar) induce food cravings and overeating, which in turn leads to overweight. They can worsen lipids (especially triglyceride/HDL ratio) and seem to increase inflammation. All these changes likely lead to increased vascular risk.

The advent of high-speed steel roller mills resulted in the creation of extremely fine flours (both whole grain and white flour) that have a high GI. Thus, bakery products made from these flours should be avoided. Instead, teach patients to choose grain products processed by traditional methods, such as stone-ground flours and old-fashioned rather than instant oatmeal. Pasta should be *al dente*. Breads made from sprouted grains or containing grain kernels and sourdough breads have a lower GI.

Carrots have a high GI, but because they contain so little absorbable carbohydrates, they have a low glycemic load. (Glycemic load = [GI × grams carbohydrate]/100). They can be eaten without problems.

13. **d.** Calories in–calories out determines weight. High-energy density foods promote excess calorie intake and weight gain. Eating a more substantial breakfast and less calories in the evening promotes healthy eating. The minimum amount of fiber is 25 to 30 g/day. Adequate fiber allows normal signaling of satiety when eating, thus controlling appetite.

14. **d.** Not all fat is created equal. Healthy fats such as monounsaturates and polyunsaturates (in the correct ratio) have a markedly different health effect than unhealthy fats such as trans fats and excess saturated fats. Increasing seed oils, which are high in omega-6 fatty acids, would worsen an already unbalanced omega-6 to omega-3 ratio, which should be approximately 1:1 to 2:1. Most Americans, as illustrated by Mr. Couchpo, have an omega-6/omega-3 ratio of 15:1 to 25:1—this worsens inflammation, a keystone of many chronic diseases. Partial hydrogenation is a main source of unnatural and mildly toxic trans fats, and it should be avoided by everyone. Flax and walnut oils are excellent sources of the omega-3 linolenic acid and should be used only unheated or, at most, with low heat since heating (especially sauteing) damages them and creates potentially toxic by-products.

15. **d.** Total protein, especially animal protein, is likely excessive for a basically sedentary person, whose protein requirements are approximately 0.8 g/kg/day. Chronic protein intake above twice the Recommended Daily Allowance has been associated with age-related decrease in kidney function (although causality is not proven), which is not seen in cultures with lower protein intakes. Protein should be mainly from plant sources such as legumes. Fish or white meat of chicken without the skin can be eaten in moderation (e.g., up to 6-ounce serving three times per week). "Industrially produced red meat" from livestock as usually raised in the United States is high in poor-quality fat (although healthier choices are becoming more available). It should be eaten infrequently (e.g., maximum 1 serving/week) or not at all. Protein requirements in exercisers are increased to 1.2 to 1.7 g/kg/day, but excess protein beyond a maximum of approximately 1.7 g/kg/day does not help build muscle even in exercisers. Protein powder drinks would simply worsen his excessive protein and are not a substitute for a healthy whole foods diet. High-protein, very low-carbohydrate diets are inappropriate, especially in exercisers, who require carbohydrate for muscle function.

16. **d.** All patients should eat (1) three to five vegetable servings/day (a serving is 1/2 cup cooked or 1 cup raw), including at least one dark leafy green (the super-veggies—kale, collards, broccoli, chard, spinach, etc.), and (2) two or three whole fruits/day (better than fruit juice or fruit drink). Iceberg lettuce, commonly used in commercial sandwiches and salads, has little nutrition. Supplements and "nutraceuticals" do not replace a whole foods diet, although a multivitamin/multimineral is not unreasonable to add to a healthy diet.

17. **c.** A reasonable quota of sweets per week in the setting of a healthy whole foods diet is unlikely to derail the patient's treatment plan. Mindfully savoring sweets allows one to fully enjoy them. Attempts to ban sweets usually backfire because patients emotionally revolt. High-fructose corn syrup, a ubiquitous commercial sweetener, is associated with overeating and elevated triglyceride levels. The fructose in whole fruit does not have this effect, however.

18. **d.** The best exercise is the one the patient will continue. Sixty percent of patients give up an exercise program within several weeks because they take on too much too fast. The earlier during the day a patient exercises, the more likely the patient will keep it up—morning or at lunch are preferable. Walking is available practically to this patient as a starting point. Although good in itself, the evening program in choice "b" is too much too fast, and it is unlikely that he would continue such a regimen for long after his late commute home from the city. He obviously has no time for travel soccer, nor is he conditioned for it. The musculoskeletal and cardiorespiratory systems have a natural pace of growth: Increase any exercise parameter such as exercise time, speed, repetition, or resistance no faster than 5% to 10% per week. There is overwhelming evidence that regular exercise improves well-being and longevity.

19. **b.** Postprandial blood sugar elevates before fasting blood sugar. Metformin may decrease the risk of progressing to diabetes, but lifestyle change is much more effective.

20. **b.** The endocannabinoid system is a newly discovered and conceptualized endocrine system that is intricately involved in a plethora of functions, including stress recovery, energy balancing, and feeding behavior. Expect breakthroughs in our understanding of eating behavior, obesity, and DM with further study of this system. One of the first canabinoid receptor antagonists to undergo clinical trials is rimonabant, which in combination with diet and exercise has been shown to reduce weight and improve HbA_{1c} as well as a number of cardiovascular risk factors in overweight patients with type 2 DM.

21. **a.** Her medical problems need better control. African Americans have poorer outcomes. It is not clear if this is due to discrimination, lower socioeconomic status, differences in diet, differences in utilization of health services, or genetic variations. Simply following any diet brochure is unlikely to change lifestyle—patients need ongoing coaching, often with the services of a dietician and fitness specialist.

As mentioned previously, this patient has type 2 DM, which accounts for 90% of all cases of DM; it is characterized by both an impairment of β cell function and a decreased sensitivity to insulin in the cells of the body.

Type 2 DM is often discovered in asymptomatic patients by finding an elevated blood sugar. It may also present with nonspecific symptoms, including fatigue, weakness, blurred vision, vaginal and perineal pruritus and candidiasis, erectile dysfunction, and paresthesias. Unlike the patient with type 1 DM, weight loss is uncommon in these patients. In fact, the majority of patients with type 2 DM are obese and many have a strong family history of obesity and DM.

A reasonable workup for the diagnosis of type 2 DM includes laboratory evaluation of fasting or random plasma glucose; HbA_{1c}; fasting lipid profile; serum creatinine; and urinalysis for ketone, glucose, protein, and microalbumin.

A diabetic diet plus weight management and exercise should be pushed to the maximum. If these are not effective, the oral hypoglycemic agent metformin should be the next step. Oral hypoglycemic agents currently available include sulfonylureas, α-glucosidase inhibitors, biguanides, meglitinides, and thiazolidinediones. The second-generation sulfonylurea agents include glyburide, glipizide, and glimepiride. These sulfonylureas work as "false sugars," stimulating the secretion of insulin in the pancreas. One member of this class, glimepiride (Amaryl), is claimed to also increase insulin sensitivity in the peripheral tissue. All sulfonylureas tend to induce weight gain and, like insulin, can induce hypoglycemia.

Biguanides inhibit gluconeogenesis; thus, they decrease the production of glucose. They also decrease the rate of glucose absorption and increase its uptake in the periphery. Because of the rare complication of lactic acidosis, biguanides should be used with caution, particularly in patients with renal insufficiency. Despite these precautions, biguanides have become the recommended first line of therapy for adult patients with type 2 DM. The only biguanide available is metformin, sold as Glucophage and Glucophage XL, a slow-release variant. Two advantages of metformin are that it should not induce hypoglycemia and it does not promote weight gain.

Meglitinides are nonsulfonylurea benzoic acid derivatives that work by stimulating insulin release from the pancreas but by a different mechanism than the sulfonylureas; they have a short half-life and have a reduced effectiveness at normal fasting glucose levels. Therefore, they are to be taken shortly before a meal (1 to 30 minutes) to reduce the postprandial hyperglycemic surge, which has been shown to play an important role in causing secondary complications. Postmeal serum glucose levels should not regularly be more than 162 mg/dL, and levels higher than 180 mg/dL are grounds for action. Prandin (repaglinide) and Starlix (nateglinide) are Food and Drug Administration-approved meglitinides. Drug interactions have been reported to enhance the activity of these drugs, possibly creating a risk of hypoglycemia. The manufacturer warns that nateglinide should not be used in the presence of other drugs that enhance insulin secretion. Similarly, a Finnish study has shown that gemfibrizol (Lopid) increases the circulating concentration of repaglinide; this effect is enhanced if itraconazole (Sporanox) is also used.

Thiazolidinedione (TZD) derivatives, such as pioglitazone (Actos) and rosiglitazone (Avandia), decrease insulin resistance and also inhibit liver gluconeogenesis. TZDs can cause elevations in hepatic enzymes, jaundice, and, in rare instances, hepatic failure. They are also contraindicated in severe cardiac heart failure because they facilitate fluid retention.

The α-glucosidase inhibitors, acarbose (Precose) or miglitol (Glyset), work by slowing the rate of disaccharide and polysaccharide hydrolysis, thereby reducing the rate of glucose absorption and the peak glucose levels. They have been associated with gastrointestinal discomfort.

Oral hypoglycemic therapy should begin with the lowest effective dose; this should then be increased every few days to achieve maximal control. Self-monitoring of blood glucose is the key to the evaluation of efficacy of an oral hypoglycemic-mediated treatment program.

Approximately 25% to 30% of patients with type 2 DM fail to respond to sulfonylurea drugs. These patients are called primary failures. In addition, approximately 5% of patients who initially responded to these drugs will lose their responsiveness. These patients are termed secondary failures. Sometimes a combination of a morning oral hypoglycemic and an evening intermediate-acting insulin can be beneficial in lowering blood sugar to normal. A subcutaneous injection of very long-acting insulin such as insulin glargine each evening can provide the basal insulin needed to enhance control.

With the several classes of agents now available, other combination therapies are available besides combination with insulin. Sulfonylureas may be combined with several different classes of agents, such as metformin, acarbose, and thiazolidinediones. Sulfonylureas may also be combined with the meglitinides. Repaglinide may be used in combination with metformin. All combination therapies require the same careful attention to side effect profiles and outcomes that monotherapies require. Nevertheless, with the increased variety and range of agents available, patients with type 2 DM now have more options for effective pharmacotherapy.

22. c. Regular insulin is not appropriate for most early type 2 diabetics.

23. d. It is important to increase exercise slowly. Lifestyle change requires ongoing coaching. Patient education handouts are important but not sufficient.

24. c. Metformin is the drug of choice in obese diabetics with dyslipidemia. Thiazolidinediones such as pioglitazone are insulin sensitizers. Because they carry a theoretical risk of liver toxicity, they require periodic monitoring of liver enzymes and are considered second line. Nonsulfonylurea insulin secretagogues such as nateglinide (Starlix) are much more expensive and would likely impose a financial burden on this patient, who has to pay out of pocket. Their main advantage is that they can be used in renal disease without dosage adjustment. Regular insulin is not generally used in early type 2 DM.

25. b. Patients with type 2 DM demonstrate the following: (1) Except for being obese, most patients are asymptomatic (identification most often occurs by screening); (2) most patients are older than age 40 years; (3) most patients develop the same complications (microvascular and macrovascular complications) as in patients with type 1 diabetes; and (4) most patients have motivational difficulties in relation to diet and exercise.

26. d. Chromium enhances glucose uptake, is found in brewer's yeast and whole grain products, and has a moderate level of evidence suggesting it might be useful in some subpopulations of diabetics. Reasonable doses are 200 to 400 μg daily. Keep in mind, however, that supplements rank a far second to proper diet in importance.

27. c. α-Lipoic acid is a potent antioxidant that enhances glucose uptake and prevents glycosylation of tissues. Randomized double-blind trials have shown that 600 mg/day improves diabetic neuropathy.

28. b. Evidence suggests that statins benefit virtually all type 2 diabetics older than 40 years of age. They have been shown to reduce cardiovascular endpoints including mortality. At least 4 g of fish oil/day (containing approximately 2 g of actual omega-3 fatty acids) is required to lower triglycerides. Omacor is a high-quality and concentrated prescription source of omega-3s.

29. e. Avoid or minimize NSAIDs whenever possible in diabetics—they aggravate progression to kidney disease. If used, be sure the patient is well hydrated. Glucosamine sulfate 500 mg (and chondroitin sulfate 400 mg) three times a day have been shown in most clinical trials to help osteoarthritis (although some trials have not shown benefit). Knee strengthening and even modest weight loss also significantly improve pain and function and are underutilized.

30. e. Sulfonylureas have no effect on insulin sensitivity.

31. b. Metformins should not be used in these circumstances.

32. a. Fluid retention is a common side effect.

33. e. The best management of diabetic foot problems involves podiatric care for careful debridement of corns and calluses that might predispose to foot ulcers. Improved glycemic control is the primary available treatment for the pathology underlying neuropathy. α-Lipoic acid and medications such as pregabalin, gabapentin, and amitriptyline may be used to help relieve neuropathy-associated chronic pain. Metformin can interfere with B_{12} (as well as folate) metabolism—check a level. Do not just assume neuropathy is related to the DM.

34. f. Because there are at least 10 patients with type 2 DM for each patient with type 1 DM, the prevalence of complications resulting from type 2 DM is higher than for type 1 DM.

35. e. Annual dilated full eye exams and tight glycemic and blood pressure control are cornerstones of good eye care. Lutein has been shown to reduce progression of macular degeneration in at least one well-designed randomized controlled trial, either alone or in combination with other antioxidants. Further trials are indicated to confirm and expand the generalizability of these results. Good sources are dark leafy green vegetables such as kale. Be sure any supplement claiming to have lutein has at least 6 mg for adequate affect. Vitamin A is necessary for retinal function, but the dose listed is excessive. The maximum tolerable limit for vitamin A is 10,000 units/day.

36. a. Calcium channel blockers have not shown much benefit in reducing vascular complications, unlike ACE inhibitors or angiotensin receptor blockers. Statins have strong evidence of benefit in DM, which is considered a cardiac disease equivalent, and if possible should be considered in virtually all type 2 diabetics older than 40 years of age regardless of lipid profile. Aspirin lowers the risk of thrombotic events such as myocardial infarction. Proper diet, including the correct omega-3/-6 ratio and plenty of vegetables and whole fruit, is a cornerstone of vascular health.

37. b. Primary care clinicians miss approximately half of the cases of depression in their diabetic patients, according to various studies. Depression is more common in diabetics, especially those with comorbid conditions, and is associated with poorer self-care and outcomes. Depressed women diabetics have increased coronary heart disease risk. Collaboration between physicians and nurse case managers who offer ongoing support and education has been shown to optimize outcome.

38. d. Sexual dysfunction is more common in male and female diabetics than in the general population. Patients will often not volunteer their concerns about sexual function unless directly asked by the physician.

39. a. Those listed are common offenders.

40. c. The patient with DM who presents with microalbuminuria already has a problem. The probability of this individual developing overt nephropathy is quite high. It has been demonstrated that progression to overt nephropathy can be prevented by the prophylactic administration of an ACE inhibitor or angiotensin receptor blocker.

41. b. Diet is an essential component of treatment in all patients with DM. In patients with insulin-dependent DM, the rate at which insulin enters the blood from an injection site is fixed, and the patients must match meals to the pattern of insulin absorption. A high-fiber diet slows the rate of glucose or fructose absorption, which decreases the initial insulin surge from the β cells—a fact of importance to the patient with type 2 DM. However, in the long term the same amount of glucose will be accessible and the total insulin demand will be the same. Thus, to the patient with type 1 DM who has nonfunctional β cells and is taking a set amount of insulin, the fiber content is not as relevant in determining his or her insulin dose.

The patient with DM undergoing insulin therapy must have three meals at fixed times each day, with a fixed distribution of calories. Frequent snacks, also with a fixed distribution of calories, are also recommended.

If a patient with DM is overweight, a weight-reducing program should be initiated. This may be facilitated by substituting complex, low GI carbohydrates

with high residue for simple sugars and high GI carbohydrates. In addition, saturated animal fats should be replaced with healthier fats. One-fifth of the daily caloric intake should be consumed at breakfast and approximately two-fifths each at lunch and dinner. These percentages may be reduced to allow for small snacks, such as crackers or fruit, in midafternoon and at bedtime. A reasonable exercise program is fundamental to the treatment of all patients with DM. Also, the patient with DM should moderate sugar and alcohol consumption and limit intake of high-sugar foods. Because carbohydrate has the greatest impact on blood glucose, its effect can be minimized by spreading carbohydrate consumption evenly throughout the day. Discourage the use of high-protein fad diets in all people with long-standing DM and with particular emphasis to those with impaired renal function.

42. c. Human insulin is the only available insulin in the United States. The average insulin doses are 0.6 to 0.8 units/kg of body weight per day.

Glargine insulin is very long acting and should be given once daily, often in the evening or at bedtime. Lispro insulin is quick acting and should be given within 30 minutes of starting a meal.

Insulin can be coadministered with oral sulfonylureas. In long-term type 2 DM, long-acting or intermediate-acting insulin can be added at bedtime to improve control.

43. c. The starting dose of insulin is usually as follows: (1) morning, two-thirds of total daily dose; (2) evening, one-third of total daily dose; (3) morning, two-thirds intermediate, one-third regular; and (4) evening, two-thirds intermediate, one-third regular.

44. a. The "abnormal gas in the stomach" is most likely the result of diabetic gastroparesis, an autonomic neuropathy variant. This is a very common complaint, and it is best treated by a prokinetic agent, such as metoclopramide, or by macrolide antibiotics.

45. d. Inhaled insulin is indicated only in adults free of lung disease or smoking. It can be used in both type 1 and type 2 DM, and it can be used with other oral diabetic medications such as sulfonylureas and metformin. If insulin is required, control of fasting insulin to a level of approximately 100 mg/dL should generally be accomplished first (such as with an evening dose of subcutaneous long-acting insulin) before using any preprandial insulin, such as inhaled insulin. The long-term side effects of inhaled insulin are unknown. Other issues with inhaled insulin include its high cost, the need for multiple inhalations to achieve a correct dose, and the possibility of severe hypoglycemia.

46. d. Approximately 38% of hospital patients have hyperglycemia, a third of whom have no history of DM. Poor glycemic control in hospitalized patients (above 110 to 120 mg/dL fasting and 180 mg/dL maximum blood sugar) is associated with increased chances of myocardial infarction, stroke, nosocomial infection, complications of surgery, prolonged length of stay, and death. Tight glycemic control in hospitalized patients is clearly associated with better outcomes in clinical trials, but it is often not addressed adequately. Evidence is especially strong for critically ill patients, but tight control also benefits general medical and surgical patients. Accomplishing this tight control may require an insulin drip and the services of a endocrinologist.

47. b. The wide breadth of knowledge and skills of primary care physicians allows them to do an excellent job as the main providers of care of diabetic patients, but only if they use these skills to organize a collaborative team to help the patients. This can include endocrinologists, podiatrists, nurse managers, social workers, fitness experts, nutritionists, and others as the clinical situation dictates. Most primary care physicians work in a medical system that undervalues their counseling skills and do not have the time to adequately counsel patients on proper diet and exercise. Group diabetic visits are one forum that has been demonstrated to improve outcomes. Tight glycemic control is difficult for both inpatients and outpatients by any physician, and it often requires a group effort. Patients should be encouraged to be an active member of the diabetic team rather than a passive "recipient of care."

Solution to the Clinical Case Management Problem

1. What is the GI? The GI is a scientifically validated comparison of the ability of various foods to raise postprandial glucose values—their so-called glycemic response. This glycemic response is compared to a control, usually 50 g of glucose given by convention a GI value of 100. The lower the GI value of the food tested, the lower the postprandial glucose peak and the lower the total area under the curve for blood glucose. High GI foods lead to high blood glucose levels, triggering high levels of insulin secretion, which stresses the β cells of the pancreas and worsens diabetic control. Although it is true that high GI foods are absorbed faster and thus result in an earlier and higher blood glucose level peak, they also raise the total amount of glucose in the bloodstream over the postprandial period more than a low GI food. This fact, often misunderstood, is crucial to understanding the real value of the GI concept. Thus, the total amount of postprandial glucose in the blood is lower with lower GI foods. Again, it is not just a matter of speed of absorption resulting in an earlier and higher peak with high GI foods but with equal amounts of glucose in the bloodstream over the postprandial time period; rather, high GI foods (compared to a low glycemic food with an identical amount of available carbohydrates) raise total blood sugar excessively. The concept of GI/load largely replaces or clarifies the outdated concept of complex versus simple carbohydrates.

2. Definitions
   a. GI is a measure of how much a food raises blood glucose level. Glucose is given by convention a GI of 100, and all other foods are measured against it.
      i. High GI = 70 to 100. Examples: bagel, white bread, "sticky" rice
      ii. Medium GI = 56 to 69. Examples: spaghetti, banana, basmati rice
      iii. Low GI = 55 or lower. Examples: lentils, apple
   b. Glycemic load (GL) = GI expressed as a percentage × amount of available carbohydrates eaten.
      i. Glycemic load per serving of food:
         A. Low GL = 10 or less. Example: 250-g serving of lentil and barley soup
         B. Medium GL = 11 to 19. Example: 50-g serving of Sara Lee pound cake
         C. High GL = >19. Example: 1 bagel (70 g)
      ii. Glycemic load per day:
         A. Low GL <80
         B. High GL >120
   c. Glycemic response is an individual's response to eating a certain food. This may vary according to the patient's age, genetic makeup, and exercise level. Some patients are more "glucose tolerant" than others. Level of fitness and exercise also affect how carbohydrates are processed.

3. How is the GI measured? Fifty grams of the food to be tested is eaten by a study subject, and his or her blood sugar levels are measured frequently for the next 2 or 3 hours. From these data, an area under the curve (AUC) is calculated. Each study subject is tested three separate times and an average is taken. The same is repeated with 50 g of glucose. Since different study subjects may have different responses to the same foods, this entire process is repeated for 10 study subjects and an average is taken. The average AUC tested food/AUC of glucose × 100 = GI.

4. Factors that increase the GI of food are complex and include the following:
   a. Finely milled flours, even if whole wheat
   b. High concentration of glucose or starch, as opposed to lactose, sucrose, and fructose levels
   c. Low soluble-fiber content
   d. Soft, overcooked, overripe food (e.g., an underripe banana has a GI of approximately 45, normal ripe banana approximately 50, and overripe banana approximately 75)
   e. Overprocessed food
   f. Possibly lack of fat in food
      i. More neutral pH: Acidic foods have a lower GI compared to their nonacidic counterparts: sourdough bread GI is approximately 50, whereas neutral pH bread made from the same flour may have a GI of 75.
      ii. Documented benefits of eating low GI/GL foods: (1) reduces food cravings and overeating, thus helping control weight; and (2) improves hyperinsulinemia and possibly insulin sensitivity, thus improving DM control. This would be expected to also lower the risk of other insulin-resistant syndromes, including HTN, polycystic ovarian syndrome, and heart disease, although clinical trials are needed to confirm this.
   g. Improves triglyceride/HDL ratio
   h. May reduce vascular risk by normalizing elasticity of blood vessels, blood clotting, and reducing plaque formation

5. What is the effect of low GI diet on diabetes control? Obviously, avoiding those foods that raise the postprandial glucose peak to a great degree would be of value to the patient with DM or metabolic syndrome. This is the same rationale as used in prescribing acarbose; in fact, a meta-analysis by Brand-Miller and colleagues in 2003 indicated that using the GI as a dietary guide provides a small but clinically usefully reduction in HbA_{1c} values, about as much as use of acarbose.

6. Do the GI and glycemic load of a food always match? Usually, a high GI food has a high glycemic load, but not always, because some foods with a high GI have little available carbohydrates. Thus, for example, the GI value of some carrots is approximately 90; at face value, eating carrots is a greater risk to the patient with DM than consuming table sugar (GI = 60). This might be true if the patient with DM ate the 50 pounds or so of carrots required to ingest the 50 g of glucose on which the index is based. To circumvent this problem, a new index, the GL, was developed. The GL is determined by multiplying the GI by the percentage available carbohydrate (approximately 7% for carrots); thus, the available carbohydrates of 100 g of carrots is only approximately 7 g, and the GL would be only 6.3 (0.90 × 7 = 6.3). Therefore, carrots are returned to the status of an acceptable food.

The real potential value of the GI and its offspring (the GL system) is in uncovering differences in the rate of digestion and absorption of foods. Again, for the most part, the GI and the older systems arrive at the same conclusions, namely that unprocessed whole foods and other foods with fiber are better for a person because the carbohydrate they contain is digested and absorbed more slowly. However, the GI system does provide a few surprises. For instance, the GI/GL value for russet baked potatoes (85) or commercial bakery products made from finely milled flour created with high-speed steel roller mills (70s to 80s) is higher than that of sucrose or table sugar (60). Of course, sugar lacks the fiber, vitamins, and minerals found in potatoes (i.e., a person cannot live on empty calories alone); no sane clinician would recommend sugar as a significant part of anybody's diet, let alone for a person with DM. However, fruits can be eaten in significant quantities because they provide many valuable nutrients besides fruit sugar (fructose), which has a low GI.

7. Practical advice for your patients
   a. Patients should include at least one low GI/GL food in each meal. They need not eliminate all high glycemic foods, but they should practice portion control of them.
   b. High glycemic foods are ok to eat during or within 2 hours after endurance exercise to help replenish muscle glycogen stores.

c. Minimize commercial processed breads, bagels, rolls, muffins, pastries, and most commercial breakfast cereals. These are the source of most of the glycemic load in most people's diet.

d. Choose minimally processed breakfast cereals made from oats, barley, and bran.

e. Decrease the amount of potatoes you eat.

f. Eat three to five servings of different color nonwhite vegetables (avoid overcooked) and two or three servings of different color fruit (avoid overripe) per day.

g. Choose Basmati, Doongara, or converted whole grain (brown) rice.

h. Pasta in moderation is ok. Cook *al dente*.

8. Key points about GI/GL

a. GI/GL is not meant to be used in isolation. It is only one important factor in healthy nutrition.

b. Some associations, such as the ADA, have expressed concern that the GI/GL system may be too complex for some patients to follow. For motivated patients, learn the system thoroughly and keep the message simple to enhance patient compliance. A registered dietician with expertise in medical nutrition therapy for DM and GI can be very helpful. The Web site www.glycemicindex.com is good resource.

c. For approximately 99.9% of humans' experience on earth, we ate a whole foods diet that was naturally low GI/GL. Thus, the low GI/GL principle is simply a new, scientifically validated description of an ancient, time-tested way of eating that our bodies are designed for. It is important to keep perspective that many high glycemic foods, even though ubiquitous in our society, such as those made from finely milled flour from high-speed steel roller mills, place an undue stress on our insulin-mediated metabolic systems. This is likely true for everyone, but it is especially true for those who have glucose intolerance-related diseases such as metabolic syndrome and type 2 DM. Their regular consumption is part of the "new malnutrition"— a malnutrition of imbalance in contradistinction to the old malnutrition of deficiency found more often in Third World countries. As part of this new malnutrition, they are likely a significant factor in much of the increasing chronic disease burden of Western societies.

Summary

TYPE 1 DIABETES MELLITUS

1. Epidemiology: 10% of all cases of diabetes

2. Signs/symptoms: polyuria, polydipsia, nocturia, weight loss

3. Etiology: genetics plus environment—an autoimmune disease:

a. Most common: HLA-DR4 plus viral exposure; vitamin D deficiency may aggravate

b. Less common: associated with other autoimmune diseases

4. Diagnosis

a. Two fasting values of 126 mg/dL or greater

b. One random blood sugar 200 mg/dL plus symptoms

c. Two blood sugars 200 mg/dL in a 3-hour, 75-g glucose tolerance test (one value at 2 hours)

5. Self-monitoring: Home blood sugar monitoring, emphasizing strict control, reduces complications. When there is a risk of hypoglycemia, recommend four values three times a week.

6. Long-term control (every 3 months; red cell turnover is 120 days): HbA_{1c} less than 7.0%. Fructosamine analysis is a newer measure (based on glycated serum protein turnover [average approximately 17 days]) that can be used to measure intermediate control (2 to 4 weeks). It is particularly useful to monitor changes in patients in which control is deteriorating and in patients with hemoglobinopathies (abnormal hemoglobin turnover times) in which HbA_{1c} values are not reliable.

7. Treatment

a. Diet

b. Exercise

c. Insulin replacement (e.g., regular/intermediate): The total initial insulin dose is 15 to 20 units using the rule of two-thirds; that is, two-thirds total dose in the morning (split 2:1, regular:intermediate) and one-third total dose in the evening (split 2:1, regular:intermediate). Other insulin regimens are possible, such as long-term (basal) insulin plus prandial dosing. The goal is establishment and maintenance of euglycemia as measured by HbA_{1c}.

8. Complications: Both macrovascular and microvascular. In both type 1 and type 2 DM, macrovascular and microvascular complications are present. Because the ratio of type 2/type 1 diabetics is 10/1, of 100 cases of

diabetic nephropathy, more than 80% of the secondary complications are the result of type 2 diabetes.

TYPE 2 DIABETES MELLITUS

1. Epidemiology: 90% of all cases of DM are type 2.
2. Signs/symptoms: Because a minority of patients with type 2 DM present with symptoms, patients are often discovered when undergoing screening in a medical setting.
3. Risk factors
   a. Poor lifestyle choices: sedentary, poor diet, obesity
   b. Type 2 DM in a first-degree relative
   c. Race (e.g., Native American)
4. Diagnosis: Diagnosis of type 2 DM is the same as for type 1.
5. Self-monitoring: Same as for type 1. However, for the patient with type 2 diabetes, also recommend at least a 2-hour postprandial determination after meals containing newer foods; in this way, the patient can self-estimate what and/or how much he or she can or cannot eat and help monitor diet.
6. Long-term control: Same as for type 1.
7. Treatment
   a. Prudent diet and weight control absolutely essential
   b. Exercise daily
   c. Oral medications as summarized in Table 41-1.
   d. A small percentage (15% to 20%) of patients with type 2 diabetes need insulin in the evening in addition to oral hypoglycemics (glyburide/glipizide) in the morning. The majority of type 2 diabetics who do not adequately improve lifestyle will eventually require insulin.
8. Complications: Same as for type 1

Table 41-1	Classes of Oral and Non-insulin Subcutaneous Injectable Glucose-Lowering Agents			
Medications	**Group/Subclass**	**Example**	**Mechanism of Action**	**Comments**
Insulin secretagogues	Sulfonylureas	Glyburide Glimepiride	"False sugars" that stimulate insulin secretion	Sulfonylureas have the potential to cause hypoglycemia and tend to cause weight gain
	Nonsulfonylureas	Repaglinide Nateglinide	Increase insulin secretion	To be taken within 30 minutes before meals and CHO-rich snacks. Can cause hypoglycemia, particularly if taken without a meal containing CHO
Delay CHO absorption	α-Glucoside inhibitors	Acarbose Miglitol	Effectively decrease glycemic load of a meal by delaying CHO absorption, when taken with the first bite of a meal	Tend to cause gas, bloating, and diarrhea; thus, not to be used by patients with intestinal disorders. Since they slow CHO absorption, any advent of hypoglycemia should be treated with glucose, not a more complex CHO. However, when used alone they will not induce hypoglycemia or weight gain
Insulin sensitizers	Biguanides	Metformin	Decreases gluconeogenesis and intestinal absorption and increases peripheral uptake	Does not promote weight gain or hypoglycemia when used alone. In rare cases, it can cause lactic acidosis
	Thiazolidinediones	Rosiglitazone Pioglitazone	PPARγ agonists that activate insulin-responsive genes	Rare hepatotoxicity requires LFT monitoring Fluid retention

Table 41-1 Classes of Oral and Non-insulin Subcutaneous Injectable Glucose-Lowering Agents—cont'd

Medications	Group/Subclass	Example	Mechanism of Action	Comments
Injectables (SC)	Incretin mimetics	Exenatide	Mimics enhanced glucose-dependent insulin secretion, other antihyperglycemic actions of incretins	Can be added to metformin, sulfonylureas, thiazolidinediones or some combinations of these to attain adequate glycemic control. May support weight loss
	Amylin mimetics	Pramlinitide	Inhibits glucagon secretion; delays gastric emptying and suppresses appetite	Approved in type 1 and 2 type diabetes mellitus inadequately controlled on insulin. Not associated with weight gain. May induce severe hypoglycemia if insulin doses are not adjusted. May cause gastrointestinal upset

CHO, carbohydrate; LFT, liver function test.

Suggested Reading

American Diabetes Association. Available at www.diabetes.org.

Bray AG, Nielsen SJ, Popkin BM: Consumption of high-fructose corn syrup in beverages may play a role in the epidemic of obesity. *Am J Clin Nutr* 79:537–543, 2004.

Diabetes Control and Complications Trial Research Group: The effect of intensive treatment of diabetes on the development and progression of long-term complications in insulin-dependent diabetes mellitus. *N Engl J Med* 329:977, 1993.

Glycemic index. Available at www.glycemicindex.com.

Hyppönen E, Lara E, Reunanen A, et al: Intake of vitamin D and risk of type 1 diabetes: A birth–cohort study. *Lancet* 358:1500–1503, 2001.

Katon W, Unutzer J, Fan M, et al: Older adults with diabetes and depression. *Diabetes Care* 29:265–270, 2006.

Khan SK: Glycemic index and glycemic load. In Rakel D, ed., *Integrative Medicine*, 2nd ed. Philadelphia: Saunders, 2007.

Kopple JD: Nutrition, diet, and the kidney. In Shils ME, Olson JA, Shike M, Ross AC, eds., *Modern Nutrition in Health and Disease*, 10th ed. Philadelphia: Lippincott Williams & Wilkins, 2006.

Linkner E: Insulin resistance and the metabolic syndrome. In Rakel D, ed., *Integrative Medicine*, 2nd ed. Philadelphia: Saunders, 2007.

Mark JD: Diabetes. In Rakel D, ed., *Integrative Medicine*, 2nd ed. Philadelphia: Saunders, 2007.

National Diabetes Information Clearinghouse. Available at www.diabetes.niddk.nih.gov.

Pagotto U, Pasquali R: The role of the endocannabinoid pathway in metabolism and diabetes. *Curr Opin Endocrinol Diabetes* 13:171–178, 2006.

Powers AC: Diabetes. In Kasper DL, Braunwald E, Fauci AS, et al, eds., *Harrison's Principles of Internal Medicine*, 16th ed. New York: McGraw–Hill, 2007.

Rakel D, Rindfleish JA: The anti-inflammatory diet. In Rakel D, ed., *Integrative Medicine*, 2nd ed. Philadelphia: Saunders, 2007.

Richer S, Stiles W, Statkute L, et al: Double-masked, placebo-controlled, randomized trial of lutein and antioxidant supplementation in the intervention of atrophic age-related macular degeneration: The Veterans LAST study (Lutein Antioxidant Supplementation Trial). *Optometry* 75(4):216–230, 2004.

Rolls B: *The Volumetrics Eating Plan*, pp. 6–12. New York: HarperCollins, 2004.

Scheen AJ, Finer N, Hollander P, et al: Efficacy and tolerability of rimonabant in overweight or obese patients with type 2 diabetes: A randomised controlled study. *Lancet* 368:1660–1672, 2006.

Shikany JM, White GL: Dietary guidelines for chronic disease prevention. *South Med J* 93(12):1157–1161, 2000.

Whaley MH, et al: *ACSM's Guidelines for Exercise Testing and Prescription*. Baltimore: Lippincott Williams & Wilkins, 2006.

Ziegler D, Ametov A, Barinov A, et al: Oral treatment with α-lipoic acid improves symptomatic diabetic polyneuropathy: The SYDNEY 2 trial. *Diabetes Care* 29:2365–2370, 2006.

CLINICAL CASE PROBLEM 1

A 38-Year-Old Female with Sweating, Palpitations, Nervousness, Irritability, and Tremor

A 38-year-old female comes to your office with a 3-month history of sweating, palpitations, weight loss, nervousness, irritability, insomnia, hand tremors, and diarrhea. She has no significant past illness. One of her sisters has rheumatoid arthritis. The patient, a stockbroker, is finding it increasingly difficult to perform her job because of profound fatigue and inability to concentrate.

On examination, her blood pressure is 140/70 mmHg. Her pulse is 120 beats/minute and regular. She demonstrates mild proptosis. You feel a smooth, diffusely enlarged, and nontender thyroid gland. Cardiovascular examination reveals a loud S1 and a loud S2 with a systolic ejection murmur heard loudest along the left sternal border. The murmur does not radiate. No other abnormalities are noted.

SELECT THE BEST ANSWER TO THE FOLLOWING QUESTIONS

1. What is the most likely diagnosis in this patient?
   a. toxic multinodular goiter
   b. Graves' disease
   c. Hashimoto's thyroiditis
   d. pheochromocytoma
   e. panic disorder

2. What is the etiology of the disorder described?
   a. idiopathic
   b. an autoimmune disease
   c. a hereditary disease
   d. viral infection
   e. iatrogenic

3. What is the best initial test to diagnose hyperthyroidism?
   a. radioactive iodine uptake test
   b. thyroid ultrasound
   c. free serum T4
   d. serum thyroid-stimulating hormone (TSH)
   e. thyroid antibodies

4. Your diagnosis of hyperthyroidism is confirmed with the appropriate test from question 3. Which test is the next most appropriate to determine the underlying etiology?
   a. radioactive iodine uptake
   b. fine needle aspiration (FNA) of thyroid
   c. free T4
   d. ultrasound
   e. TSH receptor antibodies

5. What treatment will be most effective to acutely alleviate the patient's symptoms?
   a. methimazole
   b. radioactive iodine
   c. propylthiouracil (PTU)
   d. atenolol
   e. diltiazem

6. Which of the following medications provides effective long-term control of the disease presented in this problem?
   a. methimazole
   b. propranolol
   c. levothyroxine
   d. prednisone
   e. indomethacin

7. The patient described here is not pregnant or breast-feeding. What is the definitive treatment of choice for her?
   a. PTU
   b. methimazole
   c. radioactive iodine
   d. subtotal thyroidectomy
   e. propranolol

8. The recommended treatment of choice is undertaken in this patient. Which of the following will be the end result of this treatment?
   a. complete cure: no further medication or other treatments necessary
   b. complete cure: hyperthyroid medication should be started immediately and continued for life
   c. complete cure: patient should be monitored every 6 months for the development of hypothyroidism
   d. partial cure: hypothyroid medication needed for 5 years
   e. partial cure: hyperthyroid medication needed for 5 years

9. Untreated hyperthyroidism can lead to
   a. increased bone density
   b. constipation
   c. atrial fibrillation

d. cold intolerance

e. thyroid nodules

10. The patient tells you that she would like to get pregnant in 2 years. Which statement is false regarding the treatment of hyperthyroidism in women of childbearing age?

a. in pregnant women with hyperthyroidism, ultrasound monitoring for fetal goiter is essential

b. women treated with radioactive iodine before pregnancy have children with a higher incidence of birth defects

c. thyroidectomy is indicated for pregnant women who cannot tolerate antithyroid medications

d. radioactive iodine treatment is contraindicated in pregnant women because it may destroy fetal thyroid tissue

e. in pregnant women, PTU is preferred over methimazole

CLINICAL CASE PROBLEM 2

25-Year-Old Female with a Higher Than Normal T4 Level

A 25-year-old female is seen for her periodic health examination. Her past history is unremarkable, but she states that she has noticed some irregularity in her menses; she is otherwise feeling well. She is currently taking an oral contraceptive pill.

On physical examination, her blood pressure is 130/75 mmHg. Examination reveals that the head and neck are completely normal; specifically, no abnormalities of the thyroid gland are noted. You decide to check thyroid function test and receive some perplexing results. TSH is normal but a total serum T4 level is elevated at 13 mg/dL (169 nmol/L).

11. What is the most likely explanation for the elevated T4 level in this patient?

a. Graves' disease

b. thyroiditis

c. toxic nodular goiter

d. an elevated thyroid-binding globulin (TBG)

e. laboratory error

12. To confirm your diagnosis in the patient just described, which of the following would you order?

a. the all-out, all-inclusive, miss-nothing workup

b. serum T3

c. serum TBG

d. serum free T4

e. estradiol level

CLINICAL CASE PROBLEM 3

A "Wonderfully Healthy" 38-Year-Old-Female

A 38-year-old female is seen in your office for a complete baseline health assessment. You have never seen this patient before. She feels well and tells you that she is "wonderfully healthy." She has had no weight loss or gain; no sweating, no tremors, no diarrhea or constipation; no anxiety or depression; no irritability; and no other symptoms.

On examination, she is found to have a 2-cm nodule in the left lobe of the thyroid gland. Her blood pressure is 120/70 mmHg. Her pulse is 90 beats/minute and regular.

13. What is the first test that should be ordered to evaluate the patient's physical exam abnormality?

a. magnetic resonance imaging (MRI) scan of the thyroid

b. thyroid ultrasound

c. radioactive iodine uptake scan

d. FNA of the nodule

e. computed tomography (CT) scan of the thyroid

14. Two suspicious thyroid nodules are identified after ordering the appropriate primary test. What is the next test in the evaluation of the patient's thyroid nodules?

a. serum T4

b. radioactive iodine uptake thyroid scan

c. FNA of the nodules

d. thyroid ultrasound

e. CT scan of the thyroid

15. Which of the following statements regarding "hot nodules" and "cold nodules," found on radioactive iodine scan, is true?

a. cold nodules are more likely to be benign than hot nodules

b. cold nodules need not be investigated any further

c. cold nodules are more likely to be associated with signs and symptoms of hyperthyroidism than hot nodules

d. cold nodules always require further investigation to differentiate benign from malignant status

e. all nodules, whether hot or cold, require further investigation to differentiate benign from malignant status

16. A FNA showed that the mass is benign and thyroid function testing is normal. What would you do now?
    a. perform a radioactive iodine uptake thyroid scan
    b. refer the patient to a surgeon for excision
    c. give a trial of suppressive levothyroxine and reevaluate in 6 months
    d. reassure the patient and provide yearly ultrasound surveillance of the nodule
    e. obtain an MRI scan of the head and neck to search for further disease

17. Which of the following statements is not an indication for performing a thyroid ultrasound examination?
    a. palpable thyroid nodule
    b. history of neck irradiation
    c. family history of thyroid carcinoma or multiple endocrine neoplasia
    d. a patient with unexplained cervical lymphadenopathy
    e. general screening exam

CLINICAL CASE PROBLEM 4

A Lethargic 65-Year-Old Male

A 65-year-old male presents with a 6-month history of lethargy, weakness, psychomotor retardation, cold intolerance, constipation, hair loss, and weight gain. You suspect hypothyroidism.

18. Which of the following investigations will provide the most useful information for diagnosing hypothyroidism in this patient?
    a. serum T4
    b. serum T3
    c. free serum T4
    d. serum TSH
    e. serum TBG

19. Which of the following statements is inconsistent with the diagnosis of hypothyroidism in this patient?
    a. his total cholesterol has been increasing along with his weight for the past year
    b. he began amiodarone therapy 1 year ago for recalcitrant atrial fibrillation
    c. it can be difficult to separate hypothyroidism from depression in the elderly
    d. there is a delay of the relaxation phase of his deep tendon reflexes
    e. his blood pressure has decreased without treatment

20. Which of the following statements is false regarding the treatment of this patient?
    a. optimal therapy for this condition can be determined by measurement of the serum TSH level
    b. the average replacement dose of levothyroxine is 1.6 μg/kg/day
    c. elderly patients and patients with significant cardiac disease should be treated cautiously
    d. a combination of T4 and T3 is the treatment of choice for hypothyroidism
    e. coadministration of levothyroxine with a proton pump inhibitor may alter its absorption

21. After starting the appropriate medication in this patient, when should his TSH be reassessed?
    a. 1 or 2 weeks
    b. 2 to 4 weeks
    c. 4 to 6 weeks
    d. 10 to 12 weeks
    e. approximately 6 months

22. What is the most common cause of hypothyroidism in the United States?
    a. Hashimoto's thyroiditis
    b. post I^{131} hypothyroidism
    c. iodine deficiency
    d. idiopathic hypothyroidism
    e. central hypothyroidism

23. Which of the following statements is false regarding Hashimoto's thyroiditis?
    a. Hashimoto's thyroiditis is more common in females than in males
    b. anti-thyroid antibodies are found in the majority of individuals with this condition
    c. this condition is also known as chronic autoimmune thyroiditis
    d. its pathophysiology is due to antibody-mediated destruction of circulating thyroid hormone
    e. symptoms of hyperthyroidism often precede symptoms of hypothyroidism

24. The patient's wife comes to see you because she's had similar symptoms as her husband during the past year and wants to know if she has the same problem. You perform thyroid function tests that show her TSH to be slightly elevated and her free T4 to be normal. Which of the following statements best describes the diagnosis and treatment of this scenario?
    a. laboratory error; repeat the thyroid function tests
    b. central hypothyroidism; perform an MRI of the brain

c. subclinical hypothyroidism; treat with low-dose replacement therapy

d. Graves' disease; treat with radioactive iodine

e. Subclinical hypothyroidism; no treatment

CLINICAL CASE PROBLEM 5

A 28-Year-Old Female with an Ongoing Upper Respiratory Infection

A 28-year-old female presents to your office for the second time in 4 weeks. You previously diagnosed her with a viral upper respiratory infection. She states that she began to improve, but her sore throat moved to the front of her neck and she began having symptoms of palpitations and profuse sweating that have since resolved. She now feels tired all the time and has become constipated. She wants to know why her cold is lasting so long. Physical exam is normal except for mild diffuse tenderness of the thyroid.

25. What is the most likely diagnosis for this patient?
    a. Graves' disease
    b. Hashimoto's thyroiditis
    c. subacute thyroiditis
    d. iodine deficiency
    e. papillary thyroid carcinoma

26. Thyroid function testing confirms a current hypothyroid state. What is the most appropriate course of action for this patient?
    a. no treatment; this will resolve on its own
    b. thyroid replacement therapy with close follow-up of thyroid function
    c. guarantee the patient that her thyroid function will normalize in a few weeks
    d. perform a radioactive iodine scan
    e. perform a thyroid ultrasound

Clinical Case Management Problem

Describe the appropriate workup for a patient with a palpable thyroid nodule.

Answers

1. **b.** This patient has Graves' disease, which is the most common cause of hyperthyroidism in the United States. It is an autoimmune-mediated stimulation of the thyroid. It usually presents with symptoms of sweating, palpitations, nervousness, irritability, tremor, diarrhea, heat intolerance, and weight loss.

Physical signs of Graves' disease include a diffusely enlarged, nontender thyroid gland; tachycardia; loud heart sounds; and a cardiac murmur. A bruit may be heard over the thyroid. Proptosis is often seen. Occasionally, patients present with severe exophthalmos accompanied by ophthalmoplegia, follicular conjunctivitis, chemosis, and even loss of vision.

Toxic multinodular goiter and toxic adenoma are other causes of hyperthyroidism. Their presentation, however, is distinguished on physical examination by the presence of a nodule or several nodules, whereas the thyroid examination in Graves' disease shows a diffusely enlarged gland.

Hashimoto's thyroiditis is a cause of hypothyroidism rather than hyperthyroidism. Its presentation is usually that of hypothyroid symptoms but can less commonly present with a short-lived hyperthyroid phase. It is also of an autoimmune origin.

Pheochromocytoma and panic disorder are not serious considerations with this presentation history.

2. **b.** Graves' disease is thought to be the result of an autoimmune process, and antibodies that stimulate the thyroid receptors are present in the serum.

3. **d.** The serum TSH level is used to measure and detect hyperthyroidism and hypothyroidism. The *sine qua non* of hyperthyroidism is a low serum TSH level, and it is the screening test that should be used. The serum free T4 should be measured after hyperthyroidism is confirmed by TSH. If the free T4 is normal, then a serum T3 should be ordered; 10% of the cases of hyperthyroidism are actually the result of a T3 toxicosis rather than a T4 problem. Radioactive iodine uptake will show hyperthyroidism in this case, but it is not the most appropriate initial test. Its use will be discussed later in the chapter. Thyroid antibodies will be present in Graves' disease and can help to confirm your suspicions, but they are not used to diagnose hyperthyroidism.

4. **a.** Radioactive iodine uptake testing is a valuable tool to narrow the differential diagnosis of hyperthyroidism. A homogeneous, diffuse uptake is consistent with Graves' disease. Different patterns are associated with other etiologies, such as multinodular heterogeneous uptake in toxic multinodular goiter, a "hot" nodule in a hyperfunctioning thyroid adenoma, and diffusely decreased uptake seen in thyroiditis. TSH receptor antibodies are helpful in the diagnosis of Graves' disease when present, but when absent, they are not helpful in differentiating the cause of hyperthyroidism. Ultrasound may be useful in identifying nodules and goiter that may not be readily

apparent, but it is not the best test to determine the cause of hyperthyroidism. FNA has a role in the investigation of thyroid nodules. Free T4 will be elevated in hyperthyroidism but does not provide diagnosis.

5. d. Patients with hyperthyroidism display symptoms of increased adrenergic tone causing tachycardia, palpitations, anxiety, and other symptoms. β-Adrenergic blocking agents, such as atenolol, are effective in alleviating many of these symptoms in the acute setting. Use of methimazole or PTU will decrease excessive production of thyroid hormone, but they take time to work and have no effect on thyroid hormone already in circulation. Diltiazem is a calcium channel blocker that may help to control tachycardia, but it is not effective at blocking increased adrenergic tone. Radioactive iodine ablation may be an appropriate definitive treatment for certain forms of hyperthyroidism, but it does not have a role in the acute setting.

6. a. See answer 10.

7. c. See answer 10.

8. c. See answer 10.

9. c. See answer 10.

10. b. The two basic treatments for Graves' disease are antithyroid drugs (propylthiouracil or methimazole) and radioactive iodine therapy.

1. Antithyroid drugs
   a. Advantage: These drugs provide the opportunity for the patient to experience a spontaneous remission and avoid lifelong medication (e.g., levothyroxine).
   b. Disadvantages: Remissions are attained in fewer than 50% of patients, and continuous or repeated courses of drug therapy are usually necessary.
   c. Rare but potentially fatal side effect of agranulocytosis.
2. Radioactive iodine therapy
   a. Advantages: Radioactive iodine therapy is curative, and managing postradiation hypothyroidism is simpler than managing most patients undergoing long-term antithyroid drug therapy.
   b. Disadvantage: Iatrogenic hypothyroidism is produced in the majority of patients within 10 years.

On the basis of weighing advantages versus disadvantages for both, the recommendation has been made that radioactive iodine is the treatment of choice for adult patients. In children and adolescents, antithyroid medication remains first-line treatment, with radioactive iodine being second-line treatment. Radioactive iodine is contraindicated in pregnant women. Women treated with radioactive iodine before pregnancy have children with no higher incidence of congenital malformation or childhood cancers than controls and no difference in fertility. When maternal hyperthyroidism is present, ultrasound surveillance for fetal goiter must be performed to monitor fetal thyroid status.

Untreated hyperthyroidism can cause atrial fibrillation, osteoporosis, diarrhea, and heat intolerance. It does not cause thyroid nodules.

11. d. See answer 12.

12. d. The most likely explanation for the elevated serum T4 in this patient is an elevated TBG secondary to the estrogen component of the oral contraceptive pill.

TBG is increased in patients with increased levels of circulating estrogen. This can result from taking the oral contraceptive pill, taking estrogen supplementation, pregnancy, and patients with infectious hepatitis. Many different medications, such as nonsteroidal antiinflammatory drugs, phenytoin, and furosemide, may affect the amount of circulating T4 bound to TBG. In circulation, there are free and bound forms of T4, with the free T4 being active. There may be increased total T4 due to increased amounts of circulating TBG, but this does not lead to hyperthyroidism since the bound form is inactive. A free T4 assay is preferred due to the previous reasons.

13. b. The initial procedure of choice is thyroid ultrasound. Despite the presence of a palpable nodule, there may be other nodules that are not clinically evident. The decision to do FNA should not be made on size alone. A thyroid ultrasound may uncover other nodules not palpated that may have features that would put them at high risk of malignancy and should receive FNA in addition to the palpable nodule. Among those receiving ultrasound for a clinically suspected thyroid nodule, 20% will have another, clinically inapparent nodule, and 10% of those will have no nodule found sonographically. Radioactive iodine uptake scanning can indicate if the nodule is functioning or not, but it does not provide as much information regarding the presence of other nodules or their internal features. CT and MRI scanning have limited value in the investigation of thyroid nodules.

14. c. After suspicious nodules are identified, FNA should be performed to further evaluate for thyroid carcinoma. Although FNA may be done blindly, the use of ultrasound-guided FNA is increasing. This allows direct visulation of the needle in the nodule, allowing accurate sampling of the desired area. This also helps to avoid accidental damage to surrounding neck structure such as the trachea and the neurovasculature. Results of FNA are reported as positive, negative, suspicious, or nondiagnostic for malignant cells. Refer to the Solution to the Clinical Case Management Problem for complete details on the management of thyroid nodules.

15. d. Cold nodules require further investigation because they carry a 5% to 15% risk of malignancy. Hot nodules are extremely unlikely to be malignant and do not require FNA.

16. d. In the past, treatment of benign nodules was TSH suppressive therapy with levothyroxine, but studies have shown that this provides little clinical benefit and may potentially be harmful. This therapy was aimed at shrinking current nodules, arresting further growth, and preventing the appearance of new nodules. Treatment with levothyroxine creates a state of subclinical hyperthyroidism that has been associated with increased rates of atrial fibrillation and morbidity and mortality from cardiovascular disease. Specific treatment is not necessary if thyroid function is normal and malignancy is excluded. Unless the nodule causes local symptoms, the patient may be reassured with clinical and ultrasound follow-up of the nodule every 1 or 2 years. Excision would only be appropriate if the size of the nodule was causing local symptoms. Radioactive iodine uptake scanning would provide little information if thyroid function was normal. There is no indication for MRI in this scenario.

17. e. Thyroid ultrasound is not to be used as a general screening exam. It is a necessary exam in the evaluation of a thyroid nodule. It is a warranted surveillance test in patients with a history of neck irradiation and in those with a family history of thyroid carcinoma, family history of multiple endocrine neoplasia type 2, and when there is unexplained cervical lymphadenopathy.

18. d. The most useful test for diagnosing hypothyroidism is the serum TSH level. Serum TSH is elevated in almost all cases of primary hypothyroidism. If hypothyroidism is suspected, the serum TSH will provide definite proof for or against the condition. Other tests, such as T3 and T4, may be helpful once the diagnosis is made, but they are not necessary in the initial diagnosis of hypothyroidism.

19. e. In hypothyroidism, systemic vascular resistance increases, and there is a rise in diastolic blood pressure. Other cardiovascular signs of hypothyroidism include an increase in low-density lipoprotein cholesterol and reduced exercise tolerance. Alterations in thought process, fatigue, and memory changes are symptoms associated with depression in the elderly, but they may also be due to effects of hypothyroidism on the central nervous system. Amiodarone therapy can predispose patients to hypothyroidism. The iodine content of the medication eventually leads to decreased thyroid hormone synthesis and release. All patients started on amiodarone therapy should have baseline thyroid function tests and should be screened periodically.

20. d. Combined T3 and T4 are not indicated.

21. c. Once hypothyroidism is diagnosed, replacement with synthetic thyroxine may begin, with the average replacement dose of 1.6 µg/kg/day. The serum TSH level should be measured 4 to 6 weeks later. This level will determine whether an increased or deceased amount of replacement therapy is needed. The TSH should be measured every 4 to 6 weeks until it is normal. In the elderly and those with underlying coronary artery disease, starting with 25 to 50 µg daily is more prudent. The complications of overreplacement with thyroid hormone increase the risk of atrial fibrillation and other cardiovascular complications. Levothyroxine is the preferred therapeutic agent. There is not enough evidence to warrant the use of T3 and T4 in combination for the treatment of hyperthyroidism. Levothyroxine is best absorbed on an empty stomach and should be taken at least 30 minutes prior to breakfast. Coadministration with other medications, such as proton pump inhibitors, antacids, phenytoin, calcium, and iron, may increase the daily requirement of thyroid replacement.

22. a. The most common cause of hypothyroidism is the autoimmune condition known as Hashimoto's thyroiditis. The patient with Hashimoto's thyroiditis may initially present in a hyperthyroid state but always progresses to a hypothyroid state. Symptoms of hypothyroidism include fatigue, lethargy, constipation, cold intolerance, dry skin, hair loss, weight gain, edema, headache, arthralgias, hoarseness, amenorrhea, and bradycardia.

23. d. Hashimoto's thyroiditis is also known as chronic autoimmune thyroiditis. The disease is due to an antibody and cell-mediated destruction of the thyroid gland, not of the circulating thyroid hormone.

It is much more common in females than in males. Anti-thyroid antibodies are present in up to 80% of patients. These constitute autoantibodies to different parts of the thyroid gland, including thyroperoxidase, thyroglobulin, the TSH receptor, and TSH blocking antibodies. In the acute thyroiditis stage of the disease, symptoms of hyperthyroidism precede symptoms of an inevitable hypothyroidism.

24. **c.** The patient has a thyroid function profile consistent with subclinical hypothyroidism. The elevated TSH in light of a normal free T4 is an indication of early thyroid failure. This patient should be treated to normalize her TSH since she has symptoms of thyroid dysfunction (fatigue, memory impairment, etc.). Some studies show that subclinical hypothyroidism is a cardiac disease risk factor. Central hypothyroidism is rare and presents with low T4 and T3 in the setting of a low, normal, or minimally elevated TSH. Graves' disease would present different clinically and have a low TSH and elevated free T4.

25. **c.** Subacute thyroiditis is often preceded by a viral illness a few weeks earlier. There is often anterior neck tenderness due to the inflamed thyroid gland. There is an initial hyperthyroid state followed by a hypothyroid phase. Hashimoto's thyroiditis may present similarly, but the presence of neck tenderness and a recent viral illness is more supportive of subacute thyroiditis.

26. **b.** The patient should be started on thyroid replacement therapy to correct her current hypothyroidism. Her TSH should be monitored because most patients will become euthyroid over a period of weeks to months and will no longer need replacement. A subset of patients will remain hypothyroid. Ultrasound and radioactive iodine scanning has little value in this setting.

Solution to the Clinical Case Management Problem

The workup of a palpable thyroid nodule can undergo a stepwise process. The first tests that should be performed are thyroid ultrasound and serum TSH. Ultrasound is recommended in any patient with a palpable nodule or a multinodular goiter. Ultrasound can help detect clinically inapparent nodules and search for characteristics within nodules that put them at high risk of malignancy. High-risk characteristics include microcalcifications, hypoechogenicity, a solid nodule, irregular nodule margins, chaotic intranodular vasculature, and a nodule that is more tall than wide. Any two of these characteristics in a nonpalpable nodule warrants FNA.

The level of serum TSH will indicate the state of thyroid function and can help tailor subsequent testing.

If the TSH is depressed and the ultrasound shows a solitary nodule or a multinodular thyroid, a radioactive iodine uptake scan can be performed to provide a diagnosis. A hot, solitary nodule confirms the presence of a hyperfunctioning adenoma, and increased uptake in a diffuse, heterogeneous pattern suggests a toxic multinodular goiter.

If the TSH is normal or elevated, FNA of the palpable nodule should be performed. If multiple nodules are found on ultrasound, the characteristics described previously should be used to determine which nodules, in addition to the palpable nodule, warrant FNA.

If FNA is performed, there are four possible results. An FNA-positive nodule is malignant and warrants appropriate referral and treatment. An FNA-negative nodule is benign and can be followed yearly with clinical and sonographic exams. An FNA-suspicious nodule does not have classic malignant features but requires referral for possible surgical excision. FNA-nondiagnostic nodules require repeat FNA. See Figure 42-1 for a stepwise approach to the evaluation of a thyroid nodule.

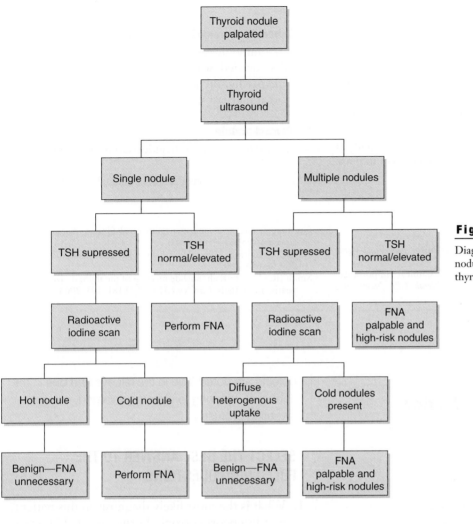

Figure 42-1

Diagnostic evaluation of a palpable thyroid nodule. FNA, fine needle aspiration; TSH, thyroid-stimulating hormone.

Summary

1. Important epidemiology

a. Hypothyroidism is one of the most commonly under-diagnosed conditions, particularly in the elderly.

b. Hypothyroidism is significantly more common than hyperthyroidism.

c. Women are more likely than men to be affected by thyroid disease.

2. Hyperthyroidism

a. Causes: The most common cause is Graves' disease. Toxic multinodular goiter and toxic adenoma are less common.

b. Signs/symptoms: The most common signs and symptoms include tremor, anxiety and nervousness, irritability, diarrhea, weight loss, sweating, palpitations, insomnia, proptosis or exophthalmos (Graves' disease), pronounced heart sounds, and cardiac murmur.

c. Investigations: A simplified initial investigation approach is to directly measure free serum T4 and serum TSH. If TSH is suppressed and free serum T4 is normal, then serum T3 should be measured as well. A radioactive thyroid scan can help to narrow the diagnosis.

d. Treatment: Radioactive iodine ablation is the treatment of choice for Graves' disease in adults. Antithyroid drugs are the treatment of choice in children and adolescents. The drugs of choice are propylthiouracil and methimazole. Subtotal thyroidectomy may be the most appropriate treatment for a toxic or solitary adenoma (nonmalignant). Radiation may sometimes be a reasonable alternative.

3. Hypothyroidism

a. Causes: The most common cause is Hashimoto's thyroiditis (chronic autoimmune thyroiditis).

Other common causes include hypothyroidism induced by thyroid surgery, radiation ablation, or drug-induced hypothyroidism.

b. Investigations: Serum TSH is the most sensitive test in diagnosing primary hypothyroidism. For the elderly patient who has become depressed, consider hypothyroidism.

c. Treatment: Levothyroxine 160 μg/kg/day. Start at 50 μg and work up slowly in the elderly and in those with underlying cardiac disease.

4. Subacute thyroiditis

a. Commonly seen after a viral infection.

b. Associated with anterior neck pain. There is a hyperthyroid phase followed by hypothyroidism that may last weeks to months.

5. Thyroid nodule

a. Initial evaluation includes serum TSH and thyroid US.

b. Perform FNA on appropriate nodules. See Figure 42-1.

Suggested Reading

Devdhar M, Ousman Y, Burman K: Hypothyroidism. *Endocrinol Metab Clin North Am* 36:595–615, 2007.

Gharib H, Papini E: Thyroid nodules: Clinical importance, assessment, and treatment. *Endocrinol Metab Clin North Am* 36:707–735, 2007.

Ginsberg J: Diagnosis and management of Graves' disease. *Can Med Assoc J* 168(5):575–585, 2003.

Nayak B, Hodak S: Hyperthyroidism. *Endocrinol Metab Clin North Am* 36:617–656, 2007.

Smith JR, Oates E: Radionuclide imaging of the thyroid gland: Patterns, pearls, and pitfalls. *Clin Nucl Med* 29(3):181–193, 2004.

CHAPTER

43 Common Endocrine Diseases

CLINICAL CASE PROBLEM 1

A 25-Year-Old Male with "Visual Problems," Headaches, Weight Gain, Sweating, and "Hands and Feet That Are Changing"

A 25-year-old male come to your office with his wife. He is very concerned about some "bizarre symptoms" that he has been experiencing. He is the chief executive officer of a family-owned manufacturing company and is "really embarrassed to go out in public any longer." He tells you that approximately 6 months ago he began to experience the following symptoms: headaches, visual spots or defects, weight gain, an appearance of his forehead growing, enlarging hands and feet (he could no longer get his gloves and shoes on), and increased sweating.

On examination, mental status examination is normal, and the apical impulse is felt in the 5th intercostal space, midclavicular line. His blood pressure is 170/105 mmHg. He does have a protruding brow, and three discrete visual field defects are noted (two in the left eye and one in the right eye). His tongue appears enlarged, and he is sweating profusely.

SELECT THE BEST ANSWER TO THE FOLLOWING QUESTIONS

1. What is the most likely diagnosis in this patient?
   a. adrenocorticotropin hormone (ACTH) excess
   b. acromegaly
   c. prolactinoma
   d. primary hypopituitarism
   e. primary hyperparathyroidism

2. The pathophysiologic lesion resides in which of the following?
   a. adrenal gland: adenoma
   b. hyperparathyroid glands: adenoma in one or more of the four glands
   c. pituitary gland: adenoma
   d. gastrointestinal ectopic tumor: adenoma
   e. none of the above

3. The treatment(s) for this patient may include which of the following?
   a. microsurgery: transsphenoidal
   b. stereotactic radiotherapy
   c. cabergoline
   d. growth hormone receptor antagonists
   e. all of the above
   f. none of the above

CLINICAL CASE PROBLEM 2

A 24-Year-Old Male with Weakness and Hyperpigmentation

A 24-year-old male comes to your office with the following symptoms: an extreme feeling of weakness, a 20-pound weight loss, a change in the color of his skin (his skin has become very hyperpigmented), and lightheadedness and dizziness.

On examination, the patient has definite skin hyperpigmentation since you last saw him 9 months ago. His blood pressure is 90/70 mmHg. He looks acutely ill.

On laboratory examination, his serum Na$^+$ is low (115 mEq/L), his serum potassium is high (6.2 mEq/L), his serum urea is elevated at 9 mg/dL, and his serum calcium is elevated (12 mg/dL).

4. On the basis of his history, physical examination, and laboratory findings, what is the most likely diagnosis of this patient?
   a. Conn's syndrome
   b. Cushing's syndrome
   c. Addison's syndrome
   d. primary hyperparathyroidism
   e. primary pituitary failure

5. What is the most likely cause of this patient's symptoms?
   a. overstimulation of the adrenal gland
   b. an adrenal adenoma
   c. autoimmune destruction of the hyperparathyroid glands
   d. autoimmune destruction of the adrenal gland
   e. a pituitary adenoma

6. What is the acute treatment of choice for this patient?
   a. prednisone orally
   b. dexamethasone orally
   c. hydrocortisone intravenously (IV)
   d. ACTH IV
   e. Depo-Provera intramuscularly

7. This patient will need chronic treatment with which of the following?
   a. hydrocortisone
   b. fludrocortisone acetate
   c. a or b
   d. a and b
   e. none of the above

CLINICAL CASE PROBLEM 3

A 25-Year-Old Female with Increased Thirst and Urination

A 25-year-old female presents with the sudden onset of increased thirst and increased urination. This began abruptly 1 week ago and has not abated since. She states that since that time, she has been thirsty all the time. The only significant illness in her life has been the recent diagnosis of bipolar affective illness that was made 12 weeks ago. She started taking lithium carbonate and currently is taking 1200 mg/day. Her serum lithium levels have been normal since the beginning.

On examination, her blood pressure is 110/70 mmHg. She has lost 5 pounds during the past week and looks somewhat dehydrated.

8. What is the most likely diagnosis in this patient?
   a. psychogenic polydipsia
   b. diabetes mellitus type 1
   c. central diabetes insipidus
   d. nephrogenic diabetes insipidus
   e. adverse drug reaction to lithium

9. What is the treatment of choice in this patient?
   a. hospitalization and complete psychiatric assessment
   b. insulin: beginning at 10 to 20 units/day
   c. glyburide
   d. discontinuation of lithium carbonate
   e. substitution of carbamazepine for lithium carbonate

CLINICAL CASE PROBLEM 4

An Overly Tired 37-Year-Old Female with Hypertension

A 37-year-old female comes to your office because she was found to be "hypertensive" by a nurse in a shopping mall screening program. She tells you that when she thinks about it, she really has not felt well for a couple of months. Her major complaint has been profound generalized fatigue and weakness. She has also been increasingly thirsty, urinating more frequently, and having to urinate frequently at night.

On physical examination, her blood pressure is 190/110 mmHg. Laboratory abnormalities include a mildly increased serum Na$^+$ (150 mEq/L), hypokalemic metabolic alkalosis, a low renin level, and increased urine potassium.

10. What is the most likely diagnosis based on the information presented?
    a. Conn's syndrome
    b. Cushing's syndrome
    c. Addison's syndrome
    d. Bartter's syndrome
    e. diabetes insipidus

11. What is the most likely pathophysiologic cause of this syndrome?
    a. benign adenoma of the adrenal gland
    b. malignant adenoma of the adrenal gland
    c. pituitary adenoma
    d. bilateral hyperplasia of the adrenal gland
    e. none of the above

12. What is the treatment of choice for the condition described here?
    a. bromocriptine
    b. transsphenoidal surgery
    c. clomiphene
    d. spironolactone
    e. surgical removal of the adenoma

CLINICAL CASE PROBLEM 5

A 22-Year-Old Female with Breast Secretions, Amenorrhea, and Decreased Libido

A 22-year-old female, married for 18 months, has been trying to get pregnant without success. Approximately 9 months ago, she developed breast secretions, amenorrhea, and decreased libido. No other symptoms are present.

On examination, there is definite galactorrhea present. Her blood pressure is 140/80 mmHg. No abnormalities are found on physical examination.

13. From the information provided, what is the most likely diagnosis?
    a. anorexia nervosa
    b. stress-induced amenorrhea
    c. pregnancy
    d. prolactinoma
    e. hypopituitarism

14. If you could order only one test, what would that test be?
    a. serum estrogen
    b. serum progesterone
    c. serum luteinizing hormone
    d. serum follicle-stimulating hormone
    e. serum prolactin

15. What is the treatment of choice for this condition?
    a. transsphenoidal resection
    b. bromocriptine
    c. clomiphene
    d. lithium carbonate
    e. thyroxine

CLINICAL CASE PROBLEM 6

A 42-Year-Old Female with Increased Body Hair and Purple Streaks on Her Abdomen

A 42-year-old female comes to your office with the following signs and symptoms: obesity (she has gained 40 pounds in the past 6 months), elevated blood pressure at her last walk-in clinic visit, increased body hair, purple streaks on her abdomen, "a fat face" (her description), and pains in her bones and joints.

She is taking no medication at present, nor has she been on any medication for the past year.

On examination, her body mass index is 35 kg/m². Her blood pressure is 160/110 mmHg; she has obvious hirsutism over her entire body, and her abdomen (which is obese) has purple stria. Her face is not only plethoric but also demonstrates a double chin. Her thoracic spine shows evidence of what is known as a buffalo hump.

16. Based on the information provided, what is the most likely diagnosis in this patient?
    a. Conn's syndrome
    b. Cushing's syndrome
    c. Addison's syndrome
    d. primary hyperparathyroidism
    e. prolactinoma

17. Of all possible causes for the condition in this patient, which of the following is the most common?
    a. adenoma of the adrenal gland
    b. adenoma of the pituitary gland
    c. hyperplasia of the adrenal gland
    d. corticosteroid therapy for suppression of inflammation
    e. small cell carcinoma of the lung

18. Which of the following tests is (are) an appropriate screening test(s) for this patient?
    a. serum cortisol
    b. low-dose dexamethasone (cortisol analogue) suppression test
    c. 24-hour urine for free cortisol

d. all of the above

e. none of the above

19. This patient has an imaging study that confirms she has the most common cause of Cushing's syndrome. Which of the following is the recommended treatment?

   a. surgery to remove the adenoma of the pituitary gland

   b. surgery to remove the adenoma of the adrenal gland

   c. surgery to remove the carcinoma of the adrenal gland

   d. chemotherapy to kill as much abnormal tissue as possible

   e. none of the above

20. Which of the following conditions is metastatic malignancy most likely to mimic?

   a. Cushing's syndrome

   b. primary hyperparathyroidism

   c. Conn's syndrome

   d. Addison's syndrome

   e. Nelson's syndrome

Clinical Case Management Problem

For hyperparathyroidism:

1. Define the condition.
2. Provide the sex predilection.
3. Provide the age predilection.
4. Explain the pathogenesis.
5. Provide the clinical symptoms.
6. Explain the mnemonic "stones, bones, abdominal groans, and psychic moans."
7. Explain the changes in blood and serum levels that characterize the condition.
8. Discuss treatment.
9. Identify the most characteristic laboratory abnormality.

Answers

1. b. The condition is acromegaly, which often goes undiagnosed for many years. Acromegaly produces many signs and symptoms, including the following:

1. General symptoms: (a) fatigue, (b) increased sweating, (c) heat intolerance, and (d) weight gain

2. Changes in peripheral and general appearance: (a) enlarging hands and feet, (b) coarsening facial features, (c) oily skin, and (d) hypertrichosis

3. Head: (a) headaches, (b) parotid enlargement, and (c) frontal bossing

4. Nose–throat: (a) sinus congestion, (b) voice change, (c) obstructive sleep apnea, and (d) goiter

5. Cardiovascular system: (a) hypertension, (b) congestive cardiac failure, and (c) left ventricular hypertrophy

6. Genitourinary system: (a) kidney stones, (b) decreased libido/impotence, (c) infertility, and (d) oligomenorrhea

7. Neurologic system: (a) paresthesias, (b) hypersomnolence, and (c) carpal tunnel syndrome

8. Muscular system: (a) weakness and (b) proximal myopathy

9. Skeletal system: (a) joint pains and (b) osteoarthritis

2. c. Acromegaly is almost always the result of a growth hormone excess caused by a pituitary adenoma.

3. e. Treatments include transsphenoidal pituitary microsurgery (treatment of choice), stereotactic radiosurgery, cabergoline (dopamine agonist), somatostatin analogues such as octreotide, and growth hormone receptor blockers such as pegvisomant. The dopamine agonist pergolide was withdrawn from the market due to adverse cardiac valvular effects. Endoscopic pituitary microsurgery achieves remission in 70% of patients.

4. c. This patient has Addison's disease or primary adrenocortical insufficiency. The prominent clinical features of Addison's disease include weakness (100%), weight loss (100%), hyperpigmentation (95%), and hypotension.

The pertinent laboratory findings include hyponatremia, hyperkalemia, increased blood urea nitrogen, hypercalcemia, increased plasma ACTH, and decreased serum cortisol level.

In Addison's disease, both the short ACTH stimulation test and the prolonged ACTH stimulation test yield no cortical response.

5. d. Most commonly, Addison's disease results from an autoimmune destruction of the adrenal gland. At least 50% of patients with Addison's disease have anti-adrenal antibodies. Other potential causes of adrenocortical insufficiency include tuberculosis, disseminated meningococcemia, and metastatic cancer.

6. **c.** Because of the acutely ill state of this patient, dexamethasone sodium phosphate 4 mg every 12 hours or hydrocortisone 100 mg IV every 6 hours for 24 hours should be administered acutely. If the patient shows adequate clinical response, the dose may be tapered gradually and changed to oral prednisone.

7. **d.** The chronic treatment of Addison's disease is a combination of hydrocortisone (15 to 25 mg/day) and fludrocortisone (0.05 to 0.3 mg/day). This combination is based on the need for a combination of glucocorticoid replacement and mineralocorticoid replacement. Dosage is increased for stressful events such as infection. Watch for activation of latent tuberculosis.

8. **d.** This patient has nephrogenic diabetes insipidus. This has resulted from the lack of renal response to antidiuretic hormone (ADH); in this case, the diabetes insipidus is of the nephrogenic subtype and caused by the drug lithium carbonate.

There are two basic types of diabetes insipidus: central (the central type is usually idiopathic) and nephrogenic (the collecting tubules of the kidney are not responsive to the ADH that is produced). The nephrogenic type is usually the result of either a drug (lithium carbonate and amphotericin B) or severe hypokalemia (which makes the renal tubules resistant to ADH).

9. **e.** The treatment for central diabetes insipidus is desmopressin either intranasally or orally; nephrogenic diabetes insipidus is best treated by discontinuation of the offending drug (if the drug is the cause, as is the most common scenario). In the case of this patient, who was started on lithium carbonate to treat bipolar affective disorder, a switch to carbamazepine would be most appropriate.

10. **a.** This patient has Conn's syndrome.

11. **a.** Conn's syndrome is primary hyperaldosteronism that results from an excess mineralocorticoid production from (in most cases) a unilateral adenoma of the adrenal cortex. If not the result of an adenoma, hyperplasia of the adrenal cortex is found. The benign adenoma is usually present in the zona glomerulosa.

The clinical signs/symptoms of Conn's syndrome are weakness (as a result of the effect of hypokalemia); hypertension; carbohydrate intolerance (as a result of increased insulin release from hypokalemia); and polyuria, polydipsia, and nocturia as the result of either hypokalemic nephropathy or nephrogenic diabetes insipidus.

Laboratory abnormalities include mild hypernatremia; hypokalemic metabolic alkalosis; low renin; increased urine potassium; and an inability to suppress aldosterone with isotonic saline load, captopril, or use of another mineralocorticoid.

12. **e.** The treatment of choice for this patient, who most likely has a benign adenoma, is laproscopic surgical removal of the adenoma. If a case of Conn's syndrome were the result of a bilateral hyperplasia of the adrenal glands, spironolactone would be the treatment of choice.

13. **d.** This patient has hyperprolactinemia, most likely from a pituitary micro- or macroadenoma. The combination of galactorrhea, amenorrhea, infertility, and decreased libido is almost certainly the result of a prolactinoma.

14. **e.** A prolactinoma can be confirmed by performing a serum prolactin level test. A level of serum prolactin of 300 ng/mL or greater is almost always the result of a pituitary adenoma (in the absence of pregnancy).

A magnetic resonance imaging (MRI) scan of the pituitary gland will confirm the diagnosis. Note that a prolactinoma is the most common overall pituitary tumor in women.

15. **b.** Treatment is controversial, but because of a high rate of recurrence with surgery, initial therapy with cabergoline or bromocriptine is the best choice. Treatment with dopamine agonists is not curative; it does, however, reduce the prolactin level, reduce the tumor mass, and increase fertility. Side effects include nausea and vomiting, an increase in liver enzymes, and an increase in serum uric acid.

16. **b.** This patient has Cushing's syndrome. The definition of Cushing's syndrome is "a manifestation of hypercorticalism due to any cause."

17. **b.** The most common cause of Cushing's syndrome is corticosteroid therapy. If steroids are excluded, the three major causes are as follows: (1) pituitary Cushing's disease (60% to 70%) as a result of an adenoma; (2) adrenal Cushing's (15%) may be from an adenoma, hyperplasia, or malignancy; and (3) ectopic Cushing's (15%) from a malignancy (small cell carcinoma of the lung).

Thus, the most likely cause of Cushing's syndrome in the patient described, who has not been taking any medication for more than 1 year, is a pituitary adenoma.

18. **d.** The clinical features of Cushing's syndrome consist of the following: (1) truncal obesity (90%); (2) hypertension (85%); (3) decreased glucose tolerance

(80%); (4) hirsutism (70%); (5) wide, purple abdominal stria (65%); (6) osteoporosis (55%); (7) plethoric face; (8) easy bruising; (9) mental aberrations; and (10) myopathy.

In terms of laboratory tests, the best overall screening tests are serum cortisol level, low-dose (1 mg) dexamethasone suppression test (in Cushing's syndrome there is no suppression), and 24-hour urine for free cortisol. Confirmation tests include high-dose (8 mg) dexamethasone suppression test (suppresses pituitary Cushing's but will not suppress adrenal or ectopic Cushing's) and plasma ACTH (normal to slightly increased in pituitary Cushing's, markedly increased in ectopic Cushing's, and very low in adrenal Cushing's; suppressed by cortisol).

19. **a.** The correct answer is surgery to remove the pituitary adenoma.

20. **b.** Metastatic malignancy is most likely to produce hypercalcemia. Hypercalcemia is most likely to mimic primary hyperparathyroidism. (Hyperparathyroidism is discussed in the Solution to the Clinical Case Management Problem.)

Solution to the Clinical Case Management Problem

Hyperparathyroidism

1. Definition: Overactivity of the parathyroid glands (one or more of the four glands)
2. Sex predilection: females > males
3. Age predilection: age 40 to 70 years
4. Pathology
   a. 82% of cases of hyperparathyroidism are the result of adenomas
   b. 15% of cases of hyperparathyroidism are the result of hyperplasia of the glands
   c. 3% are malignant
5. Clinical symptoms
   a. Renal stones (calcium oxalate): most common symptomatic presentation
   b. Peptic ulcer disease: calcium stimulates gastrin release
   c. Acute pancreatitis: calcium activates phospholipases
   d. Constipation: most common gastrointestinal complaint
   e. Band keratopathy: metastatic calcification in the limbus of the eye
   f. Nephrocalcinosis: polyuria, loss of concentrating ability, and diluting capability the result of metastatic calcification of the renal tubules
   g. Pruritus: metastatic calcification in the skin
   h. Short QT interval; bradycardia
   i. Hypertension: calcium increases muscular contraction in the resistance vessels
   j. Osteitis fibrosa cystica: late finding, commonly found in jaw, called "brown tumor" because of hemorrhage into cysts
   k. Pseudogout: calcium pyrophosphate; positively birefringent crystals
   l. Mental changes: personality changes, psychosis, and depression
   m. X-ray changes
      i. "Salt-and-pepper skull" on x-ray
      ii. Subperiosteal resorption of bone from the second and third middle phalanges and lamina dura around the teeth
      iii. Distal resorption of clavicle
6. The mnemonic "stones, bones, abdominal groans, and psychic moans"
   a. Stones: calcium oxalate renal stones
   b. Bones: osteitis fibrosa cystica, salt-and-pepper skull, resorption of clavicle, subperiosteal resorption of bone from the second and third phalanges and the lamina dura around the teeth
   c. Abdominal groans: abdominal pain resulting from acute pancreatitis
   d. Psychic moans: psychosis, depression
7. Changes in blood and serum
   a. Hypercalcemia (most common characteristic)
   b. Hypercalciuria
   c. Hypophosphatemia
   d. Hyperphosphaturia
   e. Normal anion gap metabolic acidosis
8. Treatment
   a. Adenoma: surgery to locate and remove adenoma (biopsy second gland to determine if atrophic)
   b. Hyperplasia: subtotal parathyroidectomy, monitor for tetany postoperatively
9. Most common laboratory abnormality: hypercalcemia

Summary

ACROMEGALY

1. Signs/symptoms: enlarged hands, feet, and head; hypertension; cardiomegaly; weight gain
2. Pathology: results from pituitary adenoma, growth hormone
3. Treatment: transsphenoidal surgery, radiation, cabergoline, somatostatin analogues, growth hormone receptor blockers

ADDISON'S DISEASE

1. Signs/symptoms: weakness, hypotension, hyperpigmentation
2. Pathology: autoimmune destruction of adrenal glands
3. Acute treatment: acutely ill: intravenous hydrocortisone or dexamethasone
4. Chronic treatment: replacement with glucocorticoid (hydrocortisone) plus mineralocorticoid (fludrocortisone)
5. Results: adrenocortical insufficiency

DIABETES INSIPIDUS

1. Signs/symptoms: polyuria, polydipsia as a result of deficiency of antidiuretic hormone
2. Subtypes: central and nephrogenic
3. Differential diagnosis: psychogenic polydipsia
4. Most common cause: nephrogenic subtype most commonly from lithium use
5. Treatment: desmopressin either intranasally or orally for central subtype

PROLACTINOMA

1. Signs/symptoms: galactorrhea, amenorrhea, infertility, decreased libido
2. Frequency: most common pituitary tumor
3. Investigation and confirmation: serum prolactin of 300 or more; MRI pituitary
4. Differential diagnosis: rule out pregnancy, hyperthyroidism, and drugs (major tranquilizers, oral contraceptive pills, IV cimetidine, opiates)
5. Treatment: transsphenoidal surgery, dopamine agonists (bromocriptine)

CONN'S SYNDROME

1. Signs/symptoms: weakness (as a result of hypokalemia), hypertension, carbohydrate intolerance (polyuria, polydipsia)
2. Most common cause: adenoma of the adrenal
3. Pathology: excess mineralocorticoid production
4. Laboratory investigations: mild hypernatremia, hypokalemic metabolic alkalosis
5. Treatment: adenoma removal; spironolactone for hyperplasia

CUSHING'S SYNDROME

1. Signs/symptoms: truncal obesity, carbohydrate intolerance, moon face, buffalo hump, abdominal stria, osteoporosis, psychic changes (depression and euphoria), easy bruising, myopathy, plethoric face
2. Pathology: pituitary adenoma, adrenal adenoma, steroid therapy
3. Most common cause: corticosteroid therapy
4. Laboratory investigation: lab tests (screen): serum cortisol, 24-hour urine for cortisol, dexamethasone suppression test (1 mg). Confirmation and differentiation between pituitary Cushing's, adrenal Cushing's, and ectopic Cushing's syndrome; plasma ACTH; high-dose dexamethasone (8 mg) suppression test
5. Treatment
   a. Exogenous Cushing's: stop steroids, decrease dose, or use steroids every other day with a drug holiday
   b. Endogenous Cushing's: removal of adenoma in pituitary and adrenal Cushing's syndrome

PRIMARY HYPERPARATHYROIDISM

1. Signs/symptoms: mnemonic: stones, bones, abdominal groans, psychic moans; renal colic (Ca oxalate); acute pancreatitis; constipation; x-ray: bone resorption, salt-and-pepper skull
2. Pathology: most commonly adenoma of the parathyroid gland
3. Laboratory abnormalities: hypercalcemia, hypophosphatemia, hypocalciuria, hyperphosphaturia. Hypercalcemia is most common metabolic abnormality; also may occur in metastatic carcinoma
4. Treatment: adenoma: removal; hyperplasia: subtotal parathyroidectomy

Suggested Reading

Akerstrom G, Hellman P: Primary hyperparathyroidism. *Curr Opin Oncol* 16(1):1–7, 2004.

Arnaldi G, Angeli A, Atkinson AB, et al: Diagnosis and complications of Cushing's syndrome: A consensus statement. *J Clin Endocrinol Metab* 88(12):5593–5602, 2003.

Findling JW, Raff H: Cushing's syndrome: Important issues in diagnosis and management. *J Clin Endocrinol Metab* 91(10):3746–3753, 2006.

Hollander-Rodriquez JC, Calvert JF: Hyperkalemia. *Am Fam Physician* 73:283–290, 2006.

Taniegra ED: Hyperparathyroidism. *Am Fam Physician* 69:333–340, 2004.

Vance ML, Laws ER, Jr: Role of medical therapy in the management of acromegaly. *Neurosurgery* 56(5):877–885, 2005.

Young WF, Jr: Clinical practice. The incidentally discovered adrenal mass. *N Engl J Med* 356(6):601–610, 2007.

Immune-Mediated Inflammatory Disorders and Autoimmune Disease

CLINICAL CASE PROBLEM 1

A 32-Year-Old Female with Pain in Her Hands and Wrists

A 32-year-old female comes into the office complaining of a swollen painful finger for 2 weeks. She otherwise feels well and has not noted any rash. On exam, her right middle finger is diffusely swollen and tender, but there are no other findings. You prescribe a nonsteroidal anti-inflammatory drug (NSAID) and have her return in 6 weeks, at which time you find silvery-scaled erythematous patches on the extensor surfaces of both elbows.

SELECT THE BEST ANSWER TO THE FOLLOWING QUESTIONS

1. Which of the following conditions is considered an immune-mediated inflammatory disorder (IMID)?
   a. asthma
   b. Crohn's disease
   c. psoriasis
   d. diabetes
   e. all of the above

2. What is this patient's most likely diagnosis?
   a. osteoarthritis
   b. parvovirus B19 infection
   c. psoriatic arthritis
   d. Reiter's syndrome
   e. rheumatoid arthritis

3. Which of the following medications have been approved by the Food and Drug Administration (FDA) for the treatment of ankylosing spondylitis, Crohn's disease, psoriatic arthritis, and rheumatoid arthritis?
   a. adalimumab (Humira)
   b. etanercept (Enbrel)
   c. infliximab (Remicade)
   d. a and c
   e. all of the above

CLINICAL CASE PROBLEM 2

A 29-Year-Old Female with Fatigue, Weight Loss, and Generalized Muscle Weakness

A 29-year-old female comes into your office with fatigue, weight loss, and generalized muscle weakness. She has not had her menses in more than 6 months and has noticed darkening of her skin in certain areas. She has also noticed that she has not had to shave her underarms as frequently as she had to in the past. Her past medical history is unremarkable.

Examination is as follows: blood pressure 90/60 mmHg; pulse 95 beats/minute; respiration 18 breaths/minute; temperature 98°F; height 66 inches; weight 108 pounds; cardiovascular, normal; lungs, normal; abdomen, normal; and skin, hyperpigmentation noted at palmar creases, buccal mucosa, elbows, and knees.

Lab results are as follows: Na^+ = 135 mEq/L, K^+ = 5.6 mEq/L, glucose = 71 mg/dL, blood urea nitrogen/creatinine = 34 mg/dL/1.3 mg/dL; white blood cell count = 2800 cells/mcL; hemoglobin = 10.4 g/dL; negative tuberculin purified protein derivative test; negative pregnancy test.

4. What is the most likely diagnosis?
   a. hypothyroidism
   b. Lyme disease
   c. anorexia nervosa
   d. Addison's disease
   e. hemochromatosis

5. Which of the following infectious diseases is not a known cause of the condition described?
   a. African trypanosomiasis
   b. histoplasmosis
   c. infectious mononucleosis
   d. syphilis
   e. tuberculosis

CLINICAL CASE PROBLEM 3

A 39-Year-Old Female with Joint Pains and a Rash

A 39-year-old female consults with you regarding joint pains and a rash on her face. She tells you that her knees and hands have been very sore and sometimes swollen during the past few months. She has always had "excellent skin," and she is upset about this "breakout" on her cheeks. Her past medical history is negative, and she takes no prescription or over-the-counter medications.

Examination reveals tenderness over the hands and wrists with no palpable swelling, erythema, or increased warmth. There is an erythematous, macular rash on her cheeks with no involvement of the nasolabial folds.

Lab tests reveal a thrombocytopenia (85,000/mm³), leukopenia (2200/mm³), and proteinuria (2+).

6. The most likely diagnosis is
a. ankylosing spondylitis
b. Lyme disease
c. progressive systemic sclerosis
d. rheumatoid arthritis
e. systemic lupus erythematosus

7. Which of the following ophthalmologic conditions is a potential manifestation of this disease?
a. keratitis
b. optic neuropathy
c. sicca syndrome
d. uveitis
e. all of the above

8. Which of the following conditions is not associated with a positive ANA sensitivity of greater than 90%?
a. mixed connective tissue disease
b. rheumatoid arthritis
c. scleroderma
d. Sjögren's syndrome
e. systemic lupus erythematosus

CLINICAL CASE PROBLEM 4

A 23-Year-Old Male with Low Back Pain

A 23-year-old male presents with a complaint of low back pain. He sometimes feels the pain in his buttocks, but there is no radiation into the legs. His back is stiff in the morning, but his pain tends to improve with exercise. He is often awakened by back pain in the early morning hours.

9. Which of the following blood tests is most likely to be useful in determining the diagnosis?
a. anti-cyclic citrullinated peptide antibody
b. anti-nuclear antibody
c. erythrocyte sedimentation rate
d. HLA-B27
e. rheumatoid factor

CLINICAL CASE PROBLEM 6

Matching Questions 1 to 12

10. Match the characteristic with the type of arthritis.

Type of Arthritis	Characteristic
1. Ankylosing spondylitis	a. Positively birefringent crystals under a polarizing microscope
2. Gonococcal arthritis	b. Negatively birefringent crystals under a polarizing microscope
3. Systemic lupus erythematosus	c. Most common cause of infective arthritis in young adults
4. Lyme disease	d. Conjunctivitis and urethritis are other features
5. Rheumatic fever	e. Erythema chronicum migrans
6. Gouty arthritis	f. Bamboo spine
7. Juvenile rheumatoid arthritis	g. Streptococcal pharyngitis usually occurs first
8. Reiter's disease	h. Arthritis may precede abdominal symptoms
9. Psoriatic arthritis	i. Renal failure is a major cause of death in this disease
10. Inflammatory bowel disease arthritis	j. Arthritis may appear before classical scaly skin lesions
11. Calcium pyrophosphate (CPPD) disease	k. Major cause of arthritis in children
12. Tuberculous arthritis	l. Lung disease is major manifestation of this disease in most patients

---

Answers

1. **e.** An IMID is in a group of conditions characterized by abnormal immune function leading to acute or chronic inflammation. The conditions share common inflammatory pathways. There are a broad range of diseases referred to as IMID that include some or all types of allergies, asthma, cardiovascular disease, chronic obstructive pulmonary disease (COPD), endocrine disease, hepatitis, inflammatory bowel disease, and inflammatory skin conditions.

Inflammatory proteins, called cytokines, are involved in these immune-mediated inflammatory conditions. Tumor necrosis factor-α (TNF-α) is a cytokine that plays an especially important role in the inflammation and pathogenesis of IMIDs.

In rheumatoid arthritis, TNF-α has been identified in the rheumatoid fluid and synovial membranes and is involved in leukocyte recruitment, synovial inflammation, and cartilage degradation. In Crohn's disease, TNF-α and other proinflammatory cytokines are responsible for inflammation of the intestinal mucosa.

2. **c.** The combination of a psoriatic rash makes psoriasis the mostly likely cause of this patient's sausage finger. A small percentage of patients get the arthritis before the rash appears. Unlike rheumatoid arthritis, psoriatic arthritis tends to be asymmetrical, have spinal involvement, and have no joint nodules. Peripheral joint involvement may be minimal in distribution but may also be very aggressive.

3. **d.** Adalimumab and infliximab are anti-TNF-α agents that are FDA approved for the treatment of ankylosing spondylitis, Crohn's disease, psoriatic arthritis, and rheumatoid arthritis. Infliximab is also FDA approved for the treatment of plaque psoriasis and ulcerative colitis. Etanercept is an anti-TNF-α agent that is FDA approved for the treatment of ankylosing spondylitis, juvenile rheumatoid arthritis, psoriatic arthritis, and rheumatoid arthritis but not Crohn's disease. Anti-TNF therapies may prove to be effective in many more conditions in which TNF-α is involved in the pathogenesis.

Interleukin-1 is another proinflammatory cytokine associated with inflammatory joint destruction seen in rheumatoid arthritis. Anakinra (Kineret) is an interleukin-1 receptor antagonist that has been approved for the treatment of rheumatoid arthritis.

4. **d.** This patient has Addison's disease. Autoimmune destruction of the adrenal glands accounts for most cases of the disease. Adrenal hemorrhage or infarction and certain infections, metastatic cancers, and drugs are less common causes of primary adrenal insufficiency. The symptoms of adrenal insufficiency usually begin gradually. Chronic fatigue, muscle weakness, loss of appetite, and nausea are the most common symptoms. Weight loss, hypotension, and hypoglycemia are common signs. Hyperpigmentation can be noted in the buccal mucosa and the skin, particularly in palmar creases, at pressure points such as at the elbows and knees, in perianal mucosa, and around the nipples. Unstimulated cortisol levels should be done between 6 AM and 8 AM, although the results may be difficult to interpret if the patient is acutely ill. The synthetic adrenocorticotropic hormone (cosyntropin) stimulation test is the usual test for primary adrenal insufficiency.

In some cases, onset can be sudden. This is known as an Addisonian crisis and is a medical emergency. Symptoms include penetrating pain in the low back, abdomen, or legs; vomiting; diarrhea; hypotension; dehydration; and eventual loss of consciousness. Abnormal laboratory findings include hyperkalemia, hyponatremia, hypoglycemia, neutropenia, anemia, and elevated blood urea nitrogen and creatinine.

Treatment involves replacement of corticosteroid and mineralocorticoid hormones. If an Addisonian crisis is suspected, do not delay treatment while waiting for confirming laboratory results. The combination of Addison's disease with either autoimmune thyroid disease or type 1 autoimmune diabetes mellitus defines autoimmune polyglandular syndrome, type II (Schmidt syndrome). The type I version of autoimmune polyglandular syndrome (Whitaker's syndrome) is rare and consists of adrenal insufficiency, hypoparathyroidism, and candidiasis.

5. **a.** As noted previously, some infections can cause primary adrenal insufficiency. These infections include African trypanosomiasis, histoplasmosis, HIV, paracoccidiomycosis, syphilis, and tuberculosis but not infectious mononucleosis (Epstein–Barr virus).

6. **e.** This patient most likely has systemic lupus erythematosus (SLE), a multisystem autoimmune disease. Patients with SLE have been shown to have autoantibodies in their blood years before the symptoms of SLE appear. SLE is much more prevalent in females and usually presents in the childbearing years.

According to the American College of Rheumatology, the diagnosis of SLE is made when 4 or more of the following 11 criteria are present:

1. Malar (butterfly) rash
2. Discoid rash
3. Photosensitivity
4. Oral ulcers
5. Polyarthritis
6. Serositis (pleuritis or pericarditis)
7. Renal disorder (persistent proteinuria or cellular casts)
8. Neurologic disorder (seizures or psychosis)
9. Hematologic disorder (hemolytic anemia with reticulocytosis or leukopenia or thrombocytopenia)
10. Immunologic disorder (positive for anti-dsDNA antibody or anti-Sm antibody or anti-phospholipid antibody lupus anticoagulant or a false-positive serologic test for syphilis)
11. Positive anti-nuclear antibody

In addition to blood and urine tests, the workup should include chest radiography and an echocardiogram to screen for pleural effusions, pulmonary infiltrates, and pericardial effusion.

Treatment options include NSAIDs; antimalarials such as hydroxychloroquine; corticosteroids; and immunosuppressant medications such as azathioprine, cyclophosphamide, and methotrexate.

7. **e.** All of the listed conditions are potential ophthalmologic manifestations of systemic lupus erythematosus. Table 44-1 lists some ophthalmologic manifestations of some other autoimmune diseases.

Table 44-1 — Ophthalmologic Manifestations of Autoimmune Diseases

	Keratitis	Optic Neuropathy	Sicca Syndrome	Uveitis
Ankylosing spondylitis				X
Antiphospholipid syndrome		X		
Behçet's syndrome				X
Dermatomyositis				X
Enteropathic arthritis	X			X
Grave's disease	X			
Juvenile rheumatoid arthritis				X
Multiple sclerosis		X		
Polyarteritis nodosa		X		
Psoriatic arthritis	X			X
Reiter's syndrome	X			X
Rheumatoid arthritis	X		X	
Sarcoidosis		X		X
Sjögren's syndrome			X	
Systemic lupus erythematosus	X	X	X	X
Takayasu's arteritis		X		
Wegener's granulomatosis		X		X

8. b. Patients with rheumatoid arthritis have a positive ANA in approximately 40% of cases.

9. d. HLA-B27 has a sensitivity of greater than 90% in ankylosing spondylitis (AS), so a positive result in a patient with suggestive history and findings can help confirm the diagnosis. This test is also at least 50% sensitive in cases of spondylitis associated with Reiter's syndrome, psoriasis, and inflammatory bowel disease.

Rheumatoid factor should be negative, making AS a seronegative spondyloarthropathy. The pain of AS tends to be worse with rotation, side bending, and rest, whereas mechanical low back pain tends to be worse with flexion, extension, and activity. AS patients often suffer from morning back stiffness and may have bamboo spine and sacroiliitis on lumbosacral radiography.

10. The matching answers are as follows:
1. **f.**
2. **c.**
3. **i.**
4. **e.**
5. **g.**
6. **b.**
7. **k.**
8. **d.**
9. **j.**
10. **h.**
11. **a.**
12. **l.**

Summary

IMIDs are conditions characterized by abnormal immune function leading to acute or chronic inflammation. The conditions in this group share common inflammatory pathways. A broad range of diseases can be referred to as IMID, including some or all types of allergies, arthritis, asthma, cardiovascular disease, COPD, endocrine disease, inflammatory bowel disease, and inflammatory skin conditions. Within the realm of arthritic conditions there are three distinct main disease targets: Osteoarthritis primarily affects the articular cartilage, rheumatoid arthritis primarily affects the synovium, and seronegative spondyloarthropathies primarily affect the enthesis (the site where ligaments or tendons attach to bone).

Inflammatory proteins called cytokines are involved in these immune-mediated inflammatory conditions. TNF-α, a cytokine, plays an especially important role in the inflammation and pathogenesis. A broad range of medications, including anti-TNF-α, interleukin-1 receptor antagonists, monoclonal antibodies, and other agents targeting specific aspects of the inflammatory cascade, have been developed and are being used in some of the conditions listed. Corticosteroids are used in some of these conditions to help control inflammation. Their use may be acute or chronic. These medications may be delivered to the site of need in many different ways. Direct applications include topical creams, lotions, and ointments; nasal sprays; inhaled powders; and various forms per rectum. Corticosteroid treatment can also be systemic through oral or parenteral forms of medication.

NSAIDs are used in some cases to help control inflammation and in other cases for their analgesic effect.

Montelukast and zafirlukast are nonsteroidal agents that help control inflammation in asthma by acting as leukotriene receptor antagonists. Montelukast is also FDA approved for use in allergic rhinitis.

Suggested Reading

Anandarajah AP, Ritchlin CT: Treatment update on spondyloarthropathy: From NSAIDs and DMARDs to anti-TNF-alpha agents. *Postgrad Med* 116(5):31–40, 2004.

Arbuckle MR, McClain MT, Rubertone MV, et al: Development of autoantibodies before the clinical onset of systemic lupus erythematosus. *N Engl J Med* 349(16):1526–1533, 2003.

Dall'era M, Davis JC: Systemic lupus erythematosus: How to manage, when to refer. *Postgrad Med* 114(5):31–40, 2003.

Gill JM, Quisel AM, Rocca PV, et al: Diagnosis of systemic lupus erythematosus. *Am Fam Phys* 68(11):2179–2186, 2003.

Guidelines for referral and management of systemic lupus erythematosus in adults. American College of Rheumatology Ad Hoc Committee on Systemic Lupus Erythematosus Guidelines. *Arthritis Rheum* 42:1785–1796, 1999.

Lane SK, Gravel JW: Clinical utility of common serum rheumatologic tests. *Am Fam Phys* 65(6):1073–1080, 2002.

Luxon BA: Autoimmune hepatitis: Making sense of all those antibodies. *Postgrad Med* 114(1):79–88, 2003.

Majerone BA, Patel P: Autoimmune polyglandular syndrome, type II. *Am Fam Phys* 75(5):667–670, 2007.

Nieman LK: Causes of primary adrenal insufficiency (Addison's disease). In: Rose BD, ed., *UpToDate*. Waltham, MA: UpToDate, 2007.

Patel SJ, Lundy DC: Ocular manifestations of autoimmune disease. *Am Fam Phys* 66(6):991–998, 2002.

Rose NR: Overview of autoimmunity. In: Rose BD, ed., *UpToDate*. Waltham, MA: UpToDate, 2007.

Shanahan JC, Moreland LW, Carter RH: Upcoming biologic agents for the treatment of rheumatic diseases. *Curr Opin Rheumatol* 15(3):226–236, 2003.

CHAPTER 45

Human Immunodeficiency Virus Infection

CLINICAL CASE PROBLEM 1

A 25-Year-Old Pregnant Female Is Referred to You by the Obstetrics/Gynecology Clinic Because Her Rapid HIV Test Is Positive

A 25-year-old woman presents to her first obstetrics/gynecology (Ob/Gyn) appointment for a routine initial visit during which an Ora-Quick Advance rapid human immunodeficiency virus (HIV) test is performed and is determined to be positive. She is gravida 1 para 0, and her last menstrual period was 20 weeks ago. She has no complaints and is exuberant about her pregnancy. She is in a monogamous relationship with her husband and he presents to the Ob/Gyn appointment with her. She denies intravenous drug use (IVDU) or blood transfusion, and her only lifetime sexual partner is her husband. Her physical exam is unremarkable and consistent with an 18-week gestation. Her husband is taken to a separate room and denies IVDU, having sex with men, and states that he has been monogamous with his wife for the past 5 years. He states that he is feeling well and has no complaints. He agrees to a rapid HIV test, which is negative.

SELECT THE BEST ANSWER TO THE FOLLOWING QUESTIONS

1. Regarding the patient's positive test, the most appropriate next step is to
   a. advise the patient that she should begin antiretroviral medications to prevent HIV transmission to the baby
   b. perform a confirmatory HIV Western blot test
   c. advise the patient that she is likely to be HIV positive and should practice safe sex
   d. begin prenatal vitamins and refer to an Ob/Gyn clinic that specializes in the treatment of HIV-infected pregnant women
   e. do not give the patient any information until the confirmatory Western blot has been performed

2. Regarding rapid HIV tests, which of the following statements is true?
   a. since false positive rapid HIV tests are known to occur, rapid HIV tests should only be performed when the answer will alter the imminent medical management
   b. the positive predictive value of the rapid HIV test is dependent in part on the HIV prevalence of the population that is being tested

c. the sensitivity of all rapid HIV tests is similar and is approximately 80%

d. All rapid HIV tests must be repeated for confirmation

e. HIV enzyme immunoassay (EIA) results are more accurate than HIV rapid tests

3. According to the new Centers for Disease Control and Prevention (CDC) guidelines for HIV testing, which of the following persons should not have an HIV test performed as part of his or her routine health care?

a. 20-year-old homosexual male in a low HIV prevalence area (i.e., <0.1% HIV prevalence)

b. 35-year-old female in a monogamous relationship in an area where the prevalence of HIV is known to be >0.1%

c. 70-year-old woman who denies high-risk behavior for HIV infection but lives in a high HIV prevalence area

d. 55-year-old sexually active heterosexual male who reports two new sexual partners and had a negative HIV test 1 year ago

e. 70-year-old widower who is being treated for pulmonary tuberculosis (TB) and denies high-risk behavior for HIV infection

4. Which of the following statements regarding routine HIV testing is false according to the CDC guidelines for HIV testing?

a. HIV-positive patients who are aware of their diagnosis are more likely to reduce high-risk behavior for HIV transmission

b. specific signed HIV consent is not required by the CDC

c. HIV testing should be repeated in individuals who report recent HIV exposure and have a negative HIV test

d. HIV demographics have changed over the years, making risk-based HIV testing more difficult

e. all of the above are correct

Clinical Case Problem 2

A 25-Year-Old Male Presents for Initial HIV Evaluation

A 25-year-old white male was recently discharged from the hospital with a diagnosis of bacterial pneumonia. His past medical history is significant for a nephrectomy following a motor vehicle accident 10 years ago, aseptic meningitis 12 months ago, and one prior episode of bacterial pneumonia 5 months ago. His physical exam is remarkable for oral thrush.

In the hospital, an HIV EIA and Western blot returned positive. A CD4 T lymphocyte cell count was 30 and HIV RNA was greater than 100,000 copies/mL. His Venereal Disease Research Laboratory test (VDRL) returned positive 1:256 and a tuberculin skin test (TST) measured 8 mm of induration. His hemoglobin was 11.7 g/dL, and he had a white blood cell count of 4000 cells/mm^3 and platelet count of 70,000 cells/mm^3.

5. All of the following should be performed as part of an initial HIV workup except:

a. genotype

b. *Toxoplasma gondii* IgG

c. hepatitis C antibody

d. cytomegalovirus (CMV) IgG

e. cryptococcal antigen

6. Antiretroviral (ARV) medication should be recommended to this patient for which of the following reasons:

a. latent TB infection (LTBI)

b. syphilis

c. multiple episodes of pneumonia

d. his HIV RNA is greater than 100,000 copies/mL

e. all of the above

7. Which of the following conditions meets the criteria for an AIDS-defining opportunistic infection in this patient?

a. aseptic meningitis

b. syphilis

c. oral thrush

d. thrombocytopenia

e. none of the above

8. The patient and his partner present for a follow-up exam. They are concerned about HIV transmission from the patient to his partner. The partner recently tested HIV negative. Which of the following is (are) reasonable advice to give?

a. the partner should have a repeat HIV test performed in 3 months

b. practices that increase the likelihood of blood contact, such as sharing of razors and toothbrushes, should be avoided

c. risks associated with specific sexual behaviors and the role of abstinence or risk reduction should be discussed

d. casual contact through closed-mouth kissing is not a risk for transmission of HIV

e. all of the above are reasonable recommendations

9. You review baseline lab results with the patient. Results are as follows: CMV IgG negative, *T. gondii* IgG positive, TST skin test 8 mm of induration,

hepatitis A IgM negative and IgG positive, hepatitis BSAg negative, hepatitis BSAb negative, and hepatitis CAb positive. Which of the following actions should be taken?
a. pneumovax immunization deferred until CD4 is greater than 200 cells/mm³
b. isoniazid prescription once a chest radiograph is performed and is normal
c. refer to ophthalmology for CMV screening
d. azithromycin 600 mg orally once a day
e. all of the above

CLINICAL CASE PROBLEM 3

A 32-Year-Old African American Female Presents with an Acute Retroviral Syndrome

A 32-year-old African American female comes to your office with a fever, lymphadenopathy, headache, and pharyngitis. Physical exam demonstrates oral thrush and hepatosplenomegaly. The patient reports unprotected sex with a bisexual male, and you suspect that this patient may have acute retroviral syndrome.

10. Which of the following signs and symptoms occur(s) with a frequency of greater than 75% in this syndrome?
a. diarrhea
b. fever
c. headache
d. hepatosplenomegaly
e. all of the above

11. What laboratory test is most useful in establishing the diagnosis of an acute retroviral syndrome in this patient?
a. mono spot test
b. gp 41 antigen
c. HIV RNA
d. HIV rapid test
e. HIV EIA

12. Regarding the acute retroviral syndrome, which of the following statements is true?
a. syphilis should be considered in the differential diagnosis
b. patients are generally less infectious during this time
c. an HIV RNA viral load of more than 500 copies/mL is diagnostic of acute retroviral syndrome
d. acute retroviral syndrome is seen infrequently—less than 30% of the time
e. The time from HIV exposure to the acute retroviral syndrome is 5 to 7 days

13. According to the CDC, which of the following messages regarding transmission of HIV from HIV-positive persons is true?
a. oral sex is not associated with HIV transmission
b. having sex with an person with undetectable HIV RNA is not associated with HIV transmission
c. the relative risk of receptive anal intercourse is 10 times higher than the risk of insertive fellatio (penile–oral sex)
d. the relative risk of HIV transmission without condom use is 20 times higher than that with condom use
e. none of the above

14. What is the most common cause of meningitis in a patient with advanced AIDS?
a. cytomegalovirus
b. herpes simplex
c. coccidioidomycosis
d. toxoplasmosis
e. *Cryptococcus*

15. The ideal time to discontinue secondary prophylaxis is present in all of the following scenarios except? (Assume that all of the patients are on an effective highly active antiretroviral therapy (HAART) regimen.)
a. patient with a history of PCP pneumonia and CD4 cell count that has increased to more than 200 cells/mm³ for 6 months
b. patient with disseminated *Mycobacterium avium* complex (MAC) whose CD4 cell count has increased to greater than 100 cells/mm³ for 6 months and who has completed 12 months of effective MAC therapy
c. patient with central nervous system (CNS) toxoplasmosis whose CD4 cell count has been greater than 200 cells/mm³ for 6 months and has completed his initial therapy for CNS toxoplasmosis
d. patient with coccidioidomycosis meningitis whose CD4 cell count has increased to greater than 200 cells/mm³ for 6 months and has completed initial therapy for coccidioidomycosis
e. patients with cryptococcal meningitis whose CD4 cell count has increased to greater than 200 cells/mm³ for 3 months and has completed initial therapy for cryptococcal meningitis

16. A 25-year-old asymptomatic person with HIV infection is diagnosed with chronic active hepatitis B. His CD4 count is 530 cells/mm³ and HIV RNA is 12,400 copies/mL. Which of the following treatments for hepatitis B is an appropriate option?

a. lamivudine
b. tenofovir
c. adefovir
d. entecavir
e. emtriva

17. The metabolic complication(s) implicated with treatment of HIV infection with HAART includes
    a. osteoporosis
    b. insulin resistance/diabetes
    c. lipoatrophy
    d. lipohypertrophy
    e. all of the above

18. Regarding drug interactions, which of the following statements is true?
    a. the dose of rifabutin should be increased when given concomitantly with kaletra
    b. the dose of kaletra should be increased when given with dilantin
    c. simvastin and kaletra may be given without dose adjustment
    d. zidovudine and zerit are antagonistic and should not be used together
    e. atazanavir and proton pump inhibitors may be used together as long as they are administered 12 hours apart

19. Which of the following scenarios places the health care worker at the highest risk for HIV transmission?
    a. A large amount of vomitus from a patient with AIDS is spewed onto non-intact skin. The patient's last HIV RNA was greater than 750,000 copies/mL 1 week ago.
    b. An HIV patient jerks while an arterial blood gas needle is inserted into the radial artery. The needle is accidentally stuck into the thigh of the physician drawing the blood. The patient has been diagnosed with the acute retroviral syndrome and a HIV RNA is pending.
    c. The gloved hand of a physician is accidentally stuck while withdrawing a spinal needle from a spinal tap procedure on a HIV patient. The patient's last HIV RNA was 30,000 copies/mL 6 months ago.
    d. After performing a bimanual exam on a HIV-positive patient, the glove on the physician's hand is noted to be broken. Her last HIV RNA was greater than 750,000 copies/mL.
    e. A needle stick injury occurs on the gloved hand of a physician who is suturing a laceration in a HIV patient. One week ago, the patient's last HIV RNA was greater than 750,000 copies/mL.

20. A patient is diagnosed with disseminated Cryptococcus and has positive cerebrospinal fluid (CSF), blood, and urine cultures for *Cryptococcus*. His CD4 is 10 and HIV RNA is greater 750,000 copies/mL. Which of the following statements is (are) true?
    a. one of the criteria for discontinuing diflucan suppressive therapy is a negative CSF cryptococcal serum antigen
    b. early therapy with prednisone has demonstrated a survival advantage
    c. increased intracranial pressure is associated with increased mortality
    d. all of the above are true
    e. none of the above are true

21. Which of the following AIDS-associated malignancies is least associated with immunosuppression (low CD4)?
    a. Kaposi's sarcoma
    b. systemic high-grade B cell lymphoma, immunoblastic
    c. primary lymphoma of the brain
    d. invasive cervical cancer
    e. systemic high-grade B cell lymphoma, Burkitt's lymphoma

Answers

1. **b.** All positive HIV rapid tests require confirmation with a confirmatory Western blot or immunofluorescent assay (IFA). Performing an HIV EIA is not required, but if it is performed and the results are negative, a confirmatory test is still required. For persons with a negative or indeterminate confirmatory test, follow-up HIV testing should be repeated 4 weeks after the initial positive rapid HIV test. Prior to performing a rapid test, patients should be counseled that they will receive the results at the same visit and, if positive, the meaning of a preliminary positive result. In the event of a positive rapid HIV test result, the provider should emphasize the importance of confirmatory testing. Providers should collect blood or saliva for the confirmatory test at the same visit and schedule an appointment for results of the confirmatory test. In 2006, the Food and Drug Administration (FDA) approved a new test, Aptima, for the diagnosis of primary HIV-1 infection, as well as for confirming HIV-1 infection when tests for antibodies to HIV-1 are positive. Aptima is a qualitative nucleic acid test that detects the RNA of HIV-1 infection and may be used as an alternative to the Western blot for confirmation. Aptima may be helpful to diagnose early HIV-1 infections before antibodies have developed, as well

as in cases in which the Western blot is indeterminate. The patient in Clinical Case Problem 1 should be counseled that there is a chance that her positive HIV rapid test could be a false positive as well as about risk reduction behaviors while awaiting the results of the Western blot. The patient and her husband had confirmatory HIV tests performed, and both were negative, including a repeat HIV test performed 4 weeks later.

2. b. Rapid HIV tests are an important tool to assess for early HIV infection in high-prevalence areas for high-risk individuals and for women in labor and delivery as well as other nontraditional settings. Rapid HIV tests have also been employed in emergency departments, inpatient hospital settings, correctional facilities, and for occupational exposures. In 2000, the CDC estimated that 31% of individuals who tested at a public-sector testing site did not return for HIV test results. There are four rapid HIV tests that have been approved by the FDA and share many common features. In all of these tests, HIV antigens are affixed to the test membrane or test strip. If the patient has HIV antibodies present, the antibodies will bind to the affixed HIV antigens. No instrumentation is required for these tests, and the tests are interpreted by visual inspection. When used according to the manufacturer's guidelines, these tests range in sensitivity from 99.3% to 100% and specificity from 98.6% to 99.9% and are similar to HIV EIA. False positive results are known to occur and are measured by the positive predictive value (PPV), which is the probability that the patient has the disease if the test is positive. PPV will decrease if the prevalence of HIV is low and will increase if the prevalence of HIV is high. All positive rapid HIV tests require confirmatory Western blot or IFA. However, a negative rapid HIV test does not require confirmation. False negative rapid HIV tests occur rarely and may be seen during acute HIV infection and before HIV antibodies have developed. Individuals with HIV exposure within 3 months prior should be instructed to retest at 6, 12, and 24 weeks after HIV exposure.

3. c. According to the CDC guidelines, all persons between the ages of 13 and 64 years should be screened for HIV as part of routine clinical care unless HIV prevalence has been documented to be less than 0.1%. Patients seeking care for treatment of sexually transmitted diseases as well as patients initiating TB treatment should also receive an HIV test. Annual HIV testing should be performed on all individuals with high-risk behavior for HIV infection; these include injection drug users and their partners, persons who exchange sex for drugs or money, men who have sex with men, and heterosexuals who have had more than one partner since their last HIV test.

4. e. In 2006, the CDC published new guidelines for HIV testing. The reasons for the new guidelines were to increase screening and early detection of HIV infection, link HIV-infected patients to earlier care and prevention, and reduce perinatal transmission. One rationale for implementing these new guidelines is the changing demographics of HIV-positive individuals. The rate of HIV infection is increasing in adolescents (15- to 24-year-olds), adults (50- to 64-year-olds), heterosexual men and women, members of racial and ethnic minorities, and individuals who live outside of metropolitan areas. Other reasons for the new HIV testing guidelines include prior success with universal testing of the blood supply and routine HIV testing in perinatal clinics. However, reduction in sexual transmission of HIV has been disappointing throughout the years. HIV-unknown individuals account for a disproportionate rate of sexual transmission compared with HIV-positive individuals who are aware of their diagnosis. According to a meta-analysis of eight studies, HIV-positive individuals have been shown to reduce unprotected vaginal or anal intercourse by an average of 68%. The CDC guidelines recommend HIV opt-out testing. Patients must be counseled in writing or verbally that a HIV test is planned and agree to the test. Oral and written material should be provided regarding the meaning of a positive and a negative HIV test result, and the patient should have an opportunity to ask questions. A signed HIV consent is no longer recommended by the CDC. For patients declining the HIV test, documentation of the refusal should be recorded. Informed consent for an HIV test is no longer a recommendation by the CDC, but many states have legislation that requires informed consent. Some states are working on legislation to reconcile the differences between the CDC recommendations and current legislation.

5. e. Initial laboratory evaluation of a new HIV-positive patient should include an HIV antibody test (if one is not available); CD4 T lymphocyte cell count; plasma HIV RNA; complete blood count; chemistry profile; transaminase levels; blood urea nitrogen; creatinine; urinalysis; rapid plasma reagin or VDRL; TST (unless there is a history of prior tuberculosis or positive skin test); *T. gondii* IgG; hepatitis A, B, and C serologies; and cervical Pap smear in women. The CD4 T lymphocyte cell count is part of the HIV staging system and identifies those patients at higher risk for life-threatening opportunistic infections. Prophylaxis for opportunistic infections is based on results of the CD4 T lymphocyte cell count. HIV RNA has been shown to be a prognostic indicator of HIV disease progression and is used to monitor response to ARV medications. Fasting blood glucose and lipids are recommended for those at risk for cardiovascular disease and for baseline evaluation prior to initiation of ARV medications. The HIV genotype test has become part of the initial HIV evaluation since transmission of HIV-resistant virus has been documented and associated with suboptimal response to initial ARV medications. The genotype assays detect mutations in the reverse transcriptase and protease portions of the genome. These mutations predict resistance to specific antiretroviral drugs and can influence the choice of initial ARV therapy. HIV genotype tests should be performed on those with HIV RNA greater than 1000 copies/mL, even if ARV therapy will be deferred. HIV genotyping should not be performed in those individuals with HIV RNA less than 1000 copies/mL because amplification of the virus is unreliable. The International AIDS Society–USA maintains a list of significant resistance-associated mutations that can be reviewed at www.iasusa.org. The cryptococcal antigen test is a latex agglutination test that measures cryptococcal polysaccharide antigen and should be reserved for symptomatic patients.

6. **c.** ARV medications should be initiated for any HIV-positive person with any AIDS-defining illness or severe symptoms of HIV infection regardless of CD4 T lymphocyte cell count or any asymptomatic HIV-positive person with CD4 T lymphocyte cell count of less than 200 cells/mm^3. There is strong evidence of improved survival and reduced disease progression in this group of individuals. ARV medication should be offered to asymptomatic HIV-positive persons with CD4 T lymphocyte cell count of 201 to 350 cells/mm^3. The optimal time to begin ARV medications is unknown, but most specialists recommend beginning ARV therapy in HIV-positive persons with a CD4 T lymphocyte cell count of 201 to 350 cells/mm^3 based on the risk of disease progression as determined by observational cohorts. For asymptomatic HIV-positive persons with CD4 T lymphocyte cell count greater than 350 cells/mm^3 and HIV RNA greater than 100,000 copies/mL, most clinicians will defer therapy; however, it is important to individualize whether or not to start ARV therapy because each situation is different. Recurrent bacterial pneumonia is one of the AIDS-defining opportunistic infections and would be an indication to begin ARV therapy. In addition, the patient's CD4 T lymphocyte cell count is 30, which also meets criteria to begin ARV therapy.

7. **e.** Oral thrush, aseptic meningitis, and thrombocytopenia may be examples of symptomatic HIV infection but are not AIDS-defining diagnosis. Other examples of symptomatic HIV infection include vulvovaginal candidiasis, cervical dysplasia, and constitutional symptoms such as fever or diarrhea for more than 1 month and oral leukoplakia. The AIDS-defining opportunistic infections are as follows:

- Candidiasis; esophagus, trachea, or bronchi
- Coccidioidomycosis; extrapulmonary
- Cryptococcosis; extrapulmonary
- Cervical cancer; invasive
- Cryptosporidiosis, chronic intestinal (>1 month)
- CMV disease retinitis, or CMV in other than liver, spleen, nodes
- HIV encephalopathy
- Herpes simplex virus infection with mucocutaneous ulcer for >1 month, bronchitis, pneumonia
- Histoplasmosis; disseminated
- Isoporiasis, >1 month
- Kaposi's sarcoma
- Lymphoma; primary CNS, Burkitt's, immunoblastic
- *Mycobacterium avium intracellulare* (MAC or MAI), extrapulmonary
- *Mycobacterium kansasii*, extrapulmonary
- *Mycobacterium tuberculosis*, pulmonary or extrapulmonary
- *Pneumocystis jirovecii* pneumonia (formerly *Pneumocystis carinii* pneumonia)
- Pneumonia, two or more episodes in 1 year
- Progressive multifocal leukoencephalopathy
- Salmonella bacteremia, recurrent
- Toxoplasmosis, cerebral
- Wasting syndrome

8. **e.** All of these recommendations are appropriate. The patient's partner should have a repeat HIV test performed in 3 months since he could have recently been infected and still have a negative HIV test result. Practices that increase the likelihood of blood contact, such as sharing of razors and toothbrushes, should be avoided. Gloves should be worn during contact with blood or other body fluids that could possibly contain blood. Casual contact through closed-mouth or "social" kissing is not a risk for transmission of HIV. High-risk sexual practices include unprotected anal receptive intercourse and unprotected vaginal receptive intercourse. HIV infection has been documented to occur in unprotected anal insertive intercourse, unprotected vaginal insertive intercourse, unprotected oral receptive intercourse, and unprotected oral insertive intercourse. Lower HIV transmission risk has been attributed to the use of latex/vinyl condoms.

The patient and partner should be advised of the risk of HIV transmission through sexual contact including ways to lower these risks of HIV transmission.

9. **b.** Although some immunizations in the HIV-infected population are still controversial, the risk of vaccination is minimal and may provide benefit. HIV-positive patients with CD4 less than 200 cells/mm³ are less likely to mount an effective humoral response to pneumovax, but the vaccination is safe and should be given. Once the CD4 cell count is greater than 200 cells/mm³, pneumococcal vaccination may be repeated. Pneumovax should be given every 5 years. Other recommended vaccinations are influenza vaccine (every year) and tetanus–diphtheria–acellular pertussis (once) or the diphtheria–tetanus booster vaccine (every 10 years). Hepatitis A and B vaccine series should be administered if hepatitis A IgG is negative and hepatitis B surface antibody is negative, respectively. Live virus vaccines such as oral polio or varicella-zoster vaccine are contraindicated. Human papillomavirus vaccination series for HIV-positive women between the ages of 11 and 26 years is recommended. The patient's TST is positive because it measures greater than 5 mm of induration. He is considered to have LTBI and should be treated with a 9-month regimen of isoniazid along with pyridoxine after TB has been excluded. The evaluation should include a review of symptoms with a focus on pulmonary and extrapulmonary forms of TB. A physical exam should be performed to evaluate the patient for lymphadenopathy, draining fistulas, localized bone pain, or hepatosplenomegaly. Further diagnostic testing should be performed based on the symptoms and physical exam. A chest radiograph is required for all patients with LTBI. Referral to an ophthalmologist for screening for CMV retinitis is part of HIV primary care for HIV-positive patients with a positive CMV IgG and a CD4 cell count less than 50 cells/mm³. Finally, all patients with a CD4 cell count less than 200 cells/mm³ require PCP prophylaxis, and Septra DS every 24 hours is an appropriate regimen if the patient is not allergic to sulfa drugs. Another infection requiring prophylaxis in this patient is prophylaxis against MAC. Options for MAC prophylaxis include azithromycin 1200 mg every week or clarithromycin 500 mg every 12 hours. Prophylaxis is also indicated for HIV-positive patients with CD4 cell count less than 100 cells/mm³ and positive *T. gondii* IgG. Septra will provide prophylaxis against both PCP and *T. gondii*. For the sulfa allergic patient, a regimen containing dapsone, pyrimethamine, and leucovorin is an option.

10. **b.** The most common symptoms seen in the acute retroviral syndrome are fever, lymphadenopathy, pharyngitis, and myalgias/arthralgias—all seen in more than 75% of cases. Other common symptoms include maculopapular rash, nausea, vomiting, and diarrhea. Up to 50% of patients will experience severe headaches and may have signs of meningitis or encephalitis.

11. **c.** The acute retroviral syndrome is frequently associated with a high HIV RNA; usually in the range of 1×10^5 to 10^8 copies/mL. The standard HIV EIA and Western blot may remain negative for several weeks after seroconversion. High P24 antigen levels may be present and could also be useful in this scenario. A mono spot test does not establish the diagnosis but may be performed to exclude Epstein–Barr virus (EBV) mononucleosis. Other common laboratory abnormalities seen include thrombocytopenia, lymphopenia, lymphocytosis, and transaminitis.

12. **a.** The differential diagnosis of acute retroviral syndrome should include EBV mononucleosis, CMV mononucleosis, toxoplasmosis, rubella, viral hepatitis, syphilis, primary herpes simplex virus infection, and drug reactions. An acute retroviral syndrome should be considered in any patient for whom you are considering EBV mononucleosis and in whom the mono spot test is negative. Patients tend to have high HIV RNA levels during acute retroviral syndrome and are highly infectious from either sexual activity or sharing needles. False positive HIV RNA levels have been reported in approximately 5% of patients who were tested and should be suspected when the HIV RNA is less than 1000 copies/mL. Acute retroviral syndrome symptoms occur in 50% to 90% of patients and usually last 1 or 2 weeks and infrequently up to 10 weeks. The time from HIV exposure to symptoms is usually 2 to 6 weeks.

13. **d.** Providing the relative risk associated with specific sex acts and condom use to HIV-positive persons allows the individuals to compare personal choices of sex acts and condom use. The absolute risk of insertive fellatio (penile–oral sex) is estimated to be 1 per 20,000 exposures. The relative risks of sex acts are as follows: insertive fellatio 1, receptive fellatio 2×, insertive vaginal sex 10×, receptive vaginal sex 20×, insertive anal sex 13×, and receptive anal sex 100×. Sex with the use of a condom is 1×, whereas sex without the use of a condom is 20×. The risks of these choices are multiplicative. For example, insertive fellatio with the use of a condom is 1 (1 × 1), whereas the risk of receptive anal sex without the use of a condom is 2000× (20 × 100). Although insertive fellatio has a relative risk of 1, there are well-documented reports of HIV transmission through unprotected oral sex. HIV transmission is reduced when the HIV RNA declines, but it is known that genital secretions may be a protected compartment for HIV that is not reflected by the serum HIV RNA. The relative risk based on HIV RNA is as follows: less than 3500 copies/mL, 1; 3500 to 9999 copies/mL, 5.8×; 10,000 to 49,999 copies/mL, 6.91×; and greater than 50,000 copies/mL, 11.87×.

14. **e.** Cryptococcal meningitis is the most common fungal infection of the CNS, most commonly presenting as meningitis. Cryptococcus may also cause a space-occupying mass or meningoencephalitis. The majority of cases develop when the CD4 cell count is less than 50 cells/mm^3, and it is the initial AIDS-defining illness in 50% to 60% of patients. The prevalence of herpes simplex meningitis ranges from 0.5% to 3.9%. Herpes simplex type 1 or 2 may be responsible for CNS disease (in the form of either meningitis or encephalitis) and is most commonly diagnosed in patients with advanced AIDS. CMV infection usually presents as an encephalitis or ventriculitis and will occasionally involve the meninges. Meningitis due to coccidioidomycosis is most commonly diagnosed in persons who live in endemic areas, mostly the southwestern United States, areas of Mexico, and Central and South America. The incidence of coccidioidomycosis varies from year to year, which may be related to weather patterns. Coccidioidomycosis disproportionately affects HIV-infected persons. Toxoplasmosis is the leading cause of focal CNS disease and is seen in 3% to 10% of patients with AIDS; it is rarely associated with meningitis.

15. **d.** Patients with coccidioidomycosis are recommended to receive lifelong suppression with fluconazole or itraconzaole. There are insufficient data to determine if prophylaxis can be discontinued safely. Discontinuation of secondary prophylaxis is recommended for PCP pneumonia after immune reconstitution with HAART and the CD4 cell count has been greater than 200 cells/mm^3 for more than 3 months. Options for PCP prophylaxis are trimethoprim-sulfa, dapsone, dapsone plus pyrimethamine, atovaquone, or aerosolized pentamidine. Prophylaxis for MAC in patients with disseminated MAC disease may be discontinued once 12 months of MAC therapy has been provided and immune reconstitution with HAART has occurred and the CD4 cell count is greater than 100 cells/mm^3 for 6 months or longer. Prophylaxis for CNS toxoplasmosis may be discontinued after a patient has completed a 6-week treatment course for CNS toxoplasmosis and immune reconstitution with HAART has occurred with a sustained increased in CD4 cell count greater than 200 cells/mm^3 for more than 6 months. Patients with cryptococcal meningitis who have completed initial therapy for cryptococcosis may have fluconazole

prophylaxis discontinued when the CD4 cell count is greater than 100 to 200 cells/mm^3 for 6 months after initiating HAART.

16. **c.** It is estimated that chronic hepatitis B affects approximately 10% of HIV-infected patients. Fibrosis progresses faster in persons co-infected with HIV and hepatitis B. For all patients co-infected with HIV/hepatitis B, anti-hepatitis B therapy should be considered. Lamivudine (Epivir, 3TC), emtricitabine (Emtriva, FTC), and tenofovir (Viread, TDF) are all HIV medications that also have activity against hepatitis B and are ideal medications for patients who also require HIV therapy. However, these drugs should be used in combination and as part of a HAART regimen to ensure adequate HIV viral suppression. For co-infected patients who do not require HIV therapy, adefovir dipivoxil (Hepsera and Preveon), interferon (IFN)-α2b, and pegylated IFN-α2a are options since they have anti-hepatitis B activity alone and will preserve HIV medications for future use. Entecavir (Baraclude) is a nucleoside/nucleotide medication that was reported to be associated with the M184V mutation in three patients in whom entecavir was used as monotherapy. M184V confers resistance to Epivir and Emtriva and reduces future options for ARV therapy. Previously, entecavir was thought to have no clinically relevant activity against HIV. As a result, entecavir is no longer recommended as monotherapy for HIV and hepatitis B co-infected persons.

17. **e.** HIV infection and HAART have been implicated in adverse metabolic effects that include alterations of glucose and lipid metabolism, lactic acidosis, osteopenia, osteoporosis, and abnormal fat distribution. These adverse effects create concern for many patients on HAART and are reasons that patients give for stopping HAART or refusing to initiate HAART. In addition, concerns raised have been raised regarding other long-term risks, including the risk of cardiovascular disease.

18. **d.** A major challenge for HIV physicians and pharmacists is to recognize and manage drug interactions. Often, HIV-infected patients are receiving multiple medications with known or potential adverse drug interactions. The cytochrome P450 enzyme system consists of many enzymes, including CYP1, CYP2, and CYP3, which are responsible for drug metabolism. The CYP3A is involved in the metabolism of a large number of drugs including protease inhibitors. Drugs may be inhibitors, inducers, or substrates of the CYP3A enzyme. Rifabutin is a substrate and kaletra, a protease inhibitor (PI), is an inhibitor of CYP3A. As a result, the levels of rifabutin will increase when the drugs are used together. One recommendation is to reduce the dose of rifabutin from the normal dose of 300 mg once per day to 150 mg once every 48 hours. Dilantin is a potent inducer of the cytochrome P450 system and will reduce the levels of kaletra, which is also a substrate for cytochrome P450. Dilantin levels may be affected by this combination. It is recommended that dilantin and kaletra combinations be avoided. This is also true for dilantin and all of the other PIs. The area under the curve (AUC) for simvastatin, a substrate of cytochrome P450, is greatly increased when simvastatin and kaletra are given together. The risk for myopathy and rhabdomyolsis is increased when simvastatin and kaletra are combined, and this drug combination should be avoided. Atazanavir solubility decreases as gastric pH increases. Coadministration of omeprazole and atazanavir has been demonstrated to reduce atazanavir AUC by 76% and should be avoided. All proton pump inhibitor medications should be avoided when atazanavir is prescribed. However, H_2-blockers may be prescribed with atazanavir when atazanavir is taken with food and 2 hours before and at least 10 hours after the H_2-blocker. Zidovudine competitively inhibits the intracellular phosphorylation of stavudine, and the two drugs are antagonistic and should not be used together.

19. b. In prospective studies of health care workers, the average risk of HIV transmission after a percutaneous exposure to HIV-infected blood has been estimated to be approximately 0.3%, and it is 0.09% after a mucous membrane exposure. HIV transmission after exposure to non-intact skin has been documented, but the risk is considerably lower than for blood exposure. Epidemiologic studies suggest that several factors may affect the risk of HIV transmission after an exposure. These factors and estimated odds ratio of increased risk are deep injury (16×), visible blood on device (5.2×), procedure involving a needle in the artery or vein (5.1×), terminal illness of the patient (6.4×), and postexposure use of zidovudine (0.2×). Biologic fluids that are infectious include blood, seminal secretions, vaginal secretions, CSF, synovial fluid, pleural fluid, peritoneal fluid, pericardial fluid, and amniotic fluid. Biologic fluids that are not considered infectious include feces, nasal secretions, saliva, sputum, sweat, tears, urine, and vomitus.

20. c. The early mortality for cryptococcal meningitis with treatment is estimated to be 10% to 25% and is fatal if not treated. The current recommended therapy for cryptococcal meningitis is 2 weeks of IV amphotericin 0.7 mg/kg/day and oral flucytosine 25 mg/kg in four divided doses. Maintenance therapy with oral fluconazole 400 mg per day for 10 weeks followed by oral fluconazole 200 mg/day is recommended after the IV amphotericin and oral flucytosine combination has been completed. The cryptococcal serum antigen is useful for diagnosis of cryptococcal infections but does not play a role in the management or decision to discontinue maintenance therapy. According the current recommendations from the CDC, the National Institutes of Health, and HIV Medicine Association/Infectious Diseases Society of America, discontinuation of maintenance therapy can be considered in patients who have completed initial therapy for cryptococcosis, have experienced immune reconstitution as a consequence of HAART, remain asymptomatic, and have a sustained increase (i.e., >6 months) in their CD4 T lymphocyte cell counts of 100 to 200 cell/mm³ after HAART. Increased intracranial pressure is a common problem and may be responsible for clinical worsening despite a microbiologic improvement. Patients with higher baseline opening pressures (>250 mmH₂O) are more likely to die than patients with lower baseline opening pressures (<190 mmH₂O). It is recommended that the opening pressure be measured when a lumbar puncture is performed, and if elevated, CSF should be removed. Lumbar punctures may be required daily and some patients may require placement of shunts for management. Prednisone plays no role in the treatment of cryptococcosis and may be harmful.

21. d. There is clear evidence that the precursor lesions to invasive cervical cancer, cervical intraepithelial neoplasia, or squamous intraepithelial lesion are present more frequently in HIV-positive women. Meta-analysis has demonstrated a four- to sixfold increase in the risk of cervical cancer for women infected with HIV. However, there is no clear relationship between the risk of cervical cancer and either CD4 cell count or progression to AIDS. Although there has been no decline in cervical cancer since the HAART era, some studies have demonstrated improvement in preinvasive lesions for women on HAART. Since the introduction of HAART, there has been a decrease in the incidence of Kaposi's sarcoma (KS). HAART has demonstrated a protective effect against the development of KS in a large cohort study. For patients with established KS, HAART has been associated with prolongation of the time to treatment failure as well as improvement in survival. These findings suggest a correlation between KS and immunosuppression. For high-grade non-Hodgkin's lymphoma (NHL), meta-analysis of cohort studies demonstrates a decrease in the incidence since HAART was begun. HAART appears to have a protective effect, and there is an association between NHL and immunosuppresion. Overall survival is improved for patients with NHL who are placed on HAART.

Suggested Reading

Benson CA, Kaplan JE, Masur H, et al: Treating opportunistic infections among HIV-infected adults and adolescents. *MMWR* 53(RR15): 1–112, 2004.

Branson BM, Handsfield HH, Lampe MA, et al: Revised recommendations for HIV testing of adults, adolescents, and pregnant women in health care settings. *MMWR* 55(RR14):1–17, 2006.

Bower M, Mazhar D, Stebbing J: Should cervical cancer be an acquired immunodeficiency-defining cancer? *J Clin Oncol* 24(16):2417–2419, 2006.

Cohen DE, Mayer KH: Primary care issues for HIV-infected patients. *Infect Dis Clin North Am* 21(1):49–70, 2007.

Crowe SM, Carlin JB, Stewart KI: Predictive value of CD4 lymphocyte numbers for the development of opportunistic infections and malignancies in HIV-infected persons. *J AIDS* 4(8):770–776, 1991.

Department of Health and Human Services: *Guidelines for the Use of Antiretroviral Agents in HIV-1-Infected Adults and Adolescents.* Accessed June 8, 2007. Available at http://aidsinfo.nih.gov.

Entecavir: A new nucleoside analogue for the treatment of chronic hepatitis B. *PMID* 17460784.

Greenwald JL, Burstein GR, Pincus J, Branson B: A rapid review of rapid HIV antibody tests. *Curr Infect Dis Rep* 8:125–131, 2006.

Incorporating HIV prevention into the medical care of persons living with HIV. Recommendations of CDC, the Health Resources and Services Administration, the National Institutes of Health, and the HIV Medicine Association of the Infectious Diseases Society of America. *MMWR* 52(RR12):1–24, 2003.

International AIDS Society–USA. Available at www.iasusa.org/resistance_mutations.

Marks G, Crepaz N, Janssen RS: Estimating sexual transmission of HIV from persons aware and unaware that they are infected with the virus in the USA. *AIDS* 20:1447–1450, 2006.

McMahon MA, Jilek BL, Brennan TP, et al: The HBV drug entecavir—Effects on HIV-1 replication and resistance. *N Engl J Med* 356(25):2614–2621, 2007.

Schambelan M, Benson CA, Carr A, et al: Management of metabolic complications associated with antiretroviral therapy for HIV-1 infection: Recommendations of an International AIDS Society–USA panel. *J AIDS* 31:257–275, 2002.

Thio CL, Locarnini S: Treatment of HIV/HBV coinfection: Clinical and virologic issues. *AIDS Rev* 9(1):40–53, 2007.

Note: HIV management is rapidly changing. Stay up-to-date by accessing Web-based information sources, including the following:

http://aidsinfo.nih.gov/guidelines (the U.S. Department of Health and Human Services/National Institutes of Health Web site with up-to-date treatment guidelines for adults and children)

http://aidsinfo.nih.gov/PDATools/Default.aspx?MenuItem=AIDSinfo Tools (provides tools that can be downloaded to PDAs)

http://hopkins-aids.edu/publications/pocketguide/pocketgd0106.pdf (a pocket guide Adult HIV/AIDS Treatment)

http://sis.nlm.nih.gov/hiv.html (the National Library of Medicine special information services site with excellent links to everywhere and everything you might ever want to know)

www.aids-etc.org (AIDS Education and Training Centers National Resource Center Web site)

www.cdc.gov/hiv/pubs/facts.htm (the CDC site with useful information regarding epidemiology and prevention)

www.hopkins-aids.edu (see the online educational resource, Medical Management of HIV Infection 2003, by Bartlett and Gallant, from the Johns Hopkins University AIDS Service)

www.iasusa.org/resistance_mutations/mutations_figures.pdf (a guide for HIV-1 drug-resistance mutations)

CHAPTER

46 Multiple Sclerosis

CLINICAL CASE PROBLEM 1

A 27-Year-Old Female with Weakness, Visual Loss, Ataxia, and Sensory Loss

A 27-year-old female comes to your office for assessment of symptoms including weakness; visual loss; bladder incontinence; sharp, shooting pain in the lower back; clumsiness when walking; and sensory loss. These symptoms have occurred during three episodes (different combinations of symptoms each time) approximately 3 months apart, and each episode lasted approximately 3 days.

The first episode consisted of weakness, bladder incontinence, and sharp shooting pains in the lower back (in both hip girdles). The second episode consisted of visual loss, clumsiness when walking, and sensory loss. The third episode (last week) consisted of sharp, shooting pains in the lower back and sensory loss (bilateral) in the upper extremities.

On neurologic examination, you find the following: swelling of the optic disc on funduscopy, inability to walk heel to toe, and slight objective weakness of both hip girdles. She has no symptoms today.

SELECT THE BEST ANSWER TO THE FOLLOWING QUESTIONS

1. Given this information, what is the most likely diagnosis in this patient?
   a. amyotrophic lateral sclerosis
   b. multiple sclerosis (MS)
   c. vitamin B$_{12}$ deficiency
   d. hysterical conversion reaction
   e. tertiary syphilis

2. There are four clinical categories of this disease. Which of the following subtypes does the patient presented fit into?
   a. relapsing–remitting
   b. secondary progressive
   c. primary progressive
   d. progressive relapsing
   e. none of the above

3. If you had the opportunity to do only one diagnostic test, which of the following would you choose?
   a. computed tomography scan of the head/spinal cord
   b. magnetic resonance imaging (MRI) scan of the brain/spinal cord

c. serum vitamin B$_{12}$ levels

d. Beck's depression scale

e. Venereal Disease Research Laboratory test for syphilis

4. The disease is most correctly described as which of the following?

   a. an uncommon neurologic disease that can be corrected by the administration of subcutaneous vitamin B$_{12}$

   b. the number one cause of disabling disease of young adults in the United States

   c. a very common psychiatric condition in which psychologic symptoms are manifested by physical symptoms

   d. a fatal neurologic condition that results in continual deterioration to the point of respiratory depression and the cessation of respiration

   e. none of the above

5. The disease described is associated with which of the following?

   a. racial predilection: whites more often than African Americans

   b. sex predilection: females more often than males

   c. high socioeconomic status

   d. environmental exposure

   e. all of the above

6. Which of the following statements regarding the behavior of the disease described is (are) true?

   a. in 80% to 90% of all cases, the first episode is followed by a cycle of relapses and remissions

   b. 50% of those with relapsing–remitting cases switch to a progressive course approximately 5 years after the onset of the first symptoms

   c. 10% of patients have progressive disease from the onset of symptoms

   d. up to 10% of patients with this disease have a relatively "benign" course

   e. all of the above

7. The disease, if diagnosed as a central nervous system (CNS) disease, has to involve how many different areas of the central nervous system?

   a. one

   b. two

   c. three

   d. four

   e. not applicable: not primarily a neurologic disease

8. Which of the following clinical findings support the diagnosis?

   a. a cerebrospinal fluid (CSF) mononuclear cell pleocytosis

   b. an increase in CSF immunoglobulin G (IgG)

c. oligoclonal banding of CSF IgG (two or more bands)

d. abnormalities in evoked-response testing (any type)

e. all of the above

9. The target of this disease process is an attack on which of the following?

   a. the neurotransmitter balance in the CNS

   b. the "oligodendrocytes" of the CNS

   c. the peripheral nerves in the posterior columns of the spinal cord

   d. the cerebral hemispheres

   e. the cerebellum

10. What is (are) the treatment(s) of choice for the disease process described?

   a. adrenocorticotropic hormone (ACTH)

   b. corticosteroids

   c. natalizumab

   d. interferon-β

   e. all of the above

11. Which of the following statements is true regarding the use of interferon in this disorder?

   a. interferon has been shown to reduce the rate of relapse

   b. interferon may delay the progression to disability

   c. interferon reduces the development of new lesions as seen by MRI

   d. interferon delays the increase in volume of lesions as seen by MRI

   e. all of the above

12. Which of the following symptoms is the least common?

   a. optic neuritis

   b. ataxia

   c. vertigo

   d. loss of bladder control

   e. impotence

Clinical Case Management Problem

What causes MS, and what cell type is the primary target?

Answers

1. **b.** This patient has MS. Although no laboratory test, symptom, or physical finding necessarily means a person has MS, the diagnosis relies on two broad criteria: (1) There must have been two attacks that were defined as the sudden appearance or worsening of an

MS symptom or symptoms that last at least 24 hours and are at least 1 month apart, and (2) there must be more than one area of damage to CNS myelin, with the damage having occurred at more than one point in time and not being attributed to any other disease process.

The differential diagnosis includes ruling out metabolic diseases such as B_{12} deficiencies; other autoimmune disorders such as Behçet's disease, lupus erythematosus, and Sjögren's syndrome; infections such as human immunodeficiency virus (HIV) myelopathy; genetic disorders such as hereditary ataxias; psychiatric disorders such as conversion reaction; and malignancies such as spinal cord tumors.

2. a. The most common pattern or clinical category of MS is the relapsing–remitting category. In relapsing–remitting MS, episodes of acute worsening are followed by recovery and a stable course between relapses.

In the secondary progressive category, gradual neurologic deteriorating occurs with or without superimposed acute relapses in patients who previously had relapsing–remitting MS.

In primary progressive MS, gradual continuous deterioration occurs from the onset of symptoms.

In progressive relapsing MS, gradual neurologic deterioration occurs from the onset of symptoms but with subsequent superimposed relapses.

A small fraction of patients have a relatively benign form that never becomes debilitating.

The patient described most likely has relapsing–remitting MS.

3. b. The most sensitive and specific investigation for this disorder is an MRI of the brain and/or spinal cord scan. The MRI scan will reveal plaque formation (a subsequent stage that results from the loss of the myelin sheath in different parts of the CNS) and spotty and irregular demyelination in the affected areas in a patient with MS.

4. b. MS is the number one disabling disease of young adults, primarily women. It is more common at northern latitudes than at southern latitudes. Other risk factors are addressed in answer 5.

5. e. The documented risk factors for MS include the following: (1) white race more like than African American race; (2) female more likely than male (2:1); (3) environmental influences (latitude north > south) and suspected but unidentified environmental toxins; (4) genetic (common human leukocyte antigen [HLA] histocompatibility antigen patterns); (5) viral infections are suspect but none has yet been identified; and (6) high socioeconomic status.

6. e. The clinical categories are described in answer 2. All of the following are correct: (1) 80% to 90% of all cases after the first symptom have relapses followed by remissions; (2) 50% of those who have relapsing–remitting cases switch to a progressive course approximately 5 years after the onset of the first symptoms; (3) 10% have progressive disease from the onset; and (4) 10% of patients have clinical courses that are benign. These patients have one or two relapses and then recover or have episodes of mild nondebilitating relapses with long-lasting remissions. These individuals have multifocal plaques at autopsy without evidence of an inflammatory demyelinating reaction.

There is a very rare type termed acute multiple sclerosis of the Marburg type with rapid progression of symptoms.

7. b. For a patient to be diagnosed as having MS, two separate areas of the CNS must be involved.

8. e. The following are laboratory findings that support the diagnosis of MS: (1) CSF mononuclear cell pleocytosis (5 cells/mL); (2) CSF IgG is increased in the absence of a normal concentration of total protein; (3) oligoclonal banding of CSF IgG is detected by agarose gel electrophoresis techniques (two or more oligoclonal bands are found in 75% to 90% of patients with MS); (4) metabolites from myelin breakdown may be detected in the CSF; and (5) evoked response testing may detect slowed or abnormal conduction in visual, auditory, somatosensory, or motor pathways. (One or more evoked potentials are abnormal in 80% to 90% of patients with MS.)

MRI scans of the brain are abnormal in a proportion of patients with MS at presentation; this is associated with more severe disease.

MRI of the brain and spinal cord is the most useful imaging method available, and abnormal MRI scans are seen in 90% of patients with definite MS.

9. b. The targeted cells in the MS disease process are the oligodendrocytes of the CNS. These cells fabricate and maintain the myelin sheaths, the material covering the axons that is necessary for the normal conduction of nerve impulses. Destruction of oligodendrocytes occurs in clusters and is accompanied by loss of oligodendrocytes and their myelin sheath appendages with axon sparing (primary demyelination).

The cluster destruction of oligodendrocytes–myelin sheaths forms multifocal plaques, the pathologic hallmark of the disease. The vast majority of these plaques are in the white matter.

10. **d.** The treatments of choice for MS are as follows:
- Corticosteroids are the mainstay of treatment for initial and acute relapses of MS. Although corticosteroid therapy can shorten the duration of a relapse, it is uncertain whether the long-term course of the disease will be altered with their use. ACTH has been replaced by high-dose intravenous methylprednisolone.
- Interferon-β remains the long-term treatment of choice for patients with relapsing–remitting MS. Interferon-β is available in two forms: 1A and 1B. Both types are generally well tolerated by most patients. Flu-like symptoms are common after each injection, and questions about different responses in different people remain. Therefore, interferon-β doses should be individualized.
- Glatiramer acetate is an alternative to interferon-β for those who have failed the latter therapy.
- Natalizumab, a recombinant monoclonal antibody against α_4-integrins, is the first selective immunomodulating drug for the treatment of MS and may be an advance over current therapies.

11. **e.** Interferon-β-1B and -1A are used in the treatment of MS. Both interferons have been shown to reduce the rate of clinical relapse, reduce the number of new lesions seen on MRI, and delay the increase in volume of new lesions seen on MRI. Interferon β-1A also may delay the progression to disability in some patients. Glatiramer acetate, mitoxantrone, and immunoglobulins also have been shown to reduce the rate of relapse, although much uncertainty remains about their precise usage.

12. **e.** The initial symptoms of MS and their frequency are outlined in Table 46-1.

Thus, of the symptoms listed in the question, the most common is optic neuritis, and the least common is impotence/other sexual dysfunction.

Table 46-1	Initial Symptoms of MS and Their Frequency
Symptom	**Percentage of Cases**
Sensory loss	37
Optic neuritis	36
Weakness	35
Paresthesias	24
Diplopia	15
Ataxia	11
Vertigo	6
Paroxysmal symptoms	4
Bladder disorders	4
Lhermitte's sign	3
Pain	3
Dementia	2
Visual loss	2
Facial palsy	1
Impotence	1
Myokymia	1
Epilepsy	1
Falling	1

Solution to the Clinical Case Management Problem

The etiologic agent(s) producing MS is (are) unknown. There is reasonable evidence that it results from an interaction between the individual (immunology) and his or her environment. The basic target of MS is the oligodendrocyte, the cell that fabricates and maintains myelin. Destruction of oligodendrocytes occurs in clusters and is accompanied by loss of the oligodendrocyte and the myelin sheaths. The cluster destruction of oligodendrocytes–myelin sheaths produces plaques, the pathologic hallmark of MS. This destruction of oligodendrocytes and myelin is patchy, leaving more areas unaffected. The axons invariably are spared.

Summary

1. Prevalence
It is a major disabling condition of young adults in the United States; in 2000, 250,000 to 350,000 people in the United States had physician-diagnosed MS.

2. Epidemiology
a. Almost all patients fit into one or more of the following categories:
  i. 80% to 90% of patients have after their first symptom a cycle of relapses and remissions.

ii. 50% of the 80% to 90% switch to a progressive course approximately 5 years after the first symptom.

iii. 10% of patients have progressive disease from the onset.

iv. Up to 10% of patients have a benign course, with one or two relapses and then a good recovery.

b. Risk factors for MS:
   i. Race: white > African American
   ii. Sex: females > males (2:1)
   iii. High socioeconomic status
   iv. Northern latitudes
   v. Other environmental factors not identified, such as toxins and viruses
   vi. HLA histocompatible antigens

3. Most common symptoms

a. Sensory loss
b. Optic neuritis
c. Weakness
d. Paraesthesias

4. Diagnosis criteria

a. Two episodes, or attacks, of symptoms
b. Two different areas of the CNS involved

5. Testing

a. MRI scan of the brain and spinal cord: This will show the areas of demyelination better than any other test.
b. CSF pleocytosis
c. Increased CSF IgG
d. Oligoclonal banding of IgG in the CSF
e. Evoked potentials: visual, auditory, somatosensory, and motor

6. Treatment

a. Pharmacotherapy
   i. Methylprednisolone for acute attacks
   ii. Long-term medication includes interferon-β-1A and -1B, glatiramer acetate, anti-integrin monoclonal antibodies, and mitoxantrone
b. General supportive treatments
   i. A regular exercise program
   ii. The pursuit of wellness and a positive attitude
   iii. Education regarding the disease
   iv. Support: family/support groups

Suggested Reading

Lublin FD: The diagnosis of multiple sclerosis. *Curr Opin Neurol* 15(3):253–256, 2002.

Medline Plus. Multiple sclerosis. Available at www.nlm.nih.gov/medlineplus/multiplesclerosis.html.

National Multiple Sclerosis Society. Available at www.nationalmssociety.org.

Noseworthy JH, Lucchinetti C, Rodriguez M, Weinshenker BG: Multiple sclerosis. *N Engl J Med* 343(13): 938–952, 2000.

Ropper AH: Selective treatment of multiple sclerosis. *N Engl J Med* 354:965–967, 2006.

Wingerchuck DM: Current evidence and therapeutic strategies for multiple sclerosis. *Semin Neurol* 28:56–68, 2008.

CHAPTER

47 Fibromyalgia

CLINICAL CASE PROBLEM 1

A 35-Year-Old Female with Total Body Muscle Pain

A 35-year-old female comes to your office with a 1-year history of "aching and hurting all over." She also complains of a chronic headache, difficulty sleeping, and generalized fatigue. When questioned carefully, she describes "muscle areas tender to touch."

Although the pain is worse in the back, there really is no place free of pain. She also describes headaches, generalized abdomen pains, and some constipation.

On examination, the most striking finding is the presence of discrete "tender points" (tender muscle areas when palpated). These are bilateral and include the mid to upper trapezius muscle, under the lower sternomastoid, the prominence of the greater trochanter, the medial fat pad of the knee, 2 cm distal to the lateral epicondyle, and the upper outer quadrant of the buttock.

The rest of the physical examination is normal. Her blood pressure is 120/70 mmHg, and her cardiovascular system, respiratory, and abdomen exams are normal.

SELECT THE BEST ANSWER TO THE FOLLOWING QUESTIONS

1. What is the most likely diagnosis in this patient?
   a. polymyalgia rheumatica
   b. masked depression
   c. fibromyalgia
   d. diffuse musculoskeletal pain, not yet diagnosed (NYD)
   e. early rheumatoid arthritis

2. Which one of the following is not usually a site of tenderness in the disorder described?
   a. the rectus abdominis muscle
   b. origin of the supraspinatus muscle
   c. 2 cm distal to the lateral epicondyle of the humerus
   d. mid upper trapezius muscle
   e. upper outer quadrant of the buttock

3. The differential diagnosis of the condition described includes which of the following?
   a. chronic fatigue syndrome
   b. hypothyroidism
   c. masked depression
   d. myofascial pain syndrome
   e. all of the above

4. The diagnostic criteria of the disorder described include tenderness at how many of 18 specific sites?
   a. 5
   b. 7
   c. 9
   d. 11
   e. 13

5. What is the most characteristic symptom of the condition described?
   a. pain in at least three or four body quadrants
   b. "pain all over my body"
   c. pain in specific bursa and tendons
   d. pain in specific joints
   e. pain in both arms, the posterior neck, and the upper back

6. Choose the statement that is true for fibromyalgia:
   a. because fibromyalgia is not rheumatologic, patients do not experience any symptoms in their joints
   b. most patients with fibromyalgia have always had nonspecific pains and it is rare for the condition to develop after a specific event, such as a flu-like illness or emotional or physical trauma
   c. most patients present in their teens or twenties

   d. laboratory testing is important to confirm the diagnosis
   e. fatigue is present in more than 90% of patients

7. What is the cause of fibromyalgia?
   a. an autoimmune process
   b. a chronic inflammatory process
   c. an acute inflammatory process
   d. a slow or chronic virus infection
   e. idiopathic

8. Which of the following statements regarding sleep disorders and the condition described is true?
   a. there is no association between this condition and sleep disorders
   b. patients with this disorder have an abnormal sleep pattern
   c. patients with this disorder have difficult sleep induction, early morning wakening, and nightmares
   d. patients with this disorder have profound insomnia
   e. patients with this disorder usually have profound hypersomnia

9. Regarding therapy for this disorder, which of the following statements is (are) true?
   a. nonsteroidal anti-inflammatory drugs (NSAIDs) have demonstrated a significant advantage over placebo
   b. antidepressants are superior to placebo
   c. muscle relaxants are superior to placebo
   d. b and c
   e. all of the above are true

CLINICAL CASE PROBLEM 2

A 54-Year-Old Female with Fatigue and Multiple Trigger Points

A 54-year-old female presents with pain in multiple points on her body, fatigue, and frustration that many physicians have told her there is nothing that can be done for her.

   Although this patient meets the diagnostic criteria for fibromyalgia, her medical records indicate that her prior physician did not inform the patient of this diagnosis because he believed that it would reinforce the pain behavior.

10. What is the best statement regarding the prognosis of fibromyalgia?
    a. patients with the diagnosis will generally deteriorate over the years and eventually be unable to work

b. patient education about this disorder generally reinforces the pain and increases the chances that the patient will eventually request disability leave from work

c. when patients are informed of the diagnosis of fibromyalgia, significantly fewer symptoms and a general improvement in health status follow

d. once treated for depression, most patients diagnosed with fibromyalgia will no longer experience fatigue and pain

11. What are the best recommendations for exercise for a patient with fibromyalgia?

a. since some types of exercise may initially increase pain in tender points, it is best to avoid those activities

b. muscle strengthening and flexibility programs will decrease pain, improve muscle strength, and decrease the number of tender points

c. patients with fibromyalgia will quickly accept a cardiovascular exercise program into their routine since the fatigue of fibromyalgia quickly disappears with exercise

d. although cardiovascular fitness training will improve aerobic capacity, it will not improve pain levels

12. Your patient is interested in trying some non-pharmacologic treatment modalities for her fibromyalgia. What is the best evidence-based recommendation you can give her?

a. traditional Chinese acupuncture would be the modality most likely to give long-lasting relief

b. electromyography (EMG) biofeedback intervention has shown no improvement in pain

c. physical therapy is more likely than hypnotherapy to improve pain, fatigue, and sleep

d. mindfulness meditation-based relaxation response programs and cognitive behavioral therapy have both been shown to be helpful in improving quality of life

13. Your patient is frustrated at being told her symptoms are "all in her head" and would like to know what has been discovered regarding the etiology of fibromyalgia. Which of the following should you share with her?

a. elevated levels of substance P were found in the cerebrospinal fluid of fibromyalgia patients compared to controls

b. an underlying CNS dysfunction is suggested by the sleep and mood disturbances noted in the majority of fibromyalgia patients

c. a strong correlation was found between cortisol levels and pain upon awakening and 1 hour

after waking in patients with fibromyalgia compared to controls

d. patients with fibromyalgia have been found to have orthostatic hypotension and increased pain in response to tilt table testing

e. all of the above

Answers

1. **c.** This patient has fibromyalgia. Fibromyalgia is characterized by chronic, generalized pain and associated features, including fatigue, sleep disturbances, headache, cognitive difficulty, and mood disturbances. Pain is aggravated by exertion, stress, lack of sleep, and weather changes. Some patients also have a variety of pain symptoms, including abdominal and chest wall pain, irritable bowel syndrome, pelvic pain, and bladder symptoms of frequency and urgency suggestive of the female urethral syndrome or of interstitial cystitis. Fibromyalgia is 10 times more common in women than in men and is usually diagnosed between the ages of 20 and 50 years.

Rheumatoid arthritis is unlikely because of the lack of objective evidence of joint warmth, swelling, or deformity and the multiple soft tissue areas. Laboratory evaluation, however, is necessary to exclude this inflammatory condition.

Polymyalgia rheumatica occurs in an older age group and is discussed in Chapter 44.

Diffuse musculoskeletal pain NYD is not a diagnosis.

A primary diagnosis of masked depression or a somatoform disorder should always be considered when vague, somatic complaints are accompanied by sleep disturbance and fatigue. The multiple tender areas, however, are not usually seen in masked depression (Fig. 47-1).

2. **a.** Fibromyalgia is associated with tender points at multiple characteristic locations. These locations include the following: (1) under the sternomastoid muscle, (2) near the second costochondral junction, (3) 2 cm distal to the lateral epicondyle of the humerus, (4) at the prominence of the greater trochanter, (5) at the medial fat pad of the knee, (6) insertion of the suboccipital muscle, (7) mid upper trapezius muscle, (8) origin of the supraspinatus muscle, and (9) upper outer quadrant of the buttock (Fig. 47-2).

The rectus abdominis muscle is not included. The sensitivity of the trigger points can be assessed by measuring the exact amount of pressure applied over a certain anatomic site. This can be measured by a dolorimeter.

3. **e.** Fibromyalgia certainly has some vague symptoms, and the trigger points are the most objective evi-

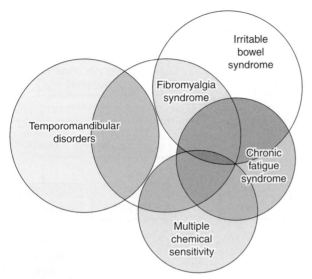

Figure 47-1

Overlap between syndromes with unexplained etiologies such as fibromyalgia, chronic fatigue syndrome (CFS), irritable bowel syndrome, temporomandibular disorder, and multiple chemical sensitivity. (Redrawn from Harris ED, Jr., Budd RC, Firestein GS, et al: *Kelley's Textbook of Rheumatology*, 7th ed., Philadelphia: Saunders, 2005.)

dence of the disorder. Many health care professionals, however, still doubt its authenticity. Hypothyroidism and chronic fatigue syndrome present with severe fatigue and share this major symptom with fibromyalgia. Myofascial pain syndrome shares the symptom of trigger points with fibromyalgia and should be considered in the differential diagnosis.

4. d. The number of trigger points identified by the American College of Rheumatology as being diagnostic of fibromyalgia is 11 or more.

5. b. The most characteristic symptom of fibromyalgia is the symptom described by patients as "total body muscle pain." This is a symptom that from clinical experience appears to have reasonable sensitivity and specificity.

6. e. Fatigue is present in most patients and is sometimes the presenting complaint. Although joint swelling and erythema are not present, joint pain is quite common. Most patients present between 30 and 55 years of age. Laboratory testing is only used to rule out other conditions. If tests have been done recently, a complete blood count, erythrocyte sedimentation rate, thyroid function tests, and muscle enzymes should be considered (Fig. 47-3).

7. e. The cause of fibromyalgia is unknown. There is no significant evidence that the process is an autoimmune process, the result of a true acute or chronic inflammatory process (although this is a possibility), or the result of any type of viral infection.

8. b. The many nonrheumatologic features of fibromyalgia include a pattern that is best described as a disorder of nonrestorative sleep (alpha non-rapid eye movement sleep anomaly). Although other sleep

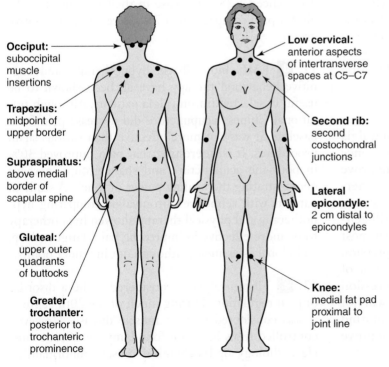

Occiput: suboccipital muscle insertions

Trapezius: midpoint of upper border

Supraspinatus: above medial border of scapular spine

Gluteal: upper outer quadrants of buttocks

Greater trochanter: posterior to trochanteric prominence

Low cervical: anterior aspects of intertransverse spaces at C5–C7

Second rib: second costochondral junctions

Lateral epicondyle: 2 cm distal to epicondyles

Knee: medial fat pad proximal to joint line

Figure 47-2

Location of specific tender points in fibromyalgia. (Redrawn from Fibromyalgia syndrome. In Schumacher HR, Jr., ed: *Primer on Rheumatic Diseases*, 10th ed., Atlanta: Arthritis Foundation, 1993.)

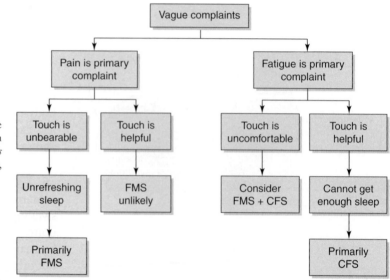

Figure 47-3

Algorithm for the diagnosis of chronic fatigue syndrome (CFS) and fibromyalgia syndrome (FMS). (Redrawn from Harris ED, Jr., Budd RC, Firestein GS, et al: *Kelley's Textbook of Rheumatology*, 7th ed., Philadelphia: Saunders, 2005.)

disorders, including sleep apnea in a small minority of patients, nocturnal myoclonus, and restless leg syndrome, are associated with fibromyalgia, a disorder of nonrestorative sleep (alpha–delta disorder) is the most common and the most diagnostic.

9. d. There is considerable controversy regarding which pharmacologic medications work and which do not. Studies have shown benefit of treatment with tricyclics, selective serotonin reuptake inhibitors, and cyclobenzaprine (Flexeril). Tramadol has a dual effect on both opiate and serotonin receptor systems and has become a popular alternative. There is evidence that the combination of 20 mg of fluoxetine in the morning and 25 mg of amitriptyline in the evening is more effective than either used alone. Inflammation is not a component of the condition and NSAIDs have not shown significant benefit over placebo. NSAIDs may be helpful in combination with a CNS active agent.

10. c. Despite the fear of some physicians that labeling people with the diagnosis of fibromyalgia will worsen their symptoms, there is actually evidence that self-reported symptoms and function improve after the diagnosis is made. The symptoms generally do not increase over time, and most patients are able to continue working. Fatigue and pain will generally persist, but it should be emphasized that most patients live normal and active lives. Depression is a coexisting condition in approximately 30% of patients with fibromyalgia. Treating the depression can help improve functioning in patients but will not eliminate pain. Even in patients without comorbid depression, the use of antidepressants can improve symptoms.

11. b. Both muscle strengthening and flexibility programs will decrease pain, improve muscle strength, and decrease the number of tender points. Strength training has also been shown to decrease depression in fibromyalgia patients. Many patients have been afraid for years that the pain they experience is a sign of tissue damage, and they have thus been avoiding exercise. Fatigue tends to increase initially in fibromyalgia patients who start an exercise program, so education and support are important to help patients be motivated to persist until they start to experience benefits. Cardiovascular fitness training will not only improve aerobic capacity (17% increase) but also decrease pain (11% decrease). Patients in the exercise group also experienced a 28% increase in their pressure threshold for pain compared to a 7% decrease in the control group.

12. d. EMG biofeedback, hypnotherapy, and cognitive behavioral therapy have all been shown to be useful in selected fibromyalgia patients. Although traditional Chinese acupuncture did decrease pain from baseline, it was not more effective than various sham procedures. It is interesting that pain improved 30% in both the acupuncture and sham groups, perhaps demonstrating the healing power of touch. A study of patients with refractive fibromyalgia comparing hypnotherapy and physical therapy showed hypnotherapy to be more effective in improving pain, fatigue, sleep, and global assessment, although not in tender points.

13. e. Fibromyalgia is considered to be a disorder of pain regulation. During much of the 20th century, it was considered to be a muscle disease. However, controlled trials have not found any significant muscle pathology or biochemical muscle abnormalities.

Muscle function, lactate production, and pain following exertion were similar in women with fibromyalgia and controls. Patients with fibromyalgia experience noxious stimuli as painful at lower thresholds compared to controls. Elevated levels of substance P were found in the cerebrospinal fluid of fibromyalgia patients. A sleep abnormality known as alpha sleep activity is common. Hyperactivity of the stress response of the neurohormonal system is present. Patients with fibromyalgia have been found to have orthostatic hypotension and increased pain in response to tilt table testing.

Summary

1. Diagnosis

Fibromyalgia is characterized by diffuse muscular pain involving many muscle groups. The pain varies in intensity but is chronic and persistent. Approximately half of cases start after a specific event (physical or emotional trauma or a flu-like illness). Fatigue is almost always present. Headaches are also commonly present, and other symptoms, including abdominal, bladder, and pelvic pain, may be present. Cognitive, mood, and sleep disturbances are often present. On physical exam, tender points are present in at least 11 of 18 specific soft tissue locations. The American Rheumatological Society has the following guidelines to establish the diagnosis of fibromyalgia:

a. Widespread musculoskeletal pain in the left and right sides of the body, above and below the waist, plus axial pain; typically described by patient as "total body muscle pain" or "I hurt all over."

b. The presence of 11 or more out of a total of 18 specifically designated tender points or trigger points.

c. The major clinical features of fibromyalgia include the following: (1) total body pain, (2) multiple tender points on examination, (3) severe fatigue, (4) nonrestorative sleep (alpha non-rapid eye movement sleep anomaly), (5) postexertional increase in muscle pain, (6) reduced functional ability, (7) recurrent headaches, (8) irritable bowel syndrome, (9) atypical paresthesia, (10) cold sensitivity (often Raynaud's phenomenon), (11) restless leg syndrome, and (12) aerobic deconditioning.

2. Pathogenesis

Much research has been done examining fibromyalgia as a muscle disorder. However, no specific muscle abnormalities are present on muscle biopsies. There is evidence of an alteration of pain processing. Elevated levels of substance P are found in the cerebrospinal fluid of patients. Genetic predisposition plays some role, with first-degree relatives 8.5 times more likely to have fibromyalgia than first-degree relatives of rheumatoid arthritis patients. Some neurohormonal changes are being investigated, including whether levels of cortisol upon awakening are associated with pain intensity. Autonomic nervous system involvement is possible because there is evidence of orthostatic hypotension and increased pain with tilt table testing.

3. Treatment

Fibromyalgia is a chronic pain condition that is difficult to treat. Patients often have the condition for years before a diagnosis is made. Patient education and reassurance that this is a real condition are therapeutic.

Multiple modalities of treatment have been shown to be effective (Fig. 47-4). Nonpharmacologic options include physical therapy (heat, cold, ultrasound, and transcutaneous electrical nerve stimulation), massage therapy, psychological counseling, biofeedback, and cardiovascular fitness training program. Pharmacologic treatments include low-dose tricyclic antidepressants (TCAs). Amitriptyline and

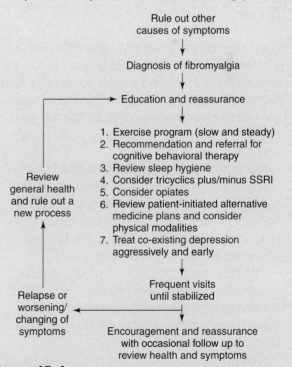

Figure 47-4

Treatment algorithm for fibromyalgia. (Redrawn from Harris ED, Jr., Budd RC, Firestein GS, et al: *Kelley's Textbook of Rheumatology*, 7th ed., Philadelphia: Saunders, 2005.)

nortriptyline are frequently used. Selective serotonin reuptake inhibitors have been found to be helpful alone and as an adjunct therapy with TCAs. NSAIDs are of limited usefulness in fibromyalgia since there is no inflammation. However, they are sometimes useful in combination with one of the CNS active medications. Muscle relaxants, such as cyclobenzaprine and a newer muscle relaxant tizanidine (Zanaflex), can be helpful. Tramadol has shown some improvement in pain, particularly when used in combination with acetaminophen. Anticonvulsants show some promise. Pregabalin, a second-generation anticonvulsant, showed a greater than 50% improvement in pain and also improved related symptoms.

Suggested Reading

Goldenberg DL: Clinical manifestations and diagnosis of fibromyalgia in adults. In: *UpToDate*. Waltham, MA: UpToDate, 2006.

Goldenberg DL: Treatment of fibromyalgia in adults. In: *UpToDate*. Waltham, MA: UpToDate, 2006.

Goldenberg DL: Pathogenesis of fibromyalgia. In: *UpToDate*. Waltham, MA: UpToDate, 2006.

Goldenberg DL, Burckhardt C, Crofford L: Management of fibromyalgia syndrome. *JAMA* 292(19):2388–2395, 2004.

Henningsen P, Zipfel S, Herzog W: Management of functional somatic syndromes. *Lancet* 369(9565):946–955, 2007.

CHAPTER

48 Chronic Fatigue Syndrome

CLINICAL CASE PROBLEM 1

A 25-Year-Old Female with Chronic Fatigue

A 25-year-old female comes to your office with a 9-month history of "unbearable fatigue." Before the fatigue began 9 months ago, she worked as a high school chemistry teacher. Since the fatigue began, she has been unable to work at all. She tells you that "one day it just hit me. I literally could not get out of bed."

Her past history is unremarkable. She has a husband and two children who have been very supportive during her 9-month illness. She has no history of any significant illnesses, including no history of any psychiatric disease. She has not expressed any signs of depression.

The other symptoms that the patient describes are difficulty concentrating, headache, sore throat, tender lymph nodes, muscle aches, joint aches, feverishness, difficulty sleeping, abdominal cramps, chest pain, and night sweats.

On physical examination, the patient has a low-grade fever (38.6°C), nonexudative pharyngitis, and palpable and tender anterior and posterior cervical and axillary lymph nodes.

SELECT THE BEST ANSWER TO THE FOLLOWING QUESTIONS

1. What is the most likely diagnosis in this patient?
   a. major depressive illness
   b. masked depression
   c. chronic fatigue syndrome
   d. fibromyalgia
   e. malingering

2. What is the etiology of the condition presented here?
   a. unequivocally related to a viral infection
   b. associated with an imbalance of neurotransmitters in the brain
   c. a factitious illness
   d. associated with major psychiatric pathology in almost all cases
   e. unknown

3. Which of the following statements regarding the condition described is (are) false?
   a. this condition is relatively new
   b. this condition is also known as epidemic neuromyasthenia
   c. this condition is also known as myalgic encephalomyelitis
   d. this condition is also known as multiple chemical sensitivity syndrome
   e. none of the above are false

4. Which of the following statements concerning the epidemiology of the condition described is (are) true?

a. patients with this condition are twice as likely to be women
b. the patients with this condition are likely to be in the 20 to 55 years age bracket
c. clusters of outbreaks of this condition have occurred in many countries during the past 60 years
d. the primary symptom of this condition may be found in up to 24% of patients attending a primary care clinic in the United States
e. all of the above

5. Which of the following best describes the onset of chronic fatigue syndrome in the majority of patients?
a. gradually increasing symptoms during a 3-month period
b. gradually increasing symptoms during a 6-month period
c. acute onset of symptoms in a previously healthy, well-functioning patient
d. chronic onset of symptoms during 1 or 2 years
e. the onset of symptoms is extremely variable; it is impossible to predict them with any degree of certainty

6. Regarding the laboratory diagnosis of the condition, which of the following statements is true?
a. no laboratory test, however esoteric or exotic, can diagnose this condition or measure its severity
b. a well-defined laboratory test that is sensitive but not specific exists for diagnostic purposes
c. a well-defined laboratory test that is specific but not sensitive exists for diagnostic purposes
d. a well-defined laboratory test that is both sensitive and specific exists for diagnostic purposes
e. a number of laboratory tests in combination are used for definite confirmation of the condition

7. Which of the following has been shown to be the most effective therapy for the condition described?
a. a tricyclic antidepressant
b. a nonsteroidal anti-inflammatory drug (NSAID)
c. a sensitive, empathetic physician who is willing to listen
d. cognitive psychotherapy
e. none of the above

8. Chronic fatigue syndrome is associated with all of the following except
a. hypothalamic dysfunction
b. conversion disorder
c. alpha-intrusion sleep disorder
d. chronic immune activation
e. myofascial pain

9. Chronic fatigue syndrome is associated with which of the following symptoms?
a. sleep disruption
b. cognitive dysfunction
c. anxiety and/or depression
d. neurologic symptoms
e. all of the above

10. Empiric evidence suggests that the best drug(s) to treat symptoms of the disorder is (are) which of the following?
a. NSAIDs
b. antidepressants
c. clarithromycin
d. tryptophan
e. a and b

11. When using antidepressant medications to treat either the sleep disorder or the mood disorder associated with chronic fatigue syndrome, what should the dose be?
a. the usual dose given to treat depression
b. One and a half times the usual dose given to treat depression
c. half the usual dose given to treat depression
d. one-fourth or less of the usual dose given to treat depression
e. twice the usual dose given to treat depression

12. Most patients with chronic fatigue syndrome
a. fully recover within 2 years
b. partially recover within 2 years
c. never recover
d. are at risk for relapse following recovery
e. b and d

CLINICAL CASE PROBLEM 2

A 44-Year-Old Woman with Chronic Fatigue

A 44-year-old woman presents to your office complaining of a 6-month history of fatigue, diffuse muscle pain, headaches, and poor sleep. She does not recall being depressed at the onset of this illness, but she has become so subsequently since she has lost her job due to the inability to complete projects. On physical exam, she has tender points bilaterally over the medial fat pads of the knee, 2 cm distal to the lateral epicondyle, the upper outer quadrant of the buttock, the mid to upper trapezius muscle, under the lower sternomastoid, and the prominences of the greater trochanter. Her laboratory results, including complete blood count, erythrocyte sedimentation rate, chemistry panel, and thyroid-stimulating hormone, are all normal.

13. Choose the statement that is true regarding this patient's condition:
    a. she meets the criterion for both fibromyalgia and chronic fatigue syndrome but not for temporomandibular joint disorder
    b. she has fibromyalgia but not chronic fatigue syndrome or temporomandibular joint disorder
    c. she has temporomandibular joint disorder but not chronic fatigue syndrome or fibromyalgia
    d. she has chronic fatigue syndrome but not fibromyalgia or temporomandibular joint disorder
    e. the diagnosis of chronic fatigue syndrome necessarily excludes the diagnosis of fibromyalgia

14. Symptoms present in chronic fatigue syndrome but not in fibromyalgia include
    a. muscle pain, aching, or discomfort
    b. difficulty concentrating or thinking
    c. problems falling or staying asleep, or sleeping too much
    d. mild fever (37.5°C to 38.6°C)
    e. abdominal pain relieved by a bowel movement

Answers

1. **c.** This patient has the clinical manifestations that support a diagnosis of chronic fatigue syndrome. Clinically evaluated, unexplained chronic fatigue cases can be classified as chronic fatigue syndrome if the patient meets both of the following criteria:

- Clinically evaluated, unexplained persistent or relapsing chronic fatigue that is of new or definite onset (i.e., not lifelong); is not the result of ongoing exertion; is not substantially alleviated by rest; and results in substantial reduction in previous levels of occupational, educational, social, or personal activities.
- The concurrent occurrence of four or more of the following symptoms: substantial impairment in short-term memory or concentration; sore throat; tender lymph nodes; muscle pain; multijoint pain without swelling or redness; headaches of a new type, pattern, or severity; nonrefreshing sleep; or postexertional malaise lasting more than 24 hours.

These symptoms must have persisted or recurred during 6 or more consecutive months of illness and must not have predated the fatigue.

The Centers for Disease Control and Prevention established a working definition of chronic fatigue syndrome in 1988, which was revised in 1993: "A thorough medical history, physical examination, mental status examination, and laboratory tests (diagram) must be conducted to identify underlying or contributing conditions that require treatment. Diagnosis or classification cannot be made without such an evaluation." The complaint of chronic fatigue accounts for 10 to 15 million office visits per year in the United States. Depression and anxiety, along with overwork, are the most common causes of chronic fatigue encountered in primary care practice. See Figure 48-1 for an algorithm for evaluating chronic fatigue.

2. **e.** The etiology of chronic fatigue syndrome is unknown. There are several common themes underlying attempts to understand the disorder. It is often postinfectious, often accompanied by immunologic disturbances, and commonly accompanied by depression. Viral agents that have been implicated as being associated with chronic fatigue syndrome include the lymphotropic herpesviruses, the retroviruses, and the enteroviruses. The real etiology, however, is unknown.

3. **a.** Chronic fatigue syndrome is not a new disease; it has been around for centuries. Certain individuals in the past have been labeled with a variety of diagnoses, such as neurasthenia, effort syndrome, hyperventilation syndrome, chronic brucellosis, epidemic neuromyasthenia, myalgic encephalomyelitis, hypoglycemia, multiple chemical sensitivity syndrome, chronic candidiasis, chronic mononucleosis, chronic Epstein–Barr virus infection, and postviral fatigue syndrome.

4. **e.** Patients with chronic fatigue syndrome are twice as likely to be women and are generally 25 to 45 years of age.

Cases are recognized in many developed countries. Most arise sporadically, but more than 30 clusters of similar illnesses have been reported. The most famous of such outbreaks occurred in Los Angeles County Hospital in 1934; in Akureyri, Iceland, in 1948; in the Royal Free Hospital, London, in 1955; in Punta Gorda, Florida, in 1945; and in Incline Village, Nevada, in 1985.

The prevalence of chronic fatigue syndrome is difficult to estimate because this is entirely dependent on case definition. Chronic fatigue is a ubiquitous symptom, occurring in as many as 24% of patients attending a primary care clinic in the United States; the syndrome is much less common.

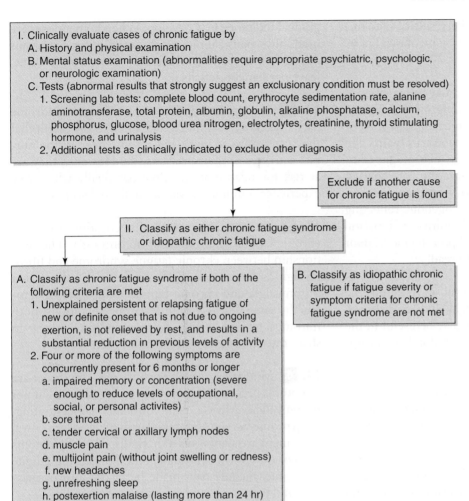

I. Clinically evaluate cases of chronic fatigue by
   A. History and physical examination
   B. Mental status examination (abnormalities require appropriate psychiatric, psychologic, or neurologic examination)
   C. Tests (abnormal results that strongly suggest an exclusionary condition must be resolved)
      1. Screening lab tests: complete blood count, erythrocyte sedimentation rate, alanine aminotransferase, total protein, albumin, globulin, alkaline phosphatase, calcium, phosphorus, glucose, blood urea nitrogen, electrolytes, creatinine, thyroid stimulating hormone, and urinalysis
      2. Additional tests as clinically indicated to exclude other diagnosis

Exclude if another cause for chronic fatigue is found

II. Classify as either chronic fatigue syndrome or idiopathic chronic fatigue

A. Classify as chronic fatigue syndrome if both of the following criteria are met
   1. Unexplained persistent or relapsing fatigue of new or definite onset that is not due to ongoing exertion, is not relieved by rest, and results in a substantial reduction in previous levels of activity
   2. Four or more of the following symptoms are concurrently present for 6 months or longer
      a. impaired memory or concentration (severe enough to reduce levels of occupational, social, or personal activites)
      b. sore throat
      c. tender cervical or axillary lymph nodes
      d. muscle pain
      e. multijoint pain (without joint swelling or redness)
      f. new headaches
      g. unrefreshing sleep
      h. postexertion malaise (lasting more than 24 hr)

B. Classify as idiopathic chronic fatigue if fatigue severity or symptom criteria for chronic fatigue syndrome are not met

Figure 48-1

The clinical evaluation and classification of unexplained chronic fatigue. The case definition for chronic fatigue syndrome was proposed by the Centers for Disease Control and Prevention in 1988 (Holmes GP, Kaplan JE, Gantz NM, et al: Chronic fatigue syndrome: A working case definition. *Ann Intern Med* 108:387–389, 1988) and refined and simplified by an international working group in 1994 (Fukuda K, Straus SE, Hickie I, et al: The chronic fatigue syndrome: A comprehensive approach to its definition and study. *Ann Intern Med* 121:953–959, 1994). (Redrawn from Behrman RE, Kliegman RM, Jenson HB: *Nelson Textbook of Pediatrics*, 17th ed., Philadelphia, Saunders, 2004.)

5. **c.** The typical case of chronic fatigue syndrome arises suddenly in a previously active and healthy individual. An otherwise unremarkable flu-like illness or some other acute stress is recalled with great clarity as the triggering event. Unbearable exhaustion is left in the wake of the incident. Other symptoms, such as headache, sore throat, tender lymph nodes, muscle and joint aches, and frequent feverishness lead to the belief that an infection persists. Then, over several weeks, the impact of reassurances offered during the initial evaluation fades as other features of the syndrome become evident, such as disturbed sleep, difficulty in concentration, and depression.

6. **a.** No laboratory test, however exotic or esoteric, can make the diagnosis of chronic fatigue syndrome. Elaborate, expensive laboratory workups should be avoided; they only make an already complicated picture even more so. However, it is reasonable to perform testing to exclude other causes of fatigue.

7. **c.** A sensitive, empathetic physician who is willing to listen is the most effective intervention that can be offered for chronic fatigue syndrome. NSAIDs alleviate headache and diffuse pain and feverishness. Nonsedating antidepressants (typically low-dose tricyclic agents) improve mood and disordered sleep and thereby attenuate the fatigue to some degree. The ingestion of caffeine and alcohol at night makes it more difficult to sleep, compounding fatigue, and should be avoided. Nothing, however, takes the place of an empathetic physician.

In terms of psychotherapy, the most effective therapy appears to be behavior-oriented therapy, not cognitive psychotherapy. If the patient is severely depressed and if tricyclic agents at full doses to treat depression have too many side effects, serotonin reuptake inhibitors or venlafaxine (Effexor) may be used.

8. **b.** Chronic fatigue syndrome is not a conversion disorder, nor is it a psychosomatic illness. Current research describes immune dysfunction in which T cells are chronically activated and hypothalamic dysfunction occurs presumably as a result of cytokine penetration of the blood–brain barrier. Alpha-intrusion sleep disorder is also probably the result of cytokine penetration and may be worsened by myofascial pain, if present.

9. e. Chronic fatigue syndrome may be classified as mild, moderate, or severe, depending on the number of symptoms present. Severe chronic fatigue syndrome may include not only fatigue, myofascial pain, and sleep disruption but also numerous neurologic complaints such as blurred vision, migrating paresthesias, and tinnitus. Mood disruption may be present; depression or anxiety or both are often endogenous, reflecting neurochemical dysequilibrium. Cognitive dysfunction may be severe, with complaints of poor memory, poor concentration, and the inability to read.

10. e. NSAIDs are often helpful in treating the symptoms of headache, diffuse pain, and feverishness. The nonsedating antidepressants may be useful in the treatment of depression, which is a predominant symptom in many patients.

11. d. Empiric evidence suggests that patients with chronic fatigue syndrome lose their tolerance to many agents, including toxins such as secondhand cigarette smoke, certain fumes, alcohol, and medications. Antidepressants, such as amitriptyline, should be given initially to patients with chronic fatigue in a dose approximately one-fourth of the usual dose, although

gradual tolerance may develop. When higher doses are used, physicians should watch carefully for symptoms of neurologic toxicity, which may, according to some, leave permanent deficits.

12. e. Most patients with chronic fatigue syndrome partially recover within 2 years, often to the extent that they can return to work and resume most of the normal activities of their previous life. However, they are at risk for relapse at any time (especially when they experience immune activation or sleep disruption).

13. a. This patient meets the criterion for both chronic fatigue syndrome and fibromyalgia. The relationship between chronic fatigue syndrome and fibromyalgia is fascinating. Some authorities believe that fibromyalgia and chronic fatigue syndrome are actually the same illness with different presentations. Both fibromyalgia and chronic fatigue syndrome appear to share the alpha-intrusion sleep disorder.

14. d. Mild fever as well as chills and sore throat are symptoms present in chronic fatigue syndrome but not fibromyalgia. Muscle pain, difficulty concentrating, sleep problems, and abdominal pain relieved by a bowel movement are symptoms of both disorders. Symptoms present only in fibromyalgia, and not chronic fatigue syndrome, include pain made better by heat or massage and pain made worse by sitting or standing.

Summary

1. Prevalence

Difficult to establish. One study suggests a prevalence of 37 cases/100,000 people. Chronic fatigue syndrome is not a new disease; it has been present for centuries. Most evidence for the disorder comes from outbreaks of the disorder, discussed previously.

2. Etiology

The etiology of chronic fatigue syndrome is unknown. Chronic fatigue syndrome has long appeared to be related to infectious agents, especially Epstein–Barr virus. However, most cases of chronic fatigue syndrome follow an influenza-like or gastroenteric-type illness, or evolve insidiously, rather than following mononucleosis. There is evidence of immune differences in patients with chronic fatigue syndrome. Circulating immune complexes and natural killer cells are present in lower than normal levels. Elevated titers of antiviral antibodies (directed against measles,

HHV-6, Epstein–Barr virus, and cytomegalovirus), lower levels of autoantibodies, and altered CD4/CD8 ratios are present. Several metabolic abnormalities, such as low serum cortisol levels, increased serotoninergic activity in the central nervous system, and increased levels of insulin-like growth factor 1, have been described, but the causal role is unclear. Alpha-intrusion sleep disorder appears to be related to cytokine involvement. Neurally mediated hypotension may play a role in chronic fatigue syndrome symptoms. Genetic studies have shown DNA sequence changes in three genes associated with brain function, stress reactions, and emotional responses.

3. Signs and symptoms

Chronic fatigue syndrome presents with a relatively sudden onset of fatigue often associated with an infection. After the infection resolves, the patient is left with an overwhelming sense of fatigue and associated symptoms, including altered sleep and cognition. The pre-chronic fatigue syndrome medical history is not one of multiple somatic complaints but, rather, of a high functioning individual. It is important to diagnose and treat other syndromes, including major depressive disorder, which may present with complaints of chronic fatigue, or others that otherwise complicate the picture. Increasing evidence shows that it may have a biologic basis and that the central nervous system and immune system are involved.

4. Course

Most patients partially recover within 2 years. All, however, are prone to relapse.

5. Treatment

a. Nonpharmacologic: An understanding physician who is prepared to spend time with the patient and listen and counsel in an empathetic fashion. The physician should help the patient reduce stress, develop a regular schedule, and maintain and gradually increase activity. Cognitive behavioral therapy has been effective. A graded exercise program can improve symptoms, although aggressive regimens can worsen symptoms.

b. Pharmacologic: No medications or special diets have proven to be uniformly effective in chronic fatigue syndrome. NSAIDs can be used to treat headaches, myalgias, and arthralgias. Low-dose tricyclic antidepressants can be used to improve the quality of sleep. For associated depression, antidepressant therapy should be used. Steroid therapy, immunomodulation, and antimicrobial therapy (acyclovir) have not been found to be helpful. Methylphenidate (10 mg twice a day) had a clinically significant improvement in fatigue in 17% of patients and on concentration in 22% of patients.

Suggested Reading

Gluckman SJ: Clinical features and diagnosis of chronic fatigue syndrome. In: *UpToDate*. Waltham, MA: UpToDate, 2006.

Gluckman SJ: Treatment of chronic fatigue syndrome. In: *UpToDate*. Waltham, MA: UpToDate, 2006.

Prins JB, van der Meer JW, Bleijenberg G: Chronic fatigue syndrome. *Lancet* 367(9507):346–355, 2006.

Viner R, Christie D: Fatigue and somatic symptoms. *BMJ* 330(7498):1012–1015, 2005.

CHAPTER

49 Rheumatoid Arthritis

CLINICAL CASE PROBLEM 1

A 35-Year-Old Female with Malaise and Vague Periarticular Pain and Stiffness

A 35-year-old female comes to your office with a 6-month history of malaise, paresthesia in both hands, and vague pain in both hands and wrists. She also has felt extremely fatigued. She tells you that the pains in her joints are much worse in the morning. She is also beginning to notice pain and swelling in both knees. The patient has a normal family history, with no significant diseases noted.

She is taking no drugs and has no allergies. On examination, vital signs are normal. There is a sensation of bogginess and slight swelling in both wrists and multiple metacarpal–phalangeal joints. Both knees also feel somewhat swollen and boggy. There are no other joint abnormalities, and the rest of the physical examination is normal.

SELECT THE BEST ANSWER TO THE FOLLOWING QUESTIONS

1. What is the most likely diagnosis in this patient?
   a. nonarticular rheumatism
   b. synovitis
   c. gonococcal arthritis
   d. rheumatoid arthritis
   e. systemic lupus erythematosus

2. What is the most characteristic symptom of this disease?
a. early morning joint stiffness
b. progressive joint pain
c. predilection for the small joints
d. joint swelling
e. rash

3. What is the most characteristic sign of this disease?
a. joint swelling
b. bilateral (symmetric) joint involvement
c. erythema surrounding the affected joints
d. joint bogginess
e. involvement of the glenohumeral joint in all cases

4. On what is the pathophysiology of this disease based?
a. bone destruction
b. bone spur formation
c. bone sclerosis
d. symmetric joint involvement
e. synovial inflammation

5. In the course of the pathophysiology of this disease, which of the following is most characteristic of the disease?
a. synovial proliferation with cartilage erosion stimulated by cytokines
b. cartilage destruction stimulated by the proliferation of proteoglycans
c. cartilage destruction stimulated by the enzymatic action of proteoglycans
d. loss of the synovial membrane
e. none of the above (the pathophysiology of the disease is not known with any certainty)

6. The disease described tends to affect which one particular part of the spine?
a. C1–C2
b. C6–C7
c. T7–T8
d. L1–L2
e. L4–L5

7. Which anemia usually accompanies this disease process?
a. microcytic, hypochromic
b. microcytic, normochromic
c. normocytic, normochromic
d. macrocytic, hyperchromic
e. normocytic, hypochromic

8. Which of the following is (are) a systemic complication(s) of the disease process?
a. vasculitis
b. pericarditis
c. pleural effusion
d. diffuse interstitial fibrosis of the lung
e. all of the above

9. Felty's syndrome is a complication of the described disorder. Which of the following is part of this syndrome?
a. hepatomegaly
b. hyperkalemia
c. proteinuria
d. splenomegaly
e. thrombocytopenia

10. For the described disorder, which of the following is a proven disease-modifying agent?
a. auranofin
b. D-penicillamine
c. hydroxychloroquine
d. indomethacin
e. methotrexate

11. The patient develops a local flare-up in her right knee. Her left knee is affected to a small degree but not nearly as severely as the right knee. Up until this time, remission had been maintained, and she was taking oral anti-inflammatory agents for suppression of inflammation. What is the treatment of choice for this local flare-up?
a. methotrexate
b. hydroxychloroquine
c. intraarticular corticosteroid injection
d. oral prednisone
e. auranofin

12. What is the drug of choice for the suppression of inflammation in a patient with this disease?
a. auranofin
b. methotrexate
c. oral prednisone
d. naproxen
e. D-penicillamine

13. Which of the following is not a classical radiological feature of rheumatoid arthritis?
a. loss of periarticular bone mass
b. narrowing of the joint space
c. bony erosions
d. subarticular sclerosis
e. all of the above are radiological manifestations

Clinical Case Management Problem

Clinic case problem matching questions 1–12.
Match the characteristic with the type of arthritis.

Type of Arthritis

1. Ankylosing spondylitis
2. Gonococcal arthritis
3. Systemic lupus erythematosus
4. Lyme disease
5. Rheumatic fever
6. Gouty arthritis
7. Juvenile rheumatoid arthritis
8. Reiter's disease
9. Psoriatic arthritis
10. Inflammatory bowel disease arthritis
11. Calcium pyrophosphate (CPPD) arthritis
12. Tuberculous arthritis

Characteristic

a. Positively birefringent under the polarizing microscope
b. Negatively birefringent under the polarizing microscope
c. Most common cause of infective arthritis in young adults
d. Conjunctivitis and urethritis are other features
e. Erythema chronicum migrans
f. Bamboo spine
g. Streptococcal pharyngitis usually occurs first
h. Arthritis may precede abdominal symptoms
i. Renal failure is major cause of death in this disease
j. Arthritis may appear before classical "silver-scaled" skin lesions
k. Major cause of arthritis in children
l. Lung disease is major manifestation of this disease in most patients

Answers

1. d. The most likely diagnosis is rheumatoid arthritis (RA).

2. a. The most characteristic symptom of RA is early morning stiffness. The total array of rheumatoid arthritic symptoms includes the following: (1) morning stiffness lasting more than 1 hour, (2) pain on motion of joints,

(3) tenderness of joints, (4) swelling (soft tissue fluid inflammation rather than bony overgrowth), (5) symmetric joint involvement, and (6) subcutaneous nodules.

3. b. The most characteristic sign of RA is symmetric joint involvement. Symptoms 3, 4, and 6 listed in answer 2 may also be confirmed as signs. The rheumatoid factor is usually positive, and characteristic histological changes will usually be found in the synovial membrane.

In most patients, RA starts out with a whimper and not a bang. The disease has an insidious start with nonspecific symptoms, such as fatigue and malaise, accompanied by arthralgia and low-grade fever. Later, symmetric polyarticular swelling begins, usually with the proximal interphalangeal, metacarpophalangeal, wrist, elbow, shoulder, knee, ankle, and metatarsophalangeal joints involved but sparing the distal interphalangeal joints. Cervical spine involvement is common at the region C1–C2, but the remainder of the spine is usually spared.

4. e. Synovial inflammation is the pathophysiological basis for this disease.

5. a. The pathophysiology of RA begins with synovial membrane swelling and synovial membrane proliferation. The synovium, which is normally only two cell layers thick, proliferates and erodes adjacent cartilage and adjacent bone. Macrophages secrete cytokines, particularly interleukin-1 and tumor necrosis factor-α, which induce chondrocyte and osteoclast stimulation, prostaglandin secretion, and endothelial activation. CD4-positive T lymphocytes promote the inflammation early in the disease and are abundant in the synovium and the synovial fluid. The macrophage/cytokine system also triggers systemic effects such as fever and anemia.

6. a. Instability of the cervical spine is a life-threatening complication of RA. The instability results from a cervical ligament synovitis in the region of the first two cervical vertebrae. This complication occurs in 30% to 40% of patients who develop RA. Of patients with RA, 5% eventually develop a myelopathy or cord injury as a result of this instability.

7. c. The anemia that most often accompanies RA is mild, normochromic, and normocytic.

The characteristics of the anemia at the cellular level include low to normal levels of iron, iron-binding protein, and erythropoietin.

8. e. RA is a systemic disease. Some of the more important complications are as follows:

- Vasculitis: From the very beginning of the synovial membrane thickening process, a microvascular vasculitis process is involved. This can progress to mesenteric vasculitis, polyarteritis nodosa, or other vascular syndromes.
- Pericarditis: Fibrinous pericarditis is present in 40% of patients with RA at autopsy. Although infrequent, this pericarditis can occasionally be constricting with resultant life-threatening tamponade.
- Pleural effusions: Rheumatic pleural effusions are extremely common.
- Rheumatic nodules in the heart may affect the conducting system and lead to conduction disturbances including heart block and bundle branch blocks.
- Rheumatic nodules in the lung can cavitate or become infected.
- Diffuse interstitial fibrosis with a restrictive pattern on pulmonary function tests and a honeycomb pattern on chest radiography may occur.

9. d. Felty's syndrome usually occurs late in the RA disease process. Neutropenia and a positive rheumatoid factor are other typical manifestations of this syndrome.

10. d. All of the other medications listed are disease-modifying drugs used in the treatment of RA.

11. c. Because the flare-up is limited to one joint, it is reasonable to treat with a localized approach. An intraarticular corticosteroid injection may temporarily help control local synovitis.

12. d. The drugs of choice for the suppression of inflammation in a patient with RA are the nonsteroidal anti-inflammatory drugs (NSAIDs). Although aspirin is still theoretically the agent of first choice, patients are more likely to take 1 or 2 pills per day rather than the 10 to 12 per day required with aspirin therapy. Thus, the answer to this question is naproxen. If an NSAID from a certain class does not work when given up to maximum dose, an agent from another class should be tried. A cyclooxygenase-2 (COX-2) inhibitor may be preferable in long-term treatment because of decreased gastrointestinal side effects, although all NSAIDs can cause gastrointestinal bleeding.

13. d. In early RA, few radiological findings are seen. Soft tissue changes in synovial fluid or capsular thickening occasionally may be seen on the radiograph but are more readily detected by physical examination. Loss of juxtaarticular bone mass (osteoporosis) is often detected near the finger joints and may be seen early in the disease. Narrowing of the joint space, as a result of thinning of the articular cartilage, is usually seen late in the disease. Bony erosions are seen best at the margins of the joint. Subarticular sclerosis is a feature of osteoarthritis, not RA.

Solution to the Clinical Case Management Problem

1. f	7. k
2. c	8. d
3. i	9. j
4. e	10. h
5. g	11. a
6. b	12. l

Summary

Rheumatoid arthritis occurs in 1% of the population. The clinical risk for developing RA is highly associated with HLA DR4 (human leukocyte antigen D-related antigen 4). Early morning stiffness is the most common symptom, and symmetric joint swelling is the most common sign. Other symptoms and signs include tenderness, swelling, and bogginess of joints; characteristic changes in the synovial membrane, including microvascular changes; positive rheumatoid factor; subcutaneous nodules; and radiographic changes including loss of juxtaarticular bone mass, joint space narrowing, and bony erosions.

The sequence and order of pathophysiological changes in RA is (a) synovial macrophage activation; (b) lymphocyte infiltration and endothelial cell proliferation; (c) neovascularization; and (d) irregular growth of inflamed synovial tissue, which invades and destroys cartilage and bone. Cytokines, interleukins, proteinases, and growth factors get released and contribute to further joint destruction as well as systemic symptoms and signs such as fever and anemia. Identification of some of these inflammatory and destructive mediators has led to newer treatments for RA.

Systemic manifestations of RA include normochromic, normocytic anemia, fever, pericarditis, pleural effusion, rheumatoid pulmonary nodules, rheumatoid cardiac nodules that can cause heart block, diffuse interstitial disease, systemic vasculitis, and Felty's syndrome.

Early and aggressive treatment will yield better long-term outcomes. Nonpharmacological treatments include systemic rest, articular rest (splints, braces, and canes), physiotherapy (both heat and cold), joint range of motion exercises, other exercise as tolerated, weight loss, and education of the patient and family.

The early use of disease-modifying antirheumatological drugs (DMARDs) for RA is beneficial. The critical question of how combination DMARD therapy compares with methotrexate plus biologic therapy is unanswered. The older DMARDs include azathioprine, cyclosporine, gold compounds, hydroxychloroquine, methotrexate, penicillamine, and sulfasalazine. Hyroxychlorquine, minocycline, or sulfasalazine are usually used initially in mild cases of RA, defined as those with no erosions visible on plain radiography. Methotrexate is typically used as first-line treatment in cases of moderate or severe RA or in addition to another DMARD in refractory cases of mild RA. It is one of the most widely prescribed disease DMARDs for RA. Its advantages include a rapid onset of action (3 or 4 weeks), dependable clinical response, and good patient tolerance when used long term. Its side effects include reversible bone marrow suppression, hepatotoxicity, pulmonary hypersensitivity, and nephrotoxicity; consider starting within 2 months of diagnosis to reduce the possibility of irreversible joint destruction.

The newest class of DMARDs is the biological response modulators that target specific cytokines (i.e., tumor necrosis factor-α and interleukin-1) that are involved in the inflammatory cascade in RA. These medications include adalimumab, anakinra, etanercept, infliximab, and leflunomide. The current recommendations are to initially treat with single conventional DMARDs and advance to combination DMARD therapy or the addition of a biological agent if necessary.

Many of the DMARDs have significant side effect profiles, and these should be considered when deciding which medication to prescribe. Pretreatment tuberculosis skin testing and baseline chest radiography should be considered, as should consultation and comanagement with a rheumatologist.

Unless contraindicated, NSAIDs should be used to treat pain and inflammation. Using a medication from the COX-2 inhibitor class or using a concurrent gastric acid-lowering medication may be necessary in some individuals with preexisting or secondary gastric complaints. Glucocorticoids can be use for refractory disease when NSAIDs and DMARDs have not been successful. This medication should be started at the lowest dose and tapered up to the lowest effective dose. When a glucocorticoid is used chronically, the use of a bisphosphonate medication to prevent osteoporosis should be considered. Injected corticosteroids are the first choice as localized remitting agents. Some rheumatologists are now using glucocorticoids earlier in the course of illness.

Some severe cases of RA require surgery such as joint replacement to relieve pain and/or provide joint stability.

Suggested Reading

Cannella AC, O'Dell JR: Is there still a role for traditional disease-modifying antirheumatic drugs (DMARDs) in rheumatoid arthritis? *Curr Opin Rheumatol* 15(3):185–292, 2003.

Furst DE, Breedveld FC, Kalden JR, et al: Updated consensus statement on biological agents for the treatment of rheumatoid arthritis and other rheumatic diseases. *Ann Rheum Dis* 61(Suppl 2):ii2–ii7, 2002.

Jenkins JK, Hardy KJ: Biological modifier therapy for the treatment of rheumatoid arthritis. *Am J Med Sci* 323(4):197–205, 2002.

Jenkins JK, Hardy KJ, McMurray RW: The pathogenesis of rheumatoid arthritis: A guide to therapy. *Am J Med Sci* 323(4):171–180, 2002.

Mochan E, Ebell MH: Predicting rheumatoid arthritis risk in adults with undifferentiated arthritis. *Am Fam Physician* 77:1451–1453, 2008.

Pisetsky DS: Progress in the treatment of rheumatoid arthritis. *JAMA* 286:2787–2790, 2001.

Rindfleisch JA, Muller D: Diagnosis and treatment of rheumatoid arthritis. *Am Fam Physician* 72:1037–1042, 2005.

CLINICAL CASE PROBLEM 1

An 80-Year-Old Female with Painful Finger Joints

An 80-year-old female presents with a 6-month history of stiffness in both hands. It is maximal upon awakening in the morning and subsides soon thereafter. She has also noticed mild pain in her lower back, hips, and knees.

On examination, the patient is obese. She has significant swelling of both the proximal interphalangeal (PIP) joints and the distal interphalangeal (DIP) joints. There is also deformity of both knees on examination. The rest of her physical examination is normal.

SELECT THE BEST ANSWER TO THE FOLLOWING QUESTIONS

1. Which of the following statements regarding this patient's condition is (are) true?
   a. the swelling present at the DIP joints may represent Bouchard's nodes
   b. the swelling present at the PIP joints may represent Heberden's nodes
   c. this patient will most likely have a positive rheumatoid factor
   d. synovial fluid analysis will probably demonstrate a low viscosity
   e. this patient will most likely have a normal erythrocyte sedimentation rate

2. Which of the following statements regarding the condition described is false?
   a. pain is the chief symptom
   b. stiffness of the involved joint is common but of relatively brief duration
   c. the pain is characteristically dull and aching
   d. a major physical finding is bony crepitus
   e. the presence of osteophytes is sufficient to make the diagnosis

3. Which of the following statements concerning the condition described is false?
   a. this condition is the most common form of joint disease in the United States

   b. 70% to 90% of people older than age 75 years have at least one affected joint
   c. this condition has both primary and secondary forms
   d. narrowing of the joint space is unusual
   e. pathologically, the articular cartilage is first roughened and then finally worn away

CLINICAL CASE PROBLEM 2

A 65-Year-Old Female with an Arthritic Hip

An obese 65-year-old female with moderately severe osteoarthritis of her left knee comes to your office requesting an exercise prescription. She wishes to "get in shape." On examination, she has genu varum and on radiography she has medial > lateral joint space narrowing.

4. Which of the following would you recommend to this patient at this time?
   a. exercise is not good for osteoarthritis; rest is much more appropriate
   b. a high-impact exercise regimen is best because it promotes new cartilage formation
   c. a passive isotonic exercise program is preferable to an active isometric exercise program
   d. any exercise program probably will hasten her need for total hip replacements
   e. swimming is the best exercise prescription you can give her; it promotes cardiovascular fitness while at the same time keeps pressure off the weight-bearing joints

5. Which of the following radiographic features is usually seen in patients with osteoarthritis?
   a. joint space narrowing
   b. osteophytes
   c. subchondral bony sclerosis
   d. subchondral pseudocysts
   e. all of the above

6. Which of the following treatment modalities is not useful in the treatment of her left knee pain?
   a. heat application
   b. laterally wedged insoles
   c. nonsteroidal anti-inflammatory drugs (NSAIDs)
   d. use of a cane in her left hand
   e. weight loss

7. Which of the following statements concerning osteoarthritis is true?
   a. 85% of the U.S. population has either clinical or radiographic evidence of osteoarthritis by age 75 years
   b. cartilaginous fraying is common
   c. mild synovitis may develop in response to crystals or cartilaginous debris
   d. the most common sites for this disease are knees, hips, and small joints of the hands and feet
   e. all of the above

8. Major goals of therapy in osteoarthritis include which of the following?
   a. minimize pain
   b. prevent disability
   c. delay progression
   d. a and b only
   e. all of the above

9. Which of the following statements regarding the use of NSAIDs given to an elderly patient with osteoarthritis is (are) true?
   a. NSAIDs are generally very safe for the treatment of the condition described in elderly patients
   b. NSAID toxicity in elderly patients is uncommon
   c. NSAID toxicity in elderly patients is unlikely to be associated with renal insufficiency
   d. the most common NSAID toxicity in elderly patients is gastrointestinal
   e. none of the above are true

10. What is the drug of first choice for the treatment of this patient's osteoarthritis pain?
    a. acetaminophen
    b. naproxen sodium
    c. diclofenac
    d. indomethacin
    e. any of the above

Answers

1. e. This patient has obvious osteoarthritis. However, the location of Bouchard's nodes represents both overgrowth and significant osteoarthritic changes at the PIP joints (not the DIP joints), whereas Heberden's nodes represent bony overgrowth and significant osteoarthritic changes at the DIP (not the PIP) joints.

Synovial fluid analysis most likely will reveal a high (not low) viscosity and normal mucin clotting. The total leukocyte count in the synovial fluid likely will be less than 1000 cells/mm^3. A significantly elevated erythrocyte sedimentation rate is seldom seen with osteoarthritis except in the unusual cases in which there is a significant inflammatory component. Similarly, the rheumatoid factor should be negative in osteoarthritis.

2. e. The most common symptom in osteoarthritis is pain. The pain is described as dull, aching, aggravated by joint use, and relieved by joint rest. Joint stiffness in weight-bearing joints is common but usually is a very transient finding, especially in the morning. It also occurs after prolonged rest.

Osteoarthritis pain is the result of movement of one joint surface against another, with both joint surfaces exhibiting characteristic articular cartilage damage including fraying and, ultimately, complete lack of cartilage. In addition, there are subchondral bone microfractures, irritation of the periosteal nerve endings, ligamentous stress, muscular strain, and soft tissue inflammation such as bursitis and tendonitis.

Bony crepitus is the most common physical finding in osteoarthritis. Osteophytes are a common radiological finding, especially with advanced age. The diagnosis of osteoarthritis, however, is clinical, and the mere presence of osteophytes on an x-ray, which can be present in asymptomatic joints, is not sufficient for the diagnosis.

3. d. Joint space narrowing is common. It is almost always associated with osteoarthritis. The primary defect in primary osteoarthritis and secondary osteoarthritis is loss of articular cartilage. In primary osteoarthritis, this is the result of "normal" wear and tear. In secondary osteoarthritis, the loss is the result of acute or chronic trauma; congenital deformities; metabolic disorders; septic and tubercular arthritis; and endocrine disorders such as acromegaly, obesity, or diabetes. The result is that the majority of people have evidence of osteoarthritis in weight-bearing joints by age 65 years, and 70% to 90% of people older than age 75 years clinically have at least one affected joint.

Cartilage changes progress as follows: (a) glistening appearance is lost; (b) surface areas of the articular cartilage flake off; (c) deeper layers of the articular cartilage develop longitudinal fissures (fibrillation); (d) the cartilage becomes thin and eventually absent in some areas, leaving the underlying subchondral bone unprotected; (e) the unprotected subchondral bone becomes sclerotic (dense and hard); (f) cysts develop within the subchondral bone and communicate with the longitudinal fissures in the cartilage; (g) pressure builds up in the cysts until the cystic contents are forced into the synovial cavity, breaking through the articular cartilage on the way; (h) as the articular cartilage erodes, cartilage-coated osteophytes may grow outward from the underlying bone and alter the bone contours and joint anatomy; (i) these spur-like bony projections enlarge until small pieces, called joint mice, break off into the synovial cavity; and (j) the process of loss of articular cartilage probably takes place through the enzymatic breakdown of the cartilage matrix (the proteoglycans, glycosaminoglycans, and collagen are involved).

4. b. Muscle spasm and muscle atrophy can be prevented in osteoarthritis by a graded exercise program. Active exercises are preferred to passive exercises; isometric exercises are preferred to isotonic exercises. Because of minimal involvement of the weight-bearing joints, swimming can be recommended as an ideal exercise.

5. e. Radiographic changes in osteoarthritis include narrowing of the joint space as a result of loss of articular cartilage, bony sclerosis as a result of thickening of subchondral bone, subchondral bone cysts, and osteophyte (bone spur) formation.

6. d. The treatments for osteoarthritis include both pharmacologic and nonpharmacologic measures. Nonpharmacologic measures include the avoidance of overuse of the affected joint; walking aids such as canes, crutches, and walkers; weight loss; heat application; exercises; and other physiotherapy techniques. Specifically, a cane should be used in the contralateral hand. Exercises should be mainly isometric (nonmovement such as quadriceps strengthening), stretching, and range-of-motion maneuvers. Heat modalities such as hot packs, soaks, and warm pools for aerobic exercise may decrease discomfort and facilitate the exercise program.

Pharmacologic measures include simple analgesics such as acetaminophen, NSAIDs, and local steroid injections. Newer concepts in the treatment of osteoarthritis that are in various stages of use or study include chondroprotective agents, which may conserve cartilage or stimulate cartilage repair within the osteoarthritic joint. These agents include chondroitan sulfate, glucosamine, tetracyclines, and intraarticular hyaluronic acid. Topical preparations such as capsaicin, DMSO, methylsalicylate, and compounded NSAID gels can be used for relief of pain. Nonnarcotic analgesics include acetaminophen, propoxyphene, and tramadol. Intraarticular corticosteroids can be used.

Anti-inflammatory agents such as NSAIDs are very effective, with limiting factors being gastric side effects and problems with renal functions. Cyclooxygenase-2

(COX-2) inhibitors are very effective and do not have the degree of gastric side effects shared by nonselective NSAIDs, although adding an acid-lowering medication or misoprostol to a nonselective NSAID may achieve the same purpose. The COX-2 inhibitors may also have renal side effects, and the possible increased risk of thrombotic cardiovascular events with both nonselective NSAIDs and COX-2 inhibitors should be taken into consideration.

Orthopedic surgery is used in severe cases. Joint replacement, especially of the knee and hip, is the treatment of choice when more conservative therapy has failed to control pain and maintain function. Osteotomy may be considered for some patients who have not yet progressed to the degree of needing total joint replacement. Arthroscopic debridement and meniscus repair may be of some benefit, but arthroscopic lavage alone has not been shown to be an effective treatment for osteoarthritis.

7. e. At least 33% of adults between the ages of 25 and 75 years have radiographic findings commonly seen in osteoarthritis. Some studies suggest that osteoarthritis begins as early as 15 or 16 years of age. In the United States, 85% of the population has either clinical or radiographic evidence of osteoarthritis by age 75 years.

The cartilaginous fraying that is associated with cartilage degeneration has been described. Associated with this may be a mild synovitis that develops in response to cartilaginous fragments ("joint mice") in the joint space.

The most common sites for osteoarthritis to develop are the small joints of the hands, the small joints of the feet, the hips, the knees, and the vertebral column where the cartilaginous degeneration is of a somewhat different type (the intervertebral discs) but nevertheless is the same basic pathologic process. With the exception of the first carpometacarpal joint, the wrists and metacarpophalangeal joints are typically not osteoarthritic.

8. e. The goals for the patient with osteoarthritis are to minimize pain, prevent disability, and delay progression. Some argue that it is not possible to delay progression in osteoarthritis; however, this is false. Weight loss in an obese individual and decreased repetitive trauma or impact to a joint with osteoarthritis will delay progression.

9. d. The most common type of toxicity associated with NSAIDs in elderly patients is gastrointestinal. This may take the form of an acute or chronic gastritis, a peptic ulcer, or a perforated ulcer. This may result in secondary anemia and other complications. NSAID toxicity is more common in elderly individuals. The risk of developing reversible renal failure while using an NSAID is greater for patients with renal disease and congestive heart failure.

10. **a.** NSAIDs, although a mainstay of treatment for osteoarthritis, have significant potential toxicity, especially when used in elderly patients with renal impairment or other diseases. Thus, ordinary acetaminophen is safer and must be considered a drug of first choice.

If an NSAID is used for the treatment of osteoarthritis in elderly patients, it is suggested that (1) the dose be kept as low as possible and (2) the drug be given with food and preferably with a cytoprotective agent such as misoprostol or an acid-lowering medication. The use of a COX-2 inhibitor can be considered.

Summary

Osteoarthritis (OA) is a typically noninflammatory joint disease characterized by its usual lack of inflammatory symptoms and signs and by the degeneration and loss of articular cartilage in synovial joints. It is the most common rheumatologic condition. Joint pain, stiffness, and swelling are the most common symptoms, and joint crepitus, swelling, and limited range of motion are typical physical exam findings. The knees, hips, and finger DIP and PIP joints are most typically affected, and the American College of Rheumatology has classification criteria for OA of these joints. Radiographic findings in OA include joint space narrowing, osteophytes, and subchondral bony sclerosis and pseudocysts.

OA is either primary or secondary. Primary OA is considered to be idiopathic, although it is typically from "wear and tear" in weight-bearing joints and therefore also called degenerative joint disease. Secondary osteoarthritis is often related to acute or chronic trauma, congenital abnormalities, and certain systemic conditions such as diabetes mellitus, hemochromatosis, and Wilson's disease. Indeed, if there are symptoms and signs of osteoarthritis in atypical joints such as the ankle, wrist, elbow, and shoulder, then a secondary cause should be considered.

The goals for the patient with osteoarthritis are to minimize pain, prevent disability, and delay progression. Treatment can be both nonpharmacologic and pharmacologic. The keys of nonpharmacologic treatment include weight loss, physiotherapy, stretching, isometric exercises, and a mild aerobic exercise program. Swimming is the single best exercise. Work should be modified to limit weight bearing on affected joints, and aids such as canes and walkers should be considered.

The most important key of pharmacologic therapy is to do no harm. Acetaminophen is the analgesic drug of choice because of its relative lack of toxicity in the elderly. Topical preparations such as capsaicin, DMSO, methylsalicylate, and compounded NSAID gels can be used for relief of pain and are quite safe. Nonnarcotic (i.e., propoxyphene and tramadol) and narcotic analgesics can be used for more severe pain. If an NSAID is needed, consideration should be given to using a cytoprotective agent or a COX-2 inhibitor.

Intraarticular corticosteroid injections should be limited to large joints that fail to respond to other measures. Treatments aimed at the articular cartilage include glucosamine, chondroitan sulfate, and intraarticular injections of hyaluronic acid. Consider surgery if all therapies fail and osteoarthritis is very severe.

Suggested Reading

American College of Rheumatology, Subcommittee on Osteoarthritis Guidelines: Recommendations for the medical management of osteoarthritis of the hip and knee. *Arthritis Rheum* 43(9):1905–1915, 2000.

Berman BM, Lao L, Langenberg P, et al: Effectiveness of acupuncture as adjunctive therapy in osteoarthritis of the knee: A randomized, controlled trial. *Ann Intern Med* 141:901–910, 2004.

Easton BT: Evaluation and treatment of the patient with osteoarthritis. *J Fam Pract* 50(9):791–797, 2001.

Hinton R, Moody RL, David AW, et al: Osteoarthritis: Diagnosis and therapeutic considerations. *Am Fam Phys* 65(5):841–848, 2002.

Kalunian KC, Brion PH, Concoff AL, et al: Nonpharmacologic therapy of osteoarthritis. In: Rose BD, ed., *UpToDate.* Waltham, MA: UpToDate, 2007.

Kalunian KC, Brion PH, Wollaston SJ: Clinical manifestations of osteoarthritis. In: Rose BD, ed., *UpToDate.* Waltham, MA: UpToDate, 2007.

Kalunian KC, Brion PH, Wollaston SJ: Diagnosis and classification of osteoarthritis. In: Rose BD, ed., *UpToDate.* Waltham, MA: UpToDate, 2007.

Kalunian KC, Concoff AL, Brion PH: Pharmacologic therapy of osteoarthritis. In: Rose BD, ed., *UpToDate.* Waltham, MA: UpToDate, 2007.

Kalunian KC, Concoff AL, Wollaston SJ: Investigational approaches to the pharmacologic therapy of osteoarthritis. In: Rose BD, ed., *UpToDate.* Waltham, MA: UpToDate, 2007.

Lo V, Meadows S: When should COX-2 selective NSAIDs be used for osteoarthritis and rheumatoid arthritis? *J Fam Pract* 55(3):260–262, 2006.

Mandelbaum B, Waddell D: Etiology and pathophysiology of osteoarthritis. *Orthopedics* 28(2 Suppl):S207–S214, 2005.

Morehead K, Sack KE: Osteoarthritis: What therapies for this disease of many causes? *Postgrad Med* 114(5):11–17, 2003.

Morelli V, Naquin C, Weaver V: Alternative therapies for traditional disease states: Osteoarthritis. *Am Fam Phys* 67(2):339–344, 2003.

Swagerty DL, Hellenger D: Radiographic assessment of osteoarthritis. *Am Fam Phys* 64(2):279–286, 2001.

CHAPTER

51 **Acute Gout and Pseudogout**

CLINICAL CASE PROBLEM 1

A 45-Year-Old Male with Excruciating
Pain in His Left Foot

A 45-year-old obese male presents to the emergency room (ER) in the middle of the night screaming and holding his left foot. He tells you that he thinks he has an "acute blood vessel blockage" in his left toe. He wakes up the entire ER observation unit with his screams. His past history is significant for essential hypertension, for which he has been treated with a thiazide diuretic for the past 5 years. He categorically relates to you that he has never had the symptoms that he is experiencing now, and he further adds that instead of all these questions he would prefer if you just got on with treatment.

On examination, the patient's temperature is 102.4°F and his blood pressure is 170/110 mmHg. He has an inflamed, tender, swollen left great toe at the metatarsophalangeal (MTP) joint. There is extensive swelling and erythema of the left foot, and his whole foot is tender. No other joints are swollen. No other abnormalities are found on physical examination.

SELECT THE BEST ANSWER TO THE FOLLOWING QUESTIONS

1. What is the most likely diagnosis?
   a. acute cellulitis
   b. acute gouty arthritis
   c. acute rheumatoid arthritis
   d. acute septic arthritis
   e. acute vasculitis

2. Which of the following statements regarding this patient's disease is false?
   a. it is more common in males than in females
   b. fever is unusual
   c. more than 50% of the initial attacks of this condition are confined to the first metatarsophalangeal joint
   d. peripheral leukocytosis can occur
   e. initial involvement is usually in a single joint

3. What is the definitive diagnostic test of choice for this patient's disease?
   a. a plasma level

b. a random urine determination
c. a 24-hour urine determination
d. a synovial fluid analysis
e. a Gram stain plus culture and sensitivity

4. What is the most common metabolic abnormality found in the disease described in this patient?
   a. increased production of uric acid
   b. decreased renal excretion of uric acid
   c. increased production of uric acid metabolites
   d. decreased renal excretion of uric acid metabolites
   e. none of the above

5. What is the pharmacologic agent of choice for the initial management of this patient's disease?
   a. indomethacin
   b. colchicine
   c. acetaminophen
   d. aspirin
   e. phenylbutazone

6. Regarding the prophylaxis recommended for the prevention of future attacks of the disease described in the patient, which of the following would adhere to the current recommendations?
   a. this patient should not be treated with a prophylactic agent
   b. this patient should be treated with a uricosuric agent as prophylaxis against future attacks of this condition
   c. this patient should be treated with a xanthine oxidase inhibitor as prophylaxis against future attacks of this condition
   d. this patient could be treated with either a uricosuric agent or a xanthine oxidase inhibitor as prophylaxis against future attacks of this condition
   e. none of the above

7. Which of the following can be used to help determine the drug of choice for the prophylaxis of the condition described?
   a. a serum blood level
   b. a joint fluid aspiration
   c. a 24-hour urine determination of uric acid
   d. a joint x-ray
   e. none of the above

8. Which of the following drugs increase(s) the excretion of uric acid?
   a. sulfinpyrazone
   b. probenecid
   c. allopurinol
   d. a and b
   e. b and c

9. Which of the following statements apply to the initiation of prophylactic therapy in this condition?
   a. the patient who is started taking a prophylactic agent should also start taking colchicine
   b. colchicine treatment should be maintained for 3 to 6 months
   c. indomethacin can replace colchicine in this instance
   d. none of the above statements are true
   e. All of the above statements are true

10. Which of the following treatments is the best choice to provide significant relief in the case of an acute attack of the condition described?
    a. oral dexamethasone
    b. oral prednisone
    c. intravenous hydrocortisone
    d. intravenous methylprednisolone
    e. intra-articular triamcinolone acetonide

11. Which of the following classes of drugs is most likely to precipitate the condition described?
    a. thiazide diuretics
    b. calcium channel blockers
    c. angiotensin-converting enzyme inhibitors
    d. beta blockers
    e. alpha blockers

CLINICAL CASE PROBLEM 2

A 55-Year-Old Male with Joint Pain

A 55-year-old male comes to your office complaining about joint pain. He states that he has had pain in both ankles for the past 4 months and it has been getting progressively worse. He has also had occasional pain in his wrists. He states that for the past 5 years he has been taking hydrochlorothiazide 50 mg each morning for hypertension with recent typical blood pressure readings in the 130s/70s mmHg. As part of your evaluation, you find that he has a serum uric acid level of 12.4 mg/dL.

12. Should the condition described be treated to reduce the serum uric acid level?
    a. yes, vigorously to prevent an acute attack of gout
    b. yes, but cautiously to prevent a too rapid release of feedback inhibition of purine synthesis
    c. no, the patient is not likely to develop gout
    d. a and c are true under certain conditions
    e. nobody really knows

CLINICAL CASE PROBLEM 3

A 65-Year-Old Male with a Swollen, Painful Knee

A 65-year-old male comes to your office with pain in his right knee. He says he fell and "banged it up fairly bad" approximately 6 months ago, but that it had since recovered spontaneously and provided no further trouble until now. He further said the pain does not get worse during the day, and, if anything, it hurts more upon awakening. His past history showed no hypertension, and he never had any other joint pain of significance.

On examination, his temperature is 37.5°C and his blood pressure is 125/70 mmHg. He has an inflamed, tender, swollen right knee. No other joints are affected. No other abnormalities are found on physical examination. A plain x-ray of the right knee reveals streaking of the surrounding soft tissue with calcium deposits (chondrocalcinosis). You remove accumulated synovial fluid for polarized light microscopic analysis and also obtain a serum sample.

13. Which of the following possible results from these laboratory studies is most consistent with the symptoms described and will confirm a diagnosis?
    a. needlelike crystals with negative birefringence and a normal serum uric acid level
    b. needlelike crystals with negative birefringence and a high serum uric acid level
    c. rhomboidal crystals with weak positive birefringence and a high serum uric acid level
    d. rhomboidal crystals with weak positive birefringence and a normal serum uric acid level
    e. none of the above

14. Which of the following conditions predispose(s) individuals toward the disease described in this case?
    a. hemochromatosis
    b. hyperparathyroidism
    c. trauma
    d. surgery
    e. all of the above

Answers

1. **b.** This patient has acute gouty arthritis. This is a very typical presentation for gout. With acute gout, a patient usually develops an acute pain in a

single joint of the lower extremity, with the most common one being the first metatarsophalangeal joint ("podagra"). The pain of acute gout often awakens a patient, and these patients often end up in the ER with pain that is described as crushing or excruciating.

The joint rapidly becomes erythematous, swollen, warm, and extremely tender. The skin surrounding the joint is usually tense and shiny. The swelling in acute gout often extends well beyond the joint and may involve the entire foot or other part of the extremity. This swelling results from periarticular edema and makes the differentiation from septic arthritis particularly difficult. Often, the patient is unable to bear weight on the affected foot.

2. b. Fever may occur in patients with gout, especially in those with polyarticular disease. The temperature may reach 103°F. Initial presentation is usually monoarticular, and more than 50% of patients experience their first acute attack in a metatarsophalangeal joint. However, gout can present in other joints such as the knee. Acute gout also may involve bursae or tendon sheaths.

Leukocytosis may also be seen. In older patients, tophi are occasionally seen with the first attack. However, there is usually a time interval, often 10 years or more, between the initial attack and the appearance of the complication of gouty tophi.

Gout is uncommon in people younger than age 30 years, and its presence in this age group should trigger a search for a hereditary purine metabolism disorder. It is more common in men than in women until the age of 60 years, after which half of newly diagnosed cases are in women. In women, gout most often occurs following menopause.

3. d. A definitive diagnosis of gout is made by demonstrating negatively birefringent, needle-shaped monosodium urate crystals under a polarizing microscope. Although an elevated serum uric acid concentration is often seen in acute gout, it is neither as sensitive nor as specific a test as the demonstration of uric acid crystals in synovial fluid under a microscope. Serum uric acid levels can be normal in patients with acute gouty arthritis. The diagnosis of septic arthritis can be ruled out by appropriate Gram stain and culture of the same specimen of synovial fluid as obtained for examination with the polarizing microscope.

4. b. Decreased renal excretion of uric acid is the cause of primary gout in 75% to 90% of patients, whereas uric acid overproduction accounts for the

other 10% to 25% of cases. Secondary causes of gout include chronic renal disease, acute ethanol ingestion, low-dose salicylates (they are uricosuric at high doses), and diuretics, especially the thiazide type. The most common cause of overproduction of uric acid is a myeloproliferative or lymphoproliferative disorder. In addition, when a patient is undergoing cancer chemotherapy there is a very significant liberation of uric acid from dying cells. The greater the responsiveness of the tumor to chemotherapy or radiotherapy, the quicker the tumor breakdown and the more extensive the breakdown of uric acid.

5. a. Nonsteroidal anti-inflammatory drugs (NSAIDs) are the drugs of first choice in most settings. There is no evidence that one NSAID is superior to another in the treatment of gout.

Colchicine has many gastrointestinal side effects, particularly diarrhea, that limit its usefulness, especially when dosed hourly, as can be done in acute gout. Dosing it every 6 hours can be beneficial and is less prone to side effects. Aspirin taken in small doses can actually aggravate the problem. Acetaminophen has no anti-inflammatory activity and is not indicated in the acute treatment of gout. Phenylbutazone is an excellent anti-inflammatory agent but has been associated with bone marrow suppression and aplastic anemia.

Systemic corticosteroid therapy can be used to treat patients with acute polyarticular gout who have not responded to other therapies as well as in patients in whom other therapies are contraindicated. Intra-articular injections of corticosteroid medication are usually very effective in patients with acute monoarticular gout.

6. a. From the history, you gather that this is the first attack of acute gout in this patient. It is not advisable to begin prophylactic therapy until the patient has had at least two or perhaps three attacks. One reason is the possibility of a precipitating secondary cause, as in this patient being treated with a thiazide diuretic, which may be able to be eliminated. Also, because a second attack may not occur for years, if ever, the risk/benefit ratio for prophylactic medication is not favorable due to potential adverse effects or drug interactions.

7. c. The choice of a prophylactic agent, if one is going to be used, can be made by determining the 24-hour secretion of uric acid. This helps determine if a patient is an overproducer or underexcreter of uric acid, and a level higher than 800 to 1000 mg indicates overproduction. This test has several limitations, and allopurinol, a xanthine oxidase inhibitor, is commonly used empirically without doing the test, even though uric acid overproduction is by far the less common etiology.

8. **d.** Probenecid and sulfinpyrazone are uricosuric medications. They should only be used in patients who have normal renal function, no history of renal stone formation, and no overproduction of uric acid. Allopurinol is indicated in patients with uric acid overproduction, severe tophi, a history of renal stones, or renal insufficiency, although the dosage should be adjusted in the latter case.

9. **e.** As previously discussed, the prophylactic agents for the prevention of gouty arthritis fall into two classes: the xanthine oxidase inhibitors, which inhibit the formation of uric acid, and the uricosuric agents, which increase the excretion of uric acid.

When prophylaxis against recurrent attacks is begun, either colchicine or an NSAID should be added to the choice of the prophylactic agent. After 3 to 6 months, the colchicine or NSAID treatment can be discontinued, and treatment with the uricosuric agent or the xanthine oxidase inhibitor can continue indefinitely.

10. **e.** A local injection of a corticosteroid such as triamcinolone acetonide into an inflamed gouty joint reliably produces a resolution of the acute gouty condition. This treatment is most beneficial in patients with acute gouty monoarthritis and multiple medical conditions, particularly if there are contraindications to other treatments.

11. **a.** Diuretics in general, and thiazide diuretics in particular, elevate the serum uric acid level. Although the vast majority of patients who are receiving thiazide diuretics do not develop gout, those who do tend to be on relatively high doses of thiazide (>25 mg) and have other coexistent reasons for the development of gout, such as acute ethanol intake. Other metabolic side effects of thiazide diuretics are hyperglycemia, hyperlipidemia, hypokalemia, hyponatremia, and hypomagnesemia. Other medications that can lead to decreased uric acid excretion include low-dose salicylates, levodopa–carbidopa, ethambutol, pyrazinamide, cyclosporine, and nicotinic acid.

12. **c.** The condition described in this case is asymptomatic hyperuricemia. The symptoms described do not sound like gout and are unlikely to be related to the elevated uric acid level. Hyperuricemia is commonly the result of renal insufficiency or pharmacologic agent such as thiazide diuretics or low-dose salicylates. Ethanol consumption and obesity can also raise serum uric acid levels. Most patients with hyperuricemia are asymptomatic and never develop gout. Thus, the treatment of asymptomatic hyperuricemia is not recommended.

13. **d.** The condition described is undoubtedly pseudogout, also known as calcium pyrophosphate deposition disease (CPDD). The symptoms are caused by calcium pyrophosphate deposition in nonosseous tissues in joints, most commonly in a knee. The differential diagnosis includes the many things that can cause swelling and pain in a knee. Considering the patient's age and history, the more likely conditions are osteoarthritis, gout, and pseudogout. The fact that the pain does not get worse during the day points away from, but certainly does not exclude, osteoarthritis. Similarly, the presence of the condition in the knee rather than an MTP joint points away from, but does not exclude, gout. The chondrocalcinosis found on x-ray is almost pathognomic for CPDD, and the presence of rhomboid-shaped crystals with weak positive birefringence in the synovial fluid confirms this diagnosis. The serum uric acid level is not elevated.

14. **e.** CPDD can be caused by any condition that provides a local nucleation site for formation of calcium pyrophosphate crystals, likely via initial precipitation of apatite with subsequent conversion, or in conditions that increase serum phosphate levels until precipitates form at vulnerable sites. Trauma and surgery are likely to create nucleation sites prone to such crystallization, whereas hemochromatosis and hyperparathyroidism tend to increase the serum phosphate level. Diabetes mellitus and hypothyroidism are other endocrine disorders associated with an increased risk for developing CPPD. Many cases appear not to be associated with any known risk factors but possibly are the result of some forgotten relatively mild trauma.

Prevalence increases with age, having been reported to be 3% or 4% in patients younger than age 60 years, as high as 25% in individuals in their 80s, and 50% in patients older than 90 years. It is also said to be seen approximately half as often as gout in the typical primary care office setting.

Symptoms tend to resolve with conservative treatment consisting of rest and use of anti-inflammatory drugs. Intra-articular steroid injections are usually helpful in otherwise intractable cases. Rarely, surgery, in which the crystals are scraped off of the soft tissues, is used as a last resort.

Summary

The diagnosis of gout is firmly established by examination of joint aspirate under a polarizing microscope and finding needlelike, negatively birefringent uric acid crystals. In contrast, the diagnosis of pseudogout (CPDD) is established by finding weakly positively birefringent rectangular or rhomboid crystals in a joint aspirate.

The primary symptom of gout is acute onset of pain in a joint of the lower extremity, most commonly the first metatarsophalangeal joint. Along with the pain there is associated tenderness, erythema, and swelling of the surrounding tissues. The most important differential diagnosis in acute gout is septic arthritis. Acute gout is associated most often with decreased renal excretion of uric acid rather than an overproduction of uric acid.

Treatment of acute attacks of gout can include an NSAID, colchicine, an intra-articular corticosteroid injection, or systemic corticosteroid orally or by intramuscular injection. Colchicine given acutely two or three times daily rather than hourly will usually avoid the previously limiting gastrointestinal side effects. Neither colchicines nor NSAIDs should be used in patients with chronic kidney disease, making an intra-articular corticosteroid injection a good option in these cases.

Prophylactic treatment of gout should not be given after only one attack. Colchicine can be used prophylactically. A uricosuric agent or xanthine oxidase inhibitor can also be used, with the choice typically based on the results of the 24-hour urine uric acid determination plus other factors. If prophylaxis with a uricosuric agent or xanthine oxidase inhibitor is given, then concurrently use either an NSAID or colchicine in low dose for the first 3 to 6 months. Asymptomatic hyperuricemia should not be treated.

Pseudogout symptoms tend to resolve with conservative treatment such as an NSAID. Clues that suggest this diagnosis versus gout include older age, presence in the knee or wrist, absence of hyperuricemia, absence of a history of uric acid nephrolithiasis, and the presence of chondrocalcinosis (calcification of articular cartilage) on radiography.

Suggested Reading

Belestocki KB, Paget SA: Inflammatory rheumatologic disorders in the elderly: Unusual presentations, altered outlooks. *Postgrad Med* 111(4):72–83, 2002.

Chokkalingham S, Velazquez C, Mody A, et al: Diagnosing acute monoarthritis in adults: A practical approach for the family physician. *Am Fam Phys* 68(1):83–90, 2003.

Johnson MW: Acute knee effusions: A systematic approach to diagnosis. *Am Fam Phys* 61(8):2391–2400, 2000.

Lockshin MD: Endocrine origins of rheumatic disease. *Postgrad Med* 111(4):87–92, 2002.

Rosenthal AK: Hyperuricemia and gout. In: Rakel RE, Bope ET, eds., *Conn's Current Therapy*, 55th ed. Philadelphia: Saunders, 2003.

Rott KT, Agudelo CA: Gout. *JAMA* 289(21):2857–2860, 2003.

Schumacher HR: Newer therapeutic approaches: Gout. *Rheum Dis North Am* 32:235–244, 2006.

Terkeltaub RA: Gout. *N Engl J Med* 349(17):1647–1655, 2003.

Winklerprins VJ, Weismantel AM: How effective is prophylactic therapy in people with prior gout attacks? *J Fam Pract* 53(10):837–838, 2004.

CLINICAL CASE PROBLEM 1

A 15-Year-Old Distressed Adolescent with "Zits"

A 15-year-old female comes to your office with a complaint of "zits." She has been attempting to treat these with frequent washings with a buff puff and avoidance of cosmetics and other facial products. She is very distressed and breaks down crying. She is afraid that "no boys will ever go out with someone with such an ugly face." Her past history is unremarkable. She is taking no medications at present. She has no allergies. Her family history is unremarkable.

On physical examination, the patient has multiple maculopapular–pustular lesions with comedones on her face and back. No other abnormalities are found on examination.

SELECT THE BEST ANSWER TO THE FOLLOWING QUESTIONS

1. What is the diagnosis in this patient?
   a. acne vulgaris
   b. polycystic ovary syndrome
   c. acne cystica
   d. rosacea
   e. folliculitis

2. What is the treatment of first choice in this patient at this time?
   a. topical tretinoin
   b. intralesional corticosteroids
   c. topical benzoyl peroxide
   d. topical erythromycin
   e. oil-based antiacne moisturizers

3. The patient returns. There has been an improvement of approximately 20% in the skin lesions since her first visit. She gradually has increased the strength of the preparation you gave her. What would you do at this time?
   a. discontinue the first agent and treat her with topical benzoyl peroxide
   b. discontinue the first agent and treat her with topical tretinoin
   c. continue the first agent and add topical tretinoin
   d. discontinue the first agent and treat her with topical clindamycin
   e. continue the first agent and add topical erythromycin

4. The patient returns again in another 8 weeks. She now has sustained an improvement of approximately 35% in the lesions since her first visit, and she continues to execute your instructions faithfully. However, she is still not satisfied, and neither are you. What would you do at this time?
   a. discontinue the first and second agents and substitute a systemic antibiotic
   b. continue the first and second agents and add a systemic antibiotic
   c. continue the first and second agents and add topical clindamycin or erythromycin
   d. continue the first and second agents and add oral isotretinoin
   e. continue the first and second agents and add a new "oil-free" product that through your local pharmaceutical detail agent you have learned "kills acne bugs dead"

5. The patient returns again in 4 weeks. She now has sustained an improvement of approximately 50% but is still not satisfied. What would you do at this time?
   a. refer her for psychiatric counseling for distorted body image perception
   b. refer her to a dermatologist
   c. tell her to "hang in there" for a little longer and if she is not satisfied then, she will start taking an oral antibiotic
   d. stop all the medication and try something else
   e. continue all three agents and add a systemic antibiotic

CLINICAL CASE PROBLEM 2

A Case of Nodular–Pustular Acne

An 18-year-old male comes to your office with moderately severe nodular–pustular acne on his face and back.

6. What would be your agent of first choice in this case?
   a. topical benzoyl peroxide
   b. topical tretinoin
   c. systemic tetracycline
   d. penicillin
   e. isotretinoin

7. The patient returns in 6 weeks with only moderate improvement. What would you now prescribe?
   a. systemic tetracycline
   b. systemic erythromycin
   c. cyproterone acetate
   d. isotretinoin
   e. none of the above

8. Choose the correct statement:
   a. a closed comedone is also known as a blackhead
   b. an open comedone is a noninflamed follicular opening containing a keratotic plug that appears black
   c. an open comedone is also known as a whitehead
   d. a papule is a round elevation of skin with a central pocket of pus
   e. mild acne is characterized by comedones, papules, and cysts

9. Acne is the result of a pathophysiologic process in the pilosebaceous unit that stems from abnormalities in
   a. sebum production
   b. follicular hyperkeratization
   c. proliferation and colonization of *Propionibacterium acnes*
   d. release of inflammatory mediators
   e. all of the above

10. Which of the following statements regarding acne is (are) true?
    a. chocolate can exacerbate acne vulgaris
    b. acne medications initially may worsen acne
    c. acne is a result of poor hygiene
    d. it is not necessary to use sunscreen with topical retinoid products but it is necessary with oral retinoid products
    e. all of the above

11. Which of the following bacteria is (are) associated with the condition described?
    a. *Staphylococcus aureus*
    b. *Streptococcus viridans*
    c. *Propionibacterium acnes*
    d. all of the above
    e. none of the above

12. Which of the following is (are) essential for a good skin care program specifically designed for patients with the described disorder?
    a. oil-free products
    b. thorough, frequent cleansing of skin with exfoliants
    c. manual manipulation of skin lesions
    d. use of gels and solutions for dry skin
    e. applying all of topical medications at bedtime

13. On further questioning, you learn that the patient in Clinical Case Problem 1 has missed several periods, but that is not unusual for her. Her skin looks a little worse. You now would
    a. inquire about excessive hair growth
    b. check a pregnancy test
    c. if no contraindications exist, prescribe an oral contraceptive
    d. after confirmatory testing, consider an antiandrogen
    e. all of the above

14. The patient in Clinical Case Problem 1 started taking oral contraceptives and tetracycline. Important information about these medications and acne is
    a. because she is taking an oral contraceptive, no risk for pregnancy exists with concomitant tetracycline therapy
    b. tetracycline is more photosensitizing than doxycycline
    c. vaginal yeast infections are rarely seen with tetracycline
    d. isotretinoin may be prescribed only by physicians enrolled in a program monitored by Roche Pharmaceutical Company
    e. adapalene is more irritating than tretinoin

15. What is (are) the absolute contraindication(s) to the use of oral isotretinoin for the treatment of acne vulgaris?
    a. children younger than age 14 years
    b. women of childbearing potential who are not adequately protected against pregnancy
    c. allergy to topical tretinoin
    d. all of the above
    e. none of the above

16. Which of the following is (are) true concerning rosacea?
    a. rosacea occurs in middle-aged individuals
    b. rosacea consists of papules and pustules on the face
    c. rosacea produces a background erythema and telangiectasias on the face
    d. all of the above
    e. none of the above

17. What is the first-line treatment of rosacea?
    a. topical benzoyl peroxide
    b. topical tretinoin
    c. topical erythromycin or clindamycin

d. topical metronidazole

e. none of the above

18. What is the second-line treatment of rosacea?
    a. topical metronidazole
    b. oral metronidazole
    c. oral tetracycline
    d. oral 13-*cis*-retinoic acid
    e. oral erythromycin

19. Other treatments for rosacea include
    a. avoidance of alcoholic beverages to reduce flushing
    b. use of permethrin cream to reduce papules and erythema
    c. use of isotretinoin in nonpregnant women
    d. use of laser therapy to eradicate telangiectasias
    e. all of the above

20. Which of the following conditions is sometimes associated with rosacea?
    a. rhinophyma
    b. cellulitis
    c. multiple carbuncle formation
    d. cavernous sinus thrombosis
    e. anaerobic septicemia

Clinical Case Management Problem

Describe the pathophysiology of acne vulgaris.

Answers

1. **a.** This patient has acne vulgaris. Acne vulgaris primarily affects teenagers but continues to affect many patients into their 20s and 30s.

2. **c.** See answer 7 for explanation.

3. **c.** See answer 7 for explanation.

4. **c.** See answer 7 for explanation.

5. **c.** See answer 7 for explanation.

6. **c.** See answer 7 for explanation.

7. **d.** The treatment of choice for acne can take many forms, but a recommended approach is outlined here. In this approach, only one drug is added at a time; this allows you to evaluate clearly the efficacy of that agent. Allow 6 to 8 weeks for treatment to work before deciding to try another regimen or add another agent. This approach may need to be amended if the patient presents with a nodular–pustular acne.

1. Treatment protocol for mild to moderate acne
   a. Begin with topical benzoyl peroxide 2.5%. Increase to 5% and 10% rapidly. Benzoyl peroxide is usually applied twice a day.
   b. Add topical tretinoin or adapalene. These are applied at bedtime. Remember to tell your patient to expect redness and irritation of the face, especially in the initial period. Urge the patient not to discontinue the product because of this side effect.
   c. Add topical erythromycin or topical clindamycin. This should be used in combination with a and b. If there are significant lesions on the back that are difficult for the patient to reach (even at the beginning of treatment), you may need to prescribe a systemic antibiotic from the beginning.
   d. Add systemic tetracycline to the topical benzoyl peroxide and topical tretinoin. Continue the topical antibiotic.

2. Moderate to severe nodular pustular acne
   a. The choices for systemic antibiotic therapy include tetracycline, minocycline, doxycycline, erythromycin, clindamycin, and trimethoprim–sulfamethoxazole.
   b. In severe cystic acne, an oral retinoid, isotretinoin, may be necessary.

8. **b.** An open comedone is a noninflamed follicular opening containing a keratotic plug that appears black (i.e., a blackhead).

9. **e.** Acne vulgaris is the result of the obstruction of sebaceous follicles by sebum and desquamated epithelial cells. An anaerobic organism, *Propionibacterium acnes*, will proliferate, which leads to inflammation. Clinically, these pathophysiologic events will lead to noninflammatory open and closed comedones and, in more severe cases, inflammatory papules, pustules, and nodules. Most patients will have a mixture of both noninflammatory and inflammatory lesions. Closed comedones are also known as whiteheads, and open comedones are also known as blackheads. Mild acne is characterized by comedones and papules. Cystic acne is moderate to severe.

The pathophysiology of acne vulgaris involves the following six steps: (1) androgen stimulation of sebum production; (2) keratinous obstruction of the sebaceous follicle outlet; (3) accumulation of keratin and sebum with the formation of open and closed comedones (blackheads and whiteheads); (4) bacterial colonization of the trapped sebum with *P. acnes*; (5) inflammatory reaction to the colonization of the trapped sebum; and (6) production of inflammatory papules, pustules, nodules, and cysts.

10. b. Acne medications can cause an initial worsening of symptoms. There is no indication that the intake of certain foods is associated with acne. This includes chocolate, nuts, and shellfish. A common acne myth is that acne is the result of poor hygiene. Retinoid products of any kind are photosensitizing, and sunscreen is mandatory with the concurrent use of these products.

11. c. Acne vulgaris is associated with the bacterium *P. acnes*.

12. a. A good skin care program includes the following: cleansing gently and nonabrasively, using oil-free products, and leaving the skin lesions alone. It is also important to match the vehicle (lotion, cream, gel, or solution) with the skin type. Gels and solutions tend to be more drying, whereas lotions and creams are somewhat more emollient.

13. e. This patient exhibits two of the three characteristics of polycystic ovarian syndrome (PCOS). The triad consists of acne, hirsutism, and irregular periods. Obesity and the metabolic syndrome may also be features of this condition. Oral contraceptives can be beneficial for acne treatment and restoration of menses to prevent endometrial proliferation. Antiandrogens (spironolactone) are useful in the management of the acne and hirsutism. Lastly, a pregnancy test must be checked in a woman with amenorrhea because pregnancy is the primary cause of amenorrhea. PCOS is the second leading cause of amenorrhea.

14. d. Broad-spectrum antibiotics may reduce the effectiveness of oral contraceptives. Certain estrogen-containing oral contraceptives may be used in the treatment of moderate acne vulgaris in females 15 years of age or older who desire contraception, have achieved menarche, and are unresponsive to topical antiacne medications. Doxycycline is slightly more photosensitizing than tetracycline. An advantage of adapalene over tretinoin is that it is less irritating. In April 2002, Roche Laboratories released the System to Manage Accutane Related Teratogenicity (SMART) program aimed at preventing pregnant women from receiving

isotretinoin. The prescriber must be enrolled in this program.

15. d. The single most important absolute contraindication to the use of 13-*cis*-retinoic acid (Accutane) is women in the reproductive years. Accutane is teratogenic and should never be used in this age group. Children younger than age 14 years and individuals with allergic reactions (not the redness that is characteristic of topical isotretinoin) also should not be given 13-*cis*-retinoic acid.

16. d. Rosacea is an acneiform condition that affects middle-aged or older patients. It is characterized by papules and pustules occurring on a background of erythema and telangiectasia of facial skin. The main area affected is the middle third of the face, from the forehead to the chin. With rosacea, comedones are typically absent. There is, however, a tendency for the facial skin of patients affected by rosacea to become thickened and to produce enlarged sebaceous glands. When this happens in the area of the nose, the condition is known as rhinophyma. Rosacea is more common in women, but affected men seem more prone to develop severe cases of rhinophyma. W. C. Fields' nose was a classic example.

17. d. The first-line treatment for rosacea is a topical antibiotic. The antibiotic of choice is metronidazole (MetroGel) applied twice daily. Topical tretinoin and topical benzoyl peroxide preparations aggravate the erythema and are usually not helpful. Topical corticosteroids also aggravate the condition.

18. c. The second-line treatment for rosacea is a systemic antibiotic. Tetracycline is the drug of choice. After the first month, the dosage can often be lowered and then ultimately discontinued. Recurrences are common, however, and repeated courses of antibiotics are often needed. Systemic antibiotics are also useful in treating the associated keratitis and blepharitis that are occasionally associated with rosacea.

Systemic therapy with erythromycin, minocycline, doxycycline, or metronidazole is effective if tetracycline is ineffective.

Rosacea that fails to respond to the treatment alternatives just outlined may respond to oral isotretinoin.

19. e. There are many lifestyle recommendations for the treatment of rosacea. Many involve avoidance of substances that may be vasoactive, such as hot beverages, cold beverages, caffeine, alcohol, or spicy foods. A study found efficacy with the use of permethrin cream to reduce papules and erythema. Laser treatments can eradicate telangiectasias.

20. **a.** Rhinophyma is hypertrophy of the soft tissue of the nose. Patients have a large, bulbous, ruddy appearance of the nose. Seen in men, usually older than 40 years of age, it is considered a severe form of rosacea. Treatment is usually surgical, often with lasers, although Accutane has been used with good results.

Solution to the Clinical Case Management Problem

The pathophysiology of acne vulgaris involves the following six steps: (1) androgen stimulation of sebum production; (2) keratinous obstruction of the sebaceous follicle outlet; (3) accumulation of keratin and sebum with the formation of open and closed comedones (blackheads and whiteheads); (4) bacterial colonization of the trapped sebum with *P. acnes*; (5) inflammatory reaction to the colonization of the trapped sebum; and (6) production of inflammatory papules, pustules, nodules, and cysts.

Summary

ACNE VULGARIS

1. Prevalence: 75% of teenagers and young adults (up to and including patients in their 20s and 30s)
2. Pathophysiology: See the Clinical Case Management Problem box
3. Causative organism: *Propionibacterium acnes*
4. Classification of acne vulgaris
   a. Obstructive acne
      i. Closed comedones (whiteheads)
      ii. Open comedones (blackheads)
   b. Inflammatory acne: Formation of lesions generally occurs in the following order: papules, pustules, nodules, cysts, and scars
5. Treatment measures
   a. Nonpharmacologic: Gentle face washing, avoidance of manipulation of acne lesions, using water-based cosmetics only, and using oil-free moisturizers only
   b. Pharmacologic: The treatment of acne vulgaris can be seen as a series of discrete steps:
      Step 1: Begin with benzoyl peroxide gel.
      Step 2: Add topical tretinoin or adapalene. (Consider using step 1 in the morning and step 2 in the evening.)
      Step 3: Add topical antibiotic (erythromycin or clindamycin). (Consider using step 3 along with a combination of steps 1 and 2.)
      Step 4: Add systemic antibiotics, such as tetracycline, minocycline, doxycycline, erythromycin, clindamycin, or trimethoprim–sulfamethoxazole. (Consider using a combination of steps 1, 2, 3, and 4.)
      Step 5: For severe nodular–cystic acne only, use oral isotretinoin (associated with serious, dose-related side effects).
6. Common myths believed by patients
   a. Acne is caused by failure to wash away dirt and oil with sufficient zeal. Not true—acne can be made worse by washing too vigorously and causing irritation. Gentle washing with normal soap is sufficient.
   b. Too much junk food causes acne. Not true—no connection between diet and acne has ever been established.
   c. "Unhealthy" sex habits, including masturbation, same-sex play, or even simple indulgence, can cause acne. Not true—sex with the wrong person can cause rashes but it will not be acne.
   d. Stress can cause acne. Not true—however, stress can increase a nervous tendency to pick, squeeze, and/or rub pimples and make them worse.
   e. Acne is a normal adolescent problem of no consequence that should be allowed to run its course. Not true—the physical and psychologic consequences of acne can be cataclysmic. Prompt treatment can prevent severe outbreaks and avoid physical and emotional scarring.
   f. Acne vulgaris always clears up after adolescence. Not true—more than 10% of individuals continue to have this form of acne well into adulthood.

ROSACEA

1. Definition: Acneiform eruption that affects middle-aged patients. It is characterized by papules and pustules occurring on a background of erythema and telangiectasia of facial skin.
2. Complications: Thick skin forms on the face (especially on nose). This condition is called rhinophyma.
3. Treatment
   Step 1: Topical metronidazole
   Step 2: Systemic therapy—tetracycline, erythromycin, minocycline, doxycycline, metronidazole, or isotretinoin

Suggested Reading

American Academy of Dermatology. Available at www.aad.org.

Blount BW, Pelletier AL: Rosacea: A common, yet commonly overlooked, condition. *Am Fam Phys* 66:435–440, 2002.

Feldman S, Careccia RE, Barham KL, Hancox J: Diagnosis and treatment of acne. *Am Fam Phys* 69:2123–2130, 2004.

Institute for Clinical Systems Improvement: *Health Care Guidelines, Acne Management.* Available at www.icsi.org, 2006.

James WD: Acne. *N Engl J Med* 352:1463–1472, 2005.

Powell FC: Rosacea. *N Engl J Med* 352:793–803, 2005.

CHAPTER

53 Common Skin Cancers

CLINICAL CASE PROBLEM 1

A 68-Year-Old Female Who Loves Sunbathing

A 68-year-old female comes to your office and asks you to examine three shiny, pearly, semitranslucent, red nodules on her upper back. She is a light-skinned individual of northwestern European descent. When asked if her back was ever exposed to the sun, she replied she had been sunbathing since her teens in as skimpy bathing suit as the law permitted. When she was younger, she believed a total body tan was sexy, and she still believed a tan was a sign of good health; even now at her age she thought sunbathing was a good way to get the vitamin D she needed for her old bones. In fact, she had just come from the beach.

SELECT THE BEST ANSWER TO THE FOLLOWING QUESTIONS

1. Which of the following is the most likely cause of the nodules on her back?
   a. squamous cell carcinoma
   b. actinic keratosis
   c. basal cell carcinoma
   d. nodular melanoma
   e. sand flea bites

2. If left untreated, the most likely outcome of the condition described here is
   a. metastasis to bone
   b. metastasis to the liver
   c. increased size

   d. a and c
   e. b and c

CLINICAL CASE PROBLEM 2

A 70-Year-Old Male Office Worker Who Surfed as a Youth

During a routine examination, you note a circular, pinkish spot with a diameter of ¼ inch on the face of a 70-year-old patient. When you rub your finger across it, you note it is dry and rough. Your patient tells you that on occasion it will become scaly and that it appeared and disappeared several times during the course of the past year before finally becoming permanent.

3. This pinkish area is most likely which of the following?
   a. squamous cell carcinoma
   b. actinic keratosis
   c. basal cell carcinoma
   d. nodular melanoma
   e. an age-related "liver spot"

4. If left untreated, the most likely outcome of the condition described is which of the following?
   a. spreading of the affected area without malignancy
   b. development of a squamous cell carcinoma
   c. development of a basal cell carcinoma
   d. development of a melanoma
   e. spontaneous remission

5. Which of the following methods is (are) used to treat the condition described here?
   a. laser surgery
   b. topical medication with or without chemical peeling
   c. curettage as desiccation
   d. cryosurgery
   e. photodynamic therapy
   f. all of the above

An African American Pipe Smoker

A 58-year-old dark-skinned African American man comes to your office worried about an open sore on the left side of his lower lip that occasionally bleeds. He says he has had this sore for approximately 3 months. However, for at least a year before developing this open sore his lip was dry, scaly, and had become paler than the surrounding area. When asked if he smoked, he said he habitually puffed on a pipe that he kept on the left side of his mouth.

6. This open sore on his lip is most likely which of the following?
   a. squamous cell carcinoma
   b. actinic keratosis
   c. basal cell carcinoma
   d. nodular melanoma
   e. a herpes infection

7. If left untreated, the most likely outcome of the condition described here is which of the following?
   a. continued intermittent bleeding from the upper skin layers with no more profound consequence
   b. penetration of the cancer into deeper layers of the skin
   c. development of metastatic cancers
   d. a and b
   e. b and c

A 49-Year-Old Female with a Funny-Looking Mole

A mammography radiology technician noted a mole in the area were her patient's bra rubbed under her left breast. She became concerned because this mole was asymmetric, had an uneven border, and was colored with various shades of brown. At the technician's recommendation, the patient made an appointment with her primary care physician to examine it further. The physician made a probable diagnosis.

8. The most probable diagnosis is which of the following?
   a. an unremarkable nonmalignant mole
   b. actinic keratosis
   c. a melanoma

d. any of the above
e. all of the above

9. Which of the following is true about the condition described in Clinical Case Problem 4?
   a. almost all of the conditions described are caused by overexposure to sun
   b. the number of cases is increasing
   c. the number of cases is decreasing
   d. most of the conditions described are located on the face
   e. White people are more prone to get the condition described in Clinical Case Problem 4 under the nails, the soles of their feet, or palms of their hands than African Americans or Asians.

10. Assuming the probable diagnosis in Clinical Case Problem 4 was confirmed and proper treatment was provided, which of the following is the most accurate statement concerning the likely outcome?
    a. a high probability of death
    b. a high probability of a cure
    c. it depends on the type of condition
    d. there is no way of predicting it
    e. it will depend on the patient's eating habits

Answers

1. **c.** Basal cell carcinoma is the most common form of skin cancer; it affects approximately 800,000 Americans annually. It can present in several ways: typically as a shiny, pearly, or translucent nodule; in fair-skinned individuals the nodule is red, pink, or white, whereas it might be tan, brown, or black in more deeply pigmented individuals. Fair-skinned individuals are more susceptible. The major cause is chronic exposure to sunlight, and the prevalence of the disease is increasing. Several decades ago, it was most commonly found in older men who spent a lifetime working outdoors, and it was usually found on the face, hands, and arms. Recently, the disease has become more common in women, and as bathing suits receded in size, the area of the body in which these cancers are found increased in both sexes. Because most sunbathing is done without shoes, it is not unusual to see basal cell carcinoma of the feet.

Besides presenting as a shiny, pearly, or translucent nodule, basal cell carcinomas can present in four additional ways: (1) as an open sore that bleeds, oozes, or crusts and remains open for at least 3 weeks (such open, nonhealing sores are a very common sign of early basal cell carcinoma); (2) as a reddish patch that might crust and that might itch or hurt or provide no discomfort; (3) as a slightly elevated area with a rolled border and a crusted indentation in the center in which, as the crust enlarges, tiny blood vessels develop in the center; and (4) as a white or yellow-tinted, sometimes waxy area with poorly defined borders, in which the skin appears shiny and tight. This is the least frequent sign but also may denote the presence of a particular aggressive type of basal cell carcinoma.

2. **c.** These cancers arise in the basal cells of the epidermis and rarely metastasize. If left untreated, they will continue to grow into an increasingly unsightly mass on the skin, but only in very rare case will they metastasize into deeper tissue and cause other morbidity or death.

Treatment may be accomplished by excision, electrodesiccation and curettage, application of liquid nitrogen, Moh's surgery, radiation, or topical 5-fluorouracil cream. An advantage of excision is that this will provide a sample for biopsy. Before using a method that will destroy the sample, a specimen must be obtained for pathologic evaluation.

3. **b.** This is actinic keratosis (AK), which usually develops as a scaly, crusty, slightly elevated spot on the skin in an area chronically exposed to the sun, leading to the pseudonym solar keratosis. Fair-skinned individuals are more susceptible, and AK is very common in such populations, especially if they live in sunny areas. Chronic exposure to ultraviolet light is the cause, and the damage accumulates over time; thus, it more commonly appears in older people. It has been claimed that the majority of people who live into their 80s will have developed AK. Typically, AK lesions appear on areas chronically exposed to the sun, such as the face, ears, neck, back of the forearms, shoulders, lips, and the scalp (the latter especially on men who are bald or shave their heads). The lesions tend to start out as small circular individual spots that develop slowly, even appearing and then disappearing and reappearing several times until fully established. These affected areas are often flat but sometimes slightly elevated, are always rough, and will develop white scales that tend to come and go. They usually have a color similar to the normal skin with slightly changed pigments. Thus, in fair-skinned individuals they usually have a light pinkish hue but sometimes are a deeper red or even a rusty brown or tannish color. In highly pigmented individuals, they are sometimes lighter in color than the surrounding area. Several AKs may appear at the same time, and as they mature they create an area of scaly patches rather than discrete little circles.

4. **a.** The most likely outcome is that the affected area will increase but it will not undergo a malignant transformation. However, approximately 5% will undergo a malignant transformation, most commonly into a squamous cell carcinoma; therefore, AK should be treated. AKs on the lip, known as actinic cheilitis, have a propensity for developing into a particularly aggressive type of squamous cell cancer and are therefore the most dangerous.

5. **f.** All the methods mentioned can be used. Cryosurgery is the most common method used when a limited number of lesions are involved. Liquid nitrogen is applied, commonly via a spraying device, although a cotton-tipped applicator can also be used. The AK becomes crusted, shrinks, and falls off within 1 or 2 weeks. Sometimes, some pigment is lost, particularly in highly pigmented people.

Curettage involves taking a biopsy specimen and is particularly valuable if a malignancy is suspected.

Topical medication is usually used if a large area is involved. A cream containing 5-fluorouracil is applied by the patient on a predetermined schedule. The AK usually crusts over and falls off within a few weeks. Chemical peeling is a variation on the previous procedure using a more corrosive agent, usually trichloroacetic acid, which is applied directly to the affected area. Within a week, the skin sloughs off to be replaced by new epidermis. This method requires local anesthesia and can cause temporary discoloration and irritation.

In laser surgery, a laser beam is focused on the AK, removing the epidermis and even some of the deeper areas. It is a particularly effective technique for treating small narrow areas on the face, scalp, or ears and in particular for actinic cheilitis of the lip.

In photodynamic therapy, topical 5-aminolevulinic acid (5-ALA) is applied to the affected area. On the following day, the medicated area is exposed to a strong light, activating the 5-ALA and selectively destroying the AK. This causes little damage to the surrounding skin.

6. **a.** The hallmark of a squamous cell carcinoma is an open sore that will not heal. Squamous cell carcinoma is the second most common form of skin cancer, with a yearly incidence of approximately 200,000 cases. As with other skin cancers, most cases occur in response to chronic exposure to the sun and are far more prevalent in the elderly, fair-skinned populations. However, they also occur in areas where skin is damaged by other agents, such as burns, petroleum byproducts, radiation, and chronic irritation such as that which might be inflicted by a hot pipe. In the latter case, the carcinogenic chemicals in the tobacco smoke probably play a synergistic role. Indeed, squamous cell carcinoma is rarely induced by sun in dark-skinned African Americans. Such highly pigmented individuals are far less likely to develop skin cancer than less pigmented people. However, when they do, approximately two-thirds of these cancers are squamous cell carcinoma, mostly induced by non-sun-related causes of skin damage, as in the case described. In addition, a small fraction of squamous cell carcinomas may arise from an inherited condition or from white patches on the tongue or inside the mouth (leukopenia).

The dry, scaly lip described as a precursor to the open sore in Clinical Case Problem 3 was actinic cheilitis. Whether caused by chronic sun exposure or other injurious factors, some form of AK is usually the precursor; on the lip, this is actinic cheilitis.

7. e. Untreated cases of squamous cell carcinoma will eventually penetrate the underlying tissue. A small but significant fraction of these will metastasize and may become fatal. This latter outcome is much more likely to occur from squamous cell carcinoma of the lip.

Treatment is the same as described for basal cell carcinoma.

8. c. This mole bore at least three of the five typical earmarks of a melanoma (the "ABCDEs"). These are asymmetry (A), border irregularity (B), coloration that is uneven (C), a diameter greater than 6 mm that is atypical of moles (D), and elevation or enlargement (E). The next step would be to arrange for a biopsy and determine if the diagnosis can be confirmed.

9. b. During the past decade, the number of melanoma cases diagnosed has increased more rapidly than that of any other cancer. The American Cancer Society estimates that there are at least 51,000 new cases each year. Although exposure to the sun is a risk factor, most melanomas appear to start from a chronic irritation of a preexisting mole, as in Clinical Case Problem 4. As a consequence, most melanomas are found on the trunk, legs, arms, and scalp—not the face. African Americans and Asians are prone to develop a variant type of melanoma that usually appears as a black or brown discoloration under their nails, the soles of their feet, or palms of their hands.

10. c. There are four types of melanomas. Of these, some tend to remain located on the uppermost part of the skin. Assuming these "*in situ*" cases are treated early and properly, they have an almost 100% cure rate. However, some are invasive and quickly metastasize to other tissues and as a consequence are likely to be fatal. The four basic variant types are (1) superficial spreading melanoma, (2) lentigo melanoma, (3) acral lentiginous melanoma, and (4) nodular melanoma.

Superficial spreading melanoma is the most common variant, accounting for approximately 70% of the total. Although these spread, they tend to do so along the top layers of skin, and they only dive deeper after a considerable time. As a consequence, the prognosis is favorable. This is the most prevalent form in young adults and generally is found on trunk or legs.

Most lentigo melanomas grow in a manner similar to the superficial spreading melanomas, but they most commonly are found on areas chronically exposed to the sun and on elderly people. Presumably, sun exposure is the precipitating factor. This form most commonly occurs in tropical/semitropical climates. A lentigo melanoma variant, called lentigo maligna melanoma, exists, which is more invasive than the more common form.

Acral lentiginous melanoma also first spreads superficially but differs from the other forms in that it appears as a black or dark brown discoloration under the nails and on the soles of the feet and palms of the hands. As mentioned previously, it rarely is found in white people.

The fourth melanoma variant is nodular melanoma. This form is invasive from the beginning, and the prognosis is not good. It is often first recognized as a bump (hence the name). As a rule, this node is black, but it can be almost any other color except green.

Melanoma *in situ* should be excised with margins of at least 0.5 cm. Melanoma less than 1.5 mm deep should be cut out with a margin of at least 1 cm. Lesions that are 1.5 to 4 mm deep should be removed with margins up to 2 cm. Still deeper melanomas should have margins up to 3 cm. Sentinel node biopsy is used in patients with lesions that are more than 1 mm in depth.

Summary

1. Most, but not all, types of skin cancer are induced by exposure to ultraviolet rays from the sun. Lightly pigmented people are more susceptible to all forms of sun-induced skin lesions, and in large part these cancers appear in late maturity but got their start during an individual's first two decades.

2. The incidence of and mortality from skin cancers have increased exponentially during the past few decades. This is in part the result of high-level atmospheric protective ozone depletion, secondary to the use of aerosolized fluorocarbons. Modern dress styles also permit exposure of greater amounts of

skin, particularly among younger people engaged in swimming and other sports.

3. The most common form of skin cancer is basal cell carcinoma. Theses cancers seldom metastasize.

4. The second most common form is squamous cell carcinoma. These cancers have a greater chance of penetrating the basal skin layer and metastasizing than do basal cell carcinomas, but this still is a relatively rare occurrence. The most dangerous are those on the lips or mucus membranes.

5. Actinic keratosis is a skin lesion largely derived from sun exposure. It is extremely common and has an approximately 5% chance of becoming malignant. As a rule, the resultant malignancy is a squamous cell carcinoma.

6. Melanomas are pigmented cancers often derived from preexisting moles. Melanomas are considered likely if the lesion meets one of the five "ABCDE" criteria: asymmetry, border irregularity, color variegation, diameter greater than 6 mm, and enlargement or elevation. There are four types: superficial spreading melanomas, lentigo maligna, acral lentiginous melanoma, and nodular melanoma. For the most part, the first three of these are *in situ* cancers; that is, although they may spread horizontally on the skin, they only penetrate to deeper layers after being present for some time. This makes them accessible for excision and permits a respectable "cure" rate, provided they are diagnosed and treated within a reasonable time. Nodular melanomas, however, immediately go deep, making metastasis likely and the prognosis poor.

7. Most melanomas are found on the trunk and legs and are not induced by exposure to the sun. The exception is lentigo melanoma, which tends to be found on the face and other sun-exposed areas and more often arises in the elderly in a manner analogous to basal cell and squamous cell carcinomas.

8. Acral lentiginous melanoma generally arises on soles of the feet, palms of the hands, or under the nails. It is most common in highly pigmented African Americans and Asians.

9. To reduce the risk of most skin cancers, sun burns should be avoided and exposure to ultraviolet radiation should be reduced by using a sunscreen rated 15 or higher. It is particularly important to ensure that light-skinned young children are protected from overexposure to the sun.

10. To avoid mortality from skin cancer, one should periodically perform a self-exam on all areas of the body.

Suggested Reading

Martinez JC, Otley CC: The management of melanoma and non-melanoma skin cancer: A review for the primary care physician. *Mayo Clinic Proc* 76(12):1253–1265, 2001.

Miller AJ, Mihm MC, Jr.: Melanoma. *N Engl J Med* 355:51–65, 2006.

Rubin AI, Chen EH, Ratner D: Basal cell carcinoma. *N Engl J Med* 353:2262–2269, 2005.

Strayer SM, Reynolds PL: Diagnosing skin malignancy: Assessment of predictive clinical criteria and risk factors. *J Fam Pract* 52(3):210–218, 2003.

CHAPTER

54 Ear, Nose, and Throat Problems

CLINICAL CASE PROBLEM 1

A 38-Year-Old Female with a Feeling of Dizziness and Imbalance

A 38-year-old female comes to your office with a 1-year history of episodic dizziness, ringing in both ears, a feeling of aural fullness, and hearing loss. The symptoms come on every 1 or 2 weeks and usually last for 12 hours. Nausea and vomiting are present. When asked to describe the dizziness, the patient says, "the world is spinning around me."

On physical examination, the patient has horizontal nystagmus. The slow phase of the nystagmus is to the left, and the rapid phase is to the right. Audiograms reveal bilateral sensorineural hearing loss in the low frequencies.

SELECT THE BEST ANSWER TO THE FOLLOWING QUESTIONS

1. What is the most likely diagnosis in this patient?
   a. vestibular neuronitis
   b. acute labyrinthitis
   c. benign positional paroxysmal vertigo
   d. orthostatic hypotension
   e. Ménière's disease

2. The treatment of this disorder includes each of the following except
   a. decreased caffeine intake
   b. decreased alcohol intake
   c. use of a thiazide diuretic
   d. salt restriction
   e. Epley maneuvers

3. All of the following are true regarding this disease except
   a. it is also known as endolymphatic hydrops
   b. surgery is a treatment option
   c. there is low-frequency sensorineural hearing loss
   d. steroids are a treatment option
   e. vertigo can be treated with benzodiazepines

CLINICAL CASE PROBLEM 2

A 23-Year-Old Female Who Is Dizzy

A 23-year-old female comes to your office with a 6-month history of dizziness. She "feels dizzy" when she stands up (as if she is going to faint). The sensation disappears within a minute.

She has a history of major depression. She started taking doxepin 6 months ago, and her depression has improved much since that time.

The patient's blood pressure is 140/90 mmHg sitting and decreases to 90/70 mmHg when she stands. There is no ataxia, nystagmus, or other symptoms.

4. What is the most likely diagnosis in this patient?
   a. vestibular neuronitis
   b. acute labyrinthitis
   c. benign positional paroxysmal vertigo
   d. orthostatic hypotension
   e. Ménière's disease

5. What is the best treatment for this patient?
   a. an antiemetic
   b. increase antidepressant dose
   c. education and reassurance
   d. Epley maneuvers
   e. prednisone

CLINICAL CASE PROBLEM 3

A 30-Year-Old Male Who Becomes Dizzy When He Rolls Over

A 30-year-old male comes to your office for assessment of dizziness. The dizziness occurs when he rolls over from the lying position to either the left side or the right side. It also occurs when he is looking up. He describes a sensation of "the world spinning around" him. The episodes usually last 10 to 15 seconds. They have been occurring for the past 6 months and occur on average one or two times per day.

6. What is the most likely diagnosis in this patient?
   a. vestibular neuronitis
   b. acute labyrinthitis

   c. benign positional paroxysmal vertigo
   d. orthostatic hypotension
   e. Ménière's disease

7. What is the treatment of choice for this patient?
   a. avoidance of alcohol and caffeine
   b. dimenhydrinate
   c. a thiazide diuretic
   d. reassurance and simple exercises
   e. endolymphatic surgery

CLINICAL CASE PROBLEM 4

A 39-Year-Old Female with Unrelenting Dizziness Associated with Nausea and Vomiting

A 39-year-old female comes to your office with a 2-day history of "unrelenting dizziness." The room feels like it is spinning and there is associated nausea and vomiting. There has been no hearing loss, tinnitus, or sensation of aural fullness. The patient has just recovered from an upper respiratory tract infection.

The patient is afebrile. On examination, nystagmus is present. The slow phase of the nystagmus is toward the left, and the rapid phase of the nystagmus is toward the right. There is a significant ataxia present.

8. What is the most likely diagnosis in this patient?
   a. vestibular neuronitis
   b. acute labyrinthitis
   c. benign positional vertigo
   d. orthostatic hypotension
   e. Ménière's disease

9. What is the treatment of choice for this patient?
   a. avoidance of alcohol and caffeine
   b. a thiazide diuretic
   c. endolymphatic surgery
   d. reassurance and antiemetics
   e. antibiotics

10. The patient returns to your office the next day saying her ear hurts and she cannot taste anything in her mouth. The vertigo has not improved. Upon examination, you notice crops of vesicles on the pinna of the left ear and a subtle left facial droop. What is the most likely diagnosis?
    a. Lyme disease
    b. impetigo
    c. otitis externa
    d. Ramsay Hunt syndrome
    e. lacunar stroke

11. What is the treatment for the diagnosis?
  a. oral antibiotics
  b. prednisone
  c. acyclovir
  d. prednisone and acyclovir
  e. hospitalization and intravenous antibiotics

CLINICAL CASE PROBLEM 5

A 26-Year-Old Female with Severe Dizziness, Ataxia, and Hearing Loss

A 26-year-old female comes to your office with a 6-day history of severe dizziness associated with ataxia and right-sided hearing loss. She had an upper respiratory tract infection 1 week ago. At that time, her right ear felt plugged.

On examination, there is fluid behind the right eardrum. There is horizontal nystagmus present, with the slow component to the right and the quick component to the left. Ataxia is present.

12. What is the most likely diagnosis in this patient?
  a. vestibular neuronitis
  b. acute labyrinthitis
  c. benign positional vertigo
  d. orthostatic hypotension
  e. Ménière's disease

13. What is the treatment of choice for this patient?
  a. avoidance of caffeine and alcohol
  b. a thiazide diuretic
  c. endolymphatic surgery
  d. rest and antiemetics
  e. none of the above

14. The patient returns to your office 2 days later stating that she had fever throughout the night. She continues to have all the symptoms she had prior but overall feels worse and woke this morning in a sweat. On examination, her temperature is 39.5°C, pulse is 122 beats/minute, and blood pressure is 96/60 mmHg. She appears ill. What is the likely reason for the change in symptoms?
  a. misdiagnosed sinusitis
  b. conversion to bacterial labyrinthitis
  c. acute otitis media
  d. worsening of her viral illness
  e. viral meningitis

15. What is the current treatment of choice?
  a. education and reassurance
  b. hospitalization and intravenous antibiotics

  c. lumbar puncture
  d. prednisone
  e. anticholinergics

16. What is the most common cause of sensorineural hearing loss in the adult population?
  a. Ménière's disease
  b. chronic otitis media
  c. presbycusis
  d. otosclerosis
  e. mastoiditis

17. What is the most common cause of conductive hearing loss in adults who have normal-appearing tympanic membranes?
  a. Ménière's disease
  b. chronic otitis media
  c. presbycusis
  d. otosclerosis
  e. mastoiditis

CLINICAL CASE PROBLEM 6

A 37-Year-Old Female with Intermittent Hearing Loss

A 37-year-old female comes to your office for assessment of hearing loss. She has had problems intermittently for the past 12 months.

On examination, the Weber tuning fork test lateralizes to the right ear, and the Rinne tuning fork test is negative in the right ear (bone conduction is greater than air conduction [BC > AC]).

18. This suggests which one of the following hearing losses?
  a. a right-sided conductive hearing loss
  b. a left-sided conductive hearing loss
  c. a right-sided sensorineural hearing loss
  d. a left-sided sensorineural hearing loss
  e. a or d

CLINICAL CASE PROBLEM 7

A 43-Year-Old Male with Hearing Loss Lateralized to the Left Ear

A 43-year-old male comes to your office for assessment of hearing loss. He has had hearing difficulties for the past 4 years.

On examination, the Weber tuning fork test lateralizes to the left ear. The Rinne tuning fork test is normal bilaterally (AC > BC).

19. This suggests which one of the following hearing losses?
   a. a right-sided conductive hearing loss
   b. a left-sided conductive hearing loss
   c. a right-sided sensorineural hearing loss
   d. a left-sided sensorineural hearing loss
   e. b or c

20. Which of the following statements is (are) true regarding the condition of acute mastoiditis?
   a. it is a complication of acute otitis media
   b. it is most likely caused by *Streptococcus pneumoniae*
   c. otalgia, aural discharge, and fever are characteristically seen 2 or 3 weeks after an episode of acute suppurative otitis media
   d. none of the above statements are true
   e. a, b, and c are true

CLINICAL CASE PROBLEM 8

A 42-Year-Old Woman with Facial Pain

A 42-year-old woman comes to your office complaining of severe facial pain in the region of her right maxilla, fever, and a purulent discharge from her right nose, all of which started after a recent upper respiratory infection. She is taking no medications and has no known drug allergies. Her temperature is elevated to 101°F. There is tenderness over the right maxillary sinus and a greenish discharge in her right nares. The rest of her examination is normal.

21. Which of the following statements concerning rhinosinusitis is (are) true?
   a. the most common causes of sinusitis are allergic sinusitis and viral sinusitis
   b. rhinovirus is the most common cause of viral sinusitis
   c. viral sinusitis is often accompanied by fever, malaise, and systemic symptoms
   d. a and b
   e. a, b, and c

22. Acute bacterial rhinosinusitis is caused most commonly by which of the following organisms?
   a. *S. pneumoniae*
   b. *Haemophilus influenzae*
   c. *Moraxella catarrhalis*
   d. *Streptococcus pyogenes*
   e. *Staphylococcus aureus*

23. Which of the following is the most predictive factor distinguishing viral rhinosinusitis and bacterial rhinosinusitis?

   a. thick and greenish nasal discharge
   b. facial pain
   c. degree of fever
   d. duration of symptoms
   e. systemic symptoms

24. What is the antibacterial drug of first choice for moderate to severe acute bacterial rhinosinusitis?
   a. amoxicillin (10- to 15-day course)
   b. Bactrim/Septra (10- to 15-day course)
   c. cefuroxime (10-day course)
   d. ciprofloxacin (10- to 14-day course)
   e. erythromycin (10-day course)

25. Which of the following is not considered criteria suggestive of chronic sinusitis?
   a. duration longer than 12 weeks
   b. nasal obstruction
   c. nasal polyps
   d. lack of response to antibiotic therapy
   e. facial pain

CLINICAL CASE PROBLEM 9

A 12-Year-Old Male with Ear Pain

A 12-year-old male is brought to your office by his mother. He is complaining of right ear pain for the past 24 hours. The mother states that he spent the past 4 days swimming in the pool and began to complain of pain in the right ear yesterday afternoon. She states that she noticed some fluid on his pillow after he woke up this morning. The patient states that he has been using cotton swabs in his ear to remove excess water. On examination, the patient is afebrile. Otoscopic exam is significant for purulent material in the ear canal with significant erythema. The tympanic membrane is erythematous, but there is no adjacent fluid. He has pain when you pull on the pinna.

26. What is the most likely diagnosis?
   a. otitis media
   b. otitis externa
   c. otitis media and otitis externa
   d. auricular cellulitis
   e. mastoiditis

27. What is the most common organism in this problem?
   a. adenovirus
   b. *Pseudomonas aeruginosa*
   c. *S. aureus*
   d. rhinovirus
   e. *Streptococcus* spp.

28. You prescribe the patient a topical solution of polymyxin, neomycin, and hydrocortisone. The patient returns 4 days later. His mother states that they lost the prescription and now he is getting worse. Otoscopic exam at this time reveals increased debris and purulent material and a 2-mm perforation in the tympanic membrane. What is the most appropriate treatment at this time?
a. referral to an ear, nose, and throat specialist
b. re-prescribe the polymyxin, neomycin, hydrocortisone otic solution
c. prescribe an otic aminoglycoside
d. prescribe an otic fluoroquinolone
e. irrigate the ear to remove excessive debris

Clinical Case Management Problem

Describe the long-term complications of otitis media.

Answers

1. **e.** This patient has Ménière's disease. The classic features of Ménière's disease are recurrent episodes of vertigo, fluctuating low-frequency sensorineural hearing loss, tinnitus (ringing or buzzing in the ears), and aural fullness in the affected ear. The vertigo typically lasts hours, not minutes or days. The fluctuating hearing may not be related temporally to the vertigo.

To make the diagnosis of Ménière's disease, the characteristic pattern of vertigo lasting a matter of hours, as well as sensorineural hearing loss, must be present. One additional factor (aural fullness or buzzing tinnitus) should also be present.

2. **e.** Epley maneuvers are used to treat positional vertigo, not Ménière's disease. *performed by physician or PTherapist*

3. **d.** Ménière's disease is also known as endolymphatic hydrops. There is a buildup of fluid in the endolymphatic system that is secondary to either excessive fluid production or decreased fluid resorption. This causes dilation of the endolymphatic system and may be responsible for the development of the acute attacks. Salt restriction and diuretic therapy are the cornerstones of medical therapy. Use of hydrochlorothiazide is a reasonable treatment (especially for patients who are having frequent attacks). Some patients with Ménière's disease are acutely sensitive to alcohol, caffeine, or both. In these patients, alcohol and caffeine should be avoided.

The use of an antinausea medication may be extremely effective in the treatment of the acute attack. Benzodiazepines have also been found to be helpful in some cases. Surgical decompression of the endolymphatic system is reserved for patients who do not respond to medical management. Epley maneuvers and steroids are not helpful in the treatment of Ménière's disease.

4. **d.** This patient has orthostatic hypotension. This case illustrates the importance of obtaining an accurate history in the patient who complains of "feeling dizzy." In any patient who has this complaint, it is important to ask four specific questions: (1) Can you describe your dizziness? (2) How much of the dizziness is a sensation of the "world spinning around you," and how much would be a sensation of "things going black in front of you and a feeling that you're about to pass out?" (3) How long does the feeling of dizziness last—seconds, minutes, or hours? and (4) Are there any other symptoms present when you feel dizzy, such as deafness, ear fullness, or ringing in the ears?

The answers to these questions are the most important clues to leading you toward a diagnosis. This patient does not have clear symptoms of vertigo, and one should focus on nonvertigo-related dizziness.

Orthostatic hypotension is typically initiated after standing up suddenly. There is a transient lack of cerebral blood flow. The feeling described is that of a subjective dizziness and the patient feels as if he or she might faint. It is not associated with any other neurologic sensations or ear symptoms. It is also characterized by a lack of symptoms when sitting or lying. Medications are the most likely culprits in this scenario, but occasionally there is no clear etiology for the autonomic disturbance.

In this clinical case problem, the orthostatic hypotension is almost certainly associated with the beginning of the tricyclic antidepressant therapy 6 months ago.

5. **c.** The most important treatment is to reassure the patient and explain how the symptom can be minimized by slowly assuming the upright position.

The orthostatic hypotension in this case developed after the initiation of the tricyclic antidepressant, doxepin. It would be reasonable to switch to an antidepressant with less alpha-adrenergic side effects. A good choice would be a selective serotonin reuptake inhibitor.

6. **c.** This patient has benign positional paroxysmal vertigo (BPPV), a disorder that consists of brief episodes (lasting 2 to 10 seconds) usually caused by turning the head.

BPPV is caused by the formation of crystalline debris in the semicircular canals that leads to labyrinthine irritation, causing vertigo and nystagmus.

7. **d.** The treatment of choice for this patient is reassurance and the prescription of canolith repositioning maneuvers. The goal of these maneuvers is to reposition the crystals into the vestibule, where they avoid further irritation of the semicircular canals. The Epley, modified Epley, and Semont maneuvers are a few forms of canolith repositioning.

Performance of these exercises can occur in the office setting but should also be taught to the patient so the patient can continue them at home. These maneuvers have an 80% success rate in relieving patients' symptoms, but approximately 15% of people will have a reoccurrence of symptoms within 1 year.

Even if the exercises are not prescribed or prescribed and not performed, the condition tends to resolve with time (usually several weeks to a few months).

8. **a.** This patient has a left vestibular neuronitis. The etiology of this disorder is commonly associated with a viral infection (such as adenovirus) following a respiratory tract infection and involves some portion of the vestibular system but with total sparing of the cochlear area. It most commonly affects young or middle-aged adults.

The disorder consists of severe vertigo with associated ataxia and nausea and vomiting. There is no hearing loss, aural pain, or other symptoms, which is helpful in distinguishing it from other causes of vertigo. Recovery usually takes 1 or 2 weeks.

9. **d.** The treatment of choice for a patient with vestibular neuronitis is rest, reassurance, and antiemetics. Antiemetics such as droperidol, chlorpromazine, or dimenhydrinate may be given for symptomatic relief of the vertigo. Some studies have shown that early use corticosteroids may shorten the duration of the illness. Symptoms are normally severe enough that patients may require bed rest during the acute attack. The course of illness is typically severe vertigo for a few days that gradually resolves over a period of weeks.

10. **d.** The patient is showing signs and symptoms of Ramsay Hunt syndrome. This is a reactivation of the varicella-zoster virus that affects the seventh and eighth cranial nerves. There can be any pattern of symptoms, from unilateral facial droop to loss of taste and hyperacusis. Vesicles may or may not be present along the pinna, auditory meatus, or the hard palate. Irritation of the vestibular portion of the eighth cranial nerve causes vestibular neuronitis and the symptoms of vertigo.

11. **d.** Treatment of Ramsay Hunt syndrome is the same as that for zoster elsewhere on the body. If caught early enough, the combination of acyclovir and corticosteroids can reduce the length and severity of the illness.

12. **b.** This patient has acute labyrinthitis. Acute labyrinthitis usually follows otitis media or an upper respiratory tract infection. The disorder probably represents a chemical irritation of the canals of the inner ear. The features of acute labyrinthitis are similar to those of vestibular neuronitis, except it includes significant sensorineural hearing loss (with a conductive component if a middle ear effusion is present) and severe vertigo that lasts several days. Fever may accompany the illness.

13. **d.** See answer 15.

14. **b.** See answer 15.

15. **b.** The treatment of choice for acute labyrinthitis includes rest, antiemetics, and, if the etiology is bacterial, antibiotics. Bacterial labyrinthitis may complicate serous labyrinthitis if antibiotics are not administered. Amoxicillin would be a good first-line agent for antibiotic prophylaxis. If symptoms do not improve, the addition of clavulanic acid to amoxicillin would be a reasonable second choice. If a patient appears very ill from presumed acute bacterial labyrinthitis, hospitalization and intravenous antibiotics are required. Occasionally, surgical drainage may be necessary.

16. **c.** Hearing loss can be divided into sensorineural hearing loss and conductive hearing loss. The most common cause of sensorineural hearing loss in adults is presbycusis, a gradual deterioration that begins after the age of 20 years in the highest frequencies and often involves all speech frequencies by the sixth and seventh decades of life. The impaired hearing associated with presbycusis stems from degenerative changes in the hair cells, auditory neurons, and cochlear nuclei. Tinnitus is a common complaint.

Sound amplification with an electrical hearing aid does benefit some patients with relatively good speech discrimination.

17. **d.** The most common cause of conductive hearing loss in adults who have normal-appearing tympanic membranes is otosclerosis. Otosclerosis is a localized disease of the otic capsule, reducing ankylosis or fixation of the stapes footplate. The resulting conductive hearing loss starts insidiously in the third and fourth decades of life and progressively involves both ears in 80% of individuals. Otosclerosis, an inherited disease, is typically found in white, middle-aged women.

18. **a.** The characterization of hearing loss can be localized by a combination of the Weber test and the Rinne test.

In the Weber test, placement of a 512-Hz tuning fork on the skull in the midline or on the teeth stimulates both cochleae simultaneously. If the patient has a conductive hearing loss in one ear, the sound will be perceived loudest in the affected ear (i.e., it will lateralize). When a unilateral sensorineural hearing loss is present, the tone is heard in the unaffected ear.

The Rinne test compares air conduction with bone conduction. Normally, AC is greater than BC. Sound stimulation by air in front of the pinna is normally perceived twice as long as sound placed on the mastoid process (AC > BC). With conductive hearing loss, the duration of AC is less than BC (i.e., negative Rinne test). In the presence of sensorineural hearing loss, the durations of both AC and BC are reduced; however, the 2:1 ratio remains the same (i.e., a positive Rinne test).

Facts for question 18: (1) Bone conduction is greater than air conduction: This indicates that this is a conductive hearing loss; (2) in conductive hearing loss, the Weber test lateralizes to the affected ear, and because the Weber test lateralized to the right ear in this patient, she has a unilateral right-sided conductive hearing loss.

19. **c.** AC is greater than BC; therefore, this is a sensorineural hearing loss. The Weber test lateralizes to the left ear, and in sensorineural hearing loss the Weber test lateralizes to the unaffected ear; therefore, in this case, the right ear is the affected ear. This is a unilateral right-sided sensorineural hearing loss.

20. **e.** Acute mastoiditis is a complication of acute otitis media that develops as a result of the retention of pus in the mastoid area. Acute mastoiditis is most commonly caused by *S. pneumoniae*. *S. pyogenes* and *S. aureus* are other recognized causes.

The inflammatory process in acute mastoiditis results in the destruction of bony septa (almost an osteomyelitis-like process), and, as a result, there is a coalescence of mastoid air cells. This leads to subsequent erosion of the mastoid process of the petrous temporal bone.

The symptoms of acute mastoiditis include otalgia, aural discharge, and fever. These symptoms usually appear 2 or 3 weeks after an episode of acute suppurative otitis media. Examination reveals severe mastoid tenderness, lateral displacement of the pinna, and postauricular mastoid swelling secondary to the periosteal abscess. The treatment of choice is ceftriaxone (with or without metronidazole) and surgical drainage (for a subperiosteal abscess).

21. **e.** The most common causes of acute rhinosinusitis are allergic and viral. It is often extremely difficult to distinguish between the two types, although a seasonal sinusitis points to allergic sinusitis, as do symptoms such as itching and redness of the eyes.

Viral rhinosinusitis may be accompanied by systemic systems including fever, chills, facial pain, malaise, and fatigue.

22. **a.** The organisms most commonly implicated in acute bacterial sinusitis include *S. pneumoniae* (the most common), *H. influenzae*, *M. catarrhalis*, and *S. pyogenes*. Other organisms implicated include *S. aureus* and anaerobic organisms.

23. **d.** Acute bacterial sinusitis should be suspected when symptoms last more than 10 days from the onset of upper respiratory symptoms or if symptoms of acute rhinosinusitis worsen after an initial improvement. Purulent rhinorrhea, facial/dental pain, and nasal obstruction are suggestive of acute viral and bacterial rhinosinusitis but should not be presumed to be bacterial unless symptoms follow the previously mentioned time pattern.

24. **a.** The antibiotic treatment of choice for moderate to severe acute bacterial sinusitis is at minimum a 10- to 15-day course of amoxicillin. Second-line antibiotics, and primary for those with penicillin allergies, include trimethoprim–sulfamethoxazole and macrolides. Antihistamines, decongestants, and intranasal steroids are also options as adjunctive or primary therapy.

25. **d.** Diagnosis of chronic sinusitis requires the following: (1) duration of 12 weeks or longer; (2) two or more of the following symptoms: facial pain, nasal obstruction/congestion, mucopurulent discharge, or decrease in sense of smell; and (3) evidence of inflammation by documentation of one of the following: purulent (not clear) mucus or edema in the middle meatus or ethmoid region, polyps in nasal cavity or the middle meatus, or radiographic imaging showing inflammation of the paranasal sinuses.

26. **b.** The patient has a classic case of otitis externa (OE). It is an infection of the external auditory meatus that typically follows swimming or local trauma. Signs and symptoms include pruritis, pain, erythema, otorrhea, and edema in the ear canal. The tympanic membrane will often be erythematous in OE, but this does not indicate a concomitant otitis media.

27. **b.** Approximately 90% of acute OE is causes by bacteria. The other 10% usually has a fungal etiology.

Of bacterial infections, *P. aeruginosa* is the most common pathogen, occurring in 50% if cases. *S. aureus* is the next most common organism. It is the overgrowth of these bacteria in the moist and/or traumatized ear canal that leads to OE.

28. **d.** There are many topical otic solutions available for the treatment of OE, but the fluoroquinolone preparations are the only one approved for use when there is perforation of the tympanic membrane. The polymyxin, neomycin, hydrocortisone preparation and the aminoglycoside have the potential of being ototoxic and should not be used unless the tympanic membrane is intact. Small tympanic perforations will likely close on their own and do not require specialty referral.

Solution to the Clinical Case Management Problem

The long-term complications of chronic otitis media in adults include the following: (1) seventh nerve paralysis, (2) labyrinthitis, (3) petrositis, (4) intracranial suppuration, and (5) cholesteatoma.

The major complication of acute otitis media in adults is acute mastoiditis.

Summary

VERTIGO

1. Ménière's disease
   a. Symptoms: vertigo (lasting hours), hearing loss, tinnitus, aural fullness
   b. Treatment: avoidance of caffeine, avoidance of alcohol, low-dose hydrochlorothiazide, antiemetics
2. Acute labyrinthitis
   a. Symptoms: vertigo (lasting days) and associated hearing loss usually follow an upper respiratory tract infection in which there is a middle ear effusion
   b. Treatment: rest, antiemetics, antibiotics if middle ear fluid is infected
3. Vestibular neuronitis
   a. Symptoms: vertigo (lasting days), no hearing loss, no ear pain, no other symptoms; may result from upper-respiratory tract infection
   b. Treatment: rest, reassurance, antiemetics
4. Positional vertigo
   a. Symptoms: vertigo (lasting for seconds), also associated with rolling over toward the left or the right when supine or when looking up
   b. Treatment: reassurance, simple exercises

ORTHOSTATIC HYPOTENSION

1. Symptoms: not true vertigo (rather a sensation of lightheadedness or faintness) on assuming the upright position; often associated with antihypertensive and antidepressant medications
2. Treatment: reassurance, change in medications to one with fewer alpha-blockade properties and fewer orthostatic side effects

HEARING LOSS

1. Sensorineural hearing loss
   a. 80% of hearing loss in the United States. The pathology is usually a disorder affecting the cochlea and auditory nerves with the perception of a "distorted sound." The deficit is usually greater in the higher frequencies. There are usually degenerative changes in the hair cells, auditory neurons, and cochlear nuclei.
   b. The most common cause is presbycusis, which is a gradual deterioration that starts with high-frequency loss and often involves all speech frequencies by the sixth or seventh decade.
   c. Treatment is provision of a hearing aid, which may benefit patients with relatively good speech discrimination.
2. Conductive hearing loss
   a. Pathologic condition/causation: Conductive hearing loss involves either chronic serous otitis media or otosclerosis. Otosclerosis results as a localized disease of the otic capsule where new spongy bone replaces normal bone, producing ankylosis or fixation of the stapes footplate.
   b. Treatment: The treatments for the chronic causes of conductive hearing loss are usually surgical.
   c. Interpretation of hearing loss: (i) audiogram and (ii) Weber test or Rinne test

RHINOSINUSITIS

1. Possible pathologic conditions include allergic, viral, bacterial; and other organisms.

a. Rhinovirus is the most common viral cause, followed by adenovirus.

b. *S. pneumoniae* is the most common bacterial cause, followed by *H. influenzae* and *M. catarrhalis*.

2. Symptoms: fever, chills, malaise, fatigue, facial pain

3. Acute bacterial rhinosinusitis is distinguished from viral rhinosinusitis mainly by the presence of symptoms longer than 10 days from the onset of upper respiratory symptoms or a worsening of rhinosinusitis after a period of improvement.

4. Treatment: Mild disease requires no antibiotics—only symptomatic therapy with antihistamines/decongestants and/or intranasal steroids. Amoxicillin (10 to 15 days) or Floxin (for recurrent diseases) are reasonable drugs of choice for moderate to severe acute bacterial sinusitis.

OTITIS EXTERNA

1. 90% of cases are bacterial, with remaining 10% being fungal in origin.

2. Erythema, pain, pruritis, and otorrhea are common signs and symptom of disease.

3. Otic fluoroquinolones are the only preparations approved for use when there is a perforation of the tympanic membrane.

Suggested Reading

Chawla N, Olshaker J: Diagnosis and management of dizziness and vertigo. *Med Clin North Am* 90:291–304, 2006.

Isaacson J, Vora N: Differential diagnosis and treatment of hearing loss. *Am Fam Phys* 68(6):1125–1132, 2003.

Osguthorpe JD, Nielsen D: Otitis externa: Review and clinical update. *Am Fam Phys* 74(9):1510–1516, 2006.

Rosenfeld R, Andes D, Bhattacharyya N, et al: Clinical practice guideline: Adult sinusitis. *Otolaryngol Head Neck Surg* 137:S1–S31, 2007.

Swartz R, Longwell P: Treatment of vertigo. *Am Fam Phys* 71(6): 1115–1122, 2005.

CHAPTER

55 Disorders of the Eye

CLINICAL CASE PROBLEM 1

A 32-Year-Old Female with Bilateral Red Eyes, a Sore Throat, and a Cough

A 32-year-old female comes to your office with a 1-week history of bilateral red eyes associated with tearing and crusting, a sore throat with difficulty swallowing, and a cough that was initially nonproductive but has become productive during the past few days. The patient displays significant fatigue and lethargy, is hoarse, and is having great difficulty performing any of her routine daily chores.

On physical examination, there is bilateral conjunctival injection. Her visual acuity is normal. There is significant pharyngeal erythema but no exudate. Cervical lymphadenitis is not present. Examination of the chest reveals a few expiratory crackles bilaterally.

SELECT THE BEST ANSWER TO THE FOLLOWING QUESTIONS

1. What is the most likely cause of this patient's "red eye" condition?

a. an autoimmune reaction secondary to the beginning of a severe systemic illness

b. bacterial conjunctivitis related to her other symptoms

c. bacterial conjunctivitis unrelated to her other symptoms

d. allergic conjunctivitis secondary to a severe eosinophilic pneumonia

e. none of the above

2. Concerning this patient's sore throat and in relation to the scenario described and the physical findings provided, what would you do?

a. perform a throat culture and order antibiotics

b. perform a throat culture and a rapid enzyme-linked immunosorbent assay (ELISA) *Streptococcus* test and treat with an antibiotic if the ELISA test is positive

c. perform a throat culture and await the results

d. order a complete blood count and total eosinophil count

e. none of the above

3. What is the most likely organism or condition responsible for the constellation of symptoms in this patient?

a. endotoxin-producing *Staphylococcus*

b. endotoxin-producing *Streptococcus*

c. exotoxin-producing *Staphylococcus*

d. activation of the autoimmune system

e. none of the above

CLINICAL CASE PROBLEM 2

A 17-Year-Old Female with a 1-Day History of Red Eye

A 17-year-old female comes to your office with a 1-day history of red eye. She describes not being able to open her right eye in the morning because of crusting and discharge. The right eye feels swollen and uncomfortable, although there is no pain.

On examination, she has a significant redness and injection of the right conjunctiva. There is a mucopurulent discharge present. No other abnormalities are present on physical examination. Her visual acuity is normal.

4. What is the most likely diagnosis in this patient?
   a. bacterial conjunctivitis
   b. viral conjunctivitis
   c. allergic conjunctivitis
   d. autoimmune conjunctivitis
   e. none of the above

5. Which of the following agents is (are) a common cause(s) of bacterial conjunctivitis?
   a. *Haemophilus influenzae*
   b. *Staphylococcus aureus*
   c. *Streptococcus pneumoniae*
   d. a and b
   e. a, b, and c

CLINICAL CASE PROBLEM 3

A 29-Year-Old Male with Bilateral Red Eyes

A 29-year-old male comes to your office with bilateral red eyes. This symptom came on quite suddenly 2 hours ago while visiting a friend's home. He describes itching and a clear discharge from both eyes. The patient mentions one previous episode that also began while visiting the same friend.

On examination, the conjunctivae are diffusely injected and edematous. On eversion of the eyelids, there are large papillae present. Visual acuity is intact.

6. What is the most likely diagnosis in this patient?
   a. chemical conjunctivitis
   b. toxic conjunctivitis
   c. allergic conjunctivitis
   d. bacterial conjunctivitis
   e. none of the above

CLINICAL CASE PROBLEM 4

A 29-Year-Old Female with a Tender, Painful, Red, and Sore Eye

A 29-year-old female comes to your office for assessment of a red eye. She describes a tender, painful, and sore right eye that began yesterday. She has had no other symptoms. On examination, the patient has a localized area of inflammation, with dilated vessels and redness, in the lateral area of the right bulbar conjunctiva. The inflammation appears to lie beneath the conjunctival surface. Visual acuity is normal.

7. What is the most likely diagnosis in this patient?
   a. localized bacterial conjunctivitis
   b. acute iritis
   c. acute angle closure glaucoma
   d. acute episcleritis
   e. none of the above

CLINICAL CASE PROBLEM 5

A 35-Year-Old Female with an Acutely Inflamed and Painful Eye

A 35-year-old female comes to your office with an acutely inflamed and painful left eye. Her symptoms began 2 days ago. There is some visual blurring associated with the symptoms. The patient wears contact lenses.

On examination, there is a diffuse inflammation of the left conjunctiva. On fluorescein staining, there is a dendritic ulcer seen in the center of the cornea. Visual acuity is intact.

8. What is the most likely diagnosis in this patient?
   a. corneal abrasion
   b. herpetic corneal ulcer
   c. contact lens stress ulcer
   d. adenoviral ulcer
   e. foreign body complicated by a viral ulcer

CLINICAL CASE PROBLEM 6

A 36-Year-Old Male with Ankylosing Spondylitis and a Painful Red Eye

A 36-year-old male with ankylosing spondylitis comes to your office for assessment of a painful, red left eye. The pain is associated with photophobia.

On examination, the redness is more pronounced around the area of the cornea. His visual acuity in the left eye has decreased to 20/60.

9. What is the most likely diagnosis in this patient?
  a. bacterial conjunctivitis
  b. viral conjunctivitis
  c. acute iridocyclitis
  d. acute episcleritis
  e. acute angle closure glaucoma

CLINICAL CASE PROBLEM 7

A 61-Year-Old Male with an Extremely Painful Eye

A 61-year-old male comes to your office with a 12-hour history of an extremely painful and red left eye. The patient complains that his vision is blurred and he is seeing halos around lights. He states that he has had similar but milder attacks in the past.

On examination, the eye is tender and inflamed. The cornea is hazy, and the pupil is semidilated and fixed. On palpation, the left eye is significantly harder than the right. Visual acuity is significantly diminished in the left eye.

10. What is the most likely diagnosis in this patient?
  a. bacterial conjunctivitis
  b. viral conjunctivitis
  c. acute iridocyclitis
  d. acute episcleritis
  e. acute angle closure glaucoma

CLINICAL CASE PROBLEM 8

A 23-Year-Old Female with a Painful Eye and Blurred Vision

A 23-year-old female comes to your office with a painful left eye, conjunctival injection, and blurred vision. On examination, the visual acuity is markedly diminished in the affected eye. The conjunctival injection is primarily circumcorneal, and there is photophobia.

11. What is the most likely diagnosis in this patient?
  a. acute conjunctivitis
  b. acute iritis
  c. acute episcleritis
  d. acute angle closure glaucoma
  e. acute corneal abrasion

12. In this patient, what will the size of the left pupil be, relative to that of the right pupil?
  a. larger than the right pupil
  b. smaller than the right pupil
  c. the same size as the right pupil
  d. indeterminate
  e. nobody really knows for sure

Clinical Case Management Problem

Compare and contrast acute conjunctivitis, acute glaucoma, acute iritis, and corneal trauma or infection with respect to the following: (1) incidence, (2) discharge, (3) vision, (4) pain, (5) conjunctival infections, (6) cornea, (7) pupil size, (8) pupillary light response, (9) intraocular pressure, and (10) smear.

Answers

1. e. See answer 3.

2. e. See answer 3.

3. e. This picture is completely consistent with adenovirus infection and a primary viral conjunctivitis. Viral agents, especially adenovirus, produce signs and symptoms of upper respiratory tract infection, with the presence of the red eye being prominent among those symptoms.

With adenovirus there is often associated conjunctival hyperemia, eyelid edema, and a serous or seropurulent discharge. Viral conjunctivitis is self-limiting, lasting 1 to 3 weeks. If the conjunctivitis is definitely caused by a virus, no antibiotic treatment is necessary.

There is no indication for performing a throat culture or any other test at this time. The only theoretic concerns are the "rales" that are present in both lung bases; you could argue that if the patient is sick enough, a chest x-ray may be indicated.

4. a. This patient has a primary bacterial conjunctivitis. Unlike in viral conjunctivitis, bacterial conjunctivitis will produce a mucopurulent discharge from the beginning. Symptoms are more often unilateral, and associated eye discomfort is common.

In bacterial conjunctivitis, normal visual acuity is always maintained. There is usually uniform engorgement of all the conjunctival blood vessels. There is no staining of the cornea with fluorescein. Bacterial conjunctivitis should be treated with antibiotic drops such as sodium sulfacetamide, gentamycin, or fluoroquinolones.

5. **e.** The most common organisms responsible for bacterial conjunctivitis are *Staphylococcus*, *Streptococcus*, and *Haemophilus*. *Pseudomonas* and *Moraxella* are other common bacterial isolates.

6. **c.** The most likely diagnosis in this patient is allergic conjunctivitis. The most common complaint with allergic conjunctivitis is itchy, red eyes. Both eyes are affected, and there is usually a clear discharge.

Examination reveals diffusely infected conjunctiva, which may be edematous (chemosis). The discharge is usually clear and stringy. Treatment can include avoidance of allergens, immunotherapy, oral antihistamine, topical antihistamine, topical nonsteroidal anti-inflammatory drugs (NSAIDs), topical mast cell stabilizer, and topical corticosteroids (use with caution).

The culprit, in this case, is most likely something in his friend's home.

7. **d.** This patient has episcleritis, which differs from conjunctivitis in that it usually presents as a localized area of inflammation. Although episcleritis may occur secondary to autoimmune disease such as rheumatoid arthritis, most cases of episcleritis are idiopathic. Episcleritis is almost always self-limiting; scleritis, however, may lead to serious complications such as loss of visual acuity and perforation of the globe.

Patients with episcleritis usually have a sore, red, and tender eye. Although there may be reflex lacrimation, there is usually no discharge. Scleritis is much more painful than episcleritis, and the signs of inflammation are usually more prominent.

In episcleritis, there is episcleral injection, which can be nodular, sectoral, or diffuse. There is no palpebral conjunctival injection or discharge like that seen in conjunctivitis.

The symptoms of episcleritis usually resolve spontaneously in 1 or 2 weeks. Chilled artificial tears can be given until the redness resolves. In cases associated with systemic disease, the underlying cause is treated appropriately.

8. **b.** This patient has a dendritic ulcer, which is almost always caused by a herpetic infection, although other viral agents, bacterial agents, or fungal agents may also be responsible. These infections may be primary or secondary to excessive contact lens wear, a corneal abrasion, or the use of corticosteroid eye drops.

The patient with a herpetic dendritic ulcer usually has an acutely painful eye associated with conjunctival injection, discharge, and visual blurring. Visual acuity, however, depends on the location and the size of the corneal ulcer. The discharge may be watery (reflex lacrimation) or purulent (bacterial). Conjunctival injection may be generalized or localized, depending on the location of the ulcer.

Treatment consists of specific anti-infective therapy (vidarabine or trifluridine for herpes simplex ulcers and topical antibiotics for ulcers suspected of being primarily or secondarily infected by bacteria) and cycloplegic drops to relieve pain caused by ciliary muscle spasm. Topical corticosteroids are absolutely contraindicated in patients with a dendritic herpetic ulcer.

In a patient with a dendritic ulcer, referral to an ophthalmologist is recommended.

9. **c.** This patient has an acute iridocyclitis or anterior uveitis. Patients at risk for anterior uveitis are those with a history of a seronegative arthropathy, particularly if they are positive for HLA-B27. Children with seronegative arthritis are also at high risk.

Symptoms of acute iridocyclitis include a painful red eye, often associated with photophobia, and decreased visual acuity.

On examination, the affected eye is red; the inflammation is particularly prominent over the area of the inflamed ciliary body (circumcorneal). The pupil is small because of spasm of the sphincter or irregular because of adhesions of the iris to the lens (posterior synechiae). Inflammatory cells may be seen on the back of the cornea (keratitic precipitates) or may settle to form a collection of cells in the anterior chamber of the eye (hypopyon).

Treatment of anterior uveitis should include topical corticosteroids to reduce the inflammation and prevent adhesions within the eye. Mydriatics should be used to paralyze the ciliary body to relieve pain.

As with scleritis and dendritic ulcers, a patient with iridocyclitis should be referred to an ophthalmologist.

10. **e.** This patient has acute angle closure glaucoma. Acute glaucoma should always be suspected in a patient who is older than age 50 years and has a painful red eye.

Unlike the more common open-angle glaucoma, acute glaucoma usually comes on rapidly. The most common symptom is severe pain in one eye, which may or may not be accompanied by other symptoms such as nausea and vomiting. The patient complains of impaired vision and halos around lights. This is caused by edema of the cornea.

On examination, the eye is tender and inflamed. The cornea is hazy, and the pupil is partially dilated and fixed. Vision is impaired because of edema of the cornea. On palpation, the involved eye often feels significantly harder than the uninvolved eye.

Untreated, the condition can lead to blindness in 2 to 5 days. Initial emergent treatment to reduce intraocular pressure includes topical beta blockers, intravenous and oral carbonic anhydrase inhibitors (e.g., acetazolamide), and hyperosmotic agents. Once intraocular pressure is under control, a peripheral laser iridectomy is performed. Ophthalmology consult is urgently indicated.

The other eye should be treated prophylactically with a laser iridotomy.

11. b. This patient has an acute iritis.

12. b. Acute iritis is characterized by the following: incidence, common; eye discharge, none; visual acuity, slightly blurred; pain, moderate; conjunctival injection, mainly circumcorneal; cornea, usually clear; pupil size, smaller than unaffected eye; pupillary light response, poor; intraocular pressure, normal; and Gram's stain and smear, no organisms.

The treatment of acute iritis is a mydriatic to relieve ciliary spasm and a corticosteroid to decrease inflammation. Again, this patient should be referred to an ophthalmologist.

Solution to the Clinical Case Management Problem

There are four major conditions that should be considered when a patient comes to the physician's office with a red eye: acute conjunctivitis, acute iritis, acute glaucoma, and corneal trauma or infection. Their differentiation and treatment are as follows:

1. Incidence: (a) acute conjunctivitis, extremely common; (b) acute iritis, common; (c) acute glaucoma, uncommon; and (d) corneal trauma or infection, common
2. Discharge: (a) acute conjunctivitis, moderate to copious; (b) acute iritis, none; (c) acute glaucoma, none; and (d) corneal trauma or infection, watery or purulent
3. Vision: (a) acute conjunctivitis, no effect on vision; (b) acute iritis, slightly blurred; (c) acute glaucoma, markedly blurred; and (d) corneal trauma or infection, usually blurred
4. Pain: (a) acute conjunctivitis, none; (b) acute iritis, moderate; (c) acute glaucoma, severe; and (d) corneal trauma or infection, moderate to severe
5. Conjunctival injection: (a) acute conjunctivitis, diffuse, more toward fornices; (b) acute iritis,

mainly circumcorneal; (c) acute glaucoma, diffuse; and (d) corneal trauma or infection, diffuse
6. Cornea: (a) acute conjunctivitis, clear; (b) acute iritis, usually clear; (c) acute glaucoma, steamy; and (d) corneal trauma or infection, change in clarity related to cause
7. Pupil size: (a) acute conjunctivitis, normal; (b) acute iritis, small; (c) acute glaucoma, moderately dilated and fixed; and (d) corneal trauma or infection, normal
8. Pupillary light response: (a) acute conjunctivitis, normal; (b) acute iritis, poor; (c) acute glaucoma, none; and (d) corneal trauma or infection, normal
9. Intraocular pressure: (a) acute conjunctivitis, normal; (b) acute iritis, normal; (c) acute glaucoma, elevated; and (d) corneal trauma or infection, normal
10. Smear: (a) acute conjunctivitis, causative organisms; (b) acute iritis, no organisms; (c) acute glaucoma, no organisms; and (d) corneal trauma or infection, organisms found only in corneal ulcers caused by infection

Summary

INFECTIOUS CONJUNCTIVITIS

1. Etiologic agents: (a) adenovirus is most common cause of conjunctivitis; and (b) bacterial conjunctivitis, most commonly caused by *S. aureus*, *S. pneumoniae*, and *H. influenzae*
2. Symptoms: (a) watery discharge with viral infection; mucopurulent discharge with bacterial infection; and (b) other symptoms as described in the Clinical Case Management Problem

3. Treatment: ciprofloxin (Ciloxan), gatifloxacin sulfacetamide, or gentamicin drops

ALLERGIC CONJUNCTIVITIS

1. Symptoms: Itching and clear discharge are main symptoms; conjunctiva are diffusely injected and may be associated with swelling (chemosis).
2. Treatment: Avoidance of allergens, immunotherapy, topical antihistamines, topical NSAIDs, topical mast

cell stabilizers, oral antihistamines, topical corticosteroids (use with caution).

CORNEAL ULCERS

1. May be bacterial, viral, or fungal in origin or also may be secondary to a corneal abrasion, contact lens wear, etc.
2. Visual acuity depends on the location and size of the ulcer. Conjunctival injection may be generalized or localized. Fluorescein must be used to stain the cornea.
3. Treatment: Cycloplegic eye drops are used to relieve ciliary muscle spasm. Trifluridine or vidarabine are used for dendritic (herpetic) ulcer; antibiotic drops are used for suspected bacterial infection. Corticosteroid eye drops are absolutely contraindicated in herpetic ulcers.

IRIDOCYCLITIS (ANTERIOR UVEITIS)

1. Iridocyclitis is often associated with seronegative arthropathy.
2. Inflammation of the iris (iritis) and inflammation of the ciliary body (cyclitis) occur together.

3. The inflammation of anterior uveitis is circumcorneal in location, and the pupil is usually small because of associated spasm.
4. Treatment: Mydriatics are used to relieve ciliary spasm; corticosteroid drops are used to decrease inflammation.

ACUTE ANGLE CLOSURE GLAUCOMA

1. Acute, unilateral, painful red eye in a patient older than 50 years of age
2. The attack usually comes on quickly, characteristically in the evening.
3. Impaired vision caused by corneal edema and halos around lights are common.
4. Palpation reveals a hard eye.
5. Emergent treatment: Topical beta blocker, intravenous and oral carbonic anhydrase inhibitors, and hyperosmotic agents are first steps. Once intraocular pressure is under control, a peripheral laser iridectomy is performed.

Suggested Reading

Leibowitz HM: The red eye. *N Engl J Med* 343(5):345–351, 2000.

Pokhrel PK, Loftus SA: Occular emergencies. *Am Fam Phys* 76: 829–836, 2007.

Rodriguez JO, Lavina AM, Agarwal A: et al: Prevention and treatment of common eye injuries in sports. *Am Fam Phys* 67(7):1481–1488, 2003.

Shingleton BJ, O'Donoghue MW: Blurred vision. *N Engl J Med* 343(8):556–562, 2000.

Vafidis G: When is red eye not just conjunctivitis? *Practitioner* 246: 469–481, 2002.

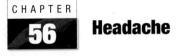

Headache

CLINICAL CASE PROBLEM 1

A 45-Year-Old Male with a Headache

A 45-year-old male comes to your office with a 4-week history of recurrent headaches that wake him up in the middle of the night. The headaches have been occurring every night and have been lasting approximately 1 hour. The headaches are described as a deep burning sensation centered behind the left eye. The headaches are excruciating (he rates them as a 15 on a 10-point scale) and are associated with watery eyes, "a sensation of heat and warmth in my face," nasal discharge, and redness of the left eye.

Before the onset of these headaches 4 weeks ago, the patient describes no more than the occasional tension headache. Headaches were

certainly never a problem. The patient describes no recent life changes and no major life stresses. He is happily married, has three children, and has a secure job that he enjoys.

On examination, his blood pressure is 120/70 mmHg. His pulse is 82 beats/minute and regular.

SELECT THE BEST ANSWER TO THE FOLLOWING QUESTIONS

1. What is the most likely cause of this patient's headache?
   a. subarachnoid hemorrhage
   b. tension-type headache
   c. brain tumor
   d. cluster headache
   e. migraine without aura

2. How would you best treat his acute headache?
   a. oral ergotamine
   b. high-flow oxygen
   c. subcutaneous sumatriptan

d. b and c

e. a, b, and c

3. He returns 3 days later and tells you that the medicine you gave him works, but he still keeps getting these awful headaches. What medication listed here would not help prevent his headaches?

a. verapamil

b. lithium

c. diazepam

d. prednisone

e. topirimate

CLINICAL CASE PROBLEM 2

A 28-Year-Old Female with a 2-Year History of Sinus Headaches

A 28-year-old female comes to your office with a 2-year history of recurrent headaches. These headaches occur three or four times per month and last 12 to 24 hours. The headaches are usually located over the right or left frontal sinuses. She often gets relief from ibuprofen and pseudoephedrine combinations. This particular headache has lasted 2 days now and she has some nausea associated with it. When questioned, she notes that the bright lights and loud music do make her head pain feel worse. The patient has been using an over-the-counter analgesic decongestant combination without significant relief and comes to you for antibiotics for her sinus infection.

On examination, the patient's blood pressure is 100/70 mmHg. Her neurologic examination is within normal limits. The optic fundi are normal, as is the rest of the neurologic examination.

4. What workup would you perform to determine the etiology of this headache?

a. computed tomography (CT) of the paranasal sinuses

b. erythrocyte sedimentation rate (ESR)

c. magnetic resonance imaging (MRI) scan of the brain

d. careful history and physical

e. c and d

5. This patient's headache is most likely a

a. migraine headache without aura

b. migraine headache with aura

c. sinus headache

d. tension-type headache

e. optic chiasm tumor

CLINICAL CASE PROBLEM 3

A 25-Year-Old Newlywed Female with a 3-Year History of Recurrent Headaches

A 25-year-old female comes to your office with a 3-year history of recurrent headaches that have gotten worse during the past year. These headaches occur approximately twice per week. She is concerned that she may be having some kind of stroke because before the headache, nausea, and severe vomiting begins she experiences a "type of odd visual feeling or sight—flashing lights, almost like a pattern in front of my eyes." With respect to the headache, it usually lasts 24 to 36 hours. It is throbbing in nature and often "switches from one side to the other" with each attack. She needs to be in a dark room and finds noise bothersome when she has these headaches. She is otherwise healthy and takes birth control pills for contraception since getting married this past year.

On physical examination, the patient's blood pressure is 110/70 mmHg. Examination of the optic fundi is completely normal, as is the rest of the neurologic examination.

6. What is the most likely diagnosis in this patient?

a. migraine headache without aura

b. migraine headache with aura

c. ophthalmoplegic migraine

d. tension-type headache

e. transient ischemic attack

7. What is the best acute treatment for this patient's headaches?

a. subcutaneous sumatriptan

b. intramuscular meperidine

c. dihydroergotamine

d. naratriptan

e. ketorolac

8. The appropriate treatment you prescribed did not work and she goes to the emergency room (ER) the next day. The ER doctor is asking what to treat her with next. You recommend

a. intravenous meperidine

b. zolmitriptan

c. dihydroergotamine and metoclopramide

d. butalbital with codeine

e. morphine

9. The patient sees you for a follow-up visit after successful treatment in the ER. She is frustrated

by these headaches and is wondering how she can feel better. You recommend all but

a. discontinuing oral contraceptives
b. exploring what is going on in her life and how she is adapting to her new marriage
c. starting daily amitriptyline
d. starting daily low-dose sumatriptan
e. keeping a headache diary

CLINICAL CASE PROBLEM 4

A 24-Year-Old Female Patient with Chronic Headaches Preceded by Nausea and Vomiting

A 24-year-old patient comes to your office for assessment of headache. She describes the onset, characteristics, duration, and associated features of a migraine headache that is preceded by nausea and vomiting, confined to the left side of the head, and characterized by a throbbing pain lasting approximately 48 hours. The unusual feature of this headache is that it always begins approximately 2 days before menstruation, and it always ends with the onset of menstruation.

On physical examination, the patient's blood pressure is 120/70 mmHg. Her optic fundi are clear, and her neurologic examination is completely normal.

10. What is the most likely diagnosis in this patient?
a. premenstrual syndrome
b. menstrual migraine
c. premenstrual dysphoric disorder
d. migraine without aura
e. complicated migraine syndrome

11. Which statement regarding preventive treatment of menstrual migraine is false?
a. prophylactic use of naproxen reduces migraine frequency
b. prophylactic use of triptans is safe and effective
c. prophylactic use of sertraline is safe and effective
d. prophylactic use of low-dose estrogen is recommended
e. none of the above statements are false

CLINICAL CASE PROBLEM 5

A 35-Year-Old Male with a 6-Month History of Recurrent Steady, Aching, "Viselike" Headaches

A 35-year-old male comes to your office with a 6-month history of recurrent headaches at least three

or four times a week, usually in the late afternoon. The headaches are described by the patient as "a vice around my head."

The headaches are not associated with nausea, vomiting, or malaise. The patient does not have photophobia or phonophobia. He smokes one pack of cigarettes per day and says he does not drink alcohol.

On examination, the patient's blood pressure is 130/70 mmHg. His optic fundi are normal. There are no neurologic abnormalities.

12. What is the likely type of headache in this patient?
a. chronic daily headache: tension type
b. episodic tension-type headache
c. migraine without aura
d. nicotine-related headache
e. cluster headache

13. The patient returns to your office a few months later complaining of daily headaches and constant heartburn since he started taking ibuprofen for his headaches. Which of the following statements best represents the current problem?
a. he has developed *Helicobacter pylori*-associated headache syndrome
b. his smoking will make it more difficult to treat his condition successfully
c. his headaches will improve with daily diazepamuse
d. he has developed analgesic rebound headache
e. b and d
f. c and d

CLINICAL CASE PROBLEM 6

A 75-Year-Old Female with a Severe Left-Sided Temporal Headache

A 75-year-old female comes to your office with a severe left-sided temporal headache. She describes a tender area in the left temple. She also describes pain in the area of the jaw while chewing her food. This headache has been present for the past 3 days.

On physical examination, the patient's blood pressure is 170/100 mmHg. Her neurologic examination is normal. There is moderate tenderness in the area of the left temple.

14. Which of the following statements regarding this patient's symptoms is (are) true?
a. this probably represents a late-onset migraine syndrome

b. simple analgesics should be prescribed before embarking on any extensive investigation of these symptoms
c. this headache is unlikely to be associated with any significant complications
d. an ESR should be ordered on this patient
e. all of the above

15. What is the appropriate treatment for this headache?
    a. acetaminophen
    b. sumatriptan
    c. cyclobenzaprine
    d. prednisone
    e. verapamil

CLINICAL CASE PROBLEM 7

A 35-Year-Old Female with Almost Constant Migraine Headaches

A 35-year-old female comes to the ER with another "migraine headache." She has had migraine headaches for the past 20 years, and during the past 4 years they have been almost constant.

She states that her headaches have required intramuscular meperidine and hydromorphone injections approximately twice per week for the past 3 years. She has made 100 trips to the ER with the same symptoms during the past year.

This patient categorically tells you that she has "tried every abortive agent and every prophylactic agent and nothing has worked."

16. Which of the following statements regarding this patient's headaches is (are) true?
    a. this headache most likely is an example of status migrainous
    b. the major component of this headache is likely an analgesic rebound headache
    c. the scenario presented here is uncommon
    d. the majority of the patients with this headache type are female
    e. all of the above

17. What is the treatment of choice for the headache described here?
    a. continue the current treatment plan: repeated injections of meperidine and hydromorphone
    b. change the treatment plan to regular injections of dihydroergotamine and metoclopramide
    c. seek immediate psychiatric consultation
    d. change the treatment plan to one that uses nonnarcotic analgesics (in fairly large doses) in place of the narcotic analgesics
    e. none of the above

CLINICAL CASE PROBLEM 8

A 62-Year-Old Male Patient with Headaches That Have Been Getting Progressively Worse

A 62-year-old patient comes to the ER with headaches that have been getting progressively worse during the past 7 days. He has not had previous problems with headache, and his only significant illness was a lobectomy and radiation therapy for carcinoma of the lung 3 years ago. He has not had any recurrence and is feeling well.

The significant features of this headache include the following: The headache appears to be significantly worse every day; the headache is absolutely constant (it never goes away and never decreases in severity to any extent); and the headache is described as a "terrible pressure within my head."

18. What is the most likely cause of this patient's headache?
    a. migraine without aura: status migrainous type
    b. tension-type headache
    c. secondary headache: cerebral edema
    d. chronic daily headache
    e. status migrainous

19. What is the drug of choice for this patient at this time?
    a. sumatriptan
    b. ergotamine
    c. meperidine and hydromorphone
    d. dexamethasone
    e. chlorpromazine

CLINICAL CASE PROBLEM 9

A 17-Year-Old Male with a Headache from Hell

A 17-year-old male comes to the ER with "a headache like I've never had before." He is brought to the ER by his mother. The patient had been completely well, healthy, and active prior to this episode (which began last night). Nausea and vomiting began soon after the headache onset. The patient and his family report no history of trauma. There is no family history of migraine or cluster headache.

On examination, there is significant neck stiffness. The patient is unable to move his neck without extreme pain. You are just about to continue with the neurological examination when a patient with a cardiac arrest is wheeled through the ER doors.

20. At this time, with this information you have to this point, what is the most likely diagnosis?
    a. acute subdural hematoma
    b. cluster headache
    c. subarachnoid hemorrhage
    d. migraine headache without aura
    e. glioblastoma multiforme

21. With the provisional diagnosis you have made on this patient, what should you do now?
    a. perform a lumbar puncture
    b. perform a CT or MRI scan of the brain
    c. administer oxygen and sumatriptan
    d. give merperidine
    e. get a gastroenterologist consultation for the profuse vomiting

---

Clinical Case Management Problem

Discuss the classification of primary headache disorders that has been proposed by the International Headache Society. Distinguish between primary headache and secondary headache.

Answers

1. **d.** This patient has developed a typical cluster headache. Although we can diagnose with considerable confidence, it is too early to predict which of the two subtypes of cluster headache the patient ultimately will develop: episodic cluster headache and chronic cluster headache.

The typical cluster headache awakens a patient from sleep, although both daytime clusters and nighttime clusters are well described. Multiple daily episodes usually lasting between 45 minutes and 1 hour may occur on a regular basis for periods of 2 or 3 weeks. Remissions may last from several months to several years. Episodic cluster headaches constitute 90% of cases. In the other 10% of patients, the headaches do not remit (chronic cluster headache). The typical description of cluster headache is a headache that has the properties of a "deep, burning, or stabbing pain." It very often is described by the patient as "excruciating" or "the worst pain I have ever had." It is almost exclusively unilateral in nature. The pain may become so bad that the patient actually becomes suicidal. Cluster headache is associated with lacrimation, facial flushing, and nasal discharge. The affected eye often becomes red, conjunctival vessels become dilated, and a Horner's-type syndrome including both ptosis and pupillary constriction develops.

2. **d.** Cluster headache is thought by many authorities to be a migraine variant. Injectable sumatriptan (Imitrex) is the only injectable triptan currently available and is the drug of choice for acute episodes of cluster headache. Also, inhalation of 7 to 15 L/minute of oxygen with a non-rebreather facial mask can be beneficial in an acute cluster attack. Ergotamine preparations have also been shown to be effective, but oxygen and subcutaneous sumatriptan have a faster onset of action and are the first line in treatment.

3. **c.** Prophylactic medications that are indicated in the treatment of cluster headache include verapamil, ergotamine, lithium, methysergide, prednisone, topirimate and other corticosteroids, indomethacin, beta blockers, tricyclic antidepressants, and selective serotonin reuptake inhibitors (SSRIs). Diazepam is not indicated as a prophylactic agent in cluster headache.

4. **d.** At this time, a careful history and physical is the only diagnostic step to take. Other tests are not indicated. For details, see answer 5.

5. **a.** This patient has migraine headache without aura. Migraine headache is a type of headache that is typically episodic, usually occurring one or two times per month. Migraine headaches are often misdiagnosed by patients and doctors as sinus headaches. The International Headache Society defines sinus headache by purulent nasal discharge, pathological sinus finding by imaging, simultaneous onset of headache and sinusitis, and headache localized to specific facial areas overlying the sinuses.

The prodromal phase of migraine consists of symptoms of excitation or inhibition of the central nervous system and can include irritability; appetite changes, food cravings, and fatigue. These symptoms may precede the migraine attack by up to 24 hours. Migraine headache is unilateral in more than 50% of patients, but bilateral migraine is more common than previously thought. In addition, it is not uncommon for a migraine headache to begin on one side and switch to the other. The character of the pain is also much more variable than previously thought: "pulsating or throbbing" in only 50% of cases and a "dull, achy" pain in the other 50%. The headache phase usually lasts between 4 and 72 hours but is occasionally longer. Migraine headache is often associated with other symptoms, including nausea and vomiting. Heightened sensory perceptions, such as photophobia, phonophobia, and increased sensitivity to smell, can occur during the attacks. A moderate level of physical activity exacerbates the migraine headache pain, distinguishing it from the pain of tension-type headache, which is not worsened by physical exertion.

The workup needed to establish the diagnosis of migraine includes a careful history and physical exam as well as focused neurologic examination to rule out other causes of headache. Blood testing and radiographic imaging are not indicated unless other causes of headache are suspected.

6. b. This patient has migraine headache with aura. The visual symptoms that this patient describes follow the classical description of an aura. An aura is usually visual, although neurologic auras consisting of hemisensory disturbances, hemiparesis, dysphasia, and changes in memory or state of consciousness can occur occasionally. Only approximately 20% of migraine headaches can be classified as migraine with aura. Also, it is quite frequent for a patient to alternate between migraine with aura and migraine without aura. The ensuing headache follows the characteristic migraine pattern.

7. a. The first-line treatment for a moderate to severe migraine headache accompanied by vomiting in the absence of contraindications is subcutaneous sumatriptan. Its nonoral route is essential in effective treatment of a patient who is vomiting.

8. c. If subcutaneous sumatriptan fails and the patient comes to the emergency department, intravenous dihydroergotamine and intravenous metachlorpropamide is an underused but highly effective treatment. There is no place for the use of meperidine in the treatment of a patient with migraine.

9. d. Sumatriptan or other drugs in the tryptan class are not indicated for the prevention of migraine. In fact, excessive use can be associated with the development of medication rebound headaches. Preventive treatment of migraine headaches includes identifying trigger factors, which can include various foods—caffeine, alcohol, monosodium glutamate, chocolate, and aged cheeses. Medications such as nitroglycerine, nifedipine, and oral contraceptive may trigger migraine headaches. Discontinuing oral contraceptives has been shown to be an important means of reducing risk of ischemic stroke in patients with migraine with aura. A headache diary noting emotional state, sleep, activity, food and beverage intake, as well as medications taken for headache can be helpful in identifying trigger factors. The first-line medications for prevention of migraine headache are tricyclic antidepressants, beta blockers, and antiepileptic medications. These medications are generally started one at a time, but combinations of the different classes can be helpful in resistant cases.

10. b. Although migraine headache without aura can occur at any time during the menstrual cycle, this patient's description of a cyclic repeatable headache that occurs between 2 days prior to menstruation and the last day of menses clearly establishes this headache as what is referred to as menstrual migraine. Estrogen withdrawal is likely the trigger for migrainous attacks.

11. c. Therapy for an acute attack is similar to that for other migraines. Prophylaxis for menstrual migraine includes low-dose estrogen supplementation, NSAIDs, and ergot and triptan drugs used premenstrually. The SSRIs do not have a role in prophylaxis of migraine headaches.

12. a. This patient has chronic tension-type headache. Chronic tension-type headaches are often described as a steady, aching, "viselike" sensation that encircles the entire head. Chronic tension-type headaches are often accompanied by tight and tender muscles at the site of maximal pain, often in the posterior cervical, frontal, or temporal musculature. Chronic tension-type headache is defined as tension-type headache occurring more than 15 days a month. Chronic daily tension-type headaches are usually related to causal factors that include stress and worry, depression, overwork, lack of sleep, incorrect posture, and marital and family dysfunction.

13. e. This patient has analgesic rebound headache and has developed gastritis as a side effect of frequent NSAID use. This condition requires prophylactic treatment. Tricyclic antidepressants are helpful in treating analgesic rebound headaches. The patient also needs to minimize his use of simple analgesics. Patients who smoke are more difficult to treat successfully for chronic daily headache and analgesic rebound headache, and they have a higher chance of success if they quit smoking.

Treatment approaches for the relief of tension-type headaches should center on the following principles: (1) Identify the causal factor(s); (2) employ stress reduction techniques such as exercise, cognitive behavioral therapy, yoga, meditation, or biofeedback; and (3) consider the use of mild analgesics such as acetaminophen or NSAIDs for acute, less frequent headaches. Codeine or other narcotic agents should be avoided.

14. d. This patient has temporal arteritis (giant cell arteritis) until proved otherwise. When an elderly patient presents with a new-onset headache, temporal arteritis must be excluded. This patient presents with a unilateral headache with a tender temporal area. This probably represents the inflamed temporal artery.

The most significant complication of temporal arteritis is sudden unilateral blindness resulting from occlusion of the terminal branches of the ophthalmic artery. This is a completely preventable complication.

Temporal arteritis is often associated with polymyalgia rheumatica.

The ESR is a highly sensitive test in a patient you suspect of having temporal arteritis. The ESR is usually elevated higher than 50 mm/hour and may exceed 100 mm/hour.

15. d. The treatment of choice for a patient with temporal arteritis is high-dose prednisone. When temporal arteritis is diagnosed or even suspected, treatment should be started immediately with at least 50 mg of prednisone. If the diagnosis is confirmed, treatment should be continued for at least 4 weeks before any gradual reduction is instituted. If ocular complications have occurred, treatment should continue for 1 or 2 years.

16. b. This case represents a common scenario in many emergency rooms, and it presents significant challenges to many physicians. It provides an excellent example of the mistakes made in treating this type of headache pattern.

This patient should not be given narcotic analgesics in the first place. Only rarely is a one- or two-time dose of morphine indicated. When a patient with migraine headache tells you that "no abortive or prophylactic agent has ever worked," she is essentially telling you that she does not have a migraine headache. We now realize the importance of the neurotransmitter serotonin in the pathogenesis of migraine headache. If none of the abortive prophylactic agents work, we can draw the reasonable conclusion that the major headache component is not dependent on serotonin. In this patient, there is no doubt that migraine headache was the beginning of the problem, but now rebound analgesic headache with migraine underlay is the most likely diagnosis and the treatment problem to be faced.

A status migrainous is defined as a prolonged migraine attack usually lasting more than 72 hours that does not resolve spontaneously.

17. e. For the treatment of this patient, the physician must be both empathetic and firm, explaining the true cause of the patient's condition and working with the patient to gradually reduce the dose of narcotics. It is suggested to reduce the total narcotic dose by 10% a week.

It would be very unwise to use large doses of nonnarcotic analgesics in this patient. The most common cause of rebound analgesic headaches is, in fact, acetaminophen. Starting a prophylactic medication such as a tricyclic antidepressant or antiepileptic medication will help to reduce the frequency of these headaches. Adjunct treatments such as cognitive behavioral therapy and biofeedback may also be beneficial.

18. c. This patient has a secondary headache (a headache resulting from a secondary disease or process). The description is a classic presentation of the headache of cerebral edema. In this case, the cerebral edema is the result of metastatic deposits related to the carcinoma of the lung that was previously resected and radiated. The classic symptoms in this case are fairly acute onset, constant headache, pressurelike sensation, and a progressively more severe headache every day.

19. d. The treatment of choice for this patient is dexamethasone. The correct starting dose is 4 mg four times a day with omeprazole to protect the gastric mucosa and prevent peptic or stress ulceration.

20. c. This headache scenario could represent a first-time migraine, but no family history of migraine or cluster and acute onset make a secondary headache possible. This description of the worst headache of his life is a classic description for subarachnoid hemorrhage. An acute subdural hematoma would be accompanied by a history of a high-impact traumatic injury. A cluster headache would be described as seen in Clinical Case Problem 1. In glioblastoma multiforme, the symptoms of headache, nausea, and vomiting gradually occur and increase over a period of a few months.

21. b. This patient should have an immediate CT scan or MRI scan, and this should be followed by angiography or magnetic resonance angiography to localize the blood vessel. The most common pathogenesis of subarachnoid hemorrhage is rupture of a saccular aneurysm in the circle of Willis.

Solution to the Clinical Case Management Problem

The classification of primary headache disorders (according to the International Headache Society) is as follows: (1) migraine without aura, (2) migraine with aura, (3) childhood periodic syndromes that are commonly precursors of migraines, (4) retinal migraine, (5) complications of migraine, (6) probable migraine, (7) infrequent episodic tension-type headache, (8) frequent episodic tension-type headache, (9) chronic tension-type headache, (10) probable tension-type headache, (11) cluster headache, (12) paroxysmal hemicrania, (13) short-lasting unilateral neuralgiform headache attacks with conjuctival injection and tearing, (14) probable trigeminal autonomic cephalalgia, (15) primary stabbing headache, (16) primary cough headache, (17) primary exertional headache, (18) primary headache associated with sexual activity, (19) hypnic headache, (20) primary thunderclap headache, (21) hemicrania continua, and (22) new daily persistent headache.

Secondary headaches are caused by another disorder. These headaches can be due to trauma; vascular disorders; intracranial disorder; substances or withdrawal from substances; infection; disorders of the ears, eyes, nose, sinuses, teeth, or mouth; or psychiatric disorders. These headaches can also be due to disorders of homeostasis.

Summary

Headaches are classified as either primary or secondary headaches. Appropriate treatment of headaches depends on the correct diagnosis. The details of the diagnosis and management of the most important forms of headaches have been discussed previously. Because headaches are among the most common problems encountered in primary care, the following are important points to remember when evaluating and treating a patient with a headache:

1. Take a complete history and perform a complete physical (especially neurologic) examination.
2. Do not rely on CT or MRI scans to make the majority of headache diagnoses.
3. Recognize that migraine headache in the same patient may have different presentations on different occasions.
4. Do not label a headache as tension headache unless the criteria for its diagnosis are met.
5. Attempt to discover the triggers or stressors that bring on both migraine-type headaches and tension-type headaches.
6. Remember that the pathophysiology of migraine is related to serotonin depletion.
7. Recognize the contraindications to 5-HT-1 agonists: (a) ischemic heart disease/angina pectoris; (b) previous myocardial infarction; (c) uncontrolled hypertension; (d) basilar artery migraine; (e) hemiplegic migraine; and (f) concomitant use of monoamine oxidase inhibitors, SSRIs, or lithium.
8. Avoid narcotics for the treatment of migraine headaches.
9. Recognize rebound analgesia headaches; these are underdiagnosed.

Suggested Reading

Dalessio DJ: Relief of cluster headache and cranial neuralgias: Promising prophylactic and symptomatic treatments. *Postgrad Med* 109(1):69–78, 2001.

Headache Classification Subcommittee of the International Headache Society: International classification of headache disorders: 2nd edition. *Cephalalgia* 24(Suppl 1):9–160, 2004.

Institute for Clinical Systems Improvement: *Health Care Guideline: Migraine Headache*, 5th ed. Bloomington, MN: Institute for Clinical Systems Improvement, 2007.

CLINICAL CASE PROBLEM 1

A 22-Year-Old Male Who Suddenly Lost Consciousness, Became Rigid, and Fell to the Ground

A 22-year-old male is brought to the emergency department by his wife. While he was raking leaves in the backyard, he suddenly lost consciousness, became rigid, and fell to the ground. His respirations temporarily ceased. This lasted for approximately 45 seconds and was followed by a period of jerking of all four limbs lasting 2 or 3 minutes. The patient then remained unconscious for 3 or 4 minutes.

On examination, the patient is drowsy. The vital signs are normal. There is a large laceration present on his tongue and a small laceration present on his lip. The neurologic examination is otherwise normal.

SELECT THE BEST ANSWER TO THE FOLLOWING QUESTIONS

1. What type of seizure is this patient suffering from?
   a. simple partial seizure
   b. complex partial seizure
   c. absence seizure
   d. grand mal (tonic–clonic) seizure
   e. myoclonic seizure

2. Which of the following medications would not be a drug of first choice for the prevention of further seizures in the patient described?
   a. phenytoin
   b. carbamazepine
   c. phenobarbital
   d. primidone
   e. ethosuximide

CLINICAL CASE PROBLEM 2

A 76-Year-Old Female with a New-Onset Seizure

A 76-year-old female with hypertension, hypercholesterolemia, coronary artery disease, and chronic obstructive pulmonary disease is transferred to your nursing home service. She is there for subacute rehabilitation after hospitalization for new-onset atrial fibrillation. During her hospitalization, a computed tomography (CT) scan of the brain demonstrated multiple old lacunar infarcts. To prevent further cerebrovascular accidents, she was started on coumadin and her international normalized ratio is therapeutic. Her rehab stay has been uneventful, her strength is improving, and she is able to ambulate without an assistive device. On day 7 during recreational activities, she experienced a 3-miniute lapse of consciousness. The nursing staff returned her to her room and evaluated her.

On examination, her blood pressure is 150/92 mmHg, her pulse is 96 beats/minute and irregular, her respirations are 16 breaths/minute, and she is afebrile. She is in no acute distress, and her neurologic examination is normal except for some increased somnolence. The rest of her examination is unchanged from admission.

3. Which of the following is the most correct statement regarding this event?
   a. there is probably no association with the abnormal CT
   b. cardiac issues are the most likely cause
   c. cerebrovascular disease is the most common cause of this event
   d. the patient has only one risk factor for cerebrovascular disease
   e. this is an unusual presentation for seizures in the elderly

4. What is the type of seizure described in this patient?
   a. a simple partial seizure
   b. a complex partial seizure
   c. an absence seizure
   d. a tonic–clonic (grand mal) seizure
   e. a myoclonic seizure

5. What is the most common cause of a new-onset seizure in a patient of this age?
   a. acute stroke
   b. alcohol withdrawal
   c. head trauma
   d. brain tumor
   e. an old stroke

6. Which of the following medications would not be a drug of first choice for the prevention of further seizures in this patient?
   a. phenytoin
   b. carbamazepine
   c. phenobarbital
   d. valproic acid
   e. none of the above

7. Which of the following is (are) a likely outcome(s) from the diagnosis of a new seizure disorder?
   a. increased falls and fractures
   b. decline in activities of daily living
   c. depression
   d. decline in cognitive function
   e. all of the above

CLINICAL CASE PROBLEM 3

A 12-Year-Old Girl Who Stares into Space

A mother comes to your office with her 12-year-old daughter. The mother states that for the past 6 months she (and the girl's teacher) has frequently noted the child staring into space. This lack of concentration usually lasts only 30 to 45 seconds. Sometimes there appears to be brief twitching of all limbs during this time. The child's neurologic examination is normal.

8. What is the most likely cause of the symptoms described here?
   a. simple partial seizures
   b. complex partial seizures
   c. absence seizures
   d. myoclonic seizures
   e. none of the above

9. All of the following may be useful in the treatment of this patient except
   a. valproic acid
   b. clonazepam
   c. ethosuximide
   d. phenytoin
   e. none of the above

10. Which of the following statements regarding beginning and stopping antiepileptic therapy is (are) true?
    a. antiepileptic therapy can be discontinued safely after a seizure-free interval of 1 year
    b. every patient who has a seizure should be started taking antiepileptic medication
    c. antiepileptic medication should be started with a combination of two or more antiepileptic agents
    d. the decision to stop antiepileptic medication should be guided by the results of the electroencephalogram (EEG)
    e. a and d

11. Which of the following investigations is (are) useful in the initial evaluation of a patient with new-onset seizures?
    a. EEG
    b. magnetic resonance imaging (MRI) scan of the brain
    c. serologic test for syphilis
    d. carotid ultrasound
    e. a, b, and c
    f. a, b, c, and d

12. Which of the following statements regarding the diagnosis and treatment of status epilepticus is (are) true?
    a. poor compliance with the anticonvulsant drug regimen is the most common cause of tonic–clonic status epilepticus
    b. the mortality rate of status epilepticus may be as high as 20%
    c. the establishment of an airway is the first priority in the management of status epilepticus
    d. intravenous (IV) diazepam is the drug of first choice in the immediate management of status epilepticus
    e. all of the above statements are true

13. Which of the following is (are) a cause(s) of non-epileptic seizures?
    a. hypocalcemia
    b. hypomagnesemia
    c. pyridoxine deficiency
    d. thyrotoxic storm
    e. a, b, and c
    f. a, b, c, and d

14. Which of the following most often is confused with petit mal seizures (absence seizures) in adults?
    a. benign rolandic epilepsy
    b. complex partial seizures
    c. myoclonic seizures
    d. simple partial seizures
    e. clonic seizures

15. Which of the following is the most common neurologic disorder?
    a. epilepsy
    b. multiple sclerosis
    c. stroke
    d. myasthenia gravis
    e. Bell's palsy

16. Which metabolic abnormality is least likely to cause a seizure?
    a. alcohol withdrawal
    b. hypoglycemia
    c. hyponatremia
    d. sepsis
    e. anemia

Clinical Case Management Problem

Discuss the pathophysiology and treatment of febrile seizures in children.

Answers

1. d. This patient has had a grand mal (tonic–clonic) seizure. Tonic–clonic seizures are often associated with a sudden loss of consciousness. The tonic phase is followed by a clonic phase characterized by generalized body musculature jerking. Following this is a stage of flaccid coma. Associated manifestations include tongue or lip biting, urinary or fecal incontinence, and other injuries. An aura may precede a generalized seizure.

2. e. As in partial (focal) seizures, the drugs of choice are phenytoin, carbamazepine, phenobarbital, primidone, and valproic acid. Ethosuximide is not an effective drug in the treatment of grand mal seizures.

3. c. The incidence of seizure disorders increases with age. In people older than age 60 years, the incidence of seizure disorders is more than double that in the 40 to 59 age group. In the older than 85 age group, the incidence of seizure disorders is more than three times that in the 65 to 69 age group.

The most common cause of seizures is cerebrovascular disease, which accounts for 40% of new-onset symptomatic seizures. Twenty-two percent of elderly patients who suffer strokes will go on to develop a seizure disorder. In addition to strokes, other acute cerebrovascular causes of seizures include subarachnoid hemorrhage, subdural hematoma, intracranial hemorrhage, and head injury.

4. b. The seizure described in this patient is a complex partial seizure. In a complex partial seizure, consciousness is impaired. Other symptoms may include amnesia, confusion, and repetitive behaviors. Outcomes are poorer for patients who have a complex partial seizure following a stroke.

5. a. Partial seizures are the most common type of seizure in the elderly. Recognition of seizures in elderly patients can be challenging. In an elderly patient, a seizure may be either the first manifestation of a problem not previously recognized or the root cause of previous symptoms not understood.

Two-thirds of elderly patients who have seizure disorder do not have convulsions. Seizures caused primarily by vascular disease frequently present only with a lapse of consciousness. These seizures may last for a very short time (2 to 5 minutes). A patient may have several seizures in one day. The postictal state may last more than 24 hours, and in some cases it may last several days or a week.

6. e. Seizures are readily controlled by medication. In addition to efficacy, however, tolerability and potential side effects should be taken into account when considering which agent to use. The three most common antiepileptic drugs are phenytoin, carbamazepine, and phenobarbital. Phenobarbital has the highest incidence of side effects and generally should be avoided. All of these medications promote osteoporosis by increasing the metabolism of vitamin D or by having direct effects on bone. They are not recommended for those with osteopenia or those at high risk for osteoporosis due to immobility.

7. e. Seizure disorders in elderly patients are associated with anxiety, a decline in the ability to perform activities of daily living, depression, diminished cognitive function and self-esteem, falls and fractures, functional dependence, and increased social isolation. Seizures are associated with greater morbidity in elderly patients than in other groups.

8. c. This patient presents with typical absence (petit mal) seizures. Petit mal seizures may present with impairment of consciousness, sometimes accompanied by mild clonic, tonic, atonic, or autonomic symptoms. These seizures, often very brief in duration, interrupt the current activity and are characterized by a description of the patient "staring into space."

Petit mal seizures that begin in childhood are terminated by the beginning of the third decade of life. A bilaterally synchronous and symmetric 3-Hz "spike-and-wave" pattern is seen on EEG.

9. d. Petit mal seizures can be treated effectively with ethosuximide, valproic acid, or clonazepam. Phenytoin is not an effective treatment for petit mal seizures.

10. d. The criteria for decision to treat or not to treat an initial seizure should include details of the seizure; adequate laboratory data including measurement of glucose, electrolytes, alcohol, and other toxins; and the presence of EEG evidence of epileptic activity at least 2 weeks after the seizure. Careful reevaluation and monitoring are essential. A consideration of discontinuation of medication can be made after a seizure-free period of 2 to 4 years. This decision should be confirmed by a lack of seizure activity on EEG.

11. e. Laboratory investigations for a patient with an initial seizure should include a complete blood count, blood glucose determination, liver and renal function tests, and a serologic test for syphilis. Initial and periodic EEG is mandatory. CT scanning or MRI scanning should be performed in patients with focal neurologic symptoms and/or signs, focal seizures, or EEG findings indicating a focal disturbance.

A chest x-ray should be performed in all patients who are cigarette smokers; a primary lung neoplasm with secondary brain metastases producing cerebral edema and seizures is not uncommon. However, a plain x-ray of the skull or a skull series is unlikely to produce any useful diagnostic information.

12. e. Status epilepticus is a medical emergency, with a mortality rate of up to 20% and a high incidence of neurologic and mental sequelae in survivors.

Status epilepticus may be caused by poor compliance with medication, alcohol withdrawal, intracranial infection, neoplasm, a metabolic disorder, or a drug overdose. Prognosis depends on the length of time from the onset of the seizure activity to effective treatment.

The management of status epilepticus includes establishing an airway, giving 50% dextrose in case of hypoglycemia, giving IV diazepam, giving IV phenytoin, and treating resistant cases with IV phenobarbital.

13. f. There are many causes of nonepileptic seizures. These are divided into the following categories:

1. Cardiogenic: (a) simple syncope, (b) transient ischemic attacks, (c) arrhythmias, and (d) sick sinus syndrome
2. Electrolyte imbalance: (a) hypocalcemia, (b) hyponatremia and water intoxication, and (c) hypomagnesemia
3. Metabolic: (a) hypoglycemia, (b) hyperglycemia, (c) thyrotoxic storm, and (d) pyridoxine deficiency
4. Acute drug withdrawal: (a) alcohol, (b) benzodiazepines, (c) cocaine, (d) barbiturates, and (e) meperidine

5. Drug intoxication: (a) cocaine, (b) dextroamphetamine, (c) theophylline, (d) isoniazid, (e) lithium, (f) nitrous oxide anesthesia, and (g) acetylcholinesterase inhibitors
6. Metals: (a) mercury and (b) lead
7. Infections: (a) gram-negative septicemia with shock, (b) viral meningitis, and (c) bacterial meningitis (gram-negative or syphilitic)
8. Hyperthermia
9. Pseudoseizures (psychogenic)
10. Malignancies
11. Idiopathic (isolated unprovoked seizure)

14. b. Absence (petit mal) seizures are often confused with complex partial seizures in adolescents and adults. An accurate diagnosis can often be made on the basis of history, the duration of the seizure, the presence of an aura and/or postictal confusion, the pattern of autonomic behavior, and the EEG.

In absence seizures, minor clonic activity (eye blinks or head nodding) is present in up to 45% of cases, the mean duration is seconds, and the EEG shows the typical bilateral symmetric three-cycle second spike and wave that may be easily provoked by hyperventilation. There is no aura or postictal confusion.

In contrast, complex partial seizures may be preceded by an aura, are followed by postictal confusion, last longer (1 to 3 minutes), and are associated with more complex automatisms and less frequent clonic components. The EEG tends to show focal slow or sharp and slow wave activity. The differentiation between these two types of seizures is important. Absence seizures tend to disappear in adulthood, but complex partial seizures do not. Furthermore, phenytoin (Dilantin) and carbamazepine (Tegretol) are effective in treating complex partial seizures but not absence attacks.

15. c. The most common neurologic disorder is stroke. Epilepsy is the second most common disorder, with the prevalence ranging between 0.6% and 3.4% in the general population.

16. e. Seizures may be caused by toxic or metabolic conditions, most commonly from hypoglycemia or hyponatremia, that are induced by diabetes, kidney or liver failure, and medication reactions. Alcohol withdrawal, electrolyte disturbances, hypoxia from cardiac causes, and infection may also provoke seizures.

Solution to the Clinical Case Management Problem

Febrile Seizures in Children

1. Age of risk: 6 months to 5 years
2. Risk factors for febrile convulsions
   a. Previous febrile convulsion: The risk of a subsequent febrile convulsion is 30% when the first seizure occurred between the ages of 1 and 3 years; 50% when it occurred first at other ages; and 50% after a second febrile seizure.
   b. Family history of febrile convulsion (25%)
3. Prognosis: The prognosis for normal school progress and for seizure remission is excellent in children with febrile seizures.
4. Chances of progression of febrile seizures to epilepsy are very small: 98% of children with febrile seizures will have no further seizures after 5 years of age.
5. Factors that increase the chance of progression of febrile seizures to epilepsy
   a. The presence of developmental delay
   b. Cerebral palsy
   c. Abnormal neurologic development
   d. History of epilepsy in a parent or sibling
   e. A seizure that has a focal onset, lasts more than 15 minutes, or recurs in the same febrile illness
6. Treatment: Usually no treatment is necessary.
   a. Usually not indicated. If you do use prophylactic anticonvulsants, it will be only to treat the febrile seizure, not to prevent later epilepsy.
   b. The drug of choice when indicated is rectal or oral diazepam.

Summary

1. Absolute rules concerning seizures
   a. Not all that seizes is epilepsy.
   b. Not all epilepsy seizes.
   c. Many "seizures" are associated with other systemic disorders.
2. Major classification causes of nonepileptic seizures
   a. Metastases to the brain
   b. Cardiogenic
   c. Electrolyte imbalance
   d. Metabolic causes
   e. Acute drug withdrawal
   f. Drug intoxication
   g. Heavy metal poisoning
   h. Infections
   i. Hyperthermia
   j. Pseudoseizures
3. Greatly simplified classification of epileptic seizures
   a. Partial seizures
      i. Simple partial seizures
      ii. Complex partial seizures
   b. Generalized seizures
      i. Petit mal (absence seizures)
      ii. Tonic–clonic (grand mal) seizures
   c. Myoclonic seizures
   d. Tonic, clonic, or atonic seizures
4. Diagnosis and investigations
   a. History (from a relative or bystander)
   b. Physical examination
   c. EEG
   d. CT and/or MRI
   e. Blood profile including complete blood count, blood glucose, liver function tests, renal function tests, human immunodeficiency virus serology (in high-risk groups), serum calcium, and serologic test for syphilis
5. Treatment
   a. Carefully evaluate whether the patient needs treatment after the first seizure. In both adults and children, risk of recurrence is increased from 33% to 50% by the presence of a focal seizure, abnormalities on neurologic examination, a preexisting neurologic disorder, and focal spikes or generalized spike waves on EEG.
   b. Monotherapy suffices for most seizure disorders. As Blume states, "Severity of the seizure disorder, not the laboratory numbers, determines the therapeutic range." Whatever serum drug level renders the patient seizure free is adequate for that patient, even if it is below the laboratory range.
   c. Both effectiveness and side effects are dependent on dosage, with small changes often having major effects. There are currently no studies to suggest that newer antiepileptic drugs are more effective than older ones. The most common side effect of most antiepileptic drugs is fatigue.
   d. Drugs for generalized tonic–clonic (grand mal) seizures or partial seizures include the following:
      i. Phenytoin (drug of choice). Phenytoin is also the only antiepileptic drug that can be started at full dose.

ii. Carbamazepine
iii. Phenobarbital
e. Once antiepileptic drug therapy is initiated, it should be maintained for a time period measured in years, not months. Patients must be considered carefully for discontinuation of therapy.
f. Febrile seizures are not necessary to treat; diazepam can be taken every 8 hours for prevention, if that has been evaluated carefully.

g. Status epilepticus: Treatment is IV diazepam; alternatively, IV phenytoin or IV phenobarbital can be used.
h. Newer nonpharmacologic treatments include implantable vagal nerve stimulation for intractable seizures.

Suggested Reading

Adams S, Knowles P: Evaluation of first seizure. *Am Fam Phys* 75(9):1342–1348, 2007.

American Medical Directors Association: *Seizures in the Long-Term Care Setting,* LTC Physician Information Tool Kit Series. Columbia, MD: American Medical Directors Association, 2007.

Blume WT: Diagnosis and management of epilepsy. *Can Med Assoc J* 168(4):441–448, 2003.

Epilepsy Foundation: Epilepsy and seizure statistics. Available at www.epilepsyfoundation.org.

Pathhak M: Stroke and seizure. Stroke Awareness for Everyone. Available at www.strokesafe.org.

Riviello JJ: Classification of seizures and epilepsy. *Curr Neurol Neurosci Rep* 3(4):325–331, 2003.

CHAPTER

58   Sleep Disorders

CLINICAL CASE PROBLEM 1

A 48-Year-Old Male with a 6-Month History of Snoring, Nocturnal Breath Cessations, and Excessive Daytime Sleepiness

A 48-year-old male comes to your office with his wife. His wife tells you that "he is constantly snoring" and she has put up with all she can. This has been going on for a number of years, but it has been getting worse lately. His wife also tells you that "sometimes he even stops breathing during the night." When you ask the patient directly, he says, "Well, I may snore a bit, but I think my wife is exaggerating." You somehow doubt the latter statement. There is a history of sleepiness during the day; he has fallen asleep at his desk at work.

On examination, the patient weighs 310 pounds. His blood pressure is 200/105 mmHg (measured with a large cuff). Head, ears, eyes, nose, and throat examination shows boggy nasal mucosa but a normal pharynx. There is a grade III/VI systolic murmur present along the left sternal edge. You believe that there is elevated jugular venous pressure when he lies at a 45-degree angle. Chest is normal

to auscultation and percussion. His abdomen is obese, and his extremities are without edema.

SELECT THE BEST ANSWER TO THE FOLLOWING QUESTIONS

1. What is the most likely diagnosis in this patient?
    a. narcolepsy
    b. obstructive sleep apnea (OSA) syndrome
    c. generalized poor physical condition
    d. central sleep apnea syndrome
    e. adult-onset adenoid hypertrophy

2. To what is the pathophysiology of this condition related?
    a. collapse of the pharyngeal walls repetitively during sleep
    b. failure of upper airway dilator muscle activity
    c. sleep-related upper airway obstruction and cessation in ventilation (apneas)
    d. a and c
    e. a, b, and c

3. This condition is accompanied by which of the following?
    a. hypoxemia
    b. hypercarbia
    c. metabolic acidosis
    d. respiratory acidosis
    e. a, b, and d
    f. a, b, c, and d

4. What is (are) the major symptom(s) of this disorder?
   a. loud snoring
   b. daytime hypersomnolence
   c. disturbed nonrefreshing sleep
   d. weight gain
   e. a, b, and c
   f. a, b, c, and d

5. What is (are) the clinical feature(s) associated with the condition described?
   a. systemic hypertension
   b. inhibited sexual desire
   c. depression
   d. a and b
   e. a, b, and c

6. What is (are) the factor(s) that predisposes to this condition?
   a. alcohol intake
   b. benzodiazepines
   c. hyperthyroidism
   d. a and b
   e. a, b, and c

7. What is the treatment of first choice for this disorder?
   a. uvulopalatopharyngoplasty surgery (UPP)
   b. tracheostomy
   c. continuous positive airway pressure (CPAP)
   d. nortriptyline
   e. alprazolam

8. Which of the following drugs is contraindicated in the treatment of the disturbed, nonrefreshing sleep that is associated with the condition described?
   a. fluoxetine
   b. sertraline
   c. alprazolam
   d. phenelzine
   e. paroxetine

CLINICAL CASE PROBLEM 2

A 76-Year-Old Female with an 8-Month History of Poor Sleep

A 76-year-old female presents to your office with a chief compliant of poor sleep during most nights for the past 8 months. On further questioning, the patient recently moved into an assisted living facility after an extended rehab stay postoperatively for a right hip fracture.

9. What is your tentative diagnosis?
   a. chronic insomnia
   b. depression
   c. physiologic aging
   d. CVA
   e. narcolepsy

10. The patient is on a total of 10 prescription medications. She is concerned that some of these could be causing her not to sleep well. Which of the following medications are not associated with insomnia?
    a. Lipitor
    b. beta blocker
    c. Synthroid
    d. corticosteroids
    e. albuterol

11. The patient states that she had been living with her husband in the same house for the past 30 years. Her husband passed away 8 months ago. At that time, she insisted on continuing to live in their house alone with minimal help. She denies being depressed. What other symptoms besides insomnia would lead you to confirm your suspicion that the patient is depressed?
    a. decreased energy
    b. poor concentration
    c. decreased appetite
    d. loss of interest
    e. all of the above

12. This patient wants some advice to improve her sleep. Which of the following are helpful tips?
    a. consider the effects of medications on sleep
    b. avoid caffeine and alcohol after lunch
    c. avoid naps or limit to one nap of less than 30 minutes in the early afternoon
    d. limit liquids in the evening, especially if urinary frequency is a problem
    e. all of the above

13. Besides sleep hygiene, are there any other nonpharmacologic modalities to treat chronic insomnia?
    a. stimulus-controlled therapy
    b. sleep-restriction therapy
    c. cognitive therapy
    d. cognitive–behavioral therapy
    e. all of the above

Clinical Case Management Problem

Discuss the principles of the use of hypnotic agents in the management of sleep disorders.

Answers

1. **b.** This patient has OSA. Polysomnography will confirm the diagnosis and will demonstrate disordered sleep with periods of apnea and hypopnea.

2. **e.** The pathophysiology of OSA syndrome includes the following: (1) The pharyngeal walls collapse repetitively during sleep, causing intermittent sleep-related upper airway obstruction and cessation in ventilation (apneas); (2) the cessation of ventilation is related to a concomitant loss of inspiratory effort; and (3) upper airway closure in OSA occurs as a result of a failure of the genioglossus and other upper airway dilator muscles and apnea results.

3. **e.** OSA produces the following acid–base balance situation: (1) Apnea causes hypercarbia, hypoxemia, and a resulting respiratory acidosis; and (2) only if there is another preexisting condition associated with OSA will metabolic acidosis be produced.

4. **f.** The major symptoms of OSA syndrome are as follows: (1) loud snoring, (2) reports of prolonged pauses in respiration during sleep, (3) daytime hypersomnolence, (4) disturbed nonrefreshing sleep, and (5) weight gain.

5. **e.** Associated clinical features of OSA include systemic hypertension; inhibited sexual desire; impotence; ejaculatory impairment; depression; deficits in attention, motor efficiency, and graphomotor ability; deterioration in interpersonal relationships; marital discord; and occupational impairment.

6. **d.** Factors that predispose to OSA include sedating pharmacologic agents such as alcohol and benzodiazepines (all are contraindicated in OSA); nasal obstruction; large uvula; low-lying soft palate; retrognathia, micrognathia, and other craniofacial abnormalities; pharyngeal masses such as tumors or cysts; macroglossia; tonsillar hypertrophy; vocal cord paralysis; obesity; hypothyroidism; and acromegaly.

7. **c.** Polysomnography demonstrates that CPAP devices reverse apnea and hypopnea. In randomized controlled trials, CPAP devices also reduce daytime somnolence and improve mood and alertness. Compliance ranges from 50% to 80%. Although a CPAP is the best choice of those listed, always recommend weight reduction in obese individuals.

8. **c.** The most established management options, in addition to weight loss, in order of preference are as follows: (1) CPAP, (2) UPP, and (3) tracheostomy. Additional measures are antidepressants that are stimulating, such as protriptyline, fluoxetine, sertraline, and paroxetine, particularly with coexistent depression. Chronic anxi-

ety, which may complicate the OSA picture, should not be managed with benzodiazepines. Instead, the non-benzodiazepine buspirone, which does not appear to aggravate OSA, should be used, along with behavioral treatments. Thus, alprazolam is contraindicated.

9. **a.** Chronic insomnia is defined as any insomnia lasting more than 6 months and is associated with a wide variety of disorders, including depression. More information is needed before depression can be diagnosed in this case.

10. **a.** Many medications are associated with insomnia (Table 58-1). However, Lipitor, a statin used to treat hyperlipidemia, does not have the side effect of insomnia.

11. **e.** Symptoms of depression include SIGECAPS:

Sleep problems
Interest lacking
Guilt
Energy
Concentration
Appetite
Psychomotor retardation
Suicidal ideation

12. **e.** Sleep hygiene rules for older adults:

- Maintain a regular wake-up time and a regular bedtime.
- Avoid caffeine and alcohol after lunch.
- Avoid naps or limit to one nap of less than 30 minutes in the early afternoon.
- Limit liquids in the evening, especially if urinary frequency is a problem.
- Spend time outdoors (without sunglasses), particularly in the late afternoon or early evening.
- Exercise daily but not too close to bedtime.
- Consider the effects of medications on sleep.
- Alerting medications at bedtime or sedating medications during the day can adversely affect sleep.

13. **e.** Table 58-2 describes nonpharmacologic treatment options for insomnia.

Table 58-1	Examples of Medications Associated with Insomnia
Type of Medication	**Example**
Central nervous system stimulants	Dextroamphetamine, methylphenidate, mixed amphetamine salts
Antihypertensives	α-blockers, β-blockers
Respiratory medications	Albuterol, theophylline,
Decongestants	Phenylephrine, pseudoephedrine
Hormones	Corticosteroids, thyroid medications
Other noncontrolled substances	Alcohol, caffeine, nicotine

Table 58-2 | Psychological and Behavioral Treatments for Primary Insomnias

Therapy	Description
Stimulus-control therapy	A set of instructions designed to strengthen the association between the bed/bedroom and sleep and to reestablish a consistent sleep-wake schedule: (1) Go to bed only when sleepy; (2) get out of bed when unable to sleep; (3) use the bed/bedroom for sleep only (no reading, watching TV, etc); (4) arise at the same time every morning; and (5) no napping.
Sleep-restriction therapy	A method designed to restrict time spent in bed as close as possible to the actual sleep time, thereby producing mild sleep deprivation. Time in bed is then gradually increased over a period of a few days/weeks until optimal sleep duration is achieved.
Relaxation training	Clinical procedures aimed at reducing somatic tension (e.g., progressive muscle relaxation and autogenic training) or intrusive thoughts (e.g., imagery training and meditation) interfering with sleep. Most relaxation requires some professional guidance initially and daily practice over a period of a few weeks.
Cognitive therapy	Psychotherapeutic method aimed at reducing worry and changing faulty beliefs and misconceptions about sleep, insomnia, and daytime consequences through Socratic questioning and behavioral experiments. Other cognitive strategies may involve paradoxical intention to alleviate performance anxiety associated with the attempt to fall asleep.
Sleep hygiene education	General guidelines about health practices (e.g., diet, exercise, and substance use) and environmental factors (e.g., light, noise, and temperature) that may promote or interfere with sleep. Sleep hygene education may also include some basic information about normal sleep and changes in sleep patterns with aging.
Cognitive-behavioral therapy	A combination of any of the previous behavioral (e.g., stimulus control, sleep restriction, and relaxation) and cognitive procedures.

Solution to the Clinical Case Management Problem

The use of hypnotic agents in sleep disorders is a subject of great controversy (mainly because of their very wide and sometimes very inappropriate use). Sedative–hypnotic agents do not cure insomnia but may provide symptomatic relief (Table 58-3). There are many factors that influence the decision of whether to prescribe a hypnotic agent and which hypnotic agent to prescribe.

The most appropriate use of these drugs is for transient and short-term insomnia in combination with nonpharmacologic modalities. Hypnotic medications should never be used as sole therapy for chronic insomnia.

The disadvantages of prescribing a hypnotic agent include the following:

1. There is a propensity for daytime somnolence with the use of an agent that has either a medium half-life or a long half-life.

2. A second factor is the propensity for the development of drug tolerance; increasingly larger quantities of the drug are needed to produce the same effect.

3. Hypnotics may produce symptoms of autonomic hyperactivity and irritability the following day. This is a particular problem with those hypnotics that have a very short half-life. Next-day tremors and nervousness are very good examples of this phenomenon.

4. In the vast majority of cases, although hypnotics are specifically indicated for only short periods, they are used for increasingly longer time periods. The result is that after approximately 3 weeks, the hypnotic agents begin working in the opposite manner to which they were intended: Instead of helping sleep, they actually hinder sleep.

Table 58-3	Food and Drug Administration-Approved Agents for the Treatment of Insomnia	
Drug	**Half-Life (hr)**	**Geriatric Starting Dose (mg)**
BENZODIAZEPINES		
Estazolam	10–24	0.5
Flurazepam	47–100	15
Quazepam	39–73	7.5
Temazepam	10–15	7.5
Triazolam	1.5–5.5	0.125
NONBENZODIAZEPINES		
Eszopiclone	6	1
Zaleplon	1	5
Zolpidem	1.4–4.5	5
Zolpidem MR	2.8–2.9	6.25
MELATONIN RECEPTOR AGONIST		
Ramelteon	1–2.6	8

Summary

1. Prevalence

The overall prevalence of sleep disorders and sleep difficulties in the U.S. population is estimated to be approximately 27% in any given year. This includes, of course, all forms of sleep disturbance, both long- and short-term.

2. Clinical issues of sleep/diagnostic criteria of insomnia (Figs. 58-1 and 58-2)

a. A complaint of difficulty initiating sleep, difficulty maintaining sleep, or waking up too early or sleep that is chronically nonrestorative or poor in quality. In children, the sleep difficulty is often reported by the caretaker and may consist of observed bedtime resistance or inability to sleep independently.

b. The sleep difficulty occurs despite adequate opportunity and circumstances for sleep.

c. At least one of the following forms of daytime impairment related to nighttime sleep difficulty is reported by the patient:
   i. Fatigue or malaise
   ii. Attention, concentration, or memory impairment
   iii. Social or vocational dysfunction or poor school performance
   iv. Mood disturbance or irritability
   v. Daytime sleepiness
   vi. Motivation, energy, or initiative reduction
   vii. Proneness for errors or accidents at work or while driving
   viii. Tension, headaches, or gastrointestinal symptoms in response to sleep loss
   ix. Concerns or worries about sleep

Figure 58-1

A model of the evolution of the insomnia disorder. (Adapted from Spielman AJ, Glovinsky PB: The varied nature of insomnia. In: Hauri PJ, ed., *Case Studies of Insomnia*. New York: Plenum, 1991, p. 12, with permission.)

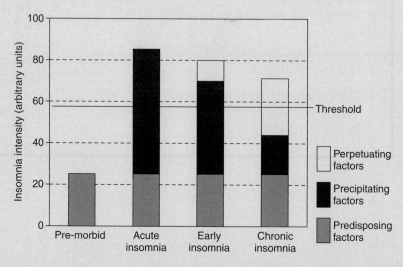

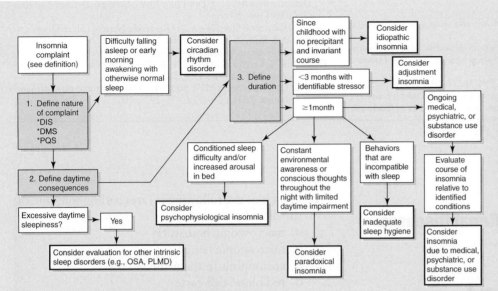

Figure 58-2

Algorithm for evaluating insomnia. DIS, difficulty initiating sleep; DMS, difficulty maintaining sleep; OSA, obstructive sleep apnea; PLMD, periodic limb movement disorder; PQS, poor quality sleep. (Adapted from American Academy of Sleep Medicine: *The International Classification of Sleep Disorders*, 2nd ed. Rochester, MN: American Sleep Disorders Association, 2005.)

3. Sleep phases and laboratory investigation

a. Human sleep: Made up of basically two types of sleep patterns: non-rapid eye movement (non-REM) sleep and REM sleep. Non-REM sleep has four stages and accounts for approximately 75% of total sleep. REM sleep occupies approximately 25% of total sleep.

b. Sleep investigations: All sleep investigations should be performed in a proper, accredited sleep laboratory. The two basic tests indicated in sleep disorders are the nocturnal polysomnogram and the multiple sleep latency test (MSLT).

4. Specific sleep disorders

a. OSA: This consists of loud snoring; prolonged pauses in breathing during sleep; daytime hypersomnolence; disturbed, nonrefreshing sleep; and weight gain.
  i. Pathophysiologic abnormalities produce apnea.
  ii. Associated conditions include obesity, systemic hypertension, sexual dysfunction, depression, and anxiety. Confirmatory test: polysomnogram
  iii. Treatment of choice for OSA is CPAP. Second and third management choices include UPP surgery and tracheostomy.
  iv. Weight loss should be encouraged in all overweight patients with OSA, alcohol should be discouraged, benzodiazepines should be prohibited, and systemic hypertension should be treated.
  v. Depression should be treated with a nonsedating antidepressant (SSRIs) or protriptyline.

b. Central sleep apnea: This is a rare syndrome characterized by cessation of ventilation related to a concomitant loss of inspiratory effort.

c. Narcolepsy
  i. Symptoms include cataplexy, hypnagogic or hypnopompic hallucinations, and sleep paralysis.
  ii. Associated conditions include persistent daytime sleepiness and restless and disturbed sleep. Confirming test: MSLT

  iii. Treatment consists of medications used to combat excessive sleepiness, including pemoline, methylphenidate, and dextroamphetamine. Mazindol is used in resistant cases. The REM-related symptoms of cataplexy and hypnagogic hallucinations are best treated with a stimulating tricyclic antidepressant such as nortriptyline or protriptyline.

d. Idiopathic hypersomnolence: A lifelong and incurable disorder that has as its most prominent feature unrelenting daytime somnolence. Patients spend lengthy periods sleeping at night only to awaken feeling more sleepy. Unlike patients with narcolepsy, they awaken from their frequent daytime naps feeling unrefreshed.

e. Periodic limb movement disorder (nocturnal myoclonus): This is characterized by repetitive (usually every 20 to 40 seconds) twitching or kicking of the lower extremities during sleep. Patients usually present with the complaint of unrelenting insomnia, most often characterized by repeated awakenings following sleep onset. Baclofen, clonazepam, and carbidopa–levodopa may relieve these symptoms.

f. Restless legs syndrome: The hallmark of this disorder is a "creeping sensation" in the lower extremities and irresistible leg kicks that affect patients on reclining prior to falling asleep. Unlike periodic limb movement disorder, the patients are very well aware of these symptoms and resort to moving the affected extremity by stretching, kicking, or walking to relieve the symptoms.

5. Hypnotic agents

In most primary care practices, the distinct disadvantages described in the Solution to the Clinical Case Management Problem outweigh any possible benefit, especially on a long-term basis.

Suggested Reading

Caples SM, Gami AS, Somers VK: Obstructive sleep apnea. *Ann Intern Med* 142(3):187–197, 2005.

Chai CL, Pathinathan A, Smith B: Continuous positive airway pressure delivery interfaces for obstructive sleep apnoea. *Cochrane Database Syst Rev1* (4):CD005308, 2006.

Feldman NT: Narcolepsy. *South Med J* 96(3):277–282, 2003.

Giles TL, Lasserson TJ, Smith BH, et al: Continuous positive airways pressure for obstructive sleep apnoea in adults. [update of Cochrane Database Syst Rev (1):CD001106, 2006]. *Cochrane Database Syst Rev* (3):CD001106, 2006.

National Center on Sleep Disorders Research: National Sleep Disorders Research Plan, NIH publication No. 03-5209, 2003. Available at www.nhlbi.nih.gov/health/prof/sleep/res_plan/sleep-rplan.pdf

Ringdahl EN, Pereira SL, Delzell JE, Jr: Treatment of primary insomnia. *J Am Board of Fam Pract* 17(3):212–219, 2004.

Schenck CH, Mahowald MW, Sack RL: Assessment and management of insomnia. *JAMA* 289(19):2475–2479, 2003.

CHAPTER 59

Common Renal Diseases

CLINICAL CASE PROBLEM 1

A 29-Year-Old Female with Fatigue, Anorexia, and Bloody Urine

A 29-year-old female comes to your office with symptoms of extreme fatigue, no appetite, and bloody urine. She developed a very sore throat 3 weeks ago but did not have it examined or treated. Her 6-year-old daughter had a similar sore throat 1 week before her. Her doctor (over the phone) said, "You probably have a viral infection from your daughter. Don't worry about it."

Three days ago, she began to have bloody urine and swelling of her hands and feet, and she felt terrible. Her past health has been excellent. There is no family history of significant illness. She has no allergies.

On examination, she has significant edema of both lower extremities. Her blood pressure is 170/105 mmHg. Her blood pressure was last checked 1 year ago, at which time it was normal.

SELECT THE BEST ANSWER TO THE FOLLOWING QUESTIONS

1. What is the most likely diagnosis in this patient at this time?
   a. hemorrhagic pyelonephritis
   b. immunoglobulin A nephropathy (Berger's disease)
   c. poststreptococcal glomerulonephritis
   d. hemorrhagic cystitis
   e. membranous glomerulonephritis

2. Which of the following is (are) pathognomonic of the disorder described?
   a. macroscopic hematuria
   b. microscopic hematuria
   c. eosinophils in the urine
   d. red blood cell casts
   e. protein 1 g/day

CLINICAL CASE PROBLEM 2

A Girl with Joint Swelling Erythema and Pain

Approximately 4 weeks after the mother develops her symptoms, her daughter comes down with an illness characterized by swelling of a number of joints with erythema and pain, bumps on both of her elbows, significant fatigue, fever, and a skin rash covering her body.

On examination, the daughter has a grade III/VI pansystolic murmur. Her blood pressure is 100/70 mmHg.

3. What is the most likely diagnosis in this case?
   a. juvenile rheumatoid arthritis
   b. Still's disease
   c. postviral arthritis syndrome
   d. rheumatic fever
   e. autoimmune complex disease

4. Which of the following statements regarding the prevention of the problems experienced by the patient and her daughter is (are) true, assuming both are treated with 10 days of penicillin?
   a. the mother's condition was preventable by penicillin; the daughter's condition was not
   b. the mother's condition was not preventable by penicillin; the daughter's condition was

c. both the mother's condition and the daughter's condition were preventable by treatment with penicillin

d. neither the mother's condition nor the daughter's condition could have been prevented by treatment with penicillin

e. prevention is variable with both conditions: penicillin may prevent both conditions, but it may not prevent either

5. What is the treatment of choice for the condition described in the mother?
   a. penicillin
   b. gentamicin
   c. prednisone
   d. a and b
   e. none of the above

6. Which of the following statements concerning prognosis of the condition described in the mother is (are) true?
   a. most patients with this disorder eventually develop end-stage renal failure
   b. the prognosis in the mother depends on how aggressively the antecedent streptococcal infection is treated
   c. most patients with the acute disease recover completely
   d. up to 20% of patients with this acute disease end up with chronic renal insufficiency
   e. c and d

7. Which of the following is (are) a complication(s) of the disease process described in the mother?
   a. hypertensive encephalopathy
   b. congestive cardiac failure
   c. acute renal failure
   d. a and b
   e. all of the above

8. Which of the following subtypes of the disease presented in the mother is associated with group A β-hemolytic streptococcus?
   a. minimal change
   b. focal segmental sclerosis
   c. membranous
   d. diffuse proliferative
   e. crescentic

9. Which of the following subtypes of the disease presented in the mother is associated most closely with nephrotic syndrome?
   a. minimal change
   b. focal segmental sclerosis

c. membranous
d. diffuse proliferative
e. crescentic

10. What is the most common cause of chronic renal failure?
    a. glomerulonephritis (acute to chronic)
    b. chronic pyelonephritis
    c. diabetes mellitus
    d. hypertensive renal disease
    e. congenital anomalies

11. What is the least common cause of chronic renal failure among the following causes?
    a. glomerulonephritis (acute to chronic)
    b. chronic pyelonephritis
    c. hypertensive renal disease
    d. diabetes mellitus
    e. congenital anomalies

12. Which of the following is true regarding angiotensin-converting enzyme (ACE) inhibitors?
    a. ACE inhibitors are contraindicated in patients with chronic renal insufficiency
    b. ACE inhibitors dilate the efferent arteriole of the kidney
    c. in patients with diabetes, ACE inhibitors prevent progression of microalbuminuria, even in patients with controlled blood pressure
    d. b and c
    e. all of the above

13. What is the major cause of death in patients with chronic renal failure?
    a. uremia
    b. malignant hypertension
    c. hyperkalemia-induced arrhythmias
    d. myocardial infarction
    e. subarachnoid hemorrhage

14. What is the anemia usually associated with chronic renal failure?
    a. hypochromic
    b. macrocytic
    c. normochromic, normocytic
    d. microcytic
    e. hypochromic, microcytic

15. Which of the following classes of medications have been shown to slow the decline in glomerular filtration rate (GFR) in patients with chronic renal failure?
    a. ACE inhibitors

b. nondihydropyridine calcium channel blockers
c. angiotensin receptor blockers
d. a and c
e. all of the above

16. Which of the following is (are) associated with nephrotic syndrome?
   a. proteinuria, 3.5 g/day
   b. edema
   c. hypoalbuminemia
   d. hypercholesterolemia
   e. all of the above

17. Which of the following is (are) a cause(s) of nephrotic syndrome?
   a. diabetes mellitus
   b. amyloidosis
   c. Hodgkin's lymphoma
   d. preeclamptic toxemia
   e. all of the above

18. Which of the following statements regarding diabetes mellitus and chronic renal failure is (are) true?
   a. diabetes mellitus is an uncommon cause of chronic renal failure
   b. diabetes mellitus type 1 is a more common cause of chronic renal failure than diabetes mellitus type 2
   c. diabetes mellitus type 2 is a more common cause of chronic renal failure than diabetes mellitus type 1
   d. diabetes mellitus type 2 does not lead to chronic renal failure
   e. diabetes mellitus type 1 does not lead to chronic renal failure

19. The treatment of nephrotic syndrome includes which of the following?
   a. corticosteroids
   b. loop diuretics
   c. anticoagulant therapy
   d. sodium restriction
   e. all of the above

20. Comparing the recommended treatment of post-streptococcal glomerulonephritis (PSGN) with the recommended treatment of non-poststreptococcal glomerulonephritis (NPSGN), which of the following statements is most accurate?
   a. the treatment protocols are the same
   b. corticosteroid treatment is indicated for both PSGN and NPSGN
   c. corticosteroid treatment is generally not indicated for PSGN, but it is for NPSGN

d. corticosteroid treatment is generally indicated for PSGN but not for NPSGN
e. the prognosis of neither PSGN nor NPSGN depends on the presence or absence of treatment

Answers

1. **c.** This patient has poststreptococcal glomerulonephritis. Poststreptococcal glomerulonephritis is the most common cause of acute glomerulonephritis. The syndrome may begin as early as 1 week after the initial streptococcal infection. Poststreptococcal glomerulonephritis predominantly affects children between the ages of 2 and 10 years. In patients with mild disease, there may be no signs or symptoms. In more severe disease, the symptoms of malaise, headache, mild fever, flank pain, edema, hypertension, and pulmonary edema may occur. Oliguria is common. The urine is often described as bloody, coffee colored, or smoky.

2. **d.** The pathognomonic clue concerning acute glomerulonephritis is red blood cell casts in the urine of patients. Other notable abnormalities include an elevated erythrocyte sedimentation rate and an elevated antistreptolysin O (ASO) titer. Some strains of streptococci do not produce streptolysin, thereby limiting the usefulness of the ASO titer in patients with recent pharyngeal infections.

3. **d.** In this case, the daughter of the patient has developed rheumatic fever. The Jones criteria for the diagnosis of rheumatic fever are outlined in Table 59-1.

Two major criteria or one major criterion and two minor criteria are virtually diagnostic of rheumatic fever.

It is important to realize that in some areas of the United States, the incidence of rheumatic fever is

Table 59-1	Jones Criteria for the Diagnosis of Rheumatic Fever	
Major Criteria	**Minor Criteria**
Carditis	Arthralgias
Polyarthritis	Fever
Chorea	Elevated erythrocyte sedimentation rate
Erythema marginatum	Elevated C-reactive protein
Subcutaneous nodules	Prolonged P-R interval on electrocardiogram

increasing, not decreasing. The increase may be the result of more virulent strains of streptococci.

4. b. Poststreptococcal glomerulonephritis is not preventable by penicillin; rheumatic fever, however, is preventable. In both conditions, the cause of complications is group A β-hemolytic streptococcus. Once the clinical or laboratory diagnosis of streptococcal pharyngitis is made, therapy with penicillin should be instituted and continued for a period of 10 days.

5. e. The primary treatment of acute glomerulonephritis associated with streptococcal infection is symptomatic. Although penicillin will eradicate the carrier state of group A β-hemolytic streptococci, it will not influence the course of the glomerulonephritis.

Symptomatic treatment should include bed rest and protein restriction (if the blood urea nitrogen or creatinine level is elevated). Fluid overload and hypertension should be treated with diuretics and other antihypertensive medications as needed. Immunosuppressive treatment may be necessary if heavy proteinuria or rapidly decreasing GFR is present. If acute renal insufficiency develops and volume overload is unresponsive to diuretics, hemodialysis should be considered.

6. e. Most patients with PSGN recover completely. However, up to 20% of patients will end up with chronic renal insufficiency. As indicated previously, the treatment of the antecedent streptococcal infection has no bearing on the prognosis.

7. e. Complications of acute PSGN include hypertensive encephalopathy, congestive cardiac failure, acute renal failure, chronic renal insufficiency, and nephrotic syndrome.

8. d. PSGN usually presents as a diffuse proliferative glomerulonephritis.

9. c. Membranous glomerulonephritis is the most common cause of nephrotic syndrome. The majority of children with nephrotic syndrome have minimal change disease.

10. c. The most common cause of chronic renal failure is diabetes mellitus, followed by hypertension and then glomerulonephritis.

11. b. Chronic pyelonephritis is the least likely cause of chronic renal failure of those listed. Chronic pyelonephritis rarely leads to chronic renal failure in the absence of obstruction.

12. d. The treatment for chronic renal failure is aggressive control of blood pressure and proteinuria. ACE inhibitors are a vital part of this treatment.

13. d. The major causes of death in patients with chronic renal failure are myocardial infarction and cardiovascular accidents (CVAs), secondary to atherosclerosis and arteriolosclerosis. Uremia can be controlled by dialysis or renal transplantation. Hypertension is usually controllable by individualized antihypertensive therapy. Arrhythmias, although they do occur in these patients, are not the major cause of death. Subarachnoid hemorrhage, as a subset of a CVA, does occur but is less common as a cause of death than myocardial infarction.

14. c. The anemia of chronic renal failure is usually normochromic, normocytic. Hematocrit often starts to decrease when the serum creatinine reaches 200 to 300 µmol/L (2 or 3 mg/dL) or when the GFR has decreased to approximately 20 to 30 mL/minute. The etiology of the normochromic, normocytic anemia is probably a decreased synthesis of erythropoietin by the kidney.

15. e. Treatment of chronic renal failure may include the following: (1) ACE inhibitors, adrenergic receptor binders (ARBs), and nondihydropyridine calcium channel blockers (diltiazem or verapamil) slow the progression of chronic renal disease; (2) limitation of dietary protein (usefulness is controversial); (3) statins (HMG-CoA [3-hydroxy-3-methylglutaryl coenzyme A] reductase inhibitors; recent studies have shown that statins slow the decline in GFR); (4) erythropoietin; (5) diuretics if significant fluid overload is present; and (6) control of renal osteodystrophy with calcium and vitamin D supplementation.

16. e. Nephrotic syndrome, as previously mentioned, is associated most closely with membranous glomerulonephritis. Nephrotic syndrome is characterized by albuminuria (>3.5 g/day), hypoalbuminemia, hyperlipidemia, edema, hypertension, and renal insufficiency.

17. e. Causes of nephrotic syndrome include the following: (1) primary glomerular diseases (all subtypes), (2) secondary to infections (including poststreptococcal glomerulonephritis), (3) drugs (e.g., nonsteroidal anti-inflammatory drugs [NSAIDs], penicillamine, and gold), (4) neoplasia (as in Hodgkin's lymphoma), (5) multisystem disease (systemic lupus erythematosus and Goodpasture's syndrome), (6) endocrine diseases (diabetes mellitus), and (7) miscellaneous (preeclamptic toxemia).

18. **c.** As stated previously, diabetes mellitus is the most common cause of chronic renal failure. Although the prevalence is less common in type 2 (20%) as opposed to type 1 (40%) diabetes, the prevalence of type 2 diabetes is actually 10 times the prevalence of type 1 diabetes. The logical conclusion from this consideration is that type 2 diabetes mellitus is a more common cause of chronic renal failure than type 1 diabetes mellitus.

19. **e.** Nephrotic syndrome is treated with nonpharmacologic symptomatic therapies, such as sodium restriction and fluid restriction, and pharmacologic symptomatic therapies, such as loop diuretics, ACE inhibitors (to reduce proteinuria), anticoagulant therapy (while patients have nephrotic proteinuria and/ or albumin level < 20 g/L), prednisone, and, in some cases, cytotoxic drugs.

20. **c.** The most important difference in therapy between PSGN and NPSGN is corticosteroid therapy (useful in NPSGN but not in PSGN).

Summary

GLOMERULONEPHRITIS

1. Classification (simplified): (a) PSGN and (b) NPSGN with many subtypes
2. More than 50% of cases involve children younger than 13 years of age
3. Symptoms and signs: (a) malaise, (b) headache, (c) anorexia, (d) low-grade fever, (e) edema, (f) hypertension, (g) gross hematuria with red blood cell casts, (h) proteinuria, and (i) impaired renal function
4. Treatment
   a. PSGN, symptomatic: protein restriction, fluid restriction, low salt intake, and loop diuretics
   b. NPSGN, symptomatic (as described for PSGN) plus corticosteroids
5. Prognosis
   a. 95% of patients with PSGN recover renal function within 8 to 12 weeks
   b. Excellent prognosis in patients with minimal change disease
   c. More than 70% of patients with mesangial capillary glomerulonephritis will develop chronic renal failure

NEPHROTIC SYNDROME

1. Etiology and prevalence: (a) many and diverse causes and (b) membranous glomerulonephritis is most common cause of nephrotic syndrome
2. Signs and symptoms: (a) edema, (b) hypoalbuminemia, (c) hypertension, (d) hyperlipidemia, and (e) renal insufficiency
3. Treatment: (a) sodium restriction, (b) fluid restriction, (c) loop diuretics, (d) ACE inhibitors, (e) anticoagulant therapy, (f) prednisone, and (g) cytotoxic agents

CHRONIC RENAL FAILURE

1. Causation: most common cause is diabetes mellitus
2. Symptoms, signs, and laboratory findings: (a) weakness, (b) fatigue, (c) headaches, (d) anorexia, (e) nausea, (f) pruritus, (g) polyuria, (h) nocturia, (i) edema, (j) hypertension, (k) congestive heart failure, (l) pericarditis, (m) anemia, (n) azotemia, (o) acidosis, (p) hyperkalemia, (q) hypocalcemia, and (r) hyperphosphatemia
3. Treatment: (a) restrict protein (insufficient evidence for routine recommendation); (b) maintain careful fluid balance (may need to restrict fluids if edema is present); (c) restrict sodium, potassium, and phosphate; (d) avoid potentially renal toxic drugs, such as NSAIDs; (e) adjust certain drug doses to correct for prolonged half-lives; (f) prescribe ACE inhibitors, ARBs, and nondihydropyridine calcium channel blockers; (g) prescribe erythropoietin for anemia; (h) prescribe loop diuretics if fluid overload; (i) correct electrolyte abnormalities; (j) prescribe HMG-CoA reductase inhibitors (get low-density lipoprotein cholesterol to less than 100 mg/dL); (k) prescribe calcium and vitamin D supplementation; (l) maintain hypertension control; (m) provide hemodialysis or peritoneal dialysis; and (n) perform renal transplantation

Suggested Reading

Del Rio M, Kaskel F: Evaluation and management of steroid-unresponsive nephrotic syndrome. *Curr Opin Pediatr* 20:151–156, 2008.

Hodson EM, Alexander SI: Evaluation and management of steroid-sensitive nephrotic syndrome. *Curr Opin Pediatr* 20:145–150, 2008.

Madaio MP, Harrington JT: The diagnosis of glomerular diseases: Acute glomerulonephritis and the nephrotic syndrome. *Arch Intern Med* 161(1):25–34, 2001.

McDonald MM, Swagerty D, Wetzel L: Assessment of microscopic hematuria in adults. *Am Fam Phys* 73:1748–1754, 2006.

Needham E: Management of acute renal failure. *Am Fam Phys* 72:1739–1746, 2005.

Snyder S, Pendergraph B: Detection and evaluation of chronic kidney disease. *Am Fam Phys* 72:1723–1734, 2005.

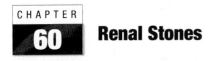

CHAPTER

60   Renal Stones

CLINICAL CASE PROBLEM 1

A 30-Year-Old Male with Flank Pain

A 30-year-old male comes to the emergency department with acute onset of severe right-side flank pain. The pain radiates down into the groin and testicle and is associated with hematuria, urinary frequency, urgency, and dysuria.

On examination, the patient is in acute distress. The patient is febrile at 101°F, pulse is 101 beats/minute, respirations 20 breaths/minute, and blood pressure 140/90 mmHg. He has significant right costovertebral angle tenderness. The rest of the examination is normal. There is 2+ blood on the urine dipstick test; no casts are seen on microscopic examination.

SELECT THE BEST ANSWER TO THE FOLLOWING QUESTIONS

1. What is the most likely diagnosis in this patient?
   a. renal colic
   b. acute pyelonephritis
   c. acute pyelitis
   d. atypical appendicitis
   e. none of the above

2. What is the most common composition of a kidney stone?
   a. calcium oxalate
   b. mixed calcium oxalate/calcium phosphate
   c. calcium phosphate
   d. struvite
   e. uric acid

3. Which of the following abnormalities is (are) usually associated with calcium oxalate stones?
   a. hypercalciuria
   b. hyperuricuria
   c. hypocitraturia
   d. all of the above
   e. none of the above

4. What is the drug of choice for the management of idiopathic hypercalciuria?
   a. cellulose sodium phosphate
   b. an orthophosphate
   c. potassium citrate
   d. hydrochlorothiazide
   e. pyridoxine

5. What is the most important component of the diagnostic workup in a patient with a kidney stone?
   a. serum calcium/serum uric acid
   b. serum creatinine
   c. intravenous pyelography
   d. 24-hour urine for volume, calcium, uric acid, citrate, oxalate, sodium, creatinine, and pH
   e. serum parathyroid hormone

6. Which of the following statements regarding uric acid stones is (are) correct?
   a. uric acid stones are formed in patients who are found to have an acidic urine
   b. uric acid stones are formed in patients with increased uric acid secretion
   c. the initial treatment for patients with uric acid stones is alkalinization of the urine
   d. patients with recalcitrant uric acid stones should be treated with allopurinol
   e. all of the above statements are correct

7. Which of the following statements regarding the treatment of nephrolithiasis is (are) true?
   a. extracorporeal shock wave lithotripsy (ESWL) has become widely used for the treatment of renal stones

b. ureteral stones, unless large, are best managed by awaiting their spontaneous passage
c. ESWL has shown its greatest benefit in patients with stones less than 2 cm in diameter
d. all of the above statements are true
e. none of the above statements are true

8. Which of the following is (are) part of the differential diagnosis of renal colic?
a. acute pyelonephritis
b. renal adenocarcinoma
c. papillary necrosis
d. all of the above
e. none of the above

9. What is the treatment of choice for metabolic stone formation?
a. hydrochlorothiazide
b. sodium potassium citrate
c. pyridoxine
d. an organophosphate
e. none of the above

10. Magnesium ammonium phosphate stones are usually secondary to urinary tract infection with which of the following?
a. *Escherichia coli*
b. *Proteus* species
c. *Klebsiella* species
d. *Enterococcus* species
e. *Enterobacter* species

Clinical Case Management Problem

A 45-year-old male comes to the emergency department with left-sided flank pain. An x-ray of the kidneys, ureter, and bladder (KUB) suggests a ureteric stone. While straining his urine, the patient discovers a stone. The pain subsides. The stone is analyzed and found to be a calcium oxalate stone. Describe the general treatment measures that you would use to prevent further stone formation in this patient.

Answers

1. **a.** This patient has renal colic. Renal colic is characterized by the sudden onset of severe flank pain radiating toward the groin. It is usually associated with hematuria, urinary frequency, urgency, and dysuria and is relieved immediately following the passage of the stone. Acute pyelonephritis, which may be associated with similar symptoms, is usually accompanied by fever and chills.

The sudden onset of severe flank pain is not typical of appendiceal disease.

2. **a.** Calcium oxalate stones are the most common type of renal stones; they constitute 60% of all stones. They are most commonly idiopathic. Other stones in order of frequency of occurrence are uric acid, mixed calcium oxalate/calcium phosphate, struvite, and cystine stones.

3. **d.** Calcium oxalate stones may be associated with hypercalciuria, hyperuricosuria, and hypocitraturia. Hypercalciuria is most common.

4. **d.** A thiazide diuretic, such as hydrochlorothiazide, is the agent of choice for the treatment of idiopathic hypercalciuria. Thiazide diuretics work by lowering urine calcium excretion. Other measures include increasing total daily fluid intake and decreasing animal protein and salt intake. Restriction of calcium intake has not been proved to be effective.

5. **d.** The basic laboratory evaluation of a patient with renal colic includes urinalysis; urine culture; blood chemistry profile including serum calcium, phosphorus, uric acid, electrolytes, and creatinine; x-ray examination of the KUB; and helical computed tomography (CT) of the abdomen. The most sensitive test for the diagnosis of metabolic abnormalities associated with nephrolithiasis, however, is the 24-hour urine collection. The 24-hour specimen should be analyzed for calcium, uric acid, citrate, oxalate, sodium, creatinine, and urine pH.

When stone composition is unknown, urine should also be obtained for qualitative cystine screening. Serum parathyroid hormone assay should be performed when hypercalcemia is present.

6. **e.** Uric acid stones, the second most common type of renal stone, are formed in patients with a persistent acidic urine or a high uric acid secretion (exceeding 1000 mg/day). The initial treatment of a patient with a uric acid stone involves alkalinization of the urine with either sodium bicarbonate or citrate. Patients with uric acid stones should be treated with allopurinol. A decreased purine intake (i.e., decreased consumption of red meat and, in particular, animal organs such as liver, sweetbreads, and kidney) is also recommended.

7. **d.** ESWL is used widely in the treatment of nephrolithiasis to break up renal stones with shock waves, permitting them to pass spontaneously.

Lithotripsy is most effective when the stone is less than 2 cm in diameter. For patients with stones larger than 2 cm, initial percutaneous nephrolithotomy followed by ESWL and a "second-look" percutaneous nephrolithotomy give the best results.

Patients with staghorn calculi, obstruction, or complex anatomy should be treated with open surgery.

Ureteral stones are best managed by awaiting spontaneous passage. If spontaneous passage is unlikely or delayed, ESWL is the first choice for stones in the upper two-thirds of the ureter; endoscopic surgery is the best alternative for lower ureteral stones.

A ureteropelvic or other obstruction, as well as stones deposited in diverticula, should be managed by endourologic techniques.

8. **d.** The major differential diagnosis of renal colic includes infection of the upper urinary tract (acute pyelonephritis or acute pyelitis), renal adenocarcinoma, and papillary necrosis. Papillary necrosis (ischemic necrosis of the renal papillae or of the entire renal pyramid) is usually secondary to excessive ingestion of analgesics, sickle cell trait (associated with hematuria), diabetes mellitus, obstruction with infection, or vesicoureteral reflux with infection.

9. **b.** Metabolic stones, including cystine stones, are best treated by giving the patient a sodium–potassium citrate solution, 4 to 8 mL four times a day. In this case, the urine pH should be monitored.

10. **b.** Magnesium ammonium phosphate stones are usually secondary to urinary tract infection with bacteria that produce urease (primarily *Proteus* species). The urease hydrolyzes the urea, producing ammonia and thereby raising the pH and providing the source of ammonia. Eradication of the infection prevents further stone formation. After calculi removal, prevention of stone growth is best accomplished by urinary acidification, long-term use of antibiotics, and the use of acetohydroxamic acid (a urease inhibitor that maintains an acid urinary pH).

Solution to the Clinical Case Management Problem

The treatment of calcium oxalate stones includes the following: (1) maintaining normal calcium intake with meals (this binds the oxalate that forms stones, increasing its loss from the gastrointestinal tract), (2) restricting dietary sodium to 2000 mg/day (6 g salt/day), (3) limiting intake of proteins and carbohydrates, (4) using oral orthophosphates to decrease stone-forming potential, (5) using thiazide diuretics to decrease urine calcium content, and (6) using allopurinol and urinary alkalinization to reduce the formation of urate crystals.

Summary

1. Classic symptoms of renal colic

Sudden, severe, flank pain with radiation to the groin; associated with hematuria, frequency, urgency, dysuria, and relief following stone passage. Diagnosis of retained stones is made by helical CT.

2. Types of stones

a. Calcium oxalate stones: (a) most frequent type of stone; (b) usually idiopathic and associated with hypercalciuria, hyperuricuria, and hypocitraturia; (c) in patients with hypercalciuria, restricted intake of animal protein and salt, combined with normal calcium intake, recommended to prevent recurrence

b. Uric acid stones: (a) second most frequent type of stone; (b) associated with urine that is persistently acidic and in conjunction with massively increased urinary uric acid secretion (>1000 mg/day); (c) prevention with alkalinization of urine with bicarbonate or citrate; in addition, may have to use allopurinol

c. Infective stones: (a) caused by urea-splitting organisms (*Proteus* species); (b) stone should be completely removed and antibiotic therapy prescribed

d. Cystine stones: occur with the inherited transport disorder cystinuria

3. Stone treatment

a. Ureteral stones: Await spontaneous passage. If not forthcoming, then use ESWL (upper two-thirds of ureter) and endoscopic techniques (lower one-third of ureter).

b. Renal stones: ESWL is the treatment of choice for stones less than 2 cm and located in the upper pole of the kidney. If stones larger than 1 cm are located in the lower pole of the kidney, a combination of ESWL and percutaneous nephrolithotomy is preferred.

Suggested Reading

Borghi L: Comparison of two diets for the prevention of recurrent stone in idiopathic calciuria. *N Engl J Med* 346(2):77–84, 2002.
Curhan GC: A 44-year-old woman with kidney stones. *JAMA* 293: 1107–1114, 2005.
Lindbloom EJ: What is the best test to diagnose urinary tract stones? *J Fam Pract* 50(8):657–658, 2001.
Miller NL: Management of kidney stones. *BMJ* 334:468–472, 2007.
Teichman JMH: Acute renal colic from ureteral calculus. *N Engl J Med* 350:684–693, 2004.

CHAPTER

61 Urinary Tract Infections

CLINICAL CASE PROBLEM 1

A 27-Year-Old Female with Spina Bifida and Bilateral Costovertebral Angle Pain

A 27-year-old female presents to the emergency room (ER) with a 4-day history of fever, chills, and bilateral costovertebral angle (CVA) pain. She has an indwelling urinary catheter and describes to you "at least 12 of these episodes before this current one." She has been seeing the same family physician since birth and has been diagnosed as having "nervous bladder and kidney syndrome." He has prescribed some over-the-counter "kidney pills" in the past for these symptoms. She tells you that they "never really worked," and she often has found herself bedbound with symptoms for several weeks before the fever broke.

You, the ER doctor on shift, are somewhat skeptical about the nervous bladder and kidney syndrome.

On examination, the patient is flushed. Her temperature is 40°C. She has intermittent shaking rigors. She has CVA tenderness bilaterally. Her abdomen is somewhat tender to palpation. There is blood in the catheter collection bag.

SELECT THE BEST ANSWER TO THE FOLLOWING QUESTIONS

1. What is the most likely diagnosis in this patient?
   a. nervous bladder and kidney syndrome
   b. acute hemorrhagic cystitis
   c. acute urethritis
   d. acute pyelonephritis
   e. spina bifida bladder spasm syndrome (SBBSS)

2. What would be the most likely organism in this patient?
   a. a gram-positive coccus
   b. a gram-positive rod
   c. an anaerobic organism
   d. a fungal organism
   e. a gram-negative organism

3. Which of the following bacteria would not likely be considered as highly probable of causing this problem?
   a. *Pseudomonas aeruginosa*
   b. *Klebsiella pneumoniae*
   c. *Enterobacter* species
   d. group A β-hemolytic streptococcus
   e. *Proteus* species

4. After obtaining a urinalysis and a urine specimen for culture and sensitivity, you now should treat the patient with which of the following?
   a. the over-the-counter kidney pills
   b. ciprofloxacin 500 mg three times a day by mouth (outpatient)
   c. Septra DS two tabs two times a day by mouth (outpatient)
   d. intravenous (IV) antibiotics in a hospital
   e. no medications are indicated at this time

5. Which of the following antibiotics would not be of first choice for this patient?
   a. IV ceftriaxone (Rocephin) or cefotaxime (Claforan)
   b. IV trimethoprim–sulfamethoxazole (TMP-SMX)
   c. IV ciprofloxacin
   d. IV ampicillin and gentamicin
   e. IV piperacillin-tazobactam

6. The investigations that should be performed on this patient at this time include which of the following?
   a. serum blood urea nitrogen (BUN) and creatinine
   b. renal ultrasound
   c. blood cultures
   d. complete blood count (CBC) with differential
   e. all of the above

7. The renal ultrasound shows small, shrunken kidneys, with no enlargement of the ureters and no stones. What is the most likely diagnosis in this patient?
   a. chronic pyelonephritis
   b. uterovesical reflux
   c. hydronephrosis
   d. vesicular diverticula
   e. none of the above

8. Which of the following statements regarding chronic prophylaxis in this patient is true?
   a. chronic prophylaxis is not indicated
   b. chronic prophylaxis is unlikely to be of any benefit
   c. chronic prophylaxis may make a significant difference in the preservation of this patient's renal function
   d. chronic prophylaxis is unlikely to be difficult because of resistant organisms
   e. none of the above are true

A 34-Year-Old Female with Hematuria, Dysuria, Increased Urinary Frequency, and Nocturia

A 34-year-old female presents with a 3-day history of hematuria, dysuria, increased urinary frequency, and nocturia. She has had no fever, chills, or back pain.

On examination, she does not look ill. Her temperature is 37.5°C. Her abdomen is nontender. There is no CVA tenderness.

9. What is the most likely diagnosis?
   a. Berger's disease (immunoglobulin A nephropathy)
   b. acute hemorrhagic cystitis
   c. acute hemorrhagic urethritis
   d. acute glomerulonephritis
   e. acute cystitis with concomitant coagulation disorder

10. What is the treatment of choice for this patient?
    a. a 10-day course of ampicillin and probenecid
    b. a 7-day course of ampicillin and probenecid
    c. a 3-day course of TMP-SMX
    d. a 1-day course of TMP-SMX
    e. a single dose of ampicillin 3.5 g and probenecid 1 g

11. You have decided on your therapeutic plan for the patient described. At what time would you implement this plan?
    a. right away: forget about the culture
    b. right away: start therapy immediately after taking the urine specimen for culture and sensitivity
    c. tomorrow: send the urine culture stat and order the pathologist to call you with the result personally
    d. tomorrow: send the urine culture and ask the pathology department for a report as soon as possible without aggravating the pathologist
    e. whenever: send the urine culture and when you get it back call the patient. If the symptoms have not cleared up, then consider starting the antibiotic

12. What is the most likely organism involved in the infection that has developed in the patient described?
    a. *P. aeruginosa*
    b. *Providencia* species
    c. *Escherichia coli*

d. *Klebsiella* species
e. *Enterococcus* species

13. The quinolone antibiotics (e.g., ciprofloxacin and levofloxacin) are a very significant advance in antimicrobial treatment. They also work by a unique mechanism. The mechanism(s) of action is (are)
    a. bactericidal mode of action
    b. inhibition of DNA gyrase
    c. blocks protein synthesis
    d. inhibition of cell wall synthesis
    e. a and b

14. All of the following statements regarding asymptomatic bacteriuria in women are false except
    a. risk is increased with sexual intercourse
    b. risk is not increased in women who use diaphragms
    c. it has been shown to lead to renal damage in normal hosts
    d. prevalence in elderly women may be as high as 75%
    e. treatment is never indicated

15. The patient returns to your office 3 days after you start her treatment and states that symptoms have not improved. What is the most appropriate next step?
    a. change the antibiotic and add pyridium
    b. check a urine culture and sensitivity and change therapy according to results
    c. send the patient for a renal ultrasound to rule out obstruction and change antibiotic
    d. collect a urine sample and check BUN and creatinine
    e. c and d

Clinical Case Management Problem

Discuss a classification of urinary tract infections in adult males and adult females.

Answers

1. d. This patient has acute pyelonephritis. First, she has very significant predisposing factors for urinary tract infections (UTIs), including an indwelling urinary catheter and a neurologic condition that increases the probability of same. Second, she seems to have had some less than optimal medical diagnoses. Third, she almost certainly has had recurrent episodes of pyelonephritis. This raises the possibilities of chronic pyelonephritis, reflux kidney damage, and resistant organisms. Fourth, the symptoms fit. Fever, chills, and CVA pain in a patient with a neurologic predisposing condition and an indwelling catheter equal acute pyelonephritis.

2. e. First, this patient is classified as having a complicated UTI. A complicated UTI occurs when any of the following are present in the patient: obstruction (stones), indwelling urinary catheter, high postvoid residual urine volume, anatomic or functional genitourinary abnormalities, renal impairment, and renal transplantation.

Although the most common organism is a gram-negative organism, it is frequently an organism that would not occur in patients without urinary tract disease. Examples include *Proteus, Providencia, Serratia, Pseudomonas,* and *Klebsiella* species. Overall, *E. coli* (one of many serotypes and one likely to be resistant to multiple antibiotics) is probably still the most common organism. Not as common but alternative causes of pyelonephritis would be gram-positive cocci including group B streptococci or enterococci (group D streptococci).

3. d. The only organism listed that is an unlikely candidate is group A β-hemolytic streptococcus. Group A streptococci, *Streptococcus pneumoniae, Staphylococcus saprophyticus,* and *Staphylococcus aureus* do not cause acute pyelonephritis.

4. d. This patient has not had proper assessment, an accurate diagnosis, or proper treatment at any time in the past.

At this time, she should be hospitalized, treated with IV fluids and IV antibiotics, and have a complete assessment of both urinary tract function and urinary tract damage. In addition, ways of preventing future infections should be considered.

5. b. Quinolones (e.g., ciprofloxacin or levofloxacin) are indicated for the treatment of complicated UTIs and will cover most, if not all, gram-negative organisms, including *Proteus* and *Pseudomonas* species. It would also be reasonable to use gentamicin, a combination of ampicillin and gentamicin, or a third-generation cephalosporin. Piperacillin–tazobactam would also be appropriate for complicated pyelonephritis.

TMP-SMX is not appropriate because resistance in uropathogenic *E. coli* is increasing.

6. e. At this time, a complete workup should be done. This should include the following (as a minimum): (1) blood—CBC with differential, serum BUN and creatinine, electrolytes, and blood cultures; (2) urine—a complete urinalysis: urine culture for bacterial sensitivity and examination for white blood cell casts and red blood cell casts; and (3) diagnostic imaging—a renal and abdominal ultrasound or an intravenous pyelogram (IVP).

7. a. This patient's abnormal ultrasound shows small, shrunken kidneys secondary to repeated UTIs that have gone untreated, causing chronic pyelonephritis. It is important from this time onward to measure renal function regularly and do everything possible to preserve this patient's renal function. Chronic pyelonephritis is treated with 4 weeks of oral antibiotics after acute pyelonephritis is treated.

8. c. First, repeated urine cultures must be done to determine the dominant organisms growing. Next, the susceptibility/resistance of these organisms needs to be determined to guide prophylactic therapy. It is difficult to determine at this time what that therapy should be; it depends on the results, but it certainly needs to be done.

9. b. This patient has acute hemorrhagic cystitis. Acute hemorrhagic cystitis is simply a variant of acute cystitis, and it is no more difficult to treat and does not have any more complications than other forms of acute cystitis. Hematuria does not signify a poor prognosis.

10. c. Patients with uncomplicated UTIs respond well to a 3-day treatment regimen. This abbreviated course of management is a good compromise between a 1-day course of therapy and the conventional 7- to 14-day regimens. The relapse rate with the 3-day regimen is comparable to that of longer courses of therapy. An abbreviated therapy is also more cost-effective and is associated with fewer adverse drug effects than the more prolonged courses of therapy.

TMP-SMX is certainly a drug of first choice for uncomplicated UTIs. The other drug of first choice would be a quinolone such as norfloxacin, ciprofloxacin, or levofloxacin.

11. b. You should not wait to begin therapy. Pretherapy urine culture in acute uncomplicated cystitis is not considered to be cost-effective. Culture is reserved instead for those who do not respond to therapy, those who have recurrent symptoms soon after therapy, and those with complicated UTIs. Ask for the result as soon as possible, but do not aggravate the pathologist.

12. c. This is a case of uncomplicated UTI. Hemorrhagic cystitis cannot really be considered a complication. With an uncomplicated infection, you are likely going to be dealing with an uncomplicated organism. Therefore, *E. coli* is the most likely organism involved in the infection.

There are many serotypes of *E. coli* that can produce UTI. Some serotypes are more likely to produce hemorrhagic cystitis; others are more likely to produce nonhemorrhagic cystitis.

13. e. The quinolone antibiotics are a significant advance in antimicrobial therapy. They use a totally unique mechanism of action. These antibiotics are extremely effective against many gram-positive and especially gram-negative organisms. The quinolone antibiotics work essentially at a molecular genetic level.

The quinolone antibiotics are bactericidal in action. Action is achieved mainly by inhibition of the DNA gyrase. This is an essential component of the bacterial DNA replication system. The inhibition of the α subunit of the DNA gyrase blocks the resealing of the nicks on the DNA strands induced by this α subunit, leading to the degradation of the DNA by exonucleases.

14. a. Asymptomatic bacteriuria has never been shown to lead to renal damage in those without anatomic abnormality or urinary obstruction. Sexual intercourse and diaphragm use both increase the risk for it (as well as for symptomatic UTI). Prevalence in postmenopausal elderly women approaches 20% to 50%. Treatment is indicated only in pregnancy.

15. b. Patients who do not respond to initial empiric 3-day treatment should have a urine culture with sensitivity done to guide change in antibiotic. Indication for renal ultrasound and laboratory tests other than culture would be a complicated infection.

Solution to the Clinical Case Management Problem

Classification of UTIs in Adult Females

1. With uncomplicated lower tract infections, it is either acute cystitis or acute hemorrhagic cystitis.
2. With complicated upper tract infections, it is either acute pyelitis or acute pyelonephritis.
3. Conditions that are likely to increase the risk of acquiring a complicated UTI include diabetes mellitus, stone disease, chronic indwelling catheterization, immunosuppression, pregnancy, neuropathic bladder, congenital anomalies (reflux), urethral stenosis, and urinary tract obstruction.
4. Sexually transmitted UTIs: Acute urethritis can be caused by *Chlamydia trachomatis*, *Mycoplasma hominis*, *Ureaplasma urealyticum*, or *Neisseria gonorrhea*.

Classification of UTIs in Adult Males

1. Uncomplicated UTI is very rare in the absence of obstruction except for acute prostatitis and epididymitis.

2. Complicated UTIs include acute cystitis (needs to be investigated with renal ultrasound), acute pyelitis, acute pyelonephritis, chronic prostatitis, or benign prostatic hypertrophy/hyperplasia.

   The most common complicating factor in males is obstruction caused by benign prostatic hypertrophy/hyperplasia. However, all males with a UTI not resulting from sexually transmitted diseases (STDs) need to be investigated. The minimal investigation is a renal ultrasound.
3. STDs
   a. Acute urethritis may be the result of infection by *C. trachomatis* (nongonococcal urethritis [NGU]), *M. hominis* (NGU), *U. urealyticum* (NGU), or *N. gonorrhea* (gonococcal urethritis)
   b. Acute epididymoorchitis is caused by *C. trachomatis*.

Summary

1. Classification: See the Solution to the Clinical Case Management Problem.
2. Signs/symptoms
   a. Lower tract dysuria: frequency, nocturia, hematuria, terminal dribbling, and discharge (STDs)
   b. Upper tract: same as lower tract plus fever, chills, and CVA pain/tenderness
3. Laboratory
   a. Urinalysis, urinalysis for culture and sensitivity (lower tract)
   b. CBC, blood cultures, 24-hour urine for creatinine clearance and protein, renal ultrasound, IVP, and computed tomography
4. To avoid complications, evaluate each patient in terms of risk factors and avoid indwelling catheterization whenever possible.
5. Treatment
   a. Lower tract UTIs in females: 3-day course of TMP-SMX plus Pyridium for analgesia
   b. Upper tract
      i. Quinolone (e.g., ciprofloxacin or levofloxacin)
      ii. Ampicillin plus gentamicin
      iii. Third-generation cephalosporin with or without gentamicin
   c. Inpatient versus outpatient: acute pyelonephritis—hospitalize those with complications or complicating diseases; otherwise, outpatient IV port therapy daily or high-dose oral therapy
   d. Prophylaxis: consider for high-risk patients; first choice—quinolones or Macrodantin
   e. STDs
      i. Gonorrhea: Rocephin intramuscularly (250 mg) plus azithromycin (1-g single dose) or doxycycline for 7 days
      ii. Nongonococcal urethritis: azithromycin (1-g single dose) or doxycycline for 7 days

Suggested Reading

Alper BS, Curry SH: Urinary tract infection in children. *Am Fam Phys* 72:2483–2488, 2005.

Bass PF: Urinary tract infections. *Primary Care* 30(1):41–61, 2003.

Bremnor JD: Evaluation of dysuria in adults. *Am Fam Phys* 65(8): 1589–1596, 2002.

Hermanides HS, Hulscher ME, Schouten JA, et al: Development of quality indicators for the antibiotic treatment of complicated urinary tract infections: A first step to measure and improve care. *Clin Infect Dis* 46(5):703–711, 2008.

Hooton TM: The current management strategies for community-acquired urinary tract infection. *Infect Dis Clin North Am* 17(2): 303–332, 2003.

CHAPTER

62 Fluid and Electrolyte Abnormalities

CLINICAL CASE PROBLEM 1

A 72-Year-Old Male with Chronic Obstructive Pulmonary Disease

A 72-year-old male with chronic obstructive pulmonary disease (COPD) is seen in the emergency room. During the past 2 days, he has experienced a worsening cough with yellow-brown sputum production and fever to 101°F. On examination, his respiratory rate (RR) is 26 breaths/minute using accessory muscles. His acid–base gas (ABG) values on room air are as follows: pH, 7.24; Pao_2, 54 mmHg; Sao_2, 88%; $Paco_2$, 60 mmHg; and HCO_3^-, 27 mEq/L.

SELECT THE BEST ANSWER TO THE FOLLOWING QUESTIONS

1. Which process is disturbing the acid–base balance?
   a. metabolic acidosis
   b. respiratory alkalosis
   c. metabolic alkalosis
   d. respiratory acidosis
   e. none of the above

CLINICAL PROBLEM CASE 2

A 22-Year-Old Female Who Is Dizzy and Has Tingling around Her Mouth and Fingertips

A 22-year-old female comes into the emergency room with dizziness and tingling around her mouth and fingertips. Her blood pressure (BP) is 140/70 mmHg, pulse (P) is 110 beats/minute, RR is 30 breaths/minute, and temperature is 98.6°F. Her ABG values on room air are as follows: pH, 7.52; Pao_2, 90 mmHg; Sao_2, 97%; $Paco_2$, 25 mmHg; and HCO_3^-, 18 mEq/L.

2. Which process is disturbing the acid–base balance?
   a. metabolic acidosis with respiratory compensation
   b. respiratory alkalosis with metabolic compensation
   c. metabolic alkalosis without respiratory compensation
   d. respiratory acidosis with metabolic compensation
   e. none of the above

CLINICAL PROBLEM CASE 3

A 28-Year-Old Pregnant Female with Persistent Vomiting

A 28-year-old female in the first trimester of pregnancy comes into the emergency room with several days of morning sickness with persistent vomiting. She is now lethargic. Her BP is 90/60 mmHg, P is 120 beats/minute, RR is 16 breaths/minute, and temperature is 99°F. Her ABG values on room air are as follows: pH, 7.5; Pao_2, 80 mmHg; Sao_2, 94%; $Paco_2$, 49 mmHg; and HCO_3^-, 38 mEq/L.

3. Which process is disturbing the acid–base balance?
   a. metabolic acidosis with respiratory compensation
   b. respiratory alkalosis without metabolic compensation
   c. metabolic alkalosis with respiratory compensation
   d. respiratory acidosis with metabolic compensation
   e. none of the above

CLINICAL CASE PROBLEM 4

A 60-Year-Old Male Resuscitated in the Cardiac Care Unit

A 60-year-old male, admitted to the cardiac care unit for chest pain, suddenly becomes unresponsive in cardiac arrest. He is resuscitated after a 20-minute code. His ABG values on 100% O_2 are as follows:

pH, 7.28; Pao$_2$, 211 mmHg; Sao$_2$, 100%; Paco$_2$, 28 mmHg; and HCO$_3^-$, 14 mEq/L. His blood test values are as follows: Na$^+$, 140 mEq/L; K$^+$, 5.6 mEq/L; Cl$^-$, 100 mEq/L; CO$_2$, 14 mEq/L; glucose, 130 mg/dL; creatinine, 1.2 mg/dL; and blood urea nitrogen, 25 mg/dL.

4. Which process is disturbing the acid–base balance?
a. metabolic acidosis with respiratory compensation
b. respiratory alkalosis with metabolic compensation
c. metabolic alkalosis with respiratory compensation
d. respiratory acidosis with metabolic compensation
e. none of the above

5. What is the calculated anion gap?
a. 8
b. 12
c. 16
d. 26
e. none of the above

Answers

1. d. Cellular function is dependent on adequate oxygenation and a normal acid–base ratio. Any deviation in acid–base balance or blood pH can be life threatening. Whereas the body's ability to correct for inadequate oxygenation is limited, its compensatory mechanisms and ability to maintain normal blood pH are not.

Normal values for an ABG are as follows: pH, 7.38 to 7.42 (average 7.4); Pao$_2$, 80 to 100 mmHg (average 90); Sao$_2$, >95%; Paco$_2$, 38 to 42 mmHg (average 40); and HCO$_3^-$, 22 to 26 mEq/L (average 24).

Clinical Case Problem 1 is an example of acute respiratory acidosis. The pH is below 7.38 and the Paco$_2$ is greater than 42 mmHg. Respiratory acidosis is the result of either decreased alveolar ventilation or increased carbon dioxide production. Decreased alveolar ventilation is seen in COPD, acute respiratory failure, neuromuscular disorders that result in peripheral muscle weakness (i.e., myasthenia gravis), and central nervous system (CNS) depression (i.e., narcotics and general anesthetics). Increased CO$_2$ production occurs in hypermetabolic states such as sepsis or fever.

Renal compensation requires several hours to develop and is maximal after 4 days. In an acute respiratory acidosis, HCO$_3^-$ increases 1 mEq/L per 10 mmHg increase in Paco$_2$. In chronic respiratory acidosis,

HCO$_3^-$ increases 4 mEq/L per 10 mmHg increase in Paco$_2$. In an acute respiratory acidosis, for every 10 mmHg increase in the Paco$_2$, the pH decreases by 0.08.

In Clinical Case Problem 1, the Paco$_2$ is increased by 20 mmHg and the pH is decreased by 0.16. HCO$_3^-$ has increased by 3 mEq/L. This is an acute respiratory acidosis.

2. b. This is a respiratory alkalosis with metabolic compensation. The pH is above 7.42 and Paco$_2$ is below 38 mmHg. HCO$_3^-$ is less than 22 mEq/L.

Respiratory alkalosis results from hyperventilation. Specific causes include a catastrophic CNS event such as a hemorrhage, drugs such as salicylates, pregnancy (especially during the third trimester), interstitial lung diseases, and anxiety.

In respiratory alkalosis, a decrease in HCO$_3^-$ compensates for the decrease in Paco$_2$. Acutely, HCO$_3^-$ decreases 2 mEq/L for every 10 mmHg decrease in Paco$_2$. In chronic cases, HCO$_3^-$ decreases 4 mEq/L for every 10 mmHg decrease in Paco$_2$. In acute respiratory alkalosis, for every 10-mmHg decrease in Paco$_2$, the pH increases by 0.08.

In Clinical Case Problem 2, Paco$_2$ has decreased by 15 mmHg and the pH has increased by 12. HCO$_3^-$ has compensated.

3. c. This is a metabolic alkalosis with respiratory compensation. The pH is above 7.42 and HCO$_3^-$ is less than 26 mEq/L.

Metabolic alkalosis is a common metabolic disturbance in hospitalized patients related to loss of H$^+$ seen in vomiting, nasogastric suction, and hypokalemia as a result of diuretics.

In metabolic alkalosis, Paco$_2$ increases 6 mmHg for every 10 mEq/L increase in HCO$_3^-$.

In Clinical Case Problem 3, HCO$_3^-$ is increased by 15 mEq/L. To compensate, Paco$_2$ has increased by 9 mmHg.

4. a. This is metabolic acidosis with respiratory compensation. The pH is below 7.38 and HCO$_3^-$ is less than 22 mEq/L.

Metabolic acidosis can be divided into anion gap acidosis and non-anion gap acidosis. The anion gap is Na$^+$ – (Cl$^-$ + HCO$_3^-$). A normal anion gap is 12. Anion gap acidosis results from accumulation of acidic metabolites. Examples of anion gap acidosis (anion gap > 14) are ketoacidosis, lactic acidosis, renal failure, and toxic doses of salicylates. Non-anion gap acidosis (anion gap < 10) results from loss of bicarbonate or external acid infusion. Examples of non-anion gap acidosis are diarrhea, renal tubular acidosis, and hyperalimentation.

In metabolic acidosis, $Paco_2$ decreases 1.2 mmHg for every 1 mEq/L decrease in HCO_3^-.

5. **d.** Anion gap is $Na^+ - (Cl^- + HCO_3^-)$. In this case, $140 - (100 + 14) = 26$. This is an elevated anion gap (>14), a result of lactic acidosis secondary to the cardiac arrest.

Summary

APPROACH TO ANALYSIS OF ARTERIAL BLOOD GASES

1. Is the pH elevated or decreased? Acidemic (pH < 7.38) or alkalemic (pH > 7.42)? Normal arterial pH is 7.40 ± 2.
2. Is the primary disturbance respiratory or metabolic? Does the problem affect primarily $Paco_2$ or HCO_3^-?
   a. $Paco_2$ (normal value, 40 mmHg; range, 38 to 42 mmHg)
   b. HCO_3^- (normal value, 24 mEq/L; range, 22 to 26 mEq/L)
3. If a respiratory disturbance, is it acute or chronic?
   a. In acute respiratory acidosis, bicarbonate increases 1 mEq/L per 10-mmHg increase in $Paco_2$.
   b. In chronic respiratory acidosis, bicarbonate increases 4 mEq/L per 10-mmHg increase in $Paco_2$.
   c. In acute respiratory alkalosis, bicarbonate decreases 2 mEq/L per 10-mmHg decrease in $Paco_2$.
   d. In chronic respiratory alkalosis, bicarbonate decreases 4 mEq/L per 10-mmHg decrease in $Paco_2$.
4. For a metabolic acidosis, determine whether an anion gap is present.
   a. Anion gap = $Na^+ - (Cl^- + HCO_3^-)$
   b. Normal anion gap = 12 ± 2
5. Assess the normal compensation by the respiratory system for a metabolic disturbance.
   a. In metabolic acidosis, $Paco_2$ decreases 1.2 mmHg per 1 mEq/L decrease in bicarbonate.
   b. In metabolic alkalosis, $Paco_2$ increases 6 mmHg per 10 mEq/L increase in bicarbonate.

SPECIFIC ACID–BASE DISORDERS AND DIAGNOSES

1. Respiratory acidosis results from either decreased alveolar ventilation or increased CO_2 production. Decreased alveolar ventilation can be caused by COPD, acute respiratory failure, neuromuscular disorders, and CNS depression.
2. Respiratory alkalosis results from hyperventilation as might be caused by a catastrophic CNS event; certain drugs, such as salicylates; pregnancy, especially in the third trimester; interstitial lung disease; anxiety; or liver cirrhosis.
3. Anion gap acidosis results from accumulation of acidic metabolites as may be induced by ketoacidosis, lactic acidosis, renal failure; or toxic doses of salicylates.
4. Non-anion gap acidosis results from loss of bicarbonate or external acid infusion as occurs in diarrhea, renal tubular acidosis, or hyperalimentation.
5. Metabolic alkalosis results from elevation of serum HCO_3^- and can be caused by vomiting, hypokalemia, nasogastric suction, excess glucocorticoids or mineralocorticoids, or Bartter's syndrome.

Suggested Reading

Hornick DB: An approach to the analysis of arterial blood gases and acid–base disorders. University of Iowa, Virtual Hospital, 2003.

Manz F: Hydration and disease. *J Am Coll Nutr* 26(5 Suppl):535S–541S, 2007.

Sirker AA, Rhodes A, Grounds RM, Bennett ED: Acid–base physiology: The "traditional" and the "modern" approaches. *Anaesthesia* 57(4):348–356, 2002.

Tommasino C, Picozzi V: Volume and electrolyte management. *Best Pract Res Clin Anaesthesiol* 21(4):497–516, 2007.

CLINICAL CASE PROBLEM 1

A 35-Year-Old Female with Fatigue

A 35-year-old female comes to your office with a 4-month history of fatigue. Her history is unremarkable; she has had no major medical illnesses. She has noticed that during the past 12 months her menstrual periods have become heavier and longer; instead of lasting for only 4 days with bleeding that was "light to moderate," she now has a 7- to 9-day period with "very heavy flow." She is the mother of three healthy children.

On examination, the patient appears pale. Her lower eyelids are pale and so is her skin. Her blood pressure is 100/70 mmHg. Her pulse is 86 beats/minute. Physical examination, including a pelvic examination, is otherwise normal. Her blood smear reads as follows: Red blood cells (RBCs) are microcytic and appear to be hypochromic. Her platelet count is 175,000/mm^3. Her hemoglobin is 9.5 g/dL.

SELECT THE BEST ANSWER TO THE FOLLOWING QUESTIONS

1. What is the most likely cause of this patient's anemia?
   a. iron-deficiency anemia
   b. hemolytic anemia
   c. folic acid-deficiency anemia
   d. pernicious anemia
   e. anemia of chronic disease

2. What treatment(s) is (are) therapeutic in this patient's condition?
   a. naproxen 375 mg twice a day (or a similar non-steroidal anti-inflammatory drug [NSAID]) during the last 2 weeks of the menstrual cycle
   b. a low-dose oral contraceptive pill (OCP) given either continuously or in a cyclic manner
   c. ferrous sulfate 300 mg once a day to 300 mg two times a day
   d. all of the above
   e. none of the above

3. The patient comes to the emergency room later during the week. Now her hemoglobin is 6 g/dL.

She is tachycardic and hypotensive. Of the treatments listed, which will be most beneficial?
   a. intramuscular (IM) medroxyprogesterone acetate
   b. intravenous (IV) conjugated estrogen
   c. cryoprecipitate
   d. fresh frozen plasma
   e. high-dose OCPs given every hour

4. The patient follows up in your office a week after hospitalization. Her hemoglobin is now 9.6 g/dL. She says she has black stools, constipation, and nausea with the Fem-Iron (ferrous fumarate) medication. Your next suggestion is
   a. prescribe Slow Fe (ferrous sulfate)
   b. prescribe an enteric-coated iron preparation
   c. prescribe weekly IM injections of iron
   d. advise her to continue her current medication with concomitant antacid use
   e. admit to the same day unit for IV iron administration

5. Which statement about the treatment of iron-deficiency anemia is false?
   a. treatment goals should be for 150 to 200 mg of elemental iron per day
   b. tea drinkers may show decreased iron absorption
   c. concurrent vitamin C administration may decrease iron absorption
   d. reticulocyte count should increase in 1 week
   e. iron therapy should continue for 6 months after hemoglobin level goal is reached

6. Which of the following investigations should be performed in this patient to rule out a secondary cause?
   a. pelvic ultrasound plus or minus pelvic laparoscopy
   b. coagulation profile
   c. computed tomography (CT) scan of the abdomen/pelvis
   d. a and b
   e. a, b, and c
   f. none of the above

7. What is the most sensitive test for the detection of the anemia described here?
   a. serum iron
   b. serum iron binding capacity
   c. serum ferritin
   d. serum transferrin
   e. reticulocyte count

8. Based on a complete blood count (CBC) and peripheral smear only, how can iron-deficiency anemia be differentiated from thalassemia?

a. thalassemia is normochromic, normocytic, and iron deficiency is microcytic, hypochromic
b. previous CBCs are normal in patients with thalassemia
c. thalassemia shows a high to normal red blood cell (RBC) count, whereas iron deficiency shows a low RBC count
d. b and c
e. a, b, and c

CLINICAL CASE PROBLEM 2

A Pregnant Woman with a Hemoglobin Level of 10.8 g/dL

A pregnant woman at 22 weeks of gestation comes to your office for her regular checkup. Her hemoglobin level is 10.8 g/dL.

9. Which of the following statements regarding anemia and pregnancy is false?
   a. iron supplementation is necessary in pregnancy to prevent microcytic anemia
   b. a "false" anemia is seen as a result of the relative expansion of the plasma volume relative to the RBC mass
   c. folic acid supplementation is necessary in pregnancy to prevent macrocytic anemia
   d. hemoglobinopathies are often first diagnosed when a woman comes for prenatal care
   e. iron deficiency is the most common anemia in pregnancy

CLINICAL CASE PROBLEM 3

A Fatigued 55-Year-Old Male

A 55-year-old male comes to your office for a periodic health assessment. His only complaint is that he has been feeling quite fatigued during the past 3 months. He does not smoke and rarely drinks.

On physical examination, the patient appears pale. His blood pressure is 100/80 mmHg. His pulse is 96 and regular. No other abnormalities are found. A CBC reveals a hemoglobin value of 10 g/dL. His blood smear also shows a decreased mean corpuscular hemoglobin count and a decreased mean corpuscular volume (MCV).

10. Until proved otherwise, what is the most likely cause of his low hemoglobin level?
    a. lymphoma
    b. gastrointestinal malignancy

c. lack of intrinsic factor
d. dietary deficiency of folic acid
e. dietary lack of iron

CLINICAL CASE PROBLEM 4

A 78-Year-Old Female Complaining of a "Lack of Energy"

A 78-year-old female with osteoarthritis comes to your office complaining of a "lack of energy" that began 8 months ago. On examination, the patient has marked pallor. Her hemoglobin level is 7.5 g/dL. A peripheral blood smear reveals hypochromasia and microcytosis. One year ago, her hemoglobin was 13 g/dL.

11. What is the most likely cause of this patient's anemia?
    a. malnutrition
    b. pernicious anemia
    c. folic acid deficiency
    d. gastrointestinal bleeding
    e. hypothyroidism

12. The anemia of chronic disease is most often which of the following?
    a. hypochromic and normocytic
    b. hypochromic and microcytic
    c. normochromic and macrocytic
    d. normochromic and normocytic
    e. hyperchromic and macrocytic

13. What is the most common cause of anemia of chronic disease?
    a. chronic hepatic failure
    b. chronic renal failure
    c. congestive cardiac failure
    d. autoimmune disease
    e. chronic neurologic disease

14. What are acceptable treatments for anemia of chronic disease?
    a. iron therapy
    b. erythropoietin
    c. treatment of the underlying condition
    d. b and c
    e. a, b, and c

15. Which of the following disorders is (are) associated with the anemia of chronic disease?
    a. rheumatoid arthritis
    b. non-Hodgkin's lymphoma
    c. chronic renal failure

d. chronic hepatic failure

e. all of the above

16. Which of the following is the most common type of anemia in the U.S. population?

a. anemia of chronic disease

b. iron-deficiency anemia

c. macrocytic anemia

d. autoimmune hemolytic anemia

e. iatrogenic anemia

CLINICAL CASE PROBLEM 5

A 75-Year-Old Female with Fatigue, Paresthesias, Weakness, and an Unsteady Gait

A 75-year-old female comes to your office with an 8-month history of increasing fatigue, paresthesias, weakness, and an unsteady gait. These are new symptoms. Her past medical history is significant for hemicolectomy for colon cancer of the terminal ileum 3 years ago.

On examination, her skin is pale, as are her lower conjunctival lids. She has a number of interesting neurologic findings on physical examination, including patchy impairment of the sensations of touch and temperature, loss of vibration and position sense, a positive Romberg sign, hyperreflexia, and bilateral up-going Babinski signs. Her hemoglobin is 6.8 g/dL.

17. Which of the following statements regarding this patient's condition is (are) true?

a. this patient has a hemolytic anemia

b. a CT scan of the brain should be performed

c. hyposegmented neutrophils will be seen on the blood smear

d. the MCV value will be above $100\,mm^3$

e. all of the above

18. If you could choose only one investigation to do next, what would it be?

a. reticulocyte count

b. serum folate

c. serum vitamin B_{12} level

d. gastroscopy

e. bone marrow biopsy

19. What is the probable etiology of this patient's condition?

a. decreased dietary intake of vitamin B_{12}

b. alcoholism

c. surgical resection of the terminal ileum

d. brain tumor

e. chemotherapy with methotrexate

20. During the first 2 weeks of therapy for the condition described here, which of the following is the most reasonable treatment regimen?

a. folic acid 5 mg/day orally

b. vitamin B_{12} 100 mg/day orally

c. vitamin B_{12} 1000 mg/day intramuscularly

d. ferrous sulfate 300 mg/day; folic acid 5 mg/day; vitamin B_{12} 100 mg/day (all orally)

e. none of the above

21. What is (are) the acceptable option(s) for the long-term treatment of this condition?

a. long-term treatment is not necessary

b. oral B_{12} at 100 μg daily

c. nasal B_{12} gel weekly

d. oral folate

e. b and c

22. Which of the following statements regarding folic acid deficiency is false?

a. folic acid deficiency demonstrates a macrocytic anemia

b. hypersegmented neutrophils are often seen on the peripheral blood smear

c. the most common cause of folic acid deficiency is an inadequate dietary intake of folic acid

d. folic acid deficiency is uncommon in patients who demonstrate alcohol abuse

e. reduced folate levels are usually seen in RBCs and in the serum

---

CLINICAL CASE PROBLEM 6

A 38-Year-Old Male with a Hemoglobin Value of 10 g/dL

A 38-year-old male with a history of a gastric bypass for morbid obesity comes to your office with a hemoglobin of 10 g/dL. His MCV is 88 mm³. His ferritin is 35 μg/L, and his red cell distribution width is high. His reticulocyte count is high.

23. Which of the following statements about his clinical presentation is (are) true?

a. his anemia is the result of iron deficiency

b. his anemia is the result of vitamin B_{12} deficiency

c. his anemia is the result of chronic disease

d. a and b

e. a and c

CLINICAL CASE PROBLEM 7

An 18-Year-Old Female with Severe Fatigue and Lightheadedness

An 18-year-old female you saw for a urinary tract infection last week comes to your office with severe fatigue and lightheadedness. She states that her last menstrual period was 3 weeks ago and that her flow was light, as usual. Her hemoglobin is 8.7 g/dL, and her MCV is 84 mm³. Last year, her CBC was normal.

24. Which of the following statements describes her condition?
    a. this is iron-deficiency anemia
    b. this is folic acid deficiency anemia probably resulting from anorexia
    c. this is hemolytic anemia secondary to Macrodantin
    d. this patient has sickle cell anemia
    e. none of the above

Clinical Case Management Problem

Distinguish between megaloblastosis and macrocytosis.

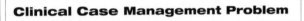

Answers

1. **a.** Iron-deficiency anemia is the most common cause of anemia. In this patient, the most likely cause of the anemia is excessive blood loss during her menstrual periods.

Pernicious anemia, folic acid deficiency anemia, hemolytic anemia, and anemia of chronic disease are not associated with the hypochromic, microcytic changes that characterize iron-deficiency anemia.

2. **d.** The OCP will accomplish the result of reducing menstrual blood flow and is the drug of choice. An NSAID drug such as naproxen may have a profound effect on decreasing the menstrual blood flow. For this patient, the appropriate symptomatic treatment to build up her iron stores is ferrous sulfate or ferrous gluconate. The initial dose of ferrous sulfate should be 300 mg twice a day. It may be necessary to use ferrous sulfate for only 1 or 2 months; at that time, the patient can stop taking iron and continue taking the OCP.

3. **b.** The patient has severe menorrhagia with hemodynamic compromise or impending hemodynamic

compromise. The treatment of choice is IV conjugated estrogen, 25 mg repeated every 4 hours until the menorrhagia subsides.

4. **a.** See answer 5.

5. **c.** Iron therapy can be associated with many gastrointestinal side effects. To minimize side effects, iron supplements should be taken with food; this may decrease iron absorption somewhat. Changing to a different iron salt or to a controlled-release preparation may also reduce side effects. Enteric-coated preparations are ineffective because they do not dissolve in the stomach. Unpredictable absorption and local complications of IM administration make the IV route preferable when it is necessary to treat with parenteral iron. Antacids and caffeinated beverages, especially tea, will reduce iron absorption. Vitamin C therapy will facilitate iron absorption.

Treatment goals for iron administration should aim for 150 to 200 mg of elemental iron per day. Iron therapy should continue for 4 to 6 months when the serum ferritin level reaches 50, indicating adequate iron replacement. Reticulocyte count does increase within 1 week of starting iron therapy.

6. **d.** Pelvic ultrasound, laparoscopy, and a coagulation profile should uncover the potential presence of uterine fibroids, endometriosis, or von Willebrand's disease, respectively. A CT scan of the abdomen/pelvis is not indicated.

7. **c.** The most sensitive test for the diagnosis of iron-deficiency anemia is the serum ferritin level. In iron-deficiency anemia, the serum ferritin level usually decreases first. Thereafter, total iron binding capacity increases and serum iron levels gradually decrease. The transferrin saturation will also decrease at this time. The reticulocyte count is not useful in assessing the degree of iron-deficiency anemia.

8. **c.** Both thalassemia and iron-deficiency anemia are hypochromic, microcytic. Thalassemia tends to be more hypochromic and microcytic than iron deficiency. A quick way to differentiate the two anemias is to examine the RBC count. In iron deficiency, the number will be low. In thalassemia, the number will be normal to high.

9. **c.** Folic acid supplementation is necessary in pregnancy to prevent neural tube defects, not macrocytic anemia. Iron supplementation is necessary in pregnancy to prevent microcytic anemia. A "false" anemia is seen because of the relative expansion of the plasma

volume relative to the RBC mass. Hemoglobinopathies are often first diagnosed when a woman comes to your office for prenatal care. Iron deficiency is the most common anemia in pregnancy.

10. b. Until proved otherwise, iron-deficiency anemia in a middle-aged or elderly male is the result of gastrointestinal blood loss, the most sinister cause of which is a gastrointestinal malignancy. Carcinomas of the colon or rectum are the most important and most common malignancies found in this situation. This patient should have fecal occult blood testing followed by colonoscopy. Air-contrast barium enema may or may not be indicated for further elucidation. If all of the investigations are normal, the upper gastrointestinal tract should be investigated by endoscopy.

Dietary iron deficiency or dietary folic acid deficiency is extremely unusual in a male without alcoholism.

A lymphoma is more likely to produce a normochromic, normocytic blood smear rather than a hypochromic, microcytic picture.

Bleeding hemorrhoids may also produce iron-deficiency anemia in middle-aged males.

Vitamin B_{12} deficiency resulting from lack of intrinsic factor would present as a macrocytic rather than a microcytic anemia.

11. d. This patient's hypochromic, microcytic blood picture, coupled with a decrease in hemoglobin from 13 to 7.5 g/dL in 1 year, is almost certainly the result of blood loss from a gastrointestinal malignancy or other bleeding source. A good bet is that she has a gastrointestinal bleed secondary to NSAID use, but colon cancer needs to also be seriously considered. The discussion in answer 10 regarding the iron-deficiency anemia in males also applies to females past menopause. The other common cause of iron-deficiency anemia in elderly patients is malnutrition.

In contradistinction to hypochromic, microcytic anemia, the most common causes of megaloblastic anemia are B_{12} and folic acid deficiencies.

12. d. The anemia of chronic disease is most often normochromic and normocytic. It can present as a mild hypochromic, microcytic anemia.

13. b. See answer 15.

14. d. See answer 15.

15. e. The anemia of chronic disease is associated most frequently with the following: (1) anemia of chronic inflammation that may be associated with infection, autoimmune connective tissue disorders, or malignancy (excluding malignancies in which blood loss is a major factor, as in colon cancer); (2) anemia as a result of chronic renal failure (this is the most common cause of anemia of chronic disease); (3) anemia as a result of endocrine failure; or (4) anemia of hepatic disease.

Treatment of anemia of chronic disease is aimed at treating the underlying condition. In some cases, particularly when chronic renal disease or cancer is the causative source, erythropoietin injections are helpful in treating the anemia.

16. b. In the United States, the most common category of anemia is iron-deficiency anemia. In order of frequency, anemia prevalence is as follows:

1. Iron-deficiency anemia as a result of blood loss from (a) excessive menstrual flow and (b) the gastrointestinal tract.
2. Anemia of chronic disease: The most common causes are (a) chronic renal failure and (b) anemia resulting from connective tissue disorders.
3. Macrocytic anemia generally is caused by (a) pernicious anemia or (b) folic acid deficiency anemia.
4. Hemolytic anemia caused by either (a) autoimmune hemolytic anemias or (b) nonautoimmune hemolytic anemias.

17. d. The signs and symptoms of pernicious anemia can be remembered well by the five Ps, namely (1) pancytopenia, (2) peripheral neuropathy, (3) posterior spinal column neuropathy, (4) pyramidal tract signs, and (5) papillary (tongue) atrophy.

The blood smear of a patient with pernicious anemia will show the following: megaloblastic anemia as demonstrated by MCV greater than 100 mm³, hypersegmented (not hyposegmented) neutrophils, and oval macrocytes.

18. c. The most significant single determination would be serum vitamin B_{12} level.

19. c. Pernicious anemia is defined as a deficiency of vitamin B_{12} resulting from lack of production of intrinsic factor by the gastric parietal cells or decreased absorption in the terminal ileum. Much less commonly, vitamin B_{12} deficiency results from inadequate intake, such as a true vegan diet. Methotrexate is a folate inhibitor and is associated with macrocytic anemia as a result of folate deficiency. Alcoholism is associated with B_{12} and folate deficiency, but the surgical resection of the terminal ileum is the most likely cause of this patient's anemia.

20. c. The acute treatment of pernicious anemia that is recommended is 1000 mg/day for 1 week followed by 1000 mg/week for 4 weeks and then followed by maintenance therapy of 1000 mg/month. Because the root cause of the disease lies in an inability to absorb the vitamin, it cannot be administered orally.

21. c. The recommended treatments for maintenance therapy of vitamin B_{12} deficiency classically have been monthly injections of 1000 µg of vitamin B_{12}. Recently, a nasal gel formulation to be used once weekly has demonstrated success. Some studies have shown successful treatment with daily large doses of oral vitamin B_{12} of 1000 to 2000 µg, but because poor absorption is the underlying problem, a dose of 100 µg daily will be insufficient.

Because the underlying cause is a B_{12} deficiency, administration of folate is not the proper treatment. Nonetheless, folate will resolve the macrocytic anemia because the anemia itself is caused by an inhibition of nucleic acid synthesis resulting from an inability to regenerate active tetrahydrofolate, one of the two functions normally provided by vitamin B_{12}. However, administration of folate will not prevent the neurologic damage, which is a direct effect of a deficiency of vitamin B_{12}, because of its second normal function as a cofactor in the methylmalonyl CoA mutase reaction. This reaction is a necessary step in the catabolism of fatty acids with an odd number of carbons and branched-chained fatty acids formed during branched-chain amino acid catabolism. (Apparently, when these unusual fatty acids are not effectively catabolized, they are incorporated into myelin sheets and cause neuropathies.) As a consequence, administration of folate in cases of megaloblastic anemia will alleviate the hematologic symptoms but will permit the neurologic symptoms to progress. Thus, megaloblastic anemia should never be treated with folate alone; it should be treated with a combination of folate and vitamin B_{12}.

22. d. The most common cause of folic acid deficiency is inadequate intake. Folic acid deficiency is most commonly seen in patients with alcoholism, patients with a malignancy, elderly patients, patients on a vegan diet, and pregnant patients.

Folic acid deficiency anemia such as vitamin B_{12} deficiency also induces a megaloblastic anemia (see answer 21). Patients with pure folic acid deficiency usually have normal vitamin B_{12} levels. Patients with folic acid deficiency anemia should be given 1 to 5 mg of folic acid/day.

23. d. This patient has a mixed-picture anemia primarily because of his gastric bypass, which is preventing him from effectively absorbing iron and vitamin B_{12}. Anemia of chronic disease would not be associated with a high reticulocyte count.

24. c. This patient has hemolytic anemia resulting from the use of Macrodantin. It is unlikely to be iron deficiency without the history of heavy menses. Her MCV is not elevated, which makes a folic acid deficiency anemia unlikely. Her CBC would have been abnormal last year if she had sickle cell anemia, which is a normochromic, normocytic anemia.

Solution to the Clinical Case Management Problem

The difference between macrocytosis and megaloblastosis is that in megaloblastosis the macrocytes are oval, whereas in macrocytosis the macrocytes are round.

Megaloblastic anemias are only one cause of macrocytosis. The differential diagnosis of macrocytosis includes the following: (1) megaloblastic anemias, (2) liver disease, (3) reticulocytosis, (4) myeloproliferative diseases (leukemia and myelofibrosis), (5) multiple myeloma, (6) metastatic disease of bone marrow, (7) hypothyroidism, (8) aplastic anemia, (9) drugs (cytotoxic agents and alcohol), and (10) autoagglutination or cold agglutination disease.

Summary

1. Normal adult hemoglobin levels are 14 to 18 g/dL for males and 12 to 16 g/dL for females.
2. Classification of anemias on the basis of cause (production, destruction, loss)
   a. Production problems include the following: (i) hemoglobin synthesis disturbances as may be caused by iron deficiency, thalassemia, chronic disease; (ii) DNA synthesis disturbances that lead to megaloblastic anemia; (iii) bone marrow infiltration in malignancies; and (iv) stem cell disease as in aplastic anemia and myeloproliferative disease.

b. Destruction problems include the following: (i) intrinsic hemolysis as in spherocytosis, sickle cell, enzyme deficiencies; and (ii) extrinsic hemolysis as in infection, immune complexes, thrombocytopenic purpura, hemolytic/uremic syndrome, or mechanical valves.

c. Blood loss problems include the following: (i) excessive menstruation, (ii) bleeding in the gastrointestinal or genitourinary tracts, and (iii) trauma.

3. Classification of anemias on the basis of cell size and appearance (microcytic, macrocytic, normocytic, hypochromic, and normochromic)

a. Microcytic anemias may be the result of the following: (i) iron deficiency, potentially caused by blood loss or nutritional deficiencies; (ii) thalassemias; and (iii) chronic disease.

b. Macrocytic anemias are either megaloblastic caused by folate or B_{12} deficiencies or nonmegaloblastic such as from chemotherapy.

4. Iron-deficiency anemia

a. This is the most common cause of anemia.

b. The most common cause in premenopausal women is excessive menstrual flow.

c. Iron-deficiency anemia in males or in post-menopausal females should be considered to be from gastrointestinal blood loss until proved otherwise; the most common secondary cause is gastrointestinal malignancy.

d. Iron-deficiency anemia is hypochromic, microcytic: Microcytosis occurs first, and hypochromasia is seen in advanced cases.

e. Serum ferritin level is usually less than 12 mg/L and is the most sensitive test for iron deficiency.

f. Most pregnant women with decreased hemoglobin are not truly anemic; they simply have a greater increase in plasma volume than in RBC mass. True anemia in pregnancy has been defined by the Centers for Disease Control and Prevention as hemoglobin in the first and third trimesters less than 11 g/dL or by hemoglobin in the second trimester less than 10.5 g/dL.

g. Investigations in women with excessive menstrual flow include pelvic ultrasound/laparoscopy (uterine fibroids and endometriosis) and coagulation disorders (e.g., von Willebrand's disease).

h. Treatment for iron-deficiency anemia: (i) Find the cause and correct if possible; (ii) administer ferrous sulfate 300 mg twice a day; for menorrhagia: prophylaxis via OCP; and severe menorrhagia with unstable vital signs use IV conjugated estrogen.

5. Anemia of chronic disease

a. Anemia of chronic disease is normochromic, normocytic.

b. Causes of anemia of chronic disease are as follows: (i) chronic renal failure (most common), (ii) connective tissue disorders (autoimmune diseases), (iii) malignancies (except gastrointestinal blood loss) such as multiple myeloma or lymphomas, (iv) inflammatory diseases, and (v) chronic hepatic disease.

c. Make the diagnosis (find the cause) and treat the cause.

6. Megaloblastic anemia as the result of a vitamin B_{12} deficiency

a. Pernicious anemia is the most common cause. It is from vitamin B_{12} deficiency caused by lack of intrinsic factor. Other causes of vitamin B_{12} deficiency are total or subtotal gastrectomy and a vegan diet.

b. Blood smear: (i) MCV greater than 100 mm³, (ii) hypersegmented neutrophils, and (iii) oval macrocytes.

c. Confirming tests are determination of the serum vitamin B_{12} level and a Schilling test.

d. The five defining Ps are as follows: (i) pancytopenia, (ii) peripheral neuropathy, (iii) posterior spinal column neuropathy, (iv) papillary (tongue) atrophy, and (v) pyramidal tract signs.

e. Treatment: (i) vitamin B_{12} subcutaneously (SC) 1000 mg/day, (ii) vitamin B_{12} SC 1000 mg/week, and (iii) vitamin B_{12} SC 1000 mg/month.

f. Remember that a vitamin B_{12} deficiency may also induce a neuropathy.

7. Megaloblastic anemia resulting from folic acid deficiency

a. Diagnosis: blood smear with hypersegmented neutrophils and macroovalocytes.

b. Confirmation: decreased serum folate or RBC folate.

c. Most common cause of folic acid deficiency is a dietary deficiency associated with alcoholism, vegan diet, and elderly patients on a "tea and toast" diet; it also results from medications such as methotrexate and OCPs, pregnancy, and malignancy.

d. Folic acid supplementation is recommended for all pregnant women (1 mg).

8. Hemolytic anemias

a. Classification: (i) autoimmune hemolytic anemias and (ii) nonautoimmune hemolytic anemias.

b. Common causes are as follows: (i) drugs (iatrogenic disease), the most common cause of hemolytic anemia; (ii) lymphoproliferative disorders (chronic lymphocytic leukemia and non-Hodgkin's lymphoma); (iii) autoimmune connective tissue disorders (systemic lupus erythematosus and rheumatoid arthritis); (iv) infections (Epstein–Barr virus, cytomegalovirus, mycoplasma pneumoniae, and human immunodeficiency virus); (v) glucose 6-phosphate dehydrogenase deficiency; and (vi) paroxysmal cold hemoglobinuria.

c. Diagnosis: (i) Coombs test (direct and indirect) and (ii) reticulocyte count (elevated).

d. Treatment: (i) corticosteroids, (ii) splenectomy (in those who do not respond), and (iii) IV immunoglobulin.

9. Miscellaneous disorders include the following: (a) aplastic anemias, (b) thalassemia, (c) sickle cell disease, (d) hemophilia, (e) platelet-associated bleeding disorders, and (f) disseminated intravascular coagulation.

Suggested Reading

Armas-Loughran B, Kalra R, Carson JL: Evaluation and management of anemia and bleeding disorders in surgical patients. *Med Clin North Am* 87:229–242, 2003.

Balducci L: Epidemiology of anemia in the elderly: Information on diagnostic evaluation. *J Am Geriatr Soc* 51(3 Suppl):S2–S9, 2003.

Brill J, Baumgardner D: Normocytic anemia. *Am Fam Phys* 62: 2255–2264, 2000.

Hermiston ML, Mentzer WC: A practical approach to the evaluation of the anemic child. *Pediatr Clin North Am* 49:877–891, 2002.

Means RT, Jr: Recent developments in the anemia of chronic disease. *Curr Hematol Rep* 2:116–121, 2003.

Tefferi A: Anemia in adults: A contemporary approach to diagnosis. *Mayo Clinic Proc* 78:1274–1280, 2003.

Weiss G, Goodnough LT: Anemia of chronic disease. *N Engl J Med* 352:1011–1023, 2005.

CHAPTER 64 Certain Hematologic Conditions

CLINICAL CASE PROBLEM 1

A 16-Year-Old Male with a Supraclavicular Mass

A 16-year-old male is brought to your office by his mother. He has noticed a significant swelling in the left supraclavicular area that has been present for approximately 4 months. According to the patient, it has not changed significantly in size during that time. He has had no fever, chills, nausea, vomiting, fatigue/malaise, weight loss, or other symptoms.

On examination, vital signs are normal. A mass measuring 2.5 × 1.5 cm is felt to be attached to the muscle above the left scapula. His chest is otherwise normal to auscultation and percussion. The abdomen is soft. There is no hepatomegaly or splenomegaly. The skin is benign. No significant lymph node enlargement is present in the cervical, axillary, or inguinal regions.

SELECT THE BEST ANSWER TO THE FOLLOWING QUESTIONS

1. What is the most appropriate definitive diagnostic step for this patient?
   a. a complete blood workup
   b. a fine needle biopsy
   c. an excisional biopsy
   d. a chest radiograph
   e. none of the above

2. The evaluation produces a report that reads as follows: "Reed–Sternberg cells present." What is the most likely diagnosis?
   a. reactive lymph-node enlargement
   b. acquired immune deficiency syndrome (AIDS)
   c. metastatic carcinoma
   d. Hodgkin's disease
   e. non-Hodgkin's lymphoma

3. What is the next step in the investigation of this patient?
   a. computed tomography (CT) scan of the abdomen
   b. radiation therapy
   c. combination chemotherapy
   d. bone scan
   e. a and d

4. In the staging of the disease from which this patient suffers, there are two distinct categories, A and B. To what do these two categories refer?
   a. the presence or absence of metastases
   b. the presence or absence of symptoms
   c. the presence or absence of bone marrow involvement
   d. the possibility or nonpossibility of cure
   e. the presence or absence of intraabdominal disease

5. The patient's disease is staged, and he is found to have disease throughout the mediastinum but not below the diaphragm. At this time, what kind of therapy is likely to be administered?
   a. no therapy is indicated at this time; await the development of symptoms
   b. combination chemotherapy
   c. radiation therapy
   d. combination chemotherapy plus radiotherapy
   e. radical surgery

6. The patient's mother asks you about his prognosis. Which of the following is not true regarding this patient's illness?
   a. most patients with this disease have an overall survival of between 80% and 90%
   b. he may be at risk for premature cardiovascular disease as a result of treatment
   c. he may be at increased risk for infertility
   d. he may be at increased risk for secondary malignancies
   e. once treated, he will have little risk of recurrence

CLINICAL CASE PROBLEM 2

A 62-Year-Old Male with Swellings in His Neck and Elbows and Chest Pains

A 62-year-old male comes to your office to reassure himself about "some swellings in my neck, elbows, as well as some chest pain." The other symptom is profound fatigue (for the past 3 months). On examination, his vital signs are normal, but he looks pale and has lost 10 pounds since a visit 1 year ago. He has multiple enlarged cervical lymph nodes (and bilateral epitrochlear nodes); they measure anywhere from 1 to 2 cm in diameter. His liver edge is palpated approximately 3 cm below the left costal edge, and the tip of the spleen can be felt when he lies on his side.

7. If you could select only one test to perform on this patient, which of the following would you select?
   a. enzyme-linked immunosorbent assay human immunodeficiency virus (HIV) screening test
   b. immunoglobulin G-viral capsid antigen (IgG-VCA) antibody titer for cytomegalovirus
   c. IgG-VCA antibody titer for toxoplasmosis
   d. CT scan of the chest
   e. excisional lymph node biopsy

8. The test you ordered is performed. The result shows diffuse small cleaved cell (diffuse poorly differentiated lymphocytic) histology. Based on what you currently know, what is the most likely diagnosis?
   a. non-Hodgkin's lymphoma
   b. Hodgkin's disease
   c. systemic toxoplasmosis: systemic immune deficiency
   d. systemic cytomegalovirus: systemic immune deficiency
   e. AIDS

9. The patient turns out to have an advanced stage (III) of a follicular form of non-Hodgkin's lymphoma. The treatment of choice may include which of the following?
   a. zidovudine (AZT)
   b. intensive chemotherapy and bone marrow transplantation
   c. interferon-α and monoclonal antibodies
   d. intensive chemotherapy and radiotherapy
   e. c and d

10. Which of the following statements is true regarding the illness seen in this patient?
    a. it is more common in younger individuals
    b. patients usually live a normal life span without treatment
    c. there appears to be a relationship with the Epstein–Barr virus in some forms of the disease
    d. it is less common than the Hodgkin's form of lymphoma
    e. there is no relationship between the disease's incidence and HIV disease

---

CLINICAL CASE PROBLEM 3

A 62-Year-Old Male with "Bone Pain" in His "Breast Bone" and Skull

A 62-year-old male comes to your office with a chief complaint of "bone pain" in "my breast bone and my head, Doc." He tells you that he is sure he is OK but is here only because "the wife kept bugging me until I gave in." The patient also appears somewhat pale and tells you that he has been feeling tired lately and a bit "weak, depressed, and maybe confused."

He had a "touch of the flu" a few months ago. His wife tells you that this "touch of the flu" was actually bacterial pneumonia (organism *Streptococcus pneumoniae*). On examination, the patient has a tender sternum, tender occipital area of the skull, and pale conjunctiva.

You perform a series of laboratory tests. The results are as follows: hemoglobin, 8.5 g/dL;

normochromic/normocytic anemia; erythrocyte sedimentation rate (ESR), 55 mm/hour; platelets, 15,000/mm^3; serum calcium, 14 mg/dL; Na$^+$, 151 mEq/L; and serum creatinine, 5.3 mmol/L.

11. Based on the information you now have for Clinical Case Problem 3, what is the most likely diagnosis?
    a. metastatic carcinoma: metastasized to bone
    b. chronic lymphocytic leukemia
    c. multiple myeloma
    d. chronic renal failure: secondary to macroglobulinemia
    e. chronic myelogenous leukemia

12. Further investigations substantiate your findings. What is the treatment of choice at this time?
    a. bone marrow transplantation
    b. total body radiotherapy
    c. adjuvant combination chemotherapy: adriamycin, vincristine, bleomycin
    d. melphalan plus prednisone
    e. none of the above

13. The patient's disease is the result of a proliferation of which of the following?
    a. myeloblasts
    b. lymphoblasts
    c. metastatic cancer cells
    d. plasma cells
    e. none of the above

MATCHING QUESTIONS

In part A, certain hematologic disorders are listed a through z. Match each numbered question (questions 14 to 23) describing a hematologic disorder in part B with an (the) appropriate disease(s) as listed in part A. Each disease may be used once, twice, three times, or not at all.

Part A: Diseases

a. Aplastic anemia
b. Secondary polycythemia
c. Hemolytic anemia
d. Drug-induced thrombocytopenia
e. Idiopathic thrombocytopenia purpura
f. Sickle cell disease
g. Sickle cell trait
h. Preleukemia
i. Acute lymphocytic leukemia
j. Disseminated intravascular coagulation
k. Hemophilia
l. Multiple myeloma
m. Chronic lymphocytic leukemia
n. Hemochromatosis
o. Acute myelogenous leukemia
p. Chronic myelogenous leukemia
q. Cutaneous T cell leukemia
r. Neutrophilia
s. von Willebrand's disease
t. Thalassemia
u. Hairy cell leukemia
v. Acute intermittent porphyria
w. Polycythemia rubra vera
x. Secondary thrombocytopenia
y. Transfusion reaction
z. Myelofibrosis

Part B: Description

14. Choice _____
    • Disease is associated with excessive proliferation of erythroid, granulocytic, and megakaryocytic precursors.
    • Splenomegaly is almost universal in this disease.
    • Disease has significantly elevated red blood cell mass.
    • Patient presents with plethora.
    • Disease characteristically has thrombocytosis.

15. Choice _____
    • Disease produces a major disorder of the bone marrow.
    • Splenomegaly is present in all patients.
    • As the disease progresses, patients experience weight loss; skin and mucous membrane bleeding; and bone pain, jaundice, and lymphadenopathy.
    • Bone marrow tap is almost always unsuccessful: It is known as a "dry tap."
    • Bone marrow biopsy reveals fibrosis of marrow spaces and osteosclerosis.

16. Choice _____
    • This disease has the presence of the Philadelphia chromosome.
    • When this disease is diagnosed, the total white blood cell count often exceeds 200,000 cells/mm^3.
    • This disease usually follows the following course: (a) chronic phase of variable duration, (b) blastic transformation, with (c) some patients experiencing a distinct intermediate accelerated phase.
    • The most consistent physical finding is splenomegaly.

- This is the most common serious hematologic disorder diagnosed in patients who survived the atomic bombs of Hiroshima and Nagasaki.

17. Choice _____
    - This form of leukemia is the most common form of leukemia in the United States.
    - The disease is usually seen in patients older than age 50 years.
    - The abnormal cells morphologically resemble mature, small lymphocytes of the peripheral blood and accumulate in the bone marrow, blood, lymph nodes, and spleen in large numbers.
    - This disease has an "indolent nature."
    - Median survival exceeds 10 years, and many patients require no treatment.

18. Choice _____
    - This disease has characteristic cells that exhibit cytoplasmic projections on their surfaces.
    - This disease is the result of an expansion of neoplastic type B lymphocytes.
    - This disease usually presents in male patients older than age 40 years.
    - Approximately 30% of patients with this disease have a vasculitis-like disorder.
    - The treatment of choice for this disease is very characteristic of the disease: cladribine.

19. Choice _____
    - This disease is a disease of children and young adults.
    - This disease is characterized by the clonal proliferation of immature hematopoietic cells.
    - The most common abnormal cells seen on bone marrow biopsy are immature lymphoblasts.
    - Infection is a nearly universal complication.
    - Approximately 50% of patients are either cured or characterized as being in long-term remission.

20. Choice _____
    - The incidence of this disease increases with increasing age.
    - The most common abnormal cells seen on bone marrow biopsy are immature myeloblasts or immature promyelocytes.
    - Some patients with this disease develop the disease after either a preleukemia syndrome or a myelodysplastic syndrome.
    - Between 10% and 30% of patients with this disease survive 5 years; most of these patients are likely to survive long term.
    - Bone marrow transplantation from either an identical twin or a human leukocyte antigen-identical sibling is a very important part of treatment.

21. Choice _____
    - This disease usually follows recovery from either a viral exanthem or a viral upper respiratory tract illness.
    - The acute form of this disease is caused by immune complexes containing viral antigens that bind to platelet receptors.
    - This disease produces a profound rapid decrease in the cell line in question.
    - Corticosteroids are the agents of choice in the treatment of this disease.
    - In severe cases of this disease, splenectomy may need to be performed.

22. Choice _____
    - This is the most common inherited bleeding disorder.
    - The factor that is missing in this disease is responsible for platelet adhesion.
    - The factor that is missing in this disease also serves as a plasma carrier for factor VIII.
    - Women with this disorder initially may be diagnosed because of severe menorrhagia.
    - The treatment of choice for this disease is cryoprecipitate.

23. Choice _____
    - This disease is associated most frequently with obstetric catastrophes.
    - Other major causes of this disease are major trauma, metastatic malignancies, and bacterial sepsis.
    - In this disease, the combination of potent thrombogenic stimuli causes the deposition of small thrombi and small emboli throughout the microvasculature.
    - Most patients with this disease have extensive skin and mucous membrane bleeding and hemorrhage from multiple sites.
    - Patients with bleeding as a major symptom should receive fresh frozen plasma as therapy for the disorder.

Answers

1. **C.** This patient should have an excisional biopsy of the mass performed as soon as possible. Although a piece of tissue could be removed (a fine needle biopsy), an excisional biopsy makes more sense because the diagnosis of a malignant disease often requires histologic identification of cell types, usually detected by lymph node biopsy. Fine needle aspirate is often inadequate to detect certain of these types of cells. Excisional node biopsy is therefore preferable to approaches that do not yield accurate and timely diagnosis. Although a chest radiograph and complete blood count (CBC) would not necessarily be incorrect to perform, even with a normal chest examination and CBC, the possibility of a malignancy must be ruled out by biopsy.

2. **d.** The anatomic pathology report of Reed–Sternberg cells present (these are large binucleate cells with a single distinct nucleoli) is pathognomonic of Hodgkin's disease. One or two unexplained, enlarged lymph nodes in a young person indicates Hodgkin's disease until proved otherwise. Hodgkin's disease most commonly presents with painless lymphadenopathy. The so-called classic symptoms of fever, weight loss, and night sweats are present in only a small number of patients and usually in those with more aggressive disease. Excisional biopsy should always be undertaken as the diagnostic procedure of choice. Fine needle aspirate is often inadequate to detect Reed–Sternberg cells, and 20% of interventional radiologic procedures performed to diagnose Hodgkin's disease give false-negative results. Hodgkin's disease is one of the most important success stories of medical oncology. It was once uniformly fatal, but now the vast majority of patients are cured.

3. **e.** After an anatomic diagnosis is made, the disease must be staged. Clinical staging of Hodgkin's disease includes physical examination of all lymph node regions; chest x-ray; CT scan of the chest, abdomen, and pelvis; nuclear imaging with gallium scans or positron emission tomography; bone scans; and bone marrow biopsy. Pathologic staging by open laparotomy is also done. The Ann Arbor Staging Classification of Hodgkin's disease is as follows: stage I, single lymph node or single extralymphatic organ; stage II, two or more lymph nodes on the same side of the diaphragm; stage III, lymph nodes involved on both sides of the diaphragm or localized involvement of spleen or extralymphatic organ or both; and stage IV, diffuse or disseminated disease or involvement of the liver or bone marrow.

4. **b.** The staging is added to further by the presence or absence of the following symptoms: fever, night sweats, and weight loss of more than 10% in the past 6 months. The presence of any of the symptoms indicates that the stage of the disease should be labeled B. The absence of any of these symptoms indicates that the stage of the disease should be labeled A.

5. **d.** Although extended radiation was very successful in the treatment of patients with early Hodgkin's disease, patients experienced an increased risk of cardiovascular disease and second cancers. To reduce these risks of therapy for early stage disease, combined therapy is now preferred. This has resulted in improved tumor control with no obvious increased risk for death from any particular cause in long-term follow-up. Unfortunately, chemotherapy alone is slightly inferior to combined therapy in disease eradication, but chemotherapy is advancing, and the search continues for treatment that obviates the need for radiotherapy, particularly in children.

6. **e.** As previously mentioned, Hodgkin's disease is one of the major success stories in cancer treatment. Survival rates exceed 80%, and patients have the potential for cure regardless of initial stage of presentation. However, successful treatment has not been without associated negative effects. Secondary cancers and coronary artery disease result in premature death for many patients, and infertility is not uncommon for many patients. Early recurrence is always a probability, but the vast majority of patients beat this cancer and go on to live productive lives.

7. **e.** The one test you should have done is excisional lymph node biopsy.

8. **a.** This patient has a non-Hodgkin's lymphoma. The characteristics that suggest this diagnosis rather than Hodgkin's disease are the presence of lymph nodes draining Waldeyer's ring, the presence of epitrochlear lymph nodes, and the presence of chest pain suggesting involvement of lung tissue. The lymph node histology involving non-Hodgkin's lymphoma is not discussed in detail. However, the lymph node pathology of diffuse small cleaved cell (diffuse poorly differentiated lymphocytic) suggests a high-grade lymphoma with extensive involvement including the liver, spleen, and bone marrow. Your physical examination confirms the possibility of the former two.

Staging is similar (although not identical) to the staging for Hodgkin's disease. Non-Hodgkin's lymphoma can be found in nodal sites, viscera, or both. Extranodal disease is often solitary. Waldeyer's ring, upper gastrointestinal tract, testes, and bone are the most common extranodal sites. The staging of non-Hodgkin's lymphoma is divided into early and late stages of indolent (follicular) disease and aggressive disease. Histologic grading differentiates tumors into low-, intermediate-, and high-grade neoplasia.

9. **e.** Treatment modalities are based on diagnosed staging and disease aggressiveness. Indolent disease in early stages (I or II) is generally treated with radiotherapy. Patients with advanced stage (III and IV) follicular lymphoma have a median survival measured in years, and the natural history is variable, leading many asymptomatic patients to reasonably choose a watchful waiting strategy. For patients with progressive or symptomatic disease, treatment approaches include radiotherapy, chemotherapy, or both. Most patients respond to chemotherapy, but duration of response is usually only 1 or 2 years. Fewer than one-third of patients remain in remission for more than 5 years. Interferon-α and monoclonal antibodies have also been demonstrated to be beneficial in primary therapy for follicular lymphoma. In aggressive disease, combined therapy is an accepted standard of care for patients with early stage disease (I and II). Combined therapy is also used for late disease stages in aggressive non-Hodgkin's lymphomas, but response rates are less than 50% despite aggressive treatment regimens. Bone marrow transplantation after aggressive chemotherapy shows promise as an effective treatment.

10. **c.** Non-Hodgkin's lymphoma is responsible for up to 80% of lymphomas, making it much more common than Hodgkin's lymphoma. Approximately 60,000 people in the United States develop non-Hodgkin's lymphoma each year, leading to more than 26,000 deaths. The disease is more common in older individuals, and prognosis for a normal life span is poor with and without treatment. There appears to be a relationship with the Epstein–Barr virus in some forms of the disease, and the disease's incidence has increased partly as a result of HIV disease, which confers greater risk.

11. **c.** The critical elements of this patient's history/physical/laboratory data are as follows:

- Signs of bone pain (sternum and skull) and anemia
- Symptoms of weakness, depression, fatigue, and confusion
- Recent history of bacterial pneumonia; possible immune suppression
- Laboratory evidence of the following: (a) anemia, usually normocytic but rouleau formation is common; (b) hypercalcemia; (c) renal failure; (d) thrombocytopenia; (e) hyponatremia; and (f) elevated ESR

The combination of bone pain (location specific), hypercalcemia, normochromic/normocytic anemia, renal failure, weakness/depression/confusion, and

history of bacterial pneumonia points to the diagnosis of multiple myeloma. The diagnosis will be substantiated by skull x-ray (showing punched-out lesions), serum electrophoresis with monoclonal peak, and demonstration of Bence–Jones protein in the urine. Multiple myeloma is a disease of older patients, with the mean age being 68 years. It appears to be more common than average in farmers, petroleum workers, wood workers, and leather workers.

12. **a.** The treatment of choice for multiple myeloma used to be a standard combination of melphalan and prednisone; more recently, chemotherapy with alkylating agents (vincristine, Adriamycin, and dexamethasone) is also being used. The median survival rate with these regimens was 36 months.

Now, newly diagnosed patients with good performance status are being treated with autologous stem cell transplantation, resulting in improved survival, particularly for patients younger than age 60 years. Thalidomide has been found to be effective in patients with refractory myeloma. Supportive care measures have also improved, including the use of bisphosphonates to prevent osteolytic lesions. Additional treatment with radiation for bone pain and aggressive treatment for hypercalcemia is important. With newer treatment regimens, patients may live long periods with virtually no symptoms.

13. **d.** Pathologically, multiple myeloma is a plasma cell malignancy or proliferation.

14. **w.**

15. **z.**

16. **p.**

17. **m.**

18. **u.**

19. **i.**

20. **o.**

21. **e.**

22. **s.**

23. **j.**

Summary

MOST COMMON SOLID HEMATOLOGIC MALIGNANCIES ARE THE LYMPHOMAS

1. Disorder types and their prevalence
   a. Non-Hodgkin's lymphoma: most common (60,000 new cases per year in the United States)
   b. Hodgkin's lymphoma: second most common (7500 new cases per year in the United States)
2. Signs and symptoms
   a. The most common sign/symptom is solitary or nonsolitary lymph node enlargement.
   b. The presence or absence of systemic symptoms is not only a staging phenomenon (A or B) but also prognostic.
   c. The most common systemic symptoms include weight loss, night sweats, fevers, and pain.
3. Differentiation of Hodgkin's from non-Hodgkin's
   a. Reed–Sternberg cells are pathognomonic to the diagnosis of Hodgkin's lymphoma.
   b. Lymph node enlargement in the supraclavicular area is very common for Hodgkin's disease.
   c. In non-Hodgkin's lymphoma, the lymph nodes drain Waldeyer's ring and epitrochlear nodes are most commonly enlarged.
   d. Non-Hodgkin's lymphoma often presents with mediastinal, abdominal, and extranodal symptomatology.
4. Prognosis
   a. Hodgkin's lymphoma has a much better prognosis than non-Hodgkin's lymphoma, with treatment of the former resulting in cure up to 80% of the time.
   b. Prognosis depends on accurate staging.
5. Treatment: Hodgkin's and non-Hodgkin's are treated with a combination of chemotherapy and radiation. Monoclonal antibodies are also used. See answers 5 and 9.

MULTIPLE MYELOMA

1. Prevalence: multiple myeloma mainly a disease of the elderly
2. Pathology: plasma cell malignancy/plasma cell proliferation
3. Signs and symptoms: (a) bone pain (sternum, skull, ribs, and back); (b) anemia (normochromic/normocytic); (c) immune suppression (history of bacterial infections); (d) renal failure; (e) hypercalcemia; and (f) weakness/confusion/depression/fatigue
4. Diagnosis: (a) serum protein electrophoresis, (b) bone marrow biopsy, and (c) Bence–Jones protein in the urine

MISCELLANEOUS IMPORTANT HEMATOLOGIC CONDITIONS

1. Polycythemia rubra vera
   a. Plethora, sometimes cyanosis
   b. Proliferation of all hematopoietic cell lines
   c. Elevated hemoglobin, red blood cell mass, and thrombocytosis
2. Myelofibrosis
   a. Weight loss
   b. Bleeding from skin and mucous membranes
   c. Bone marrow biopsy: dry tap, normal bone marrow replaced by fibrotic material
3. Chronic myelogenous leukemia
   a. Atomic bomb survivors (or other radiation victims)
   b. Philadelphia chromosome
   c. White blood cells at diagnosis often greater than 200,000/mm³
   d. Chronic phase followed by blastic phase
4. Chronic lymphocytic leukemia
   a. Most common leukemia in the United States
   b. Disease of older patients
   c. Indolent nature; no treatment needed in many patients; median survival 10 years
5. Hairy cell leukemia
   a. Cytoplasmic projections give disorder its name
   b. Remarkably effective treatment with cladribine usually presents with pancytopenia
6. Acute lymphocytic leukemia
   a. Disease of children
   b. Immature lymphoblasts
   c. Infections very common
   d. Up to a 70% cure rate at present
7. Acute myeloblastic leukemia
   a. Most common acute leukemia of adults
   b. Auer rods pathognomonic
   c. Immature myeloblasts on smear
   d. Infections very common
   e. Bone marrow transplantation essential for survival (10% to 30%)
   f. May follow myelodysplastic disorder or preleukemia
8. Idiopathic thrombocytopenic purpura
   a. Acute onset after viral exanthem or viral infection
   b. Rapid drop in platelet count
   c. Corticosteroids treatment of choice: splenectomy in resistant cases
9. von Willebrand's disease
   a. Most common inherited bleeding disorder
   b. Results from a factor VIII deficiency
   c. Often presents as severe menorrhagia in women
   d. Factor VIII concentrates treatment of choice
10. Disseminated intravascular coagulation
    a. Follows obstetric catastrophes, major trauma, metastatic malignancies, or bacterial sepsis
    b. Microemboli or microthrombi in vasculature
    c. Profuse bleeding from many sites
    d. Treatment: fresh frozen plasma for severe bleeding

Suggested Reading

Cheson BD: Clinical management of T-cell malignancies: Current perspectives, key issues, and emerging therapies. *Semin Oncol* 34(6 Suppl 5):S3–S7, 2007.

Diehl V: Hodgkin's disease—From pathology specimen to cure. *N Engl J Med* 357:1968–1971, 2007.

Fermé C, Eghbali H, Meerwaldt JH, et al: Chemotherapy plus involved-field radiation in early-stage Hodgkin's disease. *N Engl J Med* 357:1916–1927, 2007.

Kyle RA, Rajkumar SV: Multiple myeloma. *N Engl J Med* 351:1860–1873, 2004.

Schwartz CL: The management of Hodgkin disease in the young child. *Curr Opin Pediatr* 15(1):10–16, 2003.

Staudt LM: Molecular diagnosis of the hematologic cancers. *N Engl J Med* 348(18):1777–1785, 2003.

CHAPTER

65 Breast, Lung, and Brain Cancer

CLINICAL CASE PROBLEM 1

A 38-Year-Old Woman with BRCA 1, Two Mutations, and Three First-Degree Relatives with Breast Cancer

A 38-year-old woman comes to the office for counseling regarding news she received from the geneticist. She has been told that she has breast cancer susceptibility genes BRCA 1 and 2, which are responsible for up to 10% of all breast cancers, and that women with these mutations have a cumulative risk of developing breast cancer of 55% to 85% up to the age of 70 years. She is at a loss of what to do and is coming to you for information and advice.

SELECT THE BEST ANSWER TO THE FOLLOWING QUESTIONS

1. Regarding the use of chemoprevention in patients with these genes, you tell her which of the following?
   a. there is nothing that can be done to prevent her from developing breast cancer
   b. her first-degree relatives are of no bearing on her risk
   c. reduction of exposure to estrogen through oophorectomy reduces risk
   d. use of tamoxifen reduces risk
   e. c and d

2. Regarding prophylactic mastectomy, which of the following is (are) true?
   a. this is a barbaric procedure of no proven value
   b. minimal benefit is gained in performing this procedure after age 60 years
   c. unilateral surgery for the right breast is recommended because incidence is highest in this location
   d. reduction in breast cancer incidence following surgery approaches 90%
   e. b and d

CLINICAL CASE PROBLEM 2

A 62-Year-Old Female with a Solitary Pulmonary Nodule

A 62-year-old woman comes to your office with her chest radiograph performed at her place of employment. She was not told the results but that she needed to see her primary care physician "pronto." She feels fine, but you know she has been a one-pack-per-day smoker for 20 years. The film reveals a 1.5-cm nodule completely surrounded by lung normal parenchyma in her right upper lobe.

3. Which of the following, if present, is suggestive of a malignancy?
   a. the presence of "corona radiata" linear strands extending out from the nodule
   b. calcifications within the lesion
   c. smooth borders to the nodule
   d. the presence of the nodule on previous films
   e. dimensions greater than 3 cm

4. Which of the following is (are) true regarding nonsurgical approaches to diagnosis?
   a. computed tomography (CT) densitometry measures attenuation values that are higher in malignant lesions
   b. contrast-enhanced spiral CT has a sensitivity of 95% and specificity of 70% to 90%
   c. specificity of transthoracic fine needle aspiration biopsy is virtually 100%
   d. bronchoscopy sensitivity for lesions 1.5 cm or less is approximately 40%
   e. b and c

5. Which of the following is not true regarding video-assisted thoracoscopic surgery (VATS)?
   a. VATS lowers morbidity in resection of nodules
   b. all patients with solitary nodules are candidates for VATS
   c. VATS shortens hospital length of stay in nodule resection
   d. VATS is especially successful for treatment of peripheral lung lesions
   e. VATS allows for intraoperative decision about whether to proceed to lobectomy

6. Which of the following is (are) true regarding lung cancer?
   a. non-small cell carcinoma is less common than small cell cancers
   b. surgery plays the major role of managing stage 1 and 2 non-small cell lung cancers
   c. adjuvant radiation increases survival time in non-small cell cancer
   d. surgery is the treatment of choice in small cell cancer
   e. single-drug chemotherapy is effective in patients with extensive small cell carcinoma

CLINICAL CASE PROBLEM 3

A 79-Year-Old Male with a Bad Headache

A 79-year-old farmer presents to your office complaining of bad headaches. They have been worsening during the past several months, and lately he has developed accompanying nausea and vomiting. He was seen in a local emergency room 2 months ago and was told he has migraines. He awakes with headaches, and yesterday he walked into a partially opened barn door. He has a big lump on the side of his head. Vital signs show blood pressure at 140/89 mmHg, a pulse of 89 beats/minute, and respiration rate of 17 breaths/minute. He is afebrile. Neurologic examination shows a partial visual field loss on the right. The rest of his examination is normal. You are concerned about the possibility of serious intracranial pathology.

7. Which of the following is the best test to perform at this time?
   a. no testing is indicated at this time
   b. CT scan of the head without contrast
   c. CT scan of the head with and without contrast
   d. magnetic resonance angiography of the head
   e. contrast-enhanced magnetic resonance imaging (MRI) of the head

8. Which of the following is (are) true regarding brain tumors?
   a. ionizing radiation is an identified risk factor for glial neoplasms
   b. use of cellular telephones is a risk factor for meningiomas
   c. headache occurs in approximately 90% of all patients with brain tumors
   d. postictal hemiparesis or aphasia known as Todd's phenomenon is helpful in localizing tumors
   e. a and d

9. This patient is found to have a brain glial malignancy. Based on his history, he is likely to have which of the following?
   a. anaplastic astrocytoma
   b. glioblastoma
   c. meningioma
   d. anaplastic oligodendroglioma
   e. primary central nervous system lymphoma

10. The described patient is started with the appropriate therapy. He experiences difficulty with the chemotherapy and radiotherapy and schedules an appointment to ask you about using various mind–body interventions (MBIs), including contingency management counseling, relaxation therapy, and guided imagery, to help with side effects. Regarding various MBIs, you can tell him which of the following?
   a. MBIs have not scientifically been proved to work
   b. MBIs have been effective in reducing acute pain from therapeutic procedures
   c. MBIs have been ineffective in treating anticipatory nausea and vomiting from therapeutic procedures
   d. MBIs have no effect on mood and can worsen coping capacity
   e. MBIs are extremely effective in postchemotherapy nausea reduction

Answers

1. **e.** BRCA 1 and 2 genes are responsible for 10% of breast cancers, and women who have these mutations have a cumulative risk of developing breast cancer up to age 70 years of 55% to 85%. Women with first-degree relatives with breast cancer are additionally at increased risk. What to do with this information is the challenge faced by patients and their primary care physicians. Strategies for surveillance and chemoprevention are in transition, but the efficacy of tamoxifen

chemoprevention and prophylactic mastectomy is now proven. In the National Adjuvant Breast and Bowel Project Prevention Trial, tamoxifen reduced the risk in high-risk women by 49%. Reducing exposure to estrogen by oophorectomy also seems to reduce risk in the population. Because stakes are high, confirmation of testing is recommended.

2. **e.** Prophylactic mastectomy reduces the risk of breast cancer by approximately 90% in women at high risk. However, minimal survival gains are seen in women older than age 60 years. Some physicians and patients find this procedure unacceptable; however, psychologic functioning in women who choose to have this procedure seems to be well maintained. The decision to undertake any prophylactic measures, be it chemoprevention or surgery, should rest with a well-informed patient aware of all the risks, benefits, and alternatives.

3. **a.** An estimated 150,000 solitary pulmonary nodules are discovered each year, and their evaluation represents a thorny clinical problem. Lesions that are greater than 3 cm have a high probability of malignancy. Although there can be many causes for a pulmonary nodule, carcinoma must be ruled out. Several characteristics seen on plain films increase the likelihood of a nodule being a malignancy: a "corona radiata" sign of fine linear strands or spiculated rays radiating out from the nodule, an irregular or scalloped border to the nodule, lack of calcification, or growth in size of the nodule within 2 years. High-resolution CT can be used to follow nodules over time for changes in appearance.

4. **b.** Several nonsurgical approaches to diagnosis are useful in distinguishing benign from malignant lesions in high-risk patients such as long-term smokers. CT densitometry involves the measurement of attenuation values, which are higher in benign lesions. Local expertise varies with this technique, and it has not been widely adopted. Contrast-enhanced spiral CT is widely available and has a sensitivity of 95% and specificity of 70% to 90%. Specificity of transthoracic fine needle aspiration biopsy is 55% to 88%, and sensitivity is 80% to 95%. However, nodules must be in the periphery to be accessible. Bronchoscopy sensitivity for lesions 1.5 cm or less is only approximately 10% but increases to 60% in larger lesions. Positron emission tomography (PET) scanning uses measures of glucose metabolism to distinguish between benign and malignant lesions, and sensitivities of 96% and specificities of 78% have been attained. However, the procedure is not widely available and requires further study. The approach to diagnosis will be guided by risk assessment, location of the lesion, and available technologies.

5. **b.** VATS has been shown to reduce morbidity in resection of nodules compared to open thoracotomy. Although available to most patients with solitary nodules, the procedure requires anesthesia with double lumen tubes for separate ventilation of each lung followed by discontinuation of ventilation and induced partial pneumothorax on the side of the nodule. VATS shortens hospital length of stay in nodule resections and is especially successful for treatment of peripheral lung lesions. The procedure allows for intraoperative frozen-section diagnosis to aid in the decision of full lobectomy. Mortality and morbidity are in part a function of volume of procedures performed, with better outcomes in high-volume centers.

6. **b.** Lung cancer is one of the most common malignancies, and primary lung cancers can be broadly classified into two forms: non-small cell and small cell carcinomas. Non-small cell carcinomas account for up to 75% of all lung cancers. Surgery plays a major role in managing stage 1 and 2 non-small cell lung cancers, whereas patients with advanced non-small cell disease are treated with combination chemotherapy. Adjuvant radiation reduces local recurrence and, when combined with chemotherapy, may confer a small survival advantage in non-small cell cancer. Surgery has only a limited role in the treatment of small cell cancer. Patients with limited small cell disease are treated with a platinum-based chemotherapeutic regimen plus radiation. Extensive small cell disease is treated with combination chemotherapy. Unfortunately, most lung cancers at the time of diagnosis are incurable.

7. **e.** The best test to confirm the diagnosis of a brain malignancy is the gadolinium contrast-enhanced MRI of the brain.

8. **e.** Approximately 17,000 new brain tumors are diagnosed each year, and 14,000 people die each year of primary cancers of the central nervous system. Ionizing radiation is an identified risk factor for glial neoplasms, whereas use of cellular telephones has not been identified as a risk factor for any brain malignancies. Headache occurs in approximately half of all patients with brain tumors, and seizures occur in up to 60% in some studies. Headache is usually diffuse, often is noticeable on awakening in the morning, and can be confused with migraines or cluster headaches. In seizures related to brain malignancy, postictal hemiparesis or aphasia known as Todd's phenomenon is helpful in localizing tumors. Other symptoms or signs that help localize tumors include hemiparesis, aphasia, and visual field losses, as is seen in this patient.

9. **b.** Brain tumors are a heterogeneous group of neoplasms. Glial tumors are divided into two main categories: astrocytic and oligodendroglial. Astrocytomas are seen predominately in young patients, and most astrocytomas progress to high-grade malignant lesions within 5 years and ultimately cause death. Malignant astrocytomas are made up of anaplastic astrocytomas and glioblastomas. Glioblastomas tend to be a disease seen later in life, usually in the sixth or seventh decades (mean age, 55 years). Oligodendrogliomas, like astrocytomas, can be low grade or anaplastic. Most of the former eventually progress to the latter. Meningiomas are not strictly brain tumors because they arise from the meninges, which cover the brain, and occur primarily at the base of the skull. Primary central nervous system lymphomas have tripled in incidence in the past two decades and are often associated with immunosuppression, particularly human immunodeficiency virus (HIV).

10. **b.** MBIs include a wide range of interventions, including contingency management counseling, stress reduction and relaxation therapy, meditation and guided imagery, hypnosis, and traditional behavioral counseling. After many years, studies have finally subjected these treatments to the scientific method. There is now considerable evidence that a wide range of mind–body therapies can be used as effective adjuncts for several common clinical conditions related to cancer treatment. For example, MBIs have been effective in reducing acute pain from therapeutic procedures and have been effective in treating anticipatory nausea and vomiting from therapeutic procedures. MBIs have had positive effects on mood and can enhance coping capacity. They are mildly effective in postchemotherapy nausea reduction. The clinician should keep an open mind regarding these and other adjunctive therapies for the cancer patient while relying on the scrutiny of the scientific method to examine their effects.

Summary

BREAST CANCER-ASSOCIATED GENE MUTATIONS

BRCA 1 and 2 genes are responsible for 10% of breast cancers, and women with these mutations have a cumulative risk of breast cancer up to age 70 years of 55% to 85%. Because stakes are high, confirmation of testing is recommended.

Strategies for surveillance and chemoprevention are in transition, but efficacy of tamoxifen chemoprevention and prophylactic mastectomy is proven.

In the National Adjuvant Breast and Bowel Project Prevention Trial, tamoxifen reduced risk in women at high risk by 49%. Reducing exposure to estrogen by oophorectomy also seems to reduce risk in the population.

Prophylactic mastectomy reduces risk of breast cancer by approximately 90% in high-risk women. However, survival gains are minimal after age 60 years.

Decisions to undertake any prophylactic measures, be it chemoprevention or surgery, should rest with a well-informed patient aware of all the risks, benefits, and alternatives.

SOLITARY LUNG NODULES

Each year, 150,000 solitary pulmonary nodules are discovered. Although there are many causes, carcinoma must be ruled out. The approach to diagnosis is guided by risk assessment, location of the lesion, and available technologies.

Characteristics on plain films associated with malignancy are as follows: lesions larger than 3 cm, "corona radiata" sign of spiculated rays, irregular or scalloped border, lack of calcification, and growth in size within 2 years. High-resolution CT should be performed to follow over time for changes in appearance.

Nonsurgical approaches to distinguish benign from malignant lesions in high-risk patients (e.g., long-term smokers) include the following:

1. CT densitometry: measures attenuation values, which are higher in benign lesions. Local expertise varies; not widely adapted.
2. Contrast-enhanced spiral CT: widely available, sensitivity 95% and specificity 70% to 90%.
3. Transthoracic fine needle aspiration biopsy: specificity 55% to 88% and sensitivity 80% to 95%. However, must be in periphery to be accessible.
4. Bronchoscopy: sensitivity (lesions 1.5 cm or smaller) 10%, but 60% in larger lesions.
5. PET scanning: measures glucose metabolism to distinguish between benign and malignant lesions; sensitivity 96%, specificity 78%. However, not widely available, and it requires further study.
6. VATS: reduces morbidity, shortens hospital length of stay, and is very successful for peripheral lung lesions. Allows for intraoperative frozen-section diagnosis to aid decision of full lobectomy. Mortality and morbidity

are a function of number performed; better outcomes in high-volume centers.

BRAIN TUMORS

Each year, 17,000 brain tumors are newly diagnosed and there are 14,000 deaths from primary central nervous system cancers.

Brain tumors are heterogeneous; the best test to confirm diagnosis is contrast-enhanced MRI.

There are two main categories of glial tumors: astrocytic and oligodendroglial. Astrocytomas are seen in young patients, and most progress to high-grade malignant lesions within 5 years and are fatal. Malignant astrocytomas are made up of anaplastic astrocytomas and glioblastomas. Glioblastomas occur in the sixth or seventh decades (mean age, 55 years). Oligodendrogliomas, like astrocytomas, are low grade or anaplastic. Most of the former progress to the latter.

Meningiomas are not strictly brain tumors (arise from meninges); they occur primarily at the base of the skull.

Primary central nervous system lymphomas have tripled in incidence in the past two decades; they are often associated with immunosuppression, particularly HIV disease.

Ionizing radiation is a risk factor for glial neoplasms; cellular telephones are not confirmed as a risk factor.

Headache occurs in 50% of all patients, and seizures occur in up to 60%. Headache is diffuse, often confused with migraines or cluster headaches. In seizures related to brain malignancy, postictal hemiparesis or aphasia known as Todd's phenomenon helps localize tumors.

Other symptoms or signs include hemiparesis, aphasia, and visual field losses.

MBIs include contingency management counseling, stress reduction and relaxation therapy, meditation and guided imagery, hypnosis, and traditional behavioral counseling. MBIs can be used as effective adjuncts for reducing acute pain from therapeutic procedures, for treating anticipatory nausea and vomiting from procedures, for positive effects on mood, and for enhancing coping capacity.

Suggested Reading

Astin JA, Shapiro SL, Eisenberg DM, et al: Mind–body medicine: State of the science, implications for practice. *J Am Board Fam Pract* 16(2):131–147, 2003.

Barfi K, Newton H, Von Roenn J: Palliative care for patients with brain metastases. *Cancer Treat Res* 136:215–233, 2007.

Cersosimo RJ: Lung cancer: A review. *Am J Health Syst Pharm* 59(7):611–642, 2002.

De Angelis LM: Brain tumors. *N Engl J Med* 344(2):114–123, 2001.

Gomez M, Silvestri GA: Lung cancer screening. *Am J Med Sci* 335:46–50, 2008.

Lim LC, Rosenthal MA, Maartens N, Ryan G: Management of brain metastases. *Intern Med J* 34:270–278, 2004.

Moulder S, Hortobagyi GN: Advances in the treatment of breast cancer. *Clin Pharmacol Ther* 83:26–36, 2008.

Ost D, Fein AM, Feinsilver SH: Clinical practice. The solitary pulmonary nodule. *N Engl J Med* 348(25):2535–2542, 2003.

Tacon AM: Meditation as a complementary therapy in cancer. *Fam Community Health* 26(1):64–73, 2003.

Tanvetyanon T, Soares HP, Djulbegovic B, et al: A systematic review of quality of life associated with standard chemotherapy regimens for advanced non-small cell lung cancer. *J Thorac Oncol* 2(12):1091–1097, 2007.

CHAPTER

66 Cancer Pain Management

CLINICAL CASE PROBLEM 1

A 75-Year-Old Male with Metastatic Bone Pain Secondary to Advanced Prostate Cancer

A 75-year-old male diagnosed with stage D cancer of the prostate 6 months ago comes to your office. He has been asymptomatic for the past 6 months, but last week he began to develop severe pain in the lower lumbar spine. He also appears quite pale.

On examination, his prostate is hard. He has tender lumbar vertebrae L2–L5. Your suspicions of metastatic bone disease are confirmed when a technetium-99 bone scan shows increased uptake of radionuclide in L2–L5 and in both femurs, both tibias, and both humeri.

SELECT THE BEST ANSWER TO THE FOLLOWING QUESTIONS

1. What is the treatment of first choice at this time?
   a. high-dose morphine sulfate
   b. high-dose hydromorphone
   c. transdermal fentanyl
   d. palliative radiotherapy to the lumbar spine
   e. acetaminophen–hydrocodone

2. You institute appropriate therapy for this patient. He quickly becomes pain free and remains that way for 6 months. He then returns with cervical, thoracic, and lumbar back pain; bilateral thigh pain; bilateral knee and leg pain; and pain in both shoulders

and both arms (diffuse). Therapeutic options at this time include which of the following?

a. intravenous (IV) chlorinate
b. IV radioactive strontium
c. morphine sulfate
d. hydromorphone
e. naproxen
f. all of the above

3. Which of the following pharmacologic agents is the drug of first choice for the treatment of mild metastatic bone pain?

a. morphine sulfate
b. hydromorphone
c. fentanyl
d. a nonsteroidal anti-inflammatory drug (NSAID)
e. carbamazepine

4. Which of the following drugs should not be used in the management of chronic pain?

a. codeine
b. meperidine
c. levorphanol
d. methadone

CLINICAL CASE PROBLEM 2

A 52-Year-Old Male with Metastatic Renal Cell Carcinoma

A 52-year-old male with metastatic renal cell carcinoma presents for assessment of a pain beginning in the buttocks and traveling down the left leg. It has a sharp, stabbing, burning, or "zingerlike" quality, according to the patient. The patient indicates that the baseline pain is 5 on a 10-point scale, with a range from 3 to 7.

5. What is (are) the drug(s) of first choice for the management of this patient's cancer pain?

a. carbamazepine
b. hydromorphone
c. morphine sulfate
d. amitriptyline
e. desipramine

CLINICAL CASE PROBLEM 3

A 66-Year-Old Female with Metastatic Renal Cell Carcinoma

A 66-year-old female patient with metastatic renal cell carcinoma presents for assessment of a pain also beginning in the buttocks and traveling down the left

leg. The only difference between this patient's pain and that of the patient in Clinical Case Problem 2 is that this patient describes the pain as dull and throbbing.

6. What is (are) the drug(s) of first choice for the management of this patient's cancer pain?

a. carbamazepine
b. hydromorphone
c. morphine sulfate
d. desipramine
e. valproic acid

7. The location of the lesions described in the two patients presented in cases 2 and 3 is best portrayed as which of the following?

a. retroperitoneal
b. lumbar–sacral plexopathy
c. intraabdominal–visceral
d. a and b
e. b and c

8. What percentage of patients with cancer pain responds well to first-line analgesic therapy such as acetaminophen or NSAIDs?

a. 1%
b. 5%
c. 10%
d. 15%
e. 20%

9. Which of the following agents would be classified as second-line analgesic therapy for the management of cancer pain?

a. hydrocodone
b. acetaminophen
c. morphine sulfate
d. levorphanol
e. hydromorphone

10. Which of the following agents is not classified as a third-line pharmacologic agent in the management of cancer pain?

a. methadone
b. morphine sulfate
c. hydromorphone
d. fentanyl
e. codeine

11. A patient comes to your office with moderately severe cancer pain. You prescribe the third-line agent (because of the description of the pain as moderately severe). Which of the following best describes the preferred approach to managing this patient's cancer pain?

a. begin with a twice daily oral dose of long-acting morphine

b. begin with a twice daily oral dose of long-acting morphine plus short-acting oral morphine for breakthrough pain

c. begin with a dose of short-acting oral morphine every 4 hours

d. begin with a transdermal fentanyl analgesic patch

e. begin with a dose of 200 mg morphine/day in any form

12. A patient who is maintained on long-acting morphine with short-acting morphine for breakthrough pain presents with a 1-week history of an increasing need for short-acting morphine. He is now taking three times the number of short-acting tablets as previously. What should you do at this time?

a. prescribe more short-acting morphine; keep the amount of long-acting morphine the same

b. transfer the increased requirement into long-acting morphine and maintain a supply of short-acting morphine

c. transfer the increased requirement into both increased amounts of long-acting morphine and increased amounts of short-acting morphine

d. switch to another third-line oral agent

e. switch to a transdermal delivery system

13. What is the average starting daily dose of morphine sulfate in the treatment of a patient with moderately severe cancer pain?

a. 10 to 15 mg

b. 15 to 30 mg

c. 30 to 60 mg

d. 60 to 120 mg

e. 120 to 240 mg

14. Which of the following statements regarding the use of morphine in the treatment of terminal cancer pain is (are) relevant to the patent in question?

a. morphine produces rapid tolerance

b. morphine produces euphoria

c. morphine produces respiratory depression

d. none of the above

e. all of the above

15. When starting a patient taking a narcotic analgesic, what is the single most important agent that should be started at the same time?

a. an agent to prevent constipation

b. an agent to prevent nausea and vomiting

c. an agent to enhance sedation

d. an agent to prevent drowsiness

e. an antidepressant

16. Which of the following is (are) essential to cancer pain management?

a. a collaborative, interdisciplinary approach to care

b. an individualized pain-control plan developed and agreed on by the patient

c. ongoing assessment and reassessment of the patient's pain

d. the use of both pharmacologic and nonpharmacologic therapies to prevent or control pain

e. all of the above

17. Which of the following is (are) an aim(s) of pain management in palliative care?

a. to identify the cause of the pain

b. to prevent the pain from recurring

c. to maintain a clear sensorium

d. to maintain a normal affect

e. all of the above

18. Which of the following factors modify the pain threshold in patients with cancer pain?

a. insomnia

b. fear

c. anxiety

d. sadness

e. all of the above

19. A patient develops severe nausea and vomiting as the dose of morphine being used for terminal cancer pain (endometrial) is increased. The patient is undergoing triple antinauseant therapy, which includes dimenhydrinate, metoclopramide, and prochlorperazine. Which of the following statements regarding this situation is (are) true?

a. you should add a fourth antinauseant to the regimen at this time, preferably a corticosteroid or ondansetron

b. you should put an IV line in place and make sure the input equals the output; do not change drugs

c. decrease the dose of the morphine by 10% for 24 hours

d. switch to another narcotic analgesic; no further investigations are necessary or desired

e. none of the above

20. A patient who is being treated for terminal cancer (esophageal adenocarcinoma) pain with oral morphine requires increased morphine doses daily. Six weeks ago, his morphine dose was 180 mg/day; it is 600 mg/day now. Which of the following

statements regarding this increased dose of morphine is (are) true?
a. the dosage increase most likely represents tolerance to the morphine
b. the dosage increase most likely represents increased requirements as a result of tumor growth
c. both a and b are true
d. either a or b could be true, but not both
e. neither a nor b

21. A patient is being treated for breast cancer with adjuvant chemotherapy following a lumpectomy. One of the drugs she is taking is cisplatin. She develops intractable nausea and vomiting while taking this drug. Which of the following antiemetics is the drug of first choice for this patient?
a. prochlorperazine
b. ondansetron
c. dimenhydrinate
d. metoclopramide
e. dexamethasone

22. A patient develops intractable nausea and vomiting secondary to carcinoma of the colon with partial bowel obstruction. She has been taking both morphine and hydromorphone by mouth but is having great difficulty keeping anything down. What would you do at this time?
a. switch to levorphanol for the pain
b. switch to methadone for the pain
c. switch from the oral medication route to a subcutaneous infusion
d. switch from the oral route to the suppository route
e. switch from the oral route to the intravenous route

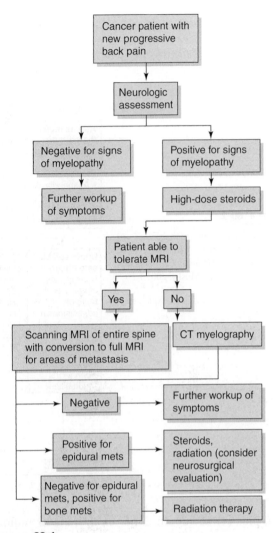

Figure 66-1

Approach to a patient with cancer and back pain. CT, computed tomography; mets, metastases; MRI, magnetic resonance imaging. (Modified from Ruckdeschel JC: Spinal cord compression. In: *Clinical Oncology*, 2nd ed. New York: Churchill Livingstone, 2000.)

Answers

1. d. This patient, who was diagnosed with stage D cancer of the prostate 6 months ago, will benefit from local treatment. A very important point in this case is that although his bone scan shows more diffuse skeletal disease, his clinical status suggests symptoms only in the lumbar spine. Thus, radiation therapy to the lumbar spine is the most reasonable course of action. Again, the reasoning is that local symptoms should receive local therapy (Fig. 66-1). (This applies to palliative situations only.)

It could also be appropriate to start morphine sulfate or hydromorphone. However, it would not be appropriate to start with high-dose morphine sulfate or high-dose hydromorphone.

2. f. There are many therapeutic options for the treatment of metastatic bone. The following treatment options have been shown to be effective: bisphosphonates, radioactive strontium, NSAIDs, and narcotic analgesics (Fig. 66-2).

A reasonable treatment plan at this time would be to begin with an NSAID (naproxen) plus short-acting morphine sulfate or short-acting hydromorphone for breakthrough pain. Then ask the patient to call you within 24 hours to ensure that pain has begun to decrease. On his next visit (in perhaps a week if you are beginning to get his pain under control), you could (1) switch him to a long-acting morphine preparation or a longer acting hydromorphone preparation, plus (2) continue the NSAID agent, plus (3) continue to supply him with short-acting narcotics for breakthrough

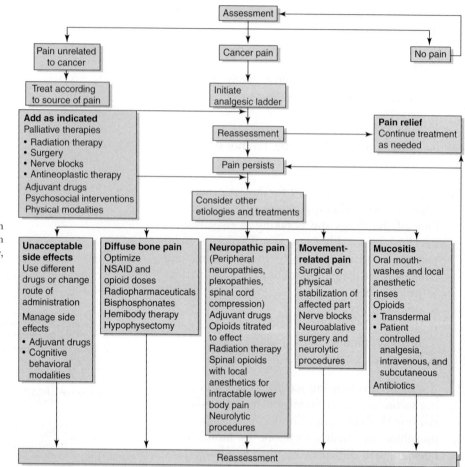

Figure 66-2

Algorithm for pain management in patients with cancer. (Redrawn from Noble J: *Textbook of Primary Care Medicine*, 3rd ed. Philadelphia: Mosby, 2001.)

pain, plus (4) decide on either clodronate or radioactive strontium as adjuvant therapy.

3. **d.** The drug class of first choice for the management of mild to moderate metastatic bone pain is the NSAID agents. If these do not work, then opioids can be added to NSAIDs for mild to moderate pain.

4. **b.** Meperidine (Demerol) is contraindicated in the management of chronic pain (both malignant and nonmalignant). The reasons for its contraindication are its relatively short half-life and its lack of efficacy.

The other drugs, levorphanol (oral) and methadone (oral), are very reasonable agents to use in the management of chronic cancer pain, as is fentanyl (transdermal, subcutaneous, or IV).

5. **a.** See answer 6.

6. **d.** These two cases illustrate the use of adjuvant analgesics in the treatment of neuropathic pain. Neuropathic pain is the most common type of cancer pain and presents diagnostic and therapeutic challenges. It is described as either a sharp, stabbing, burning, ("zingerlike") pain or as a dull, aching pain. Both types of neuropathic pain respond better to adjuvant analgesics than to narcotic analgesics. However, in response to typical adjuvant agents, the sharp, stabbing, burning pain responds better to anticonvulsant medications; the first choice is carbamazepine, and the second choice is valproic acid. In contrast, the dull, "aching" pain responds better to tricyclic antidepressants; the first choice is desipramine, and, generally, the second choice is amitriptyline. However, if sedation would be of benefit to the patient, amitriptyline may be the agent of choice.

7. **d.** The greatest number of neuropathic pains seen in cancer pain management result from retroperitoneal lesions either infiltrating or pressing on the lumbar–sacral plexus.

8. **e.** See answer 10.

9. **a.** See answer 10.

10. **e.** The World Health Organization (WHO) has developed an analgesic ladder for the treatment of cancer pain. Although it is not necessarily always in the patient's best interest to start with a first-line agent (the pain may be too severe), many patients can be managed with first-line agents such as acetaminophen or NSAIDs. In fact, 20% to 25% of patients with cancer pain can have their pain totally or almost totally controlled with these agents.

The WHO's analgesic ladder is summarized as follows: (1) First-line agents are acetylsalicylic acid (aspirin), other NSAIDs, or acetaminophen; (2) second-line agents are hydrocodone or codeine; and (3) third-line agents are morphine sulfate, hydromorphone, fentanyl, levorphanol, or methadone (Fig. 66-3).

11. **c.** The best approach to the management of moderately severe cancer pain is to begin with an every 4-hour dose of short-acting morphine sulfate (the drug of first choice in the third-line group) and have the patient use the analgesic as needed to attain complete pain control. Once the dose is established, you may switch to a longer acting preparation (twice a day) and maintain for the patient a supply of short-acting morphine for breakthrough pain.

12. **b.** What the patient needs at this time is an increased supply of long-acting morphine as well as the maintenance of a supply of short-acting morphine for breakthrough pain.

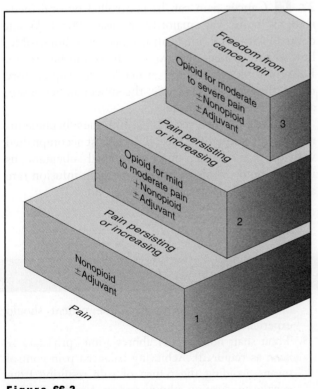

Figure 66-3

The World Health Organization three-step analgesic ladder.

13. **c.** The average daily starting dose of morphine sulfate (oral) in a patient with moderately severe cancer pain is 30 to 60 mg.

14. **d.** Although the use of morphine may cause tolerance, euphoria, and respiratory depression, these are not a significant concern in those who are in the terminal or palliative phase of their illness.

There is no maximum morphine or other analgesic equivalent dose. Each patient requires the dose to be individualized. This should be done by starting at lower doses and increasing the dose until you have achieved total pain control and are able to prevent further pain.

15. **a.** Any patient who is started taking a narcotic analgesic should also be started on a regimen to prevent constipation. The drugs most commonly used include lactulose, an osmotic agent, and a combination of a stool softener and a peristaltic stimulant (e.g., docusate sodium and senna). An antiemetic such as dimenhydrinate, prochlorperazine, or metoclopramide may be indicated for the first 2 or 3 weeks to prevent nausea and vomiting that sometimes accompany the initiation of a narcotic.

16. **e.** Clinical practice guidelines have been issued by the Agency for Healthcare Research and Quality, a branch of the Department of Health and Human Services. The purpose of these guidelines is to correct the problem of inadequate (or underdosing) pain treatment for cancer. These guidelines call for the following: (1) a collaborative, interdisciplinary approach to the care of patients with cancer pain; (2) an individualized pain-control plan developed and agreed on by the patient (the patient must be regarded as the head of the health care team); (3) an ongoing assessment and reassessment of the patient's pain; (4) the use of both nonpharmacologic and pharmacologic therapies to prevent or control pain; and (5) explicit institutional policies on the management of cancer pain, with clear lines of responsibility for pain management and for monitoring its effectiveness.

17. **e.** The aims of pain management in palliative care are as follows: (1) to identify the cause of the pain, (2) to prevent the pain from occurring again, (3) to erase the memory of the pain, and (4) to maintain a clear sensorium and a normal affect. Remember that palliative care is active treatment, not passive treatment.

18. **e.** Cancer pain is a complex entity that requires treatment of not only the somatic source(s) but also the other aspects, including depression, anxiety, anger, and isolation. Pain threshold is raised by relief of symptoms, sleep, rest, empathy, understanding, diversions, elevation of mood, effective analgesic therapy, anxiolytic therapy, and antidepressant therapy.

Pain threshold is lowered by discomfort, insomnia, fatigue, anxiety, fear, anger, sadness, depression, mental isolation, introversion, and past painful experiences.

Cancer pain should be considered as a complex consisting of a physical component, a psychological component, a social component, and a spiritual component. Unless each one of these areas is addressed in the overall cancer pain management strategy, therapy will not be effective (Fig. 66-4).

19. e. At this time, the first priority is to determine the cause of the nausea. The narcotic analgesic may not

be the cause. A thorough search for all other serious and potential causes of the nausea must be undertaken. In this case, a likely cause is hypercalcemia. Another common cause is the production by the tumor of emetic substances. Once causes such as these are ruled out, it is then reasonable to switch to another narcotic analgesic (e.g., hydromorphone) and/or to institute effective antiemetic therapy.

20. c. The increase in the dose of morphine during the 6-week period most likely represents a combination of tolerance to morphine and increased requirements resulting from growth of the tumor. As noted previously, rapid tolerance is usually not seen when the patient is being given a narcotic for cancer pain. However, tolerance can be developed over time and must be considered.

21. b. Chemotherapy that includes the drug cisplatin is very likely to produce very severe nausea and vomiting. Therefore, it is mandatory to treat this aggressively. Ondansetron, a serotonin antagonist, has been found to be extremely useful for the control of chemotherapy-induced nausea and is recommended (other serotonin antagonists include granisetron and dolasetron). In other cases in which control is difficult despite combination antinauseant therapy, ondansetron should also be used.

22. c. Cancer pain can be controlled by oral medications in the vast majority of cases (90%). When control with oral medications becomes impossible, however, it is necessary to switch to another route. Four possible routes are available: the suppository route, the intravenous route, the subcutaneous route, and the transdermal route.

With a patient in severe discomfort, the subcutaneous route is the route of choice. This is best accomplished with the use of a computer-controlled subcutaneous infusion pump. This provides a constant infusion rate and boluses whenever needed.

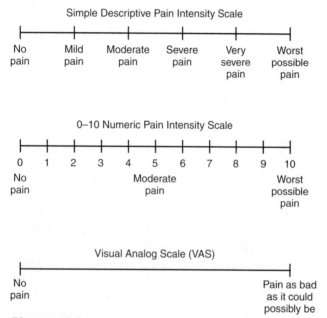

Figure 66-4

Pain intensity scales. (Redrawn from Jacox A, Carr D, Payne R, et al: *Management of Cancer Pain*, Clinical Practice Guideline No. 9, AHCPR Publication No. 94-0592. Rockville, MD: U.S. Department of Health and Human Services, Public Health Service, Agency for Health Care Policy and Research, 1994.)

Summary

THE TEN COMMANDMENTS OF CANCER PAIN MANAGEMENT

1. Thou shall not assume that the patient's pain is a result of the malignant process. Always begin with steps aimed at making a specific, anatomic, and pathologic diagnosis.
2. Thou shall consider the patient's feelings. Pain threshold varies with mood and morale. Given the

opportunity to express fears, the patient should experience less pain.
3. Thou shall not use the abbreviation "prn" (*pro re nata*, as required). Achieving balanced pain control means avoiding the return of pain resulting from gaps in medication administration. Less medication will be required if given around the clock.

4. Thou shall prescribe adequate amounts of medication. The right dose of medication is not dictated by recommendations from a book but, rather, by the patient's level of pain. Use what it takes to relieve the pain, titrating for effect.

5. Thou shall always try nonnarcotic medications as the first step unless your clinical judgment deems the patient to be in moderately severe or severe pain. Mild to moderate pain in many cases will respond to acetaminophen or NSAIDs. NSAIDs are particularly useful for bony metastases.

6. Thou shall not be afraid of narcotic analgesics. When nonnarcotic agents fail, move to a narcotic agent quickly.

7. Thou shall not limit thyself to using only drug therapies. Nondrug therapies, such as hypnosis, imagery techniques, biofeedback, physiotherapy, individual psychotherapy, group psychotherapy, and family psychotherapy, are very beneficial.

8. Thou shall not be reluctant to seek a colleague's advice. If you have exhausted your skills or run out of ideas, ask someone else to evaluate your patient.

9. Thou shall provide support for the entire family. Treatment of anticipatory grief experienced by the family will help to prevent isolation and loneliness. Be able to intervene quickly when a crisis arises.

10. Thou shall maintain an air of quiet confidence and cautious optimism. Aim for "graded relief," choosing small goals that can be accomplished to build the patient's trust and hope. Exhibit a determination to succeed.

WAYS TO ADMINISTER MEDICATIONS FOR CANCER PAIN

1. Oral: Most patients can be managed with oral medications.

2. Rectal: This can be a relatively simple way to administer medications at home to patients who cannot tolerate oral dosing. Morphine, oxymorphone (Numorphan), and hydromorphone (Dilaudid) are available for rectal use.

3. Transdermal: Fentanyl is the only narcotic available for transdermal use. It can be convenient; however, it does carry the risk of overdosage because the analgesic effect remains for 16 to 24 hours even after removal of the patch.

4. Oral transmucosal: Fentanyl is available in the form of a "lollipop" ("Acted"). Compounding pharmacies can also make concentrated solutions of morphine, oxymorphone, or hydromorphone for sublingual usage. The injectable form of methadone is also absorbed sublingually very well.

5. Topical: Topical morphine gel can be used on malignant ulcers.

6. Parenteral: Injectable narcotics are useful for rapid titration of the dose. Frequent dosing is required. For longer term use, patient-controlled analgesia devices are useful for efficient titrate dosing. They may be safer to use because patients will not administer more medication when they are sedated (they will be unable to press the button for an additional dose).

CLASSIFICATION OF CANCER PAIN

1. Somatic pain (including bone pain)
2. Neuropathic pain
   a. Type I is a sharp, stabbing, burning, "zinger" pain. Adjuvant analgesics to use are anticonvulsants, such as carbamazepine (Tegretol), oxcarbazepine (Trileptal), and gabapentin (Neurontin).
   b. Type II is a dull, aching pain. Adjuvant analgesics of choice are tricyclic antidepressants such as amitriptyline or desipramine.
3. Visceral pain: Corticosteroids are used as adjuvant therapy, especially in visceral pain where there is swelling around a visceral capsule (e.g., the hepatic capsule). These can also provide anti-inflammatory action, stimulate appetite, and decrease cerebral or spinal cord swelling.
4. NSAIDs are used for somatic pain (metastatic bone).
5. Benzodiazepines have very little utility in pain management, but muscle relaxants may help muscle spasms and neuralgias.

PATHOPHYSIOLOGY OF CANCER PAIN

1. Physical (biologic) component: 25%
2. Psychological (emotional) component: 25%
3. Social component: 25%
4. Spiritual component: 25%

Unless all four components are addressed, the treatment of cancer pain will be unsuccessful.

CONVERSION OF ONE NARCOTIC ANALGESIC TO ANOTHER

1. Calculate equianalgesic doses between drug 1 (the drug to be discontinued) and drug 2 (the drug to be started).
2. Begin drug 2 at no more than 20% of equianalgesic dose. The reasons for this are that there is tolerance built up to the first drug and that different narcotics react on different receptors in the brain.

METHOD OF BEGINNING NARCOTIC ANALGESIC FOR MODERATE TO SEVERE CANCER PAIN

1. Choice drug is usually morphine sulfate.
2. Begin morphine sulfate with short-acting morphine (morphine 5- or 10-mg tabs).
3. The daily starting dose is 30 to 60 mg/day.
4. After 1 week, switch total daily dose to long-acting morphine, and continue short-acting morphine for breakthrough.
5. Begin a bowel-regulating regimen at the same time as narcotic is begun using lactulose or a stool softener (Colace) plus peristaltic stimulant (senna alkaloid).

6. Consider antiemetic therapy for the first few weeks of narcotic therapy (prochlorperazine, dimenhydrinate, and metoclopramide).

CANCER PAIN

Optimal management combines pharmacologic management with nonpharmacologic management. Nonpharmacologic therapies include relaxation techniques, support groups, biofeedback, mental imagery, physiotherapy, transcutaneous electrical nerve stimulation, physical activity, individual psychotherapy, group psychotherapy, and family psychotherapy.

OTHER FORMS OF PALLIATIVE CANCER PAIN THERAPY

1. Palliative radiotherapy, which is especially useful for metastatic bone pain and neuropathic pain (lumbosacral plexopathy and brachial plexopathy)
2. Palliative surgery
3. Palliative chemotherapy

Suggested Reading

Bajwa ZH, Warfield CA: Nonpharmacologic therapy of cancer pain. *UpToDate*, version 14.3. Waltham, MA: UpToDate, 2006.
Bajwa ZH, Warfield CA: Overview of cancer pain. *UpToDate*, version 14.3. Waltham, MA: UpToDate, 2006.
Bajwa ZH, Warfield CA: Pharmacologic therapy of cancer pain. *UpToDate*, version 14.3. Waltham, MA: UpToDate, 2006.
Fallon M, Hanks G, Cherny N: Principles of control of cancer pain. *BMJ* 332(7548):1022–1024, 2006.
Morrison LJ, Morrison RS: Palliative care and pain management. *Med Clin North Am* 90(5):983–1004, 2006.

CHAPTER 67 Developmental Disabilities

CLINICAL CASE PROBLEM 1

A 55-Year-Old Female with a 6-Month History of "Acting Out," Increased Moodiness, and Weight Loss

A new patient, a 55-year-old female with Down syndrome, is brought to your office by her caretaker for a health maintenance visit. She lives in a residential group home with three other individuals and is cared for by in-home staff provided by a residential care company under contract with the state Department of Human Services, Division of Developmental Disabilities. The caretaker reports that for the past 6 months the patient has become increasingly "moody." She normally is quite active; she works part-time at a local supermarket and participates in activities such as hiking and arts and crafts at home. However, slowly she has become withdrawn, refusing to go out, and sometimes "acts out" by throwing things at staff when encouraged to participate in meals and laundry chores. She recently has had to be coached to perform activities of daily living in which she was formerly independent. Her appetite has diminished, and her clothes are loosely fitting, whereas before they were snug.

SELECT THE BEST ANSWER TO THE FOLLOWING QUESTIONS

1. Appropriate areas of particular inquiry regarding this behavior should include
   a. any recent changes in staff or residents in the home
   b. any recent changes at work or in her family
   c. new and current medications and recent health care events
   d. any other declines in normal functioning
   e. all of the above

2. You are unable to obtain records of her previous health care. If you were, particular areas of interest might include
   a. previous residential history
   b. immunization record
   c. sexual history
   d. a and b
   e. a, b, and c

3. You call her legal guardian for additional information. Appropriate issues to discuss with the guardian at this time include
   a. sterilization and contraception
   b. any advance directives
   c. the appropriateness of the patient's deinstitutionalization
   d. any suspicion of neglect or abuse in the residential setting
   e. b and d

4. You attempt to examine the patient, but she refuses. At this time, an appropriate method to deal with this behavior is
   a. physically restrain the patient so you can perform the examination
   b. reschedule several more brief visits before performing an examination
   c. give the patient chloral hydrate
   d. administer a dose of haloperidol
   e. give the patient a short-acting benzodiazepam

5. You see the patient at a later date to finish the evaluation. Appropriate health maintenance interventions at this time would include
   a. vision and hearing screening
   b. obtaining a serum thyroid-stimulating hormone (TSH) measurement
   c. obtaining an osteoporosis assessment
   d. colon cancer screening
   e. a, c, and d
   f. a, b, c, and d

6. Despite no obvious findings of illness and behavioral intervention by the group home staff and clinical psychologists, the patient's behavior deteriorates. She is now very withdrawn and refusing most meals. She has little interest in and interaction with those around her, including her good friend and housemate of 10 years. At this time, you decide to give a trial of which of the following medications?
   a. risperidone
   b. valproic acid
   c. carbamazepine
   d. depot medroxyprogesterone acetate (Depo-Provera)
   e. sertraline

Clinical Case Management Problem

Discuss the principles of the use of psychotropic medications in the management of behavioral disorders in the developmentally disabled.

Answers

1. **e.** Developmental disability (DD) is a chronic mental or physical impairment that results in the delay or failure to achieve normal developmental milestones. By federal statute, developmental disabilities are defined as a group of conditions that include mental retardation, autism, cerebral palsy, spina bifida, and others. Individuals with mental retardation make up the largest group of those with DD. In the past 30 years, many individuals with DD have been deinstitutionalized to group residential settings. Family physicians are often called to care for these individuals in community settings. There can be many challenges and rewards in rendering care to patients with DD. Among them is the challenge of interpreting and diagnosing behavioral changes. Changes in behavior in the developmentally disabled are a form of communication and a clue to an underlying disturbance. The disturbance can range from something as minor as a social or environmental change to a major physiologic event such as illness. Appropriate areas of particular inquiry regarding acute behavior change should include the search for social, physical, and temporal clues:

1. Any recent changes in staff or residents in the home: Residents of group homes, like all of us, are sensitive to changes in the social order. This includes not just other residents in the home but also changes in staff who could have become like family to the resident.
2. Any recent changes at work or in the family: Likewise, the patient's work environment or birth family can be a source of stress. Deaths are particularly difficult events in the developmentally disabled. Usual methods of sense-making may be absent or impaired and cause behaviors that are a reflection of insecurity, fear, and all the other emotions concomitant with loss.
3. Medications are a frequent cause of behavioral change in DD. Similarly, recent or past health care events or experiences can be a cause of trauma and result in behavioral change.
4. Any other declines in normal functioning are also clues to what may be causing the behavioral change. Staff and family should be questioned for key insights into what they believe has contributed to the behavioral change in patients with DD.
5. Changes in vital signs: Although crude measures, they point to underlying illnesses and should always be attended to carefully.

2. **e.** The past history in initial data collection is of major importance and unfortunately is often unavailable or limitedly available. If available, particular areas of interest might include previous residential history; past medical, surgical, and reproductive history; immunization record including hepatitis, tetanus, and varicella status; guardianship; history of tuberculosis testing; and current medications and allergies.

3. **e.** Legal guardians vary according to circumstance and can range from family members to state professionals, but in all states a court-appointed guardian for individuals with DD should exist. Clinicians should not presume that caretakers are necessarily the legal guardians of the patient. Appropriate issues to discuss with guardians include, at a minimum, all health status-related issues, acute and crisis care anticipation, advanced directives in the event of life-threatening illness, and any concerns about abuse or neglect. Physicians should be careful about fostering prejudices concerning the quality of life for patients with DD. Issues such as reproductive rights, if relevant, should be approached sensitively and with respect for the patient and probably after a relationship has been established with both the patient and the guardian.

4. **b.** An appropriate approach is to schedule a series of brief visits to familiarize the patient with the routine and thereby desensitize the patient to the potential trauma of the examination and visit. The use of restraints is inappropriate in most situations, but they may be used briefly in situations of potential self-harm. The use of medications is a last resort, and short-acting anxiolytics are used most often, usually administered just before the visit. Occasionally, the patient must be examined under general anesthesia, but this is necessarily limited in frequency. Given sufficient time and patience, most examinations, including pelvic examinations, can be accomplished in the office.

5. **f.** In this patient, given her age, appropriate health maintenance interventions at this time would include vision and hearing screening; dental screening; thyroid screening via a serum TSH; an osteoporosis assessment; breast, cervical, and colon cancer screening; alcohol, tobacco, and drug use counseling; safe sex counseling; diet and exercise counseling; and immunization updates including tetanus, hepatitis, varicella, and influenza as needed.

6. **e.** This patient more than likely is suffering from depression. Factors that point to this include the many behavioral changes during the past 6 months, age older than 50 years, loss of interest in daily activities that formerly gave pleasure, withdrawn behavior, and loss of appetite. Behavioral disorders are common in patients with DD, particularly depression in the aging patient. Patients with Down syndrome are particularly susceptible; they can experience age-related declines in functioning seen much later in patients with Alzheimer's disease. Consultation with a psychiatrist and a psychologist experienced with treating behavioral disorders in patients with DD is often helpful.

Solution to the Clinical Case Management Problem

The use of psychotropic agents in DD is a subject of great controversy (mainly because of their wide and sometimes inappropriate use). There are many factors that influence the decision of whether to prescribe a pharmacologic agent and which agent to prescribe. In general, nonpharmacologic measures should be tried first unless there is clear and present danger to the patient or those in the vicinity. Positive reinforcement of desirable behaviors is effective; punishment or limit setting is best accomplished by "time-outs" or privilege restriction. However, should medication become necessary, the general rule is to start low and titrate slowly. The following medications may be considered as alternatives to traditional neuroleptics: (1) Selective serotonin reuptake inhibitors can help reduce self-injurious and aggressive behaviors, (2) buspirone is effective in mild chronic agitation and generally free of most side effects, (3) trazodone can be used for moderate agitation and irritability, (4) beta blockers can help with aggressive behaviors and tremulousness, (5) newer anticonvulsants (valproic acid and carbamazepine) may control mood swings and impulsivity, and (6) risperidone is preferred over older antipsychotics because of less incidence of tardive dyskinesias.

Summary

DD is a chronic mental or physical impairment that results in the delay or failure to achieve normal developmental milestones. By federal statute, DD is defined as a group of conditions that include mental retardation, autism, cerebral palsy, spina bifida, and others.

Individuals with mental retardation make up the largest group of those with DD.

In the past 30 years, many individuals with DD have been deinstitutionalized to group residential settings. Family physicians are often called to care for these individuals in community settings. There can be many rewards and challenges in caring for patients with DD.

Changes in behavior in the developmentally disabled are a form of communication and a clue to an underlying disturbance. The disturbance can range from something as minor as a social or environmental change to a major physiologic event such as illness.

In general, health maintenance protocols are identical to those for other adults and children, but the problems associated with aging are being seen more often now as adults live longer, and aging effects occur earlier particularly in patients with Down syndrome.

Psychotropics must be used with particular caution and with careful attention to their effects. They can be over-prescribed and generally should be used after a trial of behavior modification. However, behavioral illnesses are seen more often in patients with DD, and a trial of medications is often indicated. See the Solution to the Clinical Case Management Problem for a discussion of agents.

Suggested Reading

Havercamp SM, Scandlin D, Roth M: Health disparities among adults with developmental disabilities, adults with other disabilities, and adults not reporting disability in North Carolina. *Public Health Rep* 119:418–426, 2004.

McDermott S, Moran R, Platt T, Dasari S: Health conditions among women with a disability. *J Women's Health (Larchmt)* 16:713–720, 2007.

McDermott S, Moran R, Platt T, Dasari S: Variation in health conditions among groups of adults with disabilities in primary care. *J Community Health* 31:147–159, 2006.

Messinger-Rapport BJ, Rapport DJ: Primary care for the developmentally disabled adult. *J Gen Intern Med* 12:629–636, 1997.

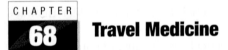

CHAPTER 68 Travel Medicine

CLINICAL CASE PROBLEM 1

A 42-Year-Old Male Filled after a Tropical Feast

A 42-year-old male and his life partner take a yachting vacation in the Caribbean. One night after a fabulous landside feast from the sea's bounty, including sea bass, red snapper, and a variety of tropical fish, the patient pays a visit to your dispensary complaining of nausea, vomiting, weakness, numbness, "lightening-like" discomfort in his face and hands, and chills. His vital signs are a temperature of 97°F orally, blood pressure of 90/50 mmHg, pulse of 110 beats/minute, and respiration rate of 20 breaths/minute. He appears ill. After supportive measures that you take, he improves in 24 hours.

SELECT THE BEST ANSWER TO THE FOLLOWING QUESTIONS

1. Which of the following is the most likely cause of his symptoms?

a. *Escherichia coli*
b. *Vibrio cholera*
c. ciguatoxin poisoning
d. Norwalk virus
e. giardiasis

CLINICAL CASE PROBLEM 2

Another Tropical Feast

He recovers, but several days later his 40-year-old partner drops by after another land excursion. He too has sampled the sea's bounty, but he carefully avoided eating what his friend had eaten the day he became sick. He stuck to mahi mahi and yellowfin tuna. After arriving back on board, he began to experience headache, flushing, hives, diarrhea, and vomiting. Physical examination reveals normal vital signs, urticarial wheals, and diffuse epidermal erythema. You take appropriate action, and he recovers.

2. The most likely cause of his symptoms is

a. ciguatoxin poisoning
b. insect bite
c. scorpion bite
d. histidine poisoning
e. *E. coli*

CLINICAL CASE PROBLEM 3

An "Ecotour" with Unintentional Sampling of the Ecosystem

A 67-year-old female comes to your office 2 weeks after she returns from an "ecotour" to the Central American rainforest. She is an infrequent visitor to your office, and her health maintenance protocols are not up-to-date, nor did she consult you prior to her trip. She tells you that she "went native," which she explains means she ate local food and drank local water, being careful to not disturb the local environment. Near the end of her trip, she developed nausea and vomiting, followed by persistent diarrhea, fever, and chills. All other symptoms have abated, but the diarrhea persists. The diarrhea is not bloody. On examination, her temperature is 99.4°F, pulse is 80 beats/minutes, respiration rate is 16 breaths/minute, and blood pressure is 140/85 mmHg. Aside from some increased bowel sounds and diffuse mild abdominal discomfort with deep palpation, the rest of her examination is normal. There is no blood or stool on rectal examination.

3. You order appropriate tests, which would include which of the following?
   a. complete blood count
   b. stool culture
   c. stool for ova and parasites
   d. b and c
   e. no tests are necessary at this time

One week later, she returns to your office complaining of passing dark urine. Examination is normal. Previous tests were negative. You order blood work to confirm your hypothesis.

4. The most likely explanation of the patient's complaints is
   a. *E. coli*
   b. hepatitis A
   c. giardiasis
   d. schistosomiasis
   e. shigellosis

CLINICAL CASE PROBLEM 4

Planning a Trip

A 35-year-old female comes in for an office visit for advice 3 months before a January departure for a 6-week trip to Thailand. She will make some day trips to some rural areas but will spend most of her time in urban areas.

5. She wonders what precautions she should take to avoid traveler's diarrhea. Which of the following is not good advice for her?
   a. avoid local sources of water that are not boiled
   b. avoid eating raw vegetables
   c. avoid drinking unpasteurized milk
   d. ice is okay for drinks because freezing kills the contaminants in water
   e. peel your own fruit

6. You review her immunization history and note that she has not received any since childhood. Which of the following immunizations would you not recommend?
   a. tetanus
   b. hepatitis A
   c. Japanese encephalitis virus
   d. inactivated poliovirus vaccine
   e. typhoid fever

7. Which one of the following statements is true for trips to mosquito-infested areas?
   a. an *N,N*-diethylmetatoluamide (DEET)-based insect repellent should be used
   b. do not use DEET on children older than age 2 years
   c. avoid insecticide use because of potential toxicity
   d. short-sleeve shirts and short pants are okay in hot weather because mosquitoes are inactive
   e. chemoprophylaxis with chloroquine works everywhere in the world

CLINICAL CASE PROBLEM 5

Another Traveler

A 51-year-old male comes to your office for a periodic health examination. He is planning on traveling to the Yucatan Peninsula in Mexico in the near future and wishes to discuss immunizations and prophylaxis against malaria. He is feeling well. He has had no major medical problems in the past, nor has he had any operations. He has no known allergies. His examination is appropriate and normal for his age. You check the Centers for Disease Control and Prevention (CDC) Web site, and there are no reports of antimalarial drug resistance in the area to which he is traveling.

8. What is the primary chemoprophylactic agent for the prevention of malaria in this area?
   a. chloroquine
   b. mefloquine
   c. pyrimethamine
   d. dapsone
   e. proguanil

9. The drug of choice you selected in question 8 should be given for the following length of time:
   a. 1 week before travel and for 4 weeks after return from travel
   b. 1 month before travel and for at least 1 month after return
   c. 2 weeks before travel and for 2 weeks after return
   d. 1 week before travel and for 1 week after return
   e. 6 weeks before travel and for at least 4 weeks after return

10. The drug of choice you selected in question 8 was chosen primarily for its activity against which of the following?
    a. *Plasmodium falciparum*
    b. *Plasmodium vivax*
    c. *Plasmodium ovale*
    d. *Plasmodium malariae*
    e. none of the above

CLINICAL CASE PROBLEM 6

A Pilgrim to Mecca

A 33-year-old male is making a return trip to Mecca for the hajj. He last made this pilgrimage 5 years ago. He is on no medications and has no allergies.

11. Which of the following immunizations is required for his entry into Saudi Arabia?
    a. yellow fever
    b. meningococcus
    c. hepatitis A
    d. cholera
    e. tetanus

CLINICAL CASE PROBLEM 7

A Bicycle Trip through Africa

A married couple of elite endurance athletes in their mid-30s will be competing in a 5-month bicycle expedition from Egypt to South Africa. They are up-to-date with tetanus, polio, and hepatitis A immunizations. They know that they will be passing through yellow fever endemic zones, and since you are an authorized yellow fever vaccination provider they have come to you for a travel medicine consultation. They also request meningococcal immunization because they will be in the sub-Saharan meningitis belt during the endemic December-to-June dry season.

12. Which of the following immunizations should you have these patients consider?
    a. cholera
    b. hepatitis B
    c. rabies
    d. a and b
    e. b and c

Answers

1. **c.** This patient is exhibiting the classic features of ciguatoxin, the most common type of biotoxin in fish. Found in such commonly ingested tropical fish as red snapper, grouper, sea bass, and a wide range of reef fish, the potential for ciguatoxin poisoning exists in all subtropical and tropical insular areas of the Caribbean Sea and the Pacific and Indian Oceans, where these species thrive. Ciguatera (ciguatoxin poisoning) is manifested by the following symptoms: gastroenteritis followed by neurological problems such as weakness, paresthesia, and dysesthesia; body temperature reversals; and, in severe cases, hypotension. Although the other choices are possibilities in gastrointestinal disturbances, the timing and history fit best with this explanation.

2. **d.** Another classic case of fish poisoning is exhibited by this patient. This time it is histidine poisoning, commonly seen after ingesting members of the scombroid family of fish (tuna, mackerel, and bonito) and sometimes also some nonscombroid fish, such as bluefish, mahi mahi, and herring. This condition is sometimes called scombroid poisoning. Occurring after ingestion of fish that has been refrigerated or preserved improperly, histidine is converted to histamine and causes headache, flushing, nausea and vomiting, diarrhea, and hives. Cases are distributed worldwide.

3. **d.** Given the patient's fever has resolved, but that it has been 2 weeks, it would be appropriate to culture the stool and check for ova and parasites. An argument might be made for watchful waiting because most domestic diarrheal illnesses resolve spontaneously, but this patient has been out of the country, which makes the possibility of parasites much more likely.

4. **b.** All prior tests are negative, and both the dark urine (consistent with bilirubin) and the incubation period suggest that she has hepatitis A. Unfortunately, hepatitis A is a common consequence of unimmunized travel to developing countries, with the virus being spread via the fecal–oral route, most commonly through ingesting contaminated food or water.

5. e. Ingestion of contaminated food and drink is the most common source of infection during travel. The list of common infections occurring secondary to ingestion includes *E. coli*, shigellosis, giardiasis, cryptosporidiosis, Norwalk-like viruses (often seen in cruise ship outbreaks), and hepatitis A. Less common infections include typhoid fever (*Salmonella typhi*), cholera, rotavirus infections, and a variety of parasites other than Giardia and cryptosporidium. To avoid illness, the CDC recommends selecting food with care. Avoid raw food such as salads and uncooked vegetables, sushi (raw fish), and unpasteurized milk and milk products such as cheese. Peel your own fruit. Avoid undercooked and raw meat and shellfish. Commercially available bottled water, preferably carbonated, is safest, and ice should not be used in drinks because it may be made from contaminated water sources and freezing does not kill all possible contaminants. On trips home, consideration should be given to the possibility that food and water on commercial aircraft may be obtained in the country of departure, where items may be contaminated.

6. c. Given this patient's age and immunization history, she is overdue for a tetanus booster. An inactivated polio vaccine booster is recommended by the CDC Committee on Immunization Practices for travel to many countries. Immunization against hepatitis A and typhoid fever should be given to protect against these illnesses transmitted by contaminated food and/or water. She should be advised to return in 6 to 12 months for a second hepatitis A immunization to make her immunity last longer. She has time to take the oral typhoid fever vaccine, the immunity from which lasts 5 years as opposed to only 3 years for the injectable typhoid fever vaccine. Japanese encephalitis virus immunization is only indicated for those individuals facing a potential prolonged stay in an endemic zone during the transmission season. It is not given more readily due to the occurrence of serious hypersensitivity reactions (urticaria, angioedema, respiratory distress, and anaphylaxis) in up to 0.6% of those receiving the vaccine. These reactions can occur immediately or up to 1 week after immunization, so those receiving the vaccine should be observed in the medical office for 30 minutes and should not travel for at least 10 days. In this case, the patient's potential rural exposure will be minimal and she will not be in Thailand during a time of peak transmission of the virus.

7. a. Mosquito and other arthropod-borne illnesses are a serious concern for travelers. Malaria, Dengue fever, West Nile fever, and various encephalitides are all capable of producing significant morbidity and mortality. Protection from the insect carriers of these diseases is important. Topical insect repellents containing DEET are most effective, but they should not be used on infants younger than age 2 months. Bed netting, proper clothing that covers skin surfaces as much as possible, and permethrin spray for clothing are all good precautions. *P. falciparum* is resistant to chloroquine in the majority of malaria-endemic countries.

8. b. Recommendations from the CDC are as follows: "For travel to areas of risk where chloroquine-resistant *P. falciparum* has not been reported, once-a-week use of chloroquine alone is recommended for prophylaxis. Persons who experience uncomfortable side effects after taking chloroquine may tolerate the drug better by taking it with meals. As an alternative, the related compound hydroxychloroquine sulfate may be better tolerated. Travelers unable to take chloroquine or hydroxychloroquine should take atovaquone/proguanil, doxycycline, or mefloquine; these antimalarial drugs are also effective against chloroquine-sensitive parasites." One of the latter three drugs should be used in areas of chloroquine resistance, with the exception of a few areas in Southeast Asia where there is mefloquine resistance that require the use of either atovaquone/proguanil or doxycycline.

9. a. The usual recommendation is that treatment should begin 1 week before traveling to the malaria-endemic area and continue for 4 weeks after the return home.

10. a. There are several strains of plasmodium that cause malaria. They are *P. falciparum*, *P. ovale*, *P. vivax*, and *P. malariae*. Most of the concern arises over *P. falciparum*, and it is crucial that treatment be directed to the most virulent and morbidity-producing strain. In addition, drug resistance has been seen primarily in *P. falciparum*; with only a few exceptions, the others remain sensitive to chloroquine.

11. b. According to the CDC, "visitors from all over the world arriving for the purpose of 'Umra' or pilgrimage or for seasonal work are requested to produce a certificate of vaccination against meningitis not more than 3 years and not less than 10 days before arrival in Saudi Arabia." Anyone older than 2 years of age must be given the quadrivalent vaccine against serogroups A, C, Y, and W135. Children between 3 months and 2 years of age must receive two doses of the A serogroup vaccine at a 3-month interval. Immunization for tetanus should be given if it has been more than 10 years since the patient's last tetanus booster. Immunization for hepatitis A should be considered if the patient has not received this in the past. Saudi Arabia is not an area where yellow fever is endemic. Cholera vaccine is not very effective and is no longer available in the United States.

12. **e.** According to the CDC, "modes of HBV transmission in areas with high or intermediate prevalence of chronic HBV infection that are important for travelers to consider are contaminated injection and other equipment used for health care-related procedures and blood transfusions from unscreened donors." These patients will be at particular risk for needing medical and surgical care due to the potential for trauma during their cycling activity. As noted by the CDC, "travelers with extensive unprotected outdoor exposure in rural areas, such as might be experienced while bicycling, camping, hiking, or engaging in certain occupational activities, might be at high risk even if their trip is brief." Pre-exposure rabies immunization consists of three doses over a 3- or 4-week period. Postexposure immunization consists of two doses for previously immunized individuals and five doses plus a dose of rabies immune globulin (RIG) for those not previously immunized. As previously noted, cholera vaccine is not very effective and is no longer available in the United States. A clinician should also check the CDC Web site (www.cdc.gov/travel/default.aspx) for the traveler's destination points to determine if additional immunizations and precautions are required.

Summary

"The world is getting smaller" is more than just a cliché. Infectious and communicable diseases respect no political boundaries, and increasingly mobile populations make the spread of once geographically limited or confined illnesses no longer unusual. The best medicine here is prevention.

Avoid areas of local epidemics and take precautions if this is unavoidable. Travel insurance is important and less costly than the alternative, particularly if air transportation/evacuation becomes necessary to access medical care.

Protection from arthropod-borne illnesses is important in warmer climates and primarily involves the use of protective clothing, protected sleep environment, and the application of the insect repellent DEET.

In rural or developing areas, avoid local drinking water supplies and food that is not thoroughly cooked.

Immunize against common infectious illnesses such as hepatitis A and B. Remember that seasonal differences may exist in travel to different hemispheres, necessitating influenza vaccination. If traveling to malaria-endemic areas, begin prophylaxis with appropriate medications.

Always check the CDC Web site for the most up-to-date, geographically specific travel-related information.

Suggested Reading

Centers for Disease Control and Prevention, Travelers' Health Web. Available at www.cdc.gov/travel/default.aspx.

Centers for Disease Control and Prevention: *Epidemiology and Prevention of Vaccine-Preventable Diseases*, 9th ed. Washington, DC: Public Health Foundation, 2006.

Kaplan DH: Holiday hazards: Common stings from New World visits. *Clin Exp Dermatol* 28(1):85–88, 2003.

Katz BZ: Traveling with children. *Pediatr Infect Dis J* 22(3):274–276, 2003.

Moore DA, Jennings RM, Doherty TF, et al: Assessing the severity of malaria. *BMJ* 326(7393):808–809, 2003.

Ryan ET, Wilson ME, Kain CK: Illness after international travel. *N Engl J Med* 347(7):505–516, 2002.

Zuckerman JN: Recent developments: Travel medicine. *BMJ* 325(7358):260–264, 2002.

WOMEN'S HEALTH

CLINICAL CASE PROBLEM 1

A 61-Year-Old Postmenopausal Female

A 61-year-old white postmenopausal female comes to your office for a routine health exam. She has a history of osteoarthritis, and she smokes one pack of cigarettes per day. She fractured her left wrist at age 50 years after falling down some stairs. Her mother has osteoporosis and fractured her hip after a fall. Her diet is low in calcium-rich foods, and she is not currently taking a calcium supplement. She is on no medications. Her blood pressure is 120/80 mmHg, her height is 5 foot 3 inches, and she weighs 115 pounds. The rest of her physical exam is normal.

SELECT THE BEST ANSWER TO THE FOLLOWING QUESTIONS

1. You believe she is at risk for osteoporosis. You initially recommend that she
   a. obtain a central dual-energy x-ray absorptiometry (DXA) scan
   b. start a bisphosphonate immediately
   c. obtain serum calcium, thyroid-stimulating hormone (TSH), and 25-hydroxy vitamin D levels
   d. obtain a lateral spine x-ray
   e. obtain a quantitative computed tomography (QCT) scan

2. The test of choice in the diagnosis of osteoporosis is
   a. quantitative ultrasound (QUS)
   b. peripheral DXA (pDXA)
   c. central DXA
   d. QCT
   e. plain x-ray of the thoracic spine

3. Which of the following is not an established major risk factor for osteoporosis?
   a. low body weight
   b. current smoking
   c. history of fragility fracture in first-degree relative
   d. low calcium intake
   e. chronic use of steroids

4. According to the National Osteoporosis Foundation (NOF), in which case would primary screening for osteoporosis be appropriate?
   a. a 28-year-old female athlete with a 5-month history of amenorrhea
   b. a 40-year-old female with regular menses who smokes two packs of cigarettes per day
   c. a 68-year-old female with no risk factors
   d. a 35-year-old female with regular menses with multiple fractures after a motor vehicle accident
   e. a 40-year-old male who smokes two packs of cigarettes per day

5. According to the World Health Organization (WHO), osteoporosis is defined as
   a. bone mineral density (BMD) between 1.5 and 2 standard deviations below the mean for young normal adults (*T* score)
   b. BMD between 1.5 and 2 standard deviations below the mean for age-matched adults (*Z* score)
   c. BMD less than 2.5 standard deviations below the mean for young normal adults (*T* score)
   d. BMD less than 2.5 standard deviations below the mean for age-matched adults (*Z* score)
   e. osteoporosis is not defined by BMD at all

6. Which of the following is not an associated risk factor for osteoporosis?
   a. low calcium intake
   b. sedentary lifestyle
   c. cigarette smoking
   d. obesity
   e. excessive alcohol intake

7. What is the most common presenting fracture in osteoporosis?
   a. wrist fracture (Colles' fracture)
   b. vertebral compression fracture
   c. femoral neck fracture
   d. tibial fracture
   e. femoral head fracture

8. Which of the following sites for osteoporotic fracture is most commonly associated with morbidity and mortality?
   a. Ward's triangle (hip)
   b. the femoral neck (hip)
   c. the thoracic vertebrae (spine)
   d. the lumbar vertebrae (spine)
   e. the distal radius (wrist)

9. Which of the following conditions is not associated with an increased risk for osteoporosis?
   a. hyperparathyroidism
   b. rheumatoid arthritis
   c. history of solid organ transplant
   d. chronic dilantin therapy
   e. history of osteoarthritis

10. You order a central DXA scan on the patient in Clinical Case 1. The scan returns with a *T* score of –1.3 for the lumbar spine and *T* score of –1.9 for the total hip. What do you recommend to the patient at this time?
    a. no action needed; her lumbar spine reading does not qualify her for treatment
    b. repeat a central DXA in 6 months
    c. recommend adequate calcium intake and weight-bearing exercise
    d. recommend adequate calcium intake, weight-bearing exercise, and a bisphosphonate
    e. recommend adequate calcium intake, weight-bearing exercise, and calcitonin

11. Which of the following is not a therapy approved by the Food and Drug Administration (FDA) for the prevention of osteoporosis?
    a. bisphosphonates
    b. selective estrogen receptor modulators (SERMS)
    c. calcium supplementation
    d. teriparatide
    e. estrogen

12. Which of the following statements regarding non-pharmacologic management for the prevention and treatment of postmenopausal osteoporosis is true?
    a. patients should obtain an adequate intake of dietary calcium (at least 1200 mg/day, including supplements if necessary)
    b. patients should obtain an adequate intake of dietary vitamin D (400 to 800 IU/day)
    c. patients should be encouraged to participate in regular weight-bearing and muscle-strengthening exercise
    d. patients should be assessed for fall risk and educated in fall prevention strategies
    e. all of the above

13. Which of the following statements about calcium supplementation is true?
    a. calcium carbonate absorption is best in an acidic environment
    b. calcium carbonate absorption is not dependent on gastric pH
    c. calcium citrate is not recommended in elderly patients
    d. calcium citrate is not recommended in patients on antacids
    e. none of the above

14. Which of the following is not recommended for treatment of established osteoporosis?
    a. estrogen
    b. calcium and vitamin D
    c. bisphosphonates
    d. SERMs
    e. calcitonin

15. Which of the following studies may be indicated in an asymptomatic patient recently diagnosed with osteoporosis?
    a. 240-hour urine calcium
    b. serum 25-hydroxy vitamin D
    c. complete blood count (CBC)
    d. TSH
    e. all of the above

16. The following statements about BMD testing are true except
    a. it is appropriate in patients who have evidence of osteopenia on plain x-ray
    b. Medicare does not cover BMD testing in any situation
    c. it is appropriate to repeat testing in order to monitor long-term treatment of osteoporosis
    d. it is appropriate to repeat testing every 1 or 2 years in at-risk patients
    e. none of the above

17. Your patient from Clinical Case 1 returns after taking a bisphosphonate for 6 months for confirmed osteoporosis. Her initial lab work was normal, including CBC, serum chemistry, and 25-hydroxyvitamin D. A baseline serum N-telopeptide

level was done prior to the initiation of bisphosphonate therapy and found to be elevated. The patient has followed your recommendations about weight-bearing exercise and calcium intake. She wants to know if the "treatments have worked." You tell her the following test may assess effectiveness of treatment at this time:

a. repeat DXA
b. plain x -ray of the hip
c. repeat serum calcium level
d. repeat serum N-telopeptide level
e. there is no test that will reflect treatment efficacy at this time

---

Clinical Case Management Problem

Discuss nonpharmacologic measures that may be employed in the prevention and treatment of osteoporosis.

Answers

1. **a.** A central DXA is the gold standard for assessment of BMD. During this procedure, two beams of different energy are directed at the patient. The difference in the absorption rate of the two energy beams by the patient's body is recorded to quantify the amount of bone mineral content. A BMD is computed at different sites, including the lumbar spine (L1–L4), femoral neck, and total proximal femur (hip); Ward's triangle is a computer-generated area and should not be used for diagnosis. At least two different sites, preferably the spine and hip, should be measured. Of all measurements, total hip BMD is the best predictor of future hip fracture. Advantages of central DXA include higher precision, minimal radiation exposure, and rapid scanning time. Disadvantages include cost and nonportability, which can make widespread screening in disadvantaged populations challenging. QCT scans can selectively measure BMD and exclude extraosseous calcium deposits. However, QCT cannot assess BMD at the proximal femur and has relatively high doses of radiation. Central DXA BMD has better correlation with fracture risk than QCT scan BMD. A lateral spine x-ray may reveal evidence of vertebral compression fractures or rarefication of bony elements, which should make one suspicious of osteoporosis; however, it is not a good screening tool in asymptomatic patients. A vertebral fracture assessment can be ordered with a DXA if a vertebral compression fracture is suspected.

Starting a bisphosphonate or performing laboratory assessments for secondary causes of osteoporosis is not appropriate for this patient until a diagnosis of osteopenia or osteoporosis has been established. The American College of Rheumatology (ACR) recommends starting a bisphosphonate in patients initiating chronic corticosteroid treatment (>5 mg/day for more than 3 months), even prior to obtaining a DXA. ACR also recommends initiating bisphosphonate therapy in patients already on chronic corticosteroid therapy if their DXA *T* score is –1.

2. **c.** As discussed previously, central DXA is the gold standard for assessment of BMD. QCT scan was discussed previously as well. Peripheral bone densitometry devices utilize a variety of techniques, including radiographic absorptiometry (RA) and pDXA). Peripheral QUS is yet another method of assessing BMD. Measurement sites include the finger, forearm, and heel. Advantages of these modalities include less expense, easier portability, and relatively low to no radiation exposure. Peripheral devices can be useful for assessing fracture risk and identifying patients unlikely to have osteoporosis. However, peripheral BMD devices lack the precision of central DXA and thus should not be used for diagnosing osteoporosis or osteopenia or for monitoring patients.

3. **d.** Of the major risk factors for postmenopausal osteoporosis, patient age older than 65 years is most consistently associated with increased risk of osteoporosis. Compared to women aged 50 to 54 years, there is a 5.9-fold higher risk of osteoporosis in women aged 65 to 69 years and a 14.3-fold higher risk in women aged 75 to 79 years. In addition to age, gender, and menopausal status, NOF lists the following major risk factors for postmenopausal osteoporosis and related fracture:

- Personal history of fracture as an adult (especially after age 45 years; not including fingers, toes, and skull)
- History of fragility fracture in a first-degree relative (especially maternal hip fracture)
- Low body weight (less than approximately 127 pounds)
- Current smoking
- Use of oral corticosteroid therapy for more than 3 months

Additional risk factors include estrogen deficiency at an early age (<45 years old), low calcium intake (lifelong), low physical activity, excessive alcohol (more than 2 drinks/day), impaired vision, dementia, poor health/frailty, and recent falls.

4. **c.** The NOF expert panel recommends that all women 65 years of age or older be screened for osteoporosis regardless of the presence or absence of risk factors. Younger postmenopausal women with one or more risk factors (other than being white, postmenopausal, and female) should also be screened for BMD (see major risk factors listed in answer 3). Although in practice these guidelines are extrapolated for all women and even men in some cases (i.e., chronic steroid use), NOF's guidelines are based on studies done primarily on postmenopausal Caucasian women only. Data on men and women of other races are insufficient to make definitive recommendations for these population groups. When deciding who to screen for osteoporosis, physicians should make recommendations that account for an individual's risk factors, willingness to start treatment, and patient preference. The U.S. Preventive Services Task Force (USPSTF) also recommends universal BMD screening for all women 65 years of age or older. For women age 60 years or older, USPSTF recommends screening if there are risk factors for osteoporotic fractures. In contrast to NOF, USPSTF makes no recommendation for or against routine screening in postmenopausal women younger than age 60 or aged 60 to 64 years without increased risk for osteoporotic fracture.

The patient described in choice a may suffer from the "female athlete triad," a condition commonly found in high-level competitive female athletes. The triad consists of eating disorder, osteoporosis, and amenorrhea. Although this patient is certainly at risk for fracture later in adult life if this condition continues, there are no formal guidelines that recommend screening women at this young age. Medical attention should be focused on correcting the underlying problem (low body weight and excessive exercise) and encouraging adequate calcium intake. The patients described in choices b and d have risk factors associated with osteoporosis but are premenopausal and are too young to recommend for screening. Of note, a "fragility" fracture is not associated with major trauma such as a motor vehicle accident.

5. **c.** Bone mineral density measurements are reported as the number of standard deviations from the mean BMD in a young healthy female reference population (*T* score) or an age-matched reference population (*Z* score). As shown in Table 69-1, WHO defines "normal" as a BMD *T* score above –1. Osteopenia is defined as a *T* score from –1 to –2.5. Osteoporosis is defined as a *T* score at or below –2.5. Osteopenia and osteoporosis are not defined by *Z* scores.

6. **d.** The major risk factors for osteoporosis and related fracture were discussed previously. Other associated risk factors for osteoporosis include certain

Table 69-1	World Health Organization Criteria for Diagnosis of Bone Status	
T* Score	**Classification**
Above or equal to –1	Normal
Between –1 and –2.5	Ostoepenia (low bone mass)
–2.5 or lower	Osteoporosis
–2.5 or lower + fracture	Severe osteoporosis

* T score indicates the number of standard deviations below or above the average peak bone mass in young adults.

medical conditions such as rheumatoid arthritis, chronic obstructive pulmonary disease (COPD), hyperthyroidism, and hyperparathyroidism, as well as the chronic use of certain medications, such as anticonvulsants, gonadotropin-releasing hormone (GnRH) agonists, immunosuppressants, aromatase inhibitors, and glucocorticoids. Obesity is not by itself a risk factor for osteoporosis.

7. **b.** Vertebral compression fractures are the most common presenting fractures in osteoporosis. However, many of these fractures are found incidentally (radiographic) in patients who are either asymptomatic or previously thought to have a different etiology for their chronic back pain.

8. **b.** Although osteoporotic vertebral fractures occur far more often, hip fractures are the most common cause of osteoporosis-related morbidity and mortality. Hip fractures can result in up to 20% excess mortality within 1 year. Ward's triangle is not an actual anatomic site.

9. **e.** Many chronic medical conditions are associated with an increased risk of osteoporosis. Examples include hyperparathyroidism, rheumatoid arthritis, hypogonadism, Cushing's syndrome, history of solid organ transplant (secondary to chronic immunosuppression), COPD, multiple myeloma, and any malabsorptive syndromes (i.e., celiac sprue). A history of osteoarthritis may mimic symptoms of vertebral compression fracture pain but is not directly a risk factor for osteoporosis.

10. **d.** The decision to treat for osteoporosis should be based on the lowest *T* score from the sites (spine, hip, or wrist) measured. NOF recommends treatment for (1) patients with *T* scores below –2 by central DXA regardless of risk factors, (2) patients with *T* scores below –1.5 by central DXA if one or more risk factors are present, and (3) all patients who have had osteoporotic fractures. These guidelines are based on central DXA BMD measurements and cannot be extrapolated to measurements made by other bone densitometry devices.

The patient in this question should be considered for pharmacological therapies FDA indicated for the prevention of osteoporosis given her T score of -1.9 at the hip as well as multiple risk factors (personal wrist fracture, family hip fragility fracture, current smoking, and low body weight). Of note, central DXA BMD measurements can be falsely elevated in the lumbar spine secondary to osteoarthritic changes (i.e., osteophytes). The patient in this case does have a history of osteoarthritis, which may account for her higher vertebral BMD reading in comparison to her hip BMD. All patients being considered for pharmacologic therapy should also be counseled on the importance of calcium, vitamin D, weight-bearing exercise, and fall prevention strategies to further reduce their risk of fracture. Prior to initiating pharmacologic treatment, patients should also be evaluated for secondary causes of osteoporosis.

Table 69-2 lists the FDA-approved medications for the prevention and treatment of osteoporosis.

First-line treatment options for prevention and treatment of osteoporosis include the bisphosphonates, such as alendronate, risedronate, and ibandronate. Bisphosphonates work by inhibiting osteoclastic activity as well as binding to hydroxyapatite to decrease bone resorption.

All three FDA-approved bisphosphonates significantly reduce the incidence of vertebral fractures. Both alendronate and risedronate have also been shown to reduce the risk of hip fractures by 30% to 50% in patients with established osteoporosis. Because a minority of patients may suffer from erosive esophagitis, the patient should be advised to take bisphosphonates with 8 ounces of water upon awakening, remain upright, and avoid food for 30 minutes afterwards. Estrogen therapy alone (ET) or with a progestin (HT) is indicated for the prevention of osteoporosis only. ET/HT has the additional benefit of reducing vasomotor and vaginal atrophic symptoms. However, because of the potential risks of estrogen, the FDA recommends that if a woman does not have symptoms, nonestrogen treatments should be carefully considered before using estrogen therapy solely for the prevention of postmenopausal osteoporosis.

Raloxifene, a SERM, demonstrates partial agonist/antagonist effects on estrogen receptors depending on the target organ site. At the bone, raloxifene selectively binds to estrogen receptors and inhibits bone resorption. Raloxifene is FDA approved for both the prevention and treatment of osteoporosis. Although raloxifene decreases the risk of vertebral fracture, there is no evidence that it decreases the risk of nonvertebral fractures including the hip. SERMs do not increase the risk of endometrial carcinoma, and they may reduce the incidence of invasive breast cancer. However, patients should be warned that use of SERMs carries the same risk of thromboembolic events as oral estrogen therapy, as well as an increased incidence of vasomotor symptoms (hot flashes). Intranasal calcitonin is only indicated for the treatment of osteoporosis in women at least 5 years postmenopausal, who cannot use estrogen. Although studies have demonstrated that calcitonin significantly reduces the incidence of vertebral fractures, there is no evidence that it reduces nonvertebral/hip fractures. Teriparatide (hPTH 1–34) is an anabolic agent indicated for the treatment of osteoporosis only. It has proven efficacy for reducing both vertebral and nonvertebral fractures in high-risk postmenopausal women. However, it is very expensive, requires daily subcutaneous injections, and its use is limited to 2 years.

Based on this patient's BMD and risk factors, bisphosonates, estrogen, or raloxifene would be an appropriate treatment option.

11. **d.** Bisphosphonates and SERMs are both approved for the prevention of osteoporosis and are discussed in question 10. Estrogen alone or combined with progestin is indicated for prevention. Calcitonin and teriparatide are indicated for osteoporosis treatment only.

12. **e.** NOF recommends that all individuals obtain at least 1200 mg of calcium per day. The specific age at which calcium supplementation should be started is unclear, but it is reasonable to begin supplementation in early to mid-adult years to maintain bone mass later in life. A general guideline may be as follows: 1000 to 1200 mg for premenopausal patients and postmenopausal patients on hormone replacement therapy (HRT), 1500 mg for postmenopausal patients not on HRT, and 1500 mg for patients with established osteoporosis or those older than age 65 years. The average postmenopausal woman consumes approximately 600 mg of dietary calcium per day, necessitating supplementation in most patients. NOF recommends 400 to 800 IU of vitamin D per day to maximize calcium absorption in patients at risk for vitamin D deficiency

Table 69-2	FDA-Approved Therapeutic Options	
Prevention (Stops Bone Loss)	**Treatment (Reduces Spine Fractures)**
Estrogen	Calcitonin (Miacalcin)
Alendronate (Fosamax)	Parathyroid hormone (Forteo)
Risedronate (Actonel)	
Ibandronate (Boniva)	
Raloxifene (Evista)	

(dark-skinned patients and patients living in northern locations). Approximately 10 to 30 minutes of sun exposure to the hands, face, and arms a few times a week is needed to receive the daily recommended allowance of vitamin D. Many calcium supplements already contain vitamin D, and most milk is fortified with vitamin D. Weight-bearing and muscle strengthening exercises may result in only small increases in bone density but can significantly improve patients' mobility and flexibility, thereby reducing pain and fall risk. Patients with osteoporosis should be advised to avoid spine flexion exercises. Poor vision, gait disturbance, frailty, sedating medications, and other factors can increase a patient's risk for falls and subsequent fracture. Specific strategies should be employed to reduce a patient's fall risk.

13. a. Calcium carbonate is generally more potent and less expensive per pill than calcium citrate. However, calcium carbonate absorption is dependent on an acidic environment and thus should be taken with food in divided doses (maximum 600 mg/dose). Patients with chronic achlorhydria may not absorb calcium carbonate as effectively. Calcium citrate is effective regardless of gastric pH/need for food, and it may be a better choice in patients with achlorhydria such as the elderly or patients on proton pump inhibitors, H_2 blockers, or antacids.

14. a. As discussed previously, bisphosphonates, SERMS (raloxifene), calcitonin, teriparatide, and calcium supplementation are recommended treatments for established osteoporosis. However, estrogen is FDA approved for prevention of osteoporosis only.

15. e. An evaluation for secondary causes of osteoporosis is appropriate in all patients diagnosed with osteopenia/osteoporosis prior to initiating pharmacologic therapy. Reasonable lab studies include CBC (malignancy/malabsorption), comprehensive metabolic panel (hypercalemia/liver disease/renal disease), 25-hydroxy vitamin D (vitamin D deficiency), 24-hour urine calcium (malabsorption/hypercalciuria), and a TSH (hyperthyroidism) if symptomatic or on thyroid hormone.

16. b. An appropriate indication for BMD testing includes confirming suspicion of osteoporosis when a patient has an incidental finding of osteopenia (rarefication of bone elements) noted on plain film x-ray. A patient may have lost approximately one-third of her bone mass before evidence of osteopenia appears on a plain x-ray. Central DXA testing is also appropriate to monitor treatment for osteoporosis at 1- or 2-year intervals (the ACR recommends repeat DXA testing every 6 to 12 months in patients on chronic corticosteroids). It is also recommended to continue BMD screening at regular intervals in patients who are at risk for osteoporosis. Medicare does cover BMD testing for patients 65 years old or older, at least every 23 months, under the following conditions: (1) hypoestrogenic women at risk for osteoporosis, (2) vertebral abnormalities, (3) chronic steroid therapy, (4) primary hyperparathyroidism, and (5) monitoring response to an approved osteoporosis drug therapy.

17. d. It is generally recommended that central DXAs be repeated no less than 1 or 2 years from initiation or change in drug therapy in order to detect significant changes in BMD. It is also important to note that drug therapy may decrease fracture risk without an apparent increase in BMD. Plain x-rays of the hip are not recommended for monitoring treatment efficacy for osteoporosis. Some experts recommend using serum or urine N-telopeptide (NTx) levels to monitor drug treatment progress. N-telopeptide is a marker of bone turnover and may decline significantly within 3 to 6 months of treatment. However, obtaining NTx levels is expensive, the results are highly variable, and this may not be covered by insurance.

Solution to the Clinical Case Management Problem

Multiple nonpharmacologic strategies should be used in conjunction with medical therapy to decrease a patient's risk of morbidity and mortality from osteoporosis. All patients should have adequate calcium and vitamin D intake. All patients should engage in weight-bearing exercise if possible. Other benefits of regular exercise include improved flexibility, strength, and agility. To minimize risk of falls, attention should be directed toward assessment of the patient's vision and gait. Any visual deficits should be corrected as best as possible. Physical therapy and/or referral to a physiatrist may be helpful for a comprehensive gait and fall risk evaluation. A home safety assessment may identify potentially correctable hazards that can lead to falls. "Hip protectors" are anatomically designed pads that can be worn in the patient's undergarment and have been shown to reduce the rate of hip fractures particularly in frail, elderly patients. However, rates of compliance can be low because of patient concerns about comfort and appearance.

Summary

1. **Major risk factors for osteoporosis**
   a. Age older than 65 years
   b. Female sex
   c. Postmenopausal status or hypoestrogenic state (menopause prior to age 45 years and bilateral oopherectomy)
   d. Low body weight (<127 pounds)
   e. White or Asian race
   f. Personal history of fracture as an adult not associated with major trauma
   g. History of fragility fracture in a first-degree relative
   h. Current cigarette smoking
   i. Oral corticosteroid therapy for more than 3 months

2. **Other risk factors associated with osteoporosis**
   a. Impaired vision
   b. Frailty/poor health
   c. Excessive alcohol intake
   d. Sedentary lifestyle
   e. Chronic use of certain medications (anticonvulsants, GnRH agonists, aromatase inhibitors, immunosuppressants, and glucocorticoids)

3. **NOF guidelines for BMD screening of postmenopausal women**
   a. All women aged 65 years or older
   b. Younger postmenopausal women with one or more risk factors (other than being white, postmenopausal, and female)

4. **Other conditions for which BMD testing is appropriate**
   a. Evidence of osteopenia on X-ray
   b. To monitor response to treatment
   c. To rescreen at-risk individuals every 1 or 2 years if initial testing is normal

5. **WHO criteria for osteoporosis and osteopenia based on central DXA BMD testing**
   a. Normal = T score above −1
   b. Osteopenia = T score from −1 to −2.5
   c. Osteoporosis = T score at or below −2.5
   d. Osteopenia and osteoporosis not defined by Z scores

6. **NOF recommendations for treatment based on central DXA BMD**
   a. Patients with T score below −2
   b. Patients with T score below −1.5 if one or more risk factors present
   c. Patients who already have had osteoporotic fracture(s)

7. **Recommended therapies for prevention and treatment of osteoporosis**
   a. For all patients
      i. Calcium (at least 1200 mg/day) supplementation and vitamin D (400 to 800 mg in individuals at risk for deficiency) supplementation
      ii. Weight-bearing exercise
      iii. Fall prevention strategies
   b. For prevention of osteoporosis only
      i. Estrogen
   c. For treatment of osteoporosis only
      i. Calcitonin (demonstrated efficacy for vertebral fracture reduction only)
      ii. Teriparatide (demonstrated efficacy for vertebral and nonvertebral fracture reduction)
   d. For prevention and treatment of osteoporosis
      i. Bisphosphonates (demonstrated efficacy for vertebral fracture reduction; alendronate and risedronate for nonvertebral and hip fracture reduction as well)
      ii. Raloxifene (demonstrated efficacy for vertebral fracture reduction only)

Suggested Reading

American Association of Clinical Endocrinologists: Medical guidelines for clinical practice for the prevention and treatment of postmenopausal osteoporosis: 2001 edition, with selected updates for 2003. Available at www.aace.com/pub/pdf/guidelines/osteoporosis2001Revised.pdf.

American College of Rheumatology: Recommendations for the prevention and treatment of glucocorticoid-induced osteoporosis. Available at www.rheumatology.org/publications/guidelines/osteo/osteoupdate.asp?aud=mem.

National Institute of Arthritis and Musculoskeletal and Skin Diseases: Osteoporosis overview. Available at www.niams.nih.gov/bone/osteoporosis.htm.

National Osteoporosis Foundation: Clinical guidelines. Available at www.nof.org.

U.S. Department of Health and Human Services, Agency for Healthcare Research and Quality: U.S. Preventive Services Task Force: Guidelines on osteoporosis screening. Available at www.ahcpr.gov/clinic/uspstfix.htm.

CLINICAL CASE PROBLEM 1

A 41-Year-Old Female with a Painless Breast Lump

A 41-year-old female comes to your office after finding a breast lump during a routine self-examination. She has been examining her breasts regularly for the past 5 years; this is the first lump she has found. On examination, there is a lump located in the right breast. The lump's anatomic location is in the upper outer quadrant. It is approximately 3 cm in diameter and is not fixed to skin or muscle. It has a hard consistency. There are three axillary nodes present on the right side; each node is approximately 1 cm in diameter. No lymph nodes are present on the left.

SELECT THE BEST ANSWER TO THE FOLLOWING QUESTIONS

1. At this time, what would you do?
   a. tell the patient that she has fibrocystic breast disease; ask her to return in 1 month, preferably 10 days after the next period, for a recheck
   b. tell the patient to see her lawyer and update her will; prognosis is grave
   c. tell the patient to go home and relax; we generally get too worked up about breast lumps
   d. order an ultrasound of the area
   e. none of the above

2. What is the first diagnostic procedure that should be performed in this patient?
   a. ultrasound of the breast
   b. mammography
   c. fine needle biopsy
   d. all of the above
   e. none of the above

3. What is the definitive procedure that should be performed in this patient?
   a. ultrasound of the breast
   b. mammography
   c. biopsy
   d. all of the above
   e. none of the above

CLINICAL CASE PROBLEM 2

A 49-Year-Old Female with a Suspicious Lesion Discovered on Mammography

A mammographic examination uncovered a very suspicious lesion in the right breast of a 49-year-old female. Clinically, the lesion is a 3-cm mass present in the left upper outer quadrant. No axillary lymph nodes are palpable. You refer her to a surgeon who books her for a surgical procedure.

4. What surgical procedure should be used in this patient?
   a. a lumpectomy
   b. a modified radical mastectomy
   c. a lumpectomy plus axillary lymph node dissection
   d. a modified radical mastectomy plus axillary lymph node dissection
   e. none of the above

5. The risk factors for carcinoma of the breast include which of the following?
   a. a first-degree relative with breast cancer
   b. nulliparity
   c. birth of a first child after age 35 years
   d. early menarche
   e. all of the above

6. Current estimates suggest that one out of every how many women will eventually develop breast cancer?
   a. 1 out of 8
   b. 1 out of 15
   c. 1 out of 25
   d. 1 out of 50
   e. 1 out of 100

7. The U.S. Preventive Services Task Force (USPSTF) recommends which of the following as the preferred mammographic screening protocol for breast cancer in women?
   a. screen all women older than age 40 years every year
   b. screen all women age 40 years or older every 1 or 2 years
   c. screen all women age 50 years or older every 1 or 2 years
   d. screen all women older than age 55 years every 1 or 2 years
   e. screen all women between the ages of 35 and 40 years with a baseline mammogram, and screen all women older than age 40 years every 1 or 2 years

8. Which of the following statements regarding breast-conserving surgery or lumpectomy for stage I or II disease is correct?
    a. lumpectomy and breast irradiation are just as effective as modified radical mastectomy (MRM)
    b. lumpectomy has not undergone enough testing to predict its efficacy relative to MRM
    c. patient preference should be followed because data are scarce for any scientific-based treatment recommendations
    d. MRM remains the treatment of choice for most women with breast cancer
    e. nobody really knows for sure

9. What is the most common histologic type of breast cancer?
    a. infiltrating ductal carcinoma
    b. medullary carcinoma
    c. invasive lobular carcinoma
    d. noninvasive intraductal carcinoma
    e. papillary ductal carcinoma

CLINICAL CASE PROBLEM 3

A 42-Year-Old Female with Painful Bilateral Breast Masses That Wax and Wane with Her Period

A 42-year-old female comes to your office with bilateral breast masses that are painful and seem to "come and go" depending on the stage of the menstrual cycle. There is significant pain with these masses during menstruation.

On examination, there are two areas of dense tissue, one in each breast, and each is approximately 4 cm in diameter. No axillary lymph nodes are palpable.

10. What is the most likely diagnosis in this patient?
    a. carcinoma of the breast
    b. mammary dysplasia (fibrocystic disease)
    c. fibroadenoma
    d. Paget's disease of the breast
    e. none of the above

11. If medical treatment is indicated and prescribed for the condition described here, which of the following should be considered as the therapeutic agent of first choice?
    a. hormone therapy: the oral contraceptive pill
    b. hormone therapy: danazol
    c. a thiazide diuretic
    d. vitamin E
    e. none of the above

CLINICAL CASE PROBLEM 4

A 23-Year-Old Female with a Firm But Mobile Mass

A 23-year-old female consults her physician because of a breast mass; the mass is mobile, firm, and approximately 1 cm in diameter. It is located in the upper outer quadrant of the right breast. No axillary lymph nodes are present.

12. What is the most likely diagnosis in this patient?
    a. carcinoma of the breast
    b. mammary dysplasia (fibrocystic disease)
    c. fibroadenoma
    d. Paget's disease of the breast
    e. none of the above

13. What is the treatment of choice for the condition described here?
    a. modified radical mastectomy
    b. lumpectomy
    c. biopsy
    d. radical mastectomy
    e. watchful waiting

CLINICAL CASE PROBLEM 5

A 33-Year-Old Female with a Small Lump and a Bloody Nipple Discharge

A 33-year-old female comes to your office with a 2-month history of a bloody unilateral left nipple discharge. She also has noted a small and soft lump just beneath the areola on the left side.

On examination, there is a 4-mm soft mass located just inferior to the left areola. No other abnormalities are present in either breast.

14. What is the most likely diagnosis in this patient?
    a. carcinoma of the breast
    b. fibroadenoma
    c. intraductal papilloma
    d. fibrocystic breast disease
    e. none of the above

Clinical Case Management Problem

The following consist of seven brief case histories describing seven patients with different combinations of stages of breast cancer using the American Joint Committee on Cancer (AJCC) classification and estrogen receptor status. The AJCC staging system is based on combinations of tumor size, nodal involvement, and metastasis (TNM). Match the numbered clinical case problem history to the preferred treatment option. Discuss the use of each of the following treatment options for each case:

   a. Tamoxifen
   b. Adjuvant combination chemotherapy
   c. Surgery and reconstruction
   d. Radiation
   e. Multimodal therapy

1. A 37-year-old premenopausal woman with an estrogen receptor-positive breast cancer at stage 2A (three positive axillary lymph nodes, no metastases)

2. A 34-year-old premenopausal women with an estrogen receptor-positive breast cancer at stage 1 (negative axillary lymph nodes, no metastases)

3. A 42-year-old premenopausal woman with a 1.5-cm estrogen receptor-negative breast cancer with negative axillary lymph nodes

4. A 61-year-old postmenopausal woman with a 3-cm estrogen receptor-positive breast cancer with positive axillary lymph nodes

5. A 63-year-old postmenopausal woman with a 2-cm estrogen receptor-negative breast cancer with positive axillary lymph nodes

6. A 58-year-old postmenopausal woman with a 2-cm estrogen receptor-positive breast cancer and negative axillary lymph nodes

7. A 72-year-old postmenopausal woman with a 3-cm estrogen receptor-negative breast cancer with negative axillary lymph nodes

Answers

1. **e.** The most likely diagnosis in this patient is carcinoma of the breast. Therefore, delay is not appropriate. However, even if that were the diagnosis, it is not a death sentence. The most common presenting symptom in breast cancer is a painless lump. Although the cause of such benign lumps is generally unknown, diabetes mellitus can induce them in a condition known as diabetic mastopathy, which most commonly occurs in women who are premenopausal and have type 1 diabetes. However, diabetic mastopathy also occurs in men and type 2 diabetics.

Other symptoms that may occur in patients with breast cancer (usually at a more advanced stage) are breast pain, nipple discharge, erosions, retraction, enlargement or itching of the nipple, redness, generalized hardness of the breast, and enlargement or shrinking of the breast.

2. **b.** On the basis of the symptoms described, the next diagnostic procedure that should be performed in this patient is a mammogram, possibly followed by an ultrasound (particularly for women younger than 35 years of age). Such imaging studies will more clearly outline the characteristics of the mass, permitting biopsy, which always must follow, using either open or fine needle. Use of the latter has improved greatly, and it currently has a very low level of false-negative diagnoses.

3. **c.** Biopsy, by either open or needle aspiration, is the surgical procedure of choice in this patient.

4. **e.** The important choice of the type of surgery and the local and regional treatment needs to be made if this is a breast cancer. This is often a difficult decision and requires considerable thought on the part of both the patient and the doctor; it also requires information (education) and time.

5. **e.** Endogenous factors associated with an increased risk of breast cancer include (1) white race (white women have approximately twice the risk of Asian women, and the risk for Ashkenazi Jewish women is again doubled [likely because this population has a high incidence of the BRCA1 and BRCA2 cancer-causing mutations]); (2) increasing age (cancer is rare among women younger than age 25 years, increases slowly thereafter, and progresses more rapidly after age 40 years); (3) a family history of breast cancer in a mother or sister increases risk up to four times and even more if the breast cancer was bilateral or premenopausal; (4) ataxia telangiectasia heterozygotes have a four times greater risk than average; and (5) risk also increases if there is a previous medical history of endometrial cancer, some forms of mammary dysplasia, cancer in the other breast, an early menarche (younger than age 12 years), a late menopause (older than age 50 years), a late first pregnancy (especially after 35 years of age), obesity, or nulliparity or not breastfeeding. For an unknown reason, risk is decreased in women who have had cervical cancer.

Exogenous, lifestyle-related risk factors include (1) hormonal replacement therapy (a selective estrogen receptor modulator [e.g., Raloxifene and Evista] may, in certain cases, be used in place of estrogen because it has little, if any, negative effect on breast tissue and endometrium while retaining estrogen agonist effects on bone and lipid metabolism), (2) estrogen-containing oral contraceptive pills, (3) use of diethylstilbestrol, (4) regular consumption of alcohol, and (5) exposure to irradiation particularly as a child.

6. a. Current estimates indicate that among U.S. women, approximately one woman in eight will develop breast cancer by the age of 80 years. It is 100 times less prevalent in men, but it does occur.

7. b. Yearly or biannual mammographic screening is recommended for all women starting at the age of 40 years. The USPSTF found evidence that mammography screening every 12 to 33 months significantly reduces mortality from breast cancer. Evidence is strongest for women aged 50 to 69 years, the age group generally included in screening trials. For women aged 40 to 49 years, the evidence that screening mammography reduces mortality from breast cancer is weaker, and the absolute benefit of mammography is less than it is for older women. Most, but not all, studies indicate a mortality benefit for women undergoing mammography at ages 40 to 49 years, but the delay in observed benefit in women younger than age 50 years makes it difficult to determine the incremental benefit of beginning screening at age 40 years rather than at age 50 years.

The USPSTF concluded that the evidence is also generalizable to women age 70 years or older (who have a higher absolute risk for breast cancer) if their life expectancy is not compromised by comorbid disease. The absolute probability of benefits of regular mammography increases along a continuum with age, whereas the likelihood of harms from screening (false-positive results and unnecessary anxiety, biopsies, and cost) diminishes from ages 40 to 70 years. The balance of benefits and potential harms, therefore, grows more favorable as women age.

8. a. The National Surgical Adjunctive Breast Project has concluded that segmental mastectomy (lumpectomy) followed by breast irradiation in all patients and adjunctive chemotherapy in women with positive nodes is appropriate therapy and is just as effective (i.e., no difference in mortality rates) as modified radical mastectomy in patients with stage I and stage II breast cancer with tumors less than 4 cm in diameter.

9. a. The most common histologic type of breast cancer is an infiltrating ductal carcinoma. This type comprises 70% to 80% of all breast cancers. The subtypes of infiltrating ductal carcinoma include medullary, colloid (mucinous), tubular, and papillary carcinoma.

10. b. This patient almost certainly has fibrocystic breast changes, also known as mammary dysplasia. All breast tissue contains cysts, and thus the term fibrocystic breast disease, as the condition previously was called, is confusing and inappropriate. The most common scenario following this label is that a woman with fibrocystic breast changes believes, in fact, that she has a serious breast disease.

Fibrocystic breast changes are most likely hormonal in origin. This may be either an estrogen or progesterone imbalance or a prolactin excess. The most common presenting symptom is pain. The pain usually begins 1 week before menstruation and is relieved following menstruation. The pain is usually bilateral and is most commonly located in the upper outer quadrants. It may be associated with breast swelling and yellow-green breast discharge.

11. a. In most women, fibrocystic breast changes do not have to be treated. If they do, the most effective treatments are a low-dose oral contraceptive pill that contains a potent progestational agent (e.g., Loestrin 1/20) or medroxyprogesterone acetate 5 to 10 mg/day from days 15 to 25 of the calendar month.

Danazol may be used to induce a pseudomenopause in patients with severe fibrocystic breast changes. It is expensive, however, and has significant side effects.

Thiazide diuretics are useful in reducing total body fluid volume and edema. In the cases of the type of "localized swelling in an enclosed cyst" that is seen in fibrocystic breast change, they are not useful.

Vitamin E has not been shown to be of value in the treatment of fibrocystic breast changes.

12. c. This patient has a fibroadenoma, or breast mouse. Fibroadenomas are the most common type of solid benign breast tumors. They are most prevalent in women younger than age 25 years. They are usually painless, well circumscribed, completely round, and freely mobile. The classic description with respect to consistency is "rubbery."

13. c. The treatment of choice for a suspected fibroadenoma is either a fine needle biopsy or an excisional biopsy. Although rare, malignancies have occasionally been found in fibroadenomas.

14. c. This patient has an intraductal papilloma, which is a small, soft tumor that is found just below the areola. If a patient has a bloody nipple discharge associated with a small, soft mass, there is a 95% probability that this is an intraductal papilloma. If physical examination reveals no mass, Paget's disease of the nipple, an adenoma of the nipple, or a breast carcinoma with ductal invasion must be considered in the differential diagnosis. The treatment of choice is surgical removal. This is often facilitated by mammography or a ductogram.

Solution to the Clinical Case Management Problem

Treatment options in breast cancer are based on staging. The National Cancer Institute (NCI) trials are based on staging, and much of the information we have on treatment is derived from these trials. Hence, staging is an important part of diagnosis and treatment. The AJCC system of TNM tumor description and staging is as follows:

Description

Tumor description is based on size, axillary node involvement, and metastasis.

Primary tumor (T)

T1: Tumor not larger than 2 cm in greatest dimension

T2: Tumor >2 cm but 5 cm in greatest dimension

T3: Tumor >5 cm in greatest dimension

T4: Tumor of any size with direct extension to (a) chest wall or (b) skin

Regional lymph nodes (N)

N0: No regional lymph node metastasis

N1: Metastasis in 1 to 3 axillary lymph nodes

N2: Metastasis in 4 to 9 axillary lymph nodes, or in clinically apparent internal mammary lymph nodes in the absence of axillary lymph node metastasis

N3: Metastasis in 10 or more axillary lymph nodes, or in infraclavicular lymph nodes, or in clinically apparent ipsilateral internal mammary lymph node(s) in the presence of 1 or more positive axillary lymph node(s); or in >3 axillary lymph nodes with clinically negative microscopic metastasis in internal mammary lymph nodes; or in ipsilateral supraclavicular lymph nodes

Distant metastasis (M)

M0: No distant metastasis

M1: Distant metastasis

Staging

Tumor staging is based on different combinations of the TNM classification.

Stage 0

T in situ, N0, M0

Stage I

T1, N0, M0

Stage IIA

T0, N1, M0

T1, N1, M0

T2, N0, M0

Stage IIB

T2, N1, M0

T3, N0, M0

Stage IIIA

T0, N2, M0

T1, N2, M0

T2, N2, M0

T3, N1, M0

T3, N2, M0

Stage IIIB

T4, N0, M0

T4, N1, M0

T4, N2, M0

Stage IIIC

Any T, N3, M0

Stage IV

Any T, Any N, M1

Treatment

The following discussion, abstracted from the NCI Web site, provides a summary of treatment options.

Stage I, II, IIIA, and operable IIIC breast cancer often requires a multimodal approach to treatment. Irrespective of the eventual procedure selected, the diagnostic biopsy and surgical procedure that will be used as primary treatment should be performed as two separate procedures. In many cases, the diagnosis of breast carcinoma using core needle biopsy or fine needle aspiration cytology may be sufficient to confirm malignancy. After the presence of a malignancy is confirmed and histology is determined, treatment options should be discussed with the patient before a therapeutic procedure is selected. The surgeon may proceed with a definitive procedure that may include biopsy, frozen section confirmation of carcinoma, and the surgical procedure elected by the patient. Estrogen receptor (ER) and progesterone receptor protein status should be determined for the primary tumor. Additional pathologic characteristics, including grade, proliferative activity, and human epidermal growth factor receptor 2 (HER2/neu) status, may also be of value.

Options for surgical management of the primary tumor include breast-conserving surgery plus radiation therapy, mastectomy plus reconstruction, and mastectomy alone. Surgical staging of the axilla should also be performed. Survival is equivalent with any of these options as documented in randomized prospective trials. Selection of a local therapeutic approach depends on the location and size of the lesion, analysis of the mammogram, breast size, and the patient's attitude toward preserving the breast. The presence of multifocal disease in the breast or a history of collagen vascular disease are relative contraindications to breast-conserving therapy.

Radiation therapy is regularly employed after breast-conservation surgery. Radiation therapy can also be indicated for postmastectomy patients. The main goal of adjuvant radiation therapy is to eradicate residual disease, thus reducing local recurrence. Different courses of therapy have been used based on clinically available data related to tumor type and size.

The age of the patient should not be a determining factor in the selection of breast-conserving treatment versus mastectomy. A study has shown that treatment with lumpectomy and radiation therapy in women 65 years or older produces survival and freedom-from-recurrence rates similar to those of women younger than age 65 years.

Whether young women with germline mutations or strong family histories are good candidates for breast-conserving therapy is not certain. The group with a positive family history, however, does appear more likely to develop contralateral breast cancer within 5 years. This risk for contralateral tumors may be even greater in women who are positive for BRCA1 and BRCA2 mutations. Because the available evidence indicates no difference in outcome, women with strong family histories should be considered candidates for breast-conserving treatment. For women with germline mutations in BRCA1 and BRCA2, further study of breast-conserving treatment is needed.

Breast-conserving surgery alone versus surgery plus radiation has been compared in six prospective randomized trials. In two trials, all patients also received adjuvant tamoxifen. Every trial demonstrated a lower in-breast recurrence rate with radiation therapy, and this effect was present in all patient subgroups. In some groups—for example, women with receptor-positive small tumors and those older than age 70 years—the absolute reduction in the rate of recurrence was small (<5%). The administration of radiation therapy may be associated with short-term morbidity, inconvenience, and potential long-term complications.

The axillary lymph nodes should be staged to aid in determining prognosis and therapy. To decrease the morbidity while maintaining accurate staging, investigators have studied lymphatic mapping and sentinel lymph node (SLN) biopsy in women with invasive breast cancer. SLN biopsy with complete dissection after a positive result is a commonly used alternative to axillary lymph node dissection. SLN biopsy alone is associated with less morbidity than axillary lymphadenectomy. Ongoing randomized trials will help to determine if both procedures yield comparable survival rates and if there is a therapeutic benefit to complete axillary lymphadenectomy in patients with SLN metastases.

Adjuvant chemotherapy is employed for most tumor types. A rich history of results from clinical trials is available to guide therapy. A variety of agents and regimens are available and used according to tumor characteristics. Most agents have their particular toxicities. CMF (cyclophosphamide, methotrexate, 5-florouracil) and anthracyclines are the mainstays of agents. All chemotherapeutic agents take advantage of the more rapid proliferation of cancer cells compared to normal cells of the body by targeting rapidly dividing cells preferentially. This mechanism also accounts for these agents' toxicities. Careful choice of oncologist is a key to effective management.

What about tamoxifen therapy? Meta-analyses of studies of early breast cancer by hormone, cytotoxic, or biologic therapy methods in women with stage I or stage II breast cancer have examined this therapy. An analysis published in 2005 showed that the benefit of tamoxifen was restricted to women with ER-positive or ER-unknown breast tumors. In these women, the 15-year absolute reductions in recurrence and mortality associated with 5 years of use were 12% and 9%, respectively. Approximately 5 years of adjuvant tamoxifen reduced the annual breast cancer death rate by 31%, largely irrespective of the use of chemotherapy, age (<50 years, 50 to 69 years, and ≥70 years), progesterone receptor status, or other tumor characteristics. Tamoxifen is also associated with an increased incidence of deep venous thrombosis and pulmonary emboli.

Stages IIIb and IV diseases are challenging to patients, oncologists, and family physicians. Multimodal therapy delivered with curative intent is the standard of care for patients with clinical stage IIIB disease. Treatment for systemic disease is palliative in intent. Goals of treatment include improving quality and, possibly, quantity of life. The family physician plays an essential role in all stages of disease but particularly can assist with patient decision making in these more challenging situations. Helping decide when curative treatment should be discontinued and palliative therapy substituted is an essential and important role that derives from the personal and longitudinal patient–doctor relationship.

Summary

1. Fibrocystic breast changes

a. Cause: hormonal factors

b. Symptoms: breast pain and fullness premenstrually, with or without discharge

c. Diagnosis: breast cyst aspiration supplemented by mammography and ultrasound

d. Treatment: supportive measures, oral contraceptives with low estrogenic activity and potent progestin, medroxyprogesterone acetate

2. Fibroadenoma

a. Prevalence: most frequent solid benign tumor of breast; painless, well-circumscribed, round, rubbery, freely mobile lesion; common in young women

b. Treatment: biopsy

3. Intraductal papilloma

a. Bloody, unilateral nipple discharge with a soft mass

b. Treatment: surgical removal

4. Carcinoma of the breast

a. Most common symptom: painless lump often diagnosed by the patient.

b. Treatment: multimodal depending on the histologic type and stage of disease. Modalities include surgery, radiation, adjuvant chemotherapy, and hormonal therapy for earlier stages (see the Solution to the Clinical Case Management Problem).

c. Screening: All women age 40 years or older should have a screening mammogram performed every 1 or 2 years (depending on risk factor status). If carcinoma is suspected, diagnosis, staging, and treatment as discussed in the Solution to the Clinical Case Management Problem.

d. The primary care physician should help manage adverse effects of therapy; monitor the response of possible metastatic disease to therapy and search for possible reoccurrence; provide psychological support; audit long- and short-term outcome of treatments; and, if necessary, provide palliative care.

Suggested Reading

Burstein HJ, Winer EP: Primary care for survivors of breast cancer. *N Engl J Med* 343(15):1086–1094, 2000.

Kornblith AB, Herndon JE, Weiss RB, et al: Long-term adjustment of survivors of early-stage breast carcinoma, 20 years after adjuvant chemotherapy. *Cancer* 98:679–689, 2003.

Maur M, Guarneri V, Frassoldati A, Conte PF: Primary systemic therapy in operable breast cancer: Clinical data and biological fall-out. *Ann Oncol* 17(Suppl 5):V158–V164, 2006.

National Cancer Institute. Available at www.cancer.gov.

Pronzato P, Rondini M: First line chemotherapy of metastatic breast cancer. *Ann Oncol* 17(Suppl 5):V165–V168, 2006.

Reeder JG, Vogel VG: Breast cancer risk management. *Clin Breast Cancer* 7(11):833–840, 2007.

CHAPTER 71

Vulvovaginitis and Bacterial Vaginosis

CLINICAL CASE PROBLEM 1

A 21-Year-Old Female with Vaginal Itching and Discharge

A 21-year-old woman comes to your office complaining of severe vulvovaginal itching and discharge. She just finished a course of antibiotics for an uncomplicated urinary tract infection, and she states that her urinary symptoms have resolved. She has been sexually active with the same male partner for more than a year. They use latex condoms, and she has been taking oral contraceptive pills for the past 3 months. She has no medical problems or history of sexually transmitted infections (STIs). Her annual Papanicolaou (Pap) tests have all been normal. On inspection of the external genitalia, you note vulvar erythema, fissures, and swelling. On speculum examination, you note a thick, white, curdy discharge adherent to the vaginal walls with no odor. She has no vulvovaginal or cervical lesions. You perform a gross and microscopic examination of the vaginal discharge. The vaginal pH is 4, the whiff test is negative, the wet mount (saline-prepped slide) reveals no evidence of clue cells or trichomonads, and the KOH prepped slide reveals several pseudohyphae.

SELECT THE BEST ANSWER TO THE FOLLOWING QUESTIONS

1. What is the most likely diagnosis in this patient?

a. physiologic discharge

b. bacterial vaginosis (BV)

c. vulvovaginal candidiasis (VVC)

d. trichomoniasis

e. an allergic vaginitis secondary to latex condoms

2. You treat the patient accordingly and her symptoms resolve. She returns 6 months later for her routine Pap smear. The Pap smear results return as "satisfactory for evaluation, negative for intraepithelial lesion or malignancy, fungal organisms morphologically consistent with *Candida* species." The patient is asymptomatic, and speculum and pelvic examination are normal. What is the next most appropriate step?

a. treat the patient for VVC only if her wet prep is positive for pseudohyphae

b. treat the patient for VVC only if a vaginal culture is positive for *Candida albicans*

c. treat the patient for VVC only if both a wet prep and vaginal culture are positive for yeast

d. no intervention is required at this time

e. repeat the Pap smear

3. Which of the following has not been shown to increase the risk for recurrence of this condition?

a. high-carbohydrate diets

b. diabetes mellitus

c. oral contraceptives

d. frequent/prolonged antibiotic use

e. immunodeficiency

4. Which of the following is an appropriate treatment for this patient?

a. metronidazole (500 mg orally twice a day for 7 days)

b. tinidazole 2 g orally in a single dose

c. yogurt with live acidophilus cultures (8 ounces orally or 1 tablespoon intravaginally, four times daily for 7 days)

d. boric acid tablets (600 mg intravaginally daily for 2 weeks)

e. fluconazole (one dose of 150 mg orally)

5. This patient returns 2 weeks later stating that she has not responded to the treatment you prescribed. What should you do next?

a. repeat the same treatment, but double the dose

b. repeat the same treatment, but double the duration of use

c. reconsider the diagnosis, and reevaluate the patient

d. apply topical metronidazole gel to her vulvar and vaginal areas

e. reassure the patient that it often takes several weeks for symptoms to resolve

6. Which of the following therapies has been shown to be useful in this patient if this condition is recurrent/chronic?

a. a high-potency topical steroid cream applied intravaginally

b. oral steroids

c. boric acid

d. Minocin (100 mg orally twice daily for 1 month)

e. vinegar and water douches

7. Which of the following statements regarding vulvovaginal candidiasis is true?

a. *C. albicans* is the most common cause of vulvovaginal candidiasis

b. *Candida glabrata* is not associated with chronic/recurrent vulvovaginal candidiasis

c. all *Candida* species are equally sensitive to imidazole antifungal agents

d. Pap tests are reliable tests for candidiasis

e. intestinal *Candida* is the major source of recurrent vulvovaginal candidiasis

8. Which of the following is not included in the classification for uncomplicated vulvovaginal candidiasis as defined by the Centers for Disease Control and Prevention (CDC)?

a. sporadic and infrequent episodes

b. mild to moderate signs and symptoms

c. occurring in pregnant women

d. *C. albicans*

e. occurring in nonimmunocompromised individuals

9. Which of the following statements regarding prophylactic antifungal therapy for recurrent VVC is true?

a. there is no evidence to support that prophylactic antifungal therapy for recurrent VVC reduces the risk of recurrence

b. prophylactic therapy for recurrent VCC is not necessary for nonimmunocompromised patients since their symptoms are not severe

c. prophylactic therapy for recurrent VCC is effective indefinitely, even after therapy has been discontinued

d. oral flucanozole therapy (150 mg orally once every 3 days for 2 weeks, followed by 150 mg orally each week for 6 months) has been shown to decrease the number of VVC episodes in women suffering from recurrent VVC

e. prophylactic therapy for recurrent VCC should be initiated in all HIV-infected women, even in the absence of symptoms

A 29-Year-Old Female with a Malodorous Vaginal Discharge

A 29-year-old woman comes to your office with a 2-week history of a persistent, malodorous vaginal discharge. The unpleasant "fishy" odor appears to worsen after sex. She denies any vaginal itching, urinary symptoms, or any other complaints. She is in a long-standing monogamous relationship with her husband, who is asymptomatic. She has no history of sexually transmitted diseases (STDs) or abnormal Pap test results. She has been douching weekly for the past several months. On examination, there is a thin, milky, off-white discharge present at the introitus without any evidence of vulvar irritation. On speculum examination, the discharge is homogeneous and pooling on the floor of the vagina with no signs of vaginal or cervical inflammation. You perform a gross and microscopic examination of the vaginal discharge: The pH is 6, the whiff test is strongly positive, the wet mount slide reveals the presence of several clue cells but no trichomonads or polymorphonuclear/white blood cells (WBCs), and the KOH slide reveals no evidence of pseudohyphae or budding yeast cells.

10. What is the most likely diagnosis in this patient?
    a. physiologic discharge
    b. trichomoniasis
    c. candidiasis
    d. atrophic vaginitis
    e. bacterial vaginosis

11. Which of the following statements regarding this patient's condition is (are) true?
    a. it is considered a sexually transmitted infection
    b. treating the partner will prevent recurrence
    c. it has no association with preterm labor
    d. it has no association with postpartum endometritis
    e. it is the result of an overgrowth of lactobacilli in the vagina

12. Which of the following is no longer an acceptable treatment for this patient's condition, according to the CDC?
    a. metronidazole (500 mg orally twice a day for 7 days)
    b. metronidazole (2 g orally for a single dose)
    c. metronidazole gel 0.75% (5 g intravaginally at bedtime for 5 days)
    d. clindamycin (300 mg orally twice a day for 7 days)

    e. clindamycin cream 2% (5 g intravaginally at bedtime for 7 days)

13. What is the most common class of organisms associated with this patient's condition?
    a. aerobic bacteria
    b. anaerobic bacteria
    c. virus
    d. fungi/yeast
    e. protozoa

14. Treatment for BV is indicated for all of the following patients except
    a. all nonpregnant women who have signs and symptoms of BV
    b. women who have evidence of BV based on Pap smear
    c. all pregnant women who have signs and symptoms of BV
    d. women who have a reported history of allergy to metronidazole
    e. women with a reported history of alcoholism, due to the potential interaction between alcohol and metronidazole

A 17-Year-Old Female with Severe Pruritus and Malodorous Vaginal Discharge

A 17-year-old woman comes to your office with her partner complaining of severe vaginal itching and malodorous discharge. She denies any vaginal bleeding or urinary symptoms. She has been sexually active with a new partner for the past 3 months. On external genital examination, you note vulvar edema and erythema. Speculum examination reveals copious, frothy, yellow-green, malodorous discharge with petechial-like lesions on the cervix. A bimanual examination reveals no cervical motion tenderness and no uterine or adnexal masses or tenderness. You perform a gross and microscopic examination of the vaginal discharge: The pH is 6, the whiff test is slightly positive, the wet mount reveals several motile flagellated organisms and many WBCs (>10/HPF) but no clue cells, and there are no pseudohyphae or budding yeast cells noted on the KOH slide.

15. What is the most likely diagnosis in this patient?
    a. candidiasis
    b. trichomoniasis
    c. bacterial vaginosis
    d. physiologic discharge
    e. atrophic vaginitis

16. All of the following statements are true regarding the patient's condition except
    a. it is a sexually transmitted infection
    b. it is a potential cause of preterm labor
    c. males with this condition are usually symptomatic
    d. Pap tests are not reliable diagnostic tests for this condition
    e. the organism that causes this condition is a protozoa

17. All of the following are acceptable treatments for her condition except
    a. clindamycin phosphate cream (5 g intravaginally at bedtime for 5 to 7 days)
    b. tinidazole (2 g orally in a single dose)
    c. metronidazole (500 mg orally twice a day for 7 days)
    d. metronidazole (2 g orally in a single dose)
    e. metronidazole gel (5 g intravaginally twice a day for 7 days)

18. Which of the following recommendations should you give her at this time?
    a. her partner should be treated for trichomonas only if he has symptoms
    b. screening for other STIs is unnecessary since trichomoniasis is not an STI
    c. she can continue with normal sexual activity during the course of her treatment
    d. her partner should be treated for trichomonas even if he is asymptomatic
    e. she can choose between metronidazole intravaginal gel or tablets because the efficacy for either route of administration is equivalent

19. Which of the following are potential noninfectious causes of vulvovaginitis?
    a. estrogen deficiency
    b. latex allergy
    c. nonoxynol-9
    d. local anesthetics
    e. all of the above

Clinical Case Management Problem

Describe the differences between the presentation of vulvovaginal candidiasis, bacterial vaginosis, and trichomoniasis based on the characteristics of vaginal discharge, pH, whiff test, and microscopic findings.

Answers

1. c. This patient has the classic symptoms, signs, and microscopic examination findings for VVC. *C. albicans* is a commensual organism in most women. When *Lactobacillus acidophilus* and specific fungal inhibitory factors are suppressed, infection can result. Vulvovaginal pruritus, irritation, and external dysuria are the most common symptoms. Vulvovaginal erythema and swelling are common findings; vulvar scaling and fissures may also be present.

The vaginal discharge may be normal or increased and usually is described as thick, white, and curdy, like cottage cheese, with no odor. It is usually adherent to the vaginal walls. The vaginal pH is usually normal (3.8 to 4.2); the whiff test is negative for an amine ("fishy") odor; and the microscopic examinations of wet mount and KOH preparations are positive for pseudohyphae, mycelial tangles, and/or budding yeast cells in 50% to 70% of patients with VVC.

2. d. It is not necessary to treat asymptomatic women who have evidence of *Candida* on Pap smear, wet prep, or vaginal culture because 10% to 20% of women normally harbor *Candida* species in the vagina. Antifungal treatment should be initiated for women who have signs and symptoms of VVC and evidence of yeast infection by KOH prep (pseudohyphae and/or budding yeast). If the KOH prep is negative, it is appropriate to obtain vaginal cultures at that time. However, if cultures cannot be obtained, empiric treatment may be initiated for women who have signs and symptoms of VCC but negative KOH preps. Women who have signs and symptoms of VCC and a positive culture for nonalbicans *Candida* species should be treated, preferably with a nonfluconazole azole drug.

3. a. Although high-carbohydrate and other diets have been suggested as causes of recurrent VVC, most studies have not supported dietary factors as a significant risk factor nor dietary restrictions as effective prevention. Frequent antibiotic use decreases the protective flora that usually prevents the proliferation of *Candida* species. The risk of a yeast infection appears to increase with the duration of antibiotic use, regardless of the antibiotic type. Hyperglycemia (diabetes mellitus), increased glycogen production, pregnancy, and altered estrogen and progesterone levels (via oral contraceptive pills) enhance the ability of *Candida* to bind to vaginal epithelial cells and facilitate their proliferation. Patients with impaired or deficient cell-mediated immunity are susceptible to vulvovaginal and systemic candidal infections. Other potential risk factors for VVC include tight-fitting/poorly ventilated clothes, mechanical vulvovaginal irritation (e.g., sexual intercourse), diaphragm/spermicide use, and use of intrauterine devices (IUDs).

4. e. A single 150-mg dose of oral fluconazole (Diflucan) is the recommended regimen by the CDC. Other over-the-counter antifungal vaginal creams and suppositories are also appropriate. Neither metronidazole (Flagyl) nor tinidazole (Tindamax) are indicated for yeast infections. *L. acidophilus* has not been proven to effectively prevent or treat vaginal yeast infections. Boric acid may be used for recurrent VVC but is not indicated for first-line therapy in uncomplicated VVC.

5. c. The patient typically should have responded to the previously mentioned treatments by this time. The most appropriate next step for this patient would be to reconsider the diagnosis and reevaluate the patient to rule out another etiology, concurrent infection, or partially treated candidiasis as a result of noncompliance or imidazole resistance. A vaginal culture should be performed at this time to assess for the possibility of nonalbicans *Candida* species. If your diagnosis is still VVC, the patient may benefit from a different antifungal treatment.

6. c. Boric acid, administered in a 600-mg vaginal suppository, has been shown to be effective as treatment and prophylaxis for recurrent/chronic VVC. However, its use is limited by significant local irritation. Oral and topical steroids, antibiotics (e.g., Minocin), and douching can actually worsen this condition.

7. a. *C. albicans* is the most common pathogen identified in patients with vulvovaginal yeast infections. *C. glabrata* is often associated with chronic/recurrent yeast infections. In fact, the number of cases of VVC caused by nonalbicans species is increasing, and they are significantly less sensitive to imidazole antifungal agents. This is probably because of the inappropriate use of over-the-counter antifungal medications.

Per CDC guidelines, a nonfluconazole azole drug is recommended as first-line treatment for nonalbicans VVC.

Pap tests are indicated for the screening of cervical dysplasia and malignancy, not vaginal infections. Pap tests provide no advantage over the microscopic examination of the wet mount and KOH preparations of the vaginal discharge. Patients should not be empirically treated for any vaginal infection based on the Pap test result alone. Studies have not found a strong association between recurrent VVC and the presence of intestinal *Candida*.

8. c. The CDC classifies VVC as uncomplicated if the episodes are sporadic and infrequent, signs and symptoms are mild to moderate, the fungal species involved is likely to be *C. albicans*, and the infection occurs in nonimmunocompromised women. In contrast, complicated VCC includes episodes that are recurrent or severe in signs and symptoms; involve nonalbicans *Candida* species; or occur in women with uncontrolled diabetes, debilitation, immunosuppression (e.g., AIDS) or pregnant women.

9. d. Prophylactic therapy should be considered for recurrent episodes of VVC (at least four episodes in the previous year), regardless of whether or not the individual is immunocompromised. HIV-infected patients do not require prophylactic treatment for VVC in the absence of signs or symptoms. A double-blind, randomized controlled trial compared oral fluconazole therapy (150 mg orally at 3-day intervals for 2 weeks, followed by 150 mg orally once a week for 6 months) to placebo among 373 women with recurrent VVC. Women treated with oral fluconazole had fewer recurrences than women treated with placebo, and this difference was more pronounced by the end of the 6-month treatment (9% versus 64%; $P < 0.001$; absolute risk reduction, 55%; number needed to treat, 2). However, the treatment effects disappeared after the drug was discontinued.

10. e. This patient's symptoms, physical examination, and vaginal discharge findings are classic for BV, the most common cause of vaginitis in reproductive-aged women in the United States. Many women with BV are asymptomatic. BV appears to occur when there is a decrease in the number of hydrogen peroxide-producing *Lactobacillus* organisms, raising the normal vaginal pH (3.8 to 4.2). Elevated vaginal pH is subsequently associated with the proliferation of organisms such as *Gardnerella vaginalis*, *Mycoplasma hominis*, and *Mobiluncus* species. These organisms produce metabolic by-products, such as amines, which are responsible for the characteristic "fishy" odor. This process is intensified by the addition of KOH, causing a positive whiff test. Risk factors for BV include douching, antibiotic use, use of an IUD, and pregnancy. "Clue cells" are vaginal epithelial cells that are coated with coccobacilli. The presence of at least three of four of the following (Amsel's criteria) establishes the accurate diagnosis of BV in 90% of affected women: the presence of a thin, homogeneous, vaginal discharge; vaginal pH above 4.5; positive whiff test; and microscopic identification of clue cells.

11. e. BV is a risk factor for premature rupture of membranes, preterm labor, and postpartum endometritis. The role of sexual transmission for BV is unclear.

Treating the male sexual partner of a woman with BV has not been shown to significantly reduce chronic or recurrent infection. BV is believed to result from a reduction of vaginal *L. acidophilus* organisms.

12. b. Because a single 2-g dose of oral metronidazole has the lowest efficacy, it is no longer recommended as treatment for BV, according to the 2006 CDC treatment guidelines. The other options are all appropriate treatments for BV.

13. b. BV is believed to be caused by a proliferation of anaerobic bacteria, including *G. vaginalis*, *Mobiluncus* species, *M. hominis*, and *Peptostreptococcus* species.

14. b. All women who have signs and symptoms of BV should be offered treatment. Symptomatic pregnant women should be treated as well to relieve symptoms. Metronidazole treatment in pregnancy has not been associated with teratogenic effects. However, treating BV in asymptomatic pregnant women has yielded mixed results. Allergy or other contraindication to metronidazole therapy is not a sufficient reason to withhold treatment for BV because there are acceptable alternative treatments, such as oral or intravaginal clindamycin.

15. b. This patient's symptoms, physical examination, and vaginal discharge findings are classic for trichomoniasis.

16. c. Trichomonas vaginalis is a sexually transmitted protozoan. Trichomoniasis is associated with, and may act as a vector for, other STIs. Risk factors for trichomoniasis include multiple sexual partners, cigarette smoking, and IUDs. Trichomoniasis is also associated with premature rupture of membranes and preterm delivery. Infected male partners are often asymptomatic.

17. e. Per the 2006 CDC treatment guidelines, recommended regimens for trichomoniasis include oral metronidazole or tinidazole (2 g orally in a single dose for both drugs). An alternative regimen is oral metronidazole 500 mg twice daily for 7 days. Metronidazole gel is not recommended given its inferior cure rate (<50%) compared to oral metronidazole; the use of other antibiotic gels is also not recommended.

18. d. Trichomonas is an STI, and sexual partners should be treated even if asymptomatic. Sexual intercourse should be avoided during treatment and until both partners are cured and asymptomatic. Trichomoniasis is associated with, and may act as a vector for, other STIs, including HIV. Patients with trichomonas infection and their partners should be offered full STI testing. Oral metronidazole is the treatment of choice given its superiority over metronidazole gel.

19. e. As many as 90% of vaginitis cases are secondary to bacterial vaginosis, VVC, and trichomoniasis. However, noninfectious causes can mimic infectious presentations (pruritus, vulvovaginal erythema and swelling, and discharge) and should be excluded. They include vaginal atrophy, allergies, and chemical irritation. Patients with these conditions are often misdiagnosed and treated for candidiasis. Vaginal atrophy usually occurs in estrogen-deficiency states, such as menopause. An elevated vaginal pH (>4.5) is usually noted, and round "parabasal" cells may be found on wet mount. Patients usually improve with estrogen supplementation. Vaginitis caused by either allergic reactions to latex condoms or other allergens or vaginal irritation from spermicides or other chemical agents do not typically demonstrate any classic physical findings or vaginal discharge characteristics. A thorough exposure history and examination to exclude infectious causes is usually required to make the proper diagnosis and to determine the offending agent.

Solution to the Clinical Case Management Problem

Signs	Vulvovaginal Candidiasis	Bacterial Vaginosis	Trichomoniasis
Vaginal discharge	Thick, white, curdish	Thin, gray, homogeneous, "fishy" odor	Copious, frothy, yellow-green
Vaginal pH	Normal (3.8–4.2)	Elevated (>4.5)	Elevated (>4.5)
Whiff test	Negative	Positive	Can be positive
Microscopic findings	Pseudohyphae, mycelial tangles, or budding yeast	Clue cells, no WBCs	Motile trichomonads, WBCs (>10/HPF)

Summary

DIAGNOSIS

See the table in the Solution to the Clinical Case Management Problem for a summary of the diagnostic features.

TREATMENT

Treatment options (based on the 2006 CDC treatment guidelines) for each condition are outlined as follows:

1. Vulvovaginal candidiasis (VVC): *C. albicans* is the most common pathogen identified in patients with VVC. For uncomplicated VVC
   a. A topical azole agent (intravaginally for 1 to 14 days)
      or
   b. Fluconazole (150 mg orally for a single dose)
   For complicated VCC (recurrent or severe or nonalbicans *Candida* species or in women with uncontrolled diabetes, debilitation, immunosuppression, or who are pregnant)
   a. A topical azole agent (intravaginally for 7 to 14 days)
      or
   b. Fluconazole (150 mg orally × two or three doses, 72 hours apart)
   For suppressive therapy
   a. Diflucan 150 mg orally every 3 days for 2 weeks, followed by 150 mg orally every week for 6 months
      or
   b. Topical clotrimazole 200 mg twice a week or other topical treatments used intermittently for 6 months
   For pregnant women, use only topical azoles for 7 days
   For nonalbicans VVC
   a. A topical or oral nonfluconazole azole agent
   b. If recurrence, boric acid (600 mg vaginal suppository twice a day for 14 days)
2. Bacterial vaginosis: Bacterial vaginosis is the most common cause of vaginitis among women of reproductive age in the United States.
   Recommended regimens
   a. Metronidazole (500 mg orally twice a day for 7 days)
      or

   b. Metronidazole 0.75% gel (5 g intravaginally once at bedtime for 5 days)
      or
   c. Clindamycin 2% cream (5 g intravaginally once at bedtime for 7 days)
   Alternative regimens
   a. Clindamycin (300 mg orally twice a day for 7 days)
      or
   b. Clindamycin ovules (100 g intravaginally once at bedtime for 3 days)
   For pregnant women with BV (Note: Several studies have shown an increase in adverse events with the use of clindamycin cream during the second trimester; therefore, clindamycin cream should be avoided in the second trimester and beyond.)
   a. Metronidazole (250 mg orally three times a day for 7 days)
      or
   b. Metronidazole (500 mg orally twice a day for 7 days)
      or
   c. Clindamycin (300 mg orally twice a day for 7 days)
3. Trichomoniasis: Trichomoniasis is an STD. Sexual partners should be treated and instructed to avoid sexual intercourse until both partners are cured and asymptomatic. Trichomoniasis is associated with, and may act as a vector for, other STDs. Patients with trichomoniasis should be screened for other STDs.
   Recommended regimens
   a. Metronidazole (2 g orally for a single dose)
      or
   b. Tinidazole (2 g orally for a single dose)
   Alternative regimen, metronidazole (500 mg orally for 7 days)
   For pregnant women, metronidazole (2 g orally for a single dose)

Studies have not demonstrated a consistent association between use of metronidazole during pregnancy and teratogenic effects in infants.

Patients should be instructed to avoid alcohol during treatment with metronidazole and for 24 hours thereafter.

Suggested Reading

Centers for Disease Control and Prevention: Sexually transmitted diseases treatment guidelines. *MMWR* 55(RR-11):1–93, 2006.

Egan ME, Lipsky MS: Diagnosis of vaginitis. *Am Fam Phys* 62: 1095–1104, 2000.

Ringdahl EN: Treatment of recurrent vulvovaginal candidiasis. *Am Fam Phys* 61:3306–3312, 3317, 2000.

Cervical Abnormalities

Author's note: A portion of this chapter reflects the most recent recommendations of the American Society for Colposcopy and Cervical Pathology (ASCCP) as of May 2007. Updated consensus guidelines for the management of cervical cytological and histological abnormalities were expected to be released in late summer of 2007 by the ASCCP. Please refer to the ASCCP Web site for any relevant updates in the consensus guidelines: www.asccp.org.

CLINICAL CASE PROBLEM 1

A 26-Year-Old Female with an "ASC-US" Pap Test Result

A 26-year-old woman comes to your office for her health maintenance examination. She is married with two children, and she has no major medical illnesses. She reports a 10 pack-year history of cigarette smoking. She has had 10 heterosexual partners in her lifetime and denies a history of sexually transmitted disease (STD). All of her Papanicolaou (Pap) tests have been normal. Her physical examination, including pelvic, is unremarkable. A week later, you receive her Pap result, which reads "satisfactory for evaluation, ASC-US."

SELECT THE BEST ANSWER TO THE FOLLOWING QUESTIONS

1. Which of the following would be appropriate as initial management for this patient?

2001 Bethesda System for Reporting Cervical Cytology and Histology

ASC, atypical squamous cells
ASC-US, atypical squamous cells of undetermined significance
ASC-H, atypical squamous cells, cannot exclude HSIL
LSIL, low-grade squamous intraepithelial lesion
HSIL, high-grade squamous intraepithelial lesion
AGC, atypical glandular cells
NOS, not otherwise specified
CIN, cervical intraepithelial neoplasia

---

a. repeat the Pap test in 1 year
b. perform an endocervical curettage only
c. perform human papilloma virus (HPV) DNA testing
d. perform cryotherapy
e. perform a loop electrosurgical excision procedure (LEEP)

2. All of the following are known risk factors for carcinoma of the cervix except
a. multiple sexual partners
b. early age of first intercourse
c. infection with "high-risk" HPV subtypes
d. smoking
e. alcohol use

3. What is the most appropriate approach to a patient who undergoes cervical cancer screening with liquid-based cytology and the Pap returns as "satisfactory for evaluation, ASC-US, positive for high-risk HPV type"?
a. repeat Pap test in 4 to 6 months
b. repeat HPV DNA testing in 4 to 6 months
c. colposcopy
d. continue annual Pap tests
e. cryosurgery or LEEP

4. According to the 2003 U.S. Preventive Services Task Force (USPSTF) guidelines, which of the following statements regarding cervical cancer screening is correct?
a. all women should begin cervical cancer screening at age 18 years
b. all women who have had a total hysterectomy for benign disease should continue cervical cancer screening
c. all women who have been sexually active and have a cervix should undergo cervical cancer screening
d. annual cervical cancer screening should continue for all women past the age of 65 years
e. pregnant women should not have Pap tests

5. According to the 2003 USPSTF guidelines, which of the following regarding cervical cancer screening intervals is correct?
a. routine cervical cancer screening via Pap test should occur at least every 3 years
b. women age 65 years or older should undergo more frequent Pap smear screening than women younger than age 65 years
c. women who are heavy smokers should have more frequent Pap tests than nonsmokers

d. pregnant women should have more frequent Pap tests than nonpregnant women

e. HPV DNA testing alone can replace conventional Pap tests as a method of cervical cancer screening

6. Carcinoma of the cervix is associated with which HPV types?
   a. 6, 11
   b. 16, 18, 31, 45
   c. 40, 42
   d. 53, 54
   e. all of the above

7. Which of the following statements is true?
   a. the risk of invasive carcinoma with ASC-US is less than 1.0%
   b. AGC is associated with endometrial neoplasia, not cervical neoplasia
   c. approximately 75% of women with LSIL have histologically confirmed high-grade cervical lesions (CIN 2/3)
   d. approximately 25% of women with HSIL have histologically confirmed high-grade cervical lesions (CIN 2/3)
   e. ASC-US is more frequently associated with histologically confirmed high-grade cervical lesions (CIN 2/3) than ASC-H

8. The nurse informs you that your patient recently had a Pap test result of "satisfactory for evaluation, consistent with AGC, NOS." You review her chart and note she is 40 years old and otherwise healthy. You discuss the results with your patient and advise that she:
   a. repeat a Pap in 1 year
   b. repeat a Pap in 4 to 6 months
   c. undergo colposcopy and endocervical curettage
   d. undergo colposcopy, endocervical curettage, and endometrial biopsy
   e. undergo cryotherapy

9. Your colleague asks your opinion about liquid-based cytology for cervical cancer screening. You explain that advantages of liquid-based cytology include
   a. it is less expensive than conventional Pap tests
   b. it permits reflex HPV testing
   c. collection of a cervical specimen is easier than with conventional Pap
   d. the patient is more comfortable during cervical sampling than with conventional Pap
   e. all of the above

CLINICAL CASE PROBLEM 2

A 33-Year-Old Female with an "LSIL" Pap Test Result

A 33-year-old female (gravida 2, para 2) comes to your office for a routine annual examination. She has never smoked and has no history of STDs. She is in a stable, monogamous relationship with her husband. Her previous Pap smears have been normal. Her physical examination is normal, including pelvic examination. You perform a Pap smear at this time. Two weeks later, the Pap smear comes back as "satisfactory for evaluation, consistent with LSIL."

10. Which of the following would be most appropriate as initial management for this patient?
    a. continue routine screening because she has no other risk factors for cervical dysplasia
    b. repeat a Pap test in 4 to 6 months
    c. perform HPV DNA typing
    d. perform colposcopy
    e. perform LEEP or cryotherapy

11. The patient returns after having a colposcopy that was satisfactory (the entire squamocolumnar junction was visualized). Her cervical biopsy was consistent with "CIN 1," and her endocervical curettage (ECC) was "negative for neoplasia." All of the following are acceptable management plans for biopsy-confirmed CIN 1 except
    a. repeat Pap smear and colposcopy at 12 months
    b. perform LEEP or cryotherapy
    c. perform HPV DNA testing at 12 months
    d. repeat Pap smears at 6 and 12 months
    e. perform total hysterectomy

12. You perform a routine screening Pap smear, which is read as "satisfactory for evaluation, negative for intraepithelial lesion or malignancy" but also notes that there is "absence of an endocervical component." Which of the following is the most appropriate method of management?
    a. perform an endocervical curettage
    b. repeat the Pap test immediately
    c. repeat the Pap test in 6 weeks
    d. repeat the Pap test in 4 to 6 months
    e. perform the next Pap smear per routine screening guidelines

13. Which part of the cervix is most vulnerable to dysplastic changes?
    a. the squamous epithelium

b. the columnar epithelium
c. the squamocolumnar junction
d. the superior lip of the cervix
e. the inferior lip of the cervix

CLINICAL CASE PROBLEM 3

A 26-Year-Old Pregnant Woman with an "HSIL" Pap Test Result

A 26-year-old female (gravida 3, para 2) who is approximately 22 weeks pregnant recently moved to the area and would like to transfer her prenatal care to you. She brings her prenatal records for your review. You note her prenatal history has been unremarkable except that her initial Pap test came back as "HSIL." She states that her last doctor recommended a colposcopy but she never followed up because she thought it would "hurt the baby."

14. At this time, you should advise her that
    a. it is not safe for pregnant women to undergo colposcopy
    b. it is safe for pregnant women to undergo colposcopy but not cervical biopsy
    c. she should delay the colposcopy to 6 weeks postpartum
    d. she should have a repeat Pap test 6 weeks postpartum
    e. she should be scheduled for colposcopy now

CLINICAL CASE PROBLEM 4

An Adolescent Girl Interested in the Human Papillomavirus Vaccine

You are seeing a 14-year-old girl today for a routine exam. She has never been sexually active. Her mother accompanies her to the visit and wants to know what your opinion is regarding the new "HPV (human papillomavirus) shot."

15. You tell her that the quadrivalent HPV vaccine
    a. is not necessary because the patient is a virgin and HPV is only transmitted sexually
    b. is not appropriate for the patient because she is too young
    c. is not appropriate for the patient because she is too old
    d. provides 99% to 100% protection from HPV types 6, 11, 16, and 18
    e. provides 99% to 100% protection from all HPV subtypes

Clinical Case Management Problem

Compare cervical cytological terms as classified in the 1991 Bethesda System with the 2001 Bethesda System. Correlate cytopathologic findings with the histologic classification system.

Answers

1. **c.** The 2001 Bethesda System subdivides ASC into ASC-US (atypical squamous cells of undetermined significance) and ASC-H (atypical squamous cells, cannot exclude high-grade squamous intraepithelial lesion). The risk of a high-grade cervical lesion is higher for ASC-H (24% to 94%) than for ASC-US (5% to 17%). Women with ASC-H should be referred for colposcopy given the increased risk of high-grade dysplasia.

According to the 2001 Consensus Guidelines for the Management of Women with Cervical Cytological Abnormalities, the management of ASC-US can involve any of the following: (1) repeat cytology at 4- to 6-month intervals until two consecutive negative Pap test results are obtained, with referral to colposcopy if repeat Pap is ASC-US or greater cytologic abnormality; (2) testing for HPV DNA type, with referral to colposcopy if the patient tests positive for "high-risk" HPV types (e.g., HPV 16 or 18); or (3) immediate colposcopy. There are advantages and disadvantages for each option. The rationale for repeat cytologic testing is based on the fact that serial Pap smears increase the sensitivity of detecting a high-grade cervical lesion. Potential disadvantages of this approach include added patient discomfort and inconvenience, risk of noncompliance secondary to multiple office visits, and delayed diagnosis of high-grade cervical lesions or cancer. Data have demonstrated that immediate HPV-based triage of ASC-US Pap tests has excellent sensitivity (90% to 96%) for the detection of high-grade cervical lesions, compared with a sensitivity of 75% to 85% for repeat Pap tests. In fact, the absence of high-risk HPV types has a high negative predictive value of at least 98%. The advent of sensitive HPV DNA tests (e.g., Hybrid Capture 2 System) facilitates "triaging" women with ASC-US into those with high-risk HPV types versus women with low-risk HPV types and women without HPV infection. Liquid-based cytology that permits "reflex HPV testing" for those Pap smears read as ASC-US may also be used.

The preferred approach to the management of ASC-US is to perform HPV DNA testing if liquid-based cytology is available. An acceptable alternative is repeat cytologic testing, as outlined previously, if HPV DNA testing is not available. There is less evidence supporting immediate referral to colposcopy for ASC-US. Advantages to this approach include the immediate confirmation of the presence or absence of significant disease. Disadvantages to this approach include creating unnecessary patient anxiety, patient discomfort, potential for overtreatment, and added expense. The other choices (performing an endocervical curettage alone or pursuing immediate ablative/excisional treatment) are not appropriate ways to manage ASC-US.

2. e. There is no known association between cervical cancer and alcohol use. Infection with "high-risk" types of HPV is a necessary but insufficient precursor to cervical carcinoma. The majority of HPV infections (90%) will resolve spontaneously within 2 years from the time of acquisition. The remaining 10% of persistent infections have the potential to advance to cervical precancerous lesions. The risk of progression depends on the HPV type, with HPV 16 having the greatest associated risk. Other host factors that increase the risk of cervical carcinoma include smoking, immunocompromised state, and high-risk sexual history (early age of first intercourse and multiple sexual partners).

3. c. There is a clear association between high-risk HPV DNA types and cervical neoplasia. As discussed previously, women with ASC-US who test positive for high-risk HPV should be referred for colposcopy. Women with ASC-US who test negative for high-risk HPV can return to routine screening. It is not acceptable to treat women with either ablative or excisional therapies without first doing further assessment with colposcopy because the vast majority of ASC-US pap smears resolve spontaneously.

4. c. The 2003 USPSTF guidelines strongly recommend that all women who have been sexually active and have a cervix should undergo cervical cancer screening. There is less evidence to support when cervical cancer screening should begin. Current USPSTF guidelines suggest that cervical cancer screening should be initiated within 3 years from the onset of sexual activity or age 21 years, whichever comes first. Data on the natural history of HPV infection suggest that the time required to develop high-grade lesions from the onset of sexual activity is delayed such that screening can safely occur within 3 years from onset of sexual activity. The USPSTF recommends against routine Pap test screening in women who have had a total hysterectomy for benign disease because there is low yield for detecting significant disease. Women who have had a supracervical (cervix-sparing) hysterectomy

should follow routine cervical cancer screening guidelines. There is little evidence to support cervical cancer screening in women older than age 65 years because the risk of high-grade cervical neoplasia decreases with age. In addition, cervical cancer in older women is not more aggressive than in younger women. Women age 65 years or older with recent normal Pap tests and no history of gynecologic malignancy may consider stopping cervical cancer screening following a discussion with their clinicians about the relative benefits and risks. Pregnant women should undergo the same cervical screening guidelines as nonpregnant women.

5. a. The USPSTF guidelines recommend cervical cancer screening at least every 3 years, citing a lack of evidence to support that annual cervical cancer screening is more effective. The American Academy of Family Physicians Recommendations for Periodic Health Exams makes the same recommendation. Other U.S. organizations recommend yearly screening until three consecutive negative Pap test results have been obtained, at which time screening can be done less frequently. Ultimately, the decision should be made on an individual basis based on the patient's risk factors, compliance, and personal preferences. Women older than 65 years of age who are otherwise low risk and have had recent negative Pap test results may stop screening per USPSTF recommendations. Although cigarette smoking is associated with an increased risk of cervical neoplasia, there is no evidence to support more frequent cervical cancer screening in these patients. The frequency of cervical cancer screening is the same for pregnant women as for nonpregnant women. There is insufficient evidence to recommend for or against HPV DNA testing alone as primary screening for cervical cancer.

6. b. There is a well-established association between persistent HPV infection and cervical dysplasia and cervical neoplasia. The type of HPV involved is important in determining the malignant potential of the virus. HPV types 6 and 11 are associated with genital warts and are believed to be of low-risk malignant potential. In contrast, HPV types 16, 18, 31, and 45 are considered to be high risk. HPV 16 alone accounts for 68% of viral types found in squamous cell tumors. HPV 40 and 42 are low-risk subtypes.

7. a. The risk of invasive carcinoma with ASC is extremely low (0.1% to 0.2%). Approximately 15% to 30% of women with LSIL have a histologically confirmed high-grade cervical intraepithelial lesion (CIN 2/3). The risk of CIN 2/3 is higher with HSIL (70% to 75%), not lower than with LSIL. AGC is associated with cervical neoplasia, not just endometrial neoplasia. The risk of histologically confirmed high-grade cervical dysplasia (CIN 2/3) is higher with ASC-H (24% to 94%) than with ASC-US (5% to 17%).

8. **d.** The 2001 Bethesda System classifies glandular abnormalities less severe than adenocarcinoma into three categories: (1) AGC-NOS; (2) AGC, favor neoplasia; or (3) AIS (endocervical adenocarcinoma in situ). As a category, AGS and AIS are associated with a substantially higher risk of cervical neoplasia than ASC or LSIL. "AGC, favor neoplasia" has an even higher risk of high-grade cervical lesions and carcinoma (27% to 96%) than "AGC-NOS" (9% to 41%). Regardless, all women with AGS or AIS should have colposcopy with endocervical sampling because the risk of cervical neoplasia is substantially higher than with ASC or LSIL. In addition, endometrial biopsy should be performed in conjunction with colposcopy in women older than age 35 years or in younger women with unexplained vaginal bleeding to rule out invasive disease. Repeat cytologic sampling is unacceptable as initial management of AGS or AIS. Cryotherapy is not appropriate as initial management without confirmation of the absence or presence of disease.

9. **b.** Conventional Pap tests have been limited by inadequate sampling, obscuring elements, delays in fixation, and random distribution of cells. Liquid-based cytology involves mixing the specimen in a liquid fixative and then transferring a thin layer of evenly distributed cells on a slide. Liquid-based cytology offers the opportunity to perform reflex HPV testing in cases of ASC-US. It is also possible to test for *Neisseria gonorrhea* and *Chlamydia trachomatis* using the same specimen collected by liquid-based cytology. There is good evidence that liquid-based cytology has improved sensitivity for detecting cervical dysplasia compared to conventional Pap tests. However, it is considerably more expensive and may have lower specificity. According to the USPSTF, there is insufficient evidence to recommend for or against the use of new technologies for cervical cancer screening (e.g., liquid-based cytology, computerized screening, and algorithm-based screening). Collection of the cervical specimen is the same as for conventional Pap, using an Ayres spatula for collection of ectocervical cells and an endocervical brush for endocervical cells. Patient comfort should not be any different during the collection of liquid-based cytology than with a conventional Pap.

10. **d.** According to the 2001 Consensus Guidelines, patients with LSIL should have colposcopy because 15% to 30% of these patients will have biopsy-confirmed CIN 2 or 3. Immediate referral for excisional or ablative procedures such as LEEP or cryotherapy

without confirmation of disease via colposcopy is unacceptable. HPV DNA typing is not useful in patients with LSIL because 83% of these women are positive for high-risk types. Repeating the Pap test in 4 to 6 months is not recommended because of the small but real risk of delaying diagnosis of invasive disease.

11. **e.** Total hysterectomy for localized disease is not recommended. According to the 2001 Consensus Guidelines for the Management of Women with Cervical Intraepithelial Neoplasia, patients with CIN 1 who had a satisfactory colposcopy (the entire transformation zone was visualized) may elect follow-up without treatment (preferred approach), which can occur in one of several ways: (1) serial Pap smears at 6 and 12 months, (2) HPV DNA testing at 12 months, or (3) Pap smear and colposcopy at 12 months. Alternatively, patients with CIN 1 may opt for ablative or excisional treatment. Ablative treatment options include cryotherapy or laser ablation. Cryotherapy is a simple, minimally invasive method that can be performed easily in the office setting. Excisional modalities include LEEP or cold-knife conization.

12. **e.** For Pap tests that are "satisfactory for evaluation," there is little evidence to suggest that lack of an endocervical component on Pap test increases the chance of missing significant disease. If endocervical cells are absent, the patient can repeat a Pap test per routine screening protocols.

13. **c.** The majority of the cervix is covered with stratified squamous epithelium. The area from the endocervix to the margin of the squamous cells is laid with columnar epithelium. At puberty, when estrogen levels increase and *Lactobacillus* species consequently colonize the vagina, the vaginal pH drops into an acidic range. Exposure of the fragile columnar epithelial cells around the cervical os to this acidic environment stimulates their transformation into squamous epithelium, a process referred to as squamous metaplasia. As this process proceeds over decades, the advancing edge of the squamous epithelium, also known as the squamocolumnar junction (SCJ), migrates centrally toward the cervical os and ultimately into the endocervical canal. Because of increased cell turnover, the SCJ is most vulnerable to dysplastic changes. There is no known anatomic preference for cervical dysplasia when comparing the superior lip to the inferior lip of the cervix.

14. **e.** Pregnancy is not a contraindication to colposcopy. The patient should be reassured that there is no increased risk of preterm labor or harm to the fetus with colposcopy or cervical biopsy. The most important goal of colposcopy in the pregnant patient is to rule out invasive carcinoma. Cervical biopsies may be performed during pregnancy, although the pregnant cervix is more vascular and may have increased incidence of minor (but not major) bleeding. Endocervical curettage is contraindicated during pregnancy because of potential risk of premature rupture of membranes, preterm labor, and bleeding. There is a high rate of spontaneous regression of cervical lesions postpartum. Hence, it is recommended that treatment for all but invasive carcinoma be delayed until postpartum reassessment.

15. **d.** The quadrivalent HPV vaccine provides 100% immunity against HPV types 6, 11, 16, and 18, which are responsible for 70% of cervical cancers (HPV 16 and 18) and 90% of genital warts (HPV 6 and 11). The vaccine consists of viral-like particles that produce high levels of neutralizing antibodies. The vaccine series consists of intramuscular shots given at 0, 2, and 6 months. The Advisory Committee on Immunization Practices recommends that the quadrivalent HPV vaccine be routinely administered to girls age 11 or 12 years. The recommendation also allows for the vaccination of girls as young as 9 years of age and women 13 to 26 years old. It is important to inform women that the vaccination is not therapeutic because it will not eradicate HPV strains that have already been acquired. However, the vaccine can prevent future infections from HPV types that have not been acquired. Therefore, women who have a history of or current cervical dysplasia and/or have tested positive for high-risk HPV types can still benefit from the quadrivalent vaccine.

Solution to the Clinical Case Management Problem

1991 Bethesda System	2001 Bethesda System	Histologic Correlate
ASC-US, favor reactive	ASC, ASC-US	Variable
ASC-US, favor neoplastic	ASC-H	Variable
Mild dysplasia, HPV infection	LSIL	CIN 1
Moderate dysplasia, severe dysplasia, carcinoma in situ	HSIL	CIN 2/3, squamous cell carcinoma
AGC-US, favor reactive	AGC	Variable
AGC-US, favor dysplasia	AGC, favor neoplasia	Variable
AGC-US, probably neoplastic	AIS	Variable

AGC, atypical glandular cells; AGC-US, atypical glandular cells of undetermined significance; AIS, adenocarcinoma in situ; ASC, atypical squamous cells; ASC-H, atypical squamous cells, cannot rule out high-grade lesion; ASC-US, atypical squamous cells of undetermined significance; CIN, cervical intraepithelial neoplasia; HPV, human papillomavirus; HSIL, high-grade squamous intraepithelial lesion; LSIL, low-grade squamous intraepithelial lesion

Summary

The 2003 U.S Preventive Services Task Force Guidelines for Cervical Cancer Screening are as follows:

1. It is strongly recommended that women who have been sexually active and have a cervix should undergo cervical cancer screening.
2. Cervical cancer screening should be initiated within 3 years of onset of sexual activity or at age 21 years, whichever comes first.
3. Cervical cancer screening should occur at least every 3 years.
4. Women older than age 65 years with recent normal Pap tests and low-risk history may stop cervical cancer screening.
5. Women who have had a total hysterectomy for benign disease may choose to discontinue cervical cancer screening.
6. There is insufficient evidence to recommend for or against the use of new screening technologies for cervical cancer.
7. There is insufficient evidence to recommend for or against the routine use of HPV DNA tests as a primary screening tool for cervical cancer.

The 2001 Consensus Guidelines for the Management of Women with Cervical Cytological Abnormalities are as follows:

1. Women with ASC-US may be managed by either repeat cytologic testing or HPV DNA typing. Those women with either ASC or greater cytologic abnormality on repeat Pap, or who test positive for high-risk HPV, should be referred for colposcopy.

2. Women with ASC-H should be referred for colposcopy.

3. Women with LSIL should be referred for colposcopy.

4. Women with HSIL should be referred for colposcopy.

5. All women with AGC or AIS should be referred for colposcopy with endocervical sampling. Endometrial biopsy should also be done for women older than age 35 years or younger than 35 years with unexplained vaginal bleeding.

6. Risk factors associated with cervical neoplasia include the following: "high-risk" HPV types 16, 18, 31, and 45 acting along with cofactors, which include cigarette smoking, early first intercourse, multiple sexual partners, and partner who has had multiple sexual partners or immunocompromised state.

7. Liquid-based cytology allows for "reflex" HPV testing in cases of ASC-US on cervical cytology.

8. Acceptable treatments for confirmed CIN 1 include follow-up without treatment, cryotherapy, or LEEP. Total hysterectomy is not acceptable for noninvasive disease.

9. The squamocolumnar junction of the cervix is most vulnerable to cervical dysplasia.

10. Pregnancy is not a contraindication for colposcopy.

11. The quadrivalent HPV vaccine provides 100% immunity against HPV types 6, 11, 16, and 18.

12. The Advisory Committee for Immunization Practices recommends universal HPV vaccination for girls ages 11 and 12 years. The recommendation also allows for the vaccination of girls as young as 9 years of age and women 13 to 26 years old.

Suggested Reading

Markowitz LE, Dunne EF, Saraiya M, et al: Quadrivalent HPV vaccine: Recommendations of the Advisory Committee on Immunization Practices (ACIP), Centers for Disease Control and Prevention. *MMWR* 56:1–24, 2007.

U.S. Preventive Services Task Force: Screening for cervical cancer. Available at www.ahrq.gov/clinic/uspstf/uspscerv.htm.

Wright TC, Cox JT, Massad LS, et al: 2001 consensus guidelines for the management of women with cervical cytological abnormalities. *JAMA* 287(16):2120–2129, 2002.

Wright TC, Cox JT, Massad LS, et al: 2001 consensus guidelines for the management of women with cervical intraepithelial neoplasia. *Am J Obstet Gynecol* 189(1):295–304, 2003.

CHAPTER 73

Premenstrual Syndrome and Premenstrual Dysphoric Disorder

CLINICAL CASE PROBLEM 1

A 23-Year-Old Female with Cyclic Physical and Affective Symptoms

A 23-year-old woman comes to your office with a 6-month history of fatigue, anxiety, emotional lability, difficulty concentrating, and insomnia. She also complains of breast tenderness, abdominal bloating, and food cravings. She denies any menstrual irregularities or prodromal life stressors. These symptoms recur on a regular basis during the week leading up to her menstrual period but completely resolve within the first 3 days of menses. She denies any suicidal ideations. However, she tearfully admits that she feels totally incapacitated when she is symptomatic and that these symptoms are adversely affecting her personal and professional life.

SELECT THE BEST ANSWER TO THE FOLLOWING QUESTIONS

1. What is the most likely diagnosis in this patient?
   a. generalized anxiety disorder
   b. dysmenorrhea
   c. major depression
   d. panic disorder
   e. premenstrual dysphoric disorder syndrome (PMDD)

2. Which of the following is not a necessary *Diagnostic and Statistical Manual of Mental Disorders*, 4th edition (DSM-IV) criteria for diagnosing this condition?
   a. symptoms must be present most of the time during the last week of the luteal phase
   b. symptoms must remit a few days after the onset of the follicular phase (menses)

c. symptoms must be present in the week post menses

d. symptoms must occur in most menstrual cycles during the past year

e. symptoms must interfere with function

3. What is the main characteristic that differentiates this condition from major depression?
   a. the type of symptoms
   b. the severity of symptoms
   c. the duration of this condition
   d. the timing of the symptoms relative to the menstrual cycle
   e. occurs in reproductive-age women

4. What is the main characteristic that differentiates this condition from premenstrual syndrome (PMS)?
   a. the type of symptoms
   b. the severity of symptoms
   c. the duration of this condition
   d. the timing of the symptoms relative to the menstrual cycle
   e. occurs in reproductive-age women

5. Which of the following is a reliable aid in the diagnosis of this condition?
   a. patient completes a prospective daily symptom rating form for two consecutive cycles
   b. follicle-stimulating hormone-to-luteinizing hormone (FSH:LH) ratio
   c. progesterone withdrawal test
   d. an empiric 4-week trial of a selective serotonin reuptake inhibitor (SSRI)
   e. estradiol and progesterone levels obtained during the patient's late luteal phase

6. Which of the following statements comparing PMS and PMDD are true?
   a. PMDD is a more common condition than PMS
   b. PMS and PMDD both include physical symptoms
   c. early menopause often exacerbates the symptoms of PMS and PMDD
   d. symptoms have to interfere with normal function in PMDD but not PMS
   e. c and d

7. Which of the following is true regarding hormone levels in patients with PMS or PMDD?
   a. they have excess levels of female sex hormones (estrogen and progesterone)
   b. they have excess levels of male sex hormones (testosterone and dehydroepiandrosterone [DHEA])
   c. they have deficient levels of female sex hormones
   d. they have deficient levels of male sex hormones
   e. they have an abnormal response to normal female sex hormone fluctuations

8. Which of the following pharmacologic treatments has demonstrated the best evidence (level 1a) to support its effectiveness for the treatment of PMDD?
   a. SSRIs
   b. any combined oral contraceptives (COCs), containing estrogen and progestin
   c. progesterone vaginal suppositories
   d. transdermal estrogen patches
   e. oral medroxyprogesterone acetate (Provera)

9. Which of the following vitamins/minerals has demonstrated the best evidence (level 1b) to support its effectiveness for the treatment of PMDD?
   a. vitamin B_6
   b. calcium
   c. magnesium
   d. vitamin A
   e. vitamin E

10. Which of the following nonpharmacologic therapies have demonstrated the best evidence (level 1c) to support their effectiveness for the treatment of PMS/PMDD?
    a. dong quai and ginseng
    b. St. John's wort and kava kava
    c. evening primrose oil and chasteberry
    d. black cohosh and blue cohosh
    e. wild yams and soybeans

Clinical Case Management Problem

Compare the diagnostic criteria for PMS and PMDD.

Answers

1. **e.** The patient's presentation is most consistent with PMDD, a cyclic disorder of reproductive-aged women characterized by a wide variety of severe emotional and physical symptoms that consistently occur during the luteal phase of the menstrual cycle. PMDD is a diagnosis of exclusion. Although the patient may have symptoms consistent with an affective disorder (anxiety, depression, and panic), the cyclic onset and remission of her symptoms, in relation to her menstrual cycle, are classic for PMDD. Dysmenorrhea is a condition characterized by pelvic pain that occurs just after the onset of menses and peaks with heaviest flow. This patient's symptoms precede the onset of menses and remit during menses.

2. **c.** The following are *DSM-IV* diagnostic criteria for PMDD: (1) Symptoms must be present most of the time during the last week of the luteal phase,

(2) symptoms must remit a few days after the onset of the follicular phase (menses), (3) symptoms must be absent in the week post menses, (4) symptoms must occur in most menstrual cycles during the past year, (5) symptoms must interfere with function, and (6) symptoms must not be an exacerbation of an existing disorder.

3. d. The affective symptoms of PMDD can be indistinguishable from those of major depression. The recurrent onset and remission of these symptoms, in relation to the menstrual cycle, help distinguish PMDD from major depression.

4. b. Like PMDD, PMS is characterized by the cyclic recurrence of psychological and physical symptoms during the late luteal phase of the menstrual cycle. The variety of potential symptoms for both of these conditions is similar and they generally begin between the ages of 25 and 35 years. Women who have more severe affective symptoms are classified as having PMDD. Both PMS and PMDD symptoms improve rapidly following the onset of menses.

5. a. PMS and PMDD can be diagnosed only after a variety of physical and psychiatric disorders have been excluded. PMS and PMDD are best distinguished from other conditions by the consistent occurrence of function-impairing symptoms only during the luteal phase of the menstrual cycle. This can be confirmed best by having the patient complete a prospective daily symptom rating form for at least two consecutive cycles. Although sensitivity to sex hormones may play a role in both of these conditions, patients with PMS and PMDD have normal estradiol, progesterone, FSH, LH, and other hormone levels. SSRIs often improve the symptoms of PMS and PMDD, although there is also a significantly high placebo effect when treating these conditions. SSRIs also alleviate the symptoms of several other similar conditions (depression, anxiety, and panic), so the response to their empiric use is nondiagnostic.

6. b. PMS and PMDD have a variety of psychological and physical symptomatology in common, which interfere with normal function. PMS (20% to 40%) is a significantly more common condition than PMDD (2% to 10%) in menstruating women. As many as 85% of menstruating women report having one or more premenstrual symptoms. Menopause usually results in cessation of these conditions.

7. e. There is no consensus regarding the etiology of either PMS or PMDD. Patients with these conditions usually have normal hormone levels. However, they appear to have an abnormal response to normal female sex hormone fluctuations.

8. a. Although numerous treatment strategies are available, few have been evaluated adequately in randomized controlled trials (RCTs). Even the results of RCTs can be difficult to apply because of the significant variability of inclusion criteria and outcome measures and the high response rate to placebo (25% to 50%). However, the systematic review of many of these RCTs has yielded some evidence-based recommendations. There is clear evidence that SSRIs can significantly improve the symptoms of severe PMS and PMDD (evidence level 1a). Fluoxetine and sertraline are the most extensively studied for the treatment of PMS and PMDD, but all SSRIs appear to be effective. SSRIs can be administered daily or only during the luteal phase. However, there are no definitive recommendations regarding how long to continue treatment because symptoms tend to return on discontinuation. Nonsteroidal anti-inflammatory drugs (NSAIDs) can be helpful for symptoms of abdominal pain and headaches. Aldactone has been shown to relieve symptoms of fluid retention. Estrogen and/or progesterone/progestin-containing products, administered via different routes (intravaginally, rectally, orally, and transdermally), have been widely prescribed for the management of PMS and PMDD. However, none have been shown to be consistently effective and actually may exacerbate symptoms in some patients. Low-dose estrogen therapy may improve some physical symptoms, but it does not appear to have a positive effect on mood symptoms. The efficacy of estrogen therapy is limited by the need for progestin/progesterone opposition, which commonly exacerbates PMS and PMDD symptoms; however, it is required to prevent endometrial hyperplasia or carcinoma. Gonadotropin-releasing hormone (GnRH) agonists (e.g., Lupron) and androgens (e.g., Danazol) are somewhat effective in alleviating the physical and behavioral symptoms of PMS and PMDD. However, their short- and long-term side effect profiles limit their use. The Food and Drug Administration approved the oral contraceptive Yaz (3 mg drospirenone/30 μg ethinyl estradiol) for the treatment of the physical and emotional symptoms of PMDD, in women who choose to use an oral contraceptive as their method of contraception, based on the results of two RCTs. Drospirenone exhibits antimineralocorticoid and antiandrogenic properties unlike any other available progestin oral contraceptives. Although YAZ has been shown to be effective for the treatment of symptoms of PMDD, it has not been evaluated for the treatment of PMS. The effectiveness of YAZ for the treatment of symptoms of PMDD has not been evaluated for more than three menstrual cycles in clinical trials. Prescribing information for Yaz is available at http://berlex.bayer-healthcare.com.

9. **b.** There is good evidence that calcium is effective for the treatment of PMS and PMDD (evidence level 1b). A large, well-conducted RCT demonstrated that 1200 mg/day of calcium carbonate administered for three consecutive menstrual cycles resulted in significant symptom improvement in 48% of women with PMS compared with 30% of women treated with placebo. Although there is evidence suggesting that vitamin B₆ may improve PMS/PMDD symptoms, most of the RCTs were of poor quality. Magnesium has only been shown to have minimal benefit in alleviating PMS-related bloating. Studies of vitamin A do not support its use for PMS or PMDD. The result of one RCT suggests that vitamin E, administered at 400 IU/day during the luteal phase, may improve both affective and somatic symptoms (especially mastalgia) in women with PMS. However, larger, better quality studies are needed.

10. **c.** Two herbal therapies, chasteberry and evening primrose oil, may be effective in alleviating breast tenderness in patients with PMS/PMDD (evidence level 1c). The other options either have been shown to be likely ineffective (dong quai) or lack sufficient data to support their use. Some even have potential severe side effects, such as kava kava (liver damage), blue cohosh (peripheral vascular constriction), and St. John's wort (decreased oral contraceptive pill efficacy). One should also keep in mind the following: (1) None of the therapies listed are approved by the Food and Drug Administration for PMS or PMDD, (2) their safety in pregnancy and lactation has not been established, and (3) the manufacturing standards for herbal products are not uniform. Recommended nonpharmacologic interventions for patients with PMS/PMDD include the following: (1) patient education regarding the biologic basis and prevalence of their condition, (2) keeping a daily symptom diary, (3) adequate rest/structured sleep schedule, (4) sodium and caffeine restriction, and (5) aerobic exercise.

Solution to the Clinical Case Management Problem

PMS

National Institute of Mental Health Criteria

A 30% increase in the intensity of symptoms of PMS (measured using a standardized instrument) from cycle days 5 to 10 compared to the 6-day interval before the onset of menses and documentation of these changes in a daily symptom diary for at least two consecutive cycles.

University of California at San Diego Criteria

At least one of the following affective and somatic symptoms during the 5 days before menses in each of the three previous cycles:

Affective symptoms: depression, angry outbursts, irritability, anxiety, confusion, and withdrawal
Somatic symptoms: breast tenderness, abdominal bloating, headache, and swelling of the extremities
Symptoms relieved from days 4 through 13 of the menstrual cycle.

PMDD

DSM-IV Research Criteria

A. In most menstrual cycles during the past year, five or more of the following symptoms were present for most of the time during the last week of the luteal phase, began to remit within a few days after the onset of the follicular phase, and were absent in the week after menses, with at least one of the symptoms being 1, 2, 3, or 4:

1. Markedly depressed mood, feelings of hopelessness, or self-deprecating thoughts
2. Marked anxiety, tension, or feelings of being "keyed up" or "on edge"
3. Marked affective lability
4. Persistent and marked anger or irritability, or increased interpersonal conflicts
5. Decreased interest in usual activities
6. Subjective sense of difficulty concentrating
7. Lethargy, easy fatigability, or marked lack of energy
8. Marked change in appetite, overeating, or specific food cravings
9. Hypersomnia or insomnia
10. A subjective sense of being overwhelmed or out of control
11. Other physical symptoms such as breast tenderness or swelling, headaches, joint or muscle pain, a sensation of "bloating," or weight gain

B. The disturbance markedly interferes with work or school, or with usual social activities and relationships with others.
C. The disturbance is not merely an exacerbation of symptoms of another disorder.
D. Criteria A, B, and C must be confirmed by prospective daily ratings during at least two consecutive symptomatic cycles.

Summary

For diagnostic criteria, see the Solution to the Clinical Case Management Problem.

Treatment options include the following:

1. Nonpharmacologic: (1) patient education, (2) daily symptom diary, (3) adequate rest/structured sleep schedule, (4) sodium restriction, (5) caffeine restriction, and (6) aerobic exercise
2. Pharmacologic: (1) SSRIs (evidence level 1a), (2) estrogen therapy/COCs (mixed outcomes; may exacerbate symptoms), (3) androgen therapy (e.g., Danazol; use limited by side effects), (4) GnRH agonists (e.g., Lupron; use limited by side effects), (5) NSAIDs (effective for physical symptoms except breast tenderness), and (6) diuretics (i.e., spironolactone; effective for breast tenderness and bloating)
3. Supplements and herbal therapies: (1) calcium carbonate 1200 mg/day (evidence level 1b), (2) vitamin B$_6$ 100 mg/day, (3) vitamin E 400 IU/ day, (4) chasteberry (level 1c), and (5) evening primrose oil

Suggested Reading

American College of Obstetricians and Gynecologists: ACOG Practice Bulletin. Clinical management guidelines for obstetrician–gynecologists. Premenstrual syndrome. *Obstet Gynecol* 95:1–9, 2000.
American Psychiatric Association: *Diagnostic and Statistical Manual of Mental Disorders*, 4th ed Washington, DC: American Psychiatric Association, 1994, pp. 715–718.

Bhatia SC, Bhatia SK: Diagnosis and treatment of premenstrual dysphoric disorder. *Am Fam Phys* 66:1253–1254, 2002.
Dickerson LM, Mazyck PJ, Hunter MH: Premenstrual syndrome. *Am Fam Phys* 67:1743–1752, 2003.
Johnson SR: Premenstrual syndrome, premenstrual dysphoric disorder, and beyond: A clinical primer for practitioners. *Obstet Gynecol* 104:845–859, 2004.

Evidence-Based Systemic Review Sources

Clinical Evidence Mental Health. Available at www.bmjjournals.com.
Cochrane Database. Available at www.cochrane.org

Medical Inforetriever/infopoems. Available at www.essentialevidenceplus. com.
Natural Medicines Comprehensive Database. Available at www.natural database.com

---

CHAPTER

74 Postmenopausal Symptoms

CLINICAL CASE PROBLEM 1

A 51-Year-Old Female with Hot Flashes

A 51-year-old woman has been experiencing progressive symptoms of profuse night sweats and frequent hot flushes occurring both day and night. She finds her emotional state increasingly labile. She is also experiencing sleep disturbances and anxiety. She denies any other complaints. Her last period was approximately 12 months ago. She has no history of medical problems or affective disorders. Her pulse is 78 beats/ minute, and her blood pressure is 122/74 mmHg. Her pelvic examination reveals atrophic external genitalia, a small anteverted uterus, and no adnexal masses. The rest of her examination is completely normal.

SELECT THE BEST ANSWER TO THE FOLLOWING QUESTIONS

1. What is the most likely diagnosis in this patient?
   a. pheochromocytoma
   b. hyperthyroidism
   c. menopause
   d. generalized anxiety disorder
   e. depression or panic attacks

2. What is the most effective treatment option for this patient?
   a. thyroid replacement
   b. estrogen with progestin (hormone therapy [HT])
   c. antidepressants
   d. estrogen alone (estrogen therapy [ET])
   e. progestin/progesterone alone

3. Alternative therapies, with demonstrated efficacy, for this patient's condition might include
   a. black cohosh
   b. soy isoflavones
   c. red clover

    d. selective serotonin reuptake inhibitors (SSRIs)/ selective serotonin and norepinephrine reup-take inhibitor (SSNRIs)

    e. all of the above

4. If this patient was also complaining of vaginal dry-ness, reasonable treatment options would include

    a. intravaginal estrogen creams/tablets

    b. an intravaginal estrogen ring

    c. vaginal moisturizers

    d. increased foreplay and intercourse

    e. all of the above

5. The HT (combined estrogen/progestin) arm of the Women's Health Initiative (WHI) random-ized, controlled trial (RCT) was stopped prema-turely primarily because patients in the treatment group demonstrated an increased relative risk for what condition?

    a. breast cancer

    b. endometrial cancer

    c. colon cancer

    d. osteoporotic fractures

    e. all of the above

6. What conclusions can be accurately made based on the findings of the WHI HT trial?

    a. combined equine estrogen (CEE) appears to cause breast cancer

    b. CEE appears to cause coronary heart disease (CHD)

    c. medroxyprogesterone acetate appears to cause breast cancer

    d. medroxyprogesterone acetate appears to cause CHD

    e. daily combined use of 0.625 mg CEE and 2.5 mg medroxyprogesterone acetate proges-terone (MPA) should not be initiated or con-tinued for the primary prevention of CHD

7. Potential limitations of the HT arm of the WHI include

    a. average age of the patients at the start of the trial was 63 years

    b. patients with significant vasomotor symptoms were excluded from the trial

    c. only one dose, combination, and route of estro-gen/progestin were studied

    d. quality-of-life indicators were not assessed

    e. all of the above

8. Current Food and Drug Administration (FDA) indications for ET/HT include

    a. urge incontinence

    b. prevention of dementia

    c. prevention of osteoporosis

    d. treatment of osteoporosis

    e. treatment of hyperlipidemia

9. Which of the following statements regarding postmenopausal osteoporosis is true?

    a. the most rapid loss of bone density occurs within the first 5 years of menopause

    b. surgical menopause is a lower risk factor for osteoporosis than natural menopause

    c. the protective effects of estrogen on bone den-sity are maintained after discontinuation

    d. all women should undergo bone density testing at menopause

    e. the U.S. Preventive Services Task Force (USPSTF) recommends against bone density testing for women older than age 65 years

10. Your patient also complains of chronic urinary urgency and frequency. She admits that she needs to wear a pad and also notes leakage of urine whenever she coughs, laughs, or sneezes. She has no history of urinary tract infections (UTIs), diabetes, or kidney problems. The most likely diagnosis for this patient is

    a. urge incontinence

    b. stress incontinence

    c. mixed incontinence

    d. overflow incontinence

    e. neurogenic bladder

11. Initial workup for this patient would include all of the following except

    a. urinalysis

    b. postvoid residual

    c. voiding diary

    d. urine culture

    e. bladder ultrasound

Clinical Case Management Problem

Discuss the latest USPSTF recommendations for HT.

Answers

1. **c.** The most likely diagnosis in this patient is menopause. Menopause is a retrospective diagnosis based on 12 or more months of amenorrhea occurring at a mean age of 51 years. The diagnosis is based on the appropriate age of a female patient for menopause (range, 45 to 55 years), symptoms of frequent classic "hot flashes," night sweats, and the association of these symptoms with the cessation of menses. Although the patient does have some symptoms associated with the other conditions listed, her lack of other complaints (hair loss, diarrhea, and palpitations) or previous history of an affective disorder (depression, anxiety, and panic) along with her normal vital signs and essentially normal physical examination make the diagnosis of these other conditions less likely. The findings of vulvovaginal atrophy are also consistent with menopause.

2. **b.** The most effective treatment for this patient's vasomotor symptoms is HT (estrogen combined with a daily or cyclic progestin/progesterone). A progestin or progesterone alone may alleviate some of this patient's symptoms, but her symptoms are related primarily to estrogen deficiency and thus respond best to ET. However, because this patient still has her uterus, ET (estrogen alone) is not recommended because of the significantly increased risk of endometrial hyperplasia/cancer with prolonged unopposed estrogen use. Antidepressants might help alleviate some of this patient's symptoms, especially if she was also clinically depressed. However, this patient's symptoms are most likely hormonally related, and HT/ET alone often alleviates both the affective and the somatic symptoms of menopause. There is no strong evidence that this patient has hypothyroidism, and there is certainly no indication for empiric use of thyroid hormone without objective evidence of hypothyroidism (i.e., thyroid-stimulating hormone and thyroid function test).

3. **d.** Although ET/HT remains the most effective therapy for this patient's vasomotor symptoms, many women will not or cannot use estrogen. All of the therapies listed have been evaluated for effectiveness in alleviating hot flushes and night sweats associated with menopause. Data for these therapies are limited, and most of the studies have been conducted on women with a history of breast cancer. Various SSRIs and particularly the SSNRI venlafaxine have been shown to reduce hot flashes 19% to 60% and were well tolerated by study participants. Small studies evaluating gabapentin have also demonstrated significant reductions in vasomotor symptoms. Clonidine patches have demonstrated some efficacy in reducing vasomotor symptoms, but dry mouth, constipation, drowsiness, and application site irritation are potential side effects. Soy isoflavones reduced hot flashes in some trials, but most trials showed no difference compared with placebo. Black cohosh and red clover have also had inconsistent results, with some trials showing benefit and some no difference compared with placebo. Other agents that have been used to alleviate hot flashes include belladonna/ergotamine tartrate/phenobarbital combination, dong quai, evening primrose oil, ginseng, mirtazapine, trazodone, vitamin E, and wild yam, but few data regarding their effectiveness have been published.

4. **e.** Symptoms of urogenital atrophy related to menopause (estrogen deficiency) include vaginal dryness, vaginitis, dyspareunia, dysuria, urinary incontinence, and recurrent UTIs. Intravaginal estrogen creams or tablets (usually inserted daily initially and then two or three times per week) and the estrogen-embedded vaginal ring, Estring (changed every 3 months), are highly effective for reducing both the signs and the symptoms of urogenital atrophy, with significantly less systemic estrogen absorption compared to oral or transdermal ET. Although this minimizes the risk of venous thromboembolic events (VTEs), there is no strong evidence that they are less likely to increase the risk of other cardiovascular events (i.e., myocardial infarct [MI] and cardiovascular accident [CVA]) or breast cancer. Vaginal moisturizers and increased vaginal sexual activity also help with vaginal lubrication and reduce atrophic symptomatology.

5. **a.** The WHI was the largest multicenter clinical investigation of postmenopausal women, having recruited more than 60,000 patients. The WHI included a randomized, double-blind, placebo-controlled set of three trials and one observational study to examine the effects of various interventions on the major causes of morbidity and mortality in postmenopausal women, namely CHD, breast cancer, colon cancer, and osteoporotic fractures. One arm of the WHI followed 16,608 healthy patients aged 50 to 79 years at baseline, with an intact uterus, taking either HT (using 0.625 mg of CEE combined with 2.5 mg of MPA) or placebo. On July 9, 2002, 5.2 years after study initiation (intended duration, 8 years), the HT portion of the trial was halted because of the findings that the overall health risks of treatment (observed increases in CHD, VTE, and breast cancer) outweighed its benefits, which were observed decreases in osteoporotic fractures and colon cancer (Fig. 74-1 and Table 74-1). However, these increases in adverse events in the treatment group were small, and there were no significant differences between groups regarding endometrial cancer and mortality from any causes.

6. **e.** The HT arm of the WHI RCT did demonstrate a higher relative risk of cardiovascular events (MI, CVA, and VTE) and breast cancer in the HT treatment group compared to the control group. However, the absolute risk of these events attributable to HT is small and no cause-and-effect conclusions should be inferred. In addition, these findings may not apply to other estrogen and/or progestin formulations, combinations,

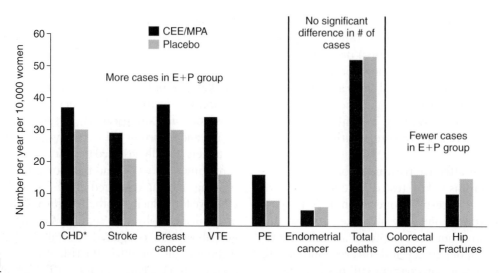

Figure 74-1

The Women's Health Initiative: Absolute risks and benefits. Risk of coronary heart disease (CHD) in first year was statistically significant; overall risk of CHD was not statistically significant. CEE, conjugated equine estrogen; MPA, medroxyprogesterone acetate progesterone; PE, pulmonary embolism; VTE, venous thromboembolism. (Adapted from National Institutes of Health, National Heart, Lung, and Blood Institute: *WHI HRT Update—2002.* Available at www.hnlbi.nih.gov/health/women/upd2002.htm.)

Table 74-1 | **Results of the Women's Health Initiative's Hormone Replacement Therapy Randomized Clinical Trial**

ABSOLUTE AND RELATIVE RISK OR BENEFIT OF CEE/MPA

Health Event	Overall Hazard Ratio	CONFIDENCE INTERVAL		Increased Absolute Risk per 10,000 Women/Year	Increased Absolute Benefit per 10,000 Women/Year
		Nominal 95%	Adjusted 95%		
CHD	1.29	1.02–1.63	0.85–1.97	7	—
Strokes	1.41	1.07–1.85	0.86–2.31	8	—
Breast cancer	1.26	1.00–1.59	0.83–1.92	8	—
VTED	2.11	1.58–2.82	1.26–3.55	18	—
Colorectal cancer	0.63	0.43–0.92	0.32–1.24	—	6
Hip fractures	0.66	0.45–0.98	0.33–1.33	—	5
Total fractures	0.76	0.69–0.85	0.63–0.92	—	44

CEE, conjugated equine estrogen; CHD, coronary heart disease; MPA, medroxyprogesterone acetate; VTED, venous thromboembolic disease. Data from Writing Group for the Women's Health Initiative Investigators: Risks and benefits of estrogen plus progestin in healthy postmenopausal women. *JAMA* 288:321–322, 2002.

dosages, and routes of administration (i.e., transdermal and intravaginal). However, it is reasonable to infer from these data that the combination of 0.625 mg/day of CEE and 2.5 mg/day of MPA does not appear to prevent CHD. Thus, the authors of the WHI HT trial data made the following recommendations: "Results from WHI indicate that the combined postmenopausal hormones CEE, 0.625 mg/day, plus MPA, 2.5mg/day, should not be initiated or continued for the primary prevention of CHD. In addition, the substantial risks for cardiovascular disease and breast cancer must be weighed against the benefit for fracture in selecting from the available agents to prevent osteoporosis."

7. **e.** To ensure that patients in the placebo arm of the WHI HT trial would continue to participate for the entire study, patients with significant vasomotor symptoms were excluded. Thus, the average participant age at the start of the study was 63 years, with an average of 6 years since the onset of menopause. In addition, quality-of-life indicators, including menopausal symptom relief, were not measured in this trial. For obvious reasons of project cost, recruitment, and statistical power, only one dose and route of one combination formulation of HT were evaluated in this study. All of these limitations may affect the generalizability of this RCT's results to other HT formulations,

dosages, and routes, and they may affect the applicability of these results to younger, symptomatic postmenopausal patients.

8. c. The current FDA indications for ET/HT include the following: (1) treatment of moderate to severe vasomotor symptoms, (2) treatment of moderate to severe symptoms of vulvar and vaginal atrophy (dryness and irritation) associated with menopause, and (3) prevention of postmenopausal osteoporosis. Despite recent studies, including the WHI HT trial, supporting the effectiveness of ET/HT for preventing osteoporotic fractures, it is not indicated for the treatment of osteoporosis. Although Postmenopausal Estrogen/Progesterone Interventions trials and other RCTs have demonstrated the overall favorable lipid effects of ET/HT, it is not indicated for the treatment of hyperlipidemia. ET/HT may benefit urinary symptoms related to urogenital atrophy, but it is not indicated for urge incontinence.

On January 8, 2003, the FDA issued a statement advising women and health care professionals about important safety changes to labeling of all estrogen and estrogen with progestin products for use by postmenopausal women. These changes reflected the FDA's analysis of data from the WHI that raised concern about risks of using these products. The FDA's labeling changes include a black boxed warning that reflects new risk information and changes to the approved indications to emphasize individualized decisions that appropriately balance the potential benefits and risks of these products.

The black boxed warning, the highest level of warning information in labeling, highlights the increased risks for heart disease, heart attacks, strokes, and breast cancer. This warning also emphasizes that these products are not approved for heart disease prevention. The FDA has also modified the approved indications for ET and HT to clarify that these drugs should be used only when the benefits clearly outweigh risks. Of the three indications, two were revised to include consideration of other therapies. The three indications are as follows:

1. Treatment of moderate to severe vasomotor symptoms (such as "hot flashes") associated with menopause. (This indication has not changed.)
2. Treatment of moderate to severe symptoms of vulvar and vaginal atrophy (dryness and irritation) associated with menopause. It is now recommended that when these products are being prescribed solely for the treatment of symptoms of vulvar and vaginal atrophy, topical vaginal products should be considered.
3. Prevention of postmenopausal osteoporosis, when these products are being prescribed solely for the prevention of postmenopausal osteoporosis. The current recommendation is that approved nonestrogen treatments should be considered carefully and estrogens and combined estrogen–progestin products should be considered only for women with significant risk of osteoporosis that outweighs the risks of the drug.

To minimize the potential risks and to accomplish the desired treatment goals, the labeling also advises health care providers to prescribe estrogen and combined estrogen with progestin drug products at the lowest dose and for the shortest duration for the individual woman. Similarly, American College of Obstetricians and Gynecologists recommends that the lowest effective estrogen dose should be used for the shortest possible time to alleviate symptoms, and the North American Menopause Society recommends that estrogen duration and dose be consistent with treatment goals.

Women who choose to take estrogens or combined estrogen and progestin therapies after discussing their treatment with their doctor should have yearly breast examinations by a health care provider, perform monthly breast self-examinations, and receive periodic mammography (scheduled based on their age and risk factors). Women should also talk to their health care provider about other ways to reduce their risk factors for heart disease (e.g., high blood pressure, poor diet, and tobacco use) and osteoporosis (e.g., an appropriate diet, use of vitamin D and calcium supplements, and weight-bearing exercise).

9. a. Osteoporosis is a systemic skeletal disease characterized by low bone mass and microarchitectural deterioration of bone tissue, with a consequent increase in bone fragility and susceptibility to fracture. There is a clear causal relationship between estrogen deficiency and osteoporosis. A woman's bone density tends to peak by age 30 to 35 years, whereas her most rapid loss of bone tends to occur during the first 5 years of menopause. Postmenopausal status, regardless of the etiology (natural or surgically/hormonally induced), or estrogen deficiency at any age significantly increases a patient's risk for osteoporosis and subsequent fragility fractures. Estrogen appears to inhibit bone resorption by reducing the production of bone-resorbing osteoclasts while promoting the activation of bone-forming osteoblasts. Estrogen deficiency leads to a rapid increase in osteoclast formation and activity, leading to accelerated bone resorption. Studies also suggest that bone loss is accelerated when ET/HT is discontinued.

Therefore, ET/HT may simply postpone the rapid bone loss associated with menopause. This is a very important point when counseling patients about ET/HT compliance and the long-term prevention of osteoporosis.

The National Osteoporosis Foundation (NOF) expert panel recommends that all women age 65 years or older be screened for osteoporosis regardless of the presence or absence of risk factors. NOF also recommends screening younger postmenopausal women with one or more major risk factor (personal history of atraumatic fracture, family history of osteoporotic fracture, smoking, and body weight less than 127 pounds). USPSTF also recommends universal bone mineral density (BMD) screening for all women age 65 years or older. For women age 60 years or older, USPSTF recommends screening if there are risk factors for osteoporotic fracture. USPSTF makes no recommendation for or against routine screening in postmenopausal women younger than age 60 years or age 60 to 64 years without increased risk for osteoporotic fracture.

10. **c.** This patient's history is most consistent with mixed urinary incontinence. However, she requires further evaluation to confirm the diagnosis and rule out other causes. Urge incontinence is usually caused by irritability and/or instability of the detrusor muscle in the bladder. Patients with this condition often present with almost constant urinary urgency, frequency, and the sensation of incomplete emptying with voiding. Patients with more severe symptoms may have frequent incontinent episodes. Patients with stress incontinence often note that they "leak urine" whenever they cough, laugh, or sneeze (Valsalva). Patients with a neurogenic bladder (e.g., patients with paraplegia or severe diabetes) have no neurologic control of their bladder and are susceptible to overflow incontinence.

11. **e.** An appropriate initial workup for this patient would include the following: (1) a urinalysis (to assess for proteinuria and glucosuria), (2) a postvoid residual (to assess for incomplete emptying or overflow incontinence), (3) a urine culture (to rule out an infection), and (4) a daily fluid intake and voiding diary (to assess potential contributing factors to patients symptoms). A bladder ultrasound would not be indicated at this point in the evaluation based on the patient's presenting complaints.

Solution to the Clinical Case Management Problem

USPSTF published its latest recommendations for HT in May 2005. It recommends against the routine use of estrogen and progestin for the prevention of chronic conditions in postmenopausal women (a D recommendation), and it recommends against the use of unopposed estrogen for the prevention of chronic conditions in postmenopausal women who have had a hysterectomy (an D recommendation).

Summary

Review the WHI HT RCT results illustrated in Figure 74-1 and summarized in Table 74-1.
Symptoms are as follows:

1. Vasomotor: (a) hot flushes/hot flashes (occur in up to 85% of postmenopausal women) and (b) night sweats
2. Urogenital: (a) dyspareunia, (b) vaginitis, (c) vaginal dryness, (d) dysuria/urgency, (e) urinary incontinence, and (f) recurrent/chronic UTIs
3. Behavioral: (a) sleep disturbances, (b) irritability, (c) emotional lability, (d) decreased libido, (e) memory loss, and (f) problems concentrating

Treatments are as follows:

1. FDA indicates use of ET/HT for (a) treatment of moderate to severe vasomotor symptoms, (b) treatment of moderate to severe symptoms of vulvar and vaginal atrophy, and (c) prevention of postmenopausal osteoporosis
2. ET/HT options
   a. Routes: oral, transdermal, intravaginal (cream/tablet/ring)
   b. Estrogen formulations: CEE, estradiol, estrone sulfate, ethinyl estradiol

c. Progestin/progesterone formulations: MPA, norethindrone, micronized progesterone. (Patients with an intact uterus should receive an estrogen combined with a daily/cyclic HT that is FDA approved for the prevention of endometrial hyperplasia.)

3. Alternative therapies: (a) SSRIs/SSNRIs, (b) gabapentin, and (c) clonidine patches

Screening tests for postmenopausal women are as follows: (1) height/weight (periodically), (2) blood pressure (periodically), (3) vision (periodically), (4) mammogram/ clinical breast examination (after 40 years; annually), (5) Pap test (every 1 to 3 years until age 65 years; stop if postabdominal hysterectomy, not because of malignancy), (6) colorectal (after 50 years; frequency depends on method—fecal occult blood test, flexible sigmoidoscopy, or colonoscopy), (7) BMD (see USPSTF and NOF screening guidelines), and (8) fasting lipid profile (after 45 years; every 5 years if previous results were normal).

Suggested Reading

American College of Obstetricians and Gynecologists Task Force on Hormone Therapy: Vasomotor symptoms. *Obstet Gynecol* 104(Suppl 4):106S–117S, 2004.

Carroll DG: Nonhormonal therapies for hot flashes in menopause. *Am Fam Physician* 73(3):457–464, 2006.

Hodis H: Estrogen and atherosclerosis: Putting WHI into perspective. *The Female Patient* 6(Suppl):2–4, 2002.

National Osteoporosis Foundation: Physician's Guide to Prevention and Treatment of Osteoporosis. Available at www.nof.org/physguide/diagnosis.htm, Accessed March 2, 2007.

North American Menopause Society: Treatment of menopause-associated vasomotor symptoms: Position statement of the North American Menopause Society. *Menopause* 11:589–600, 2004.

Speroff L: Hormone replacement and breast cancer: Putting WHI into perspective. *The Female Patient* Suppl:6–7, 2002.

Suckling J, Lethaby A, Kennedy R: Local oestrogen for vaginal atrophy in postmenopausal women. *Cochrane Database Syst Rev* (4): CD001500, 2006.

U.S. Department of Health and Human Services: U.S. Food & Drug Administration approves new labels for estrogen and estrogen with progestin therapy for postmenopausal women following review of WHI. *FDA News* P03–01, January 8, 2003.

U.S. Preventive Services Task Force: Postmenopausal hormone replacement therapy for primary prevention of chronic conditions: Recommendations and rationale. USPSTF guide to clinical preventive services. *Ann Intern Med* 137(10):834–839, 2002.

U.S. Preventive Services Task Force: *Screening for Osteoporosis in Postmenopausal Women: Recommendations and Rationale*. Available at www.ahrq.gov/clinic/3rduspstf/osteoporosis/osteorr.pdf.

Weiss BD: Selecting medications for the treatment of urinary incontinence. *Am Fam Physician* 71(2):315–322, 2005.

Writing Group for the Women's Health Initiative Investigators: Risks and benefits of estrogen plus progestin in healthy postmenopausal women. *JAMA* 288(3):321–333, 2002.

CHAPTER

75 Dysmenorrhea

CLINICAL CASE PROBLEM 1

A 14-Year-Old Female with Painful Menses

A 14-year-old female comes to your office with a 6-month history of lower midabdominal pain. The pain is colicky in nature, radiates to the back and upper thighs, begins with onset of menses, and lasts for 2 to 4 days. She has missed several days of school during the past 2 months because the pain was so severe. Menarche began 18 months ago, and her menses became regular 6 months ago. The patient is not sexually active. Physical examination, including abdomen and pelvis, is normal. The patient has normal secondary sexual development.

SELECT THE BEST ANSWER TO THE FOLLOWING QUESTIONS

1. What is the most likely etiology of this patient's pain?
   a. primary dysmenorrhea
   b. pelvic inflammatory disease (PID)
   c. secondary dysmenorrhea
   d. endometriosis
   e. premenstrual syndrome

2. The etiology of this patient's conditions is related to
   a. increased levels of prostaglandin
   b. decreased levels of prostaglandin
   c. increased levels of cyclic adenosine monophosphate (cAMP)
   d. decreased levels of cAMP
   e. none of the above

3. What would you recommend as initial treatment of choice?
   a. nonsteroidal anti-inflammatory drugs (NSAIDs)
   b. oral contraceptive pills (OCPs)
   c. gonadotropin-releasing hormone (GnRH) agonist
   d. acetaminophen
   e. intrauterine device (IUD) placement

4. The pathophysiology of this patient's pain is associated with
   a. vasodilation of the uterine arteries
   b. vasoconstriction of the uterine arteries
   c. vasodilation of the pelvic veins
   d. vasodilation of the uterine veins
   e. none of the above

5. When does the disorder described usually begin?
   a. 13 to 16 years of age
   b. within 3 years of onset of thelarche (breast development)
   c. within 5 years of onset of thelarche
   d. within 3 years of onset of menarche (first menses)
   e. within 5 years of onset of menarche

6. Which of the following is not usually associated with primary dysmenorrhea?
   a. pain beginning with onset of menses
   b. pain peaking during heaviest flow
   c. pain responsive to NSAIDs
   d. endometriosis
   e. pain responsive to OCPs

7. Which of the following is more consistent with premenstrual syndrome (PMS) than with primary dysmenorrhea?
   a. symptoms that interfere with patient's daily function
   b. symptoms that are cyclic in nature
   c. abdominal symptoms associated with menses
   d. symptoms with onset during late luteal phase
   e. diagnosis based generally on history alone

8. The patient returns 6 months later. She has tried several different NSAIDs, using the correct doses and regimens you prescribed. She had partial relief of her pain but still experiences such bothersome symptoms that she still misses school occasionally. At this time, you recommend that she
   a. continue the NSAIDs only
   b. discontinue the NSAIDs and begin oxycodone
   c. add OCPs
   d. switch to danazol
   e. undergo laparoscopic presacral neuroectomy

CLINICAL CASE PROBLEM 2

A 24-Year-Old Female with Infertility and Painful Menses

A 24-year-old nulligravida woman comes to your office with an 18-month history of cyclic, debilitating pelvic pain related to menses. Her menses is regular and heavy, requiring 10 to 15 thick pads on the days of heaviest flow. She denies ever being diagnosed with a sexually transmitted infection (STI). She and her husband have been engaging in regular intercourse without contraception for 1 year in an attempt to conceive. On pelvic examination, you find a normal-sized, immobile, retroverted uterus with nodularity and tenderness on palpation of the uterosacral ligaments.

9. You inform the patient that the most likely diagnosis is
   a. uterine fibroid
   b. endometriosis
   c. adenomyosis
   d. PID
   e. endometrial carcinoma

10. You further explain that her pain is described most accurately as
    a. primary dysmenorrhea
    b. secondary dysmenorrhea
    c. premenstrual syndrome
    d. psychogenic pain
    e. none of the above

11. Which of the following studies would establish a diagnosis in this condition?
    a. hysteroscopy
    b. ultrasound
    c. laparoscopy
    d. hysterosalpingogram (HSG)
    e. magnetic resonance imaging (MRI)

12. Which of the following is not an appropriate medical therapy for this condition?
    a. danazol
    b. GnRH agonist
    c. continuous OCPs
    d. medroxyprogesterone acetate (Depo-SubQ Provera 104)
    e. clomiphene

13. Which of the following is least consistent with secondary dysmenorrhea?
    a. normal pelvic examination
    b. onset of pain after the age of 25 years

c. onset of pain during adolescence
d. pain relief with NSAIDs
e. pain relief with OCPs

14. Other causes of secondary dysmenorrhea include all of the following except
   a. PID
   b. chronic use of OCPs
   c. uterine fibroids
   d. IUD
   e. adenomyosis

Clinical Case Management Problem

Discuss proposed etiologies of endometriosis.

Answers

1. a. This young woman has primary dysmenorrhea. Primary dysmenorrhea is the most common gynecologic complaint of young women, with reported prevalence rates as high as 90%. It is one of the leading causes of absenteeism in young women. Primary dysmenorrhea usually begins within 6 to 12 months of menarche. The pain is described as sharp spasms in the lower abdomen and suprapubic area. Associated symptoms include nausea, vomiting, diarrhea, headache, and fatigue. The timing of the pain in relation to menses is key to the diagnosis. The onset of pain is usually within hours of menstrual flow onset and peaks on the day of heaviest flow. Secondary dysmenorrhea is defined as dysmenorrhea with identifiable pelvic etiology. PID and endometriosis are two causes of secondary dysmenorrhea. PMS is characterized by symptoms of bloating, fatigue, and breast tenderness just prior to menses.

2. a. Women with primary dysmenorrhea have ovulatory cycles and produce progesterone during the luteal phase. Progesterone stimulates prostaglandin production in the endometrium. After progesterone withdrawal, the endometrium sloughs and releases prostaglandins. Prostaglandins stimulate myometrial contractions, leading to decreased blood flow and local ischemia. These physiologic changes result in increased production of vasoconstrictive prostaglandins, causing uterine hypoxia and pain. Women with primary dysmenorrhea have been found to have elevated levels of prostaglandin, particularly $PGF_{2\alpha}$. Hence, first-line therapy for dysmenorrhea is NSAID therapy, which decreases prostaglandin levels.

3. a. NSAIDs are the treatment of choice. They inhibit cyclooxygenase, thus decreasing prostaglandin levels. Oral contraceptives may be used in conjunction with NSAIDs for the treatment of dysmenorrhea and are particularly ideal in women who desire contraception. However, OCPs are not considered first-line treatment because they do not address directly the problem of elevated prostaglandin levels. The other answers listed are not first-line treatment for primary dysmenorrhea.

4. b. Primary dysmenorrhea is mediated pathologically by an increase in the level of the enzyme prostaglandin synthetase. Elevated levels of the enzyme produce vasoconstricting prostaglandins that are responsible for uterine hypoxia, or uterine angina, which produces the pain of dysmenorrhea. The vasoconstriction takes place in the branches of the uterine artery. Venous vasodilation is not responsible for dysmenorrhea.

5. d. Primary dysmenorrhea almost always begins within 3 years of the onset of menstruation. Exact age of onset for primary dysmenorrhea will vary depending on the age of menarche. If dysmenorrhea begins at a later time, one should suspect secondary dysmenorrhea. The definition of primary dysmenorrhea is related to menarche, not thelarche (breast development).

6. d. As discussed previously, primary dysmenorrhea is painful menses coinciding with onset of menses, peaking during heaviest flow, and is responsive to NSAIDs and OCPs. Endometriosis is associated with secondary dysmenorrhea.

7. d. Both PMS and primary dysmenorrhea may involve abdominal symptoms associated with menses and are cyclic in nature. Both conditions may be so severe that they interfere with quality of life and daily function. However, PMS is characterized by symptoms occurring in the late luteal phase, just prior to the onset of menses, and resolve soon after menstrual flow begins. PMS symptoms include abdominal bloating, breast tenderness, irritability, and fatigue.

8. c. NSAIDs are the drugs of choice for the treatment of primary dysmenorrhea. If there is no significant change in pain after a reasonable duration (approximately 3 months) of one NSAID regimen, it is sometimes helpful to try an NSAID from a different category. Some cyclooxygenase-2 (COX-2) inhibitors have the Food and Drug Administration (FDA) indication for dysmenorrhea. However, they have not demonstrated superior efficacy to other NSAID therapy. Although COX-2 inhibitors may provide reduced risk of gastrointestinal (GI) bleeds, they are more expensive and recent concerns regarding their cardiovascular safety profile have resulted in either FDA withdrawals (i.e., Vioxx and Bextra) or restrictions in their use (i.e., Celebrex). Most patients only use NSAIDS during the time of menses for dysmenorrhea, limiting their risk of GI irritation and bleed.

With each prescribed regimen, it is important to assess patient compliance, such that maximum daily frequency and dose have been reached. If the patient has only partial relief from NSAIDs, switching directly to a narcotic is not appropriate until other alternatives have been explored. Second-line treatment for primary dysmenorrhea includes a trial of oral contraceptives. The use of OCPs is particularly advantageous if the patient also desires a method of birth control. OCPs help alleviate symptoms of dysmenorrhea by both reducing menstrual flow and inhibiting ovulation, and they have been shown to be 90% effective within 3 or 4 months of use. Continuous use of oral contraceptives can be very helpful by reducing the number of menstrual cycles. During continuous OCP use, the patient takes "active" hormone pills for up to 12 weeks straight, eliminating the placebo pills and subsequent withdrawal bleeding. Seasonale (levonorgestrel/ethinyl estradiol tablets) 0.15 mg/0.03 mg is an extended cycle oral contraceptive formulation that provides 84 days of active pills. Studies have evaluated the safety and efficacy of longer use of active combined oral contraceptives as well as continuous use of transdermal (OrthoEvra) and intravaginal (NuvaRing) hormonal contraceptives for dysmenorrhea. An alternative treatment is Depo-Provera, which induces amenorrhea in half of all patients by the third injection and thus eliminates dysmenorrhea. Observational data from users of the levonorgestrel intrauterine device (Mirena) showed a decrease in prevalence of dysmenorrhea from 60% before use of the device to 29% after 36 months of use. Danazol, a synthetic androgen, can also induce amenorrhea but is associated with unpleasant side effects, including acne, hirsutism, and virilizing symptoms. Laparoscopic presacral neuroectomy is reserved for refractory cases of dysmenorrhea and is not appropriate until conservative measures have been exhausted.

9. **b.** Endometriosis is a condition in which ectopic endometrial tissue implants are found in extrauterine sites, most commonly the ovaries, fallopian tubes, cul-de-sac, and uterosacral ligaments. Patients with endometriosis complain of dysmenorrhea that often begins years after pain-free cycles. Other associated symptoms include dyspareunia (painful intercourse), dyschezia (painful defecation), and low back pain. A history of infertility is also common. Pelvic examination can reveal a fixed, retroverted uterus and masses or nodularity along the uterosacral ligaments. A normal-sized uterus is less supportive of a diagnosis for uterine fibroid or adenomyosis. PID and endometriosis could both cause infertility and painful menses. However, the negative history for STIs makes PID less likely. Endometrial carcinoma is more closely associated with irregular bleeding than with painful menses.

10. **b.** Secondary dysmenorrhea is defined as dysmenorrhea with an identifiable pelvic abnormality. Dysmenorrhea, whether primary or secondary, is not psychological in origin as once was believed.

11. **c.** The diagnosis of endometriosis can be strongly suspected on the basis of a careful history and physical examination. However, confirmation of the diagnosis requires direct surgical visualization of lesions, which is usually performed by laparoscopy. Hysteroscopy and HSG are not helpful diagnostically because they assess only the internal uterine anatomy, not the external pelvic cavity and peritoneal surfaces. Ultrasound and MRI may give useful information in differentiating solid from cystic lesions, but they cannot be used for the primary diagnosis of endometriosis.

12. **e.** The primary goal of hormonal treatment of endometriosis is to reduce dysmenorrhea or dyspareunia because medical therapy has not been shown to restore fertility. Medical therapy is directed at induction of amenorrhea, which, it is hoped, will result in atrophy of the ectopic endometrial tissue. Combination OCPs reduce menstrual volume and theoretically decrease retrograde flow. Symptoms of endometriosis are relieved in three-fourths of patients. Continuous use of OCPs as described in question 8 can be employed to achieve longer periods of amenorrhea. OCPs are an optimal choice in patients who also desire a method of contraception. Progestins (oral or injectable) are also effective at reducing the symptoms of endometriosis. Depo-subQ provera 104 (medroxyprogesterone acetate injectable suspension 104 mg/0.65 mL for subcutaneous use) is FDA approved for the management of endometriosis-associated pain. Other therapies include GnRH agonists (i.e., Lupron), which suppress gonadotropin secretion with a secondary decrease in ovarian estrogen production. A pseudomenopausal state is effectively induced such that patients may experience hypoestrogenic side effects (i.e., vasomotor symptoms and a decrease in bone density). Danazol, a synthetic androgen that inhibits luteinizing hormone and follicle-stimulating hormone, is also effective in the treatment of endometriosis. Like GnRH agonists, danazol has a problematic side effect profile, which includes both hypoestrogenic symptoms (hot flushes and night sweats) and androgenic symptoms

(acne, hirsutism, and weight gain). The response rate is approximately 90% for both GnRH and danazol. The only answer listed that is not medical treatment for pain related to endometriosis is clomiphene, which is used for ovulation induction in patients being treated for infertility. Surgical therapy is reserved for patients with symptoms refractory to medical treatment or for patients who are infertile with advanced disease.

13. **c.** Primary dysmenorrhea usually begins within 6 to 12 months of menarche and thus is likely to be associated with onset of pain during adolescence. Answers a, b, d, and e are more consistent with a patient presenting with secondary dysmenorrhea. Presentation of pain later in adulthood or pain completely unresponsive to NSAIDs or OCPs should make you suspect secondary amenorrhea. The next step is to determine the etiology of the patient's secondary amenorrhea.

14. **b.** Secondary dysmenorrhea can be caused by any condition that affects the pelvic region. Commonly associated disorders include PID, endometriosis, and adenomyosis or the presence of an IUD. Copper IUDs (ParaGard) are more commonly associated with dysmenorrhea than the progestin-releasing intrauterine system (Mirena), which tends to reduce menstrual flow and cramping. OCPs are beneficial in some cases and are not a cause of secondary dysmenorrhea.

Solution to the Clinical Case Management Problem

The etiology of endometriosis is not completely understood and is likely multifactorial. The classic theory links endometriosis to "retrograde menstruation." According to this theory, fragments of endometrium are passed in a retrograde manner through the fallopian tubes, into the pelvic cavity, and subsequently implant onto various uterine and extrauterine structures. These tissue implants have the ability to respond to hormonal cues, such that cyclic proliferation and sloughing occurs just as in native endometrial lining. Although an attractive explanation, it does not completely explain how endometrial tissue has been found in remote sites such as lung and brain.

Some have proposed that endometrial tissue travels via hematogenous or lymphatic spread to distal sites. The theory of "coelomic metaplasia" is based on the fact that peritoneal tissue shares the same origin as endometrial tissue in the primitive coelomic wall. It is hypothesized that peritoneal tissue has the potential to transform into endometrial tissue via "metaplasia" under the influence of certain environmental triggers. A third theory suggests that remnants of Müllerian cells in the pelvis retain their ability to differentiate into endometrial tissue under hormonal stimulation. Finally, alterations in cell-mediated and humoral immunity may play a role in the pathogenesis of endometriosis.

Summary

1. Diagnosis

a. Primary dysmenorrhea: Begins within 3 years of the onset of menarche. Presents with mid- to lower abdominal pain, spasmodic in nature, starting within hours of menstrual flow onset and usually lasting 2 to 4 days.

b. Secondary dysmenorrhea: Dysmenorrhea associated with pelvic pathology. Onset is usually later in relation to menarche.

2. Etiology

a. Primary dysmenorrhea: Caused by increased levels of prostaglandin.

b. Secondary dysmenorrhea: Causes include endometriosis, adenomyosis, endometrial polyps, myomas, cervical stenosis, PID, and the presence of an IUD.

3. Treatment

a. Primary dysmenorrhea: First line treatment is NSAIDs. If a drug from one class is not effective, try a drug from the other class. If this is not successful, proceed to an OCP. Although an OCP is considered a second-line option, it may be used as an initial treatment in conjunction with NSAIDs if the patient desires contraception.

b. Secondary dysmenorrhea: Establish and treat the cause.

Endometriosis is classically associated with dyspareunia, dyschezia, lower back pain, and infertility. A definitive diagnosis is based on laparoscopy. Medical treatment options include OCPs, progestins (i.e., Depo-SubQ Provera 104), danazol, or GnRH agonists.

Suggested Reading

Audet MC, Moreau M, Koltun WD, et al: Evaluation of contraceptive efficacy and cycle control of a transdermal contraceptive patch vs. an oral contraceptive: A randomized controlled trial. *JAMA* 285: 2347–2354, 2001.

Baldaszti E, Wimmer-Puchinger B, Loschke K: Acceptability of the long-term contraceptive levonorgestrel-releasing intrauterine system (Mirena): A 3-year follow-up study. *Contraception* 67:87–91, 2003.

Davis AR, Westhoff CL: Primary dysmenorrhea in adolescent girls and treatment with oral contraceptives. *J Pediatr Adolesc Gynecol* 14:3–8, 2001.

Depo-subQ provera 104 prescribing information. Available at www.depo-subqprovera104.com/pdf/deposubqPI.pdf.

Dickerson LM, et al: Premenstrual syndrome. *Am Fam Physician* 67:1743–1752, 2003.

Frackiewicz EJ: Endometriosis: An overview of the disease and its treatment. *J Am Pharm Assoc (Wash)* 40:645–657, 2000.

French L: Dysmenorrhea. *Am Fam Physician* 2005;71:285–91, 292.

Hatcher RA, Trussell J, Stewart F, et al, eds: *Contraceptive Technology*, 18th ed. New York: Ardent Media, 2005.

Mounsey AL, Wilgus A, Slawson DC: Diagnosis and management of endometriosis. *Am Fam Physician* 74(4):594–600, 2006.

Proctor M, Farquhar C: Dysmenorrhoea. *Clin Evidence* Jun(9):1994–2013, 2003.

Proctor ML, Farquhar CM, Sinclair OJ, Johnson NP: Surgical interruption of pelvic nerve pathways for primary and secondary dysmenorrhoea. *Cochrane Database Syst Rev* (3):CD001896, 2004.

Proctor ML, Roberts H, Farquhar CM: Combined oral contraceptive pill (OCP) as treatment for primary dysmenorrhoea. *Cochrane Database Syst Rev* (3):CD002120, 2001.

Seasonale prescribing information. Available at www.seasonale.com/pdf/Seasonale_prescribing_info.pdf.

Sulak PJ, Kuehl TJ, Ortiz M, Shull BL: Acceptance of altering the standard 21-day/7-day oral contraceptive regimen to delay menses and reduce hormone withdrawal symptoms. *Am J Obstet Gynecol* 186:1142–1149, 2002.

CHAPTER

76   Abnormal Uterine Bleeding

CLINICAL CASE PROBLEM 1

A 35-Year-Old Female with Heavy Menses

A 35-year-old female presents to your office with concerns about heavy menstrual periods for the past year that occur at irregular intervals. She explains that sometimes her menses comes twice a month but other times will skip 2 months in a row. Her menses may last 7 to 10 days and require 10 to 15 thick sanitary napkins on the heaviest days. She admits to some fatigue, but she denies any lightheadedness. She has no pain with menses or intercourse. She denies any vaginal discharge or any other symptoms. She is a nonsmoker. She has had normal Pap smears in the past. She is in a stable monogamous relationship with her husband and denies a history of sexually transmitted infections (STIs). On physical examination, her blood pressure is 120/80 mmHg and her body mass index (BMI) is 32. Her physical examination is normal, including pelvic exam.

SELECT THE BEST ANSWER TO THE FOLLOWING QUESTIONS

1. The patient's bleeding pattern is best described as
   a. menometrorrhagia
   b. polymenorrhea
   c. menorrhagia
   d. metorrhagia
   e. oligomenorrhea

2. Which of the following should initially be considered in the differential diagnosis of this patient's problem?
   a. dysfunctional uterine bleeding (DUB)
   b. pelvic inflammatory disease (PID)
   c. endometrial carcinoma
   d. bleeding dyscrasia
   e. all of the above

3. Which of the following tests is not appropriate for the initial workup of this patient?
   a. complete blood count (CBC)
   b. assessment for history of bleeding dyscrasia
   c. free testosterone and dehydroepiandrosterone sulfate (DHEAS)
   d. urine pregnancy test
   e. all of the above

4. The most likely diagnosis is
   a. DUB
   b. PID
   c. endometrial carcinoma
   d. bleeding dyscrasia
   e. none of the above

5. What is the most likely underlying mechanism for this patient's abnormal bleeding?
   a. a coagulation defect
   b. anovulation
   c. uterine pathology
   d. cervical pathology
   e. none of the above

6. Your patient returns to discuss test results. Her hemoglobin is 10.8 g/dL. She does not desire future fertility and has no method of birth control at this time. Which of the following therapies would not be an appropriate medical management option for this patient?

a. iron supplementation

b. cyclic progestin

c. medroxyprogesterone acetate injection (Depo-Provera)

d. combined oral contraceptives

e. levonorgestrel intrauterine system (LNG-IUS)

CLINICAL CASE PROBLEM 2

A 25-Year-Old Female with Amenorrhea

A 25-year-old female (gravida 0, para 0) presents to your office complaining of not having her period for the past 6 months. She previously had regular cycles since menarche at age 13 years. Her blood pressure is 100/70 mmHg, and her BMI is 19. Her physical exam is unremarkable, including pelvic exam. She has normal secondary sexual development. Upon further questioning, she reveals that she has been training for a marathon and has lost approximately 10 pounds in the past 2 months. She does not have an eating disorder. She is currently sexually active with one partner and desires contraception.

7. Which of the following best describes this patient's bleeding pattern?

a. primary amenorrhea

b. secondary amenorrhea

c. dysmenorrhea

d. oligomenorrhea

e. polymenorrhea

8. Which of the following would be the least likely cause for this patient's bleeding pattern?

a. pregnancy

b. hypothyroidism

c. hypothalamic amenorrhea

d. hyperprolactinemia

e. Turner's syndrome

9. You perform a urine pregnancy test, which is negative. Which of the following laboratory studies should be done as initial workup for this patient?

a. thyroid-stimulating hormone (TSH)

b. free testosterone and DHEAS

c. CBC

d. comprehensive metabolic panel

e. all of the above

10. What is the most appropriate initial step in the evaluation of this patient's condition?

a. progestin challenge

b. hysteroscopy

c. pelvic ultrasound

d. Depo-Provera shot

e. none of the above

11. The patient's laboratory studies come back normal. She had a positive response to a progestin challenge. At this time, what would be the most beneficial medical therapy for this patient?

a. combined oral contraceptives

b. monthly progestin pills on days 1 through 10

c. monthly progestin pills on days 18 through 28

d. NSAIDs

e. all of the above are acceptable

CLINICAL CASE PROBLEM 3

A 55-Year-Old Female with Postmenopausal Bleeding

A 55-year-old postmenopausal woman with a history of type II diabetes presents to your office for her annual gynecological exam. She experienced menopause approximately 3 years ago. She mentions to you that she has had recurrent episodes of irregular "menstrual-like" vaginal bleeding, occurring every 4 to 8 weeks, for the past 6 months. She describes the bleeding as lasting from 1 to 7 days, requiring one to five pads a day. The patient has never been on hormone therapy (HT). She complains of some fatigue but is otherwise feeling well. Her Pap smears have always been normal. Sexual history is significant for a new sexual partner for the past 6 months. Her blood pressure is 130/80 mmHg and her BMI is 42. The rest of her physical exam, including pelvic, is normal.

12. You perform a Pap smear and a gonorrhea/chlamydia screen. You also check a CBC and TSH. What else do you recommend to the patient at this time?

a. transvaginal ultrasound

b. dilation and curettage (D&C)

c. combined oral contraceptives

d. oral progestin challenge

e. any of the above

13. A transvaginal ultrasound is performed and is read as "no structural abnormalities, normal

sized uterus and ovaries, 7 mm endometrial stripe noted." What should be the next step in this patient's management?
a. repeat the ultrasound in 6 months
b. give cyclic progestin
c. perform an endometrial biopsy
d. give cyclic oral contraceptives
e. observation only

CLINICAL CASE PROBLEM 4

A 27-Year-Old Female with Oligomenorrhea

A 27-year-old nulligravida female presents to your office for routine exam. Upon gynecological history, you discover that she has a 5-year history of oligomenorrhea, with only approximately two or three menses a year. She denies intercycle spotting or premenstrual symptoms. Her last menses was 3 months ago. Her blood pressure is 120/75 mmHg and her BMI is 34. Her physical exam reveals a moderate amount of facial hair and facial acne. Her pelvic examination is unremarkable.

14. What condition do you suspect in this patient?
   a. adrenal tumor
   b. polycystic ovary syndrome (PCOS)
   c. hypothyroidism
   d. hyperprolactinoma
   e. none of the above

15. All of the following laboratory studies are appropriate for initial evaluation except
   a. TSH
   b. luteinizing hormone (LH)
   c. follicle-stimulating hormone (FSH)
   d. pregnancy test
   e. transvaginal ultrasound

16. The patient returns after 2 weeks to discuss her blood test results. Her pregnancy test is negative and her prolactin, TSH, and 17-hydroxyprogesterone levels are normal. Her LH : FSH ratio is 4:1, and her testosterone level is mildly elevated. Which of the following treatment options has (have) been found to be beneficial in the treatment of PCOS?
   a. weight loss
   b. combined oral contraceptives
   c. metformin
   d. spironolactone
   e. all of the above

Clinical Case Management Problem

A 24-year-old obese female with a history of irregular periods presents to the emergency room with a 10-day history of heavy bleeding. She is soaking through 20 pads a day. Her hemoglobin is 9 g/dL: It was 14 g/dL 6 months ago. Her vital signs are stable. Discuss the medical management of emergent DUB.

Answers

1. **a.** This patient has menometrorrhagia, which is defined as excessive menstrual bleeding (>80 mL/cycle) that occurs at irregular intervals. Metorrhagia is defined as irregular, frequent bleeding of varying amounts, but not excessive. Menorrhagia is excessive bleeding (>80 mL/cycle) that occurs at regular intervals. Polymenorrhea is regular bleeding at intervals less than 21 days. Oligomenorrhea is bleeding at intervals greater than every 35 days.

2. **e.** All of the listed answers could be causes of the patient's bleeding. DUB refers to uterine bleeding for which no specific genital tract lesion or systemic cause is found. If there is a secondary cause, it should be corrected if possible. The secondary causes that should be considered include the following: (1) uterine (especially submucous) fibroids, (2) endometriosis, (3) adenomyosis, (4) chronic pelvic inflammatory disease, (5) endometrial/endocervical polyps, (6) coagulation defects, (7) morbid obesity, (8) ovarian abnormalities, (9) severe hypothyroidism, (10) adenomatous hyperplasia, and (11) endometrial carcinoma.

3. **c.** The first and most important condition to rule out is pregnancy. A urine pregnancy test is quick and inexpensive to perform and should be done as part of initial evaluation. Once pregnancy has been ruled out, one can proceed with a further workup. A pelvic exam should be performed to assess for structural lesions such as a cervical polyp or uterine fibroid. A CBC should be done to assess for anemia. Other labs, such as chemistry panel and liver function tests, can be done if there is suspicion for systemic hepatic or renal disease. Routine performance of these studies in otherwise healthy patients generally does not reveal useful information. TSH and/or serum prolactin should be considered in women deemed anovulatory. A thorough history should be sought for bleeding dyscrasia (history of easy bruising, epistaxis, bleeding gums, and family history), particularly in adolescents presenting with menorrhagia. Bleeding disorders have been demonstrated in up to 10.7% of women presenting with menorrhagia, the most common being von Willebrand's disease. Laboratory assessment for an inherited coagulation disorder should be done if indicated by history. A transvaginal ultrasound is not necessary in the initial evaluation unless pelvic examination reveals abnormalities or an adequate pelvic exam was unable to be performed (due to body habitus or patient discomfort). Testosterone and DHEAS levels should be considered if there is evidence of androgen excess (hirsutism or acne) or virilization (male pattern baldness, deepening voice, and clitoromegaly), but these are not routinely indicated in the evaluation of irregular bleeding.

4. **a.** The most likely cause for bleeding in this patient is DUB. Her history of normal Pap smears and low-risk sexual history makes PID and cervical carcinoma unlikely. Given her age (younger than 35 years), endometrial carcinoma is unlikely but should always be considered in the differential diagnosis. There should be a low threshold to perform endometrial biopsy if her bleeding is not responsive to medical therapy.

5. **b.** The most common cause of DUB is anovulatory bleeding. Ovulatory DUB accounts for less than 10% of all DUB. When the uterine lining is sequentially proliferated by estrogen and then ripened with progesterone (secretory phase), the endometrium is structurally stable. Sloughing of the endometrium does not occur unless progesterone withdrawal takes place. When progesterone is withdrawn, the tissue breakdown is orderly and progressive. Bleeding is limited in both amount and duration by spiral arteriolar vasoconstriction. Menstrual shedding is simultaneous in all endometrial segments. This is why ovulatory cycles are regular and predictable from month to month. When the uterine lining is proliferated by estrogen alone without progesterone to stabilize it, the endometrium continues to thicken. When the endometrial proliferation reaches a given thickness, it starts to shed, but this bleeding is not accompanied by spiral arteriolar vasoconstriction. Therefore, it is not limited in either amount or duration and can occur at any time. Endometrial shedding occurs at random times from random sites within the uterus. This is why anovulatory bleeding is irregular and unpredictable.

In the evaluation of abnormal uterine bleeding, it is often helpful to consider the patient's reproductive status:

1. Premenopausal women: The majority of abnormal bleeding in patients of this age group with otherwise normal exams is DUB and anovulation. A careful history and physical examination is usually all that is required in the evaluation. OCPs and NSAIDs are of particular therapeutic benefit.
2. Perimenopausal and postmenopausal women: Endometrial carcinoma must be excluded early in the investigation in this age group. Endometrial sampling and/or transvaginal ultrasound are recommended.

6. **b.** Progestins in various forms directly address the problem of an inadequate luteal phase in women with anovulatory cycles. Oral progestins may be administered in a cyclical manner. However, although cyclic progestins may effectively control her bleeding, they are not indicated for contraception. Initial medical therapies for DUB may include the following:

1. Iron therapy for excessive blood loss.
2. NSAIDs can be beneficial in patients with menorrhagia.
3. Combined oral contraceptive pills (COCs) to shorten menses and decrease blood flow. COCs also impose a cycle in patients with irregular menses and provide effective contraception.
4. Intramuscular injections of medroxyprogesterone acetate (Depo-Provera) will eventually induce amenorrhea, which can decrease anemia and provides highly effective contraception.
5. An LNG-IUS has been shown to be efficacious in the treatment of menorrhagia, with up to 96% of women reporting reduction in blood loss at 12 months. The IUD releases a low level of levonorgestrel into the uterine cavity, inducing gland atrophy and decreased menstrual flow. Approximately 50% of users become amenorrheic at 12 months of use. Of note, clinical experience with LNG-IUS is limited to women with ovulatory abnormal uterine bleeding (AUB). LNG-IUS also provides up to 5 years of highly effective contraception.
6. Tranexamic acid, an antifibrinolytic, reduces bleeding volume by 40% to 60%. Although not a standard treatment for menorrhagia in the United States, tranexamic acid is widely used in Europe.
7. Danazol, a synthetic androgen, directly suppresses ovulation and has been shown to decrease menstrual flow more effectively than NSAIDs. However, its adverse side effect profile (i.e., weight gain and acne) may limit its use.
8. GnRH agonists effectively induce a hypoestrogenic pseudomenopausal state, resulting in amenorrhea. It has been shown to be effective treatment for ovulatory and anovulatory AUB. Side effects include vasomotor symptoms and an increased risk of osteopenia, which are often treated with "add-back" cyclic estrogen/progestin therapy.

For cases of DUB refractory to medical treatment, surgical intervention may be necessary (endometrial ablation, D&C, and hysterectomy).

7. **b.** This patient has secondary amenorrhea, which is defined as either (1) the absence of menses for 6 months in women with previous regular cycles or (2) the absence of menses for three consecutive cycles in women with prior oligomenorrhea. Primary amenorrhea is defined as either (1) no menses by age 14 years in the absence of secondary sexual development or (2) no menses by age 16 years in the presence of secondary sexual development. Secondary amenorrhea is much more common, with a prevalence of 1% to 3%. Dysmenorrhea is defined as painful menses that occurs with onset of menstrual flow. Oligomenorrhea and polymenorrhea are defined in answer 1.

8. **e.** Pregnancy is the most common cause of secondary amenorrhea and should be excluded first. Once pregnancy has been excluded, a TSH and prolactin should be done to assess for hypothyroidism or hyperprolactinemia. If there is evidence of thyroid disease, it should be treated appropriately. Signs and symptoms of hyperprolactinemia (i.e., galactorrhea, headache, or visual field deficits) should be sought. Medications that cause hyperprolactinemia (e.g., metoclopramide, antidepressants, and methyldopa) should be excluded as potential causes. It is recommended to order pituitary imaging (MRI) if prolactin levels are elevated (usually >80 mcg/L) to exclude a pituitary adenoma.

This patient most likely suffers from hypothalamic amenorrhea secondary to her recent weight loss and increased level of exercise. Functional hypothalamic amenorrhea is characterized by abnormal secretion of GnRH, resulting in low LH levels and the absence of a midcycle LH surge. This leads to anovulation and low estradiol levels. There are multiple causes of hypothalamic amenorrhea, including stress, weight loss, anorexia nervosa, poor nutrition, and strenuous exercise. This patient should be counseled that her amenorrhea may correct with weight gain and return to routine levels of exercise. She should also be advised that prolonged amenorrhea may put her at risk for accelerated bone loss and osteoporosis later in life. Turner's syndrome is a cause of primary amenorrhea, not secondary amenorrhea. It is associated with delayed puberty, short stature, and the 45 XO karyotype.

9. **a.** Thyroid function should be evaluated in patients presenting with amenorrhea, as discussed previously. The other answer choices are not appropriate as initial evaluation for this patient.

10. **a.** In order for a woman to have regular menses, the following factors must be present: (1) an unobstructed outflow tract, (2) a mature and intact hypothalamic–pituitary–ovarian axis, (3) functional ovaries, and (4) a functional uterus with a responsive endometrium. Disruption at any of these levels can result in amenorrhea or irregular menses. Once the initial evaluation has excluded pregnancy, thyroid dysfunction, and hyperprolactinemia, one should assess the previous factors in a logical, stepwise manner. First, assessment of estrogen status is accomplished with a progesterone challenge test. A standard protocol is to administer 10 mg of medroxyprogesterone (Provera) daily for 10 days. A positive test is indicated by the presence of menses within 2 to 7 days of progestin withdrawal. If there is no menses, there is either (1) an obstructed outflow tract or (2) inadequate estrogen stimulation of the endometrium. At this time, a challenge of combined estrogen and progesterone should be offered. A typical regimen consists of 1.25 mg of conjugated equine estrogen on days 1 through 21, followed by 5 to 10 mg of progesterone on the last 7 days of the 21-day cycle. Alternately, a standard cycle and dose of COCs may be used. If the patient has withdrawal bleeding within 2 to 7 days of the last dose of progestin (or COCs), it confirms a competent outflow tract and a responsive endometrium. If a patient fails to have menses, outflow tract obstruction should be suspected. Asherman's syndrome (extensive scarring of the uterine cavity) can usually be suspected by history (uterine infection, obstetric complication, and repeated D&C). Congenital vaginal and uterine anomalies should be suspected in all patients presenting with primary amenorrhea. Outflow tract obstruction can be confirmed with imaging and/or hysteroscopic evaluation. Initial evaluation with ultrasound and hysteroscopy in this patient presenting with secondary amenorrhea is not indicated. The workup as outlined previously is more appropriate because it is less invasive and likely to confirm the suspected diagnosis of hypothalamic amenorrhea. Depo-Provera would not be helpful in evaluating the cause of this patient's amenorrhea because it is likely to promote amenorrhea, not correct it.

11. **a.** Cyclic progestins will help establish regular menses but do not address any contraceptive needs. In this patient, a COC may be more appropriate because it will regulate her cycles and also address her desire for contraception. Other combined hormonal contraceptive options may also be appropriate. She should also be encouraged to maintain normal body weight and levels of exercise because this will usually correct the underlying problem. NSAIDs have no role in the management of amenorrhea.

12. **a.** Evaluation of AUB is tailored specifically to age group and reproductive status of the woman. In postmenopausal women, AUB includes vaginal bleeding 12 months or more after the cessation of menses or unpredictable bleeding in postmenopausal women who have been receiving HT for 12 months or more. The evaluation of AUB in reproductive age women younger than the age of 35 years is outlined in Clinical Case Problem 1. In this case, the patient is postmenopausal and does not need a pregnancy test, unless there is a suspicion that the history is unreliable and the postmenopausal status is questionable. In postmenopausal women, AUB includes vaginal bleeding 12 months or more after the cessation of menses or unpredictable bleeding in postmenopausal women who have been receiving HT for 12 months or more. Checking a CBC and TSH is reasonable in this patient given the duration of her irregular bleeding and complaints of fatigue. A prolactin level can be considered if indicated by history, although hyperprolactinemia usually presents as amenorrhea and not as irregular or excessive bleeding. Other routine tests include a Pap smear to evaluate for cervical dysplasia as a cause for bleeding. Infection can also cause abnormal bleeding, as in active cervicitis caused by gonorrhea or chlamydia. Given the patient's recent new sexual partner, checking cervical cultures would be prudent. Ultimately, the most serious condition to assess for is endometrial carcinoma. Of all postmenopausal women with bleeding, 5% to 10% are found to have endometrial carcinoma. A transvaginal ultrasound is a reasonable first step in this evaluation. An ultrasound may reveal structural abnormalities, such as submucous fibroids, adenomyosis, or polyps. In a postmenopausal woman, an endometrial stripe of less than 5 mm on transvaginal ultrasound has a high negative predictive value such that endometrial biopsy can be avoided. In a meta-analysis comparing transvaginal ultrasound to endometrial biopsy in postmenopausal women presenting with vaginal bleeding, 96% of women with endometrial cancer had an endometrial stripe thickness greater than 5 mm. Based on this information, it has been recommended that postmenopausal women with irregular bleeding undergo a transvaginal ultrasound first to determine endometrial stripe thickness. An endometrial stripe less than 5 mm can exclude endometrial disease in the majority of women. If the endometrial stripe is greater than 5 mm, the patient should have an endometrial biopsy to confirm the presence or absence of atypia.

In general, an ultrasound is less specific for endometrial carcinoma in women on HT and in perimenopausal women. Hence, endometrial biopsy is recommended in premenopausal women older than age 35 years (some sources cite age 40 years) who present with irregular bleeding or postmenopausal women on HT for more than 6 months with irregular bleeding. Risk factors for endometrial cancer include a history of chronic anovulation, obesity, diabetes, and infertility. A D&C would not be part of the initial evaluation given its greater expense and invasiveness. Cyclic progestins or oral contraceptives should not be administered until a complete evaluation for endometrial cancer has been undertaken. Hysterectomy is never accepted as first-line treatment without confirmation of invasive disease.

13. **c.** Endometrial biopsy should be performed on all postmenopausal patients with an endometrial stripe greater than 5 mm on transvaginal ultrasound. Administering HT without confirming the presence or absence of disease is not appropriate. Repeating the ultrasound in 6 months will only delay the diagnosis. Observation is not appropriate.

14. **b.** The most likely diagnosis in this patient is PCOS. This condition is characterized by chronic anovulation and hyperandrogenism. PCOS is a diagnosis of exclusion and based largely on history and physical exam. Classic presentation includes amenorrhea, signs of androgen excess (i.e., hirsutism and acne), and polycystic ovaries. Other common findings include obesity and a history of infertility. Twenty percent of patients are asymptomatic. Physical exam should focus on assessment for obesity (increased waist-to-hip ratio >0.85), hirsutism, acne, virilizing signs (i.e., male pattern baldness, deepening voice, clitoromegaly, and increased muscle mass), stigmata of Cushing's disease, a pelvic exam for ovarian enlargement, and a breast exam to assess for galactorrhea. This patient has classic features of PCOS. An androgen-secreting tumor is unlikely given that the patient has no virilizing symptoms or signs. Adult-onset congenital adrenal hyperplasia may cause oligomenorrhea and hirsutism but is much less common than PCOS. Although it is reasonable to evaluate for hyperprolactinemia given this patient's history of anovulatory cycles, her presentation is far more consistent with PCOS than prolactinoma. Of note, prolactin levels may be mildly elevated in patients with PCOS. Hypothyroidism may cause irregular bleeding, but it should not cause signs of androgen excess.

15. **e.** PCOS is a diagnosis that can generally be made based on a careful history and exam. The National Institutes of Health has proposed that diagnostic criteria include (1) chronic anovulation and (2) signs of hyperandrogenism (i.e., acne, hirsutism, and elevated testosterone) in women in whom secondary causes have been excluded. A summary of recommended initial testing in patients with amenorrhea/oligomenorrhea and signs of androgen excess includes (1) urine or serum pregnancy test; (2) TSH; (3) prolactin; (4) LH, FSH—the LH:FSH ratio in PCOS patients is classically greater than 3:1; and (5) a testosterone level is normal to moderately elevated in PCOS (a serum testosterone level higher than 200 should make one suspicious of a virilizing tumor).

Some sources recommend testing for adult-onset congenital hyperplasia only in select cases. The American College of Obstetrics and Gynecology (ACOG) recommends testing for this condition in all women (based on expert opinion). If screening is to be performed, a morning serum 17-hydroxyprogestone level should be obtained, with basal levels higher than 5 ng/mL suggestive of adult-onset congenital adrenal hyperplasia. A serum DHEAS level may be checked to evaluate for a virilizing tumor in select patients with rapid onset of virilizing symptoms. Polycystic ovaries are present in more than 90% of women with PCOS, but they are also found in up to 25% of women in the general population. Polycystic ovaries are a sign of PCOS, as a result of chronic anvoulation, rather than a cause of this condition. Hence, a transvaginal ultrasound is not routinely indicated in patients suspected to have PCOS unless there is persistent pelvic pain or an abnormal pelvic finding.

16. e. The etiology of PCOS is complex and not completely understood. There is emerging evidence that the underlying mechanism is insulin resistance, with resultant high insulin levels stimulating excessive ovarian androgen production. The increased level of ovarian androgens is believed to be responsible for chronic anovulation. The long-term sequelae of chronic anovulation includes unopposed estrogen stimulation of the endometrium, putting women with PCOS at a three times higher risk for endometrial carcinoma than normal women. In addition, PCOS has been associated with a higher risk of lipid abnormalities, cardiovascular disease, and diabetes. All women identified to have PCOS should be screened for hyperlipidemia and diabetes. ACOG recommends that screening for diabetes should consist of a fasting glucose followed by a 2-hour glucose level after a 75-g glucose load. Treatment for women with PCOS should ultimately address (1) chronic anovulation; (2) androgen excess; (3) insulin resistance, and (4) lipid abnormalities, if present. Weight loss and exercise should be emphasized in all patients. Up to 70% of PCOS patients are overweight, and it has been shown that even a modest weight reduction can decrease insulin resistance and improve menstrual regularity. COC pills are inherently anti-androgenic and will impose regular cycles, addressing the problems of both chronic anovulation and androgen excess. COCs are an ideal first-line treatment for patients who also desire contraception. Clomiphene ovulation induction is recommended for PCOS patients suffering from infertility. Metformin, a second-generation biguanide, should also be considered a first-line treatment option for PCOS because it addresses the underlying problem of insulin resistance. Clinical studies have shown that women on metformin (500 mg three times a day or 850 mg twice a day) have increased frequency of ovulation, normalization of menses, and ovulatory response to clomiphene. Metformin can be continued during pregnancy because there has been no reported association with fetal anomalies in observational human trials or controlled animal trials. Spironolactone, in a dose of 25 to 100 mg a day, has been commonly used for problematic hirsutism.

Solution to the Clinical Case Management Problem

Attention first should be directed at the patient's vital signs and symptoms, and assessment of whether transfusion or surgical intervention is needed. Provided the patient is stable without significant symptoms, the treatment of choice for this type of heavy DUB is intravenous (IV) estrogen (Premarin 25 mg IV every 4 hours for three or four doses). In this patient, the endometrial lining that is remaining (the basal layer) will be less responsive to progestin therapy. The high-dose estrogen rapidly proliferates the thinned basal endometrium, stopping the bleeding. The estrogen administration must be followed by 10 days of a progestin to allow a normal withdrawal bleed to occur. As an alternative to IV Premarin, a standard dosed COC can be given four times per day for 5 to 7 days. This therapy may be limited by significant nausea.

Summary

ABNORMAL UTERINE BLEEDING

1. Definitions
   a. Metorrhagia: irregular, frequent bleeding of varying amounts, but not excessive
   b. Menorrhagia: excessive bleeding (>80 mL/cycle) that occurs at regular intervals
   c. Menometorrhagia: excessive menstrual bleeding (>80 mL/cycle) that occurs at irregular intervals
   d. Polymenorrhea: regular bleeding at intervals less than 21 days
   e. Oligomenorrhea: regular bleeding at intervals more than every 35 days
2. Initial evaluation of abnormal uterine bleeding
   a. Thorough history and physical
   b. Urine pregnancy test
   c. CBC if heavy bleeding suspected
   d. TSH/prolactin if indicated by history
   e. Pituitary imaging if elevated prolactin
   f. Evaluation for coagulation disorder if indicated by history
   g. Transvaginal ultrasound if abnormal pelvic exam or inadequate pelvic exam
   h. Endometrial biopsy in perimenopausal patients or postmenopausal patients on HT for more than 6 months with irregular bleeding to exclude endometrial carcinoma
   i. Transvaginal ultrasound in postmenopausal patients with irregular bleeding; perform endometrial biopsy if endometrial stripe > 5 mm
3. Secondary causes of abnormal uterine bleeding: fibroids, endometriosis, adenomyosis, chronic pelvic inflammatory disease, coagulation defects, severe hypothyroidism, renal failure, liver failure, endometrial carcinoma
4. DUB: abnormal uterine bleeding that cannot be attributed to any specific genital tract lesion or systemic disease; usually anovulatory, although less than 10% of DUB is ovulatory
   e. Treatment for DUB: NSAIDs, OCPs, progestins, tranexamic acid, danazol, GnRH agonists, LNG-IUS; surgical intervention for refractory cases—endometrial ablation and hysterectomy

AMENORRHEA

1. Primary amenorrhea: (1) no menses by age 14 years in the absence of secondary sexual development or (2) no menses by age 16 years in the presence of secondary sexual development.
2. Secondary amenorrhea: (1) the absence of menses for 6 months in women with previous regular cycles or (2) the absence of menses for three cycles in women with prior oligomenorrhea.
3. Causes of primary amenorrhea: Turner's syndrome, outflow tract obstruction.
4. Causes of secondary amenorrhea: pregnancy, thyroid dysfunction, hyperprolactinemia, hypothalamic amenorrhea (stress, weight loss, excessive exercise).
5. Evaluation of secondary amenorrhea: history and exam, pregnancy test, TSH, prolactin. If preliminary evaluation is unrevealing, administer progestin challenge. If there is no response to progestin challenge, give combined estrogen and progestin to exclude outflow tract obstruction.
6. Treatment: Correct underlying cause. Administer cyclic progestins, or administer OCPs if contraception is desired and there are no contraindications.

PCOS

1. Definition: PCOS is a condition characterized by chronic anovulation and hyperandrogenism. PCOS is a diagnosis of exclusion.
2. Laboratory evaluation: pregnancy test, TSH, prolactin, LH, FSH (LH:FSH level classically > 3:1), 17-hydroxyprogesterone, testosterone. DHEAS if suspect a virilizing tumor. Evaluation for diabetes and hyperlipidemia if diagnosis of PCOS is confirmed. Transvaginal ultrasound not routinely indicated unless there is pelvic pain or abnormality.
3. Treatment options: OCPs, metformin, spironolactone, clomiphene for infertility patients.

Suggested Reading

Albers JR, Hull SK, Wesley RM: Abnormal uterine bleeding. *Am Fam Physician* 69(8):1915–1926, 2004.
American College of Obstetrics and Gynecology: ACOG practice bulletin: Management of anovulatory bleeding. *Int J Gynaecol Obstet* 73: 263–271, 2001.
Hunter MS, Sterrett JJ: Polycystic ovary syndrome: It's not just infertility. *Am Fam Physician* 62:1079–1088,1090, 2000.

Master-Hunter T, Heiman DL: Amenorrhea: Evaluation and treatment. *Am Fam Physician* 73:1374–1382, 2006.
Oriel KA, Schraeger S: Abnormal uterine bleeding. *Am Fam Physician* 60:1371–1382, 1999.
Prentice A: Medical management of menorrhagia. *West J Med* 172:253–255,2000.

CLINICAL CASE PROBLEM 1

A 37-Year-Old Female with Pelvic Pain and Vaginal Spotting

A 37-year-old G1P1001 female comes to your office with a 3-day history of progressive pelvic pain. She notes some vaginal spotting but no frank bleeding. She denies any fevers, chills, diarrhea, vaginal discharge, or urinary symptoms. Her last menstrual period was 6 weeks ago. She is married and has been trying to conceive for the past 6 months. She and her husband have one child already, a result of in vitro fertilization (IVF). She is afebrile, and her pulse and blood pressure are normal. On speculum examination, her os appears closed and there is a small amount of dark brownish-red blood pooled in the fornix. There is no mucopurulent discharge or cervical motion tenderness. On bimanual examination, her uterus feels slightly enlarged and boggy, and the left adnexa is tender without any obvious mass. A wet prep is normal except for many red blood cells.

SELECT THE BEST ANSWER TO THE FOLLOWING QUESTIONS

1. Which of the following is the most likely diagnosis?
   a. acute cervicitis
   b. ectopic pregnancy
   c. acute pelvic inflammatory disease (PID)
   d. completed spontaneous abortion
   e. endometriosis

2. What is the most appropriate initial test that should be performed to support your diagnosis?
   a. urine or serum β-human chorionic gonadotropin (β-hCG)
   b. hysterosalpingogram
   c. culdocentesis
   d. pelvic/transvaginal ultrasound
   e. laparoscopy

3. A serum β-hCG is ordered and is reported soon thereafter to be 5000 mIU/mL. Based on this level of serum β-hCG, you would expect which of the following?
   a. an intrauterine pregnancy visible on transvaginal ultrasound only

   b. an intrauterine pregnancy visible on transabdominal ultrasound only
   c. an intrauterine pregnancy visible on both transvaginal and transabdominal ultrasound
   d. no intrauterine pregnancy yet because it is still too early
   e. none of the above

4. A transvaginal ultrasound reveals a mass in the adnexal and no evidence of an intrauterine pregnancy. Which of the following medical treatments is appropriate for this condition?
   a. intravenous estrogen
   b. combined oral contraceptives (contain estrogen and progestin)
   c. progestin-only pills
   d. intramuscular (IM) medroxyprogesterone acetate
   e. IM methotrexate

5. Which of the following situations could explain a serum β-hCG titer below the "discriminatory threshold" and an absence of an intrauterine gestational sac on ultrasound?
   a. early, normal pregnancy
   b. ectopic pregnancy
   c. heterotopic pregnancy
   d. early pregnancy failure
   e. all of the above

6. Which of the following is not a risk factor for ectopic pregnancy?
   a. intrauterine devices (IUDs)
   b. previous ectopic pregnancy
   c. PID
   d. endometriosis
   e. cigarette smoking

7. In which anatomic site do most ectopic pregnancies occur?
   a. the ampulla of the fallopian tube
   b. the isthmus of the fallopian tube
   c. the interstitial portion of the fallopian tube
   d. the interstitial portion of the ovary
   e. the endometrial lining

8. Which of the following statements is true regarding the clinical presentation of ectopic pregnancy?
   a. the majority of women present with fever higher than 100.4°F
   b. the majority of women report vasovagal symptoms
   c. the majority of women report amenorrhea or abnormal menses
   d. the majority of women have peritoneal signs
   e. the majority of women present with hemorrhage

9. Major complications of ectopic pregnancy include which of the following?
   a. intraabdominal hemorrhage
   b. hypovolemic shock
   c. fetal death
   d. a and b
   e. a, b, and c

10. Which of the following statements is true regarding ectopic pregnancy?
    a. the number of cases has markedly increased in the United States during the past 20 years
    b. the incidence decreases with age
    c. it occurs more commonly in nulligravida women
    d. there is no significant difference in incidence between different ethnic groups
    e. infertility patients have a lower risk of ectopic pregnancy

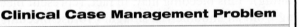

Clinical Case Management Problem

Discuss the reason(s) for the marked increase in number of ectopic pregnancies in the United States during the past two decades.

Answers

1. **b.** The most common presentation of ectopic pregnancy in symptomatic patients is abdominal pain with spotting, usually occurring 6 to 8 weeks after the last menstrual period. In a patient of childbearing age, any of the three As (amenorrhea, abdominal pain, and abnormal uterine bleeding) should suggest the possibility of an ectopic pregnancy. The patient's history of IVF should also alert the clinician that this patient is at higher risk for an ectopic pregnancy. An ectopic pregnancy is any pregnancy in which the fertilized ovum implants outside the intrauterine cavity. A ruptured ectopic pregnancy is a true medical emergency. It is the leading cause of maternal mortality in the first trimester and accounts for 10% to 15% of all maternal deaths. Ectopic pregnancy is more common in women older than age 35 years and in nonwhite ethnic groups. The differential diagnosis of ectopic pregnancy includes the following: spontaneous abortion, molar pregnancy, ruptured corpus luteum, acute PID, adnexal torsion, degenerating leiomyoma, acute appendicitis, pyelonephritis, diverticulitis, regional ileitis, and ulcerative colitis. The absence of mucopurulent discharge,

cervical motion tenderness, and white blood cells on wet prep makes a diagnosis of cervicitis or PID less likely. A complete, spontaneous abortion should be associated with resolving abdominal cramping, not increasing abdominal pain. Endometriosis classically presents as dysmenorrhea, dyspareunia, and dyschezia, which is not consistent with this patient's history.

2. **a.** Based on this patient's history and physical examination, the probability of an ectopic pregnancy is high. Therefore, a high-sensitivity urine pregnancy test or serum β-hCG should be performed at this time. If the pregnancy testing is negative, then ectopic pregnancy is essentially ruled out. If the tests indicate the patient is pregnant, it is vital to establish whether the pregnancy is intrauterine or extrauterine. This is accomplished by a combination of serial, quantitative serum β-hCG testing and abdominal/transvaginal ultrasonography.

3. **c.** This patient had a serum β-hCG of 5000 mIU/mL; an intrauterine pregnancy should be visible by either transvaginal or transabdominal ultrasound. The discriminatory threshold is the critical serum quantitative β-hCG titer above which an intrauterine pregnancy (e.g., normal-appearing gestational sac) should be seen in the uterus by ultrasonography. The discriminatory threshold is 1500 mIU/mL when using transvaginal ultrasonography or 3600 mIU/mL with abdominal ultrasonography. Failure to find a gestational sac in the uterus when either of these thresholds is reached is presumptive evidence of an ectopic pregnancy.

4. **e.** The medical management of choice for ectopic pregnancy is IM methotrexate. Methotrexate is a folic acid antagonist that destroys rapidly growing tissue, including chorionic villi. It does have the potential for serious toxicity. A single dose is successful in resolving 90% of ectopic pregnancies. Declining serum β-hCG titers indicate success. Failure of titers to decrease at least 15% by days 4 to 7 posttreatment indicates the need for an additional dose or surgery. The cumulative success rate is 95%, with subsequent evidence of tubal patency in 80% and fertility in almost 70%. These rates are similar to those reported with treatment of unruptured tubal pregnancy by salpingostomy. Methotrexate is optimal for small (<3.5-cm mass), unruptured ectopic pregnancies and should be considered only if the following conditions apply: (1) early gestation (preferably <8 weeks); (2) patient desires future fertility; (3) nonlaparoscopic diagnosis; (4) patient is hemodynamically stable without signs of hemoperitoneum; (5) patient has normal hemoglobin, liver function, and renal function; and (6) patient is able to return for follow-up care.

5. e. There are several situations in which the serum β-hCG titer may be below the discriminatory threshold and no intrauterine gestational sac is visualized: (1) an early, normal pregnancy; (2) an ectopic pregnancy; (3) a heterotopic pregnancy; or (4) an early pregnancy failure (threatened or incomplete or complete spontaneous abortion). To differentiate a normal pregnancy from an abnormal pregnancy, one can obtain serum quantitative β-hCG titers; in normal pregnancies, the β-hCG titer should approximately double every 48 hours. Once the discriminatory threshold is reached, a repeat ultrasound can be performed. If the β-hCG titer fails to double in 48 hours, an uterine aspiration procedure or uterine curettage can determine the presence (nonviable intrauterine pregnancy) or absence (probable ectopic pregnancy) of chorionic villi. Culdocentesis (aspiration of fluid from the cul-de-sac) is rarely performed when ultrasonography is readily available. A heterotopic pregnancy (coexistence of an intrauterine pregnancy and an ectopic pregnancy) is rare and extremely difficult to diagnose. The incidence of heterotopic pregnancy is higher among women receiving fertility treatments.

6. a. Major risk factors for ectopic pregnancy include previous ectopic pregnancy, PID, endometriosis, previous tubal surgery, previous pelvic surgery, infertility and infertility treatments, uterotubal anomalies, history of in utero exposure to diethylstilbestrol (DES), and cigarette smoking. These risk factors all interfere with fallopian tube function. Other possible indirect risk factors include multiple sexual partners, early age at first intercourse, and vaginal douching. Contraceptive intrauterine devices do not increase the absolute risk of ectopic pregnancy. In fact, IUD users have a lower rate of ectopic pregnancy (0.2/1000 woman-years) than non-IUD users (3 to 4.5/1000 woman-years). However, IUDs provide excellent protection from intrauterine pregnancy, and in the rare circumstance when pregnancy does occur, it is more likely to be an ectopic pregnancy.

7. a. The most frequent site of extrauterine implantation is the ampulla of the fallopian tube (78%), where most fertilizations occur. The isthmus of the fallopian tube is the next most common site of implantation (12%). Cornual pregnancies are uncommon, representing only 2.5% of the total. Abdominal, ovarian, and cervical pregnancies are rare.

8. c. There are no absolutely pathognomonic signs or symptoms of an early ectopic pregnancy. The most common symptoms noted are the three As (abdominal pain, abnormal vaginal bleeding, and amenorrhea). Between 96% and 100% of patients with ectopic gestation complain of pain, even before rupture. No specific type of pain is diagnostic. With tubal rupture, the pain becomes more severe. Amenorrhea or a history of abnormal menses is reported in 75% to 95% of patients with ectopic pregnancy. A careful history with respect to the character and timing of the last two or three menstrual cycles (amount of flow and number of days of flow) is important. Initially, patients may state that they have not missed a period; however, when questioned carefully, they may describe the period as being different (lighter than usual or irregular in timing). This bleeding may, in fact, represent bleeding from an endometrial slough. Profuse bleeding is uncommon. Common symptoms of early pregnancy, such as nausea and breast tenderness, are present in only 10% to 25% of patients with ectopic pregnancies. Vasovagal symptoms (dizziness and fainting) are present in 20% to 35% of patients. Abdominal tenderness is present in most patients (80% to 95%). Rebound tenderness may or may not be present. A mass is palpable in 50% of patients with ectopic pregnancy. If there is uterine enlargement, it is not to the degree that would be expected for the duration of amenorrhea. A few patients will state that they, in fact, passed tissue (a decidual cast). Most patients are afebrile.

9. d. The major complications of ectopic pregnancy are intraabdominal hemorrhage and hypovolemic shock secondary to rupture. Rupture of the ectopic pregnancy is responsible for almost all maternal morbidity and mortality. Fetal death cannot be classified as a major complication because of its inevitability in ectopic pregnancy.

10. a. There has been a fivefold increase in the number of ectopic pregnancies in the United States during the past two decades. There is a marked increase in the rate of ectopic pregnancies with increasing age. Most ectopic pregnancies occur in multigravida women, with only 10% to 15% occurring in nulligravida women. Rates of ectopic pregnancies are up to 30% higher in nonwhite women. Ectopic pregnancy rates are higher in women who have undergone fertility treatments.

Solution to the Clinical Case Management Problem

The significant increase in the number of ectopic pregnancies in the United States during the past 20 years is mainly the result of improved early diagnosis, including some ectopic pregnancies that previously would have resolved spontaneously without detection. Increases in certain risk factors (e.g., PID and infertility treatments) may also contribute to the increase in cases of ectopic pregnancy. However, the case fatality rate has also declined dramatically in the past 20 years.

Summary

1. **Incidence**

   There has been a 5-fold increase in the past 20 years, likely a result of improved early diagnosis. Maternal death rates have declined almost 10-fold during the same time period.

2. **Risk factors**

   a. Strong association: (1) previous ectopic pregnancy, (2) PID, (3) endometriosis; (4) previous tubal surgery, (5) previous pelvic surgery, (6) infertility and infertility treatments, (7) uterotubal anomalies, (8) history of in utero exposure to DES, and (9) cigarette smoking.

   b. Weaker association: (1) multiple sexual partners, (2) early age at first intercourse, and (3) vaginal douching.

   c. The IUD does not increase the absolute risk of an ectopic pregnancy. In fact, the incidence of ectopic pregnancy is lower in IUD users than in non-IUD users. However, if in the rare chance an IUD user does become pregnant, the pregnancy is more likely to be extrauterine.

3. **Signs and symptoms**

   a. The three As—abdominal pain, amenorrhea, and abnormal vaginal bleeding—indicate an ectopic pregnancy until proven otherwise.

   b. Vasovagal attacks and orthostatic hypotension are strong indicators of tubal rupture.

4. **Major complications**

   Tubal rupture is indicated by intraabdominal hemorrhage or hypovolemia and shock.

5. **Diagnosis**

   a. Perform qualitative urine or serum β-hCG. Know the discriminatory threshold levels above which an intrauterine pregnancy should be visualized (>1500 mIU/mL for transvaginal ultrasound and >3600 mIU/mL for an abdominal ultrasound).

   b. Other: Abdominal/transvaginal ultrasound, diagnostic uterine aspiration procedure or uterine curettage, and culdocentesis (rarely needed).

   c. Situations in which the serum β-hCG titer may be below the discriminatory threshold and no intrauterine gestational sac is visualized: (1) an early, normal pregnancy; (2) an ectopic pregnancy; (3) a heterotopic pregnancy; or (4) an early pregnancy failure (threatened and incomplete or complete spontaneous abortion).

   d. To differentiate a normal pregnancy from an abnormal pregnancy, obtain serum quantitative β-hCG titers. In normal pregnancies, the β-hCG titer should approximately double every 48 hours.

6. **Treatment**

   a. Medical management: Criteria for methotrexate therapy include the following: (1) hemodynamically stable patient, (2) small ectopic mass (early gestation), (3) lack of fetal cardiac motion, (4) normal hemoglobin, (5) normal liver function tests, (6) normal renal function, and (7) close patient follow-up is possible.

   b. Surgical management: Laparotomy with salpingectomy, tubal sterilization, and fallopian tube conservative surgery, which can include salpingostomy, segmental resection and anastomosis, and fibril evacuation.

Suggested Reading

American College of Obstetricians and Gynecologists: Medical management of tubal pregnancy, Practice Bulletin No. 3. Washington, DC: ACOG, 1998.

Tay JI, Moore J, Walker JJ: Ectopic pregnancy. *West J Med* 173:131–134, 2000.

Tenore JL: Ectopic pregnancy. *Am Fam Physician* 61:1080–1088, 2000.

CLINICAL CASE PROBLEM 1

A 23-Year-Old Female Presents for Her Annual Gynecologic Examination

A 23-year-old healthy, nulliparous female comes to your office for her annual physical and Papanicolaou (Pap) test. Her last menstrual period was 7 days ago. She has been on oral contraceptive pills (OCPs) for several years and tells you that she stopped taking them recently to "give her body a break." She heard from friends and relatives that using OCPs for a long time increases the risk of future health problems, including infertility. She is currently sexually active with one male partner for the past 6 months. They use condoms and withdrawal inconsistently. The patient reports a history of chlamydia several years ago for which she and her partner were treated. She does not want to be pregnant anytime in the near future. She smokes a pack of cigarettes a day. On examination, her blood pressure is 120/80 mmHg, her weight is 200 pounds, and she is 5 feet 5 inches tall (body mass index is 33). The rest of her examination is unremarkable except for some mild facial acne. You perform a pelvic examination, a Pap test, and gonorrhea and chlamydia cultures.

SELECT THE BEST ANSWER TO THE FOLLOWING QUESTIONS

1. What would you tell your patient regarding the use of the "withdrawal method?"
   a. it is a highly effective method of contraception but not sexually transmitted disease (STD) protection
   b. it is a highly effective method of STD protection but not contraception
   c. it has a less than 1% failure rate with "perfect use"
   d. it has up to a 24% failure rate with "typical use"
   e. it has a failure rate similar to that of not using any contraceptive method at all

2. Which of the following methods would provide both effective contraception and STD protection?

   a. nonlatex male condoms made from animal products
   b. nonlatex female condoms made from polyurethane
   c. a diaphragm
   d. OCPs
   e. the sponge with embedded spermicide

3. Which of the following statements is true regarding the use of any estrogen-containing hormonal contraceptive method for this patient?
   a. estrogen is contraindicated because she is a smoker
   b. estrogen may increase her risk of endometrial cancer
   c. estrogen is contraindicated because of her history of chlamydia
   d. estrogen is contraindicated because of her obesity
   e. estrogen may improve her acne

4. You counsel the patient about her contraceptive options. All of the following are true except
   a. she cannot get an intrauterine device (IUD) because she has never had a child
   b. she may have an increased risk of contraceptive failure on the transdermal contraceptive patch (OrthoEvra)
   c. local skin irritation is the most common side effect experienced by transdermal contraceptive patch users
   d. the vaginal contraceptive ring (NuvaRing) is a soft, flexible ring that is self-inserted and removed by the patient
   e. the depo-medroxyprogesterone shot (Depo-Provera) is associated with irregular bleeding and spotting that progressively decreases over time

5. Your patient decides that she wants to restart combined oral contraceptives (COCs) since she has used the pills in the past and would like to have regular and predictable menstrual cycles. Which option would not be ideal for this patient?
   a. progestin-only pills (POPs)
   b. COCs containing 35 µg of ethinyl estradiol
   c. COCs containing 20 µg of ethinyl estradiol
   d. monophasic COCs
   e. triphasic COCs

6. You counsel your patient about starting COCs. Which of the following statements regarding COC initiation in this patient is true?
   a. she must wait until the first Sunday after her period begins to start her COCs

b. nausea and breast tenderness are uncommon side effects of COCs

c. if she develops any breakthrough bleeding, she should stop the COCs immediately

d. weight gain is an unlikely consequence of COC use

e. if she misses a pill, she should wait until her next menses and then start a new pack

7. Your patient contacts you 6 weeks after starting her COCs. She is complaining about some mid-cycle spotting and is concerned. Which of the following statements is true regarding COC use and breakthrough bleeding (BTB) in this patient?

a. smoking and cervicitis are potential causes of her BTBb. BTB is rare after the first cycle of COCs

c. use of nonsteroidal anti-inflammatory drugs will likely exacerbate her BTB

d. BTB is a reliable indicator of noncompliance during the first few cycles of use

e. BTB is a sign of inadequate contraceptive protection

8. Which of the following statements regarding long-term COC use is true?

a. there is strong evidence that long-term COC use increases ovarian cancer risk

b. there is strong evidence that long-term COC use increases breast cancer risk

c. there is strong evidence that long-term COC use decreases cervical cancer risk

d. there is strong evidence that long-term COC use decreases osteoporotic fracture risk

e. there is strong evidence that long-term COC use decreases endometrial cancer risk

9. All of the following conditions may be improved with the use of estrogen-containing hormonal contraceptives except

a. iron-deficiency anemia

b. cholelithiasis

c. dysmenorrhea

d. ectopic pregnancy

e. mittelschmerz

CLINICAL CASE PROBLEM 2

A 40-Year-Old Postpartum Female

A 40-year-old female (gravida 2, para 2) comes to your office for her 6-week postpartum visit. She had an uncomplicated pregnancy, normal spontaneous vaginal delivery, and routine postpartum course. She and her baby are doing well. She has not gotten her period yet. She is breast-feeding and supplementing with formula intermittently. She does not want to get pregnant again, at least not for another few years. The patient has no major medical problems, does not smoke, and has already returned to her aerobics class. She has no history of STDs or abnormal Pap tests. She desires a reliable birth control method that she does not have to remember to take every day or remember to use every time she has sex with her husband. Her examination is completely normal.

10. Of the following choices, which would be the most appropriate contraceptive method for this patient at this time?

a. bilateral tubal ligation (BTL) or vasectomy

b. transdermal contraceptive patch or vaginal contraceptive ring

c. COC pills

d. a levonorgestrel IUD or Depo-Provera

e. continue with the lactation amenorrhea method (LAM) only

11. Which of the following statements is true regarding the use of estrogen-containing hormonal contraceptives in this patient?

a. estrogen is contraindicated in women older than 40 years of age

b. estrogen may increase the patient's breast milk production

c. estrogen may delay the onset of menopause

d. estrogen will promote the development of fibroids and/or increase their size

e. estrogen may help regulate menses and/or reduce perimenopausal symptoms

12. Which of the following statements is true regarding the use of Depo-Provera in this patient?

a. she will have rapid return to fertility following cessation of use

b. Depo-Provera will not adversely affect her quantity or quality of breast milk

c. Depo-Provera is contraindicated if she has a seizure disorder

d. Depo-Provera will accelerate her age of onset of menopause

e. Depo-Provera will increase her risk of post-menopausal osteoporosis

13. Which of the following statements is true regarding the use of a copper IUD (ParaGard T 380A) in this patient.

a. she will have an increased risk of ectopic pregnancy

b. there is usually a long delay in return to fertility following removal of the copper IUD

c. the copper IUD is contraindicated in breast-feeding mothers

d. the copper IUD may increase her symptoms if she suffers from dysmenorrhea or menorrhagia

e. the copper IUD should not be inserted until she begins menstruating again

14. Your patient asks you about sterilization options in the future. Which of the following statements about vasectomies and tubal ligations is true?
    a. vasectomies are usually performed in an outpatient office under local anesthesia
    b. current vasectomy and tubal ligation procedures are easily reversible
    c. vasectomies increase prostate cancer risk
    d. tubal ligations increase the risk of ectopic pregnancy
    e. vasectomies reduce libido, erectile function, and penile sensation

CLINICAL CASE PROBLEM 3

A 34-Year-Old Female with a History of Obesity, Hypertension, and Diabetes

A 34-year-old female who is a long-term patient of yours presents to the office for a routine blood pressure check. She was recently diagnosed with hypertension and diabetes. Her medications include metformin, hydrochlorothiazide, and a multivitamin. Her blood pressure today is 150/100 mmHg, and her body mass index is 30. She is currently sexually active with her husband, and they use the "rhythm" method only. She reports that her menses have been irregular and vary from 20 to 45 days apart. The patient is worried about the risks of hormonal contraception given her medical conditions. She does not want to be pregnant for several years.

15. You advise her to do all the following except
    a. exercise on most days of the week for 30 minutes
    b. eat a high-fiber, low-fat diet
    c. continue to use the rhythm method (calendar method) only
    d. consider an IUD
    e. consider a progestin implant

16. Which of the following statements about barrier methods is true?
    a. the diaphragm must be inserted at least 24 hours prior to intercourse

b. the cervical cap (FemCap) is less effective in parous women compared to nulliparous women

c. the cervical cap has a lower pregnancy failure rate compared to the diaphragm

d. barrier methods are not safe for medically complicated patients

e. women with latex allergies should not use the FemCap or Lea's Shield

CLINICAL CASE PROBLEM 4

A 21-Year-Old Female Who Had Unprotected Sex 3 Days Ago

A very tearful 21-year-old female (gravida 0, para 0) walks into your office on a Tuesday morning. She tells you that she had sexual intercourse with her boyfriend Friday night. They used a condom, but it broke. They previously had intercourse with a condom the week before. Her last menstrual period was approximately 3 weeks ago and was normal in flow and duration. She had been given a sample pack of Ortho-Tri-Cyclen during her initial gynecologic examination 2 weeks ago, but she did not have a chance to start them yet. She would be devastated if she got pregnant. She is a heavy smoker (two packs per day) but otherwise has no medical problems, denies bleeding or other symptoms, and her examination is normal. Her most recent Pap smear and gonococcus/chlamydia results were normal.

17. Which of the following statements regarding the use of emergency contraceptive pills (ECPs) in this patient is true?
    a. ECPs are contraindicated because it has been longer than 72 hours
    b. ECPs are contraindicated because she is a heavy smoker
    c. ECPs could have been prescribed to this patient over the phone without an examination
    d. ECPs would be contraindicated if either her Pap or her gonococcus/chlamydia test was abnormal
    e. ECPs are contraindicated in pregnancy because they are abortifacients

18. Which of the following ECP options is not appropriate for this patient?
    a. Ovral: two white pills now; repeat 12 hours later
    b. Plan B (levonorgestrel 0.75 mg): one pill now; one pill 12 hours later

c. Plan B (levonorgestrel 0.75 mg): two pills at once right now

d. a ParaGard (copper IUD) inserted within 5 days

e. all of the above options are appropriate

19. Which of the following best describes the effects of giving women advance supplies of ECPs?

a. women are more likely to stop routine birth control

b. women are less likely to use condoms

c. women are more likely to use ECPs when needed

d. the rate of unintended pregnancy declines

e. women have higher rates of STDs

Clinical Case Management Problem

List the important user characteristics to assess to help patients select the most appropriate contraceptive method for them.

Answers

1. **d.** Contraceptive failure rates are expressed as the percentage of women who experience pregnancy during the first year of use. The rate of contraceptive failure is largely dependent on the level of compliance to a method. With "perfect use" of the withdrawal method, the failure rate is 4% within the first year of use. However, the average user of withdrawal has a significantly higher risk of pregnancy because the failure rate with "typical use" is 24%. Compared to withdrawal, the failure rate when no birth control method is used is much higher (85%). Withdrawal is a poor form of STD protection.

2. **b.** The female condom is an effective barrier method of contraception, and it also provides excellent protection against STDs. It is made of polyurethane, but it does not contain a spermicide, which can be added. Male condoms made from animal products (usually lamb cecum) have pore sizes too large to prevent STD transmission (especially viruses such as the human immunodeficiency virus [HIV], human papillomavirus [HPV], herpes simplex virus, or hepatitis B). Diaphragms, with or without nonoxynol-9, may reduce the risk of cervicitis, pelvic inflammatory disease (PID), and cervical dysplasia, but they are not effective at preventing STD transmission (especially viral).

The active ingredient of spermicides is nonoxynol-9, which acts to disrupt the cell membranes of sperm. Spermicides are available in many formulations, including foams, gels, films, and suppositories. A spermicide-embedded sponge (the Today sponge) is available without a prescription; women self-insert the sponge and leave it in the vagina for at least 6 hours postintercourse. The sponge, even with spermicide, does not provide effective STD protection alone. Studies regarding the efficacy of nonoxynol-9 as a method of STD prevention have provided conflicting results, with some reporting a decreased risk and others reporting no effect or even an increased risk. The World Health Organization (WHO) has recommended that nonoxynol-9 not be used for protection against STDs in individuals at high risk for HIV (category 4; Box 78-1) based on some studies that demonstrated an increased risk of HIV infection in this population (sex workers and women at STD clinics). It is hypothesized that nonoxynol-9 may have a disruptive, irritative effect on the vaginal/cervical mucosa, allowing for increased risk of HIV infection. It is important to note that these findings have not been demonstrated in average- to low-risk women. Although oral contraceptives may reduce the risk of PID, there is no associated significant reduction in STD transmission.

3. **e.** COCs contain both ethinyl estradiol and a progestin. All COCs may reduce acne vulgaris, mainly through the estrogen-mediated increase in sex hormone-binding globulin, which binds free testosterone. As expressed by this patient, a common concern among patients is that long-term use of COCs incurs significant health risks. For the majority of healthy women, the benefits of COCs outweigh the risks. COCs offer

---

Box 78-1   World Health Organization medical eligibility criteria for contraceptive use

Category 1: A condition in which there is no restriction in the use of a contraceptive method

Category 2: A condition in which the advantages generally outweigh the risks or theoretical risks of using a contraceptive method

Category 3: A condition in which the risks or theoretical risks generally outweigh the advantages of using a contraceptive method

Category 4: A condition that represents an unacceptable health risk if the contraceptive method is used

several potential noncontraceptive benefits, which may improve patient satisfaction and compliance. COCs are associated with a 50% reduction in the risk of endometrial cancer after 12 months of use; this risk reduction increases to 80% after 10 years of use. WHO has rated COC use in female smokers age 35 years or older as a category 3 (the risks likely outweigh the benefits) because of the increased risk of premature cardiovascular disease. COC use in female smokers younger than age 35 years is a WHO category 2 (the benefits generally outweigh the risks) given the extremely low incidence of cardiovascular disease in younger women. However, all smokers are at an increased risk for venous thromboembolic events (VTEs) and should be encouraged to quit. Epidemiologic studies have found an association between chlamydial cervicitis and COC use. COCs can cause cervical ectopy, a broadening of the area on the ectocervix covered by the mucus-secreting columnar cells that normally line the cervical canal (ectropion), which may make the cervix more vulnerable to *Chlamydia trachomatis* infection. Some experts have suggested that enhanced cervical ectopy may allow for better detection of *Chlamydia*, introducing detection bias in these studies. Interestingly, COC use is associated with a significantly decreased risk of PID, probably because of cervical mucus thickening. Regardless, this patient's previous history of a chlamydial infection is not a contraindication to COC use (WHO category 1), although she should be offered STD screening and strongly encouraged to use an effective method of STD protection (i.e., male latex or polyurethane condoms or female condoms) in addition to OCPs. Obesity is not a contraindication to COC use, although one may consider screening these patients for diabetes and hyperlipidemia. There is no evidence that overweight women need to be prescribed a higher-dose COC to ensure contraceptive efficacy. There is no evidence supporting the common claim that estrogen-containing hormonal contraceptives cause significant weight gain. However, all COC users should be encouraged to exercise and eat a well-balanced diet.

4. **a.** Widespread confusion among patients and clinicians about the IUD and its association with infertility and pelvic inflammatory disease has led to underutilization of this excellent, user-independent method of contraception. The popular belief that IUDs cause PID is an unfortunate consequence of the U.S. experience with the Dalkon Shield, a defective IUD used in the 1970s and 1980s. Current IUDs available in the United States (the copper IUD and the levonorgestrel-releasing IUD) are extremely safe for use in the majority of women, including nulliparous women. The risk of uterine infection is higher in the first 20 days after IUD insertion,

presumably from local contamination during the insertion procedure. However, after this peri-insertion period, the risk of PID in an IUD user is directly related to sexual behavior, not the IUD device. The Food and Drug Administration (FDA) has revised patient eligibility for the copper IUD (ParaGard T 380A) to reflect current evidence regarding the IUD; it is no longer contraindicated to place an IUD in a nulliparous patient or a patient with a history of PID. It is still contraindicated, however, to place an IUD in patients with a recent history of PID (within the past 3 months) or current PID.

The major established advantage of the weekly transdermal estrogen patch (OrthoEvra) and the monthly vaginal contraceptive ring (NuvaRing) compared to COCs is the potential for improved compliance, especially in younger patients. Women with a body weight of more than 198 pounds should not be prescribed the transdermal estrogen patch (OrthoEvra) because of the increased associated risk for contraceptive failure. The most commonly reported side effect of the transdermal contraceptive patch is local skin irritation, which can be minimized by rotating patch sites every week. The vaginal contraceptive ring releases 15 μg of ethinyl estradiol and 120 μg of etonorgestrel in a controlled-release manner. It is a thin, flexible ring that is self-inserted and removed by the patient each month. Patients who are not comfortable inserting devices into their vagina are not good candidates for the vaginal contraceptive ring. The depo-medroxyprogesterone shot (Depo-Provera) provides excellent contraceptive efficacy and its infrequent dosing schedule (every 11 to 13 weeks) is one of its major benefits. All patients using Depo-Provera should be counseled to expect irregular bleeding that subsides with each injection, such that 30% to 50% of users are amenorrheic after 1 year, and 80% are amenorrheic by the fifth year of use. All of these methods should also be combined with an effective means of STD protection in this patient.

5. **a.** POPs are not the ideal contraceptive choice for this patient because of the potential for irregular bleeding (she desires regular, predictable menses) and the possibility of decreased efficacy with less than perfect use. In contrast, all COC pill types usually provide most users with regular and predictable menstrual cycles within the first 3 months of use and are more "forgiving" if a pill is missed. POPs reduce the frequency, duration, and amount of menses in most users and may cause amenorrhea. POPs have a higher potential for contraceptive failure with typical use than COCs because gonadotropins are not consistently suppressed. POPs may be preferred for certain women: (1) breast-feeding women (POPs will not decrease breast milk supply in contrast to COCs), (2) women who have

medical contraindications to estrogen (e.g., migraines with aura), or (3) women who do not want estrogen-containing contraception. Women who are prescribed POPs should be counseled about the importance of taking the pills at the same time every day.

6. **d.** There is no evidence supporting the common claim that estrogen-containing hormonal contraceptives cause significant weight gain. However, all COC users should be encouraged to exercise and eat a well-balanced diet, and their weight should be monitored during periodic follow-up visits. Traditionally, women were told to wait until the Sunday after their next menses to begin oral contraception. These instructions were largely based on cultural norms (to be able to have intercourse on the weekends) rather than any physiologic indications. These instructions are not only confusing but also can put women at risk for unintended pregnancy while they are waiting to start oral contraception. The use of the "quick start" method to initiate COC use is gaining clinical popularity based on studies demonstrating that patients who start the first pill on the day of the office visit have higher adherence at 3 months than women who do a traditional delayed start. A randomized controlled trial showed that women who initiate oral contraception between periods do not have a higher incidence of BTB than women who do a traditional start. In the quick start method, women are assessed for the risk of pregnancy based on clinical history and a urine pregnancy test if necessary. If the risk of pregnancy is ruled out or unlikely, the COCs can be initiated that day.

Nausea and breast tenderness are common side effects of estrogen-containing hormonal contraceptive methods, which usually subside within the first 3 months of use. Using a lower estrogen dose COC and/or having the patient take the pill after dinner may reduce these side effects. BTB is one of the most common side effects of all hormonal contraceptive methods and one of the most common reasons for discontinuation. The most common cause of BTB in new COC users is noncompliance. Patients should be counseled about common side effects of COCs, including BTB, and the importance of compliance. They should be provided with verbal and written instructions on proper use, compliance tips, and what to do if they miss a pill and/or develop side effects. Patients should be instructed not to stop taking pills if they develop BTB or miss a pill without speaking with their health provider first because discontinuing COCs only worsens BTB and puts them at risk for an unintended pregnancy.

7. **a.** Smoking and cervicitis are potential causes of BTB and should be considered, especially in COC users with persistent BTB or who develop BTB after

having had regular bleeding cycles while taking them. Although BTB usually decreases after the first cycle of proper COC use, it is not uncommon for it to occur until after the third cycle. Nonsteroidal anti-inflammatories are effective first-line therapy for reducing BTB for all methods of hormonal contraception. Although noncompliance is the most common cause of BTB in COC users, there are other potential causes that health providers should also consider, especially if the BTB is persistent or develops after the COC user previously had regular bleeding cycles. Pregnancy, infection, and structural causes of bleeding should be ruled out in patients with persistent BTB. However, the presence of BTB is not an indicator that any hormonal contraceptive method is subtherapeutic or ineffective.

8. **e.** There is strong evidence that long-term COC use is associated with a significant reduction of both endometrial and ovarian cancer risk and that this protective effect is sustained years after use. This is thought to be the result of the effect of COCs on reducing endometrial hyperplasia and incessant ovulation. Although some studies have suggested a potential association between COC use and breast cancer, there is no strong evidence to support this. In fact, one large study found no significant increased risk in long-term COC users, including women older than 40 years of age. However, COCs are contraindicated in women with a history of estrogen-dependent malignancies. There is evidence that COC use may be associated with an increased risk for cervical cancer, but several potential confounding variables exist, including lack of condom use in COC users compared with nonusers. COCs do not provide adequate protection against STD transmission, including HPV. COCs may be associated with higher bone densities in users than in aged-matched nonusers, but there is no evidence that this provides protection against postmenopausal osteoporosis and subsequent fractures later in life.

9. **b.** Although COCs are not associated with the development of gallstones, they may actually accelerate the progression of cholelithiasis in patients who are already susceptible. COCs do not increase the risk for gallbladder cancer. COCs promote regular, predictable menses and often reduce menstrual duration and blood loss. This may help prevent or correct iron-deficiency anemia, especially in patients with excessively heavy menses (i.e., menorrhagia). COCs are an effective treatment for primary and secondary causes of dysmenorrhea, especially when given continuously (without a pill-free/placebo period). Because the primary mechanism of action for COCs is ovulation suppression, they are highly effective for preventing ectopic pregnancies and for eliminating ovulatory symptoms (mittelschmerz). Other noncontraceptive benefits of COCs include the following: (1) prevention of functional ovarian cysts, (2) improvement of acne, (3) improvement of hirsutism, (4) decreased incidence of benign breast disease (fibrocystic disease and fibroadenoma), and (5) reduced risk of endometrial and ovarian cancer.

10. d. Estrogen-containing hormonal methods (e.g., the transdermal contraceptive patch, vaginal contraceptive ring, or COC pills) can decrease milk production and flow, which may not be ideal for this currently nursing mother. Progestin-only methods do not have an adverse effect on milk quantity and, in fact, may improve milk supply. Depo-Provera provides up to 3 months of excellent pregnancy protection with every injection. Patients should be informed that it may take up to 1 year or more for fertility to return after cessation of use. The levonorgestrel (Mirena) IUD provides up to 5 years of contraception after insertion and is therefore most cost-effective for patients who desire contraception for at least several years, despite its high upfront cost. Fertility should return rapidly after IUD removal. Sterilization procedures (bilateral tubal ligation or vasectomy) should be recommended only for patients who desire permanent methods of contraception. Sterilization reversals are rarely successful, are expensive, and are susceptible to complications (e.g., ectopic pregnancy). The LAM may provide up to 6 months of effective contraception, but only in mothers who are breast-feeding their babies exclusively and have not experienced their first menses. The patient should be asked about her reasons for formula supplementation to identify any potential problems with breast-feeding that require support or intervention.

11. e. Estrogen-containing hormonal contraceptives may help regulate menses and reduce other perimenopausal symptoms (i.e., hot flashes and night sweats) in women older than 40 years of age. They may also reduce the risk of endometrial and ovarian cancer later in life. However, they will neither delay nor accelerate the age of onset of menopause. Estrogen-containing hormonal contraceptives are not contraindicated in nonsmoking women older than 40 years of age unless they have an estrogen-dependent malignancy, undiagnosed abnormal vaginal/uterine bleeding, an undiagnosed breast mass, cardiovascular disease, a history of or high risk for thromboembolic events, uncontrolled hypertension or diabetes, significant hypertriglyceridemia, gallbladder disease, active liver disease, headaches with focal neurologic symptoms, or known or suspected pregnancy. Estrogen-containing hormonal

contraceptives should not be used in breast-feeding women until the weaning process has begun because estrogen can decrease the patient's milk production. Estrogen-containing hormonal contraceptives do not promote the development of fibroids and, in fact, may be effective treatments for abnormal uterine bleeding or dysmenorrhea caused by uterine fibroids. All estrogen-containing hormonal contraceptives are combined with a progestin, which helps prevent or slow down endometrial hyperplasia and fibroid growth.

12. b. Depo-Provera and other progestin-only methods are safe and effective for breast-feeding patients. It can take up to 1 year or more for a patient to return to fertility following cessation of Depo-Provera use, even after only one injection. It is very important to counsel all patients about this, especially if they desire a rapidly reversible contraceptive method. Depo-Provera appears to actually increase seizure thresholds and reduce seizure frequency in patients with seizure disorders, possibly because of its sedative effect on the brain. Other noncontraceptive benefits of Depo-Provera include decreased pain and bleeding in women with endometriosis and decreased risk of sickle cell crisis in women with sickle cell disease. Depo-Provera is administered via an intramuscular injection and does not require first-pass metabolism for activity; therefore, its effectiveness is not compromised by drugs (i.e., anticonvulsants and antifungals) that are actively metabolized by the liver (unlike COCs). Neither Depo-Provera nor any other hormonal contraceptive method will significantly alter a patient's age of onset of menopause. Although women may experience some loss in bone mineral density while using Depo-Provera, bone mineral density appears to return to baseline following cessation of use. In addition, there is no evidence that Depo-Provera users are at a higher risk for postmenopausal osteoporosis and subsequent fractures later in life.

13. d. The copper IUD (ParaGard T 380A) contains no hormones. It does not significantly affect menstrual flow or pain in most patients. However, it does create a sterile inflammatory reaction in the uterus, which may exacerbate bleeding and pain in patients who already suffer from significant dysmenorrhea or menorrhagia. The copper IUD actually decreases the risk of ectopic pregnancy, as long as it remains properly inserted. The copper IUD provides up to 10 years of highly effective contraception, with a rapid return to fertility following its removal. It does not interfere with breast milk and may be inserted immediately postpartum or postabortion. The copper IUD can be inserted at any time during the menstrual cycle as long as pregnancy has been ruled out. Regimens that require women to come in during their menses for an IUD insertion are inconvenient and logistically difficult to coordinate for most women and offices, prolonging timely initiation of contraception.

14. **a.** One of the advantages of vasectomies over BTLs is that they are usually performed in an outpatient office with local anesthesia and therefore carry a lower risk of complications than BTLs. Neither procedure is easily reversible, so patients need to be counseled to ensure that they desire and are prepared for permanent contraception. Despite many studies on this subject, there is no convincing evidence that vasectomies increase the risk of prostate cancer or reduce male libido, cause erectile dysfunction, or reduce penile sensation. Properly performed BTLs may actually reduce the risk of ectopic pregnancy. However, reversal attempts can lead to narrowed and scarred fallopian tubes, increasing the risk of ectopic pregnancy. An alternative to traditional BTL is a tubal occlusion device (Essure) that is hysteroscopically placed into the fallopian tubes; the coil device stimulates a fibrotic growth reaction that effectively occludes the tubes. Patients should be informed that tubal occlusion must be confirmed 3 months after placement via hysteroscopy, and that another method of birth control needs to be used in the interim.

15. **c.** The rhythm method, also referred to as periodic abstinence or the calendar method, is based on the assumption that the menstrual cycle is consistent. Patients record the length of six cycles and then determine the beginning of the fertile period by subtracting 18 days from the length of the shortest cycle and the end of the fertile period by subtracting 11 days from the length of the longest cycle. The contraceptive failure rate of the rhythm method with "perfect use" is 9%, and it is as high as 20% with "typical use." Given this patient's irregular cycles, this method is less than optimal. Patients who want to practice natural family planning can increase the effectiveness of such methods by combining various techniques to determine the fertile period, such as (1) tracking basal body temperature (a rise in temperature by at least 0.4°F indicates ovulation), (2) monitoring cervical mucus changes (clear, stretchy, or slippery mucus indicates ovulation), or (3) using home ovulation predictor kits.

Highly effective, nonestrogen, reversible contraceptives that are appropriate for women with medical comorbidities include the IUD (either copper IUD or the levonorgestrel IUD); Depo-Provera; or the single-rod progestin-only implant (Implanon), which is now available in the United States. The single-rod progestin-only implant is inserted subdermally in the inner aspect of the nondominant arm between the biceps and triceps muscle. Once inserted properly, the implant provide up to 3 years of contraception. Upon removal of the implant, fertility returns rapidly. The most common side effect is irregular bleeding that may persist for the duration of the implant's use.

This patient should be given exercise and nutrition counseling because even modest weight loss can improve her hypertension and diabetes.

16. **b.** Barrier devices prevent pregnancy by blocking the passage of sperm into the cervix. Barrier methods may be less effective in parous women, who generally have larger cervices. The diaphragm is a dome-shaped, latex rubber cup that can be filled with spermicide. The device should be inserted into the cervix and placed over the cervix immediately before or up to 6 hours prior to intercourse, and it must remain in place for 6 hours after intercourse. The diaphragm should not remain in the vagina for longer than 24 hours because of the increased risk of toxic shock syndrome. Two new types of cervical caps are available in the United States—the FemCap and Lea's Shield. The FemCap is a nonlatex cervical cap that comes in three sizes; it is associated with a two times higher rate of pregnancy compared with the diaphragm. The Lea's Shield is a one-size-fits-all, nonlatex device that is placed over the cervix. The main advantage of barrier methods is safety of use in medically complicated patients.

17. **c.** Emergency contraception (EC) is defined as any method of preventing pregnancy after inadequately or unprotected intercourse. Because EC works better the earlier it is initiated, timely access for patients should be facilitated. Patients can receive prescriptions for ECPs over the phone after simple screening questions to determine the last episode of unprotected intercourse and last menstrual period. Per the American College of Obstetrics and Gynecology (ACOG), no clinician examination or pregnancy testing is necessary prior to the provision of EC. In fact, individuals (male or female) age 18 years or older can purchase Plan B, a dedicated progestin-only EC product, without a prescription in pharmacies that carry the medication.

Patients should be advised to check a pregnancy test if there is a strong suspicion of pregnancy (missed menses) to facilitate the diagnosis of pregnancy. However, if ECPs are taken inadvertently by a pregnant patient, there are no known teratogenic effects. Common contraindications for OCP use (smoking, hypertriglyceridemia, etc.) are not believed to be significant concerns with ECP given its short duration of use. Cervical dysplasia and STDs are not contraindications to ECP use. Some experts suggest that history of thromboembolic disease should be a relative contraindication to ECP use, but there have been no reported cases of thromboembolic events resulting from ECP use. In fact, women who become pregnant are at far greater risk of thromboembolic event than nonpregnant women.

Methods of EC include COCs, POPs, and IUD placement. The "Yuzpe regimen" involves two doses of 100 μg of ethinyl estradiol and either 1 mg of norgestrel or 0.5 mg of levonorgestrel administered 12 hours apart. The progestin-only method involves the administration of two doses of 1.5 mg of norgestrel or 0.75 mg of levonorgestrel 12 hours apart. As noted previously, the progestin-only method packaged as Plan B is the only FDA-approved, dedicated EC product currently available in the United States. Clinically, the progestin-only regimen is preferred to the Yuzpe method, given its lower incidence of nausea and vomiting and its greater efficacy (decreases the risk of pregnancy by up to 85%). The efficacy of ECPs is maximized if they are initiated as soon as possible after unprotected intercourse, with standard protocols citing effectiveness up to 72 hours postintercourse. However, an international WHO trial demonstrated that a single combined dose of 1.5 mg levonorgestrel (two 0.75-mg levonorgestrel pills combined) showed excellent efficacy up until 120 hours after unprotected intercourse, without an increase in side effects. A copper IUD (ParaGard T 380A) can be inserted within 5 days of unprotected intercourse and then left in to provide up to 10 years of effective contraception in appropriate patients.

The mechanism of action of ECPs likely differs depending on when the ECPs are administered in relation to the menstrual cycle; the predominant effect has been attributed to inhibition of ovulation. ECPs have not been shown to adversely affect or disrupt an implanted embryo and thus are not considered abortifacients.

18. **e.** There is one FDA-approved, dedicated EC product available in the United States—a progestin-only method packaged as Plan B that contains two pills of levonorgestrel 0.75 mg each. The Preven EC kit (Yuzpe method) is no longer produced in the United States, mainly because of its higher incidence of side effects and inferior efficacy compared to the progestin-only method. Commonly used COC and POP brands can also provide effective EC when administered in the correct doses. A copper T IUD could be considered for this patient, absent other contraindications (e.g., current or recent PID).

19. **c.** Advance provision of ECPs has not been shown to promote unsafe sexual practice or discourage regular contraception, even among adolescents. Women who receive advance supplies of ECPs are more likely to use ECPs when necessary because the barriers to access are eliminated. Interestingly, studies of advance provision of ECPs have not shown a significant decrease in the rate of unintended pregnancy. Experts believe this is a result of gross underutilization of EC among women at highest risk for unplanned pregnancy.

All sexually active women should be counseled about the availability of EC. In 2006, the FDA approved Plan B for nonprescription purchase by individuals age 18 years or older. Patients younger than age 18 years still require a prescription to obtain Plan B. The American College of Obstetrics and Gynecology recommends that patients be provided with an advance prescription for ECPs. Patients can also call the EC hotline number (888-NOT-2-LATE) or visit the Emergency Contraception Web site (http://ec.princeton.edu) to find a provider who can prescribe EC. Advance provision of ECPs can help overcome barriers to access (pharmacy not open late hours/weekends or not able to get a doctor's appointment) and allow patients to start EC in a timely manner.

Solution to the Clinical Case Management Problem

Important user characteristics for contraceptive selection include the following:
- Gender preference
- Frequency of intercourse
- Number of past/current partners
- Problems with past/current methods
- Method of STD prevention
- Partner's willingness to participate in pregnancy/STD prevention
- Ability to cope with contraceptive failure
- Ability to use method correctly and consistently

- Personal beliefs about methods
- Contraindications to certain methods
- Medical conditions that may be adversely affected by certain methods
- Medical conditions that may be improved by certain methods
- Risk factors that may be modified by certain methods
- Desire for future fertility (long term versus short term)
- Financial ability to pay for contraception

Summary

BARRIER METHODS

1. Mechanism of action: Barrier devices block the passage of sperm into the cervix.
2. STD protection: Latex or polyurethane male condoms and the polyurethane female condom offer the most effective means of STD prevention, next to abstinence. Latex and polyurethane condoms offer protection against bacterial and viral STDs; natural (animal skin) membrane condoms do not.
3. Other barrier methods: Diaphragm and cervical caps (FemCap and Lea's Shield).
4. Advantages: They are safe for medically complicated patients and patients with contraindications to hormones.
5. Disadvantages: Contraceptive failure rates are as high as 40% (cervical cap) with "typical use," and they require patient motivation and partner cooperation.

SPERMICIDES

1. The active ingredient in spermicides is nonoxynol-9.
2. Mechanism of action: Disruption of cell membrane of sperm.
3. Spermicides are available in many formulations, including foams, gels, suppositories, and films.
4. A spermicide-containing sponge (the Today sponge) is available without prescription.
5. Advantages: They are safe for medically complicated patients and patients with contraindications to hormones.
6. Disadvantages: They require patient motivation and partner cooperation.
7. Per WHO guidelines, nonoxynol-9 should not be used for STD protection in individuals who are at increased risk of HIV infection.

ORAL CONTRACEPTIVE PILLS

1. Combined oral contraceptives: Ethinyl estradiol + a progestin.
2. Mechanism of action: Ovulation suppression, thicken cervical mucus, alter endometrial receptivity.
3. Advantages: There are many noncontraceptive benefits, including improvement of dysmenorrhea, ovulatory pain (mittelschmerz), iron-deficiency anemia, menses regulation, and acne vulgaris. They decrease the risk of ovarian and endometrial cancers and PID.
4. There is no convincing evidence that COCs increase the risk of breast, cervical, or liver cancer.
5. Potential complications: Thromboembolic events, arterial thrombotic events (stroke and myocardial infarction), hypertension, hepatic adenoma.
6. Adverse effects: Breakthrough bleeding (most often the result of noncompliance), nausea, and breast tenderness. These usually resolve within the first three cycles of use.
7. Contraindications: Estrogen-dependent malignancy, classic migraines, known or suspected pregnancy, a history of VTEs, or unexplained vaginal bleeding. Also, women who are 35 years of age or older and smoke (women younger than age 35 years who smoke can still use OCPs). Common migraines (no aura) and obesity are not contraindications.

ORAL CONTRACEPTIVE INITIATION

1. Quick start method: Initiate oral contraceptive pills on the day of the office visit.
   a. Assess risk of pregnancy by last menstrual period and recent sexual activity and urine pregnancy testing as needed
   b. Associated with higher pill adherence at 3 months compared to traditional delayed start
   c. No higher incidence of irregular bleeding
2. The quick start method can be considered for other contraceptive methods (e.g., vaginal ring and transdermal patch).

OTHER ESTROGEN-CONTAINING CONTRACEPTIVES

1. The mechanism of action, noncontraceptive benefits, adverse effects, and complications are essentially the same as for COCs.
2. Transdermal contraceptive patch (OrthoEvra): A patch is self-applied by the patient and changed each week for 3 weeks; then there is a patch-free week during which withdrawal bleeding occurs.
   a. Major advantage: Less frequent dosing schedule to increase compliance.
   b. The patch may be less effective in women who weight more than 198 pounds.
   c. Side effects are similar to those for COCs. Local skin irritation is the most common complaint. Partial or complete detachment is another side effect.
3. Contraceptive vaginal ring (NuvaRing): A small, flexible ring made of ethylene vinyl acetate that releases 15 µg of ethinyl estradiol and 120 µg of etonorgestrel in a controlled-release manner. It is self-inserted by the patient, left in for 3 weeks, and then taken out for 1 week, during which withdrawal bleeding occurs.
   a. Major advantage: Less frequent dosing schedule to increase compliance
   b. Side effects are similar to those for COCs. Device-related events (slipping and dislodging) occur.

PROGESTIN-ONLY METHODS

1. Mechanism of action: Thickens cervical mucus, inhibition of ovulation (less so than with COCs).

2. Major advantage: Can be used safely in breast-feeding women, medically complicated patients, and patients with contraindications to estrogen.
3. Progestin-only pills: Must be taken at almost the same time daily for contraceptive efficacy.
4. Depo-Provera: 150 mg intramuscularly every 11 to 13 weeks.
   a. Side effects include irregular spotting and bleeding that progressively decreases. Amenorrhea occurs in 80% of women by 5 years of use.
   b. Delayed return in fertility up to 1 year or more after cessation of use.
   c. Noncontraceptive benefits: Improves seizures, anemia, endometriosis.
   d. Associated with decrease in bone mineral density that returns to baseline following cessation of use.
5. Levonorgestrel IUD: Provides 5 years of continuous contraception.
   a. Permits a rapid return to fertility following removal.
   b. Associated with irregular spotting and bleeding. Twenty percent of users become amenorrheic at 1 year.
6. Single-rod progestin (Implanon): Provides 3 years of continuous contraception.
   a. It is inserted subdermally between biceps and triceps muscle of nondominant arm.
   b. It permits a rapid return to fertility following removal.
   c. The most common side effect is irregular bleeding that may persist for the duration of the implant's use.

COPPER INTRAUTERINE DEVICE

1. Mechanism of action: Creates sterile inflammatory reaction that is essentially spermicidal.
2. FDA revision of eligibility criteria: Nulliparity and history of PID no longer contraindications.
3. Contraindications: Current or recent PID, copper allergy, Wilson's disease.
4. Major advantage: Safe for use in medically complicated patients and patients with contraindications to estrogen.
5. Side effects: It can increase the duration and amount of bleeding in some woman. It is not ideal choice for women with heavy, painful menses.
6. Rapid return to fertility following removal.

NATURAL FAMILY PLANNING METHODS

1. Mechanism of action: No intercourse or protected intercourse on days of possible ovulation.
2. Rhythm (calendar) method: Patients calculate fertile days based on their own cycles.
3. Standard days method: Patients avoid sex on days 9 through 19 of their menses.

4. Symptothermal method: Assess for cervical mucus and temperature increase of 0.4°F.
5. Home ovulation predictor kits
6. Advantages: They are safe in medically complicated patients and patients with contraindications to estrogen. They are also inexpensive (with the exception of ovulation kits).
7. Disadvantages: They are not practical or effective for women with irregular menses. They require patient motivation and partner cooperation.

LACTATIONAL AMENORRHEA METHOD

1. Provides excellent pregnancy protection (nearly 98% effective) if the following criteria are met:
   a. The infant is exclusively or almost exclusively breast-fed.
   b. The first postpartum menses has not occurred.
   c. It is within the first 6 months after birth.

STERILIZATION: BTL, VASECTOMY, TUBAL OCCLUSION

1. Should be limited to patients who truly desire permanent contraception.
2. Reversals are difficult, expensive, and can lead to complications (e.g., ectopic pregnancy).
3. There is no conclusive evidence that vasectomies are associated with prostate cancer, cardiovascular disease, decreased libido, erectile dysfunction, or decreased penile sensitivity.
4. Vasectomies can be performed in the outpatient setting and thus have a relatively lower risk of complications than BTLs.
5. The tubal occlusion method involves hysteroscopic placement of coil devices into the fallopian tubes; the coil device stimulates a fibrotic growth reaction that effectively occludes the tubes. Patients must use an alternative contraceptive method until complete tubal occlusion has been confirmed approximately 3 months postinsertion.

EMERGENCY CONTRACEPTION

1. Mechanism of action: Inhibit or delay ovulation. Other possible mechanisms include altering endometrial receptivity and alterations in tubal transport.
2. EC does not disrupt implantation and is therefore not an abortifacient.
3. Yuzpe method: Two doses of 100 μg of ethinyl estradiol and either 1 mg of norgestrel or 0.5 mg of levonorgestrel administered 12 hours apart within 72 hours of intercourse. Can use ordinary OCPs to make up these doses (e.g., two pills of Ovral in two doses).
4. Progestin-only method: 0.75 mg levonorgestrel orally in two doses, 12 hours apart, up to 72 hours after intercourse. An alternative, evidence-based method is to take both 0.75 mg levonorgestrel tabs at once; this method can be used up to 120 hours after intercourse.

This method has less nausea and vomiting and better effectiveness than the Yuzpe method.

5. Plan B (two pills of 0.75 mg levonorgestrel each): FDA-approved progestin-only EC product. It is available without a prescription to individuals (male or female) age 18 years or older. Women younger than age 18 years still require a prescription from a clinician.

6. Per ACOG recommendations, an advance prescription for EC should be provided when necessary to eliminate barriers to timely access.

7. All sexually active women should be counseled about EC and provided with either a prescription for ECPs or information about EC. Resources include the EC hotline (888-NOT-2-LATE) and the Emergency Contraception Web site (http://ec.princeton.edu).

Suggested Reading

Hatcher RA: *Contraceptive Technology*, 18th ed. New York: Ardent Media, 2004.

Lesnewski R, Prine L: Initiating hormonal contraception. *Am Fam Physician* 74:105–112, 2006.

Raymond E, Trussell J, Chelsea B: Population effect of increased access to emergency contraceptive pills: A systematic review. *Obstet Gynecol* 109(1):181–188, 2007.

Schrager S: Abnormal uterine bleeding associated with hormonal contraception. *Am Fam Physician* 65:2073–2083, 2002.

Speroff L, Darney PD: *A Clinical Guide for Contraception*. Philadelphia: Lippincott Williams & Wilkins, 2006.

Weismiller DG: Emergency contraception. *Am Fam Physician* 70: 707–714, 717–718, 2004.

CHAPTER

79   Spontaneous and Elective Abortion

CLINICAL CASE PROBLEM 1

Bleeding in the Middle of the Night

You receive a call at 3 AM from your prenatal patient who is worried about bleeding and cramping that began several hours ago. This is the fourth pregnancy for your patient, which was a planned pregnancy. She has had two uncomplicated, spontaneous vaginal deliveries and one elective abortion in the past. Her prenatal course to date has been uncomplicated. Two weeks ago, you obtained a first trimester ultrasound for dating purposes that revealed a 6-week intrauterine pregnancy. She denies any fever, nausea, vomiting, dizziness, lightheadedness, shortness of breath, or arm or chest pain. Her cramps are becoming more intense, but she is managing to control the pain with a heating pad. She reports using approximately three sanitary pads in the past 6 hours for bleeding, none of which were soaked through. The patient is home with her husband, who is a well-known patient of yours as well. They are very anxious and want to know what to do next.

SELECT THE BEST ANSWER TO THE FOLLOWING QUESTIONS

1. You advise your patient to
   a. come to your office first thing in the morning for an evaluation
   b. take some ibuprofen and see you at her next scheduled prenatal visit
   c. rush to the emergency room because of suspected ectopic pregnancy
   d. rush to the emergency room for an immediate dilation and curettage (D&C)
   e. call an obstetrician–gynecologist to schedule an outpatient consultation

2. She follows your advice. The next day you see the patient and her husband in your office. She appears tearful, though calm. Her temperature is 98.4°F, blood pressure is 120/80 mmHg, pulse is 80 beats/minute, and respiratory rate is 16 breaths/minute. She reports that since she spoke to you, she has passed a few dime-sized clots but no obvious tissue. She continues to have lower abdominal cramping. You perform a speculum exam, which reveals some blood in the vaginal vault and a small amount of tissue protruding from an open, dilated cervical os. A bimanual exam reveals a 6-week-size uterus with minimal tenderness but no peritoneal signs. The most likely diagnosis is
   a. missed abortion
   b. recurrent spontaneous abortion

c. complete abortion
d. incomplete abortion
e. inevitable abortion

3. All of the following would be appropriate management strategies except
   a. expectant management
   b. uterine aspiration
   c. medical management with vaginal misoprostol
   d. exploratory laparoscopy
   e. serial β-human chorionic gonadotropin (β-hCG) measurements

4. The patient chooses expectant management. She returns to your office in 2 weeks for another evaluation. She reports passing tissue 48 hours after you examined her in the office. Since then, she has had only minimal spotting and her pregnancy symptoms of nausea and breast tenderness have resolved. An ultrasound reveals a thickened, heterogeneous endometrial stripe and no evidence of an intrauterine pregnancy. What issues should be discussed during this office visit?
   a. the need for uterine aspiration to remove retained products of conception
   b. the need for a high-sensitivity urine pregnancy test to confirm completion of the miscarriage
   c. the patient and her husband's emotions about the pregnancy loss, whether or not they want to be pregnant again, and a review of contraceptive options if appropriate
   d. a full genetic evaluation is needed to assess the cause of the miscarriage
   e. it is better not to discuss the pregnancy loss because it will take the patient longer to "get over" the event

CLINICAL CASE PROBLEM 2

An Unplanned Event

A 23-year-old female graduate student presents to the office for a "personal problem" as reported by your nurse. When you enter the room, she is noticeably tearful. She has regular menses, and her last menstrual period was approximately 6 weeks ago. Today, she denies fever, vaginal bleeding, and abdominal pain. You perform a high-sensitivity urine pregnancy test, which is positive. On examination, the uterus is approximately 6 weeks in size with no adnexal tenderness or masses. You tell the patient that she is approximately 6 weeks pregnant. The patient is quiet and will not make eye contact with you.

5. Which the following is the most appropriate next step in management?
   a. congratulate the patient and schedule her initial prenatal visit
   b. ask the patient how she feels about being pregnant
   c. state that the urine pregnancy test is probably a false positive and a serum beta β-hCG test is necessary to confirm the diagnosis
   d. tell her to go home and come back after she is ready to talk
   e. send her for an ultrasound for an accurate estimate of gestational age

6. The patient's pregnancy options could include all the following except
   a. continuing the pregnancy and becoming a parent
   b. continuing the pregnancy and pursuing adoption for the baby
   c. ending the pregnancy by medication abortion (e.g., mifepristone and methotrexate)
   d. ending the pregnancy by surgical (aspiration) abortion
   e. pursuing any of the above options based solely on what her partner wants

7. The following statements about mifepristone (the medication abortion pill) and emergency contraceptive pills (ECPs) are true except
   a. mifepristone disrupts an implanted pregnancy, whereas ECPs prevent pregnancy
   b. mifepristone causes heavy bleeding and cramping, whereas ECPs may be associated with light spotting and early or delayed menses
   c. mifepristone is available without prescription to women age 18 years or older
   d. ECPs are available by prescription only to women younger than age 18 years
   e. parental consent is necessary for the use of mifepristone in some states but not for the use of ECPs

8. Which of the following is true regarding unintended pregnancy and elective abortion in the United States?
   a. the United States has a relatively low abortion rate compared to most other Western, industrialized countries
   b. one in four pregnancies in the United States ends in elective termination

c. one in four pregnancies in the United States is unintended (unplanned)

d. the mortality rate from a legal, first trimester abortion in the United States is approximately 1/10,000

e. the majority of abortions in the United States occur in the second trimester

---

Clinical Case Management Problem

Compare and contrast the differences between medication abortion and aspiration abortion with respect to efficacy, patient experience, and provider role.

Answers

1. a. This patient is most likely experiencing an early pregnancy loss (also called a spontaneous abortion, nonviable pregnancy, or early pregnancy failure), which is defined as a spontaneous pregnancy loss at less than 20 weeks of gestation based on the last menstrual period. Because the patient appears to be hemodynamically stable based on your phone conversation, it is reasonable to have her evaluated first thing in the morning in your office. Furthermore, you already have preexisting documentation of an intrauterine pregnancy, which makes the possibility of an ectopic pregnancy highly unlikely. The concomitant presence of an ectopic and intrauterine pregnancy (referred to as a heterotopic pregnancy) is possible but is a very rare occurrence, with an incidence of 1:30,000 pregnancies. Reports estimate that heterotopic pregnancies are on the rise, with an incidence as high as 1:2600 pregnancies among certain high-risk subgroups, such as women who have undergone assisted reproductive interventions (e.g., in vitro fertilization). Although sending the patient to the emergency room immediately is a possible option, this will likely cause unnecessary waiting and anxiety for the couple. An immediate D&C is not necessary, given the fact that the patient is stable and not bleeding excessively. The vast majority of early pregnancy losses can be managed safely and effectively in the family medicine setting; a consultation with a obstetrician–gynecologist is not mandatory and will depend on the clinician's level of clinical comfort. Telling the patient to take ibuprofen and follow up at her next prenatal visit is not appropriate in the setting of undiagnosed first trimester bleeding.

2. d. The patient is experiencing an incomplete abortion. The terminology to describe nonviable pregnancies was devised prior to the advent of ultrasonography and can be confusing. Traditionally, nonviable pregnancies are divided into different categories based on physical examination findings: (1) A threatened abortion refers to vaginal bleeding, with or without cramping, in the presence of a closed cervix; (2) an inevitable abortion refers to a dilated cervical os without the passage of tissue; (3) an incomplete abortion refers to a dilated cervical os with the passage of some, but not all, products of conception; and (4) a complete abortion refers to the complete expulsion of the products of conception. Recurrent spontaneous abortions refers to three or more consecutive pregnancy losses. In clinical trials, an embryonic or fetal demise has been sonographically defined as an embryonic pole or crown–rump length between 5 and 40 mm without cardiac activity. An anembryonic pregnancy (commonly called a "blighted ovum") refers to a gestational sac with a mean diameter between 16 and 45 mm without evidence of a fetal pole, inadequate growth of the gestational sac, or an increase in β-hCG levels of less than 15% during a 2-day period in the presence of a yolk sac visualized on ultrasound.

3. d. Traditionally, clinicians performed immediate D&Cs to treat spontaneous abortions. Recent evidence provides support for the role of expectant management and medical management instead of surgical intervention. Expectant management allows the patient time to complete the process of spontaneous abortion on her own. This process can occur over the course of 2 to 4 weeks, depending on the patient's clinical symptoms and the patient/clinician's level of comfort with waiting. Clinicians can monitor the progress of an ongoing pregnancy loss with serial β-hCG levels and/or ultrasound. The β-hCG level should double approximately every 48 hours in a viable intrauterine pregnancy. A rise of less than 50% is associated with an abnormal pregnancy. A change of less than 15% is considered to be a plateau, which is most predictive of an ectopic pregnancy. For incomplete spontaneous abortions, the success rate of expectant management is excellent at 82% to 96%. However, the success rate of expectant management declines with anembyronic pregnancy or fetal or embryonic death (25% to 76%).

Medical management with misoprostol is another option for women. Misoprostol is a prostaglandin that causes cervical softening and uterine contractions. Based on a large, randomized trial, an initial dose of 800 µg of misoprostol via vaginal insertion was associated with a complete expulsion rate of 84% by day 8. Women with an anembryonic pregnancy or embryonic or fetal demise required a second dose of misoprostol for successful completion more often than women with incomplete or inevitable abortions.

If the patient desires a surgical evacuation of the uterus for emotional reasons, providers who are trained in doing uterine aspiration (either with a handheld manual vacuum aspirator or an electrical vacuum aspirator) can do so safely in the outpatient setting with local anesthesia. An exploratory laparoscopy would be inappropriate in the setting of an uneventful incomplete spontaneous abortion.

4. c. Women and their partners may experience a range of emotions following an early pregnancy loss. If the pregnancy was a desired one, feelings of grief, guilt, and loss are common. Clinicians should inquire about these emotions and assure patients that they are not "responsible" for the miscarriage occurring. If the pregnancy was not a desired one, women may feel a sense of relief because they have avoided the need for an elective termination. Regardless of the situation, clinicians should offer support and appropriate preventive care at the time of the follow-up visit. Women and their partners should be asked about whether another pregnancy is desired and, if so, how soon. A tailored contraceptive plan or preconception counseling should be offered, if appropriate. A thickened endometrial stripe is commonly seen after a medication abortion and does not require intervention if the patient is otherwise asymptomatic. Genetic counseling is not necessary after a single spontaneous abortion. Recurrent spontaneous abortion (three or more consecutive abortions) deserves further investigation. Avoiding discussion about the pregnancy loss is unlikely to help the patient "get over" the event any quicker.

5. b. The most appropriate next step is to inquire how the patient is feeling about being pregnant. Given her body language and tearfulness, it would be presumptive to assume she is happy about the pregnancy and wants to begin prenatal care. Simple, open-ended questions asked in a nonjudgmental manner are useful for engaging the patient in a discussion (e.g., "How are you feeling about this?" and "What does being pregnant right now mean for you and those involved in your life?"). There is good reason to believe that the patient is 6 weeks pregnant based on the history, exam, and urine pregnancy test. A serum β-hCG level is not necessary to confirm pregnancy diagnosis. A false-positive result from a high-sensitivity (able to detect as low as 25 mIU/mL of β-hCG) urine pregnancy test is rare. Although ultrasound may be indicated at some point depending on the patient's clinical course, it is not the next most appropriate step in management.

6. e. Clinicians who care for women of reproductive age should be knowledgeable about various pregnancy options and resources for patients who present with unintended pregnancy. Potential options include (1) continuing the pregnancy and becoming a parent; (2) continuing the pregnancy and pursuing adoption for the baby; (3) undergoing a medication abortion; and (4) undergoing a surgical, or aspiration, abortion. There are several medication abortion agents currently in clinical use, including methotrexate (an antimetabolite), mifepristone (an antiprogestin), and misoprostol (a prostaglandin analogue). A detailed comparison of medication abortion protocols is beyond the scope of this chapter. In 2000, the Food and Drug Administration (FDA) approved a medication abortion protocol using oral mifepristone (RU-496) and oral misoprostol in women who are up to 49 days pregnant. Based on large, randomized controlled trials, several evidence-based medication abortion protocols have extended the gestational age limit up to 56 to 63 days depending on the route of misoprostol administration. Traditionally, D&C was used to perform first trimester abortions. This procedure has largely been replaced by aspiration abortion, which involves removal of the pregnancy through suction with either a handheld syringe (manual vacuum aspirator) or an electric vacuum. Aspiration abortion has provided a safe alternative to D&C because there is no sharp curettage of the endometrium involved. It is unethical to force a woman to pursue a pregnancy option (regardless if it is continuing or ending a pregnancy) based solely on her partner's desires. In ideal circumstances, the decision should involve both the patient and her partner (if there is a partner actively involved).

7. c. Mifepristone (RU-486) is not available without a prescription. Providers must register with the distributor of RU-486 in order to obtain the pills. In contrast, Plan B, a progestin-only dedicated ECP product, was approved in 2006 by the FDA as a dual-status medication for emergency contraception, meaning that it is available without prescription to consumers age 18 years or older and by prescription only to females younger than age 18 years. ECPs do not disrupt an implanted pregnancy and are therefore not abortifacients as defined by the FDA, National Institutes of Health, the American Medical Women's Association, and the American College of Obstetrics and Gynecology. Mifepristone, an antiprogestin, is an abortifacient and causes bleeding (that can be heavy and associated with clots) and cramping. Progestin-only ECPs are associated with mild side effects, including nausea, vomiting, and menstrual changes. Most commonly, ECPs may cause early onset or delayed menses, depending on when they were taken in the menstrual cycle. Intermenstrual spotting is less commonly associated with ECPs. For more information about ECPs, please refer to Chapter 78.

Adolescents living in certain states need to obtain parental consent prior to using mifepristone for medication abortion. Currently, there are no state or federal laws that require minors to obtain parental consent prior to using contraception (including emergency contraception). In fact, Title X and Medicaid, two federal programs that fund family planning services in the United States, prohibit parental consent requirements for teens seeking contraception.

8. **b.** The United States has one of the highest abortion rates (23/1000 women of reproductive age) among developed countries, which can be attributed in large part to relatively high rates of unintended pregnancy and a lack of widespread contraceptive use among those at highest risk for unplanned pregnancy. Half of all pregnancies in the United States are unintended, and half of unintended pregnancies end in elective abortion. Therefore, one out of four pregnancies in the United States ends in an elective termination. In 2002, approximately 1.3 million abortions were performed. The majority of abortions (88%) occur in the first trimester (12 weeks gestational age or less). The mortality rate from abortion in the United States has decreased significantly since the legalization of abortion in 1973 to approximately 1 in 1 million for early abortions (8 weeks or less). To place this risk in perspective, the risk of death associated with carrying a pregnancy to term is 12 times greater. The risk of mortality from a legal abortion increases with increasing gestational age (e.g., 1/11,000 at 21 or more weeks).

Solution to the Clinical Case Management Problem

Feature	Mifepristone Abortion	Aspiration Abortion
Efficacy	95–99%	99%
Procedure	No instrumentation required (except in cases of incomplete abortion)	Involves uterine instrumentation
Number of visits	Two visits minimum	One visit minimum

Gestational age limit	Varies depending on protocol
	    FDA protocol: up to 49 days
	    Evidence-based regimens: up to 56 days (buccal misoprostol) or up to 63 days (vaginal misoprostol)
		Up to 13 6/7 weeks from last menstrual period

Pain management	Oral analgesics (ibuprofen, Tylenol with codeine)	Conscious sedation can be offered, if necessary
Provider/patient involvement	Provider gives instructions, patient initiates the process at home	Provider performs procedure in the office
Time	90% of women complete the process in 24 hours	5- to 10-minute procedure
Bleeding pattern	Same amount of blood loss as an aspiration abortion; more bleeding "seen" by the patient. Light bleeding, sometimes with clots, for 1 or 2 weeks after.	Light bleeding for approximately 1 week; can continue on and off for 1 month
Common reasons for patient preference	May feel more "natural;" can be done in privacy of home	Requires only one visit; can leave office knowing she is not pregnant
Cost	Varies: average cost in 2001, $490	Varies: average cost in 2001, $372

Summary

SPONTANEOUS ABORTION

1. Defined as pregnancy loss at less than 20 weeks of gestation based on last menstrual period. Also referred to as early pregnancy loss, nonviable pregnancy, and early pregnancy failure.

2. Classification based on history and physical exam
   a. Threatened abortion: vaginal bleeding, with or without cramping, in the presence of a closed cervix
   b. Inevitable abortion: dilated cervical os without the passage of tissue

c. Incomplete abortion: dilated cervical os with the passage of some, but not all, products of conception

d. Complete abortion: complete expulsion of the products of conception

3. Classification based on ultrasound findings
   a. Embryonic or fetal demise: embryonic pole or crown–rump length between 5 and 40 mm without cardiac activity
   b. Anembryonic pregnancy ("blighted ovum"): gestational sac with a mean diameter between 16 and 45 mm without evidence of a fetal pole, inadequate growth of the gestational sac

4. Recurrent, spontaneous abortions: three or more consecutive pregnancy losses

5. Heterotopic pregnancy: the concomitant presence of an ectopic and intrauterine pregnancy; a relatively rare occurrence, although the incidence is increasing, particularly among women who have undergone assisted reproductive technologies

6. Treatment: traditionally managed by D&C only. Recent evidence and clinical practice support the role of expectant management and/or medical management:
   a. Monitor progress with serial β-hCG levels and/or ultrasound.
   b. The β-hCG level should double approximately every 48 hours in a viable intrauterine pregnancy.
   c. Misoprosotol, a prostaglandin, can be used to treat early pregnancy failure.
   d. Women with incomplete or inevitable abortion may have a higher rate of success than women with an embryonic pregnancy or embryonic or fetal demise.

7. Treatment with uterine aspiration may be preferred by some patients and necessary in cases of failed medical or expectant management:
   a. Uterine aspiration can be accomplished with a handheld 60-mL syringe (manual vacuum aspiration) or an electrical vacuum machine.
   b. Uterine aspiration can be done safely with local anesthesia in the outpatient setting.

8. Comprehensive management of early pregnancy loss includes addressing the emotions of women and their partners, inquiring about future plans for pregnancy, and offering contraceptive or preconception planning as appropriate.

ELECTIVE ABORTION

1. Comprehensive pregnancy options counseling for women who present with an unintended pregnancy include discussion of the following:
   a. Continuing the pregnancy and becoming a parent
   b. Continuing the pregnancy and pursuing adoption for the baby
   c. Undergoing a medication or aspiration abortion

2. Medication abortion offers an alternative to aspiration abortion for appropriate candidates.

3. The FDA-approved medication abortion protocol (mifepristone and misoprostol) is approved for use in women who are up to 49 days pregnant.

4. There are alternative, widely used evidence-based regimens for medication abortion with mifepristone and misoprostol that demonstrated excellent efficacy and safety in women up to 56 to 63 days pregnant.

5. Half of all pregnancies in the United States are unintended, and half of these pregnancies end in elective abortion.

6. The mortality rate of a legal, first trimester elective abortion is approximately 1 in 1 million, and it increases with increasing gestational age.

7. Mifepristone (RU-486) disrupts an implanted pregnancy and is medically defined as an abortifacient. In contrast, emergency contraceptive pills do not disrupt an implanted pregnancy.

8. Plan B, a FDA-approved progestin-only emergency contraceptive product, is available without prescription to consumers age 18 years or older and by prescription only to females younger than age 18 years.

9. The majority of elective abortions in the United States are performed in the first trimester.

Suggested Reading

Alan Guttmacher Institute: Facts on induced abortion in the United States. Available at www.guttmacher.org/pubs/fb_induced_abortion.html.

Creinin MD, Moyer R, Guido R: Misoprostol for medical evacuation of early pregnancy failure. *Obstet Gynecol* 89(5 Pt 1):768–772, 1997.

Emergency Contraception Web site. Available at http://ec.princeton.edu/questions/ec-review.pdf.

Grieble CP, Halvorsen J, Golemon TB, Day AA: Management of spontaneous abortion. *Am Fam Physician* 72:1243–1250, 2005.

Henshaw S: Unintended pregnancy in the United States. *Fam Planning Perspect* 30:24–29, 1998.

Ibis Reproductive Health: Medication abortion: Facts and information for health professionals. Available at www.medicationabortion.com/index.html.

Schaff EA, Eisinger SH, Stadalius LS, et al: Low-dose mifepristone 200 mg and vaginal misoprostol for abortion. *Contraception* 59(1):1–6, 1999.

Trussell J, Raymond E: Emergency contraception: A cost-effective approach to unintended pregnancy. Available at http://ec.princeton.edu.

Zhang J, Gilles JM, Barnhart K, et al: A comparison of medical management with misoprostol and surgical management for early pregnancy failure. *N Engl J Med* 353:761–769, 2005.

CHAPTER 80

Sexually Transmitted Diseases

CLINICAL CASE PROBLEM 1

A 24-Year-Old Female with Diffuse Abdominal Pain

A 24-year-old female comes to the emergency room with a 2-day history of lower abdominal pain, fever, chills, and malaise. The patient also complains of nausea and multiple episodes of vomiting in the past 24 hours. On physical examination, there is bilateral adnexal tenderness, mucopurulent cervical discharge, and cervical motion tenderness. The patient has a temperature of 40°C. Her last menstrual period was 4 weeks ago, and her pregnancy test is negative. She admits to being sexually active but denies a history of any sexually transmitted diseases (STDs). She is currently not using birth control.

SELECT THE BEST ANSWER TO THE FOLLOWING QUESTIONS

1. What is the most likely diagnosis in this patient?
   a. acute appendicitis
   b. acute pelvic inflammatory disease (PID)
   c. uncomplicated cervicitis
   d. ectopic pregnancy
   e. threatened abortion

2. What is the most appropriate intervention for this patient?
   a. hospitalize the patient for parenteral treatment
   b. hospitalize the patient for immediate laporoscopy
   c. begin outpatient treatment with follow-up within 24 hours
   d. begin outpatient treatment with follow-up in 1 week
   e. begin outpatient treatment with follow-up if her condition worsens

3. If hospitalization was chosen for this patient, which of the following is an acceptable first-line parenteral regimen for her condition?
   a. intravenous (IV) ampicillin and gentamicin
   b. IV cefoxitin and oral doxycycline
   c. IV ceftriaxone only
   d. IV ciprofloxacin only
   e. IV ampicillin only

4. If outpatient management was chosen for this patient, which of the following is an acceptable first-line treatment for mild to moderate PID according to 2006 Centers for Disease Control and Prevention (CDC) guidelines?
   a. levofloxacin 500 mg orally once daily for 14 days with or without metronidazole 500 mg orally twice a day for 14 days
   b. ceftriaxone 250 mg intramuscularly (IM) in a single dose
   c. ceftriaxone 250 mg IM in a single dose, plus doxycycline 100 mg orally twice a day for 14 days if chlamydial infection is not ruled out, with or without metronidazole 500 mg orally twice a day for 14 days
   d. ofloxacin 400 mg orally twice a day for 14 days with or without metronidazole 500 mg orally twice a day for 14 days
   e. doxycycline 100 mg orally twice a day for 14 days

5. Which of the following statements regarding the relationship between combined oral contraceptive pills (OCPs) and this patient's condition is true?
   a. OCPs decrease the risk of this condition
   b. OCPs increase the risk of this condition
   c. OCPs have no influence on this condition
   d. OCPs are contraindicated in patients with this condition
   e. OCPs should be discontinued temporarily in patients with this condition

6. Which of the following organisms is not associated with the condition described in this case?
   a. *Neisseria gonorrhea*
   b. *Chlamydia trachomatis*
   c. *Gardnerella hominis*
   d. *Bacteroides fragilis*
   e. group A β-hemolytic streptococcus

7. All of the following are direct risk factors for PID except
   a. having new or multiple sexual partners
   b. living in an area with a high prevalence of *N. gonorrhea* and/or *C. trachomatis*
   c. being age 25 years or younger
   d. prior or current use of an intrauterine device
   e. a previous history of STD or PID

8. Which of the following is (are) a complication(s) of disseminated gonococcal infection (DGI)?
   a. arthritis
   b. tenosynovitis
   c. bacteremia
   d. endocarditis
   e. all of the above

CLINICAL CASE PROBLEM 2

A 19-Year-Old Female with Complaints of Vaginal Discharge

A 19-year-old sexually active female presents to your office with complaints of yellow vaginal discharge and intermittent postcoital vaginal bleeding for 1 week. She otherwise feels well. Her blood pressure is 120/60 mmHg, and her temperature is 37°C. On examination, there is purulent discharge visible in the endocervical canal. After you collect vaginal fluid for a wet prep and cervical samples for gonorrhea and chlamydia cultures, you note bleeding at the cervical os. Upon bimanual exam, the patient complains of tenderness upon cervical palpation but denies uterine or adnexal tenderness. Wet prep reveals vaginal pH 4; negative whiff; 20 white blood cells (WBCs) per high power field; and no clue cells, trichomonads, or pseudohyphae.

9. As recommended by the April 2007 update to the CDC's STD treatment guidelines (2006), which of the following is first-line treatment for this patient's condition?
   a. levofloxacin 250 mg orally in a single dose
   b. ciprofloxacin 500 mg orally in a single dose
   c. ceftriaxone 125 mg IM in a single dose plus appropriate treatment for chlamydia if chlamydial infection is not ruled out
   d. levofloxacin 250 mg orally in a single dose plus appropriate treatment for chlamydia if clamydial infection is not ruled out
   e. ciprofloxacin 500 mg orally in a single dose plus appropriate treatment for chlamydia if chlamydial infection is not ruled out

10. The U.S. Preventive Services Task Force (USPSTF) recommends the following women be screened for chlamydial disease:
    a. all sexually active women age 25 years or younger, and any other asymptomatic women at increased risk for chlamydial infection
    b. only women who have risk factors for chlamydial infection
    c. only women who have proven infection with *N. gonorrhea*
    d. only women with signs and symptoms of active cervicitis
    e. only pregnant women with signs and symptoms of active cervicitis

CLINICAL CASE PROBLEM 3

A 24-Year-Old Male with Dysuria

A 24-year-old heterosexually active male comes to your office with complaints of a 2-day history of dysuria. He denies fever, urgency, frequency, or hematuria. Physical examination reveals no suprapubic or costovertebral tenderness. Urologic examination reveals mucupurulent urethral discharge, nontender testes, normal prostate, and no penile lesions. Urine analysis is positive for leukocyte esterase, but it is negative for nitrite and blood. You send a swab of his urethral discharge for gram stain.

11. The patient's urethral gram stain reveals 20 WBCs per high power field. There are no intracellular gram-negative diplococci seen. What is the most likely diagnosis in this patient?
    a. gonorrhea
    b. acute prostatitis
    c. epididymitis
    d. nongonococcal urethritis (NGU)
    e. bacterial cystitis

12. What is the most likely organism causing this condition?
    a. *C. trachomatis*
    b. *Ureaplasma urealyticum*
    c. *Trichomonas vaginalis*
    d. *N. gonorrhea*
    e. Herpes simplex virus

13. What is first-line treatment for this patient's condition?
    a. levofloxacin 500 mg orally daily for 7 days
    b. doxycycline 100 mg orally twice a day for 7 days
    c. erythromycin base 500 mg orally four times a day for 7 days
    d. ofloxacin 300 mg orally twice a day for 7 days
    e. ceftriaxone 125 mg IM in a single dose

14. You prescribe an appropriate antibiotic regimen for this patient and his current sexual partner. He returns to your office stating that he and his partner have completed the recommended treatment. They have been in a monogamous relationship since then. His symptoms have resolved completely. He wants to know if further testing can be done to make sure the "infection is gone." You advise him that
    a. he should have a "test of cure" in 2 weeks
    b. he should have a test of cure in 6 months

c. both he and his partner should have a test of cure in 2 weeks

d. both he and his partner should have a test of cure in 6 months

e. none of the above

CLINICAL CASE PROBLEM 4

A 23-Year-Old Female Graduate Student Presents for Her Annual Exam

A 23-year-old female graduate student presents to your office for her annual gynecologic examination. She has been sexually active for 4 years with the same partner. She is up-to-date with cervical cancer screening, and her Papanicolaou (Pap) smears have all been normal. The patient appears worried and says she wants to be checked for "that HPV virus." Several of her friends have had abnormal Pap smears and were told that the human papillomavirus (HPV) was responsible for these findings. She asks how to prevent getting HPV and whether there are treatments to "get rid of it." On examination, her external genitalia and cervix appear normal without evidence of lesions. Bimanual examination reveals a small, anteverted uterus with no masses.

15. You inform the patient that
    a. there is nothing she can do to prevent getting HPV except stay in a monogamous relationship
    b. consistent condom use will protect her from HPV transmission
    c. she is a candidate for the HPV vaccine
    d. she is not eligible for the HPV vaccine because she is already sexually active
    e. she and her boyfriend should be tested for HPV immediately

16. Which of the following statements is true about HPV?
    a. the majority of cervical cancers can be attributed to HPV 16 and 18
    b. the majority of cervical cancers can be attributed to HPV 6 and 11
    c. the majority of genital warts can be attributed to HPV 16 and 18
    d. it is a rare STD predominantly seen in sex workers
    e. it is a rare STD predominantly seen in homosexual men

CLINICAL CASE PROBLEM 5

A 25-Year-Old Female with Vulvar "Growths"

A 25-year-old sexually active female comes to your office with a 2-week history of "growths" in the vulvar region. On examination, you find multiple "cauliflower" verrucous lesions on the labia majora and minora.

17. What is the most likely diagnosis in this patient?
    a. condyloma lata
    b. condyloma acuminatum
    c. herpes simplex type 1
    d. herpes simplex type 2
    e. genital acrochordon (skin tags)

18. All of the following are acceptable treatments for this condition except
    a. podophyllin
    b. trichloracetic acid
    c. carbon dioxide laser
    d. interferon
    e. acyclovir

19. The patient should be counseled that
    a. treatment for genital warts prevents further recurrences
    b. treatment for genital warts prevents transmission to her partner
    c. she should have a Pap smear every 6 months from now on
    d. recurrence of genital warts is common
    e. she should be suspicious of partner infidelity

20. Which of the following statements about syphilis is true?
    a. primary syphilis is associated with a single, painful chancre
    b. secondary syphilis is associated with skin lesions and lymphadenopathy
    c. latent syphilis is associated with constitutional symptoms
    d. treatment for primary syphilis is oral penicillin
    e. the recommended treatments for early latent and late latent syphilis are the same

21. Which of the following statements about syphilis testing is true?
    a. dark field microscopy of lesion exudates is the most convenient way to confirm *Treponema pallidum*
    b. nontreponemal tests (e.g., rapid plasma reagin [RPR]) can be falsely positive in certain medical conditions

c. treponemal-specific test (e.g., fluorescent treponemal antibody absorption test [FTA-ABS]) titers decline after syphilis treatment

d. RPR titers can be used interchangeably with Venereal Disease Research Laboratory (VDRL)

e. treponemal test antibody titers can be used to monitor treatment response

22. What is the treatment of choice in patients who are not allergic to penicillin for primary, secondary, or early latent syphilis (syphilis acquired within the preceding year without evidence of disease)?
    a. benzathine penicillin G 2.4 million units IM in a single dose
    b. benzathine penicillin 2.4 million units IM in three doses doses, at 1-week intervals
    c. aqueous crystalline penicillin G IV 18 to 24 million units/day for 10 to 14 days
    d. levofloxacin 250 mg orally a day for 7 days
    e. doxycycline 100 mg orally twice a day for 7 days

CLINICAL CASE PROBLEM 6

A 24-Year-Old Female with Genital Lesions

A 24-year-old female comes to your office with a 2-day history of dysuria accompanied by painful genital lesions that have coalesced to form ulcers. The patient also has fever, malaise, myalgias, and headache. There is no previous history of this condition. She has had three sexual partners in the past and inconsistently uses barrier contraceptive methods.

23. You tell the patient the most likely diagnosis is
    a. herpes simplex infection
    b. chancroid
    c. lymphogranuloma venereum
    d. granuloma inguinale
    e. primary syphilis

24. Which of the following statements concerning the patient's condition is false?
    a. transmission of infection can occur during asymptomatic periods
    b. duration of viral shedding may be reduced with appropriate therapy
    c. time needed to heal lesions may be reduced with appropriate therapy
    d. frequency of recurrent episodes can be reduced with appropriate suppressive therapy
    e. subclinical viral shedding can be eliminated with appropriate suppressive therapy

25. Which of the following statements about human immunodeficiency virus (HIV) is false?
    a. HIV testing should be offered to all patients seeking evaluation for STDs
    b. the HIV-2 strain is endemic to the United States
    c. HIV testing is available through urine, oral mucosal, and blood samples
    d. initial positive screening test should be followed by a more specific confirmatory test
    e. if initial testing was done less than 3 months from the time of exposure, a repeat test should be done

26. Strategies for the screening and diagnosis of HIV should include
    a. mandatory testing
    b. consent for HIV testing with an opportunity to decline
    c. further testing for STDs only if symptoms are present
    d. a chest radiograph
    e. a tuberculin skin test

27. Which of the following accurately describes the natural history of HIV?
    a. acute retroviral syndrome is usually asymptomatic
    b. antiretroviral therapy has no effect on the rate of immune system decline
    c. the median time between HIV infection and AIDS is 10 years in untreated patients
    d. opportunistic infections generally occur when CD4 counts are greater than 1000
    e. in untreated HIV-infected individuals, only 50% will develop AIDS

Clinical Case Management Problem

Discuss risk factors for hepatitis B and preventive strategies to reduce transmission.

Answers

1. **b.** This patient meets diagnostic criteria for acute PID. The clinical diagnosis of acute PID is imprecise, and episodes of PID often go unrecognized. Clinicians need to maintain a low threshold of suspicion and consider epidemiologic factors when diagnosing PID. Patients who are young, have multiple sexual partners, live in high-prevalence areas for gonorrhea or chlamydia, do not use barrier contraception, and have

a history of prior PID are at highest risk. According to the 2006 CDC STD treatment guidelines, empiric treatment for PID should be initiated in young sexually active women who report pelvic or lower abdominal pain and no other etiology can be identified as the cause of pain and the following minimal diagnostic criteria are met: cervical motion tenderness, or uterine tenderness, or adnexal tenderness. Supportive criteria include the following: (1) oral temperature higher than 101°F (>38.3°C), (2) abnormal cervical or vaginal mucopurulent discharge, (3) the presence of WBCs on wet prep, (4) elevated erythrocyte sedimentation rate (ESR), (5) elevated C-reactive protein (CRP), or (6) documentation of cervical infection with *N. gonorrhea* or *C. trachomatis*. More invasive studies, such as endometrial biopsy to document endometritis, laparoscopy, or transvaginal ultrasound to document tubal disease, are sometimes necessary in select cases to confirm diagnosis.

The differential diagnosis of acute PID is broad and includes disorders of any of the three organ systems within the pelvis: (1) the reproductive tract (adnexal torsion, ectopic pregnancy, and threatened abortion), (2) the gastrointestinal tract (appendicitis, diverticulitis, and regional ileitis), and (3) the urinary tract (cystitis and pyelonephritis). The patient in Clinical Case Problem 1 most likely has acute PID given her history and examination. The presence of vaginal discharge and pelvic findings makes acute appendicitis less likely. Uncomplicated cervicitis does not present with systemic symptoms. The negative pregnancy test makes ectopic pregnancy or threatened abortion unlikely. Pregnancy should be excluded in all women of reproductive age presenting with abdominal and pelvic symptoms.

2. a. Early treatment of acute PID decreases the probability of tubal scarring and subsequent infertility. The incidence of infertility is 15% after one episode of untreated or inadequately treated PID. In the past, it was generally advocated to hospitalize all patients for parenteral antibiotics to ensure successful eradication of infection. However, there are no data available to support that inpatient treatment results in better outcomes than outpatient treatment or that benefits exceed cost. In practice, the decision for hospitalization is made on an individual basis depending on severity of disease and patient factors such as compliance. The CDC suggests hospitalization in the following circumstances: (1) observation for potential surgical emergencies that cannot be excluded (e.g., appendicitis); (2) pregnant patients; (3) failed outpatient treatment; (4) severe illness such as high temperature, nausea, or vomiting; or (5) the presence of a tuboovarian abscess. In this patient's case, her high fever, nausea, and vomiting would be an indication for hospitalization for parenteral antibiotics. Laparoscopy is not performed routinely for suspected PID.

3. b. The treatment for acute PID should include broad-spectrum coverage for *N. gonorrhea*, *C. trachomatis*, anaerobes, gram-negative bacteria, and streptococci. The 2006 CDC STD treatment guidelines recommend the following as acceptable regimens for parenteral treatment of PID: (1) cefotetan 2 g IV every 12 hours or cefoxitin 2 g IV every 6 hours plus doxycycline 100 mg orally or IV every 12 hours or (2) clindamycin 900 mg IV every 8 hours plus gentamicin loading dose IV or IM (2 mg/kg of body weight) followed by a maintenance dose (1.5 mg/kg) every 8 hours. Parenteral therapy should continue for at least 24 hours after clinical improvement, at which time the transition can be made to oral antibiotics.

4. c. In April 2007, the CDC issued new guidelines for the outpatient treatment of gonococcal infections and associated conditions. Based on epidemiologic data from 2006 that revealed an alarming rise in the incidence of fluoroquinolone-resistant strains of gonorrhea, the CDC no longer recommends fluoroquinolones as first-line treatment for gonorrhea infections and associated conditions. Therefore, the preferred treatment of uncomplicated adult gonococcal urethritis, cervicitis, or proctitis is as follows: (1) ceftriaxone 125 mg IM in a single dose or (2) cefixime 400 mg orally in a single dose plus treatment for chlamydia if chlamydia infection is not ruled out (e.g., azithromycin 1 g orally in a single dose or doxycycline 100 mg orally twice a day for 7 days).

Following the same logic, recommended outpatient regimens for PID include the following:

1. Ceftriaxone 250 mg IM (or other parenteral third-generation cephalosporin) in a single dose plus doxycycline 100 mg orally twice a day for 14 days with or without metronidazole 500 mg orally twice a day for 14 days, or
2. Cefoxitin 2 g IM in a single dose and probenecid 1 g orally in a single dose plus doxycycline 100 mg orally for 14 days with or without metronidazole 500 mg orally twice a day for 14 days, or
3. Other parenteral third-generation cephalosporin (e.g., ceftizoxime or cefotaxime) plus doxycycline 100 mg orally for 14 days with or without metronidazole 500 mg orally twice a day for 14 days

As noted, outpatient PID regimens may be given with or without metronidazole if coverage for anaerobic bacteria or concomitant treatment for bacterial vaginosis is desired. The choice to add metronidazole to these regimens is based on the assumption that PID involves a broad spectrum of organisms, including anaerobes. Empiric treatment should be initiated in all male sex partners who had sexual contact during the 60 days preceding the patient's onset of symptoms. In cases in which cephalosporin therapy is not appropriate or feasible, fluoroquinolone therapy can be considered based on local prevalence rates, individual risk, and gonorrhea testing results.

5. a. Past epidemiologic studies have demonstrated that OCPs have a protective effect against PID. The proposed mechanism is believed to be multifactorial: (1) Progestin-induced thickening of cervical secretions inhibits bacterial ascent into the upper genital tract; (2) decreased menstrual blood flow, which may decrease the risk of menstrual blood potentially acting as a culture medium; (3) decreased cervical dilation at midcycle and menstruation; and (4) decreased strength of uterine contractions. Interestingly, OCPs do not decrease the risk of lower genital tract disease against chlamydia but, in fact, have been associated with an increased risk of cervicitis. One theory to explain these epidemiologic findings is that OCPs promote cervical ectopy, the eversion of delicate columnar cells from the cervical os onto the portio (outer surface) of the cervix, which in turn leaves columnar cells vulnerable to infection. On the other hand, some experts argue that the association between OCPs and lower genital tract infection may be a result of a detection bias, such that cervical ectopy could facilitate better collection of chlamydial organisms. Regardless, all OCP users need to be advised that OCPs alone do not prevent transmission of STDs. Counseling should focus on abstinence, consistent condom use, and/or engaging in a stable, monogamous relationship to minimize risk.

6. e. The most common organisms associated with acute PID are *N. gonorrhea* and *C. trachomatis*. Many episodes of PID are polymicrobial and involve anaerobic organisms such as *Bacteroides fragilis* and *Peptostreptococcus*. Microorganisms that include vaginal flora such as *Gardnerella vaginalis* and *Streptococcus agalactiae* have also been associated with PID. Group A β-hemolytic streptococcus (the streptococcus associated with bacterial pharyngitis) is not associated with acute PID.

7. d. Overall, the incidence of PID for IUD users is similar to that of the general population. There is an increased risk of PID limited to the first 20 days after insertion of an IUD, suggesting that placement of the device may promote ascension of bacterial into the upper genital tract. Specifically, the incidence of PID is

9.6/1000 women-years during the peri-IUD insertion period but then decreases to an incidence similar to that of non-IUD users (1.3/1000). After the immediate postinsertion period, the risk of PID is not related to IUD use but, rather, to sexual behavior. Choices a, b, c, and e are known risk factors for PID.

8. e. Gonococcal arthritis–dermatitis syndrome is the most common clinical manifestation of DGI and consists of tenosynovitis, arthritis, and a pustular or papular rash. Meningitis and endocarditis are rare complications of bacteremic gonococcal infection. Gonococcal infection at other sites in adults includes gonococcal conjunctivitis and gonococcal epididymitis.

9. c. As discussed in answer 4, the preferred treatment of uncomplicated adult gonococcal urethritis, cervicitis, or proctitis no longer includes fluoroquinolones. First-line regimens include (1) ceftriaxone 125 mg IM in a single dose or (2) cefixime 400 mg orally in a single dose. If chlamydia infection is not ruled out, azithromycin 1 g orally in a single dose or doxycycline 100 mg orally twice a day for 7 days should be added to the previous regimens. Ceftriaxone provides excellent cure rates for uncomplicated gonorrhea, eradicating 99% of infections in clinical trials. Cefixime has excellent efficacy as well (97.4%) but less than that of ceftriaxone. The advantage of cefixime is that it can be orally administered; however, the oral formulation is not currently available in the United States. The prevalence of fluoroquinolone-resistant gonorrhea (QRNG) has risen at an alarming rate, and it is no longer a disease limited to certain regions (e.g., Hawaii and California) or subpopulations (e.g., men who have sex with men). In June 2006, the estimated national prevalence of QRNG was 13%. Therefore, fluoroquinolones are no longer considered first-line therapy for gonorrheal infections. Patients with gonorrhea often have coinfection with chlamydia; this has led to the recommendation that dual treatment therapy be performed. All treatment regimens as noted previously should include either azithromycin or doxycycline if chlamydial infection is not ruled out.

10. a. The USPSTF strongly recommends screening all women age 25 years or younger and other asymptomatic women at risk for infection (multiple sexual partners, inconsistent use of barrier contraceptives, and prior history of STD/PID) for chlamydia. These recommendations are based on epidemiologic data showing that the prevalence and risk of chlamydia infection is greater in women age 25 years or younger, as well as evidence that community-based screening reduces the prevalence of disease. Because chlamydia infections are often asymptomatic, screening based on symptoms and signs alone would be inadequate. Chlamydia infections can occur in the absence of gonorrheal disease; therefore, it would be inappropriate to only screen gonorrhea-positive women for chlamydia. For gonorrhea screening, the USPSTF recommends that all sexually active women, including pregnant women, be screened if they are at increased risk for infection.

11. **d.** This patient has NGU. Urethritis can be associated with dysuria or mucopurulent discharge or can be completely asymptomatic. Patients presenting with urethritis should be investigated thoroughly for other urologic etiology, such as cystitis, prostatitis, or epididymitis. The patient's normal testicular and prostate examinations make epididymitis and prostatitis less likely. A diagnosis of urethritis can be made on any of the following signs: (1) mucopurulent or purulent urethral discharge; (2) gram stain of urethral secretions revealing five or more WBCs per oil immersion field; or (3) positive leukocyte–esterase test on first-void urine or microscopic examination revealing 10 or more WBCs per high power field. Testing for both *N. gonorrhea* and *C. trachomatis* is recommended to confirm the diagnosis. NGU can be diagnosed if a patient has urethritis with no evidence of gonorrhea infection, as evidenced by the absence of gram-negative diplococci on urethral gram stain.

12. **a.** *C. trachomatis* is the most frequent cause of NGU (15% to 55% of cases), although the prevalence varies by age groups. Other organisms that may be associated with NGU include *U. urealyticum* and *Mycoplasma genitalium*, which are difficult to detect. Less frequent causes of NGU include *T. vaginalis* and herpes simplex virus. All individuals who have had sexual contact with the index case within the past 60 days should be identified and referred for evaluation and treatment.

13. **b.** First-line treatment for uncomplicated urethral *C. trachomatis* infection includes doxycycline 100 mg orally twice a day for 7 days or azithromycin 1 g orally in a single dose. The advantage of azithromycin is that a single-dose regimen enhances patient compliance. If taken as directed, azithromycin and doxycycline have equal efficacy. Alternative second-line treatments include oral erythromycin, levofloxacin, or ofloxacin for 7 days. Female patients with chlamydial cervicitis should undergo the same treatment regimen as for males with NGU. Patients should abstain from sexual intercourse for 1 week after therapy has been initiated. After 1 week, they may resume provided that their symptoms have resolved and their partners have received appropriate treatment. Ceftriaxone is not indicated for treatment of NGU.

14. **e.** The CDC does not recommend routine "tests of cure" in patients who have completed recommended regimens for uncomplicated chlamydia infections unless symptoms persist, reinfection is suspected, or the patient is pregnant. Most posttreatment infections are a result of reinfection and not failed therapy. Because repeat infection is associated with higher morbidity and an increased risk of PID, the CDC recommends that clinicians consider rescreening all patients for chlamydia 3 months after treatment.

15. **c.** Following the 2006 release of the quadrivalent vaccine for HPV, there has been growing public interest in HPV infection as a sexually transmitted infection and a causative agent for cervical cancer. The quadrivalent HPV vaccine (Gardasil) consists of noninfectious viral-like particles and provides immunity to HPV 6, 11, 16, and 18; collectively, these viruses are responsible for two-thirds of cervical cancers (HPV 16 and 18) and 90% of genital warts (HPV 6 and 11). The vaccine consists of three shots given at 0, 2, and 6 months. The combined efficacy of the quadrivalent HPV vaccine ranged from 98% to 100% in phase III trials. All sexually active patients should be encouraged to maintain stable, monogamous relationships. The Advisory Committee on Immunization Practices (ACIP) recommends that clinicians target girls 11 or 12 years of age for routine HPV vaccination, and vaccination of women age 13 to 26 years is also recommended. Although the patient is already sexually active, it is unlikely that she has been exposed to all four serotypes (6, 11, 16, and 18); therefore, vaccination at this time can potentially provide protection from new HPV infections. Testing for HPV in the patient and boyfriend is not recommended at this time for several reasons: (1) They are both asymptomatic, (2) the patient's most recent cervical cytology was normal, and (3) the majority of HPV infections are transient and resolve spontaneously.

16. **a.** The burden of HPV disease is enormous. The CDC estimates that approximately 20 million Americans are DNA positive for anogenital HPV at any given time (15% of the population, excluding children). An estimated 75% of the reproductive-age population in the United States has had HPV infection. HPV disease is not limited to homosexual men or sex workers. The prevalence of HPV is particularly high in sexually active adolescents and young adults aged 15 to 24 years, regardless of sexual orientation. Two-thirds of all cervical cancers can be attributed to HPV 16 and 18.

HPV 6 and 11 are responsible for the vast majority of genital warts and cases of laryngeal papillomatosis (a rare but devastating disease). Furthermore, 88% of anal cancers are associated with high-risk types of HPV.

17. b. This patient has condyloma acuminatum, or "genital warts." External genital warts are caused by HPV, most commonly types 6 and 11. These HPV subtypes are considered "low risk" because they are rarely associated with cervical neoplasia. HPV types 16, 18, 31, 33, and 45 are considered "high-risk" types associated with cervical cancer precursors. Patients with external condyloma are likely infected with multiple subtypes of HPV and need to be counseled about the importance of routine cervical cancer screening. Patients with condyloma acuminatum should be screened for other STDs. Condyloma lata are painless genital lesions associated with primary syphilis. This patient's genital lesions are not consistent with genital herpes.

18. e. The primary goal of treatment for genital warts is removal of visible and symptomatic warts. There is no known definitive cure for genital warts. The treatment that has been reported to have the highest cure rate is carbon dioxide laser. Cure rates with this form of therapy approach 90%. Current treatments probably do not significantly affect the natural history of HPV infections or prevent the development of cervical carcinoma. Other treatment options include topical therapy, which can be patient applied (podofilox 0.5% gel or imiquimod 5% cream) or provider administered (podophyllin resin 10% to 25% in benzoin or trichloroacetic acid). Destructive procedures include cryotherapy, electrodesiccation, and surgical excision for recalcitrant or larger lesions. Immunotherapy with intralesional injection of interferon is reserved as second-line therapy. Acyclovir is treatment for primary or recurrent genital herpes infection, not genital warts. As discussed in case 4, patients should be informed about the availability of the quadrivalent HPV vaccine and its ability to prevent new HPV infections.

19. d. Extensive counseling about the natural course of HPV should be provided to patients with HPV infection. Recurrence of genital warts is common, even after treatment. It is unclear whether treatment reduces the risk of transmission to sexual partners. Condoms can provide some protection from HPV transmission, although areas that remain exposed (vulva, scrotum, and anus) are still vulnerable. The presence of HPV infection alone does not change the frequency of cervical cancer screening. Because of the variable incubation period of HPV, it is difficult to determine the time of infection; recently diagnosed HPV infection does not necessarily imply partner infidelity.

20. b. The causative agent of syphilis is the spirochete *T. pallidum*. Primary syphilis is characterized by a single, painless genital ulcer that develops an average of 3 weeks after exposure. Secondary syphilis is associated with skin lesions (maculopapular rash that may involve palm and soles), lymphadenopathy, condyloma lata (soft verrucous plaques), and involvement of other organ systems (renal, hepatic, and musculoskeletal). Tertiary syphilis involves gummatous syphilis, cardiovascular syphilis, or neurosyphilis. Latent syphilis by definition is serologic evidence of syphilis without any clinical manifestations. Early latent syphilis is defined as latent syphilis that was acquired within the preceding year. Early latent syphilis cannot be distinguished reliably from late latent syphilis by serologic testing alone and often requires documentation of prior seroconversion or a consistent history. The significance of making this distinction is that treatment therapy differs for early latent versus late latent syphilis. The treatment for syphilis is IM benzathine penicillin G, not oral penicillin.

21. b. Although dark field microscopy is the most specific technique for diagnosing syphilis, it is not convenient to perform in the typical office setting. It involves the collection of exudate from an active chancre or condyloma lata and examining it under a microscope with a dark field condenser. The characteristic shape of *T. pallidum* is a corkscrew appearance. Given the need for an active lesion, the proper equipment, and sufficient experience to interpret specimens, most clinicians turn to serologic tests to confirm the diagnosis. Nontreponemal studies such as VDRL and RPR test for a nonspecific antibody reaction to *T. pallidum*. VDRL and RPR titers should not be used interchangeably because RPR titers may be slightly higher than VDRL titers. Quantitative nontreponemal titers should be repeated 6 and 12 months after treatment for primary and secondary syphilis. Nontreponemal titers are used to monitor response to treatment, with a fourfold reduction in titers indicating treatment response. False-positive nontreponemal tests can often occur in the elderly, pregnant women, and patients with autoimmune disorders. Positive nontreponemal titers should be confirmed with treponemal-specific tests, which detect antibodies specific to *T. pallidum*, such as FTA-ABS or *T. pallidum* hemagglutination test (TPHA). Treponemal-specific tests tend to remain reactive for life, whereas nontreponemal test titers decline after treatment. Therefore, treponemal-specific antibody tests should not be used to monitor treatment response.

22. a. The treatment of choice for primary, secondary, and early latent syphilis is benzathine penicillin G 2.4 million units IM in a single dose. For late latent syphilis and tertiary syphilis, the treatment of choice is benzathine penicillin G 7.2 million units total, administered as three doses of 2.4 million units IM at 1-week intervals. For neurosyphilis, the treatment of choice is aqueous crystalline penicillin G 18 to 24 million units per day, administered as 3 or 4 million units every 4 hours or continuous infusion for 10 to 14 days. Oral doxycycline (100 mg orally twice daily for 14 days) is preferred for patients allergic to penicillin. Levofloxacin is not a recommended treatment for syphilis. All patients should be warned of a possible localized "Jarisch–Herxheimer reaction" after treatment for syphilis. It is characterized by an acute febrile illness with headache and myalgia and occurs within the first 24 hours of initiating therapy. This phenomenon should be treated with salicylates (acetaminophen in pregnant women) or, in severe cases, prednisone.

23. **a.** The patient's symptoms are consistent with herpes simplex virus (HSV) type 2 infection. Given her systemic symptoms, it is likely a primary infection. Classic symptoms of genital herpes infection include a prodrome of tingling or itching, followed by eruption of painful vesicular or ulcerative genital lesions. Systemic symptoms such as fever, malaise, and inguinal adenopathy may occur. Most recurrent genital herpes cases are caused by HSV-2, although HSV-1 has been identified in genital lesions in up to 50% of first-episode cases. Culture of genital ulcers can confirm diagnosis, although the sensitivity of cultures declines as lesions start to heal. False-negative HSV cultures are common. Per the 2006 CDC STD treatment guidelines, type-specific HSV serologic testing should be considered in the following situations: (1) to confirm a clinical diagnosis of genital herpes, (2) when patients present with recurrent genital symptoms or atypical symptoms and HSV cultures are negative, or (3) to determine herpes exposure for patients with infected partners.

The genital lesions of chanchroid caused by *Haemophilus ducreyi* are characterized by painful ulcers and tender inguinal adenopathy. The presence of suppurative inguinal adenopathy is almost pathognomonic for *H. ducreyi* infection. The CDC recommends that diagnosis of chancroid be based on (1) the presence of painful ulcer(s), (2) negative serologic tests for syphilis, and (3) negative HSV testing of ulcer exudates. Genital lesions caused by primary syphilis are usually painless. Granuloma inguinale (donovanosis) is a genital ulcerative infection caused by an intracellular gram-negative bacteria, *Klebsiella granulomatis* (formerly known as *Calymmatobacterium granulomatis*). It is characterized by painless, progressive ulcerative genital lesions without regional lymphadenopathy. The disease is endemic to tropical and developing areas, such as India and southern African, but is extremely rare in the United States. Lymphogranuloma venereum (LGV) is cause by *C. trachomatis* serotypes L1, L2, or L3. In the first phase of infection, a shallow, painless ulcer appears that is extremely transient and usually disappears by the time of presentation. In the second stage, patients experience painful, often unilateral inguinal and/or femoral lymphadenopathy. Multiple swollen lymph nodes may coalesce to form "buboes," which can rupture in up to one-third of patients. Advanced or tertiary LGV is characterized by protocolitis that can progress to severe scarring and damage to the perirectal area.

24. **e.** Patients and their partners should be educated about the natural history of HSV, with emphasis on the possibility of recurrent episodes and transmission of virus during asymptomatic shedding. Barrier contraceptive methods should be encouraged to prevent transmission. Physicians should inform patients that treatment of the first episode of genital herpes can shorten the duration of viral shedding and time for lesion healing. Recommended regimens for first clinical episodes include (1) acyclovir 400 mg orally three times a day for 7 to 10 days, (2) acyclovir 200 mg orally five times a day for 7 to 10 days, (3) famciclovir 250 mg orally three times a day for 7 to 10 days, or (4) valacyclovir 1 g orally twice a day for 7 to 10 days. Patients can be treated for recurrent episodes either with continuous suppressive therapy (for more than six episodes a year) or episodically for less frequent occurrences. HSV-1 is associated with fewer recurrent episodes than HSV-2. Episodic treatment initiated within a day of lesion onset can reduce the severity and duration of lesions. Chronic, suppressive therapy can decrease the number of symptomatic outbreaks a year, but subclinical viral shedding is not completely eliminated.

25. **b.** HIV testing should be offered to all patients seeking evaluation for STDs and to patients with risk factors. Urine and oral mucosal tests are available but need to be confirmed with more specific serologic testing if positive. In the United States, the HIV-1 strain is responsible for most HIV infections. The HIV-2 strain is endemic to West Africa, and patients from this region or who have sex partners from this region should have testing that will include HIV-2 detection. Standard serum screening tests (enzyme immunoassay [EIA]) detect both HIV-1 and HIV-2 antibodies. Positive EIA tests should be followed with more specific tests (Western blot) to confirm HIV. If testing was done within 3 months of exposure and there is concern about a false-negative result, repeat serologic testing may be performed at least 3 months after the time of exposure. Of patients with HIV, 95% will seroconvert within 3 months of infection. However, there have been rare documented cases of seroconversion 6 to 12 months after infection.

26. **b.** HIV screening should be voluntary. Verbal or written consent should be obtained prior to screening. A radiograph and tuberculin skin test are appropriate after a diagnosis of HIV has been made but not for routine screening. Patients should be offered the full range of STD testing, even if they are asymptomatic.

27. **c.** In untreated patients, the median time from HIV infection to AIDS is 10 years. Left untreated, nearly all HIV infections will progress to AIDS. Early detection of HIV is important because early initiation of antiretroviral therapy can slow immune function decline. The acute retroviral syndrome is characterized by fever, lymphadenopathy, malaise, and rash that occur 6 to 8 weeks after infection. Opportunistic infections, such as pneumocystis carinii (now known as *Pneumocystis jiroveci*), toxoplasmosis, and candidiasis, typically occur when CD4 levels have dropped below 200.

Solution to the Clinical Case Management Problem

Hepatitis B is an STD caused by hepatitis B virus (HBV). Patients with chronic HBV infection are at risk for cirrhosis or hepatocellular carcinoma (15% to 25% chance). An effective vaccination exists for hepatitis B, but the majority of patients diagnosed with hepatitis B were not offered immunization prior to infection. The CDC's national immunization strategy focuses on (1) preventing perinatal transmission through universal maternal screening and postexposure prophylaxis of at-risk infants (with hepatitis B immune globulin [HBIG]), (2) universal infant immunization, (3) universal immunization of previously unvaccinated children age 11 or 12 years, and (4) vaccinations of at-risk adolescents and adults. High-risk groups who should receive vaccination include the following: (1) sexually active adolescents and adults, (2) patients with a history of other STDs, (3) IV drug users, (4) household contacts or partners of patients with hepatitis B, (5) health care workers, (6) staff and residents at long-term care facilities and institutions, (7) patients undergoing hemodialysis, (8) recipients of clotting-factor concentrates, (9) people from HBV endemic areas, and (10) international travelers. Vaccination consists of three doses at 0, 1, and 6 months. If a dose has been missed, there is no need to start the series over. Other preventive measures include counseling on barrier contraceptive use, practicing universal precautions (health care workers), and not sharing toothbrushes/razor blades with infected individuals (or household contacts). In addition, postexposure prophylaxis with HBIG should be administered when appropriate.

Summary

PID

1. Diagnosis: Complaints of pelvic or lower abdominal pain and no other etiology can be identified as the cause of pain and the following minimal diagnostic criteria are met: cervical motion tenderness, uterine tenderness, or adnexal tenderness. Supportive criteria include (a) oral temperature >101°F (>38.3°C), (b) abnormal cervical or vaginal mucopurulent discharge, (c) the presence of WBCs on wet prep, (d) elevated ESR, (e) elevated CRP, or (f) documentation of cervical infection with *N. gonorrhea* or *C. trachomatis*.
2. Causative agents include *N. gonorrhea*, *C. trachomatis*, anaerobes, gram-negative bacteria, and streptococci.
3. Risk factors for PID include young age, multiple sexual partners, living in high-prevalence areas for gonorrhea or chlamydia, not using barrier contraception, and having a history of prior PID.
4. The risk of PID with IUD use is limited to the first 21 days postinsertion. After that, the risk of PID is related to sexual behavior, not the IUD device.
5. Situations that may require hospitalization for inpatient treatment include the following: (a) observation for potential surgical emergencies that cannot be excluded; (b) pregnancy; (c) failed outpatient treatment; (d) severe illness such as high fever, nausea, and vomiting; (e) the patient is unable to follow or tolerate an oral regimen; and (f) the presence of a tuboovarian abscess.

6. First-line treatment of PID
   a. Inpatient regimen: (1) IV cefotetan or IV cefoxitin plus doxycycline (orally or IV) or (2) IV clindamycin and IV gentamicin
   b. Outpatient regimen: (1) IM ceftriaxone plus oral doxycycline with or without oral metronidazole, (2) IM cefoxitin and oral probenecid plus oral doxycycline with or without oral metronidazole, or (3) other parenteral third-generation cephalosporin plus doxycycline with or without oral metronidazole

UNCOMPLICATED GONOCOCCAL CERVICITIS

1. Causative agent: *N. gonorrhea*
2. Symptoms: dysuria, postcoital bleeding, vaginal discharge, or asymptomatic
3. Signs: cervical bleeding upon contact, cervical erythema, mucopurulent discharge, tender cervix
4. The prevalence of fluoroquinolone-resistant gonorrhea strains is rising dramatically in all regions of the United States.
5. Fluoroquinolones are no longer recommended as first-line treatment for gonorrhea infections and associated diseases (e.g., PID, epidydimitis, proctitis, pharyngitis, and cervicitis).
6. Treatment for uncomplicated gonorrhea and associated complicated infections (patients and their sexual partners) is as follows: (a) IM ceftriaxone or (b) oral cefixime plus (c) oral doxycycline or oral azithromycin if chlamydia infection is not ruled out.
7. U.S. Preventive Services Task Force screening recommendations
   a. Gonorrhea: Routinely screen all sexually active women, including pregnant women, if at increased risk for infection (multiple sexual partners, no barrier contraceptive use, or prior history of STD/PID).
   b. Chlamydia: Routinely screen all sexually active women age 25 years or younger and other asymptomatic women at increased risk for infection.

NGU

1. Organism: *C. trachomatis, U. urealyticum, M. genitalium*
2. Symptoms: dysuria, frequency, mucopurulent or purulent urethral discharge
3. Diagnosis based on any of the following signs: (a) mucopurulent or purulent urethral discharge, (b) gram stain of urethral secretions revealing 5 or more WBCs per oil immersion field, (c) positive leukocyte–esterase test on first-void urine or microscopic examination revealing 10 or more WBCs per high power field, or (d) the absence of intracellular diplococci on urethral gram stain
4. Treatment (patients and their partners): oral doxycycline or oral azithromycin

5. A "test of cure" is not routinely indicated. Rescreening can be performed if reinfection is suspected.

GENITAL WARTS AND HPV

1. HPV 6 and 11 are responsible for 90% of genital warts.
2. HPV 16 and 18 are responsible for 70% of cervical cancers.
3. Symptoms of genital warts include the following: usually asymptomatic, sometimes pruritic, painful.
4. Signs include soft, sessile lesions that can appear flat or cauliflower-like on the penis, perivulvar, perirectal, or vaginal areas.
5. External condyloma is not directly associated with cervical dysplasia.
6. Patients with genital warts are at risk for infection with multiple HPV subtypes and need routine cervical cancer screening.
7. Treatment
   a. Topical (patient applied): podofilox or imiquimod
   b. Topical (provider administered): podophyllin resin in benzoin or trichloroacetic acid
   c. Surgical: cryosurgery, surgical excision, electrodesiccation, carbon dioxide laser therapy, immunotherapy
8. Prevention
   a. Abstinence, monogamy
   b. Quadrivalent HPV vaccine provides excellent immunity to HPV 6, 11, 16 and 18. (1) ACIP recommends routine vaccination for girls age 11 or 12 years; (2) can also vaccinate adolescents and women age 13 to 26 years; and (3) sexually active women can still benefit from the vaccine.

SYPHILIS

1. Organism: *T. pallidum*
2. Definitions
   a. Primary syphilis: single, painless genital ulcer
   b. Secondary syphilis: skin lesions, lymphadenopathy, condyloma latum, may be multisystem involvement
   c. Tertiary syphilis: gummatous syphilis, cardiovascular syphilis, or neurosyphilis
   d. Latent syphilis: serologic evidence of syphilis without any clinical manifestations
   e. Early latent syphilis: latent syphilis that was acquired within the preceding year
3. Laboratory diagnosis: (a) dark field microscopic confirmation of *T. pallidum*; (b) nontreponemal tests, such as VDRL and RPR; and (c) treponemal-specific tests, such as FTA-ABS and TPHA
4. Treatment for primary, secondary, and early latent syphilis
   a. Benzathine penicillin G 2.4 million units IM in a single dose

b. Repeat nontreponemal test titers at 6 and 12 months; should see at least fourfold reduction

5. Treatment for late latent and tertiary syphilis is three doses of benzathine penicillin G 2.4 million units.

6. Treponemal-specific tests generally remain reactive for life.

7. With Jarisch–Herxheimer reaction, an acute febrile illness occurs within 24 hours of syphilis treatment.

GENITAL HERPES AND HSV

1. Organism: HSV-2 is responsible for most genital herpes; HSV-1 is associated with fewer recurrences.

2. Symptoms and signs include prodrome of tingling, itching, followed by eruption of painful vesicular ulcers in genital area. Primary infection may be associated with systemic symptoms.

3. Laboratory diagnosis includes viral culture and serologic HSV type-specific antibody tests.

4. Treatment includes oral acyclovir, famciclovir, and valacyclovir.

5. Patient counseling: Emphasize risk of recurrence and asymptomatic shedding.

6. Episodic treatment can decrease severity and duration of lesions.

7. Suppressive therapy can decrease frequency of outbreaks and severity of symptoms.

HIV

1. Organism: human immunodeficiency virus

2. Presentation: acute retroviral syndrome (fever, malaise, lymphadenopathy, and rash occurring 6 to 8 weeks postinfection)

3. Natural history: 10 years median time from HIV infection to AIDS in untreated patients

4. Antiretroviral therapy can slow disease progression.

5. The HIV-1 strain is responsibly for the majority of HIV cases in the United States.

6. The HIV-2 strain is endemic to West Africa.

7. HIV testing should be voluntary; verbal and/or written consent should be obtained first.

8. Diagnosis: EIA serum testing, followed by more specific Western blot test if initially positive. Urine and oral mucosal testing also available.

9. If testing was done within 3 months of exposure and there is concern about a false-negative result, repeat serologic testing may be performed at least 3 months after the time of exposure.

OTHER STDS

1. Chanchroid
   a. Caused by *H. ducreyi*
   b. Manifests as painful ulcer(s) and tender inguinal adenopathy
   c. Diagnosis based on the presence of painful ulcers, negative tests for syphilis and HSV

2. Granuloma inguinale (donovanosis)
   a. Caused by *K. granulomatis* (formerly known as *C. granulomatis*)
   b. Manifests as painless, highly vascular, ulcerative genital lesions without regional lymphadenopathy
   c. Very rare in the United States

3. Lymphogranuloma venereum
   a. Caused by *C. trachomatis* serotypes L1, L2, or L3
   b. Manifests as unilateral painful inguinal and/or femoral lymphadenopathy, buboes
   c. Painless shallow ulcer usually gone by the time of presentation

Suggested Reading

Beerthuizen RJ: Pelvic inflammatory disease in intrauterine device users. *Eur J Contracept Reprod Health Care* 1(3):237–243, 1996.

Brown DL, Frank JE: Diagnosis and management of syphilis. *Am Fam Physician* 68:283–290, 2003.

Brown DR, Shew ML, Qadadri B, et al: A longitudinal study of genital human papillomavirus infection in a cohort of closely followed adolescent women. *J Infect Dis* 191(2):182–192, 2005.

Centers for Disease Control and Prevention: Sexually transmitted diseases treatment guidelines. *MMWR* 51(RR-6):7–61, 2006.

Centers for Disease Control and Prevention: Update to CDC's sexually transmitted diseases treatment guidelines, 2006: Fluoroquinolones no longer recommended for treatment of gonococcal infections. *MMWR* 56(14):332–336, 2007.

Koutsky L: Epidemiology of genital human papillomavirus infection. *Am J Med* 102(Suppl 5A):3–8, 1997.

Miller KE, Graves JC: Update on the prevention and treatment of sexually transmitted diseases. *Am Fam Physician* 61:379–386, 2000.

Speroff L, Darney PD: Contraception in the U.S.A. In: Snyder AM, Dernoski N, eds., *A Clinical Guide for Contraception.* Philadelphia: Lippincott Williams & Wilkins, 2006, pp. 1–19.

CLINICAL CASE PROBLEM 1

A 27-Year-Old Female Comes to Your Office with Her Husband

A 27-year-old nulligravida female comes to your office with her husband. They are concerned about not having conceived after a year of regular, unprotected intercourse.

The patient denies any major medical illnesses, and she takes no medications. The husband reports he is healthy and has never fathered a child. Both the patient and her husband are visibly upset and somewhat tearful while discussing their frustrations about not being pregnant yet. They express that they are anxious to begin "all the tests necessary" as soon as possible so they can have a child without further delay.

SELECT THE BEST ANSWER TO THE FOLLOWING QUESTIONS

1. What is the most appropriate diagnosis for this couple's condition?
   a. primary sterility
   b. secondary sterility
   c. primary infertility
   d. secondary infertility
   e. diminished fecundity

2. Infertility is defined as failure to conceive with unprotected regular sexual intercourse after
   a. 1 month
   b. 3 months
   c. 6 months
   d. 1 year
   e. 2 years

3. What is the most appropriate initial step in this couple's evaluation?
   a. basal body temperature charting
   b. history and physical examination of both partners
   c. semen analysis
   d. referral to a reproductive specialist
   e. urine ovulation predictor kit testing

4. The patient reveals that menarche occurred at age 12 years. Her periods have always been irregular, with menses occurring every 2 or 3 months and lasting 5 days with normal flow. Her last menstrual period was 2 months ago. Her sexual history is significant for six total sexual partners, although she has been monogamous with her husband for the past 3 years. She has had no pelvic surgeries, no history of sexually transmitted infections (STIs), and her Papanicolaou (Pap) test results have always been normal. Physical examination reveals she is normal height for weight. She has normal secondary sexual characteristics, and there are no signs of androgen excess. Physical examination is normal, including thyroid, breast, and pelvic examination. Appropriate initial workup in the patient may include all of the following except
   a. gonorrhea and chlamydia screen
   b. serum thyroid-stimulating hormone (TSH)
   c. serum prolactin level
   d. pelvic/transvaginal ultrasound
   e. urine pregnancy test

5. The patient's initial evaluation does not reveal any abnormalities. You discuss with the patient that the next step is to confirm the presence of ovulation. All of the following are acceptable methods for assessing ovulation except
   a. basal body temperature charting
   b. urine luteinizing hormone (LH) levels
   c. urine follicle-stimulating hormone (FSH) levels
   d. mid-luteal phase progesterone serum levels
   e. cervical mucus changes

6. All of the following may be direct causes of female infertility except
   a. previous uncomplicated abortion
   b. pelvic inflammatory disease (PID)
   c. endometriosis
   d. polycystic ovarian syndrome (PCOS)
   e. hyperprolactinemia

7. Evaluation for tubal patency or "pelvic factor" is best accomplished by
   a. transvaginal ultrasound
   b. hysteroscopy
   c. hysterosalpingogram (HSG)
   d. pelvic magnetic resonance imaging (MRI)
   e. pelvic computed tomography (CT) scan

8. The postcoital test is performed to assess which of the following?
   a. interaction of sperm with cervical mucus prior to ovulation
   b. interaction of sperm with cervical mucus after ovulation
   c. interaction of sperm with cervical mucus anytime during the cycle

d. interaction of sperm with cervical mucus in mid-luteal phase

e. none of the above

9. Which of the following statements about the etiology of infertility is true?

a. male factor is associated with up to 40% of cases

b. male factor is associated with only 5% of cases

c. no etiology is found in the majority of cases

d. tubal factors are more common than ovulatory dysfunction

e. none of the above

10. Which of the following is not considered a cause of male infertility?

a. varicocele

b. obstructive azoospermia

c. hypogonadism

d. testicular cancer

e. tight-fitting underwear

11. Appropriate initial screening for male infertility includes which of the following?

a. two semen analyses done at least 1 month apart

b. serum testosterone and FSH levels

c. postejaculatory urinalysis

d. scrotal ultrasonography

e. transrectal ultrasonography

12. It is appropriate to initiate an infertility evaluation after 6 months of trying to conceive in which of the following conditions?

a. the woman is older than age 35 years

b. the man is older than age 40 years

c. the woman has used Depo-Provera within the previous year

d. the woman has used oral contraceptive pills for at least 10 years

e. the woman has a history of recurrent vaginitis

Clinical Case Management Problem

Discuss and define the various treatments in reproductive technology available for infertile couples.

Answers

1. **c.** This couple's condition is most consistent with primary infertility. Secondary infertility refers to couples who currently are experiencing infertility but have conceived in the past. Sterility is defined as an intrinsic inability to conceive, whereas infertility implies a decreased ability to conceive. Fecundity is a term used to express the likelihood of pregnancy per month of exposure and is not generally used as a diagnostic term. The average fecundity of a young, healthy couple having frequent intercourse is approximately 20% in a given month.

2. **d.** Infertility is defined as failure to conceive after 1 year of unprotected regular sexual intercourse.

3. **b.** Couples with infertility ideally should be assessed together, if possible. A woman who comes to your office with concerns about infertility should be encouraged to bring her partner for evaluation as well. During a couple's first office visit for infertility, reasonable and realistic goals regarding evaluation and timeline should be discussed. Emotional support should be provided by the physician because couples often experience significant anxiety and frustration when coping with infertility. Referral to infertility resource groups may be appropriate for couples searching for additional support. Couples should be questioned about timing and frequency of sexual intercourse. History of the female partner can be extensive but should focus on the following: (1) general medical health (diet, weight, tobacco use, and caffeine use), (2) medications, (3) detailed menstrual history (onset, length, frequency, and flow), (4) history of pubertal development, (5) history of in utero diethylstilbestrol (DES) exposure, (6) contraceptive history, (7) history of pelvic surgery, (8) history of sexually transmitted disease or PID, (9) history of abnormal Pap test results and treatments (i.e., cold knife conization), and (10) prior pregnancies and outcomes. Physical examination of the female should search for secondary sexual characteristics, signs of androgen excess (i.e., hirsutism and acne), galactorrhea, and thyroid disorder (i.e., goiter). Body mass index should also be determined. Pelvic examination should assess for signs of infection, congenital anomalies (e.g., absent vagina or uterus), uterine size, and signs of endometriosis (e.g., nodularities or fixed uterus).

History of the male patient also should include general medical health, history of STIs, health habits, surgical history, and medications. Additional history about the male partner should include (1) history of congenital abnormalities, (2) toxin exposure, (3) prior paternity history, and (4) history of infection (e.g., mumps/prostatitis) or trauma to the genitals. Examination of the male should assess for endocrine stigmata consistent with hypogonadism (e.g., small testes and gynecomastia). Testicular examination should assess size, firmness, masses (e.g., varicoceles and hydroceles), and confirm the presence of both testes. Choices a, c, and e are reasonable steps to perform once a history and physical examination of both partners have been completed. The initial evaluation for infertility can be managed by a primary care physician, and direct referral to a specialist should be reserved for women older than age 35 years or those at high risk for infertility based on medical history.

4. **d.** This patient has oligomenorrhea defined as cycles greater than every 35 days. The approach to this patient initially should be the same as for other patients with oligomenorrhea. A urine pregnancy test should be done. If pregnancy is excluded, serum TSH and prolactin levels should be measured to detect thyroid dysfunction and/or hyperprolactinemia. A low or normal FSH level is most consistent with hypothalamic amenorrhea and PCOS. An assessment for PCOS (an LH:FSH ratio of 3:1 is suggestive) should be completed if indicated by history or physical examination (oligomenorrhea and androgen excess). Patients with evidence of androgen excess may have additional testing, such as dehydroepiandrosterone sulfate and serum testosterone levels, to rule out a virilizing tumor, as well as 17α-hydroxyprogesterone to rule out late-onset congenital adrenal hyperplasia. Given the patient's past sexual history, occult PID should be ruled out with a gonorrhea/chlamydia screen. A pelvic/transvaginal ultrasound should be reserved for patients in which pelvic examination is difficult to interpret (e.g., body habitus) or to evaluate any abnormal pelvic examination findings. If this patient was older than age 35 years, testing of FSH and estradiol levels on day 3 of her menstrual cycle could be performed to assess ovarian reserve. An FSH level of less than 10 mIU/mL (10 IU/L), combined with an estradiol level of less than 80 pg/mL (294 pmol/L), suggests favorable follicular potential.

5. **c.** The presence of ovulation can be confirmed a number of ways. Basal body temperature (BBT) is an inexpensive and simple method but requires careful patient instruction and compliance. Patients record their temperature in the resting state, just before rising in the morning. An increase in body temperature of 0.5 to 0.8°F (0.3°C) occurs just after ovulation. BBT is not useful in predicting ovulation and can confirm ovulation only in retrospect. BBT is not sensitive in all women because some women will not have a temperature change. BBT measurements can be combined with cervical mucus assessment for greater accuracy. At the time of ovulation, cervical mucus becomes thin, clear, and abundant under the influence of estrogen. Immediately after ovulation, cervical mucus becomes thick and scant under the influence of progesterone.

BBT and cervical mucus assessment can be time-consuming and may not be ideal for some women. Another method of confirming ovulation is to measure mid-luteal phase serum progesterone level, with serum levels of more than 6 ng/mL (19 nmol/L) providing presumptive evidence of ovulation. Commercial over-the-counter ovulation predictor kits provide the greatest accuracy in predicting ovulation by measuring urinary LH and detecting LH surge. A "positive test" indicates that ovulation will occur in 24 to 36 hours. Urine FSH levels are not used for predicting ovulation.

6. **a.** Common causes of female infertility may be classified in the following manner:

1. Ovulatory disorders (40%): PCOS, hypothyroidism, hyperprolactinemia, hypothalamic amenorrhea, diminished ovarian reserve, premature ovarian failure, etc.
2. "Pelvic factors": PID, tubal scarring, endometriosis, fibroids, polyps, congenital anomalies
3. "Cervical factors": history of conization, DES exposure, infection, poor cervical mucus quality/quantity
4. Other: immunologic, systemic disease (e.g., diabetes)

History of previous uncomplicated abortion has no known direct association with infertility.

7. **c.** Evaluation of tubal patency is best accomplished by HSG. During this procedure, radiographic liquid dye is injected into the uterine cavity and multiple x-rays are taken. Spillage of dye into the pelvic cavity confirms tubal patency.

Hysteroscopy involves the use of a light, flexible telescope that is passed through the vagina and into the uterine cavity. Hysteroscopy is useful to visualize anatomic defects such as fibroids and polyps, and it is often used to complement HSG. However, it cannot directly determine tubal occlusion or patency. Transvaginal ultrasound, pelvic MRI, and pelvic CT scan do not directly assess tubal patency.

8. **a.** The postcoital test can be used to assess what role the "cervical factor" plays in a couple's infertility. The postcoital test determines the quality of interaction between sperm and cervical mucus just prior to ovulation. The couple engages in intercourse at midcycle and then presents to the office 12 to 24 hours later to evaluate cervical mucus collected from the female partner. The cervical mucus is then examined under a microscope to determine the number of sperm and the quality and extent of motility. A satisfactory test reveals large numbers of forward-moving sperm. The test is inaccurate if performed after ovulation because cervical mucus thickens postovulation and is inherently inhospitable to sperm at this time. Postcoital testing is no longer commonly performed because of logistical barriers and lack of evidence that it significantly impacts pregnancy outcome.

9. a. A male factor accounts for approximately 24% and can be a contributing factor in up to 40% of infertility cases. Therefore, it is imperative that male factors be assessed early in the evaluation of infertility. Ovulatory dysfunction accounts for 21% of cases, whereas tubal factors (i.e., tubal scarring) account for 14% of cases. Approximately 28% of cases have no identifiable etiology.

10. e. Male infertility can result from a variety of conditions. Causes of male infertility may be divided into the following categories:

1. Possibly reversible conditions: varicocele, obstructive azoospermia (complete absence of sperm from ejaculate)
2. Irreversible conditions but in which viable sperm are available: inoperable obstructive azoospermia, ejaculatory dysfunction
3. Irreversible conditions in which there are inadequate or no viable sperm available (i.e., hypogonadism)
4. Serious potentially life-threatening conditions: testicular cancer, pituitary tumor
5. Genetic abnormalities that affect fertility: cystic fibrosis, chromosome abnormalities

Although environmental exposures, such as prolonged heat exposure, may cause male infertility, there is no strong evidence that wearing tight-fitting underwear adversely affects sperm production.

11. a. The initial screening of the male should include (1) a comprehensive reproductive history; (2) general physical examination, including the genitalia; and (3) two semen analyses performed at least 1 month apart. Patients should abstain from sexual activity for 2 or 3 days prior to collection. The specimen should be kept at room or body temperature and examined within 1 hour of collection. The semen is analyzed for the following parameters: volume, sperm concentration, motility, and morphology. Specific additional procedures should be considered if abnormalities are noted during the initial evaluation. A postejaculatory urine analysis is used to evaluate for the presence of retrograde ejaculation. A transrectal ultrasound may assess for ejaculatory duct obstruction. A scrotal ultrasound is performed if examination of the scrotum is limited or to evaluate testicular masses.

12. a. An infertility evaluation should be performed earlier than 1 year if (1) female infertility risk factors exist (e.g., age older than 35 years), (2) male infertility risk factors exist (e.g., a history of bilateral cryptorchidism), and (3) the couple questions the man's fertility potential. In addition, men who are concerned about the fertility status and who do not have a current partner should undergo an evaluation.

Solution to the Clinical Case Management Problem

Detailed discussion of the full range of reproductive technology options and indications is beyond the scope of this chapter. The following is a brief summary of the most common treatments:

1. Ovulation induction with clomiphene citrate: For patients with anovulation, clomiphene citrate therapy is usually a standard first-line approach for ovulation induction. Clomiphene citrate acts by binding to estrogen receptors in the hypothalamus, resulting in decreased perception of endogenous estrogen by the hypothalamus. In response, the hypothalamus increases secretion of gonadotropin-releasing hormone, facilitating FSH release and ovarian follicular development.

2. Human menopausal gonadotropins: Injection of gonadotropins can be used in sequential combination with clomiphene for those women who do not generate or sustain adequate FSH in response to clomiphene alone.

3. In vitro fertilization (IVF): This technique involves retrieval of eggs via ultrasound-guided transvaginal aspiration. The eggs are then fertilized with sperm under laboratory conditions, and the fertilized egg is then placed in the uterus. To increase the success of IVF, "superovulation" is attempted with ovulation-induction agents to allow for retrieval of multiple eggs.

4. Intrauterine insemination (IUI): IUI is less invasive than IVF because it does not involve retrieval of eggs. In IUI, washed sperm are deposited directly in the uterus, bypassing cervical mucus and placing the sperm at closer proximity to the fallopian tubes. Patients with a history of tubal damage are not good candidates for IUI.
5. Gamete intrafallopian transfer (GIFT): As in IVF, sperm and egg are retrieved from the couple.

GIFT differs from IVF in that fertilization takes place *in vivo*, not *in vitro*. Egg and sperm are then transferred into the fallopian tubes in the hopes that natural fertilization will take place.

6. Intracytoplasmic sperm injection (ICSI): A technique that directly addresses male infertility factors, ICSI involves the direct injection of a single sperm into a collected egg. If successful fertilization takes place, the fertilized egg is implanted into the female patient.

Summary

1. Definitions
a. Infertility: failure to conceive after 1 year of regular, unprotected intercourse
b. Primary infertility: refers to couples who have never conceived
c. Secondary infertility: refers to couples who may have conceived in the past
d. Fecundity: likelihood of pregnancy in a given cycle

2. Evaluation—female partner
a. History and physical examination
b. Evaluation of ovulatory status: basal body temperature, cervical mucus changes, ovulation predictor kits, mid-luteal phase progesterone
c. Complete workup of amenorrhea or oligomenorrhea if necessary: TSH, prolactin, evaluation for PCOS, if indicated
d. Evaluation of "cervical factor": postcoital test
e. Evaluation of "pelvic factor" or tubal patency: HSG

3. Evaluation—male partner
a. History and physical examination
b. Semen analysis twice, 1 month apart
c. Referral for further testing if abnormal semen analysis or abnormal physical examination findings

4. Causes of infertility—female
a. Pelvic factor: PID, tubal scarring, endometriosis, congenital abnormalities
b. Ovulatory dysfunction: PCOS, hyperprolactinemia, hypothyroidism
c. Cervical factor: history of conization, DES exposure, infection
d. Other: immunologic, systemic disease

5. Causes of infertility—male
a. Possibly reversible: varicocele, obstructive azoospermia
b. Irreversible conditions, possibly with viable sperm: inoperable obstructive azoospermia, ejaculatory dysfunction
c. Irreversible conditions, no viable sperm: hypogonadism
d. Testicular cancer, pituitary tumor
e. Genetic abnormalities: cystic fibrosis, chromosome abnormalities

6. Indications for referral
a. Women older than age 35 years
b. Identified infertility risk factor in male or female
c. Abnormal semen analysis in men

Suggested Reading

De Kretser DM: Male infertility. *Lancet* 349:787–790, 1997.
Hull MG, Glazener CM, Kelly NJ, et al: Population study of causes, treatment, and outcome of infertility. *Br Med J* 291:1693–1697, 1985.
Jose-Miller AB, Boyden JW, Frey KA: Infertility. *Am Fam Physician* 75(6):849–856, 2007.
Male Infertility Best Practice Policy Committee of the American Urological Association for the Practice Committee of the American Society for Reproductive Medicine: Report on optimal evaluation of the infertile male. *Fertil Steril* 82(Suppl 1):S123–S130, 2004.
Practice Committee of the American Society for Reproductive Medicine: Optimal evaluation of the infertile female. *Fertil Steril* 82(Suppl 1):S169–S172, 2004.
Rowe PJ: *WHO Manual for the Standardized Investigation and Diagnosis of the Infertile Couple.* New York: Cambridge University Press, 1993.
Sharlip ID, et al: Best practice policies for male infertility. *Fertil Steril* 77:873–882, 2002.

MATERNITY CARE

CHAPTER
82 Family-Centered Maternity Care

CLINICAL CASE PROBLEM 1

A 22-Year-Old Primigravida Comes for Her First Prenatal Visit

A 22-year-old woman comes to your office at 10 weeks of gestation for her initial prenatal visit. She has been referred to you by friends who are your patients. She would like you to be her physician, deliver her baby, and then care for her child. Her uterus feels 10 weeks by size on bimanual exam, and her blood pressure is 100/70 mmHg. All other aspects of the initial complete physical examination are normal.

SELECT THE BEST ANSWER TO THE FOLLOWING QUESTIONS

1. The patient asks you about birth plans during her initial visit and inquires as to your attitudes toward pregnant couples who wish to participate in decision making regarding the conduct of labor and delivery. How would you respond?
   a. birth plans are not a good idea; usually something goes wrong and the couple is disappointed
   b. birth plans are not a good idea; they frequently lead to unresolved guilt in the couple
   c. birth plans should be avoided; perinatal morbidity and mortality are usually increased
   d. birth plans are an excellent idea; everything always goes according to plan
   e. birth plans are a good idea; they involve the couple in the planning for their baby's delivery and can be a very important part of the prenatal, postnatal, and postpartum care

2. On the next prenatal visit, the couple wishes to discuss your feelings concerning a number of issues. The first issue is electronic fetal monitoring (EFM). The couple is aware that in some hospitals and with some physicians, continuous EFM during labor is standard procedure. Which of the following statements regarding continuous routine EFM is true?
   a. the perinatal mortality rate in laboring patients who undergo continuous EFM is lower than in those who do not
   b. the perinatal morbidity rate in laboring patients who undergo EFM is lower than in those who do not
   c. the incidence of cesarean section in laboring patients undergoing EFM is not statistically different from that of those who do not
   d. there is no significant difference in perinatal outcomes between those patients who undergo EFM and those who do not
   e. the incidence of admission to the intensive care nursery is greater in those infants who do not undergo EFM

3. The couple then asks you about routinely ordering ultrasound in pregnancy. Which of the following statements regarding the use of routine ultrasound in pregnancy is false?
   a. routine prenatal ultrasound has been shown by U.S. studies to be justified from a cost–benefit standpoint
   b. repetitive studies by independent researchers have not found any consistently adverse effects of obstetric ultrasound on perinatal outcome
   c. first-trimester ultrasound gestational age assessment should be performed on patients scheduled for elective repeat cesarean section
   d. vaginal bleeding in pregnancy should be assessed by ultrasound examination
   e. a size–date discrepancy in fundal height of 3 cm or more is an indication for obstetric ultrasound

4. The couple inquires about the routine administration of intravenous (IV) fluids during labor. Concerning this issue, which of the following statements is false?
   a. the use of routine IV fluids does not limit ambulation in the first stage of labor
   b. if epidural analgesia is to be administered, an IV line must be in place
   c. if the first stage of labor is prolonged, an IV line should be in place to prevent dehydration
   d. if a patient has a history of a severe postpartum hemorrhage, an IV line should be established
   e. none of the above statements are false

5. The patient tells you it is very important to her that she has a "natural" delivery and does not want any narcotics or medications that will "hurt the baby." How do you respond?
   a. many women think they do not want narcotics or an epidural, but most change their mind
   b. intravenous narcotics are totally safe and have no complications
   c. epidural analgesia is no longer associated with any complications and is completely safe
   d. massage, standing in a warm shower, alternating position, and walking with intermittent monitoring can all be used to decrease the need for pain relief during labor
   e. leave that decision to the doctor

6. Which of the following statements regarding epidural analgesia is (are) true?
   a. maternal hypertension is a common side effect of epidural analgesia
   b. high spinal anesthesia is one of the most serious complications of epidural analgesia
   c. unintentional dural puncture occurs in 10% of attempted epidural analgesia
   d. prolongation of all stages of labor by epidural analgesia has been established
   e. fetal bradycardia is seen consistently with epidural analgesia

7. The couple has some specific requests that they add to their birth plan at the 36-week visit, suggested by a friend. Which of the following would not be advisable?
   a. having the patient's mother present for support
   b. allowing the father to cut the umbilical cord
   c. putting the baby to breast before giving vitamin K and eye ointment

   d. allowing all birth plan actions to take place regardless of any unexpected emergencies
   e. delaying 30 seconds to clamp the umbilical cord

8. The couple's final question concerns "routine episiotomy." They have been told that the medical profession is "cut happy" and that the vast majority of episiotomies are unnecessary. Which of the following statements regarding routine episiotomy is true?
   a. episiotomy pain may be more severe and last longer than the pain from perineal lacerations
   b. episiotomy repairs heal more rapidly than do vaginal and perineal tears
   c. dyspareunia is more common after vaginal lacerations and perineal tear than after episiotomy
   d. episiotomy reduces the rate of subsequent pelvic relaxation problems
   e. episiotomy reduces the rate of third- and fourth-degree perineal lacerations

9. Which of the following is (are) an indication for the performance of an episiotomy?
   a. nonreassuring fetal heart rate in the second stage of labor
   b. significant maternal cardiac disease
   c. operative delivery using obstetric forceps
   d. delivery of the fetus with shoulder dystocia
   e. all of the above

10. Which of the following statements regarding the presence or absence of a supportive person (or coach) in labor is true?
    a. the presence of a support person or coach decreases the need for analgesia in labor
    b. the presence of a support person or coach decreases the need for operative interventions such as forceps or vacuum extraction
    c. the presence of a support person or coach decreases the cesarean delivery rate
    d. the presence of a support person increases the risk of malpractice-related lawsuits
    e. the presence of a support person makes the patient more anxious

---

Clinical Case Management Problem

A 29-year-old recently married woman comes for her yearly physical, and while you are discussing her overall health, she mentions her plans to conceive in the next 6 months. What issues would you want to address with her to provide the best preconceptual care?

Answers

1. e. Birth plans are an integral component of what has become known as family-centered maternity care. Family-centered maternity care allows pregnant couples the opportunity of going through labor and delivery in an informal setting, preferably with minimal medical intervention. Family-centered maternity care involves the husband or significant other as a coach in labor and allows for immediate bonding of infant to both parents.

Breast-feeding is encouraged, and rooming-in is available. A trusting doctor–patient relationship is essential to family-centered maternity care. If the couple is confident in their doctor, they feel secure that any intervention that is considered will obviously be discussed with them. If the couple is involved in the decision-making process throughout labor and delivery, any unresolved guilt related to the birth process will be avoided.

2. d. Well-controlled studies have shown that intermittent auscultation of the fetal heart rate is equivalent to EFM in assessing fetal condition when performed at specific intervals with a 1:1 nurse:patient ratio. EFM is associated with a small but significant increase in the incidence of cesarean delivery because of presumed "fetal distress." Perinatal outcomes as assessed by intrapartum stillbirths, low Apgar scores, need for assisted ventilation of the newborn, admission to neonatal intensive care unit, and the onset of neonatal seizures are similar with both intermittent auscultation and EFM.

3. a. Although obstetric ultrasound studies are performed routinely in many countries, the routine use of ultrasonography has not been supported from a cost–benefit standpoint. However, a 1984 consensus development conference convened by the National Institute of Child Health and Human Development proposed 27 indications for ultrasonography in pregnancy. These indications include estimation of gestational age for patients scheduled for elective cesarean delivery, identification of the cause of vaginal bleeding in pregnancy, and evaluation of significant uterine size–clinical dates discrepancy. Ultrasound exposure at intensities usually produced by diagnostic ultrasound instruments has not been found to cause any harmful biologic effects on fetuses. Infants exposed in utero have shown no significant differences in birth weight or length, childhood growth, cognitive function, acoustic or visual ability, or rates of neurologic deficits. The use of diagnostic obstetric ultrasound on an as-needed basis is supported by the American College of Obstetricians and Gynecologists.

4. a. An IV line can limit ambulation in the first stage of labor. Although it is customary in many hospitals to start IV infusions early in labor, there is seldom any real need to do so in women with uncomplicated pregnancies, at least until analgesia is administered. IV hydration is indicated for the following reasons: (1) for prehydration when epidural analgesia is about to be administered, (2) to prevent dehydration and acidosis in the presence of a prolonged first stage of labor, and (3) to administer oxytocin prophylactically to prevent postpartum hemorrhage.

5. d. Many women do not want pain relief in labor, and with changes in position, massage, standing in the shower (especially in early labor), rocking, or other nonnarcotic or invasive maneuvers, they may do well, especially with the assistance of a doula. Any narcotics or epidural anesthesia have potential complications. Obviously, a patient such as this needs to understand that it is fine if she changes her mind. Providing her with reading materials and encouraging her to have a doula will help give her all the options for nonnarcotic pain relief.

6. b. One of the most serious immediate complications of epidural analgesia is a high or total spinal anesthesia. Signs and symptoms include numbness and weakness of upper extremities, dyspnea, inability to speak, and, finally, apnea and loss of consciousness. Maternal hypotension, not hypertension, is common and can be minimized by prophylactic intravascular volume expansion with 500 to 1000 mL of non-glucose-containing isotonic crystalloid solution. Unintentional dural puncture, resulting in a spinal headache, occurs in less than 2% of cases. Randomized controlled trials have shown conflicting results regarding the effect of epidurals on progress of labor. Fetal bradycardia may occasionally be seen with epidural analgesia, but it is usually easily treated by IV fluid administration and conservative management.

7. d. All of these requests are reasonable except choice d. Patients must understand that if there is an emergency requiring resuscitation of the infant or mother, birth plans may be ignored. Most patients are aware of this, but it is best to specify prior to any emergencies. Putting the baby to breast immediately is recommended to promote breast-feeding, and delaying cord clamping for 30 seconds has not been found to be harmful (and is, in fact, helpful in some cases of preterm infants). Allowing a support person and the father's participation in cutting the umbilical cord are good ideas.

8. **a.** Episiotomy pain may be more severe and long-lasting than the pain of vaginal and perineal lacerations. Healing time for vaginal and perineal lacerations is generally shorter than the healing time for an episiotomy. Dyspareunia is more common after episiotomy than after vaginal and perineal tears, resulting in a prolongation of time before return to normal sexual activity.

Routine episiotomy neither increases nor decreases the incidence of subsequent pelvic relaxation. All randomized prospective studies have shown the rates of third- and fourth-degree perineal lacerations are increased rather than reduced by routine episiotomy.

9. **e.** Indications for episiotomy include nonreassuring fetal heart rate findings in the second stage of labor, significant maternal cardiac disease, prophylactic forceps, shoulder dystocia, and infants in the breech presentation when vaginal delivery is anticipated.

Contraindications to episiotomy include the presence of inflammatory bowel disease, lymphogranuloma venereum, or severe perineal scarring or malformation. Complications of episiotomy include excessive blood loss and increased rates of lacerations into the anal sphincter and anal mucosa and infections.

Episiotomy rates can be reduced by following these indications and contraindications and by not performing an episiotomy routinely. Vaginal and perineal tears may be avoided by perineal massage and stretching exercises before delivery. Communication with the patient during perineal stretching will help reduce the degree and number of tears during childbirth. Also, controlling professional urgency for rapid delivery provides extra time for the fetal head to stretch the perineum, resulting in an increased possibility for an intact perineum.

Episiotomy does shorten the second stage of labor, but that in and of itself is not a reason for its performance.

10 **a.** The presence of a support person or coach decreases the need for subsequent analgesia in labor. This does not, however, apply to subsequent operative interventions including forceps delivery, vacuum extraction, or cesarean section.

Solution to the Clinical Case Management Problem

This case management problem emphasizes the fact that family physicians have a good opportunity to intervene, possibly resulting in decreased rates of the 12% of infants born prematurely, 3% with major birth defects, and 8% with low birth weight. Since most women do not receive care until the critical stage of embryogenesis is complete, some of the important preventive measures we could take are impossible at later stages in the pregnancy. Since 11% of women smoke during pregnancy and 10% drink alcohol, it is hoped that your advice could cause these women to stop, thus decreasing the occurrence of placental insufficiency, growth retardation, and fetal alcohol syndrome that may result. Morbid obesity and poorly controlled diabetes both need to be addressed prior to conception to decrease risk to mother and fetus, particularly for birth abnormalities associated with hyperglycemia. Approximately 3% of women consume prescription or nonprescription drugs that are known teratogens; some, such as antiepileptic drugs and coumadin, can be devastating to the fetus. Identification of thyroid disease, hypertension, congenital heart disease, HIV, high-risk sexual behaviors, and sexually transmitted diseases is important prior to conception.

Summary

1. Birth plans: If prudently developed and open to negotiation and change, they may be of benefit in a couple's pregnancy. They have the potential to foster good doctor–patient communication.

2. Continuous EFM is no more effective than intermittent auscultation in reducing perinatal morbidity and mortality in low-risk pregnancies.

3. Current recommendations are that obstetric ultrasound should be used only for specific indications, although no adverse perinatal outcomes have been demonstrated in repetitive studies.

4. Intravenous therapy: Specific indications include long labor with ketones, use of epidural analgesia, and

history of severe postpartum hemorrhage; it is not routinely needed in low-risk pregnancies.

5. Anesthesia: An epidural is the analgesic of choice and should be available should women choose it. Prepared childbirth classes may increase the number of women seeking unmedicated childbirth.

6. Episiotomy: An episiotomy does not heal more quickly than a perineal tear, is more painful, has greater incidence of dyspareunia, increases the risk of third-degree and fourth-degree lacerations, and does not change the incidence of later pelvic relaxation. Although it does shorten the second stage of labor, that shortening in and of itself offers no definitive benefit to either mother or baby.

Suggested Reading

American College of Obstetricians and Gynecologists (ACOG): ACOG Practice Bulletin no. 71. Episiotomy. *Obstet Gynecol* 107(4):957–962, 2006.

Banta DH, Thacker SB: Historical controversy in health technology assessment: The case of electronic fetal monitoring. *Obstet Gynecol Surv* 56(11):707–719, 2001.

Campbell DC: Parenteral opioids for labor analgesia. *Clin Obstet Gynecol* 46(3):616–622, 2003.

Hadar A, Scheiner E: Abnormal fetal heart rate tracing patterns during the first stage of labor: Effect on perinatal outcome. *Am J Obstet Gynecol* 185(4):863–868, 2001.

Harman CR, Baschat AA: Comprehensive assessment of fetal wellbeing: Which Doppler tests should be performed? *Curr Opin Obstet Gynecol* 15(2):147–157, 2003.

Johnson K, Posner SF, Bierman J: Recommendations to improve preconception health and health care in the United States. *MMWR* 55(RR06):1–23, 2006.

Thallon A, Shennan A: Epidural and spinal analgesia and labour. *Curr Opin Obstet Gynecol* 13(6):583–587, 2001.

CHAPTER 83 Preconception Care

CLINICAL CASE PROBLEM 1

A Chance for Pregnancy Planning

A 35-year-old woman, on her first office visit, expresses her wish to become pregnant. She has never been pregnant, denies any chronic health conditions, is not overweight, and exercises regularly. As you seek further information to assist you in providing care, the following issues arise.

SELECT THE BEST ANSWER TO THE FOLLOWING QUESTIONS

1. You discuss with your patient the risk factors for adverse pregnancy outcome. Which of the following would increase the risk during her pregnancy?
   a. sexually transmitted disease (STD)
   b. obesity
   c. current use of isoretinoins
   d. elevated cholesterol
   e. a and c

2. Which of the following presents a risk during the pregnancy?
   a. history of smoking with discontinuation 2 months ago
   b. history of spousal abuse
   c. family history of cardiovascular disease
   d. current use of one or two drinks after work three or four times a week
   e. none of the above

3. During the physical examination, which of the following findings increase(s) the risk of the pregnancy?
   a. elevated blood pressure
   b. a retroverted uterus
   c. a thrombosed hemorrhoid
   d. all of the above
   e. none of the above

4. The patient relates to you that her sister had a baby who suffered from spina bifida. She questions the efficacy of folic acid:
   a. folic acid is known to reduce the occurrence of neural tube defects (NTDs) by 60% to 70%
   b. the amount of folic acid found in prenatal vitamins is sufficient in this case
   c. the fetus of this patient has a high risk of developing NTDs; therefore, she should start taking folic acid 12 months before intended pregnancy
   d. folic acid reduces the recurrence of NTDs but does not prevent first occurrences
   e. the use of folic acid in pregnancy is controversial

5. Epidemiological studies reveal that
   a. the number of NTDs has declined in the United States by 25% since folic acid has been used to fortify certain cereals
   b. there has been an increase in NTDs in the United States due to an increase in immigration from Southeast Asia
   c. low levels of folic acid are not implicated in the development of cardiac defects during fetal life
   d. megaloblastic anemia in pregnancy is usually caused by lack of vitamin B_{12} and not folic acid
   e. folic acid can be easily acquired by eating peanuts and legumes

6. Your patient is concerned about the need for vaccinations during pregnancy. You note that
   a. at present, no guidelines have been established regarding preconception vaccines
   b. it is accepted practice to offer childbearing age females both hepatitis B virus (HBV) vaccine if they are at higher risk for acquiring hepatitis B and rubella vaccine if they are seronegative
   c. the practitioner should offer varicella as well as influenza vaccines to the patient as part of her preconception counseling
   d. palivizumab (Synagis) is a pregnancy category C drug, and its use is recommended for premature infants and pregnant women during the winter season
   e. patients who will be in their third trimester during the winter season should be offered pneumococcous vaccine

CLINICAL CASE PROBLEM 2

A Chance of Counseling before Conception

A 37-year-old female sees you for her first office visit. She is interested in having a yearly Pap and mammogram.

7. During this first visit, you do which of the following?
   a. ask the patient if she intends to become pregnant in the future
   b. describe to the patient the effects of pregnancy on her general health
   c. discuss with her medications that should not be consumed during pregnancy
   d. explain to the patient that yearly Pap smears and mammograms are rarely required
   e. all of the above

8. A comprehensive preconception care counseling will include which of the following?
   a. a complete discussion of contraception in the event the patient does not wish to have children and is of reproductive age
   b. the patient should be aware of the risk of alcohol consumption during pregnancy (fetal alcohol syndrome) and the risk of smoking during pregnancy (a common cause of preterm labor, low-birth-weight infants, etc.)
   c. a screening for STDs because they can be a causative agent in preterm labor and ectopic pregnancy
   d. developing good oral hygiene because dental interventions can reduce the incidence of prematurity and low birth weight
   e. all of the above

9. Your patient asks you if she has to "hurry up" and get pregnant since she is 38 years old. With regard to age
   a. maternal age and not paternal age is the major contributor to genetic disorders of the newborn
   b. preeclampsia and toxemia affect the very young, usually nulliparous women, and spare older women
   c. diabetes mellitus is more commonly found in advanced maternal age
   d. the incidence of fetal anomalies increases with age, whereas the number of stillbirths decreases
   e. as long as your patient is in good health, exercises regularly, and does not have a chronic ailment, her age does not affect her fertility

10. Prepregnancy interventions that have shown proven benefits include which of the following?
   a. treating anti-phospholipid antibody syndrome with aspirin
   b. tight glycemic control in diabetic women
   c. maximal levothyroxine supplementation in patients suffering from hypothyroidism
   d. reducing the incidence of fetal disorders by actively restricting maternal phenylalanine-containing food products in mothers suffering from hyperphenylalanemia
   e. all of the above

11. Your patient suffers from epilepsy. She currently uses dilantin and valproic acid. She and her husband have decided to have another child. She wants to do all that she can to ensure this pregnancy will result in a child without anomalies because her daughter suffers from cleft palate and developmental delay. Which of the following is true regarding anticonvulsants and pregnancy?
   a. the kind of anticonvulsant is the only cause of fetal malformation

b. developmental delay is associated solely with the amount of anticonvulsants that the mother took

c. lomotrigine, when taken alone, may have a lower incidence of fetal malformations

d. the practitioner has to choose the drug that is best for his or her epileptic patient and "stick with it"

e. women on antiepileptic drugs should discontinue them unless they are using them for their anticonvulsants effects only

Answers

1. e. Isotretinoins, anticoagulants, and anticonvulsive drugs are recognized as extremely hazardous to a developing fetus. The Centers for Disease Control and Prevention (CDC) guidelines for improving preconception health in the United States recommend that patients taking isotretinoins use contraception. Women who use anticonvulsants that are considered teratogens (e.g., valproic acid) should be counseled to have their dose decreased. Oral anticoagulants such as warfarin, a known teratogen, should be stopped and changed to heparin or lovenox before the onset of pregnancy. STDs are a risk factor and should be diagnosed and treated. Obesity and elevated cholesterol, although considered detrimental to the patient's health, are not risk factors in pregnancy.

2. b. Current smoking is the risk for a pregnancy. A family history of cardiovascular disease may contribute to her long-term health but is not a risk for the pregnancy. Assuming that she is with the same spouse, spousal abuse often escalates during pregnancy, increasing her risk during this pregnancy. Unless she is unwilling to discontinue the alcohol, drinking prior to the pregnancy is not the risk; drinking during pregnancy is the risk.

3. a. An elevated blood pressure needs to be addressed and the best possible control obtained for optimum pregnancy outcome. A retroverted uterus presents no risk, and although you may need to address the hemorrhoid to increase her comfort, it is not a risk to the pregnancy.

4. a. Neural tube deficits include anencephaly and spina bifida. The majority are caused by a genetic defect causing a decrease in the enzyme MTHFR. This enzyme plays a key role in folate metabolism. Use of folic acid supplementation can prevent the majority of NTDs. It is recommended that women with a prior or family history of NTDs take 4 mg of folic acid daily starting 3 months prior to pregnancy and throughout the first trimester. Folic acid reduces both recurrences and the de novo occurrence of NTDs.

5. a. The Food and Drug Administration started mandatory fortifications of certain cereals with folic acid in 1988. The CDC estimates that there has been a 25% decrease in the occurrence of NTDs due to this action. Folic acid is found in leafy vegetables, broccoli, and animal liver. Lower levels of folic acid are the major cause of megaloblastic anemia in pregnancy and NTDs, and they contribute to the formation of cardiac defects.

6. b. The CDC recommendation to improve preconception health suggests that all women of childbearing age be counseled about receiving HBV vaccine if they are at a higher risk and rubella vaccine if they are seronegative. These are to be given 3 months prior to future pregnancy since they are live attenuated viruses. (Although research has failed to show a negative outcome in the mother when the vaccine is given in the pregnant state.)

Varicella virus vaccine is occasionally offered by practitioners to patients who are at high risk for chickenpox outbreaks (e.g., day care workers with a negative history of previous chickenpox disease). Pregnant women follow the general recommendation for influenza and pneumonia vaccine (give flu vaccine to females who will be pregnant during the flu season and pneumococcous vaccine if they are immunosuppressed, asplenic, etc.). There are no recommendations regarding the usage of polivzumab in adults.

7. e. Part of preconception counseling is to discuss pregnancy with any fertile female patient. Determining the need for contraception is part of preconception counseling. The physician should inform the patient that certain conditions or medications can have deleterious outcomes on her pregnancy as half of all pregnancies are unintended. Unless there is a physical finding or family history that suggests it should be performed, the patient's age of 37 years does not indicate a mammogram; mammogram screening usually begins at age 40 years. Many sources suggest that Pap smears can be done as infrequently as every 3 years if they are all normal.

8. e. The CDC has developed a list of preconception risk factors for adverse pregnancy outcomes. Clinical guidelines were developed using evidence for the effectiveness of preconception care. They include alcohol and tobacco cessation counseling as well as screening and treating (gonorrheal and chlamydial) STDs. The discussion of future fertility is an important part of preconception counseling. One of the preventive measures noted by the CDC is improvement of oral care before pregnancy.

9. c. Advanced maternal age is a leading cause of infertility, fetal anomalies, stillbirths, and diabetes mellitus. Preeclampsia occurs in women at the extremes of the age range—both younger and older pregnant patients are at risk.

10. e. The emphasis in preconception counseling is partly on improving chronic maternal conditions, diabetes mellitus, hypothyroidism, as well as genetic disorders such as hyperphenylalanemia. Therefore, a complete history is the essence of the counseling session.

11. e. More than 1 million women in their reproductive years have epilepsy. However, it is estimated that twice this number take anticonvulsant medications for headaches, chronic pain, and mood disorders. Anticonvulsants are teratogenic and carcinogenic. Fetal hydantoin syndrome results from intrauterine exposure to phenytoin and possibly other drugs. The following are keys to decreasing these teratogenic effects:

1. Stop polytherapy and monotherapy if possible.
2. Decrease the amount of anticonvulsant medication to the minimal dose.
3. Choose the least teratogenic drug; currently, lamotrigine is the most promising. Valproate poses the highest risk to the fetus.

Summary

There are proven benefits to preconception counseling, including seeking changes in behavior and promoting healthy living.

Preconception counseling is a set of interventions that aim to identify and modify biomedical, behavioral, and social risks to a woman's health or pregnancy outcomes through prevention and management. It is important to discuss preconception issues and recommendations even when women are not "planning" a pregnancy as 50% of pregnancies are "unplanned" and unplanned pregnancies have a higher complication rate than planned pregnancies.

When evaluating a patient in her reproductive years, the practitioner should offer preconception counseling. Some physicians recommend a single visit targeted to preconception counseling, risk assessment, and recommendations. Other physicians recommend using every well woman visit and primary care visit to reiterate and emphasize aspects of preconception care.

The Academy of Pediatrics and the American College of Obstetricians and Gynecologists identify four categories of assessment:

1. Physical assessment
    a. Screen and treat: STDs, HIV/AIDS
2. Risk screening
    a. Teenage patients will often suffer from anemia, preterm labor, toxemia, growth restricted fetus, higher STD prevalence, and increased infant mortality.
    b. Pregnancy in advanced maternal age is often complicated by toxemia, diabetes mellitus, preterm delivery, and fetal anomalies.
    c. Start folic acid; stop anticoagulant (replace coumadin), Accutane. Evaluate and modify to reduce risk: antiepileptic (one drug with the lowest dose and lowest side effects).
    d. General health: Chronic medical conditions such as hypertension, diabetes mellitus, thyroid disease, and epilepsy should be brought under excellent control before pregnancy in order to decrease negative outcomes.
3. Vaccinations
    a. Offer rubella testing and also HBV and varicella vaccination if warranted (high risk).
4. Counseling
    a. Smoking, alcohol consumption, and recreational drugs should be discouraged.
    b. Ask mother about domestic violence and spousal abuse because these behaviors typically increase with pregnancy.
    c. Genetic counseling and testing: Mothers with prior history of genetic malformations should be carefully evaluated. Offer Tay–Sachs testing to all Ashkenazi Jewish couples and cystic fibrosis carrier screening to both partners of Caucasian European and Ashkenazi Jewish couples. Thalassemia screening is commonly performed in couples of Mediterranean heritage, and sickle cell testing should be performed in all black patients.
    d. Discuss environmental toxins at work and at home. Dioxin-type products can increase fetal malformations, as can methylmercury, a neurotoxin (organic solvents should be avoided).

Suggested Reading

Curtis M: Do we practice what we preach? A review of actual clinical practice with regards to preconception care guidelines. *Matern Child Health J* 10(Suppl 1):53–58, 2006.

Dunlop AL, Jack B, Frey K: National recommendations for preconception care: The essential role of the family physician. *J Am Board Fam Med* 20(1):81–84, 2007.

Graham L: CDC releases guidelines on improving preconception health care. *Am Fam Physician* 74:1967–1968, 1970, 2006.

Johnson K, Posner SF, Biermann J, et al: Recommendations to improve preconception health and health care—United States. CDC/ATSDR. *MMWR Recommendations Rep* 55:1–23, 2006.

Kirkham C, Harris S, Grzybowski S: Evidence based prenatal care. Part I: General prenatal care and counseling issues. *Am Fam Physician* 71(7):1307–1316, 2005.

Posner SF, Johnson K, Parker C, et al: The National Summit on Preconception Care: A summary of concept and recommendations. *Matern Child Health J* 10(Suppl 1):199–207, 2006.

Tough S: What do women know about the risks of delayed childbearing? *Can J Public Health* 97(4):330–334, 2006.

CHAPTER

84 Routine Prenatal Care

CLINICAL CASE PROBLEM 1

A 24-Year-Old Primigravida at 8 Weeks of Gestation

A 24-year-old primigravida comes to your office at 8 weeks of gestation for her first prenatal visit. She has asked you to be her family doctor and to look after her during the entire pregnancy. You agree to provide her pregnancy care. During your first visit, you explain your general philosophy regarding prenatal care and perinatal care.

SELECT THE BEST ANSWER TO THE FOLLOWING QUESTIONS

1. Which of the following statements are true concerning prenatal care in the United States?
   a. only 70% of women in the United States receive prenatal care
   b. reducing the number of prenatal visits in low-risk women has been shown to increase pregnancy risk
   c. black women, teenagers, women with drug addictions, and the poor have the lowest rates of prenatal care in the United States
   d. only approximately 50% of women in the United States receive prenatal care in their first trimester
   e. a and b

2. The Department of Health and Human Services Expert Panel on Prenatal Care (DHHSEPPC) has recommended which of the following regarding routine prenatal care?
   a. that the number of routine office visits be significantly reduced for women at low risk
   b. that focus should be on the total health and well-being of the family, including medical, psychological, social, and environmental barriers affecting health
   c. that provision of systematic health care start long before pregnancy because it was proved to be beneficial to the physical and emotional well-being of the prospective mother and child
   d. all of the above are true
   e. a and c only are true

3. Your patient had the first day of her last menstrual period on September 9, 2006. According to Nägele's rule, what is the patient's estimated date of delivery (assume a 28-day cycle)?
   a. June 2, 2007
   b. June 16, 2007
   c. July 2, 2007
   d. July 9, 2007
   e. June 23, 2007

4. Which of the following tests are not recommended at her initial prenatal visit?
   a. complete blood count (CBC)
   b. rapid plasma reagin (screening for syphilis)
   c. screening for gestational diabetes
   d. hepatitis B virus screen
   e. blood typing (Rh and ABO)

5. Which of the following tests are recommended at her 26- to 28-week prenatal visit?
   a. screening for gestational diabetes
   b. screening for rubella immunity
   c. screening for neural tube defects
   d. screening for group B streptococcal infection
   e. screening for hepatitis C

After discussion of the visits and tests that will be done during the pregnancy, your patient indicates that she is concerned about "getting fat." She has been a smoker since age 16 years in an attempt to remain thin and she assumes she will continue to smoke after she delivers. She is concerned about breast-feeding for the same reason since people have told her that she would "have to eat for the baby" if she breast-feeds.

6. She is 5 feet 5 inches tall and weighs 130 pounds. How much weight gain do you recommend?
   a. 5 to 15 pounds
   b. 10 to 20 pounds
   c. 15 to 25 pounds
   d. 25 to 35 pounds
   e. 28 to 40 pounds

7. In counseling your patients on weight, which of the following is not a complication associated with excessive weight gain?
   a. infant macrosomia
   b. gestational diabetes
   c. shoulder dystocia
   d. intrauterine growth retardation
   e. postpregnancy obesity

8. Which of the following statements would not be regarded as reasonable nutritional advice for your patient?
   a. supplementation with iron if anemia is detected
   b. supplementation with folic acid 1 mg daily throughout pregnancy
   c. supplementation with vitamin A
   d. supplementation with calcium (Recommended Dietary Allowance, 1000 to 1300 mg/day)
   e. supplementation with vitamin D if sunlight exposure is limited

9. Which of the following statements regarding smoking in pregnancy is (are) true?
   a. the risk of spontaneous abortion is increased significantly
   b. perinatal mortality rates are increased significantly
   c. abruptio placenta rates are increased significantly
   d. birth weights are decreased significantly
   e. all of the above are true

10. Which of the following statements regarding alcohol consumption in pregnancy and fetal alcohol syndrome is (are) true?
    a. limit alcohol intake to one or two glasses of wine
    b. abstain completely from alcohol during pregnancy
    c. fetal alcohol syndrome is decreasing in the United States
    d. a and c
    e. b and c

CLINICAL CASE PROBLEM 2

A 35-Year-Old Primigravida

A 35-year-old woman and her husband have been attempting to get pregnant without success. They had considered pursuing a fertility workup but were concerned about the expense. They had begun the process for adoption, but she has had a positive home pregnancy test, and based on her last menstrual period (LMP) she is 6 weeks pregnant. She is in good health and takes no medication except for a multivitamin.

11. Which of the following is true concerning your advice and care of this patient?
    a. she has a higher risk of having a child with trisomy 21 than does a younger woman
    b. she must have an amniocentesis or chorionic villus sampling (CVS) due to her age and risks
    c. she should have checkups more often than a younger woman
    d. a triscreen (triple screen) is a serum screen for aneuploidy and neural tube defects that is generally performed
    e. a and d

12. She and her husband are quite happy about the pregnancy. She tells you that she is not interested in any invasive tests, such as an amniocentesis or CVS, but she is not sure about the blood test. She asks you for more information concerning the triscreen or similar tests. All of the following are correct except
    a. the triple screen or triscreen includes α-fetoprotein, human chorionic gonadotropin, and unconjugated estriol
    b. some cases of neural tube defects, trisomy 18, and trisomy 21 can be detected by the triscreen
    c. the most common cause of an elevated α-fetoprotein level is an inaccurate gestational age
    d. the triscreen is extremely sensitive and specific. Fetuses with abnormal results are almost always abnormal
    e. unconjugated estriol levels are decreased in trisomy 18 and trisomy 21

13. Which of the following statements is (are) true concerning current recommendations on routine prenatal visits?
    a. clinical components of routine prenatal visits are agreed upon by everyone
    b. most guidelines recommend routine assessment with fundal height, maternal weight, blood

pressure measurements, fetal heart auscultation, urine testing for protein and glucose, and questions about fetal movement
c. some authors recommend screening for domestic violence with brief questions
d. a and b
e. b and c

CLINICAL CASE PROBLEM 3

Sexually Transmitted Diseases and Pregnancy

An 18-year-old primigravida who has seen you since 16 weeks of gestation comes for a visit at 32 weeks. She found out that her boyfriend (the father of the baby) has herpes. She has "broken up" with him but does not know when he contracted the herpes virus. She does not recall ever having herpes, but she is worried about the baby.

14. Which of the following statements is not true concerning herpes infection in pregnancy?
    a. rates of vertical transmission at the time of delivery are highest for a primary herpes simplex virus (HSV) infection and lowest for a recurrent HSV infection
    b. genital herpes acquired during pregnancy does not increase rates of neonatal illness if the HSV seroconversion has completed by the time labor begins
    c. women with recurrent HSV infection should not use acyclovir or other medications because they may be teratogenic
    d. neonatal HSV infection acquired in the birth canal can cause localized disease or central nervous system disease
    e. all patients and their partners should be asked about a history of genital and orolabial HSV infection

15. The patient is concerned that she might have another sexually transmitted disease. She is not having any fever or vaginal discharge. What do you recommend?
    a. repeat her Venereal Disease Research Laboratory, gonorrhea, and chlamydia screens
    b. reassure her that there is nothing to worry about
    c. perform a screen for group B strep at 35 to 37 weeks
    d. both a and c
    e. both b and c

16. Which of the following options is (are) correct regarding intrapartum antibiotic prophylaxis of group B β-streptococcus (GBBS) sepsis?
    a. antibiotics are not effective in decreasing GBBS sepsis
    b. antibiotics are administered only to women with risk factors
    c. antibiotics are administered to women with positive late pregnancy GBBS vaginal cultures, previous GBS bacteriuria, or previous GBS positive infant
    d. antibiotics can completely prevent GBBS sepsis
    e. b and c

17. The patient presents at 40 weeks of gestation. She has a normal exam, and other than being tired, she has no complaints. She asks you, "Are you going to induce me?" Which of the following statements is (are) correct?
    a. you explain that as long as she has good fetal movements, you will wait until 42 weeks to induce her
    b. you offer to "strip" her membranes to try to start her labor
    c. you explain that you plan to induce her if she does not deliver by 41 weeks
    d. both a and b
    e. both b and c

Answers

1. c. Nearly 98% of women in the United States receive some prenatal care, and 84% receive care in the first trimester. Recent studies, as well as recommendations by the World Health Organization, show that reducing the number of prenatal visits does not adversely affect outcome. Black women, those with addictions, and the poor still have the lowest rates of prenatal care and, of course, the highest risks.

2. d. The DHHSEPPC has suggested that women at low risk can reduce the number of prenatal visits significantly. The recommendation is that office visits be limited to those necessary for indicated procedures and intervals for the first 6 months of pregnancy. This is based on the results of randomized controlled trials that found there was no difference in demonstrated quality-of-care outcomes between low-risk women who had regular monthly office visits and women who had prenatal visits at the time of recommended intervals for indicated tests and procedures.

Detailed recommendations have also been made regarding preconception care beginning within a year of a planned pregnancy. There should be an emphasis on prenatal care that provides an opportunity to focus on the total health and well-being of the family, including medical, psychologic, social, and environmental barriers affecting health. Systematic health care beginning long before pregnancy proves beneficial to the prospective mother and infant (e.g., folate supplementation).

The American Academy of Family Physicians suggests that the pregnant patient not only see her physician at the first indication that she is pregnant but also visit for preconception counseling during the year before she plans to get pregnant to ensure the healthiest possible outcome. Exercise, a healthy diet, and other healthy lifestyles should be encouraged many months before attempting to conceive.

3. **b.** Nägele's rule identifies the estimated date of delivery for women who have a 28-day menstrual cycle. The mean duration of pregnancy calculated from the first day of the last normal menstrual period (LNMP) for a large number of healthy women has been identified to be very close to 280 days or 40 weeks. Nägele's rule estimates the expected date of delivery by adding 7 days to the date of the first day of the LNMP and counting back 3 months. If a woman's menstrual periods are 35 days apart, add 14 days rather than 7 days. If her periods are 21 days apart, add 0 days rather than 7 days.

4. **c.** On the first prenatal visit, the following investigations should be performed: hemoglobin and hematocrit (or CBC), urinalysis (urine culture is recommended by most), blood group, Rh type, antibody screen, rubella antibody titer, syphilis screen, culture for gonorrhea and chlamydia, hepatitis B virus screen, and cervical cytology. Human immunodeficiency virus (HIV) testing should be offered for all pregnant women; purified protein derivative (PPD) screening should be offered for women at risk of tuberculosis.

If LMP is uncertain, obstetric ultrasound may be performed during the first trimester, but routinely it is recommended by the American College of Obstetricians and Gynecologists (ACOG) at 18 weeks of gestation (although this recommendation is not based on improved outcomes). The triscreen is generally offered at 18 or 19 weeks but may be done between 15 and 20 weeks.

At 26 to 28 weeks of gestation, the patient should have the following procedures performed: consideration for routine screen for diabetes mellitus, repeat hemoglobin or hematocrit, and repeat antibody test for unsensitized Rh-negative patients. Also at this time, prophylactic administration of Rho(d) immunoglobulin can be administered to patients who are Rh negative.

At 32 to 36 weeks of gestation, testing for sexually transmitted diseases and repeat hemoglobin or hematocrit may be performed, if indicated. Screening for group B streptococcus is performed at 35 to 37 weeks.

5. **a.** See answer 4.

6. **d.** The Institute of Medicine recommends a pregnancy weight gain of 25 to 35 pounds (11.5 to 16 kg) for women of normal body mass index/weight prepregnancy. Caloric requirements increase by 340 to 450 kcal/day in the second and third trimesters. The National Academy of Sciences summarized the published studies on weight gain during pregnancy and found that the amount of ideal weight gain varied inversely with the prepregnancy weight of the woman. Its pregnancy weight gain recommendations, based on percentage of ideal body weight (IBW), are as follows: underweight women (<90% of IBW) should gain 28 to 40 pounds (12.5 to 18 kg), normal weight women (90% to 135% of IBW) should gain 25 to 35 pounds (11.5 to 16 kg), and overweight women (>135% of IBW) should gain 15 to 25 pounds (7 to 11.5 kg). Of the recommended weight gain, approximately 9 kg comprises the normal physiologic events and features of pregnancy. These include the fetus, placenta, amniotic fluid, uterine hypertrophy, increase in maternal blood volume, breast enlargement, and dependent maternal edema as the consequence of mechanical factors. The remaining 1 to 3 kg is mostly fat.

7. **d.** All of those listed, as well as shoulder dystocia, are associated with excessive weight gain and maternal obesity. Intrauterine growth retardation is a complication of inadequate weight gain.

8. **c.** Some authorities recommend universal prenatal iron supplementation (27 to 30 mg/day), and because iron-deficiency anemia is associated with adverse outcomes, supplementation is generally recommended. The U.S. Preventive Services Task Force, however, found insufficient evidence to recommend this routinely. Calcium supplementation (1000 to 1300 mg/day) has been shown to decrease blood pressure and preeclampsia in some studies but not perinatal mortality. Supplementation of folic acid 0.4 to 0.8 mg/day prior to conception or up to 4 mg/day is recommended for those patients who have a history of an infant with a neural tube defect. Folate deficiency is associated with low birth weight, placental abruption, congenital cardiac, and orofacial cleft anomalies. Vitamin D supplementation is not routinely recommended, but it has been linked to neonatal hypocalcemia and should be considered in women with limited exposure to sunlight; however, high doses are toxic. Vitamin A in high doses may be teratogenic and is associated with cranial–neural crest defects. In industrialized countries, pregnant women should limit intake to less than 5000 IU/day.

9. **e.** Pregnancy outcomes are adversely affected by maternal cigarette smoking: Spontaneous abortion rates are doubled, perinatal mortality rates are significantly increased, placental abruption is almost twice as common in smokers, and mean birth weights of infants of smokers are almost 200 g less than those of infants of nonsmokers. This decrease in birth weight is a combined result of preterm deliveries and growth restriction of term babies. It is estimated that 4600 infants die annually in the United States because of maternal smoking. Other conditions linked with maternal smoking include placenta previa, premature rupture of the membranes, chorioamnionitis, placental calcifications, and placental hypoxia.

The pathophysiology of maternal smoking includes (1) carbon monoxide and its functional inactivation of fetal and maternal hemoglobin; (2) vasoconstrictor action of nicotine, causing reduced placental perfusion; (3) reduced appetite and, in turn, reduced caloric intake; and (4) decreased maternal plasma volume.

10. **b.** The safest policy for maternal alcohol use is no use. No safe level of alcohol intake during pregnancy has been identified. Even a few drinks at a critical time in organogenesis can be teratogenic. The incidence of fetal alcohol syndrome in the United States is increasing. Fetal alcohol syndrome is the most common preventable cause of mental retardation in the United States.

11. **e.** According to ACOG, women who will be older than age 35 years at the time of delivery should be offered amniocentesis or CVS, and women of all ages should be offered the triscreen—human chorionic gonadatropin (hCG), α-fetoprotein (AFP), and unconjugated estriol—to screen for NTDs and trisomy 18 and 21. The overall risk of having a child with Down syndrome is 1 in 1000 live births and 1 in 270 for women age 35 to 40 years and 1 in 100 for women older than 40 years. Many women, even knowing the increased risk of an affected fetus, do not want to risk damage (limb defects with CVS) or loss (spontaneous abortion) due to amniocentisis or CVS. The family physician is in an excellent position to present options and be sensitive to the woman's decision to accept or reject testing. Older age is not an indication for more frequent visits.

12. **d.** The most common reason for an abnormal serum AFP is an inaccurate estimated gestational age. It can detect 90% of anencephalic and 80% of spina bifida cases. An increased hCG level is the most sensitive marker for detecting trisomy 21. Unconjugated estriol levels are decreased in both trisomy 18 and trisomy 21. The triple screen should be done during weeks 16 to 18, but it may be done between 15 and 20 weeks. A risk cutoff of 1 in 190 on the triple screen gives a detection rate of 70% for trisomy 21, 60% for all trisomies, and a false-positive rate of 20%. Patients should understand the limitations of the triple screen prior to having it done.

13. **e.** There is disagreement among various groups and authors on what are the best and most cost-effective clinical components of routine prenatal visits. Most guidelines do recommend all of the choices given; however, the evidence supporting these practices is not consistent. Domestic violence affects many pregnant women, and studies show that integrating a screening protocol can increase identification of these patients. There is insufficient evidence that screening for domestic violence and early intervention result in improved health outcomes; however, there is minimal cost and potential benefit for this intervention.

14. **c.** Women with recurrent HSV infection should be counseled and treated with acyclovir (or other antivirals) at term to decrease the risk of cesarean delivery as well as educated in the role of cesarean delivery in decreasing vertical transmission. Rates of vertical transmission at the time of delivery are 50% for a primary HSV infection, 0% to 3% for a recurrent HSV infection, and 33% for a nonprimary first episode (preexisting antibodies to the other HSV type).

15. **d.** This patient has a high risk of having acquired an STD during her pregnancy, after her initial screen, so rescreening is wise. All patients should be screened for group B strep at 35 to 37 weeks.

16. **c.** GBBS is a part of normal human bacterial flora with reservoirs of colonization in otherwise healthy individuals. Vaginal colonization can be as high as 35%. Without prophylaxis, GBBS sepsis attacks two infants per 1000 births, with a 50% mortality rate. The highest risk is found in GBBS carriers with preterm delivery, rupture of membranes greater than 12 hours, onset of labor or rupture of membranes at less than 37 weeks of gestation, or intrapartum fever. With such a serious impact on newborns, prophylactic antibiotics, generally penicillin or clindamycin, have been used successfully to decrease the GBBS attack rate. However, concerns have been raised that widespread intrapartum prophylaxis

will lead to the emergence of resistant pathogens. In 1996, the Centers for Disease Control and Prevention (CDC) issued the following recommendations for the active prevention of GBBS: that antibiotic prophylaxis should be used with penicillin, that prophylaxis should be provided based on either positive late prenatal culture or a strategy based solely on clinical risk factors, and that all women with a previous GBBS-infected infant be prophylactically treated. In 2002, updated recommendations were issued by the CDC. Differences from the previous recommendations are as follows: recommendation of universal prenatal screening for vaginal and rectal GBS colonization of all pregnant women at 35 to 37 weeks of gestation and that prophylaxis be based on results; recommendation against routine intrapartum antibiotic prophylaxis for women who are GBS colonized and undergoing planned cesarean deliveries and who have not begun labor or had rupture of membranes; a suggested algorithm for management of patients with threatened preterm delivery; and an updated algorithm for management of newborns exposed to intrapartum antibiotic prophylaxis. Women with GBS bacteriuria or a previous infant with GBS infection should be offered intrapartum antibiotics routinely and therefore do not need culture.

17. **e.** The risk of stillbirth increases with gestational age from 1 per 3000 at 37 weeks of gestation to 3 per 3000 at 42 weeks and 6 per 3000 at 43 weeks. Routine induction of labor at 41 weeks has been shown to decrease perinatal death without increasing the rate of cesarean delivery. If dates are uncertain, or the patient is resistant to induction, tests for fetal well-being using nonstress testing and amniotic fluid volume should be begun at 41 weeks. Stripping or sweeping of membranes reduces the need for labor induction according to some trials, and it has not been shown to cause harm.

Summary

1. Routine checkups during pregnancy in low-risk patients are not indicated nearly as frequently as commonly practiced, especially in the first trimester.
2. The following are recommended as initial screening (as soon as possible after diagnosis): (a) CBC, (b) blood group and atypical antibody screen, (c) Rh status, (d) rubella antibody status, (e) syphilis, (f) HIV testing, (g) PPD for tuberculosis (consider), (h) hepatitis B surface antigen virus screen, (i) urinalysis (culture recommended by some), (j) gonococcus and chlamydia screen, and (k) Pap smear.
3. The following are recommended as initial 18-week screening: (a) obstetric ultrasound screening for fetal anomaly and (b) triscreen.
4. The following are recommended as initial 28-week screening:
   a. Gestational diabetes screening: 1-hour, 50-g glucose tolerance test; if results are ≥140 mg, perform 3-hour, 100-g glucose tolerance test
   b. Repeat antibody screen for women who are Rh negative, and administer Rh immunoglobulin, if indicated
   c. Repeat CBC
5. A GBBS rectovaginal culture is recommended at 35 to 37 weeks.
6. Prenatal surveillance (every prenatal visit) involves the following:
   a. Fetal: (i) fetal heart rate; (ii) fundal height, actual and amount of change; (iii) presenting part and station (late in pregnancy); and (iii) fetal activity
   b. Maternal: (i) blood pressure, actual and extent of change; (ii) weight, actual and amount of change; and (iii) symptoms, including epigastric pain, headache, and altered vision
7. Other prenatal factors
   a. Nägele's rule estimates the date of delivery: first day of LNMP plus 7 days, then count back 3 months
   b. Weight gain: ideal amount based on maternal prepregnancy weight
   c. Calories: 300 additional calories in pregnancy; 400 additional calories during lactation
   d. Supplementation: iron 30 to 60 mg after 4 months; folic acid 1 mg/day starting before and continuing throughout the pregnancy
   e. Smoking: stop; 4600 perinatal deaths per year in United States as a result of smoking
   f. Alcohol: none
8. Postdates: Delivery of the fetus preferably by 41 weeks, and no later than 42 weeks, is recommended due to the increased risk of stillbirth and poor perinatal outcomes. If a decision is made to continue the pregnancy, antepartum testing with nonstress testing and amniotic fluid index should be done after 41 weeks.
9. Postpartum depression (postnatal depression) or postpartum blues complicates 30% to 70% of pregnancies and is severe in up to 15%. Discussion about hormonal changes during the postnatal period and symptoms of postpartum depression during the antepartum period is essential. High-risk patients need to be identified and followed closely.

Suggested Reading

American College of Obstetricians and Gynecologists: ACOG committee opinion No. 55. Management of postterm pregnancy. *Obstet Gynecol* 104:639–646, 2004.

American College of Obstetricians and Gynecologists: ACOG Committee Opinion No. 354. Treatment with selective serotonin inhibitors during pregnancy. *Obstet Gynecol* 108(6):1601–1603, 2006

Kirkham C: Evidence-based prenatal care: Part I. General prenatal care and counseling issues. *Am Fam Physician* 71(7):1307–1316, 2005.

Kirkham C: Evidence-based prenatal care: Part II. Third trimester care and prevention of infectious diseases. *Am Fam Physician* 71(8):1555–1560, 2005.

Miller LJ: Postpartum depression. *JAMA* 287:762–765, 2002.

Nonacs R: Postpartum mood disorders: Diagnosis and treatment guidelines. *J Clin Psychiatry* 59(Suppl 2):34–40,1998.

Schrag S, Zywicki S, Farley MM, et al: Prevention of perinatal group B streptococcal disease: Revised guidelines from CDC. *MMWR Recomm Rep* 51(RR11):1–22, 2002.

Ward R: Benefits and risks of psychiatric medicines during pregnancy. *Am Fam Physician* 66(4):629–636, 2002.

Wisner KL: Clinical practice: Postpartum depression. *N Engl J Med* 347:194–199.2002.

CHAPTER

85

Immunization and Consumption of Over-the-Counter Drugs during Pregnancy

CLINICAL CASE PROBLEM 1

A Mother Moving to Nepal

A 26-year-old primagravida who has seen you for prenatal care once comes to your office asking for advice and immunizations. Based on your initial history and physical, she is 18 weeks gestation. Her husband has just accepted a position with a U.S. government agency in Nepal, and she will be moving there with him in 4 weeks. She is very anxious about possible infectious diseases she could contract, including tuberculosis. She recently moved to the area and had been unable to tell you her immunization status at the previous visit because she misplaced her records. She knows she received all the "childhood vaccines" and had a booster of some kind before entering college.

SELECT THE BEST ANSWER TO THE FOLLOWING QUESTIONS

1. Which of the following immunization combinations would be acceptable for administration to this pregnant woman if she needs them due to exposure risk?
   a. tetanus and diphtheria toxoids (Td); bacillus Calmette–Guerin (BCG); hepatitis A; measles, mumps, rubella (MMR) vaccine; varicella
   b. Td, hepatitis A, hepatitis B
   c. Td, hepatitis A, hepatitis B, MMR, varicella
   d. Td, hepatitis A, meningococcal polysaccharide, varicella
   e. MMR, hepatitis B

2. Your patient does not know about the risk of influenza in Nepal, but she will be in her second and third trimester during the influenza season. Which of the following statements is true about influenza vaccination in pregnancy?
   a. the immunization should not be given to high-risk patients (those with asthma, cardiovascular disease, or diabetes) within the first trimester
   b. the vaccine should be administered to all pregnant women who will be in the second or third trimester of pregnancy during the influenza season
   c. pregnant women have the same severity risk level of influenza as nonpregnant women
   d. immunization of pregnant women for influenza is not safe
   e. the live attenuated vaccine may be given to pregnant women

3. Your patient has studied communicable diseases and asks about the new Tdap vaccine to protect her from transmitting pertussis to her newborn infant. You suggest:
   a. she avoid contact with people who might have pertussis
   b. she receive Tdap rather than the Td booster because it is approved for pregnancy
   c. she receive the Tdap postpartum unless the vaccine is not available where she will be living
   d. she receive the Tdap vaccine after the infant is 6 months old since she can have viral shedding, which could infect the infant
   e. she need not worry about pertussis since nearly all cases have been eliminated

A Pregnant Woman Concerned about Consuming Ibuprofen

A newly pregnant woman who comes to the office is very concerned about the fact that she took ibuprofen for a headache during the past week. She is asking whether it is safe to take during pregnancy.

4. Which of the following statements about taking ibuprofen during pregnancy is true?
   a. ibuprofen is considered safe during all stages of pregnancy
   b. ibuprofen is considered relatively safe during the first and second trimester but should be avoided if possible in the third trimester
   c. ibuprofen should never be taken during pregnancy; the patient should be counseled to consult a geneticist
   d. ibuprofen can be taken in the third trimester but should be avoided if possible in the first trimester
   e. ibuprofen can be taken in the first trimester but should be avoided if possible in the second trimester

A Pregnant Patient with 2 Days of Flu-like Symptoms, Nausea, and Vomiting

A 22-week gestation primigravida patient of yours presents with a 2-day history of low-grade fever, myalgias, and vomiting once or twice. She received the influenza vaccine (killed) 1 month ago. Her physical examination is unremarkable except for slightly dry mucus membranes, and her laboratory examination is normal.

5. In addition to close follow-up and warnings about dehydration, which of the following over-the-counter (OTC) medications would you not recommend now or later during her pregnancy?
   a. chlorpheneramine
   b. pseudoephedrine
   c. aspirin
   d. acetaminophen (Tylenol)
   e. diphenhydramine (Benadryl)

6. On the way out the door, she mentions she had a loose stool and wants to know which medications she could take if she has diarrhea. Which of the following would you consider least desirable due to her pregnancy?
   a. kaolin and pectin (Kaopectate)
   b. bismuth subsalicylate (Pepto-Bismol)
   c. loperamide (Imodium)
   d. atropine/diphenoxylate (Lomotil)
   e. Maalox

7. Which of the following statements is true concerning medications for vaginal yeast infections during pregnancy?
   a. most of the OTC antifungal vaginal preparations have been studied, and although the largest studies are on clotrimazole, all are thought to be safe
   b. prescription antifungals, particularly oral medications such as fluconazole, have been directly linked to fetal anomalies
   c. vaginal yeast infections should not be treated at all in the first trimester due to unknown effects of the OTC medications
   d. vaginal yeast infections should not be treated until delivery of the fetus unless severe
   e. OTC antifungal vaginal preparations are category B

Clinical Case Management Problem

A 35-year-old primagravida accompanied by her husband comes to your office for her first prenatal visit. She has lost 6 pounds in the past week and is nauseated all the time. Based on her last menstrual period, she is 8 weeks pregnant. She adamantly tells you that she does not want to risk the health of her baby taking any medications, but she is having difficulty even getting out of bed because she is so dizzy. What is your response?

Answers

1. **b.** Varicella and MMR vaccines contain live attenuated virus. Such vaccine is contraindicated in pregnancy because the effects on the fetus are unknown. Varicella and rubella immunity status should have been ascertained on a prepregnancy counseling visit and administered at least 1 and ideally 3 months prior to the woman attempting a pregnancy. Immunity can be tested during pregnancy, and there is a good chance that the patient would have been previously exposed, permitting you to inform her that she has no worry with respect to these diseases. If a susceptible pregnant woman is exposed to varicella, administration of immune globulin should be strongly considered. Based on her history, it is likely that she has been fully immunized.

In contrast to live virus, administration of inactivated virus during pregnancy is considered to be safe. Tetanus and diphtheria toxoids are recommended routinely for susceptible pregnant women. Waiting until the second trimester of pregnancy to administer Td is considered a reasonable precaution. Hepatitis B contains noninfectious hepatitis B surface antigen particles and should cause no risk to the fetus. Since she is moving to a developing country, hepatitis A vaccine may be given if she has not received it because the consequences of infection are greater than any theoretical risk with a killed vaccine. Because she is not moving to an area with a high risk of meningococcal disease, or the meningococcal belt, this vaccine may be delayed. Were she going to an area considered a significant risk for exposure, this vaccine can be safely given during pregnancy. BCG vaccine is not recommended routinely for adults moving to developing countries, particularly during pregnancy (Table 85-1).

Table 85-1	Guidelines on Vaccination for Pregnant Women		
Vaccine	Should Be Considered if Otherwise Indicated	Contraindicated during Pregnancy	Special/Conditional Recommendation
Hepatitis A			Safety not determined but likely low risk. If high risk of exposure, consider giving it
Hepatitis B	X		
Human papillomavirus			Not recommended for use in pregnancy but data limited
Influenza , live attenuated		X	
Influenza, killed	X		
Measles, mumps, rubella		X	
Pneumococcal (PPV23)			Has not been evaluated for first trimester, but no adverse effects reported
Polio (IPV)			Should theoretically be avoided but if a woman must be protected immediately, could be used
Td	X		Second or third trimester preferred
Tdap			Pregnancy is not a contraindication, but data are not available; if given, second or third tremeter is preferred
Varicella		X	
Travel and other vaccines			
Anthrax			No studies published; only vaccinate if risks of disease outweigh potential fetal risks
BCG			No harmful effects to fetus associated, but not recommended during pregnancy
Japanese encephalitis			No specific information but vaccination poses a theoretical risk and should not be routinely administered
Meningococcal (MPSV4)	X		
Rabies	X		
Typhoid (oral and parenteral)			No data available during pregnancy
Vaccinia		X	
Yellow fever			Safety during pregnancy not established and should only be administered if travel to an endemic area is unavoidable and increased risk for exposure exists
Zoster		X	Not known if it can cause fetal harm, but should not be administered and pregnancy should be avoided for 3 months following vaccination

2. b. The inactivated influenza vaccine is a killed virus preparation and is therefore safe to administer. It should be administered annually between October and December to all pregnant women who will be in the second or third trimester of pregnancy during the influenza season. High-risk groups, such as women with asthma, diabetes, and cardiovascular disease, should be given the vaccine regardless of their trimester. Pregnant women in their second or third trimester of pregnancy during influenza season have higher morbidity, similar to other high-risk patients. The live vaccine should not be given to pregnant women.

3. c. Pregnancy is not a contraindication for the use of Tdap; however, data on the safety, immunogenicity, and outcomes of pregnancy are not available. There is a possibility that transplacental maternal antibodies could interfere with the infant's immune response to infant doses of Tdap, but they might also protect the infant against pertussis in early life. In this patient, since pertussis is an even greater threat in a developing country, she should be advised to receive the vaccine immediately postpartum, even if it has been less than 2 years since her last Td booster. If used, it should be given in the second or third trimester, like Td, and reported to the vaccine registry.

4. b. Ibuprofen, ketoprofen, and naproxen are associated with oligohydramnios, premature closure of the fetal ductus arteriosus with subsequent persistent pulmonary hypertension of the newborn, fetal nephrotoxicity, and periventricular hemorrhage if taken during the third trimester of pregnancy (category D). These nonsteroidal anti-inflammatory drugs are considered relatively safe in the first and second trimester (category B);

however, due to their danger later in pregnancy, most clinicians advise against their use.

Table 85-2 outlines the Food and Drug Administration (FDA) rating system.

5. c. Aspirin is associated with neonatal hemorrhage, decreased birth weight, prolonged gestation and labor, and possible teratogenicity. As mentioned previously, ibuprofen is particularly dangerous in the third trimester. Chlorpheneramine, diphenhydramine, and acetaminophen are thought to be safe during pregnancy. Pseudoephedrine is category B, but one study has shown increased gastroschisis. Guaifenisin is category B, but it is not recommended in the first trimester, and dextromethorphan is thought to be safe.

6. b. Bismuth subsalicylate can result in the absorption of salicylate and should be avoided, especially in the third trimester. Salicylates have been associated with increased perinatal mortality, neonatal hemorrhage, decreased birth weight, prolonged gestation and labor, and possible birth defects. Bismuth subsalicylate is considered category C in the first and second trimesters and category D in the third trimester (positive evidence of human fetal risk but the benefits from use in pregnant women may be acceptable despite the risk). Kaolin and pectin (Kaopectate) and loperamide (Imodium) are considered category B (animal reproductive studies show no fetal risk, but there are no controlled studies in pregnant women). Atropine/diphenoxylate (Lomotil) is category C (studies on animals show adverse effects on the fetus and there are no controlled studies in women, or studies on women and animals are not available). Aluminum hydroxide/magnesium hydroxide (Maalox)

Table 85-2	Food and Drug Administration Rating System	
Category	**Interpretation**
A	*Controlled studies show no risk*: Adequate, well-controlled studies in pregnant women have failed to demonstrate a risk to the fetus in any trimester of pregnancy.
B	*No evidence of risk in humans*: Adequate, well-controlled studies in pregnant women have not shown increased risk of fetal abnormalities despite adverse findings in animals, or, in the absence of adequate human studies, animal studies show no fetal risk. The chance of fetal harm is remote but remains a possibility.
C	*Risk cannot be ruled out*: Adequate, well-controlled human studies are lacking, and animal studies have shown a risk to the fetus or are lacking as well. There is a chance of fetal harm if the drug is administered during pregnancy, but the potential benefits may outweigh the potential risks.
D	*Positive evidence of risk*: Studies in humans, or investigational or postmarketing data, have demonstrated fetal risk. Nevertheless, potential benefits from the use of the drug may outweigh the potential risk. For example, the drug may be acceptable if needed in a life-threatening situation or serious disease for which safer drugs cannot be used or are ineffective.
X	*Contraindicated in pregnancy*: Studies in animals or humans, or investigational or postmarketing reports, have demonstrated positive evidence of fetal abnormalities or risks that clearly outweigh any possible benefit to the patient.

is category B, whereas calcium carbonate (Tums) is category C; both are generally considered safe.

7. **a.** All of the preparations are listed as category C, although there are studies of all preparations and all are believed to be safe. A large number of excellent studies exist on clotrimazole. There are no data on tiaconazole. Fluconazole is used by many clinicians, and studies have demonstrated that it is safe in the first trimester. There is no reason to withhold treatment of vaginal yeast infections during pregnancy due to fear of side effects.

Solution to the Clinical Case Management Problem

During your history and physical examination, you must consider causes of severe hyperemesis, such as multiple gestation, gestational trophoblastic disease, or superimposed infections. If her exam is normal and you believe that outpatient treatment is feasible, you must educate the patient on the danger to her pregnancy and the fetus due to dehydration and ketosis. Having "hard" data such as ketonuria, abnormal electrolytes, or a high specific gravity in the urine sometimes helps patients understand that this is more than normal pregnancy-associated nausea. If the patient is adamantly against use of medications, and you believe she can be adequately hydrated orally, use of pyridoxine (vitamin B_6), acupressure, and small and frequent meals are usually appropriate. If, however, she has orthostasis, as do many patients with hyperemesis gravidarum, she will improve more quickly with intravenous hydration in the hospital, allowing you to provide good care while avoiding medications she fears will harm her baby. Often in cases such as this, the patient needs more education, but we must also respect her concern since there are not adequate studies on many of the medications we use in early pregnancy for hyperemesis. Presenting it as a harm–benefit ratio is useful as well.

Summary

1. Ideally, vaccination status should be determined prior to attempting pregnancy and brought up to date at least 1 month prior to possible pregnancy.
2. If a patient has not been immunized prior to pregnancy, immunization with killed virus can be done. However, live attenuated vaccines should not be used. Thus, immunization against varicella and MMR (or individual components) is not recommended. Only the killed influenza vaccine should be used. Many vaccines have no clear danger but should be used only if the risk of exposure is greater than the potential harm to the fetus when there are no data concerning use in pregnancy.
3. Patients should be counseled about the potential dangers of OTC and prescription drugs. The effects on the fetus of many common OTC drugs are unknown, and a reasonable plan is to use as few medications as possible during pregnancy, particularly the first trimester.
4. The FDA categorizes pharmaceuticals and OTC drugs according to potential or known hazards. The categories A, B, C, D, and X are listed and defined in answer 4. Additional data should be reviewed since the FDA categories do not reflect more recent findings.

Suggested Reading

Advisory Committee on Immunization Practices: Guidelines for vaccinating pregnant women. Available at www.cdc.gov.

American College of Obstetricians and Gynecologists: Immunization during pregnancy, Committee Opinion No 282. *Obstet Gynecol* 101:207–212, 2003.

Black R, Hill D: Over-the-counter medications in pregnancy. *Am Fam Physician* 67:2517–2524, 2003.

Czeizel AE, Toth M, Rockenbauer M: No teratogenic effect after clotrimazole therapy during pregnancy. *Epidemiology* 10:437–440, 1999.

Jewel D: Nausea and vomiting of early pregnancy. *Am Fam Physician* 68:121–128, 2003.

Sur DK, Wallis DH, O'Connell TX: Vaccinations in pregnancy. *Am Fam Physician* 68(2):299–304, 2003.

Exercise and Pregnancy

A 37-Year-Old Pregnant Woman with Severe Back Pain

A 37-year-old pregnant woman comes to your office with low back pain that has been getting worse as her pregnancy has progressed. This is her third pregnancy; the previous two were uncomplicated except for chronic back pain, and this one has also been without any other difficulty. She has tried bed rest, acetaminophen, and heat pads—all without relief. She has no symptoms of dysuria or sensory/motor complaints; she says she is willing to try anything for relief. Examination is that of a normal early third trimester pregnancy.

CLINICAL CASE PROBLEM 1

A 34-Year-Old Primigravida Aerobic Dance Instructor

A 34-year-old aerobics dance instructor sees you for advice regarding her pregnancy. She is 6 weeks pregnant and wonders if she should continue her current work. Her work consists of 3 or 4 hours of exercise daily. She currently has no problems performing this activity but wonders if all the "bouncing and stepping" will cause a miscarriage or otherwise harm the baby.

SELECT THE BEST ANSWER TO THE FOLLOWING QUESTIONS

1. Regarding her current physical activity, you tell her which of the following?
   a. any exercise during pregnancy is not advisable
   b. aerobic and strength training exercises are likely to increase her chance of miscarriage
   c. the pregnancy-associated physiologic changes in her body make dance aerobics inadvisable
   d. continuing moderate exercise during pregnancy is desirable and not harmful
   e. she should decrease to 30 minutes of exercise a day to prevent intrauterine growth restriction (IUGR)

2. Which of the following is an absolute contraindication to exercise during pregnancy?
   a. a history of incompetent cervix or cerclage
   b. a history of a sedentary lifestyle
   c. poorly controlled type 1 diabetes
   d. a heavy smoker
   e. morbid obesity

3. Which of the following is correct concerning cardiovascular changes during pregnancy?
   a. after the first trimester, the supine position results in relative obstruction of venous return, decreased cardiac output, and orthostatic hypotension
   b. motionless standing is associated with an increase in cardiac output during pregnancy
   c. core temperatures during exercise increase 2 degrees more than in nonpregnant women
   d. heart rate decreases with exercise in pregnancy
   e. exertion at altitudes higher than 2500 feet cause significant cardiac compromise in pregnant women

4. Regarding her chronic pregnancy-related back pain, you state the following:
   a. step aerobics should be of therapeutic value in relieving the pain
   b. water aerobics has been shown to relieve back pain in pregnant women
   c. therapeutic massage is of no value in her condition
   d. stationary bicycling should help her discomfort
   e. bed rest is best

5. Your patient decides to try water aerobics, and her symptoms improve. Her mother-in-law, however, has told her that swimming is harmful to the baby. She seeks your advice. You tell her
   a. water immersion late in pregnancy is often complicated by an increased rate of urinary tract infections
   b. water immersion late in pregnancy is often complicated by an increase in vaginal discharges
   c. water immersion late in pregnancy is dangerous because of the possibility of inducing an amnionitis
   d. water immersion late in pregnancy is associated with preterm onset of labor
   e. water immersion late in pregnancy is safe

CLINICAL CASE PROBLEM 3

A 22-Year-Old Primigravida with Recent Onset of Abdominal Tightness While Exercising on the Treadmill

A 22-year-old primigravida in her second trimester returns to your office saying that she had an episode of abdominal tightness that occurred while exercising on her treadmill. Normally, she power walks for 20 minutes each day. She had failed to drink water, as she normally does before and during exercise, and after she rested and drank two bottles of water, her symptoms resolved. Evaluation included a normal nonstress test with minimal uterine irritability that resolved after another liter of oral rehydration and a normal hemoglobin. She asks when she can resume her exercise activity.

6. Reasons to discontinue exercise include all of the following except
   a. preterm labor
   b. dizziness or lightheadedness during exercise
   c. vaginal bleeding
   d. dyspnea prior to exertion
   e. mild dyspnea during exertion

7. Which of the following forms of exercise is (are) considered safe during pregnancy?
   a. scuba diving
   b. gymnastics
   c. basketball
   d. field hockey
   e. water aerobics

8. Women who engage in moderate aerobic exercise regularly during pregnancy
   a. are at greater risk for preterm labor
   b. may derive significant physical and mental health benefits
   c. are at risk for fetal IUGR
   d. reduce their risk for preeclampsia
   e. are at greater risk for hypertension

Answers

1. **d.** Despite the importance of regular exercise in daily life, there are relatively few good studies that examine this issue. A Cochrane evidenced-based review concluded that regular aerobic exercise during pregnancy appears to improve (or maintain) physical fitness and body image. The American College of Obstetricians and Gynecologists (ACOG) recommendations suggest 30 minutes a day of regular exercise for pregnant women without complications, but athletes with uncomplicated pregnancies can remain active during pregnancy unless there are medical contraindications. No teratogenic effects have been found related to exercise-induced hyperthermia. If a very physically active woman has findings suggestive of IUGR, this would, of course, be a contraindication to continued exercise.

2. **a.** ACOG released a consensus recommendation regarding absolute and relative contraindications to exercise in pregnancy. Absolute contraindications include a history of incompetent cervix or cerclage, placenta previa after 26 weeks of gestation, persistent second or third trimester bleeding, hemodynamically significant heart disease, restrictive lung disease, multiple gestations at risk for premature labor, ruptured membranes, and preeclampsia/eclampsia. ACOG guidelines for relative contraindications include severe anemia, chronic bronchitis, unevaluated maternal arrhythmia, poorly controlled type 1 diabetes, morbid obesity, extreme underweight (body mass index <12), history of sedentary lifestyle, IUGR, poorly controlled hypertension, orthopedic limitations, poorly controlled seizure disorder or hyperthyroidism, and heavy smoking.

3. **a.** Cardiovascular changes associated with pregnancy are important to consider when discussing exercise. After the first trimester, pregnant women should avoid supine positions during exercise as much as possible because of the obstruction of venous return. Motionless standing is also associated with a significant decrease in cardiac output. Exercise, as always, causes an increase in heart rate. Exertion at altitudes of up to 6000 feet appears to be safe; however, it depends on the exercise performed and the conditioning of the woman. There are no reports of hyperthermia associated with exercise causing teratogenic effects, and core temperatures increase no more than in the nonpregnant state.

4. **b.** Chronic back pain is a common problem in pregnancy. Conditioning the back muscles with stretching and strength training before pregnancy is a good prophylactic strategy. However, during pregnancy, water aerobics has been found in controlled trials to reduce the discomfort of low back pain in many patients. Some women feel self-conscious about exercising during pregnancy, particularly in public pools. However, many health clubs take this into account and schedule specific times for pregnancy water aerobics classes. Bed rest is likely to make muscular pain worse.

5. **e.** There are many common misconceptions regarding immersion and pregnancy. Among them are that water immersion is often complicated by urinary tract infections, vaginal discharges, leakage into the amniotic sac, and an association with preterm onset of labor. None of these are correct. Swimming and water aerobics are perfectly safe and usually easily performed because of the buoyancy effect of water.

6. e. Mild dyspnea during exertion, particularly if able to comfortably talk, is not an absolute reason to terminate exercise if not accompanied by symptoms. The prepregnant state of conditioning is most important to assess. Reasons to discontinue exercise in pregnancy include vaginal bleeding, dyspnea prior to exercise, dizziness, headache, chest pain, muscle weakness, unilateral calf or leg swelling (thrombophlebitis should be ruled out), preterm labor, decreased fetal movement, and amniotic fluid leakage.

7. e. Although physiologic and morphologic changes of pregnancy may interfere with the ability to engage in some forms of physical activity, the patient's health status should be evaluated before prescribing an exercise program. Each sport should be reviewed individually for its potential risk, and activities with a high risk of abdominal trauma should be avoided during pregnancy. These include all contact sports and scuba diving. Scuba diving increases the fetal risk for decompression sickness during this activity. Sports associated with falls or trauma, such as gymnastics, downhill skiing, horseback riding, or vigorous racquet sports, should be avoided as well.

8. b. Women who engage in moderate aerobic exercise regularly during pregnancy may derive significant physical and mental health benefits. To date, there appears to be little or no risk for adverse outcomes, such as preterm labor or fetal IUGR, and there is no effect on the risk of preeclampsia or hypertension. Generally, participation in a wide range of recreational activities appears to be safe during pregnancy and should be encouraged by clinicians.

Summary

1. For most patients, continuing moderate exercise during pregnancy is desirable and not harmful and should be encouraged by the physician. There are virtually no large trials on which to base our advice to patients.
2. The ACOG consensus is that absolute contraindications for exercise during pregnancy include a history of incompetent cervix or cerclage, placenta previa after 26 weeks of gestation, persistent second or third trimester bleeding, hemodynamically significant heart disease, restrictive lung disease, multiple gestations at risk for premature labor, ruptured membranes, and preeclampsia/eclampsia.
3. The AGOG consensus is that relative contraindications for exercise during pregnancy include severe anemia, chronic bronchitis, unevaluated maternal arrhythmia, poorly controlled type 1 diabetes, morbid obesity, extreme underweight (body mass index <12), history of sedentary lifestyle, IUGR, poorly controlled hypertension, orthopedic limitations, poorly controlled seizure disorder or hyperthyroidism, and heavy smoking.
4. Controlled trials have found that pregnant women who engage in vigorous exercise at least two or three times per week improve or maintain their physical fitness, and they have improved emotional well-being as well.
5. Symptomatic reasons for discontinuing exercise in pregnancy include vaginal bleeding, dyspnea prior to exercise, dizziness, headache, chest pain, muscle weakness, unilateral calf or leg swelling (thrombophlebitis should be ruled out), preterm labor, decreased fetal movement, and amniotic fluid leakage.
6. Although, in general, participation in a wide range of recreational activities during pregnancy is safe, may provide significant physical and mental health benefits, and should be encouraged by clinicians, the patient's health status and types of exercise should be evaluated before prescribing an exercise program. Participation in any sports involving abdominal contact should be discouraged, as should scuba diving. Scuba diving increases the fetal risk for decompression sickness.

Suggested Reading

American College of Obstetricians and Gynecologists Committee on Obstetric Practice: Exercise during pregnancy and the postpartum period, Committee Opinion No. 267. Ob*stet Gynecol* 99:171–173, 2002.

Clapp JF: Exercise during pregnancy. A clinical update. *Clin Sports Med* 19:273–286, 2000.

De Ver Dye T, Fernandez I, Rains A, Fershteyn Z: Recent studies in the epidemiologic assessment of physical activity, fetal growth, and preterm delivery: A narrative review. *Clin Obstet Gynecol* 46(2):415–422, 2003.

Kramer MS, McDonald SW: Aerobic exercise for women during pregnancy. Cochrane Pregnancy and Childbirth Group. *Cochrane Database Syst Rev* (3):CD000180, 2006.

Young G, Jewell D: Interventions for preventing and treating pelvic and back pain in pregnancy. Cochrane Pregnancy and Childbirth Group. *Cochrane Database Syst Rev* (3):CD001139, 2003.

*An 18-Year-Old Primigravida Presents
for Prenatal Care*

An 18-year-old primigravida comes to your office for her initial prenatal visit. The pregnancy was unanticipated and she is quite disconcerted. She denies any medical problems or prior surgery. Her body mass index is 29. She has been taking prenatal vitamins for 1 month. Her mother hands you a list of symptoms that are bothering her daughter. The patient is quite nauseated and "throws up constantly." She dramatically states that she has lost "at least 10 pounds in the past 6 weeks." Neither "preggie pops" nor the "wrist bands she bought at the pharmacy" help. She desires other options for ending the nausea. Other complaints include blurred vision, bleeding gums, and a vaginal discharge. Her mother is concerned that she contracted a sexually transmitted disease from her boyfriend. The patient informs you that she had a well woman exam 2 months ago. The Pap exam was normal and cultures for gonorrhea and chlamydia were negative.

On physical examination, the patient is well hydrated and has actually gained 6 pounds. The uterus is 10 weeks' size. The cervix is closed, firm, and not effaced. There is a whitish copious discharge but no odor or cervical motion tenderness. The remainder of her physical exam, including a urinalysis, is normal.

SELECT THE BEST ANSWER TO THE FOLLOWING QUESTIONS

1. Which of the following hormones is thought to have the greatest influence on nausea and vomiting in pregnancy (NVP)?
   a. progesterone
   b. estrogen
   c. thyroid-stimulating hormone
   d. human chorionic gonadotropin (hCG)
   e. human placental lactogen

2. Which of the following statements about hyperemesis gravidarum is true?
   a. hyperemesis gravidarum is diagnosed when nausea and/or vomiting cause severe fatigue in a pregnant patient
   b. the incidence of hyperemesis gravidarum in pregnancy is approximately 10%
   c. women with hyperemesis gravidarum are less likely to be coinfected with *Helicobacter pylori*
   d. pregnancies complicated by hyperemesis gravidarum have altered sex ratios in favor of male offspring
   e. maternal tobacco use is associated with a decreased risk for hyperemesis gravidarum

3. Which of the following would not be indicated as initial advice or treatment for women with NVP?
   a. eating dry, carbohydrate-rich foods and drinking clear liquids may help alleviate symptoms
   b. providing the patient with a prescription for an antiemetic (i.e., promethazine)
   c. avoiding foods with strong seasoning or odors
   d. informing the patient that symptoms usually resolve at approximately 14 weeks of gestation
   e. counseling the patient that taking prenatal vitamins may help prevent NVP

4. Which of the following remedies is no more effective than placebo in reducing symptoms of NVP?
   a. pyridoxine (vitamin B$_6$)
   b. P6 acupressure
   c. ginger capsules
   d. antiemetics (promethazine)
   e. antihistamines (meclizine, diphenhydramine)

5. How should the patient be counseled regarding her vaginal discharge?
   a. she was likely exposed to gonorrhea or chlamydia in the past 2 months
   b. decreased estrogen and vaginal blood flow in pregnancy contributes to leukorrhea of pregnancy
   c. foul-smelling discharge, dysuria, and pruritis are not associated with leukorrhea
   d. leukorrhea of pregnancy is usually blood tinged and of thick consistency
   e. none of the above

6. Which of the following physiologic changes is not associated with pregnancy?
   a. the cornea decreases in thickness, leading to blurred vision
   b. the thyroid increases in size by approximately 15%
   c. nasal mucosa becomes hyperemic/edematous, leading to nasal congestion
   d. increased splitting of the first and second heart sound in combination with an S3 gallop
   e. increase in maternal pulmonary tidal volume by 30% to 40%

7. On examination of the patient's gums, you note a smooth, soft, red-purple mass that is pedunculated. It is located on the interdental papilla and the patient states that it often bleeds. Which of the following statements is true?
   a. the lesion usually develops during the first month of pregnancy
   b. the patient should be referred to a dentist immediately for biopsy of the lesion
   c. this condition occurs in 10% of pregnancies
   d. these lesions generally regress after delivery
   e. the lesion occurs less often in pregnant women with extensive gingivitis

CLINICAL CASE PROBLEM 2

Chili Dogs and Chest Pain

A 30-year-old nullipara comes to the office for a routine prenatal visit. She is at 28 weeks of gestation and thus far has had an uncomplicated pregnancy. During the past month, she has developed heartburn. It is worse when she eats spicy or greasy foods for dinner, especially if she goes to bed within 2 hours of eating. She also complains that her bowel movements are much harder. She notices some blood when she wipes, and she is concerned because her mother was diagnosed with colon cancer at age 60 years.

On physical examination, her blood pressure is 110/70 mmHg and she has gained 2 pounds. Her abdominal exam is unremarkable except for numerous stretch marks. Fundal height is 28 cm. Rectal exam shows a 1-cm nonthrombosed hemorrhoid.

8. Which of the following statements is inappropriate advice for heartburn/gastroesophageal reflux disease (GERD) during pregnancy?
   a. consumption of chocolate, citrus juices, fatty foods, or mint worsens symptoms
   b. nocturnal symptoms are improved by elevating the head of the bed 15 cm
   c. alcohol and smoking worsen symptoms
   d. fluid and food should not be consumed at least 4 hours prior to bedtime
   e. medications for the treatment of heartburn/GERD in pregnancy are considered safe based on numerous randomized controlled trials (RCTs)

9. Which of the following statements about heartburn in pregnancy is true?
   a. heartburn symptoms are rare during the first trimester

   b. elevated progesterone levels increase the lower esophageal sphincter tone and allow reflux of stomach acid into the esophagus
   c. progesterone increases bowel smooth muscle motility and decreases transit time for food in the gut
   d. heartburn is worse in women of lower parity
   e. the prevalence of heartburn in pregnancy is similar among white, black, and Asian women

10. Which of the following medications is (are) contraindicated for treating heartburn/GERD in pregnancy?
    a. H$_2$ blockers (cimetidine)
    b. aluminum containing antacids
    c. Proton pump inhibitors (omeprazole)
    d. bismuth subsalicylate
    e. sucralfate

11. The patient has numerous red-purple striae across her abdomen and breasts. She is quite upset by the change and wants advice on how to make the marks disappear. She has tried more than $100 of products promising to cure stretch marks but sees no results. Which of the following statements about striae gravidarum is true?
    a. certain prescription creams and lotions improve stretch marks in pregnancy
    b. stretch marks are more likely to develop in older gravidas than in younger pregnant women
    c. women whose mothers had striae gravidarum have increased rates of developing stretch marks
    d. abdominoplasty or laser therapy after delivery will not improve the appearance of stretch marks
    e. less than 20% of pregnant women are affected by stretch marks

12. Which of the following statements about hemorrhoids in pregnancy is false?
    a. women with a history of multiple vaginal deliveries are less likely to have hemorrhoids after age 60 years than nulliparous women
    b. increased venous pressure in the rectal plexus causes hemorrhoids
    c. hemorrhoids are the most frequent anorectal disease of pregnancy and the puerperium
    d. the most common symptoms of hemorrhoids during pregnancy are rectal bleeding and pain
    e. hemorrhoids usually improve or resolve after delivery

13. Initial treatment for hemorrhoids during pregnancy includes all of the following except
    a. stool softeners
    b. laxatives

c. increasing fluid intake

d. high fiber diet

e. rutoside flavonoids

CLINICAL CASE PROBLEM 3

"Oh, My Aching Back!"

RL is a 36-year-old multigravida at 34 weeks of gestation. She works as a stockbroker at a large brokerage house. During the past 2 weeks, she has developed worsening edema in her bilateral lower extremities. It is worse at the end of the day and generally resolves somewhat by the next morning. Although RL has made some lifestyle changes (she no longer wears high heels to work), the symptoms are getting worse. At her routine visit, she is concerned about "severe abdominal pain." She describes the pain as inguinal, stabbing, and intermittent. RL comments that she also has significant low back pain. The pain is dull, constant, and located over the lower lumbar spine. She has no loss of bladder or bowel function and no neurologic abnormalities on exam. The low back pain is not related to the inguinal pain.

14. Which of the following statements about lower extremity edema during pregnancy is true?
    a. avoiding standing for long periods of time improves symptoms
    b. decreased sodium and water retention leads to fluid shifts
    c. decreased vascular permeability worsens dependent edema
    d. lower extremity pitting edema late in pregnancy is highly suggestive of preeclampsia
    e. symptoms often do not resolve after delivery

15. What is the appropriate management of the patient's severe inguinal pain?
    a. nonstress test to rule out an abruption
    b. reassurance
    c. emergency ultrasound for fetal well-being
    d. nonsteroidal anti-inflammatory medication
    e. venous compression stockings

16. Which of the following statements about low back and pelvic pain in pregnancy (LBPP) is true?
    a. a general decrease in the mobility of joints in late pregnancy may contribute to LBPP
    b. changes in serum procollagen and reproductive hormones are associated with LBPP
    c. younger women have a decreased risk for back pain in pregnancy

d. larger fetal weight or twin pregnancy have little impact on the risk of LBPP

e. the influence of relaxin on LBPP is well understood

Answers

1. **d.** hCG is thought to have the greatest influence on NVP. A temporal relationship exists between the peak of NVP and maternal hCG levels. The severity of NVP is worse in multifetal or molar pregnancies, both of which are associated with increased hCG levels. A review of 17 studies found an association between NVP and hCG in 13 of the trials. Although estradiol and progesterone are also causally linked to NVP, hCG is thought to have the greatest influence.

2. **e.** NVP affects approximately 80% of pregnant women. Hyperemesis gravidarum is a more extreme form of NVP, occurring in 0.3% to 2% of pregnancies. Characterized as severe NVP that interferes with oral intake and causes fluid and electrolyte abnormalities, hospitalization is sometimes necessary for intravenous hydration. Risk factors for hyperemesis include young maternal age, a previous pregnancy with hyperemesis, high or low body mass index, psychiatric conditions, and carrying a female fetus. Pregnancies complicated by fetal anomalies or multiple gestation are also at increased risk. Women who smoke are less likely to have hyperemesis. There is an altered sex ratio in favor of female fetuses, possibly due to increased maternal hormone levels. Several studies support a link between infection with *H. pylori* and increased risk of hyperemesis, although more definitive studies are needed.

3. **b.** Management of NVP depends on the severity of symptoms and the impact on quality of life. Pregnant women are encouraged to take prenatal vitamins containing folate because they may help prevent NVP. Lifestyle changes are initially recommended, including eating frequent small, bland meals, getting adequate rest, and avoiding spicy and greasy foods. First-line pharmacologic therapy for NVP is pyridoxine alone or in combination with doxylamine. Although most women experience some symptoms of NVP by 5 weeks of gestation, symptoms generally subside by week 12.

4. **b.** The P6 acupuncture point is located approximately 3 cm proximal to the wrist. Also known as the Neiguan point, P6 regulates the internal organs and calms the spirit according to traditional Chinese medicine. A Cochrane review found that P6 acupressure is no more effective than sham acupressure or standard dietary and lifestyle changes.

Pyridoxine is a water-soluble B-complex vitamin. It has a good safety record, minimal adverse effects, and is readily available. Several randomized, double-blind trials have demonstrated that pyridoxine significantly improves symptoms in women with severe NVP. It is a reasonable first-line treatment, either alone or combined with doxylamine.

One trial compared ginger capsules with placebo for NVP. Benefits were seen for both vomiting (odds ratio [OR] 0.31) and nausea (OR 0.06). Because the active agent in ginger is unknown and composition varies significantly based on the method of growth and harvesting, more research is needed to determine optimal dosing.

A meta-analysis of antiemetics in NVP showed a beneficial reduction in the incidence of nausea, although these drugs cause sleepiness.

Antihistamines inhibit the action of histamine at the H_1 receptor and indirectly affect the vestibular system. In a meta-analysis of data from seven RCTs, antihistamines were effective in reducing NVP.

5. c. Leukorrhea results from increased estrogen levels and vaginal blood flow during pregnancy. The discharge is variable in consistency and whitish to clear in color. Leukorrhea is normal in pregnancy and women should be reassured that it is not caused by sexually transmitted infections. Dysuria, pruritis, or foul-smelling vaginal discharge necessitate an evaluation for infectious causes.

6. a. Numerous physiologic changes occur during pregnancy. The cornea increases in thickness, causing blurred vision in some women. Changes usually revert to normal by the sixth week postpartum. Nasal mucosa becomes engorged, resulting in epistaxis and congestion. Although the thyroid increases in size by 15%, this is not noticeable on physical exam. Tidal volume increases during pregnancy and splitting of the heart sounds, an S3 gallop, and systolic murmur along the left sternal border are commonly noted on exam.

7. d. Pregnancy tumor, or epulis gravidarum, occurs in approximately 2% of pregnancies. It usually develops between the second and fifth months of gestation. Pregnancy tumor resembles a pyogenic granuloma and is usually smooth, semifirm, and shiny with a reddish-purple or pink hue. The most common location is the interdental papilla, although tumors are also found on the buccal and lingual gingival surfaces. After delivery, pregnancy tumor typically regresses spontaneously. It is more common in women with severe gingivitis. Minor trauma often results in hemorrhage or ulceration. Epulis gravidarum tumors are generally removed several months postpartum because of the high rate of spontaneous regression.

8. e. There are no published RCTs on GERD management during pregnancy. Medications used for heartburn and GERD are considered safe based on retrospective cohort studies and case reports. Initial treatment of heartburn involves conservative measures such as dietary and behavioral changes. Numerous foods worsen symptoms, as do alcohol, tobacco, and nonsteroidal anti-inflammatory medications. Pharmacologic treatment of heartburn/GERD is recommended only for refractory symptoms.

9. e. Heartburn is a very common complaint during pregnancy. It is not limited to the third trimester. Prevalence increases from 22% in the first trimester to 39% in the second and 60% to 72% in the last trimester. Elevated progesterone levels relax the lower esophageal sphincter and increase the transit time for food in the small bowel. Symptoms usually worsen with increasing gestational age. Heartburn increases with higher parity and is worse in women who had heartburn before becoming pregnant. Differences in prevalence are not noted when comparing pregnant women of white, black, or Asian ethnicity.

10. d. Chronic use of salicylates by gravid women may result in intrauterine growth restriction, premature ductus closure, and other congenital defects. Use is best avoided during pregnancy. H_2 blockers have the longest history of use in pregnancy and show demonstrated safety in large registry studies. They are pregnancy class B. Proton pump inhibitors (PPIs; class C) are considered safe, although they have not been as extensively used in patient care as the H_2 blockers. Antacids containing bicarbonate may cause metabolic alkalosis in the mother and fetus. Calcium, aluminum, and magnesium antacids in therapeutic doses are acceptable during pregnancy. Sucralfate is poorly absorbed and causes no risk to the fetus.

11. c. No therapy is definitively proven to decrease the development of stretch marks. The incidence of striae gravidarum in pregnancy is 55% to 90%. The lesions usually fade after delivery and become less noticeable with time. Curiously, advancing age is inversely proportional to development of striae. Half of women with stretch marks during pregnancy have mothers with similar histories. Women with prepregnancy stretch marks on the breasts or thighs are particularly likely to develop striae. Both laser therapy and abdominoplasty are options for nonpregnant women with severe striae. Abdominoplasty is most effective in women with redundant abdominal tissue.

12. a. Women who have one or more vaginal deliveries are more likely to develop hemorrhoids after age

60 years. Symptoms include itching or burning of the anus combined with intermittent bleeding and pain. Pelvic venous congestion caused by uterine compression exacerbates this condition. Although hemorrhoids are the most frequent anorectal cause of bleeding, they generally improve or resolve after delivery. Individuals with a first-degree relative diagnosed with colon cancer should be counseled on screening recommendations for colonoscopy.

13. e. Constipation is more common during pregnancy and predisposes women to developing hemorrhoids. Increasing dietary fiber and fluid intake improves both conditions. Laxatives and stool softeners also help relieve symptoms of hemorrhoids and constipation, although large randomized trials have not been conducted on pregnant women. Rutosides are a type of plant flavonoid. They possess phlebotonic activity, which involves increasing rectal venous tone and possibly decreasing rectal mucosal capillary fragility. Outside of pregnancy, hydroxyethylrutosides are useful for treating first- and second-grade hemorrhoids. Their use and safety in pregnancy are not established.

14. a. During late pregnancy, pitting edema in the lower extremities occurs in up to 70% of pregnancies. High hormonal levels enhance sodium and water retention as well as increase capillary permeability. The pressure of the gravid uterus compresses the inferior vena cava and causes engorgement of the pelvic venous system. Avoiding prolonged standing, using compression stockings, and elevating the feet appear to improve symptoms, although, randomized trials proving that these measures improve symptoms have not been conducted. Lower extremity edema alone is unlikely preeclampsia in the absence of proteinuria and blood pressure abnormalities. Edema usually resolves rapidly after delivery.

15. b. The patient has round ligament pain, which is characterized as sharp, sporadic pain in the inguinal area. Caused by spasm of the round ligaments, the condition is worse in multiparous women. Although uncomfortable, round ligament pain is not harmful to the patient or fetus. Exercise, warm soaks, a pregnancy girdle, and acetaminophen may help her symptoms. The diagnosis of round ligament pain is clinical; nonstress tests and ultrasound are not indicated. Nonsteroidal anti-inflammatory drugs are contraindicated in late gestation. Venous stockings do not help reduce round ligament pain.

16. b. LBPP is common, with a prevalence of 24% to 90% in various studies. Younger women actually have increased rates of back pain, as do women with a prepregnancy history of back pain. Multiple gestation pregnancies, first pregnancies, and larger fetal size are all associated with LBPP. The etiology of LBPP is not well understood. Decreased stability of the pelvic girdle and increased joint mobility are both implicated. Reproductive hormones and procollagen are also involved. Although relaxin was initially thought to be important in LBPP, recent studies have been contradictory. Future studies should clarify the role of relaxin on LBPP.

Summary

Pregnancy is a time of significant change for women and their families. Most women experience specific physical symptoms throughout pregnancy. The majority of these problems are benign and self-limited. Counseling women about common problems empowers them to proactively manage issues as they arise. Anticipatory guidance reassures patients that most pregnancy changes are normal and not dangerous to mother or fetus.

More than 80% of women experience NVP. Symptoms are generally worst during the first trimester, although many women suffer throughout pregnancy. NVP is thought to be related to the β-hCG surge that occurs at approximately 7 weeks of gestation. Estradiol and progesterone also likely play a role. Higher levels of β-hCG in multifetal gestations and molar pregnancies are associated with worse NVP. In evolutionary terms, NVP may provide a protective advantage for the fetus by preventing maternal ingestion of harmful substances during organogenesis. Conservative management through dietary and behavioral changes is usually all that is necessary. Medications are indicated when symptoms are severe and lifestyle changes fail to improve NVP. Pyridoxine (vitamin B_6) either alone or in combination with doxylamine improves symptoms of NVP. Several antihistamines and phenothiazines also are effective for treating NVP. Some studies demonstrate that ginger and acupressure at the P6 Neiguan point improve NVP, but further RCTs are needed.

Gastrointestinal issues are common to pregnancy. Alterations in hormones, especially progesterone, result in relaxation of the lower esophageal sphincter, increased bowel transit time, and changes in bowel function. Heartburn is common and occurs during all three trimesters of pregnancy. Symptoms tend to worsen as the pregnancy progresses and resolve after delivery. Lifestyle and dietary changes are recommended as first-line therapy. H$_2$ blockers have a good safety profile and extensive clinical use in treating heartburn/GERD during pregnancy. Antacids are generally considered safe; bicarbonate-based formulations should be avoided secondary to risks of metabolic alkalosis. PPIs are also likely safe, although they have not been as widely used as H$_2$ blockers in the clinical setting.

Exercise and increasing fluid and fiber intake help to prevent constipation. Sitz baths, steroid creams, and witch hazel are likely safe during pregnancy, although no large RCTs have been conducted. Hydroxyethylrutosides are plant flavonoids thought to decrease rectal mucosal capillary fragility and improve hemorrhoids. Their safety profile in pregnancy is unknown and more research is needed before rutosides are recommended.

Musculoskeletal and skin changes impact many expectant women. Striae gravidarum are often quite disconcerting. No current therapies definitively prevent stretch marks. Women should be reassured that striae usually fade to some degree after delivery. Laser therapy, abdominoplasty, and 1% tretinoin cream are treatment options after delivery in severe cases.

LBPP is common, especially late in gestation. Women with prepregnancy low back pain and younger parturients tend to be at higher risk for LBPP. The etiology and pathophysiology are still poorly understood. A combination of postural changes, joint mobility, and hormonal alterations is likely responsible. Little research has been done on LBPP, and encouraging good posture, reasonable footwear, and water aerobics may improve symptoms.

Pregnancy is a period of multiple physical and emotional changes. The majority of these changes are normal and expected. Anticipatory counseling early in pregnancy allows women to be proactive in understanding and dealing with these common but self-limited issues.

Suggested Reading

Badell M, Ramin S, Smith J: Treatment options for nausea and vomiting during pregnancy. *Pharmacotherapy* 26(9):1273–1287, 2006.

Choby BA:*Pregnancy Care*, FP Essentials No. 292, AAFP Home Study. Leawood, KS: American Academy of Family Physicians, 2003.

Fell D, Dodds L, Joseph K, et al: Risk factors for hyperemesis gravidarum requiring hospital admission during pregnancy. *Obstet Gynecol* 107(2):277–284, 2006.

Jewell D, Young G: Interventions for nausea and vomiting in pregnancy. *Cochrane Database Syst Rev* (4):CD000145, 2003.

Mogren IM, Pohjanen AI: Low back pain and pelvic pain during pregnancy. *Spine* 30(8):983–991, 2005.

Nussbaum R, Benedetto A: Cosmetic aspects of pregnancy. *Clin Dermatol* 24:133–141, 2006.

Quijano CE, Abalos E: Conservative management of symptomatic and/ or complicated haemorrhoids in pregnancy and the puerperium. *Cochrane Database Syst Rev* (3):CD004077, 2005.

Thukral C, Wolf J: Therapy insight: Drugs for gastrointestinal disorders in pregnant women. *Gastroenterol Hepatol* 3(5):256–266, 2006.

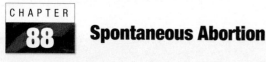

CHAPTER

88 Spontaneous Abortion

CLINICAL CASE PROBLEM 1

Evaluating Bleeding in Early Pregnancy

A 34-year-old female (gravida 2, para 1) presents to the clinic with bleeding during pregnancy. She reports that it has been 6 weeks since her last menstrual period. She had a positive home pregnancy test 1 week ago and is scheduled for her first obstetrical appointment in 3 weeks. She is complaining of light vaginal bleeding without abdominal cramping or backache. She states that her symptoms began this morning. She has no orthostatic symptoms. There are no other systemic symptoms, including fever, abdominal pain, or vomiting. Her previous medical and obstetrical history is uncomplicated. Physical examination shows that she is tearful. Vital signs reveal temperature 97.8°F, pulse 76 beats/minute, blood pressure 126/78 mmHg, and respiratory rate 20 breaths/minute. Her vital signs do not significantly change with orthostatic testing. Her abdomen is soft and flat. She has active bowel sounds. Pelvic exam shows a small amount of bright red bleeding coming from the cervical os. The uterus is parous and consistent with her dating history. Adnexal structures are normal to bimanual exam. Her urine pregnancy test is positive.

1. Vaginal bleeding in pregnancy before 20 weeks of gestation is defined as
   a. complete abortion
   b. threatened abortion

c. incomplete abortion
d. inevitable abortion
e. missed abortion

2. Which of the following conditions is the most common complication of a recognized pregnancy in the United States?
a. diabetes
b. threatened abortion
c. incomplete abortion
d. hypertension
e. inevitable abortion

3. In the management of this patient, you decide she is clinically stable. The local hospital is able to provide timely testing for you. Which of the following tests is least helpful at this time?
a. complete blood count
b. quantitative human chorionic gonadotropin (β-hCG) level
c. vaginal probe ultrasound examination
d. vaginal pH testing
e. progesterone level

4. During a follow-up visit at your clinic, this patient notes that bleeding has stopped. She has no pain or cramping. Her testing shows a quantitative β-hCG level of 950 mIU/mL, and no gestational sac is noted on pelvic ultrasound. You decide to do the following:
a. refer to surgery for ectopic pregnancy
b. repeat quantitative β-hCG level in 48 hours
c. inform the patient that she likely has completed her miscarriage, and no further workup is needed
d. inform the patient that she has a nonviable pregnancy
e. refer the patient for a dilation and curettage procedure for missed abortion

CLINICAL CASE PROBLEM 2

Follow-Up of Spontaneous Abortion

A 28-year-old (gravida 1, para 0) patient comes to see you for a follow-up clinic visit. She experienced vaginal bleeding in early pregnancy. Initially, she presented with light vaginal bleeding at 10 weeks of gestation. Her initial ultrasound was reassuring, with normal fetal growth and definite heartbeat. A few days later, she began having heavy bleeding. Follow-up testing showed an incomplete abortion. You discussed surgical, medical, and expectant management. She chose expectant management and is here for follow-up.

5. Fetal heartbeat seen on ultrasound testing has been noted to be reassuring. What percentage of pregnancies with early bleeding and documented fetal heartbeat on ultrasound testing have eventual miscarriage?
a. 50%
b. 33%
c. 20%
d. 10%
e. 5% or less

6. Many women choose expectant management for spontaneous abortion. Which of the following statements is true when comparing expectant management with surgical management of a spontaneous abortion?
a. most women who choose expectant management of spontaneous abortion will eventually require a surgical procedure
b. women tend to experience more bleeding with surgical treatment of spontaneous abortion
c. women with very heavy bleeding and orthostatic symptoms can be managed expectantly as long as good follow-up is available
d. more women undergoing expectant management will experience incomplete abortion
e. women report significantly more days of sick leave after surgical management of spontaneous abortion

7. Medical regimens exist as treatment options for spontaneous abortion. Misoprostol is part of many of these regimens. Which of the following statements is (are) true regarding use of misoprostol in the medical management of spontaneous abortion?
a. misoprostol is Food and Drug Administration (FDA) approved for labor induction of term pregnancies
b. misoprostol is FDA approved for medical management of spontaneous abortion
c. misoprostol can cause gastrointestinal side effects, including nausea and diarrhea
d. there is a minimal risk of pelvic cramping when using oral misoprostol for medical management of spontaneous abortion
e. all of the above

8. In an uncomplicated pregnancy, which of the following factors does not increase the risk for spontaneous abortion?
a. cigarette smoking
b. sexual activity
c. alcohol use

d. advanced maternal age

e. uncontrolled diabetes mellitus

9. Chromosomal abnormalities are the most common cause of first trimester spontaneous abortion. Which chromosomal abnormality is most commonly found when investigating spontaneous abortion?
a. polyploidy
b. autosomal trisomy
c. autosomal monosomy
d. sex chromosome polysomy
e. sex chromosome monosomy

10. The patient continues to be managed expectantly and experiences a completed spontaneous abortion without need for surgical instrumentation. She is now concerned that she will experience recurrent abortion. What is the definition of recurrent abortion?
a. any number of spontaneous abortions that concern a patient
b. two or more consecutive spontaneous abortions
c. two or more nonconsecutive spontaneous abortions that occur during a patient's lifetime
d. three or more consecutive spontaneous abortions
e. three or more nonconsecutive spontaneous abortions that occur during a patient's lifetime

11. Which of the following conditions is (are) a known cause(s) of recurrent spontaneous abortion?
a. celiac disease
b. antiphospholipid antibody syndrome
c. hypothyroidism
d. hypertension
e. all of the above

12. In the 6 months following miscarriage, women are at increased risk for which of the following disorders?
a. depressive disorder
b. anxiety disorder
c. obsessive–compulsive disorder
d. all of the above
e. a and b

Clinical Case Management Problem

List the differential diagnosis of first trimester vaginal bleeding.

Answers

1. a. Threatened abortion is defined as any vaginal bleeding that occurs in pregnancy before 20 weeks of gestation. Complete abortion is the spontaneous and complete passage of all products of conception. Incomplete abortion is the spontaneous but incomplete passage of the products of conception. By definition, retention of products of conception, which may include the fetus, placenta, or membranes, is seen in an incomplete abortion. Missed abortion is the retention of all products of conception after the death of the fetus. This condition may exist for days or weeks without significant symptoms. Inevitable abortion is the spontaneous rupture of membranes or dilation of the cervix before 20 weeks of gestation.

2. b. Threatened abortion is the most common complication of recognized pregnancies in the United States. Approximately 20% of recognized pregnancies in the United States will be complicated by first trimester bleeding. Fifty percent of pregnancies complicated by early vaginal bleeding will abort. The remaining pregnancies have a higher risk of preterm labor, low birth weight, and perinatal morbidity.

Early complete abortion has been detected in up to 30% of pregnancies. However, most of these pregnancies are unrecognized. These pregnancies are only detected by β-hCG testing. Women with very early spontaneous abortions usually report a painful or heavy period without recognition of the pregnancy.

3. d. Vaginal pH testing is not used clinically in the evaluation of first trimester vaginal bleeding. Although this patient is clinically stable, most clinicians would order a complete blood count at presentation. This test can rule out clinically significant occult bleeding and gives a baseline reference value if the patient continues to bleed. The quantitative serum β-hCG level and vaginal probe ultrasound are used together to determine the presence of viable pregnancy. Serum β-hCG is detectable when it reaches a level of 5 mIU/mL. In a normal pregnancy, the serum β-hCG doubles every 1.8 to 2.1 days and peaks at 100,000 mIU/mL. Vaginal probe ultrasound can detect signs of intrauterine pregnancy when the β-hCG level reaches the discriminatory zone. The discriminatory zone is different for each institution but usually correlates with a quantitative β-hCG level of approximately 1500 mIU/mL. Vaginal probe ultrasound can also detect signs of ectopic pregnancy or significant abnormalities consistent with a nonviable pregnancy. Serum progesterone levels can also help determine the viability of a pregnancy. The serum progesterone level remains stable in the first trimester, and a serum progesterone level higher than 25 ng/mL is highly suggestive of a viable intrauterine pregnancy.

4. b. The patient described is clinically stable. Her bleeding has stopped. Because her quantitative serum β-hCG level is below the discriminatory zone, it is impossible to determine if she has a viable intrauterine pregnancy. As long as she remains clinically stable and has adequate support and transportation options, she can be observed and managed expectantly. However, she should be informed of the risk of ectopic pregnancy when an empty uterus is seen on ultrasound. She needs to seek emergency care if heavy bleeding or severe pelvic pain occur.

A repeat quantitative β-hCG level in 48 hours will help determine prognosis. Most viable pregnancies show doubling of the serum β-hCG level every 48 to 72 hours. If the quantitative serum β-hCG level is following such a pattern and she remains stable, a repeat ultrasound should be ordered when her β-hCG level is above the discriminatory zone. If the β-hCG level drops slowly or plateaus, she is at risk for ectopic pregnancy. Referral to surgery is strongly recommended.

5. e. Transvaginal ultrasound examination of early pregnancy can give prognostic information for the patient with vaginal bleeding. A normal intrauterine gestational sac, normal fetal anatomy, and fetal heartbeat on ultrasound examination increase the probability that the pregnancy will continue. For patients with vaginal bleeding in early pregnancy, a normal intrauterine fetal heartbeat seen on ultrasound examination decreases the risk of spontaneous abortion from approximately 50% to 3%.

6. d. Numerous studies have compared surgical and expectant management of spontaneous abortion. Expectant management of spontaneous abortion involves supporting women throughout the process of expelling products of conception. Serial quantitative β-hCG levels are needed to document the complete passage of tissue. A quantitative β-hCG level should be tested every few days to verify that it is dropping at an adequate rate. Surgical treatment involves the dilation and curettage of the uterus. Ultrasound examination and repeat quantitative serum β-hCG testing can document adequate treatment.

Comparison studies have shown that women managed expectantly have an increased risk of incomplete abortion and increased bleeding. Surgical intervention may increase the risk of pelvic infection. A review of randomized controlled trials shows no clear benefit to either surgical or expectant management of spontaneous

abortion with regard to pain or days of work missed. As long as the risks and benefits of treatment options are understood and bleeding is not worrisome, a woman's preference should guide treatment options. Medical treatment options are an alternate choice for many women.

7. c. Misoprostol is a synthetic prostaglandin E₁ analogue. It can cause significant gastrointestinal side effects. Misoprostol is FDA approved for the prevention and treatment of peptic ulcers. Although it has been widely used for labor induction and medical management of spontaneous abortion, it has not received FDA approval for these health issues. It has been included in many medical regimens for management of first trimester incomplete abortion and missed abortion. Misoprostol has been used vaginally and orally for these purposes and can cause uterine contractions and pelvic cramping.

8. b. Sexual activity does not increase the risk of spontaneous abortion. Factors that have been associated with spontaneous abortion include advanced maternal age, alcohol use, heavy caffeine use (three or more cups of coffee a day), poorly controlled diabetes, celiac disease, autoimmune disease, cigarette smoking, cocaine use, maternal infections, certain medication use, and uterine abnormalities.

9. b. Autosomal trisomy is the most commonly identified genetic abnormality associated with early pregnancy loss. Most of these chromosomal abnormalities are spontaneous events. Autosomal trisomy is more frequent with advanced maternal age. Paternal or maternal chromosomal defects (e.g., translocations) are rarely the cause of an isolated spontaneous abortion. Some studies have demonstrated that the rate of maternal and paternal chromosomal abnormalities among couples with recurrent abortion is higher than that of couples with no such history. However, this rate is still relatively rare at approximately 6%.

Polyploidy is defined as the presence of more than two haploid complements. It is thought to be caused by dispermy. Autosomal monosomy is rarely seen. Sex chromosome monosomy (Turner X) and sex chromosome polysomy are compatible with life. Although sex chromosome monosomy is frequently encountered in the chromosomal evaluation of fetal loss, sex chromosome abnormalities are not as frequent as somatic trisomies.

10. d. Recurrent pregnancy loss or recurrent abortion is defined as three consecutive pregnancy losses. Approximately 15% of couples will experience a single recognized pregnancy loss. Two percent of couples will experience two consecutive pregnancy losses. The risk of three consecutive pregnancy losses is less than 1%. Couples who experience isolated loss should be counseled on the usual causes of spontaneous abortion and the recurrence rates. Although a previous miscarriage increases the risk of miscarriage in subsequent pregnancies, most women who have a first trimester spontaneous abortion will not experience consecutive losses.

11. **b.** Antiphospholipid syndrome is an important cause of recurrent miscarriage. The prevalence of this disease in patients with recurrent spontaneous abortion is approximately 15%. The disease state is associated with a 90% spontaneous abortion rate if untreated. Interestingly, early descriptions of antiphospholipid syndrome included recurrent spontaneous abortion

as part of the clinical criteria. Treatment of antiphospholipid antibody syndrome with aspirin and heparin greatly increases the chance of viable pregnancy. Hypothyroidism, hypertension, and celiac disease have not been shown to be significant causes of recurrent spontaneous abortion.

12. **d.** Women undergoing formal psychiatric testing and follow-up after miscarriage show higher rates of depression, anxiety, and obsessive–compulsive disorder. Women who have had a previous history of these psychiatric disorders, are childless, or have lost a wanted pregnancy are at particular risk. Because of these issues, it may be beneficial to screen for the presence of these disorders. Supportive counseling, including acknowledgment and legitimization of grief issues and guilt, may be helpful. Referral for psychological counseling or psychiatric treatment may be necessary.

Solution to the Clinical Case Management Problem

The differential diagnosis of first trimester vaginal bleeding includes the following:

Bleeding associated with implantation
Spontaneous abortion
Ectopic pregnancy
Cervicitis

Vaginal or cervical trauma
Idiopathic
Subchorionic hemorrhage
Molar pregnancy
Cervical cancer or dysplasia
Cervical polyp

Summary

1. Classification of spontaneous abortion

Threatened abortion is defined as any vaginal bleeding that occurs in pregnancy before 20 weeks of gestation. See answer 1 for the complete definition of the various types of spontaneous abortion.

2. Occurrence

Threatened abortion is the most common complication of recognized pregnancy in the United States. It occurs in approximately 20% of recognized pregnancies. Pregnancy loss occurs in approximately 10% to 15% of recognized pregnancies.

3. Diagnosis and evaluation

Evaluation of early pregnancy bleeding must take into account the clinical stability of the patient. Ectopic pregnancy and bleeding associated with spontaneous abortion remain a common cause of maternal morbidity and mortality. Patients who are clinically unstable

must be treated with resuscitation efforts and immediate surgical consultation. Clinically stable patients may undergo diagnostic measures to determine the location and viability of pregnancy. Testing of quantitative β-hCG hormone levels and ultrasound imaging help determine the viability of the pregnancy. Viable pregnancies are visible on ultrasound imaging when the β-hCG level is above the discriminatory zone. Serum β-hCG levels should increase by at least 66% every 48 hours in viable pregnancies.

4. Management

Surgical, medical, and expectant management are options for the stable patient with spontaneous abortion. Surgical treatment with dilation and curettage has been shown to decrease the risk of incomplete abortion. Because each treatment option has advantages and disadvantages, a woman's preference should be taken into consideration.

Suggested Reading

Brier N: Anxiety after miscarriage: A review of the empirical literature and implications for clinical practice. *Birth* 31(2):138–142, 2004.

Griebel CP, Halvorsen J, Golemon TB, Day AA: Management of spontaneous abortion. *Am Fam Physician* 72(7):1243–1250, 2005.

Nanda K, Peloggia A, Grimes D, et al: Expectant care versus surgical treatment for miscarriage (review). *Cochrane Database Sys Rev* 19(2):1–24, 2006.

Neilson JP, Hickey M, Vazquez J: Medical treatment for early fetal death (less than 24 weeks). *Cochrane Database Syst Rev* (3) CD002253, 2006.

Rai R, Regan L: Recurrent miscarriage. *Lancet* 368(9535):601–611, 2006.

Sotiriadis A., Paptheodorou S, Makrydimas M: Threatened miscarriage: Evaluation and management. *BMJ* 329(7458):152–159, 2004.

CHAPTER

89 Thyroid Disease in Pregnancy

CLINICAL CASE PROBLEM 1

Pregnancy, Fatigue, and an Enlarged Prostate

A 27-year-old female (gravida 2, para 1) presents to your office for prenatal care. She is approximately 6 weeks pregnant based on her last menstrual period. Her first pregnancy was uncomplicated and she had a spontaneous vaginal delivery. Past medical history is unremarkable. She has been taking prenatal vitamins for the past month. She has no major complaints except fatigue and constipation. The fatigue is more pronounced than with her first pregnancy. She attributes this to working full-time and raising a 12-month-old infant.

On physical examination, she has an elevated body mass index (33) and pulse of 55 beats/minute. The conjunctiva are pale, the oropharynx is normal, and the neck is supple. The thyroid gland is diffusely enlarged and tender; no bruits or nodules are noted. The remainder of the exam is unremarkable except for a 6-week size uterus.

1. Which of the following is the best option at this time?
   a. order a hemoglobin/hematocrit to evaluate for anemia
   b. reassure the patient that changes are a normal part of pregnancy
   c. order thyroid-stimulating hormone (TSH)
   d. order thyroxine (T4) level
   e. ask her to discontinue iron therapy

A prenatal panel and TSH are drawn. The hemoglobin and hematocrit are within normal range. The TSH is 4.5 mIU/L (reference range, 0.45 to 4.5 mIU/L).

2. What is the appropriate next step?
   a. the test should be repeated in 30 to 60 days
   b. no further workup is indicated
   c. a free T4 should be drawn
   d. an increase in serum TSH is normal in early pregnancy because of cross-reactivity with β-human chorionic gonadotropin (β-hCG)
   e. TSH levels are unreliable during pregnancy

3. Which of the following changes in thyroid function is expected during the first trimester?
   a. inhibition of the thyroid by β-hCG
   b. decrease in thyroid binding globulin (TBG)
   c. increase in iodine availability due to decreased renal clearance
   d. increase in TSH levels during the first trimester that mirrors the rise in β-hCG
   e. decline in iodine availability due to increased fetal and placental needs

4. The patient's T4 is 0.6 μg/dL (reference range, 0.7 to 1.8 μg/dL). You diagnose her with hypothyroidism. Which of the following labs is most helpful at this time?
   a. liver function tests
   b. fasting lipid panel
   c. thyroid peroxidase antibody (TPO Ab) levels
   d. fasting blood glucose
   e. cortisol level

5. Pregnancy complications associated with maternal hypothyroidism include which of the following?
   a. cervical insufficiency
   b. gestational hypotension
   c. macrosomia
   d. preterm delivery
   e. postterm pregnancy

6. Which of the following statements about treatment of hypothyroidism in pregnancy is false?
   a. levothyroxine sodium is the recommend first-line therapy

b. the starting dose of levothyroxine ranges from 1 to 2 µg/kg/day (average, 100 µg daily)

c. the therapeutic TSH goal is 0.5 to 2.5 mIU/L

d. combination T4/triiodothyronine (T3) therapy is useful in women who fail to respond to levothyroxine alone

e. TSH levels are checked 4 to 6 weeks after dosage adjustments

7. Which of the following medications does not interfere with T4 absorption?
   a. calcium carbonate
   b. carbamazepine
   c. ferrous sulfate
   d. cholestyramine
   e. colestipol

8. What is the most common cause of primary hypothyroidism in pregnancy?
   a. chronic autoimmune thyroiditis
   b. history of thyroidectomy
   c. Graves' disease
   d. Sheehan's syndrome
   e. iodine deficiency

9. Which of the following statements regarding screening pregnant women for hypothyroidism is false?
   a. all women with hypothyroidism should be screened with TSH in the preconception period
   b. all pregnant women should be screened using TSH during the first trimester
   c. universal screening for thyroid function during pregnancy is not recommended by the American Thyroid Association (ATA) or the American Association of Clinical Endocrinologists (AACE)
   d. women at high risk for developing hypothyroidism in pregnancy include those with type 1 diabetes, autoimmune disorders, or a personal or family history of thyroid dysfunction
   e. maternal subclinical hypothyroidism in the first trimester is linked to deficits in neurologic and psychological development in offspring

CLINICAL CASE PROBLEM 2

"Doctor, My Heart Is Fluttering"

A 33-year-old female (gravida 3, para 2) at 28 weeks of gestation presents to the office for a routine prenatal visit. She complains about feeling "more nervous and jittery" during the past month. Her heart "flutters" if she walks more than 5 minutes. On physical examination, her pulse is 110 beats/minute

and her weight has decreased by 5 pounds during the past month. Her neck exam shows nontender thyromegaly. No bruit or nodule is noted. Fundal height is 27 cm. Results of laboratory testing show a TSH less than 0.1 mIU/L and a free T4 level of 2 µg/dL (range, 0.7 to 1.8 µg/dL).

10. What is the most likely diagnosis at this time?
    a. subclinical hypothyroidism
    b. gestational transient thyrotoxicosis
    c. overt hyperthyroidism
    d. pheochromocytoma
    e. T3 thyrotoxicosis

11. Maternal complications of untreated hyperthyroidism include
    a. postterm pregnancy
    b. hypotension
    c. spontaneous pregnancy loss
    d. cervical insufficiency
    e. placenta accretia

12. Which of the following statements regarding treatment of hyperthyroidism during pregnancy is correct?
    a. thioamide medications are no longer considered first-line therapy
    b. treatment with radioactive iodine improves maternal symptoms with limited fetal risk
    c. thyroidectomy is contraindicated in pregnant women
    d. methimazole and propylthiouracil (PTU) are the two most commonly used thioamides for therapy in the United States
    e. overtreatment of hyperthyroidism has no adverse fetal consequences

13. Which of the following statements regarding thioamide use is untrue?
    a. some case studies report fetal choanal atresia with the use of methimazole in early pregnancy
    b. serial white blood cell monitoring is essential when using thioamides
    c. PTU is less likely than methimazole to cross the placenta
    d. women taking thioamides should be counseled to discontinue the medication immediately if they develop fever or sore throat
    e. transient leucopenia occurs in 10% of women taking thioamides

14. Which of the following statements concerning postpartum thyroiditis is correct?
    a. 15% to 20% of recently delivered women are affected

b. there is an association with human leukocyte antigens HLA-DRB, -DR4, and -DR5
c. symptoms most often develop during postpartum weeks 2 to 6
d. elevated levels of anti-thyroid peroxidase antibodies are uncommon
e. 10% of women develop permanent hypothyroidism within a decade

Answers

1. c. Between 1 and 3/1000 pregnancies are complicated by hypothyroidism. Vague, nonspecific symptoms are frequently attributed to signs of early pregnancy. Fatigue, cold intolerance, constipation, and myalgia are common complaints. Although the thyroid gland increases in size by approximately 15% during pregnancy, this is not usually detectable on clinical exam. Findings of thyroid enlargement or tenderness warrant further workup. Serum TSH is more sensitive for detecting hypo- or hyperthyroidism than T4.

2. c. Although the patient's TSH is technically within lab reference range, true "normal" ranges for TSH are unclear. Research shows that 95% of healthy individuals have TSH levels below 2.5 mU/L. Those with TSH between 2.5 and 4.5 mU/L are at increased risk for progressing to overt thyroid disease. Laboratory references are based on the range of values found in large patient populations. Many individuals have occult thyroid disease (i.e., subclinical hypothyroidism), which skews the reference range for TSH. A more narrow range (0.45 to 3 mIU/mL) may better detect thyroid abnormalities, although there is an increased risk for diagnosing individuals with asymptomatic subacute hypothyroidism.

Repeating the TSH in 30 to 60 days is an appropriate option for a nonpregnant patient. Untreated hypothyroidism during pregnancy results in adverse outcomes, so checking free T4 is important. TSH levels in early pregnancy decrease due to cross-reactivity with β-hCG. TSH levels in pregnancy vary by trimester; the upper limit of normal in the first trimester is 3 mIU/L.

3. e. TSH levels decrease in early pregnancy due to the weak thyrotropic effects of β-hCG. High β-hCG levels increase thyroid hormone production and cause feedback inhibition of TSH. A threefold increase in thyroid binding globulin is maintained throughout pregnancy. Increased iodine requirements result from preferential iodine uptake by the fetus and placenta and increased renal clearance.

4. c. Specific antibodies are common in pregnant women who have hypothyroidism. The presence of TPO Ab may increase the risk of pregnancy complications, postpartum thyroiditis, and eventual thyroid failure. Half of women with TPO Ab at 16 weeks of gestation develop postpartum thyroid problems. Fasting lipid levels are often spuriously elevated during pregnancy. Liver function tests and fasting blood glucose are also affected by hypothyroidism.

5. d. Several complications are noted in pregnant women with uncontrolled hypothyroidism. Spontaneous pregnancy loss, preterm delivery, low birth weight, gestational hypertension, and fetal distress are associated outcomes. Postterm pregnancy is not related to hypothyroidism in pregnancy.

6. d. Levothyroxine is the drug of choice for hypothyroidism in pregnancy. Starting with a full replacement dose of 1 or 2 µg/kg/day is safe in pregnant women with negative cardiac histories. TSH should be rechecked after 4 to 6 weeks of therapy. Adjustment of the dose to maintain TSH levels between 0.5 and 2.5 mIU/L is recommended. The 6- or 7-day half-life of levothyroxine permits once daily dosing and causes no significant fluctuations if an occasional dose is forgotten. T3 has a short half-life and requires multiple daily doses. Neither T3 nor T3/T4 combination therapy is recommended in pregnancy secondary to safety concerns and lack of superiority over levothyroxine.

7. b. Gastrointestinal T4 absorption is influenced by foods and medications that affect the uptake and metabolic clearance of T4. Absorption levels decrease slightly when T4 is taken with food. Carafate, calcium carbonate, iron supplements, cholestyramine, and colestipol all reduce T4 absorption. Medications that enhance the metabolism and clearance of T4 include phenytoin and carbamazepine.

8. a. Chronic autoimmune thyroiditis (Hashimoto's disease) is the most common cause of primary hypothyroidism in pregnancy. It is associated with painless thyroid enlargement and inflammation. Fibrosis, lymphocytic and eosinophilic infiltration of the thyroid, and parenchymal atrophy are common. Anti-TPO and anti-microsomal antibodies are associated with Hashimoto's thyroiditis. Both thyroidectomy and iodine deficiency are less common causes of primary hypothyroidism. Sheehan's syndrome results from obstetric hemorrhage and pituitary infarction. Considered a type of secondary hypothyroidism, Sheehan's syndrome causes deficiencies in several pituitary hormones. Graves' disease is a cause of hyperthyroidism.

9. **b.** Screening guidelines from ATA and AACE are based on expert consensus. ATA and AACE recommend "aggressive case finding" in certain women considered high risk for thyroid disorders. Insulin-dependent diabetes, autoimmune disease, a personal or family history of thyroid problems, or signs and symptoms of thyroid dysfunction are all considered risk factors. These screening guidelines are based on expert consensus. In a prospective trial, targeted case-finding missed one-third of pregnant women with overt or subclinical hypothyroidism during the first trimester of pregnancy.

Maternal T3 and T4 are the only sources of thyroid hormone available to the fetus in the initial 12 weeks of gestation. Fetuses exposed to hypothyroidism in the first trimester are at higher risk for adverse sequelae. Women with preexisting thyroid abnormalities are best screened during the preconception period.

10. **c.** Hyperthyroidism affects 2 out of 1000 pregnancies and is most commonly caused by Graves' disease. Other causes include toxic nodular goiter, thyroiditis, intake of excessive thyroid hormone, and functional adenoma. Pheochromocytoma is not consistent with the laboratory findings. A mildly elevated TSH with low-normal T4 is indicative of subclinical hypothyroidism. Gestational transient thyrotoxicosis is a form of hyperthyroidism associated with hyperemesis gravidarum and molar pregnancy. High β-hCG levels cross-react with the TSH receptor and cause temporary hyperthyroidism. Patients are rarely symptomatic and pharmacologic therapy is not necessary. Symptoms generally abate by the end of the first trimester, although TSH levels may remain spuriously decreased for several weeks. Gestational thyrotoxicosis is not associated with untoward pregnancy outcomes.

11. **c.** Untreated hyperthyroidism places pregnant women at risk for preterm labor, gestational hypertension, eclampsia, abruption, preterm labor, spontaneous pregnancy loss, congestive heart failure, and thyroid storm. It is not associated with cervical insufficiency, placenta accretia, or postdate pregnancy.

12. **d.** Thyrotoxicosis during pregnancy is controlled using thioamides such as methimazole and propylthiouracil. Overtreatment with these medications results in maternal and fetal hypothyroidism. In women who develop drug toxicity or are unable to comply with therapy, thyroidectomy may be considered after the first trimester. Ablative radioactive iodine therapy is contraindicated in pregnancy because of damage to the fetal thyroid. Nongravid women should avoid pregnancy for 6 to 12 months after receiving this therapy.

13. **b.** Ten percent of pregnant women taking thioamides develop leukopenia that generally does not require termination of therapy; 0.2% of women develop acute agranulocytosis. Due to the rapid onset of this condition, serial leukocyte counts are not useful. All pregnant women taking thioamides must discontinue the medication immediately if they develop fever or sore throat. Urgent evaluation for agranulocytosis should follow.

PTU inhibits peripheral conversion of T4 to T3 to some extent. It is less likely than methimazole to cross the placenta. First trimester use of methimazole may be associated with fetal aplasia cutis and choanal and esophageal atresia.

14. **b.** Postpartum thyroiditis affects between 5% and 7% of women after delivery. A firm, nontender goiter usually appears 2 to 6 months postpartum. Postpartum thyroiditis and Hashimoto's disease are both associated with HLA-DRB, -DR4, and -DR5. Elevated levels of antithyroid peroxidase (TPO) are noted in 80% of women. Although the majority of women are euthyroid by 1 year following delivery, 30% to 50% of these women will develop permanent hypothyroidism within a decade.

Summary

The function of the thyroid gland during pregnancy is dynamic. Alterations in levels of TBG, T4, T3, and TSH begin during the first trimester. Whereas levels of T4 and T3 are similar to those in a nonpregnant state, TSH levels vary by trimester. In the first trimester, β-hCG weakly stimulates thyroid receptors, causing an inhibitory feedback mechanism on TSH. TBG increases two- or threefold in order to accommodate increases in T4. Increased amounts of iodine are needed due to increased fetal uptake and increased maternal renal clearance.

Adequate levels of thyroid hormone are essential to healthy fetal development.

Thyroid dysfunction affects significant numbers of women during pregnancy.

One or two per 1000 pregnant women develop hypothyroidism. Maternal complications of untreated hypothyroidism include spontaneous pregnancy loss, preterm delivery, low birth weight, and gestational hypertension. Fetal complications include preterm delivery and impaired neurologic development. Symptoms of hypothyroidism include constipation, cold intolerance, fatigue, and myalgia. Complaints are often attributed to normal changes of pregnancy.

Universal screening for thyroid disorders during pregnancy is not currently recommended by ATA or AACE (expert opinion). Both groups recommend "aggressive case finding" in certain women at risk for thyroid disorders. Insulin-dependent diabetes, autoimmune disease, a personal or family history of thyroid problems, or signs and symptoms suggestive of thyroid dysfunction are considered at-risk categories.

In women with risk factors or symptoms, TSH is the recommended screening test.

TSH levels vary during pregnancy, and an abnormal result must be interpreted according to gestational age. The range of TSH in normal pregnancies is generally estimated to be between 0.5 and 2.5 mIU/L. Free T4 is evaluated if the TSH is abnormal.

Hypothyroidism is diagnosed when TSH is elevated and free T4 is decreased. Levothyroxine is the treatment for hypothyroidism during pregnancy. Initial dosage of this medication is 1 or 2 μg/kg/day. Levothyroxine has a long half-life and extensive clinical use in pregnancy. Neither T3 nor T4/T3 combinations are currently recommended for use in pregnancy.

Hyperthyroidism is characterized by tremors, nervousness, tachycardia, and weight loss. Congestive heart failure and thyroid storm occur in extreme cases. Characterized by depressed levels of TSH and elevated T4, hyperthyroidism is managed using the thioamides PTU and methimazole. Transient leukopenia occurs in 10% of women taking thioamides. The condition usually resolves over time, and the medication need not be discontinued. A total of 0.2% of women develop severe agranulocytosis. Because agranulocytosis occurs rapidly and without warning, serial white blood cell counts are not helpful with this diagnosis. Patients should be counseled to stop taking the drug if a fever or sore throat develops. Some case studies note fetal anomalies, such as choanal and esophageal atresia, in fetuses of women taking methimazole during the first trimester. In women unable to tolerate thioamides secondary to toxicity or compliance issues, thyroidectomy sometimes becomes necessary.

Postpartum thyroiditis affects 5% to 7% of women after delivery. Incidence is highest in the second to sixth month postpartum. The majority of women revert to a euthyroid state within 1 year after delivery; 30% to 50% of affected women will develop permanent hypothyroidism within a decade.

Suggested Reading

Bindra A, Braunstein GD: Thyroiditis. *Am Fam Physician* 73(10):1769–1776, 2006.

Casey BM, Leveno KJ: Thyroid disease in pregnancy. *Obstet Gynecol* 108(5):1283–1292, 2006.

Tan TO, Cheng YW, Caughey AB: Are women who are treated for hypothyroidism at risk for pregnancy complications? *Am J Obstet Gynecol* 194:e1–e3, 2006.

Thien-Giang B, Jonklaas J: Thyroid medications during pregnancy. *Ther Drug Monit* 28(3):431–441, 2006.

Vaidya B, Anthony S, Bilous M, et al: Detection of thyroid dysfunction in early pregnancy: Universal screening or targeted high-risk case finding? *J Clin Endocrinol Metab* 92:203–207, 2007.

Wartofsky L, Van Nostrand D, Burman KD: Overt and "subclinical" hypothyroidism in women. *Obstet Gynecol Rev* 61(8):535–542, 2006.

90 Gestational Diabetes and Shoulder Dystocia

CLINICAL CASE PROBLEM 1

23-Year-Old Female with Family History of Diabetes

The patient is a 23-year-old woman whose family has a history of diabetes mellitus. She is currently 28 weeks of gestation.

SELECT THE BEST ANSWER TO THE FOLLOWING QUESTIONS

1. Which of the following statements concerning gestational diabetes screening is correct?
   a. the U.S. Preventive Services Task Force (USPSTF) states that there is insufficient evidence to recommend for or against routine screening for gestational diabetes (I recommendation)
   b. the USPSTF strongly recommends that clinicians routinely provide screening to eligible patients (A recommendation)
   c. the USPSTF recommends that clinicians routinely provide screening to eligible patients (B recommendation)
   d. the USPSTF makes no recommendation for or against routine provision of gestational diabetes screening (C recommendation)
   e. the USPSTF recommends against routinely providing screening to asymptomatic patients (D recommendation)

2. Which of the following is (are) not a major risk factor(s) for gestational diabetes mellitus (GDM)?
   a. family history of diabetes
   b. history of GDM in a previous pregnancy
   c. increased pregravid body mass index (BMI)
   d. young maternal age
   e. advanced maternal age

3. Which of the following populations is most at risk for developing GDM?
   a. Asian women
   b. Hispanic women
   c. white American women
   d. Russian women
   e. Australian women

4. Which of the following statements regarding the 50-g 1-hour glucose challenge test (GCT) done on your patient at 28 weeks is considered true?
   a. half of those with an abnormal GCT will also have a positive 100-g 3-hour oral glucose tolerance test (OGTT)
   b. a threshold of 140 mg/dL detects 90% of those with gestational diabetes when followed by a 100-g 3-hour OGTT
   c. false-negative 50-g GCT is rare (less than 2%)
   d. a venous plasma glucose cutoff of 130 mg/dL detects more than 90% of all women with a positive 100-g 3-hour OGTT
   e. all the above choices are true

5. Your patient has a positive 50-g 1-hour GCT, and her 100-g 3-hour OGTT is also positive. Which of the following is considered a risk factor for macrosomia besides her GDM?
   a. primigravida status
   b. her weight gain of 30 pounds
   c. her BMI of 25
   d. her gestational age of 42 weeks
   e. her height of 5 feet 2 inches

6. Which of the following statements regarding gestational diabetes is true?
   a. the 50-g GCT can only be given to a person who is fasting
   b. women with previous infants of birth weights greater than 9 pounds are at decreased risk of gestational diabetes
   c. metformin therapy is approved by the Food and Drug Administration for treatment of gestational diabetes
   d. insulin therapy should begin when a woman's fasting blood sugar is greater than 105 mg/dL after medical nutrition therapy has been tried
   e. insulin therapy is indicated only when fasting blood sugar levels exceed 140 mg/dL

7. Your patient has "researched the Internet" and calls you because she is concerned about birth trauma. Which of the following statements do you tell her?
   a. two forms of birth trauma encountered in GDM are clavicular fractures and brachial plexus injury
   b. cesarean section will prevent birth trauma and brachial plexus injury
   c. the majority of brachial plexus injuries will resolve within the first year of life
   d. aggressive therapy of birth trauma enhances resolution
   e. induction of labor will decrease the rate of birth trauma

8. Which of the following is not considered a complication of fetal macrosomia?
   a. third- and fourth-degree maternal lacerations
   b. shoulder dystocia
   c. facial nerve injury
   d. increased rate of cesarean delivery
   e. postpartum hemorrhage

9. Of the following, which is the least accurate predictor of macrosomia?
   a. multiparous mother's estimate of fetal weight
   b. ultrasound assessment of fetal weight
   c. clinician's Leopold maneuver
   d. choices a and c have an equivalent predictive value, which is less than that of choice b
   e. none of the above have any predictive value

Your patient goes into labor at 40 weeks of gestation, gradually increasing to fully dilated. She then pushes for 3 hours until you elect to do a vacuum extraction because of maternal exhaustion. You notice immediate "turtling" of the infant's head.

10. The following are appropriate steps in using a vacuum extractor except
    a. applying the cup over the sagittal suture 3 cm in front of the posterior fontanelle
    b. applying continuous pressure against the vacuum until it disengages three times
    c. halting the procedure if there is no progress after three consecutive pulls
    d. releasing the vacuum when the jaw is reachable
    e. none of the above are appropriate steps

11. Which of the following is considered an appropriate measure at this time?
    a. performing slow gradual infant nasopharyngeal suctioning
    b. requesting the nurse to do fundal pressure
    c. performing the Zavanelli procedure (replacing the infant into the uterine cavity)
    d. requesting the nurses do maternal external rotation and flexion at the hip (McRoberts' maneuver)
    e. immediately going to the nurse's station to phone the OB/GYN backup

12. Elements of the Wood's screw maneuver include all of the following except
    a. rotating the infant's head in a counterclockwise manner
    b. applying pressure against the posterior portion of the anterior shoulder, pressing the infant's arm closer to his or her chest
    c. applying pressure on the anterior portion of the posterior shoulder in an attempt to rotate the infant 180 degrees
    d. rocking the infant's shoulder from side to side by pushing on the mother's lower abdomen
    e. pushing the posterior shoulder back up into the pelvis slightly

13. Which of the following is true regarding the incidence of shoulder dystocia?
    a. 22% of infants weighing 4000 to 4500 g will have shoulder dystocia
    b. more than 50% of shoulder dystocia cases occur in normal-weight infants
    c. 5% of infants weighing 2500 to 4000 g will have shoulder dystocia
    d. elective cesarean delivery is considered the delivery method of choice in infants who have an estimated fetal weight of more than 3800 g
    e. all of the above are true

14. The reason for neonatal hypoglycemia is
    a. lack of maternal insulin transfer to the baby after delivery
    b. lack of maternal glucose transfer after delivery
    c. overproduction of fetal blood sugars
    d. overproduction of fetal insulin with lack of maternal sugars
    e. most babies of diabetic mothers suffer from hyperglycemia

15. Your patient is concerned about the future: "What will happen after the delivery?" You assure her that
    a. she will be euglycemic in the future
    b. her child's health is assured: "Your child will be fine"
    c. she and her child are at increased risk for diabetes mellitus as well as obesity in the future
    d. her future pregnancy will be normal
    e. she should not have been screened since screening and treatment for gestational diabetes do not improve the outcome

---

Clinical Case Management Problem

1. Name at least four risk factors for developing gestational diabetes.
2. Name at least four abnormalities that maternal gestational diabetes puts the fetus at greater risk of developing.

Answers

1. **a.** The most current available literature for and against routine screening for gestational diabetes shows that there is insufficient evidence. The USPSTF gives it an I rating. The USPSTF rates its final recommendation for screening tests as A, B, C, D, or I. The A recommendation means that the USPTF found good evidence that screening improves important health outcomes and concludes that benefits substantially outweigh potential harm. B recommendation states that the USPSTF found at least fair evidence that screening improves important health outcomes and concludes that benefits outweigh potential harm. C recommendation states that the USPSTF makes no recommendation for or against routine screening because the balance of benefits and harm is too close to justify a general recommendation. D recommendation states that the USPSTF recommends against routinely providing the service to asymptomatic patients because there is fair evidence that the screening is ineffective or that the potential harm outweighs the benefits. An I recommendation means there is insufficient evidence to make a recommendation for or against screening.

2. **d.** According to the USPSTF, all of the listed choices except young maternal age are major risk factors for developing GDM.

3. **b.** The prevalence of GDM varies in direct proportion to the prevalence of type 2 diabetes in a given population or ethnic group. GDM is more common among African American, Hispanic, and American Indian women.

4. **d.** There is still a great deal of confusion and debate about what is or should be considered a "positive" 1-hour GCT. Lowering the threshold of what is considered positive increases the false-positive rate. A threshold of 140 mg/dL detects only 80% of those with gestational diabetes. A threshold of 130 mg/dL detects more than 90% of those with a positive 100-g 3-hour OGTT but significantly increases the false-positive rate. The reliability of GCT is questionable for one-third of women who eventually are identified as having GDM, and even screening performed on two successive days often produces different results. As with all screening, the question arises as to whether screening makes a difference in outcomes, and the evidence in this regard is mixed.

5. **d.** Only her prolonged gestation and her GDM are considered risk factors for macrosomia. Other risk factors include impaired glucose tolerance, multiparity, previous macrosomic infant, maternal obesity, excessive weight gain, prolonged second stage, parental stature, male infant, and need for labor augmentation.

6. **d.** Some women with GDM may be able to control their disease by strict dietary management and glucose testing four times a day. If the woman's fasting glucose is frequently higher than 105, insulin therapy should be initiated. A 50-g GCT can be done nonfasting, and women with infants weighing more than 4500 g are at an increased risk of gestational diabetes. Metformin is not recommended in pregnancy.

7. **a.** The two major forms of birth trauma encountered in gestational diabetes are clavicular fractures and brachial plexus injuries. Performing cesarean sections in general does not lower the risk of birth trauma. The majority of brachial plexus injuries will resolve within the first year of the patient's life; this will account for 80% to 90% of all cases. Most of them will not need any therapy. Binding the arm with a sling will suffice.

8. **e.** Postpartum hemorrhage is not considered a common complication of fetal macrosomia, although it may occur independently as a result of a prolonged second stage. Other complications of macrosomia include brachial plexus injury and asphyxia.

9. **b.** The average weight variance for Leopold's maneuvers is 300 g (11.6 ounces). The average weight variance for ultrasound is 300 to 550 g (11.6 to 19.2 ounces). In a study of multiparous mothers' estimations of fetal weight, clinicians' clinical estimates, and ultrasound, the ultrasound estimation was the least accurate of the three methods.

10. **b.** The traction should be halted between contractions, at which time the pressure should be released from the vacuum as well.

11. **d.** In the case of shoulder dystocia, following known protocols decreases potential morbidity and mortality of both infant and mother. Most hospitals have a set procedure for calling emergency backup. Optimally, this should involve nursing staff calling the backup physician. Because time is of the essence, gradual suctioning should be abandoned. Suprapubic, not fundal, pressure should be applied by an experienced staff person. Fundal pressure is more likely to continue jamming the obstructing shoulder into the suprapubis. The Zavanelli procedure should be avoided unless episiotomy has been done. The McRoberts' maneuver, the Wood's screw, removal of the posterior shoulder, and getting the woman into a hands and knees position are procedures that have been successful.

12. **a.** All of the choices listed except rotating the infant's head are considered part of the Wood's screw maneuver. This maneuver allows the infant's shoulders to be delivered much like turning a threaded screw. If the shoulder is extremely impacted, it may be necessary to push either the anterior or the posterior shoulder back up into the pelvis to accomplish the maneuver. Rotating the infant's head is ineffective and may increase the likelihood of brachial nerve palsy.

13. **b.** The majority of cases of shoulder dystocia occur in normal-weight infants. Elective cesarean delivery of infants with macrosomia is not considered the delivery method of choice. To prevent one case of permanent brachial plexus injury, 3700 women with infants with macrosomia would have to undergo elective cesarean delivery at a cost of $8.7 million per case prevented. Only 5% to 7% of infants weighing 4000 to 4500 g will have shoulder dystocia; the risk of shoulder dystocia in infants weighing 2500 to 4000 g is 0.3%.

14. **d.** During pregnancy, maternal glucose crosses the placenta to the fetus, but insulin does not. The baby produces insulin in response to maternal glucose. At birth—with cessation of transfer of maternal glucose and relative slowness of the baby to generate his/her own glucose—fetal insulin production can cause severe hypoglycemia.

15. **d.** It is clear that patients with gestational diabetes have an almost 50% chance of suffering from obesity and developing type II diabetes mellitus in the future. Research confirms that the risk of suffering from glucose intolerance is markedly increased among these patients' children.

Solution to the Clinical Case Management Problem

1. Risk factors for developing gestational diabetes include obesity, a family history of type 2 diabetes, maternal age older than 35 years, and a previous history of gestational diabetes.

2. Fetal risks that are increased in gestational diabetes include fetal macrosomia, intrauterine growth restriction, spontaneous abortion, neural tube defects, skeletal abnormalities, gastrointestinal malformations, and cardiac malformations.

Summary

Figure 90-1 provides a diagnosis and treatment algorithm for gestational diabetes.

1. Known risk factors for gestational diabetes, a common condition in pregnancy, are obesity, family history of type 2 diabetes, maternal age older than 35 years, and a previous history of gestational diabetes.
2. The cutoff value for the 50-g GCT is considered controversial, with some practitioners using 130 mg/dL and others using 140 mg/dL.
3. Patients with positive 3-hour GTT need to undergo strict dietary management and learn to monitor their own blood sugars four times a day. Insulin management is usually suggested for those with fasting blood sugars of more than 105 mg/dL.

4. The risk factors for shoulder dystocia include macrosomia, prolonged second stage of labor, prolonged first stage of labor, prior shoulder dystocia, high pregnancy weight and weight gain, gestational diabetes, and an instrument-assisted delivery.
5. For a shoulder dystocia, it is wise to call for extra assistance (optimally prior to delivery), consider an episiotomy, and have your assistants help the patient with a McRoberts' maneuver. Other measures to assist the delivery may include having the assistant apply suprapubic pressure, performing the Wood's screw maneuver, removing the infant's posterior arm, or having the patient roll into a hands and knees position.

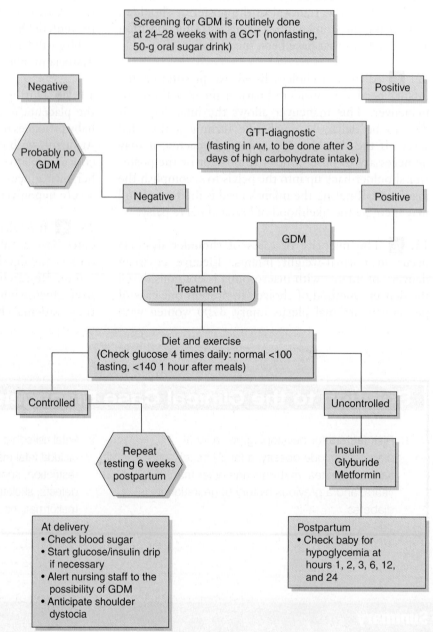

Figure 90-1

Diagnosis and treatment algorithm for gestational diabetes. GCT, glucose challenge test; GDM, gestational diabetes mellitus; GTT, glucose tolerance test.

Suggested Reading

Baxley EG, Gobbo RW: Shoulder dystocia. *Am Fam Physician* 69(7):1707–1714, 2004.

Gherman RB: Shoulder dystocia: An evidence-based evaluation of the obstetric nightmare. *Clin Obstet Gynecol* 45(2):345–362, 2002.

Norwitz ER, et al: Shoulder dystocia. In: Gabbe SG, Niebyl JR, Simpson JL, eds., *Obstetrics—Normal and Problem Pregnancies*, 4th ed. Philadelphia: Churchill Livingstone, 2002.

U.S. Preventive Services Task Force: Screening for gestational diabetes mellitus: Recommendation and rationale. *Am Fam Physician* 68(2):331–335, 2003.

Zamorski MA, Biggs WS: Management of suspected macrosomia. *Am Fam Physician* 63:302–306, 2001.

Hypertension in Pregnancy

CLINICAL CASE PROBLEM 1

A 35-Year-Old Primigravida with Hypertension

A 35-year-old pregnant woman (gravida 2, para 1) comes into the office for her 18-week prenatal appointment. Her blood pressure is 140/94 mmHg when taken by your nurse and is confirmed by your own measurement. She has no protein in her urine and has no headaches, blurred vision, nausea, or vomiting. The rest of the examination is consistent with dates; there is no lower extremity edema.

SELECT THE BEST ANSWER TO THE FOLLOWING QUESTIONS

1. Her diagnosis is
   a. chronic hypertension
   b. preeclampsia/eclampsia
   c. gestational hypertension
   d. labile hypertension
   e. none of the above

2. The patient wants to know if she has an increased risk in this pregnancy. Your explain that
   a. pregnancy complicated by chronic hypertension can be easily managed
   b. she has an increased risk of preeclampsia, eclampsia, intrauterine growth restriction (IUGR), cesarean section, and bleeding
   c. with ultrasound monitoring as well as frequent benign prostatic hyperplasia (BPH) symptom index scores she will be safe
   d. chronic hypertension is not related to eclampsia
   e. her age does not increase the risk to this pregnancy

3. The appropriate course of action to evaluate her elevated blood pressure includes
   a. blood clotting studies, lactic acid dehydrogenase level
   b. starting her on an angiotensin-converting enzyme (ACE) inhibitor
   c. starting her on Aldomet (methyldopa)
   d. inducing her labor immediately
   e. watchful waiting

4. Your patient calls you at night complaining of a severe headache and thinks she is seeing "double." She is now 30 weeks pregnant. You tell her to go to the emergency room. Your presumptive diagnosis is
   a. transient ischemic attack in pregnancy
   b. preeclampsia superimposed on chronic hypertension
   c. eclampsia
   d. hemolysis, elevated liver enzymes, low platelet count (HELLP) syndrome
   e. hepatorenal syndrome of pregnancy

5. The patient's blood pressure in the emergency room is 160/110 mmHg, and she has severe pedal edema and hyperflexia. You will
   a. hospitalize the patient, start her on hydralazine, and draw lab tests
   b. hospitalize her for observation and start her on hydralazine intravenously (IV); do a complete ultrasound and biophysical profile
   c. at this time, there is no laboratory evidence of preeclampsia, so she should be treated as an outpatient
   d. her edema and hyperflexia are sufficient evidence of her severe preeclampsia
   e. draw stat lactate dehydrogenase in the emergency room; if it is positive, preeclampsia is evident

6. Appropriate indications for induction of labor in this patient include having
   a. preeclampsia, which is an indication by itself
   b. a "kick count" of 20
   c. a biophysical profile of 10
   d. persistent severe headaches
   e. a protein count of 300 mg/24 hours noted on her first urine collection last week

7. Fetal indications for delivery of this patient's baby include all the following except
   a. signs of IUGR
   b. suspected abruptio placentae
   c. oligohydramnios
   d. an amniotic fluid index of 10
   e. fetus being at 40 weeks of gestation

8. Treatment of acute severe hypertension (sustained blood pressures higher than 160 systolic and 105 diastolic) in pregnancy include the following except
   a. labetalol (Normodyne) 20 mg
   b. nifedipine (Procardia) 10 mg orally
   c. hydralazine (Apresoline) 5 mg IV
   d. hydralazine (Apresoline) 10 mg intramuscularly (IM)
   e. methyldopa (Aldomet) 250 mg orally

9. The patient complains of a severe headache during labor, her blood pressure climbs to 150/100 mmHg, and she now has 3+ protein on a urine sample collected by the nurse. The most appropriate treatment for your patient at this time would be
   a. labetalol (Normodyne) 20 mg IV
   b. magnesium sulfate 2-g loading dose and then run at 1 g/hour
   c. magnesium sulfate 4-g loading dose and then run at 2 g/hour
   d. hydralazine (Apresoline) 10 mg IM
   e. immediate cesarean delivery

10. Which of the following statements regarding eclampsia is true?
   a. eclampsia should be treated with intravenous diazepam
   b. eclampsia may occur with a diastolic blood pressure less than 90 mmHg
   c. eclamptic seizures frequently occur during delivery
   d. phenytoin may be administered intravenously to a patient having a preeclamptic seizure
   e. none of the above are true

11. Which one of the following intrapartum conditions is associated with preeclampsia/eclampsia?
   a. postpartum hemorrhage
   b. postdates pregnancy with induction
   c. maternal hyperglycemia
   d. prolonged first stage of labor
   e. venous thromboembolism

12. Which of the following are risks for recurrence of preeclampsia?
   a. onset of preeclampsia before 30 weeks of gestation
   b. African American ethnicity
   c. previous preeclampsia as a multipara
   d. a and c
   e. all of the above

13. All of the following are criteria for HELLP syndrome except
   a. lactate dehydrogenase greater than 600 IU/L
   b. aspartate aminotransferase (AST or SGOT) greater than 70 IU/L
   c. abnormal peripheral blood smear
   d. platelet count less than 150,000
   e. increased alkaline phosphatase

14. The patient delivers vaginally. The following are considered steps to use in the active management of the third stage of labor except
   a. administration of a uterine tonic prior to delivery of the infant

b. administration of a uterine tonic prior to delivery of the placenta
   c. relatively rapid cord clamping and cutting
   d. application of controlled traction to the cord
   e. all of the above are steps to use in the active management of her labor

15. Risk factors for postpartum hemorrhage include
   a. prolonged first stage
   b. multipara
   c. large babies
   d. assisted delivery (vacuum/forceps)
   e. all of the above

16. When the patient returns for postpartum examination, she asks you if she is at risk of continued hypertension now or in the future. Your response is
   a. there is no correlation between having a hypertensive problem during pregnancy (gestational hypertension or preeclampsia) and developing hypertension later
   b. data suggest that there is a measurably higher risk of developing later hypertension if a patient had a hypertensive problem during pregnancy
   c. although gestational hypertension does pose an increased risk for later development, preeclampsia does not
   d. although gestational hypertension does not pose an increased risk for later development of hypertension, preeclampsia does
   e. most woman who develop a hypertensive problem during pregnancy remain hypertensive throughout the remainder of their lives

---

Clinical Case Management Problem

How is pregnancy-induced hypertension distinguished from preeclampsia and preeclampsia distinguished from eclampsia?

Answers

1. **c.** Chronic hypertension is a blood pressure higher than 140/90 mmHg presenting before 20 weeks of gestation. Preeclampsia/eclampsia has associated proteinuria. Gestational hypertension is defined as elevated blood pressure without proteinuria in the second half of pregnancy.

2. **b.** This woman has two risk factors: chronic hypertension, which increases her likelihood of preeclampsia, and "extreme of ages" (younger age

than 20 years or older than 35 years). Preeclampsia (which can complicate chronic hypertension in pregnancy) commonly affects primiparas younger than age 20 years or older than 35 years. It is one of the leading causes of maternal morbidity and mortality, surpassed only by trauma and deep vein thrombosis.

3. **e.** The patient has no protein in her urine and therefore does not have preeclampsia. ACE inhibitors are contraindicated in pregnancy. Most clinicians start methyldopa if the patient's blood pressures are consistently higher than 150 mmHg systolic and 100 to 110 mmHg diastolic and if there are signs of end organ damage. She is not considered a candidate for immediate induction. Watchful waiting, including seeing the patient back within 1 week or less, is the most that is indicated at this time.

4. **b.** The patient has developed preeclampsia. In her case, it is superimposed on her chronic hypertension, as is often the case. Preeclampsia has two presentations: (1) blood pressure 140/90 mmHg and proteinuria or (2) blood pressure 140/90 mmHg with end organ presentation, double vision, and headache secondary to central nervous system involvement, right upper quadrant (RUQ) pain secondary to liver capsule distention, etc. Preeclampsia, whether presenting with proteinuria or other organ system signs, is a common complication of gestational hypertension.

5. **b.** A pregnant patient with RUQ pain, double vision, and headache needs to be brought in for observation and evaluation. This will include nonstress test, BPH score, and, if not done recently, estimated fetal weight. Although edema and hyperflexia are often used as clinical assessment tools, they are not a part of the diagnostic criteria for preeclampsia. Answer d merits special attention; there is no one lab test that is diagnostic of preeclampsia. The routine labs for preeclampsia include a serum uric acid, hemoglobin, hematocrit, and platelet count; a 24-hour urine test for protein; and a serum creatinine level. Serum magnesium level is useful to monitor a patient who is taking magnesium sulfate for her preeclampsia, but it is not considered part of the early evaluation process.

6. **d.** Indications for delivery of a patient with preeclampsia include the following: favorable cervix at term, platelet count less than 100×10^3 per microliter, progressive deterioration in liver or kidney function, suspected abruptio placentae, persistent severe headache or visual changes, and persistent severe epigastric pain with nausea and vomiting. Fetal indications for delivery include being at term, signs of IUGR, abruptio placentae, and oligohydramnios.

7. **d.** See answer 6.

8. **e.** Although methyldopa is the drug of choice for chronic hypertension, its use is not recommended in the acute situation; it takes too long to become effective, is not as strong as other medications, and dosing and titration are not as flexible as for other available drugs. The other agents listed in the question are considered drugs of choice for the pregnant patient with acutely severe hypertension. In addition, nitroprusside (Nipride) can be used if the other medications have failed. Nitroprusside should not be used for more than 4 hours and should be started at a dose of 0.25 mg/kg/minute and titrated up to a maximum of 5 mg/kg/minute.

9. **c.** At this point, the patient has preeclampsia. The definition of preeclampsia is as follows: blood pressure elevated higher than 140/90 mmHg, proteinuria exceeding 300 mg/24 hours, or a concentration of 0.1 g/L (dipstick 1+) in at least two random urine specimens collected 6 hours or more apart. Patients with blood pressures 160/110 mmHg or higher should be treated with an antiepileptic medication as well as an antihypertensive medication. The appropriate loading dose of magnesium sulfate is 4 g, followed by a 2- to 4-g/hour infusion.

10. **b.** Of eclamptic seizures, 20% occur in patients whose diastolic blood pressure is less than 90 mmHg. Diazepam and phenytoin should not be administered to a patient having a seizure. Eclampsia most frequently occurs before a delivery (79%) or within the first 24 hours after a delivery (29%) but rarely occurs during the delivery.

11. **a.** Of all the conditions listed, only postpartum hemorrhage is an associated intrapartum complication of preeclampsia.

12. **e.** All of the these, along with having a different father from the previous gestation, increase the risk of recurrent preeclampsia.

13. **e.** All of the answers listed except increased alkaline phosphatase are part of the criteria of HELLP syndrome. If the platelet count is less than 50,000/mm³ or active bleeding occurs, fibrinogen, fibrin split products, prothrombin, and partial thromboplastin times should be checked to rule out disseminated intravascular coagulation. Alkaline phosphatase is elevated in normal pregnancies.

14. **a.** According to studies reviewed by the Cochran Collaboration, active management of the third stage of labor decreases maternal blood loss, decreases the rate of postpartum hemorrhages more than 500 mL, and decreases the rate of a prolonged third stage of labor (category A recommendation). Administration of a uterine tonic should be performed prior to delivery of the placenta, not prior to delivery of the infant. Delivery of the infant is the end of the second stage of labor.

15. **d.** Postpartum hemorrhage is classically defined as blood loss of more than 500 mL in the first 24 hours postdelivery. Clinically, it may be defined as blood loss sufficient to cause hemodynamic instability. Risk factors for postpartum hemorrhage include preeclampsia, nulliparity, multiple gestation, previous postpartum hemorrhage, previous cesarean delivery, prolonged third stage, mediolateral or midline episiotomy, arrest of descent, augmented labor, and assisted delivery. Lacerations of the cervix, vagina, or perineum may also cause a postpartum hemorrhage.

16. **b.** Women who had hypertension or preeclampsia/eclampsia were significantly more likely than control subjects to have evidence of later hypertension, even after adjustment for risk factors for hypertension.

Solution to the Clinical Case Management Problem

Hypertension, preeclampsia, and eclampsia all are marked by systolic pressure greater than 140 mmHg and diastolic pressure greater than 90 mmHg. Pregnancy-induced hypertension can occur anytime, but preeclampsia generally occurs after the fifth month and eclampsia occurs near term. Moreover, proteinuria accompanies preeclampsia and eclampsia but is not found in pregnancy-induced hypertension. Eclampsia is distinguished from preeclampsia by the onset of seizures not attributable to other causes. (Fig. 91-1).

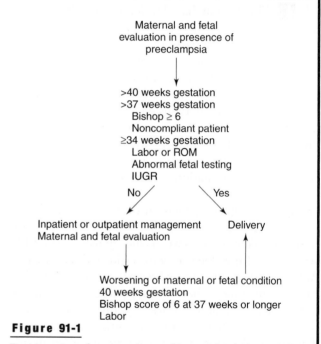

Figure 91-1

Decision tree for managing mild gestational hypertension–preeclampsia. IUGR, intrauterine growth restriction; ROM, rupture of membranes.

Summary

1. Definitions
   a. Chronic hypertension: blood pressure higher than 140/90 mmHg presenting before 20 weeks of gestation
   b. Gestational hypertension: elevated blood pressure without proteinuria in the second half of pregnancy
   c. Preeclampsia/eclampsia: elevated blood pressure plus proteinuria. (See Solution to the Clinical Case Management Problem.)
2. Treatment of choice for chronic hypertension in pregnancy: methyldopa as first line. Calcium channel blockers are also used. ACE inhibitors should be avoided, as should angiotensin II inhibitors. Thiazide

diuretics can exacerbate the intravascular fluid depletion of preeclampsia if chronic hypertension becomes complicated by superimposed preeclampsia.

3. Treatment of severe acute hypertension in pregnancy: Acceptable treatments for acute severe hypertension (sustained blood pressures higher than 160 systolic and 105 diastolic) in pregnancy include labetalol, hydralazine IV or IM, or Procardia.

4. "Gestational hypertension" should replace the term "pregnancy-induced hypertension." It is a provisional diagnosis used for a heterogeneous group of women including (1) those who will eventually develop proteinuria during the pregnancy and be diagnosed with preeclampsia, (2) those who will have persistent hypertension after 12 weeks postpartum and be diagnosed with chronic hypertension, and (3) those who do not develop preeclampsia and whose blood pressures normalize postpartum. Women in this last group are ultimately diagnosed as having had "transient hypertension of pregnancy."

5. Preeclampsia: blood pressure higher than 140/90 mmHg and proteinuria exceeding 300 mg/24 hours or a concentration of 0.1 g/L (dipstick 1+) in at least two random urine specimens collected 6 hours or more apart. Patients with blood pressure 160/110 mmHg or higher should be treated with an antiepileptic as well as an antihypertensive medication. The appropriate loading dose of magnesium sulfate is 4 g, followed by a 2- to 4-g/hour infusion.

6. Indications for delivery of a patient with preeclampsia include the following: favorable cervix at term, platelet count of less than 100×10^3 per microliter, progressive deterioration in liver or kidney function, suspected abruption placentae, persistent severe headache or visual changes, and persistent severe epigastric pain with nausea and vomiting. Fetal indications for delivery include being at term, signs of IUGR, abruptio placentae, and oligohydramnios.

7. HELLP syndrome: If the platelet count is less than $50,000/mm^3$ or active bleeding occurs, fibrinogen, fibrin split products, prothrombin, and partial thromboplastin times should be checked to rule out disseminated intravascular coagulation.

8. Eclampsia: 20% of seizures occur in patients with diastolic blood pressure of less than 90 mmHg. Eclampsia most frequently occurs before a delivery (79%) or within 24 hours after a delivery (29%). It rarely occurs during the delivery.

Suggested Reading

Duley L, Henderson-Smart DJ: Drugs for treatment of very high blood pressure during pregnancy. *Cochrane Database Syst Rev* (4):CD001449, 2002.

Hirshfeld-Cythron: Late postpartum eclampsia. *Obstet Gynecol Surv* 61(7):471–480, 2006.

Leeman L, Dresang L, Fontaine P: Medical complications of pregnancy. In: *Advanced Life Saving in Obstetrics*. Leawood, KS: American Academy of Family Physicians, 2006.

Nothnagle M, Taylor JS: Should active management of the third stage of labor be routine? *Am Fam Physician* 67:2119–2120, 2003.

Sibai BM: Diagnosis and management of gestational hypertension and preeclampsia. *Obstet Gynecol* 102(1):181–192, 2003.

Wilson BJ, Watson MS, Prescott GJ, et al: Hypertensive diseases of pregnancy and risk of hypertension and stroke in later life: Results from cohort study. *BMJ* 326:845–849, 2003.

Zamorski MA, Greene LA: NHBPEP report of high blood pressure in pregnancy: A summary for family physicians. *Am Fam Physician* 64:263–270, 273–274, 2001.

CHAPTER

92 Intrauterine Growth Restriction

CLINICAL CASE PROBLEM 1

Fetal Weight Falling Behind Gestational Age

MB is a 24-year-old (gravida 1, para 0) female who is 30 weeks pregnant. Her last menstrual period is certain. She presented for care at 9 weeks of gestation and has kept her monthly follow-up appointments. Her initial body mass index was 21, and she has gained 7 pounds during the past 8 weeks. Fundal height has been consistent with dates, but today the fundal measurement is 25 cm. She smokes one and a half packs of cigarettes a day and is unable to cut down. She denies alcohol or other substance use. She denies any recent infections. An ultrasound at 16 weeks was consistent with her last menstrual period and showed normal fetal anatomy. A repeat ultrasound shows estimated fetal weight consistent with a 25-week gestation (fetal weight below the 10th percentile for 30-week gestation). The amniotic fluid index is normal.

SELECT THE BEST ANSWER TO THE FOLLOWING QUESTIONS

1. Which of the following statements regarding intrauterine growth restriction (IUGR) is true?
   a. the term describes a fetus with an estimated weight that is less than expected for gestational age
   b. the 3rd percentile is generally the cutoff used to define IUGR
   c. IUGR is interchangeable with the term small for gestational age (SGA)
   d. IUGR is a term for infants with genetic anomalies whose weight is at the low end of the growth curve
   e. all of the above

2. What is the leading cause of fetal growth restriction in human pregnancies?
   a. poor maternal weight gain
   b. placental insufficiency
   c. maternal diabetes
   d. maternal toxoplasmosis exposure
   e. gestational hypertension

3. In the United States, what is the most commonly used definition for SGA?
   a. birth weight below the 1st percentile for gestational age
   b. birth weight below the 3rd percentile for gestational age
   c. birth weight below the 5th percentile for gestational age
   d. birth weight below the 10th percentile for gestational age
   e. birth weight below the 20th percentile for gestational age

Additional history may be helpful in attempting to identify causes contributing to MB's diagnosis of IUGR. Maternal history of chronic and acute illness may contribute to developing IUGR.

4. Which of the following adult disorders is not associated with fetal growth restriction?
   a. coronary heart disease
   b. hypertension
   c. type 2 diabetes mellitus
   d. stroke
   e. hypothyroidism

5. Which of the following types of infection need not be considered as a possible cause of fetal growth restriction?
   a. bacterial infections
   b. fetal rubella
   c. fetal cytomegalovirus
   d. syphilis
   e. *Toxoplasma gondii* infection

6. Which of the following medications is unlikely to cause fetal growth restriction?
   a. phenytoin
   b. antineoplastic agents
   c. methotrexate
   d. warfarin
   e. ondansetron

7. All of the following types of maternal substance use are linked with IUGR except
   a. marijuana
   b. tobacco
   c. methadone
   d. cocaine
   e. heroin

The care of MB over the remaining weeks until delivery will be directed at confirming estimated date of confinement, selecting the most propitious time for delivery, and confirming fetal well-being.

8. Which of the following statements regarding the use of ultrasound for diagnosis of IUGR is true?
   a. an abdominal circumference within normal range for gestational age reliably rules out growth restriction
   b. a single fetal measurement is adequate to diagnose growth restriction
   c. fetal biparietal diameter and femur length are the most important ultrasound measurements in the evaluation of IUGR
   d. estimated fetal weight below the 3rd percentile suggests possible IUGR
   e. routine second trimester anatomic survey is adequate in a fetus with suspected IUGR

9. All of the following tests are indicated for routine surveillance of IUGR except
   a. nonstress testing
   b. biophysical profile
   c. Doppler velocimetry studies
   d. fetal blood sampling via cordocentesis
   e. amniotic fluid index

10. Which of the following statements regarding management of IUGR is true?
    a. two-thirds of IUGR-affected pregnancies require delivery by cesarean section
    b. antenatal steroids are indicated for any fetus with IUGR that is expected to deliver prior to 34 weeks
    c. several effective therapies are available for fetal growth restriction

d. fetal glucose supplementation is beneficial for treating IUGR-associated acidosis

e. early delivery decreases fetal risk of morbidity and mortality in the majority of cases of IUGR

11. Which of the following complications is often seen in SGA infants?
  a. hyperthermia
  b. hyperglycemia
  c. apneic episodes
  d. anemia
  e. none of the above

Answers

1. a. The term SGA is used to describe infants with lower than expected birth weight for gestational age at delivery. IUGR refers to fetuses and is generally defined as less than 10th percentile weight for gestational age. It includes normal fetuses at the lower end of the fetal growth curve as well as fetuses that fail to grow because of maternal, placental, or fetal causes.

2. b. Placental insufficiency is the leading cause of fetal growth restriction. Decreased uteroplacental blood flow and placental infarcts are common. Maternal complications such as diabetes, hypertension, and infection may cause growth restriction. Although poor maternal weight gain warrants monitoring of fetal growth, placental insufficiency is the most common cause of IUGR.

3. d. SGA refers to infants, whereas IUGR is used when describing fetuses. Infants with birth weight at the lower extreme of the normal birth weight tables are described as SGA. In the United States, SGA is defined as a birth weight below the 10th percentile for expected gestational age.

4. e. According to the developmental origins hypothesis, epidemiological evidence links IUGR with specific adult medical conditions. Hypertension, type 2 diabetes, coronary artery disease, and stroke are all associated with IUGR.

5. a. Viral infections are estimated to cause 5% of cases of IUGR. Sixty percent of fetal rubella infections result in growth restriction. Forty percent of fetuses exposed to varicella show growth delay. Cytomegalovirus, syphilis, and protozoan infections such as toxoplasmosis and Chagas' disease are also linked with IUGR. Bacterial infections are not associated with growth restriction.

6. e. Ondansetron is used for nausea and vomiting in pregnancy and is not considered to cause fetal growth abnormalities. Antineoplastic agents, folic acid antagonists (methotrexate), and anticonvulsive agents such as phenytoin and trimethadione are linked with fetal growth restriction.

7. a. Several illicit drugs impair fetal growth. Fetal alcohol exposure significant enough to result in fetal alcohol syndrome usually causes marked growth restriction. Smoking causes a 3.5-fold increase in SGA infants. Women who quit smoking before the third trimester may decrease risk to their fetuses. Thirty-five percent of patients treated with methadone have SGA infants, as do 50% of women with heroin addiction. One-third of mothers who abuse cocaine will deliver infants that are SGA.

8. a. Ultrasound is widely used to evaluate growth restriction. Measurements routinely obtained include the head circumference, biparietal diameter, abdominal circumference, and femur length. Serial combinations of these measurements are useful to determine if growth is adequate. Numbers are then converted into an estimated fetal weight using published formulas. Abdominal circumference is especially useful in later pregnancy. A measurement greater than the 10th percentile for gestational age largely rules out IUGR; fetuses less than the 10th percentile need further evaluation for growth restriction. Diagnosis of IUGR is made using serial ultrasound measurements. Since IUGR is often associated with genetic and/or structural abnormalities, a detailed anatomic ultrasound is recommended in fetuses with growth delay.

9. d. Noninvasive assessment of fetal condition is possible using nonstress testing and ultrasound. Nonstress testing has high sensitivity for fetal acidemia and hypercarbia. Doppler waveforms of the umbilical arteries demonstrate abnormal blood flow in fetuses with IUGR. The biophysical profile (BPP) uses five categories to assess fetal well-being, although it is not ideal as a single assessment tool in IUGR. Similar to the nonstress test, marked inter- and intraobserver disparities are noted with BPP. Oligohydramnios is very suggestive of growth failure and increases the risk of fetal death. Combinations of these tests likely provide a more accurate diagnostic and management strategy. Fetal blood sampling by cordocentesis identifies acid–base abnormalities in a fetus. It is less commonly used because it is invasive and carries a procedure-related risk of approximately 1%.

10. b. There are no specific treatments proven to improve fetal growth restriction. Maternal nutritional supplements, low-dose aspirin, and fetal glucose supplements have been used without success. The most important decision in treating IUGR is determining the correct time for delivery. Gestational age, fetal well-being, maternal health, and severity of IUGR must all be considered. Fetuses delivered prior to 34 weeks of gestation benefit from steroid administration.

Only one-third of fetuses with IUGR require cesarean delivery.

11. **C.** Neonatal complications in SGA infants include hypothermia, hypoglycemia, apnea, and hyperbilirubinemia. Polycythemia is more common than anemia.

Summary

The diagnosis and treatment of IUGR is complicated by a lack of consensus regarding its definition. Much confusion stems from the terms IUGR and SGA. IUGR describes a fetus whose estimated weight is less than expected for a given gestational age. Less than the 10th percentile is traditionally classified as fetal growth restriction, although statistically, 10% of normal infants in any population fall into this category. Since the majority of adverse fetal outcomes occur in fetuses below the 3rd to 5th percentile, the 10th percentile may not have strong clinical significance.

SGA refers to infants with birth weights at the lower end of normal. The most common definition in the United States is birth weight at delivery below the 10th percentile for expected gestational age. The terms IUGR and SGA are often used interchangeably, further complicating diagnosis.

Risk factors for IUGR are diverse. Causes are classified into the broad categories of maternal, fetal, and placental. Maternal medical conditions predisposing to IUGR include renal disease, collagen–vascular disease, diabetes with underlying microvascular disease, and hypertension. Maternal abuse of tobacco, alcohol, or illicit drugs also contributes to IUGR. Specific viral infections, chromosomal abnormalities, and teratogenic medications are linked to IUGR.

Several medical problems affect SGA infants. Apneic episodes, hyperbilirubinemia, hypoglycemia, polycythemia, and hypothermia are sometimes seen after delivery with severe IUGR. Seizures, sepsis, and death are more common in SGA infants.

Establishing accurate clinical dates is essential for diagnosing IUGR. A key physical finding in IUGR is a discrepancy between the fundal height and the expected gestational age. If the fundal height is significantly less than expected in a patient with accurate dates, an ultrasound for fetal growth and biometry is indicated.

Biometry measurements performed include the fetal abdominal circumference, femur length, head circumference, and biparietal diameter. Humeral measurements are increasingly used to predict growth abnormalities in later pregnancy. When IUGR is suspected, serial ultrasounds are used to determine growth velocity during a 2- to 4-week period.

Surveillance options available for IUGR include nonstress testing, amniotic fluid index, contraction stress test, biophysical profile, and Doppler velocimetry. Although randomized controlled trials demonstrate a risk reduction in perinatal mortality with Doppler, comparable studies for the other options are not available.

Management of IUGR depends on the health of the mother, fetal well-being, and gestational age. Since there is no effective treatment for IUGR, the most critical decision is the timing of delivery. Determining the ideal time for delivery is controversial. The fetus should be delivered if the risk of intrauterine death exceeds that of neonatal mortality, although this is challenging to assess. Many fetuses are delivered because of nonreassuring fetal assessment or no growth during a 2- to 4-week period. Delivery plans must be individualized, and fetuses less than 34 weeks of gestation benefit when given corticosteroids.

Suggested Reading

Alberry M, Soothill P: Management of fetal growth restriction. *Arch Dis Child Fetal Neonatal Ed* 92:F62–F67, 2007.

American College of Obstetricians and Gynecologists Committee on Practice Bulletins: *Intrauterine Growth Restriction*, ACOG Practice Bulletin no. 12: Clinical management guidelines for obstetrician–gynecologists. Washington, DC: American College of Obstetricians and Gynecologists, 2000.

Sifianou P: Small and growth-restricted babies: Drawing the distinction. *Acta Pediatr* 95:1620–1624, 2006.

Tan T, Yeo G: Intrauterine growth restriction. *Curr Opin Obstet Gynecol* 17:135–142, 2005.

CHAPTER 93

Post-term Pregnancy

CLINICAL CASE PROBLEM 1

"Will I Ever Have a Baby?"

A 35-year-old (gravida 1, para 0) female visits your office at 40 weeks of gestation. Her last menstrual period (LMP) is "certain." Her history is significant for regular menstrual cycles and no oral contraceptive use within 3 months of becoming pregnant. A 13-week ultrasound was consistent with her LMP. The pregnancy has been unremarkable. The patient is quite concerned because today is her due date and she is not in labor. She states that her mother did not "go into labor until after 44 weeks" and she is worried that "late babies run in the family." On physical examination, fundal height is 39 cm. Her weight has increased by 1 pound and vital signs are stable. Fetal heart tones are 140. The cervix is closed, thick, and high. Estimated fetal weight is 8 pounds.

SELECT THE BEST ANSWER TO THE FOLLOWING QUESTIONS

1. Which of the following gestational ages is considered post-term?
   a. 270 days
   b. 280 days
   c. 287 days
   d. 294 days
   e. 301 days

2. Which of the following conditions is not associated with increased risk of post-term pregnancy?
   a. placental sulfatase insufficiency
   b. fetal anencephaly
   c. female gender of fetus
   d. primiparity
   e. history of previous post-term pregnancy

3. What is the most common cause of post-term pregnancy?
   a. incorrect dating
   b. fetal anencephaly
   c. genetic predisposition
   d. multiparity
   e. fetal macrosomia

4. Which of the following statements about fetal dysmaturity syndrome is true?
   a. 40% of post-term fetuses have dysmaturity syndrome
   b. post-term infants are at significant risk of long-term neurologic sequelae
   c. post-term pregnancies are at increased risk for oligohydramnios and meconium aspiration
   d. nonreassuring antepartum and intrapartum tests are uncommon with this condition
   e. post-term infants have mild decrements in their intelligence quotient (IQ) and attainment of physical milestones

5. Which of the following statements about ultrasound and post-term pregnancy is true?
   a. early ultrasound dating does not significantly reduce the number of post-term pregnancies
   b. routine ultrasound before 24 weeks of gestation provides more accurate gestational age estimates and earlier detection of fetal anomalies
   c. a certain LMP is as accurate as a 13- to 24-week ultrasound for determining gestational age
   d. ultrasound after 24 weeks most effectively detects multifetal pregnancies
   e. ultrasound after 20 weeks is as accurate in determining dates as a first trimester ultrasound

6. Which of the following statements about post-term pregnancy is false?
   a. 15% of pregnancies continue to at least 42 weeks of gestation
   b. the perinatal mortality rate at 40 weeks of gestation is 2 or 3 deaths/1000 deliveries
   c. the perinatal mortality rate increases sixfold after 43 weeks
   d. perinatal mortality per ongoing pregnancies is the best estimate for the risk of fetal death at the end of pregnancy
   e. recent epidemiologic studies suggest that the risk of stillbirth beyond 41 weeks of gestation is greater than previously reported

7. When is the most appropriate time to institute fetal monitoring in a low-risk prolonged pregnancy?
   a. weekly testing beginning at 40 weeks
   b. biweekly testing beginning at 40 weeks
   c. weekly testing beginning at 41 weeks
   d. biweekly testing beginning at 43 weeks
   e. there is insufficient evidence to indicate if routine antenatal testing of low-risk patients at 40 to 42 weeks of gestation improves outcome

8. Which of the following methods of fetal monitoring is not recommended for surveillance of the post-term fetus?
   a. nonstress test (NST)
   b. biophysical profile (BPP)
   c. Doppler velocimetry
   d. contraction stress testing (CST)
   e. modified biophysical profile

9. You perform a BPP on a 32-year old gravida 1 para 0 at 41 weeks and 5 days of gestation. Fetal breathing is seen for 10 seconds. The amniotic fluid index (AFI) is greater than 9 cm. The fetal hand opens and closes. Three gross body movements are noted during the 30-minute exam. The NST is reactive. What is the score of this BPP?
   a. 2
   b. 4
   c. 6
   d. 8
   e. 10

10. Which of the following statements about antenatal testing and post-term pregnancy is not correct?
    a. a reactive NST has a very high negative predictive value for predicting fetal well-being
    b. a modified BPP is the combination of an NST and AFI
    c. a BPP score of 8 to 10 is considered normal
    d. an abnormal modified BPP has stronger positive predictive value than a nonreactive NST for predicting fetal compromise
    e. oligohydramnios is an indication for labor induction

11. The patient progresses to 41 weeks. She now wants to be managed expectantly because she heard that the risk of cesarean is higher if she is induced. Which of the following statements about labor induction at 41 weeks is not true?
    a. induction at 41 weeks does not increase the risk of cesarean
    b. post-term induction of labor reduces the risk of perinatal death
    c. the reduction in risk of perinatal death with induction is very small compared to that of expectant management
    d. induction at 41 weeks is associated with decreased risk of meconium aspiration syndrome
    e. induction at 41 weeks increases the risk for cesarean

12. The patient agrees to proceed with labor induction. Her cervical exam at this time is as follows: 2-cm dilation, 60% effacement, −2 station, firm consistency, and posterior. Which of the following statements is correct?
    a. an oxytocin induction is indicated
    b. the Bishop score indicates a high likelihood of vaginal delivery with induction
    c. cervical ripening with prostaglandins is indicated
    d. the chance of successful induction with prostaglandins is low
    e. a Bishop score of more than 10 indicates that the probability of vaginal delivery after induction is similar to that of spontaneous labor

13. Which of the following statements about the use of prostaglandin for cervical ripening is incorrect?
    a. pitocin is contraindicated if prostaglandins are used during an induction for post-term pregnancy
    b. prostaglandin E_2 (dinoprostone) and prostaglandin E_1 (misoprostol) are two options for post-term induction
    c. no standardized dosing regimen is established for these medications
    d. higher doses are associated with uterine hyperstimulation
    e. fetal heart rate monitoring is necessary with prostaglandin induction

Answers

1. **d.** Post-term pregnancy refers to gestations that are 42 weeks (294 days) or greater calculated from the first day of the LMP. It is approximated as the estimated date of delivery (EDD) + 14 days.

2. **c.** Several factors are linked with post-term pregnancy. Primiparity, a history of post-term pregnancy, and inaccurate dating all increase the risk of post-term delivery. Placental sulfatase deficiency and anencephaly are other etiologies. Male gender is associated with an increased risk of post-term delivery.

3. **a.** The most frequent cause of post-term pregnancy is inaccurate dating. Primiparity, rather than multiparity, is a risk factor. Post-term pregnancy is rarely associated with anencephaly. Genetic predisposition has an influence; fetal macrosomia is not associated with post-term gestation.

4. **c.** Twenty percent of post-term fetuses have dysmaturity syndrome. Uteroplacental insufficiency causes an intrauterine growth restriction-like pattern. Intrapartum complications include meconium aspiration and an increased risk of cord accidents secondary

to oligohydramnios. Nonreassuring ante- and intra-partum fetal testing requires further investigation. It is unclear whether post-term infants face an increased risk of neurological problems. No significant differences are noted in IQ or physical milestones when post-term 2-years-olds are compared with those born at or before term.

5. **b.** A Cochrane review found that routine ultrasound prior to 24 weeks of gestation provides better gestational age estimates and earlier detection of both multifetal pregnancies and fetal anomalies. The use of ultrasound reduces the percentage of post-term pregnancies by an estimated 70%. One large retrospective study of women with a "sure" LMP demonstrated that the due date is more accurately predicted by a 13- to 24-week ultrasound than by the LMP. Ultrasound accuracy in pregnancy dating is highest in the first trimester and decreases with advancing gestational age.

6. **a.** A total of 5% to 10% of pregnancies continue to 42 weeks of gestation. Perinatal mortality rate (PMR) is traditionally used to describe fetal risk in post-term pregnancy. PMR is 2 or 3 deaths/1000 deliveries at 40 weeks and increases sixfold after 43 completed weeks. It is calculated as follows: [number of fetal deaths at a specific gestational age/number of live births + fetal deaths during the same period]. The risk of stillbirth from post-term pregnancy is likely underestimated because the majority of pregnancies deliver before 42 weeks. Only ongoing pregnancies are at continued risk for death. The perinatal mortality rate by ongoing pregnancy is more representative of actual risk. It is calculated from the number of fetal deaths at a specific gestation divided by the number of fetuses in all ongoing pregnancies. Recent epidemiologic studies using the adjusted PMR estimate that the actual risk of stillbirth after 41 weeks of gestation is greater than previously reported.

7. **e.** No conclusive recommendations are available regarding either type or frequency of antenatal testing in post-term pregnancy. Current studies lack adequate power to demonstrate a benefit for monitoring. Still, there is no evidence that fetal monitoring is harmful in post-term cases. Antenatal surveillance is commonly used because of universal acceptance. Many providers begin biweekly testing at 41 weeks of gestation, although this is based on expert opinion.

8. **c.** Doppler velocimetry is not beneficial in monitoring the post-term fetus and is not recommended. It may be of use in pregnancies complicated by intrauterine growth restriction. Recommended options include NST, BPP, modified BPP, and CST. No single test is demonstrated to be superior, and monitoring protocols vary widely by provider. Most begin biweekly testing at 41 weeks.

9. **d.** The biophysical profile is scored using five categories (Table 93-1). Each category is scored as either 0 or 2, for a composite score of 0 to 10. The score for this test is 8/10. Two points are deducted because of insufficient fetal breathing.

A total score of 8 to 10 on the BPP is normal. A score of 6 is equivocal; further evaluation is warranted. A score of 4 or less is abnormal and the fetus likely should be delivered promptly. The presence of oligohydramnios is worrisome even if the total score is 8. If the largest vertical pocket of amniotic fluid is 2 cm or larger, the fetus is at increased risk for cord accidents and delivery should be planned.

10. **d.** Fetal monitoring in a low-risk post-term gestation is most often done biweekly starting at 41 weeks of gestation. No specific test is superior to another, and choice of test is usually by physician preference. A reactive NST has a negative predictive value (NPV) of 99.8%. Modified biophysical profile combines the NST with an AFI. It has an NPV of 99.9%. If oligohydramnios is

Table 93-1	**Scoring Criteria for the Biophysical Profile**	
Category	**Score of 0**	**Score of 2**
Nonstress test	Nonreactive	Reactive
Amniotic fluid index	Largest vertical pocket ≤2 cm	Single vertical fluid pocket >2 cm
Fetal breathing	Abnormal or absent	≥1 episode of fetal breathing lasting ≥30 sec during 30-min test
Fetal movement	Abnormal or absent	≥3 gross body or limb movements during 30-min test
Fetal tone	Abnormal or absent	≥1 flexion/extension movement of extremity or opening/closing of hand

noted on the modified BPP, delivery should be considered. A full BPP includes an assessment of AFI, fetal tone, breathing, and movement in combination with an NST. A score of 8 to 10 is considered normal. Positive predictive values (PPVs) for both NST and modified BPP are lower than the NPV. Modified BPP has a 40% PPV; NST has a 10% PPV.

11. **e.** A Cochrane review of 19 trials involving 7984 patients found that routine induction at 41 weeks or beyond is associated with fewer perinatal deaths. The decrease in absolute risk is very small. No evidence suggests that 41-week induction increases the risk of cesarean compared to expectant management. Less meconium aspiration is noted in the induction group. Practice recommendations from this meta-analysis are that labor induction should be offered to low-risk women by 41 completed weeks.

12. **c.** The Bishop scoring system predicts the likelihood of success of labor induction. Based on five categories, the possible score ranges from 0 to 13 (Table 93-2). A score higher than 8 suggests that the probability of vaginal delivery with induction is similar to that of spontaneous labor. This patient has a Bishop score of 4. Cervical ripening with prostaglandin is indicated. Several trials report improvements in Bishop score, shorter labor duration, and lower total doses of oxytocin when prostaglandin cervical priming is used.

13. **a.** Prostaglandin preparations used for cervical ripening include dinoprostone and misoprostol. Although numerous studies use prostaglandins for labor induction, standardized doses and dosage protocols are not widely agreed upon. Dinoprostone is Food and Drug Administration (FDA) approved for cervical ripening; misoprostol lacks approval for this indication. Dinoprostone is available in gel form or as a vaginal insert. Misoprostol is available as 100- or 200-μg tablets, which are broken into 25- or 50-μg doses. Misoprostol is either taken orally or placed intravaginally. Higher doses of misoprostol occasionally cause uterine hyperstimulation. Fetal heart rate monitoring is prudent when prostaglandins are used. Oxytocin is usually started once the Bishop score is favorable. Starting oxytocin several hours (4 or more) after the last dose of prostaglandin is thought to decrease the risk of uterine hyperstimulation.

Table 93-2	Bishop Score for Labor Induction				
Score	Cervical Consistency	Cervical Position	Dilation (cm)	Effacement (%)	Station (−3 to +3)
0	Firm	Posterior	Closed	0–30	−3
1	Medium	Mid	1–2	40–50	−2
2	Soft	Anterior	3–4	60–70	0–1
3	N/A	N/A	5–6	>80	+1 to +2

A score higher than 8 indicates that the success of induced vaginal delivery is similar to that of spontaneous labor.
N/A, not applicable.

Summary

Post-term pregnancy affects 5% to 10% of pregnancies and is defined as a pregnancy lasting beyond 294 days (42 weeks or EDD + 14 days). The majority of cases are related to inaccurate calculation of the due date. Routine ultrasound prior to 24 weeks of gestation provides the best estimation of due date. It also allows for earlier detection of multifetal pregnancies and fetal anomalies. Ultrasound use reduces the percentage of pregnancies considered post-term by an estimated 70%. Ultrasound accuracy for dating is best early in pregnancy and decreases with advancing gestational age.

Several conditions are associated with post-term pregnancy. A history of previous post-term pregnancy and primiparity both increase risk. Placental sulfatase deficiency, anencephaly, and male sex of the fetus are also linked with pregnancies that are post-term. Genetic predisposition is thought to play a role, although the strength of the association is unknown.

Fetal mortality increases past term. The PMR at 40 weeks is 2 or 3 deaths per 1000 deliveries. This risk doubles by 42 weeks and increases four- to sixfold at 44 weeks. Adjusted perinatal mortality calculated using only ongoing pregnancies may provide a more accurate risk for fetal demise than does PMR alone.

Surveillance of prolonged pregnancy generally begins at 41 weeks of gestation and is done biweekly. Options for monitoring include the NST, BPP, modified BPP, and CST. No single test has been shown to be superior to another. No conclusive recommendations specify either the type or the frequency of testing. Although definitive proof that testing decreases fetal mortality is scant, there is no evidence that it is harmful. Testing is widely accepted and considered standard of care. Fetuses with nonreassuring studies or oligohydramnios require close surveillance and consideration for delivery. A description of the BPP is provided in Table 93-1.

A Cochrane meta-analysis shows that routine induction at 41 weeks or beyond is associated with fewer perinatal deaths, although the absolute risk reduction is quite small. Routine induction is also not proven to increase the risk for cesarean delivery. In women past 41 weeks who desire induction, the Bishop score is helpful for predicting the success of vaginal delivery (see Table 93-2). Women with a Bishop score higher than 8 have a probability for successful vaginal delivery with induction similar to that of spontaneous labor.

The prostaglandins dinoprostone and misoprostol are available for cervical ripening in women with an unfavorable Bishop score. Dinoprostone is FDA approved for this indication and is available as either a gel or an insert that is placed intravaginally. Misoprostol is not approved for labor induction, but it is widely used either orally or intravaginally. Standardized doses and protocols for prostaglandin use are not well-defined. High doses of the medication occasionally result in uterine hyperstimulation; fetal monitoring is recommended with prostaglandin induction. Oxytocin is often used once the Bishop score is favorable. Starting oxytocin several hours after the last dose of prostaglandins may reduce the risk of uterine hyperstimulation.

Suggested Reading

American College of Obstetricians and Gynecologists: ACOG Practice bulletin. Management of postterm pregnancy. *Obstet Gynecol* 104:639–646, 2004.

American College of Obstetricians and Gynecologists: ACOG Practice bulletin. Antepartum fetal surveillance, Number 9, October 1999. In: *Compendium of Selected Publications.* Washington DC: American College of Obstetricians and Gynecologists, 2006.

Briscoe D, Nguyen H, Mencer M, et al: Management of pregnancy beyond 40 weeks' gestation. *Am Fam Physician* 71:1935–1942, 2005.

Cleary-Goldman J, Bettes B, Robinson J, et al: Postterm pregnancy: Practice patterns of contemporary obstetricians and gynecologists. *Am J Perinatol* 23(1):15–20, 2006.

Gülmezoglu A, Crowther C, Middleton P: Induction of labour for improving birth outcomes for women at or beyond term. *Cochrane Database Syst Rev*(4):CD004945, 2006.

Hofmeyr GJ, Gülmezoglu AM: Vaginal misoprostol for cervical ripening and induction of labour. *Cochrane Database Syst Rev* (1):CD000941, 2003.

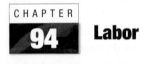

CHAPTER 94   Labor

CLINICAL CASE PROBLEM 1

"Is It Time to Have the Baby?"

MB is an 18-year-old (gravida 1) female at 39 weeks and 5 days gestation. The pregnancy has been uneventful. She arrives on the floor with her mother, boyfriend, and two friends. Her presenting complaint is contractions for 3 hours. The contractions are 5 minutes apart and irregular. She denies bleeding, fluid leakage, or decreased fetal movement. On physical examination, her cervix is dilated to 3 cm and is 20% effaced, firm, and posterior. A nonstress test is reassuring. She is monitored for 2 hours and has no significant cervical change.

SELECT THE BEST ANSWER TO THE FOLLOWING QUESTIONS

1. Women admitted to labor and delivery in this patient's stage of labor are at increased risk for all of the following except
   a. cesarean delivery
   b. shoulder dystocia
   c. amnionitis
   d. intrauterine pressure catheter placement
   e. oxytocin use

2. What is the working diagnosis at this time?
   a. active labor
   b. failure to progress
   c. latent labor

d. Braxton–Hicks contractions

e. oligohydramnios

3. Which of the following outcomes is not associated with continuity of care during pregnancy?

a. women require less medication for pain relief in labor

b. neonates are less likely to require resuscitation at delivery

c. women are more likely satisfied with their intrapartum care

d. episiotomy use is less common

e. operative vaginal delivery is more common

The patient is sent home. She returns 2 days later with continued contractions that are now 3 minutes apart and regular. On sterile vaginal exam, her cervix is 4 cm dilated, 50% effaced, –2 position, midstation, and soft. The patient is admitted to labor and delivery. Her mother and boyfriend are quite excited and want to know exactly when the baby will deliver. The patient wants to talk about whether an epidural is a good idea. Her mother wants to know when her daughter will receive an enema and "be shaved." She also warns the patient that an episiotomy is required for the baby to deliver safely.

4. What is the expected rate of cervical dilatation during active labor in nulliparous women?

a. 0.2 cm/hour

b. 0.5 cm/hour

c. 1 cm/hour

d. 1.5 cm/hour

e. 2 cm/hour

5. Which statement regarding active management of labor is false?

a. early amniotomy and oxytocin are performed to correct prolonged labor

b. it reduces the duration of labor

c. interventions are triggered if cervical progress deviates more than 2 hours from the normal progress line

d. it reduces the risk of cesarean delivery

e. interventions are indicated in primiparas without adequate cervical change after a 4-hour period

6. Which of these types of general care during labor is supported by evidence-based studies?

a. perineal shaving

b. routine enemas

c. restriction of oral fluid and food intake

d. supine positioning in the bed

e. continuous support during labor

7. Which of the following statements regarding amniotomy is true?

a. numerous studies support the benefit of amniotomy for augmentation of labor

b. it is associated with increased need for oxytocin

c. more mild and moderate variables are noted on external fetal monitoring in patients who undergo amniotomy

d. it is associated with a 30-minute reduction in the duration of labor

e. it decreases the risk for operative delivery

8. Use of continuous electronic fetal monitoring (EFM) decreases the risk for which one of the following?

a. neonatal seizures

b. 1-minute Apgar scores below 4

c. cerebral palsy

d. perinatal death

e. cesarean delivery

9. Which of the following statements about epidural anesthesia during labor is true?

a. it is associated with an increased risk of cesarean delivery

b. it significantly increases the likelihood of an instrumented vaginal delivery

c. epidural anesthesia is ineffective for pain control during labor

d. use is associated with an decreased length of the second stage of labor

e. epidural use is associated with an decreased need for oxytocin during labor

10. How should expectant women be counseled regarding episiotomy?

a. routine episiotomy facilitates delivery and is indicated to avoid perineal damage

b. extension of the episiotomy into the rectum is very rare

c. mediolateral episiotomy is superior to a midlateral approach

d. episiotomy should only be performed for specific indications

e. routine episiotomy results in less blood loss and less dyspareunia than no episiotomy

11. Which of the following is not included in active management of the third stage of labor?

a. administration of oxytocin after delivery of the anterior shoulder

b. controlled cord traction to expedite delivery of the placenta

c. use of McRoberts' maneuver to expedite delivery of the fetal head

  d. immediate clamping and cutting of the umbilical cord
  e. delivery of the placenta by maternal pushing

Answers

1. b. The first stage of labor ends with complete cervical dilatation and is divided into latent and active phases. The latent phase is of varying duration and generally defined as cervical dilatation less than 4 cm. The active phase is diagnosed when cervix dilatation is 4 cm, there are regular contractions, and cervical change is noted. Determining if a patient is actually in labor can be difficult. Many women present in latent labor and are admitted either for pain control or for further observation. These women are at increased risk for cesarean delivery. More active phase arrest, oxytocin use, intrauterine pressure catheter use, fetal scalp electrode use, and amnionitis are found in this group of women. It is not well understood if poor outcomes result from dysfunctional labor or whether being admitted in latent labor causes poor outcomes due to increased interventions.

2. c. The patient is in latent labor. She has regular contractions without evidence of cervical change. Since her cervix dilatation is less than 4 cm and shows no progression, active labor is unlikely. Observing her for 2 hours helps clarify this. Braxton–Hicks contractions are usually irregular and occur earlier in gestation. They are not associated with cervical dilatation. Oligohydramnios is less likely with a reactive nonstress test and term gestation. Failure to progress does not appropriately describe this presentation.

3. e. Continuity of care involves having one provider or a small group of individuals provide coordinated prenatal, intrapartum, and postpartum care. A Cochrane review examined whether continuity of care has an influence on delivery. It was found that women with the same care provider require less pain medication in labor, are less likely to have an episiotomy, and tend to be more satisfied with care. Neonates are less likely to require resuscitation. Increased need for forceps or vacuum delivery is not associated with continuity of care.

4. c. Nulliparas generally dilate 1 cm per hour during the active phase of labor. Multiparas have an expected cervical dilatation of 1.2 to 1.5 cm per hour during the active phase.

5. e. Partograms are pictographic representations of progress in labor that graph cervical change over time. Most contain a "normal" labor line, an alert line, and an action line. The alert line serves as a prompt that labor is progressing slowly, whereas the action line signifies a need to intervene. The time at which alert and action lines occur is a function of the specific partogram used.

Active management involves early identification of prolonged labor and early intervention with amniotomy and oxytocin augmentation. Intervention is triggered when cervical progress differs from the alert line by 2 hours. There is no evidence that active management reduces the need for cesarean, but it does reduce the duration of labor. The World Health Organization (WHO) partogram recommends action only after 4 hours elapse past the alert line. In recent studies, the 2-hour partogram increased the need for intervention without improving maternal or neonatal outcomes compared to the 4-hour approach.

6. e. Continuous support during labor is extensively described in evidence-based literature. Women with continuous support are less likely to need analgesia during labor, to require delivery by cesarean or vacuum/forceps, or to be dissatisfied with their delivery experience. Benefits are greatest if support occurs early in labor and when the support person is not a hospital staff member. Perineal shaving, supine positioning, routine enemas, and nothing per os are not supported by today's literature.

7. c. Amniotomy is frequently performed with induction or augmentation of labor. Few randomized controlled trials describe the efficacy of amniotomy, however. A Cochrane review examined the use of amniotomy in the first stage of labor. Amniotomy decreases the duration of the first stage of labor by 1 or 2 hours, although the impact on the second stage of labor is minimal. Amniotomy results in less need for oxytocin, although more fetuses develop variable decelerations during the active phase. There are no differences in operative delivery rates or nonreassuring fetal heart rate tracings with amniotomy.

8. a. A reduction in neonatal seizures is noted with continuous electronic fetal monitoring. No benefit is seen in improved Apgar scores, rate of admission to neonatal intensive care units, cerebral palsy, or perinatal death. The use of EFM is positively associated with increases in operative vaginal delivery and cesarean delivery.

9. b. Epidural anesthesia during labor controls pain more effectively than other forms of nonepidural pain control. Approximately 58% of women in the United States receive an epidural during labor. Epidural use is not thought to increase the risk of cesarean delivery, although it does increase the risk of instrumented vaginal delivery with forceps or vacuum. Both the length of the second stage of labor and the need for oxytocin augmentation are increased in women who receive epidurals.

10. **d.** Episiotomy should be performed on a restrictive, rather than routine, basis. Reserving episiotomy for delivery emergencies or operative vaginal deliveries avoids several untoward effects associated with this procedure. Extension of the incision can result in fourth-degree lacerations and anal sphincter damage. Increased blood loss is more common with episiotomy. Postoperative pain and swelling are more common with episiotomy, as is dyspareunia 6 weeks after delivery. The current literature is insufficient to determine whether a midlateral or mediolateral episiotomy is superior.

11. **c.** Active management of the third stage of labor involves administration of prophylactic oxytocin after delivery of the anterior shoulder, immediate clamping/cutting of the umbilical cord, and delivery of the placenta using maternal pushing and cord traction. McRoberts' maneuver is the flexion of the maternal thighs onto the abdomen and is used as an initial intervention when shoulder dystocia is encountered. WHO recommends that the cord not be immediately clamped or cut and that bimanual uterine massage should be performed after delivery of the placenta.

Summary

Labor is the process of progressive cervical dilatation and effacement leading to delivery of the fetus. It is divided into three stages. The first stage of labor ends with complete cervical dilatation. It is divided into latent and active phases. The latent phase is of variable duration and defined by cervical dilatation of less than 4 cm in the presence of contractions. Women who are admitted to labor and delivery while in the latent phase are at increased risk for cesarean delivery, internal monitoring, operative vaginal delivery, and amnionitis. Active labor occurs when the cervix is dilated more than 4 cm and regular contractions result in cervical change. Most nulliparas dilate 1 cm per hour, whereas multiparas generally dilate approximately 1.2 to 1.5 cm per hour. When patients do not follow these patterns, dysfunctional labor is suspected. Partograms are used to track progress in labor. Studies indicate that waiting 4 hours before intervention (amniotomy or oxytocin) in nulliparous women does not increase risk to either mother or fetus. Historically, interventions were begun after 2 hours without progress.

The second stage is the period between complete cervical dilatation and the delivery of the fetus. Pushing generally takes up to 2 hours in primiparas and 1 hour in multiparas. Women who receive epidurals for pain control in labor are at increased risk for a lengthened second stage of labor and the need for oxytocin augmentation. Epidural use does not increase the risk of cesarean delivery.

The third stage of labor is the delivery of the placenta. Active management of the placenta is increasingly used to decrease the risk of maternal blood loss and postpartum hemorrhage. It involves giving oxytocin immediately after delivery of the anterior shoulder, early cord clamping/cutting, controlled cord traction, and maternal pushing to deliver the placenta. WHO recommends against early cord clamping in order to maximize fetal hemoglobin. WHO also recommends use of bimanual uterine massage after delivery of the placenta.

Maternity care is an actively changing field. Evidence-based medicine has examined the efficacy of several routine practices traditionally used in obstetrical care. Perineal shaving, routine episiotomy, enemas, and supine laboring position are not demonstrated to provide a benefit in routine labor management. Women benefit from continuity of care and continuous support in labor. External fetal monitoring does not positively impact rates of cerebral palsy, neonatal intensive care admission, or perinatal death. Although EFM does decrease rates of neonatal seizures, adverse effects include increased risks of cesarean and operative vaginal delivery. Discussions with patients regarding interventions in labor empower couples and physicians to use evidence-based care to maximize birth outcomes.

Suggested Reading

Amin-Soumah M, Smyth R, Howell C: Epidural verses non-epidural or no analgesia in labour. *Cochrane Database Syst Rev* (4):CD000331, 2005.

Bailit J, Dierker L, Blanchard M, et al: Outcomes of women presenting in active versus latent phase of spontaneous labor. *Obstet Gynecol* 105:77–79, 2005.

Hofmeyr G: Evidence-based intrapartum care. *Best Practice Res Clin Obstet Gynecol* 19(1):103–115, 2005.

Prendiville W, Elbourne D, McDonald S: Active versus expectant management in the third stage of labor. *Cochrane Database Syst Rev* (1):CD000007, 2000.

Thacker S, Stroup D, Chang M: Continuous electronic heart rate monitoring for fetal assessment during labor. *Cochrane Database Syst Rev* (1):CD000063, 2001.

b. operative vaginal delivery using forceps
c. operative vaginal delivery using a vacuum extractor
d. manual elevation of the presenting fetal part
e. instillation of 500 mL of normal saline into the bladder

CLINICAL CASE PROBLEM 1

"Is My Baby Ok?"

A 27-year-old female (gravida 2, para 1) at 39 weeks of gestation presents to labor and delivery in active labor. Her pregnancy has been uncomplicated and her prior two deliveries were vaginal. Her cervix is checked by the nurse and judged to be 6 cm, 90% effaced, midposition, and soft. The fetus is not engaged and is thought to be vertex. Initial fetal monitoring shows a heart rate in the 140s with good accelerations and is reassuring. Contractions are 4 minutes apart and the patient is comfortable. Twenty minutes later, the patient experiences a large gush of clear fluid, and severe variable decelerations appear on the fetal heart rate monitor.

1. What is the most likely diagnosis at this time?
   a. uterine rupture
   b. placental abruption
   c. placenta previa
   d. cord prolapse
   e. vasa previa

2. Which of the following conditions is not considered a risk factor for cord prolapse?
   a. grand multiparity
   b. female fetus
   c. abnormally long umbilical cord
   d. prematurity
   e. twin gestation

3. Which of the following statements about cord prolapse diagnosis is false?
   a. cord prolapse is likely when prolonged fetal bradycardia is seen in the presence of ruptured membranes
   b. ruptured membranes are a prerequisite
   c. mean cervical dilatation at diagnosis is 7 cm
   d. the diagnosis is confirmed when the umbilical cord is palpable in the vagina ahead of the fetal presenting part
   e. repetitive moderate to severe variable decelerations are commonly seen with this condition

4. What is the recommended immediate management of this patient?
   a. emergent primary cesarean delivery

CLINICAL CASE PROBLEM 2

No Prenatal Care, Now She's Bleeding

A 23-year-old female (gravida 6, para 3114) presents to labor and delivery with severe abdominal pain. She has no prenatal care, and she thinks her last menstrual period was approximately 9 months ago. She denies a history of medical problems or surgery. All previous deliveries were vaginal. She smokes one and a half packs of cigarettes a day and admits to remote "crank" use. Fundal height measures 39 cm, and there is copious bleeding from the vagina. The fetal monitor shows contractions every minute with elevated baseline uterine tone. Fetal tachycardia at 180 beats/minute, and late decelerations are also present.

5. What is the most likely diagnosis?
   a. uterine rupture
   b. placenta previa
   c. placental abruption
   d. vasa previa
   e. gestational hypertension

6. Maternal risks associated with this diagnosis include all of the following except
   a. death
   b. hysterectomy
   c. disseminated intravascular coagulation
   d. renal failure
   e. myocardial infarction

7. Which gestational age has the highest incidence of placental abruption?
   a. 24 to 26 weeks
   b. 30 to 32 weeks
   c. 32 to 34 weeks
   d. 38 to 40 weeks
   e. more than 40 weeks' gestational age

8. Which of the following conditions is not strongly associated with placental abruption?
   a. maternal smoking
   b. maternal opiate use
   c. chorioamnionitis
   d. history of previous placental abruption
   e. paternal smoking

CLINICAL CASE PROBLEM 3

"Doctor, What's a Turtle Sign?"

A 37-year-old female (gravida 2, para 1001) at 39 weeks of gestation progresses to complete and pushing. Her pregnancy has been complicated by type 2 diabetes, for which she takes metformin. She has gained 45 pounds during the pregnancy, despite both nutritional consultation and repeated counseling. She is 5 feet 2 inches tall and has a prepregnancy body mass index of 34. Descent of the fetal head is slower than anticipated with "positive turtle sign" during contractions. The head is delivered after 2 hours of pushing. The anterior shoulder is difficult to deliver without increased traction. Sixty seconds pass without successful delivery.

9. What is the most important action to take at this time?
   a. flex the maternal hips and bring the knees up to the chest
   b. ask the nurse to apply suprapubic pressure
   c. call for additional help
   d. perform an episiotomy
   e. begin pitocin infusion at 3 mU/minute

10. Which of the following statements about shoulder dystocia is true?
    a. clavicular fracture occurs in approximately 1% of cases
    b. a previously well-oxygenated fetus can tolerate 4 or 5 minutes of severe hypoxia without residual damage
    c. brachial plexus injuries usually involve the C3 and C4 nerve roots
    d. fractures involving the growth plate usually heal well with little or no long-term problems
    e. brachial plexus injuries occur in 30% of cases of shoulder dystocia

11. Which of the following statements regarding macrosomia and shoulder dystocia is true?
    a. diabetes and maternal obesity have strong positive predictive value for shoulder dystocia
    b. 30% of macrosomic infants deliver without shoulder dystocia
    c. fetal macrosomia is suspected when the estimated fetal weight is more than 4000 g
    d. most cases of shoulder dystocia are predictable using risk factors
    e. 40% to 60% of cases of shoulder dystocia occur in infants who weigh less than 4000 g

CLINICAL CASE PROBLEM 4

Hypotension and Bleeding after Delivery

The patient in Clinical Case Problem 3 delivers atraumatically using a combination of McRoberts' maneuver, suprapubic pressure, and an episiotomy. Profuse vaginal bleeding is noted both prior to and following delivery of the placenta. The patient becomes lightheaded and tachycardic. Blood pressure drops to 60/40 mmHg.

12. Which of the following is the least likely cause of this problem?
    a. uterine atony
    b. uterine rupture
    c. retained placental parts
    d. vaginal or cervical lacerations
    e. maternal thrombin or bleeding abnormalities

13. Which of the following steps is not included in active management of the third stage of labor?
    a. administration of pitocin immediately following delivery of the anterior shoulder
    b. controlled cord traction
    c. immediate uterine massage after delivery of the placenta
    d. early cord clamping
    e. administering 400 to 600 µg of misoprostol orally

Answers

1. **d.** The most likely diagnosis is cord prolapse. Cord prolapse occurs in approximately 2/1000 deliveries. Three types of prolapse can occur. Overt cord prolapse is diagnosed when the membranes are ruptured and the umbilical cord falls through the cervix into the vagina ahead of the fetal presenting part. Funic presentation describes loops of umbilical cord between the presenting part and the cervical os prior to rupture of membranes. Occult cord prolapse is diagnosed when the cord is palpable alongside the presenting part on digital cervical exam.

In this case, uterine rupture is less likely since the patient has no history of cesarean delivery.

Abruption is often associated with tetanic contractions and bleeding. An increase in uterine tone is seen between contractions. Vasa previa usually presents with painless bleeding at rupture of membranes. The cervical exam is not consistent with a diagnosis of placenta previa.

2. **b.** Having a male fetus is a significant risk factor for cord prolapse (odds ratio, 1.4; 95% confidence

interval, 1.2 to 1.7). Grand multiparity, an abnormally long umbilical cord, prematurity, polyhydramnios, and multiple gestation pregnancies also carry an increased risk for cord prolapse.

3. c. Mean cervical dilatation at diagnosis of umbilical cord prolapse is 5 cm. Prolonged fetal bradycardia and repetitive moderate to severe variable decelerations are common. Since ruptured membranes are necessary for the cord to prolapse through the cervix, a careful digital exam prior to amniotomy is important to rule out funic presentation. The diagnosis is confirmed when the cord is palpable in the vagina ahead of the fetal presenting part.

4. d. Immediate management of cord prolapse includes manually elevating the presenting part of the fetus to decompress the cord. One study showed a perinatal mortality rate of 1.5% when elevation was performed. Preparation for an emergent primary cesarean is necessary because the cervix is not fully dilated. Instillation of 500 to 700 mL of saline into the bladder has been tested in two small case series of cord prolapse as a bridge until surgery.

5. c. Placental abruption is defined as complete or partial separation of the placenta prior to delivery. The incidence of abruption is 5 or 6 out of 1000 deliveries. Obvious vaginal bleeding occurs if the hemorrhage develops between the membranes and the uterus. Concealed presentations occur when blood collects behind the placenta. Abruption is a leading cause of second and third trimester bleeding, and it causes significant maternal and neonatal morbidity and mortality. The classically described symptoms for abruption are vaginal bleeding and abdominal pain, although the clinical presentation can vary widely.

Although hypertensive disorders of pregnancy are associated with abruption, this is not likely the reason for the patient's condition. Placenta previa and vasa previa are usually not associated with severe pain. Uterine rupture is less common in women with no prior surgical deliveries.

6. e. Maternal risks associated with placental abruption include hemorrhage, need for blood transfusion, hysterectomy, disseminated intravascular coagulation, acute renal failure, and death. Myocardial infarction is not commonly associated with this condition because most women of childbearing age are at lower risk for cardiac disease.

7. a. The incidence of abruption is greatest at 24 to 26 weeks' gestational age. Risk declines sharply with advancing fetal age.

8. b. Maternal opiate use is not strongly associated with placental abruption. A meta-analysis demonstrated that smoking increases the risk of abruption by 90%. Maternal and paternal smoking increases the risk of abruption twofold. Risk increases fivefold when both parents smoke. Women with a history of abruption have a 15% increased risk during future pregnancies. Placenta previa, cocaine use, preeclampsia, and preterm premature rupture of membranes are also associated with placental abruption.

9. c. This delivery is complicated by shoulder dystocia. Shoulder dystocia results from a size discrepancy between the bony maternal pelvis and the fetal shoulders. Infants of diabetic mothers tend to have larger shoulder and extremity circumferences and higher percentages of body fat. The incidence of shoulder dystocia ranges from 0.2% to 3% of deliveries. Management of shoulder dystocia should be performed using a standardized, choreographed procedure (Tabel 95-1). Calling for additional help is the essential first step. The American Academy of Family Physicians' (AAFP) Advanced Life Support in Obstetrics course provides excellent hands-on training for managing shoulder dystocia.

10. b. Previously well-oxygenated fetuses can tolerate 4 or 5 minutes of severe hypoxia without residual damage. Permanent damage is more common with delays in delivery of more than 10 minutes. Clavicular fractures occur in approximately 15% of cases. Humeral fractures are less common at 1%. Fractures that do not involve the growth plate usually heal without sequelae. Brachial plexus injuries occur in 5% to 15% of cases. The C5 and C6 nerve roots are most commonly involved, resulting in an Erb's palsy. Most injuries resolve by 6 to 12 months.

11. e. Risk factors, both alone and in combination, have low positive predictive value for shoulder dystocia. Only 25% of shoulder dystocia cases in one large study had one significant risk factor. Although higher birth weight is often linked to dystocia, 40% to 60% of cases of shoulder dystocia occur in infants less than 4000 g; 70% to 90% of macrosomic infants deliver without incident. Maternal diabetes doubles the risk of shoulder dystocia; the contribution of obesity per se is less understood.

12. b. The patient is experiencing postpartum hemorrhage. Postpartum hemorrhage is defined as blood loss in excess of 500 mL following vaginal delivery or more than 1 L during cesarean. The most common causes of postpartum hemorrhage include uterine tone (atony), retained products of conception, vaginal or cervical lacerations, and maternal

Table 95-1 **Protocol for Shoulder Dystocia Management**

Intervention	Description
Call for help	Additional physician, nursing, and anesthesia help should be urgently summoned
Consider episiotomy	Episiotomy may create more room for maneuvers and reduce maternal trauma
Perform McRoberts' maneuver	Flex maternal hips on abdomen; creates increased anterior to posterior diameter in pelvis; many physicians routinely employ this initially because it is simple and noninvasive
Apply suprapubic pressure	Have assistant apply pressure over the maternal suprapubic area to the posterior aspect of the fetal shoulder; if initial pressure is unsuccessful, rocking motion may be attempted (Rubin I)
Attempt internal maneuvers: Rubin II	Place fingers behind anterior fetal shoulder; apply pressure to adduct shoulder and rotate fetus to oblique position
Perform Woods' screw	Place fingers in front of posterior shoulder; rotate toward pubic symphysis; if not successful, may reverse direction with fingers behind posterior shoulder (reverse Woods' screw/Rubin II)
Attempt to deliver posterior arm	Place hand in posterior vagina and attempt to sweep posterior arm out over fetal torso
Roll patient/ all-fours technique	Increases anterior–posterior diameter of pelvis by 1 or 2 cm; favored by midwives
Attempt cephalic replacement (Zavanelli maneuver)	Attempt if all usual methods unsuccessful; manually replace fetal head into maternal pelvis and proceed with emergent cesarean delivery
Symphysiotomy	Uncommon outside developing countries
Intentionally fracture fetal clavicle	Hook clavicle and break outward and away from thoracic vessels/nerves; performed only in extreme cases

bleeding abnormalities such as disseminated intravascular coagulation. Uterine rupture is unlikely in this clinical scenario.

13. e. Management of the third stage of labor reduces the incidence of postpartum hemorrhage by increasing uterine contractions and minimizing uterine atony. Steps in active management include administering intramuscular or intravenous pitocin with delivery of the anterior shoulder. Immediate cord clamping is combined with controlled traction on the cord to augment placental delivery. Uterine massage after delivery of the placenta is the final step in this process. Misoprostol and ergotamine are both options if oxytocin is not available. Oxytocin is preferred because of its rapid effect and minimal secondary effects.

Summary

The majority of deliveries progress uneventfully. Although complications during labor and delivery are uncommon, most require a prompt and decisive response to minimize maternal and fetal compromise. Understanding the diagnosis and management of these situations is essential to optimal maternity care.

Cord prolapse occurs in 2 out of 1000 deliveries. It is diagnosed when severe variable decelerations or bradycardia occur after membrane rupture. The cord is often palpable in the vagina. Cord prolapse happens most often at 5-cm cervical dilatation and in nonvertex presentations. Immediate delivery is essential to prevent fetal compromise. Cesarean delivery is generally preferred when the cervix is not fully dilated. Vacuum or forceps delivery may be attempted if the cervix is completely dilated, although manual elevation of the fetal part and emergent cesarean are the most common management.

Placental abruption occurs in 1% of births and is a leading cause of vaginal bleeding in the second and third trimester. It occurs when the placenta prematurely separates from the uterine wall. The hemorrhage is either concealed behind the placenta or tracks down between the membranes and uterine wall, causing vaginal bleeding. Separation ranges from mild and asymptomatic to complete, which results in significant morbidity and mortality. Risk factors for abruption include maternal and paternal smoking, preeclampsia, chorioamnionitis, preterm premature rupture of membranes, and cocaine use. Women with a history of placental abruption have a 15% increased risk in a subsequent pregnancy; the risk increases to 20% after two previous abruptions. The diagnosis is made clinically in women presenting with vaginal bleeding and abdominal pain, a history of trauma, or in women with unexplained preterm labor. Ultrasound fails to diagnose at least 50% of abruptions and is less useful in finding nonconcealed abruption. Management depends on gestational age and the severity of presentation in both mother and fetus. Emergent cesarean is generally indicated when the patient is not in labor and hemodynamic compromise is present. If delivery is imminent and the abruption is mild, vaginal delivery may be attempted.

Shoulder dystocia is a frightening delivery complication occurring in 0.2% to 3% of deliveries. Resulting from a size discrepancy between the maternal pelvis and the fetal shoulders, the anterior shoulder becomes wedged against the pubic symphysis. Severe shoulder dystocia increases both maternal and fetal morbidity/mortality. The definition of shoulder dystocia is not well described. A head-to-body delivery delay of more than 60 seconds or the need for additional maneuvers to deliver the shoulder is one standardized definition. Fetal complications of shoulder dystocia include clavicular fracture, humeral fracture, and brachial plexus injuries (Erb's palsy). Most well-oxygenated fetuses can survive for 4 or 5 minutes despite severe hypoxia;

risk of permanent hypoxic injury increases greatly after 10 minutes. Maternal complications of shoulder dystocia include trauma, hemorrhage, and, rarely, hysterectomy.

Risk factors for predicting shoulder dystocia have low positive predictive value. Infants of diabetic mothers have a twofold increase in shoulder dystocia regardless of fetal weight. The influence of fetal macrosomia is less understood; 70% to 90% of macrosomic infants deliver without complications. The most important preparation for shoulder dystocia is having standardized protocols in place to actively manage this situation (see Table 95-1). The AAFP's Advanced Life Support in Obstetrics course provides excellent hands-on training in the management of shoulder dystocia.

Postpartum hemorrhage is a leading cause of maternal morbidity and mortality worldwide. The basic definition is more than 500 mL of blood loss at vaginal delivery or more than 1000 mL blood loss during cesarean delivery. Active management of the third stage of labor is thought to decrease the risk of postpartum hemorrhage by lessening uterine atony. Pitocin administration after delivery of the anterior shoulder, early cord clamping, cord traction, and uterine massage after placental delivery are considered important components in the active management protocol.

Suggested Reading

Carlin A, Alfirevic Z: Intrapartum fetal emergencies. *Semin Fetal Neonatal Med* 11:150–157, 2006.

Enakpene CA, Omigbodun A, Arowojolu A: Perinatal mortality following umbilical cord prolapse. *Int J Gynecol Obstet* 95:44–45, 2006.

Gherman R, Chauhan S, Ouzounian J: Shoulder dystocia: The unpreventable obstetric emergency with empiric management guidelines. *Am J Obstet Gynecol* 195:657–672, 2006.

Lalonde A, Daviss B, Acosta A: Postpartum hemorrhage today: ICM/FIGO initiative 2004–2006. *Int J Gynecol Obstet* 94:243–253, 2006.

Lin MG: Umbilical cord prolapse. *Obstet Gynecol Surv* 61(4):269–277, 2006.

Oyelese Y, Ananth C: Placental abruption. *Obstet Gynecol* 108(4):1005–1016, 2006.

Tikkanen M, Nuutila M, Hiilesmaa V, et al: Clinical presentation and risk factors of placental abruption. *Acta Obstet Gynecol* 85:700–705, 2006.

CHAPTER

96 Postpartum Blues, Depression, and Psychoses

CLINICAL CASE PROBLEM 1

A 26-Year-Old Primigravida Who Is Tearful and Depressed 4 Days Postpartum

A 26-year-old primigravida delivers a healthy male infant at 40 weeks of gestation who she breastfeeds on demand. She was doing fairly well until day 4 postpartum. At that time, she develops insomnia, fatigue, and feelings of sadness and depression.

The patient has a history of bipolar disorder, but she has not had an episode of either hypomania or depression for the past 5 years. Despite your concern regarding her history of bipolar disorder, she begins to improve on the day 8 postpartum and returns to her normal mental state at 2 weeks postpartum. When you see her in the office in 6 weeks she is well.

SELECT THE BEST ANSWER TO THE FOLLOWING QUESTIONS

1. What is the most likely diagnosis in this patient?
   a. postpartum depression
   b. postpartum blues

c. a mild depression, definitely associated with her previous disease

d. postpartum anxiety

e. postpartum psychosis

2. What is the best initial choice of treatment for this patient?
   a. a tricyclic antidepressant
   b. lithium carbonate
   c. a monoamine oxidase inhibitor
   d. a selective serotonin reuptake inhibitor (SSRI)
   e. supportive psychotherapy alone

3. Considering this patient's history of bipolar disorder, which of the following statements is true?
   a. the probability of a recurrence is no greater after pregnancy than in the nonpregnant state
   b. the probability of a recurrence is actually decreased in the postpartum state
   c. the probability of a recurrence is increased in the postpartum state
   d. none of the above
   e. nobody knows for sure

CLINICAL CASE PROBLEM 2

"I Should Be Happy, Not Exhausted..."

A 24-year-old primigravida is 3 months postpartum with a healthy female infant. The mother is exhausted, cries easily, and feels guilty that she does not enjoy her baby as much as she had expected. She saw her obstetrician for the 6-week postpartum exam and is due back for a physical when the baby is 6 to 9 months of age. The patient has not yet resumed any of her predelivery social outings and is often ready for bed when her husband returns from work to assume care for the baby. She is so tired that she wishes she had never begun breast-feeding.

4. When surveying for depression, the physician should extend his or her vigilance for
   a. 6 weeks postpartum
   b. 6 months postpartum
   c. 2 weeks after delivery
   d. 1 year after delivery
   e. There are no rules regarding the detection of postpartum depression (PPD)

5. The role of detecting PPD falls to
   a. the obstetrician during the first postnatal visit
   b. the pediatrician, who typically sees the mother and baby during the first 12 months postpartum
   c. the family physician

d. social workers who work in close proximity to the family

e. all of the above

6. When considering risk factors for PPD
   a. PPD occurs overwhelmingly in grand multiparas
   b. the occurrence is common in certain cultures and certain ethnic groups
   c. the etiology, in addition to the accepted risk factors, includes disappointment in developing countries with regard to the newborn's gender
   d. past history of mental illness but not hormonal factors plays a role in PPD
   e. history of depression plays a role only in late-onset postpartum depression

7. When evaluating and assessing patients for PPD
   a. the majority of patients can be identified only in the postnatal period
   b. the majority of patients can be identified during the pregnancy
   c. psychological and psychosocial interventions are the standard of care
   d. group therapy is as efficient as intensive therapy
   e. there is no role for either psychosocial or psychological interventions; antidepressants are the superior therapy

8. Regarding diagnosis and prevention of PPD
   a. the Edinburgh Postnatal Depression Scale is an accepted tool for depression screening in the postpartum period
   b. any adult depression scale can be used
   c. if the caregiver has no time, he or she can use two questions to rule out depression
   d. prevention through the goal of detection can be rarely achieved
   e. all of the above

9. Which of the following is the initial treatment of choice for this patient?
   a. intensive observation alone
   b. lithium carbonate
   c. antipsychotic medication
   d. an SSRI
   e. diazepam

10. Woman who are breast-feeding while using antidepressants should be advised to
    a. stop taking their medications
    b. continue the medications in a reduced regimen
    c. change from tricyclics to SSRIs
    d. "pump and dump"
    e. await serum levels of antidepressants before continuing

CLINICAL CASE PROBLEM 3

"Will This Depression Happen Again?"

A 29-year-old woman has begun feeling better since you discovered and treated her PPD. However, she wants more children and is concerned about future pregnancies and the impact of depression on this child and future children. Your patient wants to know whether she has to worry about her next pregnancy.

11. You tell her that
    a. her pregnancy might be complicated by depression
    b. she might be at an increased risk for preterm labor
    c. her next pregnancy might result in a low-birth-weight baby
    d. any pregnancy complication can increase the probability of depression
    e. all of the above

CLINICAL CASE PROBLEM 4

"Can I Take This Medicine While I'm Pregnant?"

Your patient has been using antidepressants for 2 years. She just found out that she is pregnant. She expresses concern regarding her "baby's health."

12. You reassure her that
    a. SSRIs and tricyclic antidepressants are safe to use in pregnancy
    b. there are rarely any side effects when ingesting antidepressants during pregnancy
    c. to the best of our knowledge, antidepressants have a transient effect on neonatal behavior
    d. all tricyclic antidepressants cause congenital malformation
    e. all of the above

Answers

1. b. This patient has postpartum blues, the common name for mild depressive symptoms that occur during this period. Postpartum blues occurs in approximately 50% to 80% of puerperal women. The syndrome is transitory, resolving spontaneously within a few days to 2 weeks. Postpartum blues usually starts with a brief period of weeping on the third or fourth day after delivery and peaks between days 5 and 10 after delivery. Symptoms include anxiety, headaches, poor concentration, and confusion.

The cause of postpartum blues is unknown, but a hormonal basis is suspected. Of the hormones involved, the most likely candidate is progesterone, and the most likely alteration is progesterone deficiency.

2. e. The treatment of choice for postpartum blues includes supportive psychotherapy; family (especially spousal) support, understanding, and reassurance; and patient education (reassuring the patient that this is completely normal). For the patient described, it is especially important to reinforce that there is no connection between the postpartum blues she is currently experiencing and her previous bipolar illness; resolution of "the blues" will occur within 2 weeks, but monitoring her condition is necessary to ensure both maternal and fetal health.

3. c. In a patient with a history of bipolar disorder, there is actually an increased chance of reoccurrence in the postpartum period.

Of the 50% to 80% of women who develop postpartum blues, only 10% will go on to have a true PPD, the common term for a major depressive disorder with postpartum onset.

4. b. Although the *Diagnostic and Statistical Manual of Mental Disorders*, fourth edition, describes PPD as occurring within 4 weeks postpartum and the *International Statistical Classification of Diseases and Related Health Problems*, 10th revision, describes it as occurring within 6 weeks postpartum, a mounting body of evidence suggests that PPD can occur even 6 months after delivery.

5. e. Many women go undiagnosed and untreated with potentially devastating consequences. It is irrelevant who detects it; all health care workers should have a level of suspicion when dealing with a patient in the postpartum period who exhibits symptoms or signs of depression after delivery.

6. c. Reports from developing countries show that in addition to the usual risk factors for PPD, a child of "unwanted" gender is an emerging risk factor. PPD is found in all cultures and across all ethnicities. Prior history of PPD is often a factor in early PPD (2 weeks postpartum). Although accepted care, evidence of the benefits of treatment with SSRIs alone or with psychotherapy is not abundant. Hormonal factors as evidenced by premenstrual dysphoric disorder as well as mood disorder during the third trimester, in addition to prior history of mental illness, are extremely important risk factors.

7. b. The incidence of third trimester depression is higher than that in the postpartum period. Studies have shown that vigilance during the third trimester will detect patients who are suffering from depression. These patients are at a higher risk for PPD. The treatment of PPD consists of both psychological and medical treatment (SSRIs mainly). Generally, only intensive behavioral therapy seems to be of benefit to these patients.

8. e. The Edinburgh Postnatal Depression Scale (EPDS) was developed for the postpartum period. In its absence, the practitioner can use any adult evaluation scale or the two cardinal questions: "During the past month did you feel depressed or hopeless?" and "During the past month, were you bothered by little interest or pleasure in doing things?" Screening is the key to treatment and possible prevention of PPD. The EPDS has been used in different countries successfully. Many physicians believe that it should be administered during pregnancy because more than 10% of PPD begins during pregnancy.

9. c. Acute treatment for this patient consists of administering an antipsychotic drug to control psychosis and agitation. A high-potency antipsychotic medication such as risperidone might be a good first choice. At the same time, the patient should be observed closely by hospital staff.

After the acute psychotic episode is under control, long-term therapy should be started. Depending on whether an underling psychiatric disorder or persistent mood symptoms are present, antidepressant or mood-stabilizing medication may be initiated. In addition, supportive individual and family psychotherapy should be given. After discharge, it is prudent to arrange regular visits by a mental health worker to measure general day-to-day coping skills immediately postpartum and for an extended time.

10. c. Antidepressants do cross to breast milk. The levels are sometimes undetectable by commercial labs. Their detection in breast milk does not signify a harmful effect on the baby. There is a paucity of randomized controlled trials regarding breast-feeding and antidepressants. Most practitioners weigh the risks of discontinuing antidepressants versus potential risks to the newborn. Fluoxetine is not commonly used. Since the peak in SSRI levels is 9 hours after ingestion, some practitioners recommend that the mother discard her breast milk collected at this time, thus reducing the infant's exposure by 20%.

11. e. Women who suffer from PPD have a higher incidence of preterm labor as well as having a child with low birth weight. The etiology is thought to involve stress as well as hormonal factors. Studies show that the woman who suffers from PPD may also suffer from antenatal depression.

12. c. Continuing antidepressants in pregnancy is extremely controversial. The risk to the mother and fetus needs to be measured against the benefit of treating depression in pregnancy. The majority of research shows transient behavioral signs in the newborn, with premature infants being the most susceptible.

Summary

1. General
   a. Many women still go undiagnosed by physicians.
   b. Pediatricians, obstetricians, and health care workers are encouraged to diagnose and detect PPD.
   c. Differential diagnosis: Before calling it depression, one must rule out thyroid dysfunction and anemia. (Five percent of women will have hypothyroidism postpartum.)
2. Postpartum blues
   a. Incidence: 50% to 80%
   b. Evolution: begins on or about the third day postpartum and resolves by 2 weeks
   c. Treatment: reassurance, supportive psychotherapy; involvement of spouse or significant other is critical

3. Postpartum depression
   a. Incidence: 13%
   b. Evolution: usually begins on the third to fifth day postpartum and lasts longer than 2 weeks; can be detected up to 12 months after delivery
   c. Treatment: psychotherapy and pharmacologic antidepressant therapy. (No studies have shown clearly that SSRIs are effective, but they are commonly used.)
   d. Impact: Maternal depression has a clear effect on growth as well as social and cognitive development of the infant. Children of depressed mothers can have developmental, language, and emotional disorders for the rest of their lives.

Babies who are born to mothers on SSRIs have transient behavioral problems. In preterm babies, these effects last longer. (Depression during pregnancy is probably a causative agent for preterm delivery, low birth rate, and PPD.)

4. Postpartum psychosis
   a. Incidence: 0.1% to 0.2%
   b. Pharmacologic treatment
      i. Acute: antipsychotic medication, close observation to prevent self-harm and harm to the infant
      ii. Long-term: mood stabilizer if underlying bipolar disorder, manic phase is present; mood stabilizer and antidepressant if bipolar disorder, depressive phase is present; antidepressant if underlying major depressive disorder is present
   c. Psychotherapy: supportive group or individual; involvement of spouse or significant other is critical
   d. Impact: Approximately 5% of psychotic mothers will commit suicide or infanticide.

5. Prevention of postpartum psychopathology
   a. Education in the prenatal period, which must include significant attention to the psychologic consequences of pregnancy, labor and delivery, and the impact of the neonate on the family
   b. Explanation of all procedures and interventions to allow the patient as much control as possible during labor
   c. Significant involvement of the husband or significant other in the process

Suggested Reading

Cooper PJ, Murray L, Wilson A, et al: Controlled trial of the short- and long-term effect of psychological treatment of post-partum depression: 1. Impact on maternal mood. *Br J Psychiatry* 182:412–419, 2003.

Cunningham FG: *Williams Obstetrics*, 22nd ed. New York: McGraw–Hill, pp. 1244–1245, 2005.

Ferreria E: Effects of SSRI and venlafaxine during pregnancy in term and pre-term neonates. *Pediatrics* 119(1):52–59, 2007.

Howard L: Clinical Evidence Concise: Postnatal depression. *Am Fam Physician* 72(7): October 1, 2005.

Wisner KL, Parry BL, Piontek CM: Clinical practice. Postpartum depression. *N Engl J Med* 347(3):194–199, 2002.

CHILDREN AND ADOLESCENTS

97 Common Problems of the Newborn

CLINICAL CASE PROBLEM 1

A Precipitous Delivery and Tachypnea

A 7-pound, 2-ounce infant delivered at 39⁶/₇ weeks arrives in the nursery with normal vital signs except for a respiratory rate of 80 breaths/minute. The labor and subsequent delivery were precipitous according to the labor and delivery nurse.

SELECT THE BEST ANSWER TO THE FOLLOWING QUESTIONS

1. Which of the following statements is (are) true?
   a. symptoms of respiratory distress in newborns include poor feeding, intercostal retraction, and nasal flaring
   b. normal respiratory rate in a newborn is less than 60 breaths/minute
   c. transient tachypnea of the newborn is the most common cause of neonatal respiratory distress
   d. cesarean section is not a risk factor for transient tachypnea of the newborn (TTN)
   e. a, b, and c

2. Which of the following is (are) manifest during the first hours after delivery?
   a. transient tachypnea of the newborn
   b. meconium aspiration syndrome
   c. sepsis
   d. asthma
   e. a and b

3. Which of the follow is not a common pathogen found in neonatal sepsis?
   a. group B streptococcus
   b. *Staphylococcus aureus*
   c. *Streptococcus pneumonia*
   d. *Bacteroides fragilis*
   e. none of the above

CLINICAL CASE PROBLEM 2

"My Baby Is Turning Yellow"

A term 8-pound infant with history of a normal postdelivery course was discharged home with mother at 40 hours of age. The infant is being fed mother's milk every 2 or 3 hours and is producing clear urine, wetting seven diapers per day. The parents call the office on the third day of life to complain that the infant appears yellow and they are concerned.

4. The most likely cause of this infant's jaundice is
   a. blood group incompatibility (ABO compatibility)
   b. sepsis
   c. physiologic jaundice
   d. breast milk
   e. dehydration

5. Serum bilirubin should be measured
   a. when jaundice is clinically evident within the first day of life
   b. in all infants who evidence jaundice
   c. in infants whose jaundice persists past 3 weeks of age
   d. a and c
   e. all of the above

CLINICAL CASE PROBLEM 3

A 1-Week-Old with Fever

A 1-week-old infant with a normal physical examination is found to have a rectal temperature of 38.1°C. The baby was born at term, weighed 7 pounds, 4 ounces, and continues to feed well and wet six to eight diapers per day. The infant interacts appropriately and is easily consoled when crying.

6. Differential diagnosis includes
a. meningitis
b. self-limited viral illness
c. pneumonia
d. urinary tract infection
e. all of the above

7. Appropriate steps to be taken include
a. complete blood count (CBC) with differential
b. blood culture
c. lumbar puncture
d. follow-up in 12 to 24 hours
e. a, b, and c

8. A 6-week-old infant has a temperature of 39°C and no abnormalities on physical examination. What are appropriate management strategies for this child?
a. CBC, blood culture, oral amoxicillin, follow-up in 10 to 14 days
b. CBC, blood culture, intramuscular ceftriaxone, follow-up in 24 hours
c. CBC, blood culture, intravenous (IV) ceftriaxone, admission to the hospital
d. acetaminophen, oral water, follow-up if fever persists
e. b and c

Answers

1. e. Infants born after cesarean section and those born after precipitous deliveries have higher rates of TTN than do infants born vaginally after labor of normal duration. Prostaglandin-driven dilatation of lymphatic vessels lags behind first breaths in infants who have not had the chest compression inherent in normal labor.

2. e. TTN and meconium aspiration syndrome are evident soon after delivery, whereas symptoms of sepsis appear several hours to a few days after birth. Asthma is not usually seen in neonates.

3. d. Most cases of neonatal sepsis are caused by *Staphylococcus* and *Streptococcus*, with *Escherichia coli* also in the differential diagnosis. Bacteroides sepsis is rare in newborns.

4. c. Physiologic jaundice manifests as jaundice without other symptoms and occurs in the first few days of life, whereas jaundice due to blood group incompatibility usually develops in the first 24 hours of life and requires more careful attention. A healthy breast-fed infant may develop some jaundice, but this is rarely a problem and normally resolves with continuation of normal feeding.

5. d. Jaundice in the first 24 hours of life is indicative of more serious problems than physiologic jaundice, and it should be evaluated with a careful clinical assessment and a total and direct bilirubin measurement. Infants whose jaundice lasts past 3 weeks of age should be assessed for cholestasis, and their newborn thyroid and galactosemia screen results should be reviewed.

6. e. Febrile infants can have serious infection even with normal examinations and no evident source of fever. Approximately 3% of these newborns have bacteremia.

7. e. All infants 0 to 30 days of age with fever should be admitted to the hospital and treated with ampicillin and either a third-generation cephalosporin or gentamicin. The workup should include CBC with differential, blood culture, lumbar puncture, urinalysis, and urine culture. A chest x-ray is optional unless physical signs indicate it.

8. e. Choices b and c are both reasonable strategies, but discharge to home with close follow-up is only appropriate if parents are reliable and communication as well as return for follow-up are highly likely. Even at 6 weeks of age, fever of unknown source has a sufficiently high risk of being associated with bacteremia that these infants should have laboratory studies and close follow-up, as well as antibiotic therapy.

Summary

1. Respiratory Distress
Newborns in respiratory distress exhibit symptoms such as apnea, cyanosis, grunting, inspiratory stridor, nasal flaring, poor feeding, and tachypnea, along with retractions of the intercostals, subcostal, and/or supracostal. Normal respiratory rate in a newborn is less than 60 breaths/minute. Approximately 7% of newborns have respiratory distress; most cases in term infants are due to transient tachypnea of the newborn, with meconium aspiration being another common cause. TTN results from residual pulmonary fluid in the neonatal lung, and it is more common after

precipitous and cesarean deliveries, when there may be delay in prostaglandin-driven dilatation of lymphatic vessels that allows removal of lung fluid with an increase in pulmonary circulation. Neonatal sepsis/infection can also be a cause; common pathogens are group B streptococcus, *S. aureus*, *S. pneumonia*, and gram-negative rods. The differential diagnosis should include anemia, congenital heart disease, neurologic abnormalities, pneumothorax, and upper airway obstruction. TTN and meconium aspiration syndrome occur immediately after delivery, but infectious etiologies manifest hours to days after birth.

Treatment for respiratory distress should first follow neonatal resuscitation protocols. Oral feedings should be delayed if respiratory rates are higher than 80 breaths/minute. Oxygen can be given by the blow-by method, nasal cannula, or mechanical ventilation as needed, and ampicillin with gentamicin or a third-generation cephalosporin can be given if sepsis or infection is suspected. Pneumothorax requires needle decompression or chest tube placement unless small enough to respond to nitrogen washout with 100% oxygen. TTN is treated with supportive measures including oxygen as needed. It is usually self-limited. Oronasopharyngeal suctioning before shoulder delivery does not prevent meconium aspiration syndrome; aspiration occurs in utero, not during delivery. Treatment is limited to oxygen and supportive care unless the baby has a heart rate less than 100 beats/minute, absence of spontaneous respirations, or low tone.

2. Hyperbilirubinemia

Common causes of hyperbilirubinemia in the newborn include physiological jaundice, blood group incompatibility, and infection. Preventive strategies against hyperbilirubinemia in newborns born at 35 weeks of gestation or more include nursing infants 8 to 12 times per day for the first several days and the avoidance of water or dextrose water in nondehydrated infants. Prenatal testing for ABO and Rh(D) blood types and maternal serum screen for isoimmune antibodies can identify infants at higher risk of neonatal jaundice. For mothers not tested prior to delivery, cord blood direct antibody test, blood type, and Rh(D) type are recommended. Newborns should be assessed for jaundice every 8 to 12 hours during the first day of life. Infants with clinical jaundice in the first 24 hours of life should have a total bilirubin level.

If there is an elevated direct (conjugated) bilirubin, urinalysis and urine are indicated, and sepsis should be considered. Ill infants and those whose jaundice that persists past 3 weeks of age should be evaluated for cholestasis with total and direct bilirubin levels,

and their newborn thyroid and galactosemia screens should be reviewed.

In cases of jaundice severe enough to require phototherapy, rising bilirubin levels suggest hemolysis. Total serum bilirubin levels of 25 mg/dL or higher (428 μM/L) should be considered a medical emergency; these infants should be admitted to the hospital for phototherapy. Exchange transfusion is recommended for infants who are jaundiced and have signs of encephalopathy (hypertonia, arching, retrocollis, opisthotonos, fever, and high-pitched cry), even if the bilirubin is falling.

Breast-fed infants should continue their feedings if they require phototherapy. Changing to formula is not necessary. If the infant has excessive weight loss or becomes dehydrated, expressed human milk (a donor's or the mother's) can be added to normal breast-feeding.

Physiologic jaundice begins on day 2 or 3 of life and usually resolves in 1 or 2 weeks. It is common and usually requires no therapy. The immature neonatal liver is initially not able to process the circulating bilirubin that results from normal red blood cell destruction. Term infants, when given adequate human milk, handle this excess bilirubin without resultant problems. Some experts call this situation "lack of breast milk jaundice" because it is more common in infants who are not fed often enough. Jaundice that begins within the first 24 hours of life is more likely to be due to infection or to ABO incompatibility.

3. Infant Feeding

Human milk is the recommended nutrition for all infants, with rare contraindications. If the contraindication to mother's milk is temporary, pumping to maintain milk production should proceed. Hospital policies and physician recommendations should facilitate normal infant feeding with human milk. Water, glucose water, formula, and other fluids are not needed by healthy newborns.

4. Neonatal Fever

Fever in the newborn can be life threatening, and clinicians should follow evidence-based guidelines for evaluation and treatment. Although parents are fairly accurate when reporting fever by touch, rectal temperature should be documented, and doctors should be aware that the magnitude of fever does not predict severity of illness. A fever is defined as a rectal temperature greater than or equal to 38°C (100.4°F). Etiologies to consider include meningitis, bone and joint infections, cellulitis, pneumonia, urinary tract infection, bacteremia, sepsis, and enteritis. The presence of lethargy, failure to interact with people or the environment, poor perfusion, acrocyanosis, mottling, capillary refill time greater than 2 seconds when warm, and hyper- or hypoventilation should be signs of concern. Without an evident source of fever, infants should have the following laboratory studies: CBC with differential white count, blood culture, urinalysis, urine culture, and lumbar puncture. In low-risk infants 31 to 60 days of age, if there is reliable follow-up in 12 to 24 hours and antibiotics will not be started, it may be acceptable to delay lumbar puncture and reexamine the infant in 12 to 24 hours. Should obtaining cerebrospinal fluid be impossible (failed tap or parental refusal), antibiotics should be begun. Other laboratory studies should be ordered based on clinical findings (e.g., chest x-ray if there are respiratory symptoms).

All infants 0 to 30 days of age with fever should be admitted to the hospital and treated with intravenous ampicillin plus a third-generation cephalosporin or gentamicin. Ampicillin covers _Listeria monocytogenes_ and _Enterococcus_. Approximately 3% of infants 0 to 30 days of age with fever of unknown source and thought to be low risk will have bacteremia. Low-risk infants 31 to 60 days of age with fever of unknown source can be managed as outpatients or inpatients depending on family needs, the judgment of the physician, and the availability of timely outpatient follow-up. Antibiotic choice should focus on third-generation cephalosporins, with IV ampicillin if urinary tract infection is suspected or if the infant is severely ill. Another option for older low-risk infants with fever is observation off antibiotics. For infants age 0 to 60 days, antibiotic therapy should continue for at least 24 to 48 hours, based on clinical response and culture results at 36 hours after incubation onset. Most positive blood, urine, and cerebrospinal fluid cultures turn positive at 16 to 18 hours.

Suggested Reading

American Academy of Pediatrics: Management of hyperbilirubinemia in the newborn infant 35 or more weeks of gestation. _Pediatrics_ 114(1):297–316, 2004.
American Academy of Pediatrics Committee on Nutrition: Policy statement: Breastfeeding and the use of human milk. _Pediatrics_ 115(2):496–506, 2005.
Cincinnati Children's Hospital Medical Center: Evidence based clinical practice guideline for fever of uncertain source in infants 60 days of age or less. Cincinnati, OH: Cincinnati Children's Hospital Medical Center, 2003.
Hermansen CL, Lorah KN: Respiratory distress in the newborn. _Am Fam Physician_ 76:987–994, 2007.

CHAPTER

98 Infant Feeding

CLINICAL CASE PROBLEM 1

A New Mother with Insecurities

A mother who just delivered her first baby 2 weeks ago comes to your office for her routine visit. She says that her milk just "isn't enough" and she plans to start supplementing since her baby cries all the time and seems unsatisfied by her milk. The mother would have given up already, but her sister breast-fed and has been giving her encouragement. In addition, her husband has encouraged her to breastfeed since it is "best for the baby." The mother appears tired, and during your interview the child is on the breast the entire time. The child is at the 50th percentile for weight and the 50th percentile for length. More important, the child has gained an average of 50 g/day since discharge from the hospital. The child is feeding every 2 hours at this time.

SELECT THE BEST ANSWER TO THE FOLLOWING QUESTIONS

1. What is the minimal appropriate weight gain (and a sign of both infant health and maternal–infant

bonding with breastfeeding) following discharge from hospital?
a. 15 g/day
b. 20 g/day
c. 30 g/day
d. 50 g/day
e. 75 g/day

2. What would be your suggestion to the mother in terms of feeding her infant?
a. reassure her that she does have enough milk, the infant's weight gain is excellent, and the infant uses the breast for comfort as well as nutrition
b. decrease the feeds of the infant to every 4 hours on a set schedule to prevent her fatigue
c. alternate every other feed breast and bottle
d. switch from breastfeeding to bottle-feeding
e. b and c

3. Regarding the feeding of infants when they cry, which of the following is the best advice to the mother?
a. feed the baby; no ifs, ands, or buts
b. let the infant cry for at least 30 minutes; if the infant is still crying, it is likely to be either a diaper problem or a food problem
c. supplement breastfeeding; crying may indicate inadequate milk supply
d. crying may or may not indicate hunger; assume that the baby needs to be fed until proved otherwise; if the baby refuses the breast, check for other causes of crying
e. crying is usually the first sign of hunger in a baby

4. Which of the following statements regarding milk production and maternal anxiety is (are) true?
a. there is little correlation between milk production and maternal anxiety
b. maternal anxiety may significantly increase milk let-down
c. maternal anxiety may significantly decrease milk let-down
d. the main determinant of a good milk supply is frequent, effective milk removal
e. c and d

5. Human colostrum is the precursor to human milk. What is (are) the major component in colostrum that offers a significant advantage to breast-fed infants?
a. macrophages that synthesize complement, lysozyme, and lactoferrin
b. bacterial antibodies that protect the infant against bacterial organisms entering through the gastrointestinal (GI) tract
c. antibodies that protect the infant against viral organisms entering through the GI tract
d. b and c
e. a, b, and c

6. Which of the following antibodies is of particular importance and is found in abundance in human colostrum?
a. immunoglobulin A (IgA)
b. IgG
c. IgM
d. IgE
e. none of the above

7. The mother returns for the infant's 2-month visit and although he is doing well, she is afraid that she might need to start infant cereal or baby food to ensure he is getting enough nutrition. Your response is which of the following?
a. go ahead and feed him cereal at night to help him sleep better
b. introduce cereal at 4 months, and then add one food of the "first foods" every day
c. introduce cereal at approximately 6 months, and then add one new food every week or two
d. introduce cereal at any time he seems to be hungry after breastfeeding
e. none of the above

8. The mother calls your nurse after the 2-month checkup because she forgot to ask you about vitamins. Her sister's baby, who was 6 weeks preterm, was given iron supplementation. Your nurse tells her, based on your answer, which of the following?
a. you will call in a multivitamin with iron and fluoride
b. because fluoride concentration in the water of your community exceeds 1 ppm, no supplementation is required
c. since breast milk has less iron than formula, you will call in some iron for supplementation
d. preterm infants have lower iron stores than term infants, so even though her sister's infant needed iron, her infant does not
e. b and d

CLINICAL CASE PROBLEM 2

A 28-Year-Old Primigravida with Mastitis

A 28-year-old primigravida develops an erythematous skin discoloration in the upper outer quadrant of the left breast. She has achy, flu-like symptoms and fever to 101°F. You suspect bacterial mastitis.

9. At this time, what would you do?
   a. stop breastfeeding and have the mother express her breast milk until the infection is cleared
   b. continue breastfeeding and treat the mother with hot compresses and antibiotics
   c. continue breastfeeding and treat both the mother and the infant with antibiotics
   d. discontinue breastfeeding for now and provide antibiotics to the mother
   e. discontinue any further breastfeeding and perform an incision and drainage immediately

10. What is (are) the organisms most likely responsible for the condition described here?
    a. *Streptococcus pneumoniae*
    b. *Staphylococcus aureus*
    c. *Escherichia coli*: subtype H-57
    d. *Bacteroides fragilis*
    e. b and d
    f. b and c
    g. a, b, and c

11. The patient is discouraged when she returns 1 month later with another bout of mastitis. She has returned to work and is pumping with a breast pump during her breaks. What is (are) the likely cause(s) of the recurrent mastitis you should explore?
    a. check her latch-on and determine if the baby is positioned properly
    b. encourage her to use different breastfeeding positions to massage different milk ducts
    c. make sure she is getting adequate rest and hydration and is not waiting too long between feeds (or pumping)
    d. check her nipples for cracks, fissures, or signs of fungal infection
    e. all of the above

12. When you are visiting with the patient, she expresses her desire to breastfeed until her child is 12 months of age. You are impressed with her perseverance and ask her what makes her willing to endure the recurrent infections. Which of the following is true concerning a woman's decision to breastfeed?
    a. most women decide to breastfeed during their third trimester
    b. the opinion of the husband/boyfriend plays little or no role in the woman's decision to breastfeed
    c. hospital practices that do not follow the Baby-Friendly Hospital Initiative have little impact on a woman's decision to breastfeed or to continue to breastfeed

   d. putting the baby to breast soon after delivery, avoiding bottles and pacifiers, and encouraging rooming in with the mother are all important in helping a woman to breastfeed successfully
   e. women who are younger with less education are more likely to breastfeed due to the cost of formula

CLINICAL CASE PROBLEM 3

A Mother with a Baby Who Spits Up Often

A mother comes to your office with her infant. Her baby is 6 weeks of age and has been "spitting up" all of her formula "since birth." She is afraid the infant is malnourished. The baby weighs 11 pounds, 3 ounces. Her birth weight was 7 pounds, 6 ounces.

13. At this time, you should advise the mother to do which of the following?
    a. return home and relax; the child will grow out of it
    b. increase the time spent burping the infant and keep the infant semiupright after feedings
    c. investigate the child for pyloric stenosis
    d. suggest the use of a GI tract motility modifier such as metoclopramide
    e. immediately refer the child to a pediatric gastroenterologist

CLINICAL CASE PROBLEM 4

A Mother with Breastfeeding Problems

A mother comes to your office with her 8-week-old infant girl. The mother is tearful and depressed. She has been trying to breastfeed, but she tells you, "I'm obviously inadequate. I'm not producing enough milk, and the baby is fussy all of the time." On examination, the infant looks thin. Since her last checkup 3 weeks ago, she has gained only 90 g. The rest of the physical examination is normal.

14. At this time, what should you not do?
    a. ask some very direct questions about the mother's feeding technique
    b. refer the mother to a lactation consultant
    c. encourage the mother to start pumping and include the baby's father or other family member in feeding her milk to the baby, adding formula if necessary until her milk supply is adequate for the baby's catchup growth

d. schedule a reassessment within 3 days after interventions have been undertaken

e. advise immediate and complete cessation of breast milk with switch to formula

15. After two more visits, the mother decides to bottle-feed. She returns when the child is 3 months old, complaining that the infant is constipated. After a careful history, you find that the infant has one hard stool a day but otherwise has no symptoms. On examination, the infant is well hydrated and has had adequate weight gain. The physical exam, including the anal sphincter tone, is normal. You advise which of the following?

a. explain to the mother that formula-fed babies generally have fewer stools than breast-fed babies. If the infant is having a stool every 1 to 3 days and has no symptoms, no treatment is needed

b. add 2 teaspoons of bran to the bottle to increase bulk

c. use glycerine suppositories twice a day

d. change to another formula

e. give mineral oil and water as needed

16. Which of the following is not true concerning differences between human milk and formula?

a. immunoglobulins constitute a sizeable portion of the protein in human milk, particularly in the first 2 to 4 days; they are not present in formula

b. breast milk contains lactoferrin, an iron-binding protein that enhances iron absorption and inhibits bacterial growth; formula has no lactoferrin

c. active leukocytes, including T cells, B cells, plasma cells, and macrophages, are present in breast milk; active leukocytes are present in the newer formulas to help the infant's immune system

d. breastfeeding provides an antigen-specific response due to the mother's ability to recognize and respond immunologically; formula has no such response.

e. human milk is metabolized more quickly than formula, resulting in more frequent feedings for breast-fed babies

17. Which of the following is not a requirement of the Baby-Friendly Hospital Initiative according to World Health Organization (WHO) criteria developed to encourage breastfeeding?

a. have a written breastfeeding policy that is communicated regularly to all staff

b. use pacifiers when infants are crying and the mother is not available to breastfeed to prevent nipple confusion

c. initiate breastfeeding within 30 minutes of birth

d. practice rooming in so mother and infant can be together

e. teach mothers how to maintain lactation even if they are separated from their infants

Clinical Case Management Problem

You are the medical director for the county indigent health system. Your budget has been decreased 15% and many on the board are suggesting that you eliminate the lactation consultant's job as well as breastfeeding classes. Their justification is that your clientele is mainly unmarried teens, and the number of girls who decide to breastfeed is minimal. What is your reply?

Answers

1. **b.** The minimal acceptable weight gain in the neonatal period and infancy is 20 g/day. If weight gain equals or exceeds this, you can be reasonably confident that the infant is thriving. Breast-fed infants should not lose more than 8% of their body weight; however, some mothers have a difficult time starting to breastfeed. If the birth weight is attained by 2 weeks or the infant is gaining 20 g/day, the mother can be assured. Electronic scales should be used and care should be taken to weigh the baby wearing a fresh diaper. Other measures of hydration, such as five or six diapers a day and two or three stools a day, may be helpful. Reminding the mother that the best way to increase her milk production is the latch-on and suck of the infant, coupled with adequate rest and nutrition for her, is important as well.

2. **a.** Often, women who are breastfeeding need reassurance that they are providing adequate nutrition to their infant. Weight gain and confirmation from the physician encourage women to continue to breastfeed. During the first few weeks and months of life, the ideal feeding schedule is feeding on demand. This will vary from infant to infant but eventually will settle into a reasonable schedule averaging 8 to 12 feedings per day. Since establishing lactation is very important early on, it is better that the mother not bottle-feed at all to avoid nipple confusion and decreased production.

In the case of this mother, the infant is likely sucking often for comfort, and encouraging her that this is not due to lack of nutrition will help prevent bottle-feeding and overfeeding. Nipple confusion is less common after the first 6 weeks, when the feeding patterns are established.

3. d. Infants cry for a variety of reasons, and crying may not always be a sign of hunger. Some infants are placid, some are unusually active, and some are irritable. Sick infants are often uninterested in food. Health care providers should encourage mothers to breastfeed for comfort and nuture, as well as nutrition. In contrast to bottle-fed babies, breast-fed babies can regulate their intake of milk at the breast by altering their suckling patterns. The mother should check for feeding cues; if the infant's cry stops when picked up or rocked, the infant may only need closeness and security.

4. e. Maternal anxiety, fatigue, postpartum depression, and stress from other causes are causal candidates for decreased milk production and let-down. The main determinant of a good milk supply is frequent, effective milk removal.

5. e. Colostrum provides macrophages that synthesize complement, lysozyme, and lactoferrin and antibodies against bacteria and viruses that protect the infant against infection through the GI tract.

6. a. Human colostrum contains antibodies of the IgA class that protect the infant from bacterial species such as *E. coli* and certain viruses. In addition, human colostrum contains macrophages that are able to synthesize complement, lysozyme, lactoferrin, and the iron-binding whey protein that is normally approximately one-third saturated with iron.

7. c. Parents often want to introduce cereal and solid foods earlier than recommended. Early introduction of foods may promote development of allergens. The American Academy of Pediatrics and the American Academy of Family Physicians recommend that solid foods should not be introduced into an infant's diet until approximately 6 months of age. New foods should not be introduced more often than one every 1 or 2 weeks. The order of food introduction appears relatively unimportant. The introduction of one food at a time will help determine if there is an allergic or atopic reaction to any particular newly introduced food. Iron-containing foods are desirable. Signs of readiness for solid foods include loss of the tongue protrusion reflex, the ability to sit unsupported, and the ability to grasp food and bring it to the mouth.

8. e. Although there is less iron in breast milk, it is better absorbed. If maternal nutrition is adequate, unless there is little sunlight, term infants younger than 6 months of age generally do not need supplementation. Some experts recommend vitamin D supplementation, particularly for dark-skinned infants not exposed to adequate sunlight. Whereas term infants who are breast-fed generally do not need iron supplementation prior to 6 months of age, preterm infants do. Only iron-fortified formula is now recommended. If the community water supply has 1 ppm of fluoride, the infant does not need supplementation.

9. b. Unless exceptional circumstances dictate otherwise, the recommended course of action with maternal mastitis is to continue breastfeeding and treat the mother with symptomatic treatments, such as hot compresses and antibiotics effective against *S. aureus* (including coagulase-positive *Staphylococcus*). The antibiotic of choice in this case is cloxacillin or dicloxacillin. Erythromycin or first-generation cephalosporins may be used for penicillin-allergic patients.

10. b. See answer 9.

11. e. Causes of recurrent mastitis are multiple. Check the latch-on and make sure the baby's nose is pointing toward the nipple and his mouth has most of the areola encircled. The mother should change positions so the infant's mouth massages different ducts. Teaching a woman to watch for clogged milk ducts prior to developing mastitis, using massage with a motion toward the nipple, as well as using warm, moist packs can often resolve the plugged duct prior to development of mastitis. Advice to "go to bed with baby" is important so the mother can relax, allow time for feeding, and prevent milk duct statis. Frequent emptying of the breast—often difficult with some of the less expensive, less effective pumps—is especially important for the working mother. The electric double-pumping system (Medela and Holister are commonly used brands) is generally more effective than hand or battery-operated pumps. An undiagnosed fungal infection of the nipple that may be due to infant thrush (or vice versa) should be treated to prevent fissuring and cracks. If a nipple has a sore or crack, the infant should begin feeding on the least sore side. Pure lanolin may be used, but otherwise breast milk may be used to soothe the crack. Other ointments and nipple shields should not be used. Generally sore, cracked nipples are due to improper positioning or prolonged suckling that is nonnutritive.

12. **d.** Most women decide to breastfeed before or during their first trimester. Preconception counseling should include discussion of the benefits of breastfeeding, and it should be part of the initial prenatal visit. The Baby-Friendly Hospital Initiative introduced by UNICEF and WHO has resulted in increased likelihood and length of time for breastfeeding in communities where the initiative is followed. Putting the baby to breast within 30 minutes after delivery, avoiding bottles and pacifiers, and encouraging rooming in with the mother are all important for helping a woman to breastfeed successfully (Box 98-1). The opinion of the husband or significant other is very important in the woman's decision to breastfeed. Women who breastfeed are typically older, more educated, and more concerned with baby benefits than those who do not.

13. **b.** Regurgitation, or spitting up, is a common problem in infants. The mechanism appears to be an incompetent gastroesophageal sphincter. Regurgitation can be reduced by adequate eructation of swallowed air during and after eating, by gentle handling, and by holding the infant against the shoulder or placing in a semi-upright position (e.g., infant car seat or

---

Box 98-1 Ten Steps to a Baby-Friendly Hospital

- Have a written breast-feeding policy that is routinely communicated to all health care staff.
- Train all health care staff in skills necessary to implement this policy.
- Inform all pregnant women about the benefits and management of breast-feeding.
- Help mothers initiate breast-feeding within one half-hour of birth.
- Show mothers how to breast-feed and maintain lactation, even if they should be separated from their infants.
- Give newborn infants no food or drink other than breast milk, unless medically indicated.
- Practice rooming in—that is, allow mothers and infants to remain together 24 hours a day.
- Encourage breast-feeding on demand.
- Give no artificial teats or pacifiers (also called dummies or soothers) to breast-feeding infants.
- Foster the establishment of breast-feeding support groups and refer mothers to them on discharge from the hospital or clinic.

Adapted with permission from UNICEF Web site. Available at www.unicef.org/programme/breastfeeding/baby.htm#10.

"bouncer") after eating. The head should not be lower than the rest of the body during rest periods. Unless the child (especially a male) demonstrates projectile vomiting, weight loss, or has a palpable mass in the pylorus, pyloric stenosis is not likely. Use of medications is generally not recommended unless the infant is having weight loss, poor weight gain, or pulmonary complications.

14. **e.** All of the answers are good suggestions except for choice e, advising cessation of breastfeeding. The mother should be questioned carefully and, ideally, observed regarding feeding technique. Before assuming that the mother has insufficient milk, other possibilities should be excluded: errors in feeding technique responsible for the infant's inadequate progress; remediable maternal factors related to diet, rest, or emotional distress; or physical disturbances in the infant that interfere with eating or with weight gain. Occasionally, infants who seem to be nursing well may not thrive because of milk insufficiency; in this case, increased frequency of feedings and increased maternal nutrition and hydration may be indicated. Usually with a demonstrated slow weight gain, insufficient maternal milk supply is strong possibility (most often because of infrequent or inadequate milk removal), and the mother needs to pump every 2 or 3 hours with a heavy-duty, double-pumping, hospital-grade electric pump to bring it back. In the meantime, there may not be enough of her milk to get this baby back from the brink. This is one of the few situations in which formula really is needed. Referral to the La Leche League or a certified lactation consultant is an alternative that can be recommended to this mother. The La Leche League is a volunteer organization composed of successfully nursing mothers willing to assist other mothers desiring to nurse. If the mother is exhausted but able to successfully express sufficient milk, the husband or significant other may be able to assist the mother in feeding. This alternative is attractive because it gives the mother time to rest and recover her strength. This infant should be reassessed soon after the previously mentioned interventions are undertaken to monitor nutritional progress. Infant formulas provide adequate nutrition for the infant and may be the last alternative. Although "breast is best," a dogmatic approach to breastfeeding should be avoided. However, remember that most breastfeeding problems can be solved without having to give up the multiple benefits of breast milk.

15. **a.** Constipation is a common problem in formula-fed infants. It is extremely rare in breast-fed babies. In most infants, parents should understand that a daily bowel movement is not required, and glycerin suppositories may be used. Mineral oil and laxatives used for adults are not appropriate. For mothers who are breast- and bottle-feeding, this is an opportunity to encourage breastfeeding. For older infants, small amounts of prune juice may be given, and in a warm climate, water may be given; however, for young infants, water is not generally recommended. Less common conditions such as Hirschsprung's disease or, in the case of meconium ileus, cystic fibrosis should be considered in severe cases.

16. **c.** Formula has no immunological properties. The benefits of breast milk immunologically in the short and long term cannot be exaggerated. Breast milk is a living fluid, packed full of healthy antibodies.

17. **b.** Using pacifiers is a major "no" according to the Baby-Friendly Hospital Initiative developed by WHO. Box 98-1 summarizes the 10 major points.

Solution to the Clinical Case Management Problem

Eliminating your breastfeeding classes and lactation consultants will likely cost your county significantly more than it will save—and there are multiple studies to support your statement.

Studies in developed countries show that formula-fed infants have higher incidences of numerous infections and higher rate of hospitalization when they become ill. Gastrointestinal infections, otitis media, bacteremia, urinary tract infections, diabetes, allergic disease, asthma, respiratory infections, and bacterial meningitis are significantly less common and less severe in breast-fed infants. Some studies suggest improved bonding and IQ in infants who are breast-fed. Maternal benefits immediately postpartum include less anemia, quicker uterine involution, and birth control. Mothers who breastfeed benefit later in life with a lower incidence of breast cancer, ovarian cancer, type 2 diabetes, hypertension, and improved bone mineralization. These cost-savings do not include the money saved from purchase of formula, bottles, and direct feeding costs.

The excess yearly medical costs for 1000 bottle-fed versus 1000 breast-fed infants are shown in Table 98-1 based on a study performed in Arizona.

Table 98-1 Excess Medical Cost Among 1000 Never–Breast-fed versus 1000 Exclusive (>3 Months) Breast-fed Infants

	Excess Services per Year/1000 Never–Breast-fed Infants	Total Excess Cost ($)
Office visits	1693	111,315
Follow-up visits	340	22,355
Medications	609	7669
Chest radiography	51	1836
Days of hospitalization	212	187,866
Total excess cost per year		331,031

Adapted from Ball TM, Wright AL: Health care costs of formula-feeding in the first year of life. *Pediatrics* 103:870, 1999. Copyright 1999 American Academy of Pediatrics, with permission.

Summary

1. Breastfeeding: Breastfeeding is best. Advantages of breastfeeding include convenience, digestibility, transfer of antiviral and antibacterial antibodies, decreased risk of allergic phenomena, maternal–infant bonding, low incidence of regurgitation, and no constipation. In addition, breastfeeding delays and reduces the incidence of infectious diseases and atopic diseases such as eczema, allergies, and asthma, and it may help prevent obesity and type 1 diabetes. Breastfeeding has increased in frequency from a low of 52% in the late 1980s to two-thirds of postpartum women at discharge today.

Breastfeeding needs to be encouraged: Education and planning should begin optimally during the early part of pregnancy. Lactation assistance by breastfeeding-knowledgeable health care professionals after birth is important for first-time mothers. After delivery, before assuming that milk production is insufficient for the infant, health care professionals should consider errors in feeding techniques, remediable maternal factors such as lack of confidence and/or lack of support, anatomic anomalies in the mother or infant, and physical disturbances in the infant. Appropriate latch-on is important to prevent nipple soreness, mastitis, and abandonment of breastfeeding (Fig. 98-1). Encouraging hospitals in our communities to follow the 10 steps for a "baby-friendly" hospital can also increase the number of successful breastfeeding mothers.

Feeding should be on demand: Although erratic in the first few months, infants tend to regulate themselves after a short time.

2. Vitamins, fluoride, and iron supplements: Vitamins are unnecessary in most babies, particularly if

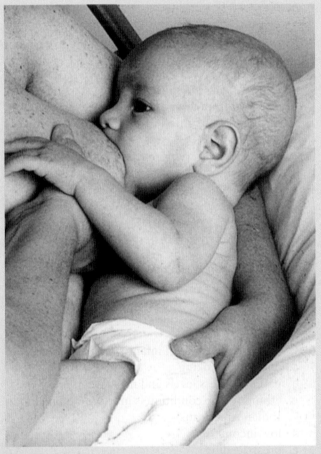

Figure 98-1

Appropriate latch-on. (Reproduced from Gabbe SG, ed: *Obstetrics: Normal and Problem Pregnancies*, 5th ed. New York: Churchill Livingstone, 2007, with permission.)

maternal supplies during pregnancy were adequate. If the baby is not exposed to sufficient sunlight or is darkly pigmented, supplemental vitamin D is recommended. Fluoride supplementation is unnecessary if the community water supply contains 1 ppm or more fluoride. Iron supplements (in the form of iron-fortified food) may be begun at the age of 6 months to reduce the possibility of anemia.

3. Solid foods: Breast milk is an excellent food through at least the first year of life, and it may be continued as long as mother and child like. Solid foods should be introduced at approximately 6 months of age; introduce one new food every 1 or 2 weeks.

4. The advantages of human colostrum and immunological benefits of human milk are innumerable; it provides macrophages as well as viral and bacterial antibodies of the secretory IgA class. Colostrum also supplies immunomodulating agents such as complement, lysozyme, lactoferrin, cytokines, and interleukins.

5. Common breastfeeding problems include difficulty with latch-on, positioning, mastitis, and inadequate milk production. Most of these problems can be prevented with good education and observation of the infant feeding prior to discharge. Close follow-up after discharge at 48 to 72 hours and availability of a health worker to counsel the mother will increase the likelihood of successful breastfeeding.

6. Growth and development: The minimum standard for the neonate is a weight gain of 20 g/day. All infants should regain their birth weight by 10 to 14 days. Frequent wet diapers and stools, coupled with return to birth weight, are good measures of adequate feeding at the 2-week visit.

7. As a general rule, any drug that can be given safely to a neonate is probably safe to use during breastfeeding. The American Academy of Pediatrics publishes a review of drugs and chemicals that can be safely used during lactation. Although the "jury is still out" in terms of studies, the prime contraindication to breastfeeding in the United States and developed countries is maternal human immunodeficiency virus infection.

Suggested Reading

Bottcher MF, Jenmalm MC: Breastfeeding and the development of atopic disease during childhood. *Clin Exp Allergy* 32(2):159–161, 2002.

Briggs GG: Drug effects on the fetus and breast-fed infant. *Clin Obstet Gynecol* 45(1):6–21, 2002.

Fulhan J, Collier S, Duggan C: Update on pediatric nutrition: Breastfeeding, infant nutrition, and growth. *Curr Opin Pediatr* 15(3):323–332, 2003.

Lawrence RA: Breastfeeding: Benefits, risks and alternatives. *Curr Opin Obstet Gynecol* 12(6):519–524, 2000.

Moreland J: Promoting and supporting breastfeeding. *Am Fam Physician* 61(7):2093–2103, 2000.

Newton E: Physiology of lactation and breastfeeding. In: Gabbe SG, ed., *Obstetrics. Normal and Problem Pregnancy*, 4th ed. Philadelphia: Saunders, 2002.

Powers N: How to assess slow growth in the breastfed infant. *Pediatr Clin North Am* 48(2):345–363, 2001.

"Make Her Stop Crying!"

A distressed mother sees you for the first time and states that her 5-week-old daughter has been crying nonstop for 2 weeks. Her husband states that he is leaving for a business trip. The father notes that their first son had to have a "stomach operation" in the fifth week of life "for vomiting and pain." The baby cries for 3 or 4 hours continuously, mainly in the afternoons, clenching his fists and pulling his legs toward the abdomen. The child is not suffering from diarrhea, and he passes flatus when he cries. You note an adequate weight gain on the growth chart.

SELECT THE BEST ANSWER TO THE FOLLOWING QUESTIONS

1. In this case, you will
   a. perform the minimum necessary laboratory tests: a complete blood count (CBC), urinalysis, and chest x-ray
   b. reassure the mother of the benign nature of the problem
   c. review all probable differential diagnoses for this age group
   d. order an ultrasound to rule out pyloric stenosis
   e. perform a thorough history and physical examination

2. After a complete history and physical, what is the first laboratory test you should undertake?
   a. CBC
   b. erythrocyte sedimentation rate (ESR) and CBC with complete white count
   c. chest x-ray followed by tympanometry
   d. urinalysis
   e. chemistry panel, CBC, and ESR

3. In order to establish the diagnosis of colic, you will use
   a. history and physical examination and the necessary laboratory workup
   b. the Wessel criteria (i.e., the rule of 3's)
   c. the Wessel criteria after organic reasons for crying have been ruled out

   d. "test for a cure" by changing from cow's milk to a hypoallergenic formula and reassessing in 7 days
   e. treat with Bentyl for 1 week to decrease abdominal spasms

4. You diagnose the child with infantile colic. A known cause for infantile colic is
   a. increase in feeding frequency or underfeeding
   b. allergy to cow's milk formula (food protein-induced enterocolitis syndrome)
   c. parental stress level as well as the number of siblings at home
   d. premature delivery or intrauterine growth slowing
   e. there are no established causes of infantile colic

5. Infantile colic is described as
   a. unprovoked, unrelieved crying, starting in the afternoon hours and accompanied by the child having clenched fists and pulling its legs toward the abdomen
   b. unpredictable crying occurring 24 hours a day and usually increasing with maternal fatigue
   c. more common in infants who are breast-fed
   d. always heralds future psychological disorders in childhood
   e. easily relieved by Phenergan and Bentyl

   The parents are exhausted and frustrated, and they ask what they can do to restore some quiet to their home. You review further history in order to make intervention recommendations.

6. Contributing factors in infantile colic are
   a. maternal smoking
   b. parental stress levels and marital status
   c. ethnicity (the condition is more common among Indian Americans)
   d. low income
   e. breastfeeding

7. Proven drug regimens in colic are
   a. antibiotics and herbal teas
   b. antispasmodics such as Bentyl and Levsin
   c. alternating Tylenol and Motrin adjusted dose
   d. "antiallergic" drugs (e.g., Benadryl) since the basis of colic is hypersensitivity to milk
   e. none of the above

8. Possible treatment strategies for infant colic are
   a. close follow-up with a physician or other medical caregiver. The patient needs to be seen every 1 or 2 weeks. Liberal use of a warm water bottle applied to the infant's abdomen is also recommended

b. avoidance of nuts, eggs, milk, and wheat in the nursing mother and (rarely) a trial of whey hydrolysate or soy formula

c. parental reassurance, providing a warm guilt-free environment in which the family can express their fears and frustration

d. hospitalization and possible sedation of mother and child in extreme cases of parental exhaustion

e. all of the above

Answers

1. **e.** The diagnosis of infantile colic (like appendicitis) is clinical and is established after a thorough history and physical examination. Although we tend to think of colic as an abdominal process, a complete evaluation of all organ systems must be performed. All other causes of inconsolable crying in an infant must be ruled out. Laboratory tests and reassurance will follow the establishment of a firm diagnosis. The history of possible pyloric stenosis with the first sibling does not change your approach. Although it predominantly affects males, pyloric stenosis has a 3% to 9% recurrence in the first-degree sibling.

2. **d.** All organic causes must be ruled out. Colic is a diagnosis of exclusion. Since children in this age group do not localize infection like adults, nonspecific signs and symptoms are very important; fever, decrease in food intake, excessive sleepiness, etc. should alert the physician. Of all the tests mentioned, a urinalysis has the highest yield (Fig. 99-1). You must rule out infections such as urinary tract infection, otitis media, pharyngitis, pneumonia, meningitis; visualize the infant eye to exclude corneal abrasion; and exclude the possibility of abdominal processes such as intussusceptions and volvulus. A complete dermatologic exam should follow because a hair tourniquet (strangulation of a toe, finger, or penis by a knot of hair) is a frequent reason for inconsolable cry.

3. **c.** After all organic reasons for inconsolable cry have been ruled out, the Wessel criteria are used (the rule of 3's). The child is described as crying more than 3 hours daily, for 3 or more days a week, during a 3-week period or longer. The infant is typically a 3-weeks to 3 months old. Remember that crying up to 2.2 hours a day is considered "normal." Colic rarely continues beyond 3 months of age.

4. **e.** The point to remember is that there is no known or established cause for infantile colic. Although over- and underfeeding, air swallowing, and cow's milk

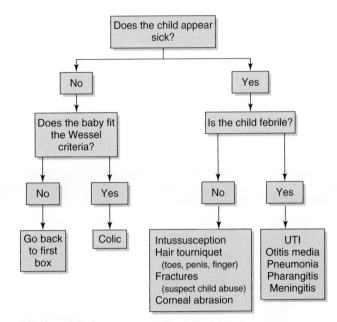

Figure 99-1

Evaluation of inconsolable crying. UTI, urinary tract infection.

have all been implicated, none have been proven as the cause of colic. Maternal food allergy has been suspected in breast-fed children, and research suggests that changing to a low-allergen diet might decrease colic. The stress encountered by the parents should be dealt with, but it not a causative factor. Cow's milk allergy causes an enterocolitis in children during their first year of life. Occasionally, these children are also allergic to soy and, unlike the patient described here, present with diarrhea, vomiting, and weight loss.

5. **a.** The key to understanding colic is the fact that holding the child, riding in a car, and changing formula may reduce actual crying time but rarely stop it. Of importance is choice e. Phenergan has a black box warning due to respiratory depression in children younger than 2 years of age with fatal consequences. Bentyl is contraindicated before the age of 6 months due to the increased risk of apnea.

6. **a.** All the other choices were speculated in the past and present as possible contributing factors to infantile colic. Studies have shown that maternal smoking doubles the occurrence of colic. Prevalence is not increased in different ethnic groups, and the average patient probably belongs to a middle-class family. It is worth noting that colic is slightly less frequent in breast-fed children.

7. **e.** Most medications are ineffective and might be dangerous. Since we do not know what causes colic, our treatment is mainly supportive. Herbal teas including vervain, licorice chamomile, and fennel are used by parents to relieve colic. They can cause malnutrition due to a decrease in formula intake, and they should be used with extreme caution.

8. **e.** Choice d is of particular interest. Colic can cause severe familial stress and may lead to child abuse. Hospitalization (of the parent and child) may be the only solution. In extreme cases, sedation may be offered. The physician should calm the parents, relieve any guilt associated with colic, and reassure them that colic usually disappears by 3 months of age. Frequent scheduled visits might be particularly helpful, and the physician should reiterate the child development, good weight gain, etc.

Summary

When faced with a child with inconsolable crying
1. Rule out organic causes—that is, fever, pharyngitis, otitis media, nausea and vomiting, rectal bleeding, and abdominal mass.
2. Think of colic: 25% of all children have it.
3. Apply the rule of 3's: the child cries for at least 3 hours daily 3 days a week for at least 3 weeks, starting before 3 months of age.
4. Males and females are affected in equal numbers, and the condition crosses social lines.
5. The etiology is unknown; however, the condition is more common among infants of smoking mothers.
6. No medication is known to help.
7. Treat the whole family with reassurance, frequent visits, and occasional warm water bottle.
8. Some research supports changing to maternal low-allergen diet in the case of the breast-fed infant (elimination of nuts, milk, soy, and fish) and possible change to whey hydrolysate in the formula-fed baby. No bacterial isolate has been associated with the condition.

Suggested Reading

Crotteau CA, Wright ST, Eglash A: Clinical inquiries: What is the best treatment for infants with colic?. *J Fam Pract* 55(7):634–636, 2006.
Fireman L: Colic (in brief). *Pediatr Rev* 27:357–358, 2006.
Heird WC: The feeding of infants and children. In: Behrman R, et al, eds., *Nelson Textbook of Pediatrics*. Philadelphia: Saunders, 2004.
Karp A: A framework and strategy for understanding and resolving colic. *Contemporary Pediatr* 21:99–114, 2004.
Shaw T, Graber MA: Pediatrics. In: Graber MA, de Almeida KN, Atkinson JC, et al, eds., *The Family Medicine Handbook*. Philadelphia: Saunders, 2006.
Wade S: Infantile colic (clinical evidence concise). *BMJ* 2006.
Woodgate P, Cook L, Webster H: Medical therapy for infantile colic. *Cochrane Database Syst Rev* (1):CD004382, 2003.

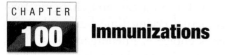

CHAPTER **100** **Immunizations**

CLINICAL CASE PROBLEM 1

A 4-Month-Old Infant Who Missed His Shots Due to a Cold at 2 Months of Age

A 4-month-old infant is brought to your office by his mother to see you for the first time. The infant and his mother recently moved to the area. When he came for a 2-month examination, the mother states that the nurse practitioner said the child had a "cold" and could not receive his immunizations. His mother is concerned since he has gotten only his first hepatitis B immunization in the hospital. He is bottle-fed and stays with a relative while the mother works. The infant has had upper respiratory symptoms for the past week, but according to the mother he is happy, interactive, afebrile, and feeding well. On physical examination, the child is appropriate weight and length for age, smiles and interacts, and the rest of the exam is completely normal with the exception of minimal clear nasal discharge.

SELECT THE BEST ANSWER TO THE FOLLOWING QUESTIONS

1. Which immunization(s) should be given to this child now, according to the Advisory Committee on Immunization Practices (ACIP) recommendations?
   a. hepatitis B, diphtheria–tetanus–pertussis (DTaP), pneumococcal conjugate vaccine (PCV),

inactivated poliomyelitis vaccine (IPV), *Haemophilus influenzae* type b (Hib)
b. hepatitis B, DTaP, PCV, IPV, Hib, rotavirus
c. DTaP, PCV, IPV, Hib
d. hepatitis B, pneumococcal polysaccharide vaccine (PPV), IPV, Hib
e. hepatitis B, DTaP, PPV, IPV, Hib, rotavirus

2. When do you ask the mother to return to give the child "catch-up" immunizations?
   a. 2 weeks and give DTaP, PCV, IPV, Hib, rotavirus
   b. 4 weeks and give DTaP, PCV, IPV, Hib
   c. 4 weeks and give hepatitis B, DTaP, PCV, IPV, Hib
   d. just have the mother return at 6 months and get the routine vaccinations—no further catch-up is required
   e. all of the above are acceptable

3. Which of the following statements regarding future immunizations for the child is true?
   a. be careful to never give an immunization with a low-grade fever because the child could react
   b. he should be given his measles–mumps–rubella (MMR) vaccine at 9 months to make sure he does not miss it
   c. reimmunize him according to the catch-up schedule and reassure the mother that a mild upper respiratory infection is no contraindication to immunization
   d. since he is late getting his first immunization, he is more likely to have a severe reaction
   e. never give an immunization if a child has an upper respiratory infection since fever could be misinterpreted as worsening illness

4. Which of the following statements regarding vaccination against poliomyelitis is true?
   a. oral polio vaccine (OPV) is a live, attenuated, trivalent vaccine known as the Salk vaccine
   b. OPV and IPV are both available for immunizations, depending on the parent preference
   c. IPV is an inactivated (killed), trivalent vaccine known as Sabin vaccine
   d. the most recent recommendation calls for an all-IPV dosing regimen
   e. OPV and IPV are both associated with a small risk of vaccine-associated paralytic poliomyelitis (VAPP)

5. Which of the following statements is true regarding hepatitis B vaccine in children?
   a. an extra dose should never be given

b. it is recommended as a routine immunization, and the first dose should not be given before the age of 2 months
c. it is recommended as a routine immunization, and the first dose should be given at 6 months
d. it is recommended as a routine immunization, and the first dose should be given prior to discharge from the hospital after birth
e. the third dose may be given within 4 weeks of the second dose, but no sooner

6. Which of the following statements is (are) true regarding the newly approved rotavirus vaccine?
   a. the first dose may be given between 8 and 32 weeks
   b. the first dose must be given between 6 and 12 weeks and is routinely given at the 2-month visit
   c. the third dose should be given between 12 and 15 months
   d. the second and third doses require an interval of 4 to 10 weeks, and they are routinely given at the 4- and 6-month visits
   e. both b and d are correct

7. Which of the following is a true contraindication to immunization?
   a. prematurity
   b. recent exposure to an infectious disease
   c. current antimicrobial therapy
   d. moderate or severe illness with or without a fever
   e. history of penicillin or other allergies

8. Which of the following statements regarding immunization against Hib is (are) true?
   a. the vaccine is known as the Hib vaccine and is available in combination with the hepatitis B vaccine
   b. the first dose of Hib vaccine should be given at age 2 months
   c. the Hib vaccine is given to protect the infant only from Hib infections that lead to meningitis
   d. all of the above statements are true
   e. a and b only

9. Which of the following vaccines is (are) recommended for first administration at age 12 to 15 months?
   a. MMR vaccine
   b. varicella and MMR
   c. varicella
   d. hepatitis A
   e. varicella, MMR, and hepatitis A

10. By the time a child reaches 7 years old, how many doses of DTaP should have been administered?
    a. 2 doses
    b. 3 doses
    c. 4 doses
    d. 5 doses
    e. none of the above

11. Which of the following statements about tetanus toxoid (Td or DT) is true?
    a. routine boosters with Td are recommended every 5 years
    b. Td is contraindicated during all trimesters of pregnancy
    c. TDaP is given to adolescents in place of one Td booster at ages 11 to 18 years and may be given to adults up to age 65 years who have contact with infants younger than 12 months
    d. TDaP may replace Td for all boosters to decrease pertussis risk in the population
    e. Td should not be given to children younger than age 7 years who have a contraindication to pertussis vaccine as they might react.

12. All of the following are true about pneumococcal infection and PCV except
    a. PCV is indicated for all children younger than 24 months and for high-risk children up to their fifth birthday (includes asplenic, other immunologic, and cardiopulmonary disorders)
    b. PCV is highly effective at preventing pneumococcal meningitis, pneumonia, sepsis, and nasal carriage (including resistant strains)
    c. the minimum interval between doses in the primary series is 8 weeks
    d. it is a heptavalent vaccine
    e. pneumococci cause more cases of otitis media than any other single pathogen

13. Which of the following is false regarding the varicella vaccine?
    a. it should not be given before 12 months of age
    b. previously two doses were recommended at least 4 weeks apart in those age 13 years or older, but now two doses are recommended in all children and adolescents
    c. it is not effective in preventing or modifying disease if given after exposure
    d. a mild varicella-like syndrome can develop in 1% to 4% of those vaccinated
    e. the vaccine is 71% to 91% effective in preventing all symptoms of this disease

14. Which of the following is true regarding the newly approved human papillomavirus vaccine?

    a. it is recommended in a two-dose schedule, with a dose interval of 4 weeks
    b. it is recommended for females as young as age 9 years, but routine vaccination is recommended for females age 11 or 12 years, with catch-up recommended for females age 13 to 26 years
    c. it cannot be given past age 18 years
    d. it is not recommended for females who are sexually active, even if they are within the recommended age range
    e. none of the above are true

Clinical Case Management Problem

Discuss some of the important changes in the immunization schedule for children and adolescents and the rationale behind them. Discuss how epidemiological data have been important in developing these recommendations.

Answers

1. a. Hepatitis B, DTaP, PCV, IPV, Hib should be given to this child, just as is recommended routinely at 2 months of age. His vaccination should not have been withheld due to a mild upper respiratory infection. Rotavirus may not be given because the child is older than age 12 weeks. PCV, not PPV, should be given routinely to infants and young children. Hepatitis B is usually given at birth and 2 and 6 months, but it is given to this child to replace the missed 2-month vaccine.

2. b. According to the catch-up immunization schedule, no vaccine may be given at an interval of less than 4 weeks. All of his previously given vaccines (DTaP, Hib, PCV, and IPV) may be given at the visit in 4 weeks except for his third hepatitis B vaccine, which requires a minimum interval of 8 weeks between doses 2 and 3 and age older than 24 weeks. In the case of this child, the final vaccine for hepatitis B must be given at his 6-month visit when he receives his third dose of the other vaccines in his primary immunization schedule. At this point, he will continue to receive immunizations as per the routine schedule.

3. c. This child should follow routine vaccination schedules once he has "caught up." MMR cannot be given prior to 12 months. A mild upper respiratory infection is not a contraindication to vaccination, and late vaccination is not a predictor of more severe adverse reactions.

4. d. Two types of vaccine are licensed in the United States for prevention of polio: OPV, a live, attenuated, trivalent poliovirus vaccine known as Sabin; and an IPV, an inactivated (killed) trivalent vaccine known as Salk. Since 2000, ACIP has recommended an all-IPV vaccine regimen scheduled at 2 months, 4 months, 6 to 18 months, and 4 to 6 years. The reason for the change was to eliminate any VAPP, which occurs in 1 case in 2.4 million doses with OPV. IPV is not known to cause VAPP. Initial recommendations changed the first doses to IPV and later doses to OPV, but this is no longer recommended.

5. **d.** Vaccination against hepatitis B is routinely recommended for all children born in the United States. The recommended schedule for hepatitis B immunization is birth, 2 months, and 6 months. In rare circumstances, if an infant's mother is known to be hepatitis B surface antigen (HBsAg) negative and the physician writes an order indicating a reason for delay, the birth dose may be given later, but it is strongly recommended that the monovalent vaccine be given prior to hospital discharge. The second dose should be given 1 or 2 months after the birth dose (minimum 4-week interval), and the third dose must be given at older than 24 weeks of age. For infants who are given the combined vaccine, giving an additional dose at 4 months of age is not a problem. Recommendations for infants of HbSAg-positive mothers are given later.

6. **e.** In 2006, the ACIP Vaccines for Children Program recommended the addition of the new rotavirus vaccine (Rota) to the routine immunization schedule. This oral vaccine is to be administered with the routine immunizations at 2, 4, and 6 months. Because safety data are not available for older infants, the initial dose may not be given after 12 weeks (range, 6 to 12 weeks), the second and thirds doses must have an interval of 4 to 10 weeks, and the final dose must be given by 32 weeks. Contraindications and precautions to use of the vaccine include allergy to components of the vaccine, moderately severe illness, acute gastroenteritis, history of gastrointestinal disease, and altered immunocompetence. Rotavirus is the most common cause of severe gastroenteritis in infants and young children worldwide.

7. **d.** There are three true contraindications to the administration of childhood immunizations: (1) an anaphylactic reaction to a vaccine, (2) an anaphylactic reaction to a vaccine constituent contraindicating the use of vaccines containing that substance, and (3) moderate or severe illness with or without a fever. Mild acute illness with or without a fever is not a contraindication. Convulsions, encephalopathy, collapse, or shocklike state within 48 hours of receipt of any vaccine is a cause for concern and may be considered a contraindication to further vaccination. Such episodes, which had been related to the whole cell DTP vaccine, are extremely rare with the acellular

DTaP vaccine. For live attenuated vaccines, known immunodeficiency and pregnancy are also contraindications.

8. **e.** Vaccination against Hib is recommended at 2, 4, 6, and 12 to 15 months of age. Three Hib vaccine conjugates are currently available. If Hib PRP-OMP (Comvax and Hebvax) is administered, a dose at 2 and 4 months only is required. Hepatitis B/Hib combinations may be used; however, DTaP/Hib combination vaccines should not be used for the primary series at 2, 4, and 6 months but may be used as booster doses with any of the Hib vaccines. The final dose in the series must be given at older than 12 months of age. *H. influenzae* vaccine is given at these times because of the age at which *H. influenzae* meningitis affects infants and children. Meningitis caused by this organism usually occurs between the ages of 1 month and 4 years. Major neurologic sequelae of Hib meningitis include behavior problems, language disorders, delayed development of language, impaired vision, mental retardation, motor abnormalities, ataxia, seizures, and hydrocephalus. Approximately 6% of patients with Hib meningitis are left with some hearing impairment. Other significant infections caused by *H. influenzae* are acute epiglottitis; pneumonia; septic arthritis; cellulitis; osteomyelitis; pericarditis; bacteremia without an associated focus; neonatal disease; and miscellaneous infections, such as urinary tract infection, cervical adenitis, uvulitis, endocarditis, primary peritonitis, periappendiceal abscess, and otitis media. The Hib immunization should be effective against all of these infections. For children 15 to 59 months of age, only one dose of Hib vaccine is recommended.

9. **e.** Three vaccinations are now given for the first time at 12 to 15 months of age: MMR, varicella, and hepatitis A. They can be administered at the same time, but if not, at least a 4-week interval needs to separate varicella and MMR. Hepatitis A was previously given at 2 years, but it is now recommended to be given at 12 months, followed by a booster dose 6 to 12 months later. Children and patients with risk factors will continue to be vaccinated under current programs.

10. **d.** By the time a child reaches 7 years of age, five doses of DTaP should have been administered. DTaP is given at 2, 4, 6, and 12 to 18 months and at 4 to 6 years of age.

11. **c.** TDaP, tetanus toxoid, reduced diphtheria toxoid, and acellular pertussis vaccine was approved in May 2005 for children age 11 or 12 years who have finished their primary series and have not received a tetanus booster. Adolescents aged 13 to 18 years who missed the 11- or 12-year booster dose should also receive a single dose of TDaP if they have completed the childhood DTaP/DPT series. Subsequent Td boosters are recommended every 10 years. TDaP is also recommended for adults up to age 65 years, especially if in contact with young infants, or for women prior to pregnancy. It may be used to replace a Td booster or may be given in an interval as short as 2 years from the tetanus booster dose to immunize against pertussis. TDaP is now preferred to be given prior to conception so the mother cannot expose the infant to pertussis. Previously, the first dose of DT was given at 11 or 12 years of age if at least 5 years had elapsed since the last dose of tetanus and diphtheria vaccine. Now that dose is replaced with TDaP. The subsequent booster of DT should be every 10 years unless a major or dirty wound is sustained, in which case the dose should be given if it has not been given in the previous 5 years. Children older than age 6 years receive DT and not DTaP. Td is not contraindicated during pregnancy. It is not teratogenic and is not a live vaccine, so it can be administered during pregnancy.

12. c. The minimal interval between doses in the primary series for the heptavalent PCV is 4 weeks. PCV is given to children younger than age 2 years, whereas PPV is given to those older than age 2 years who are high risk, such as those with asplenia, sickle cell disease, diabetes, chronic cardiac and pulmonary disease, human immunodeficiency virus, and congenital immune deficiency. PPV is not effectively immunogenic in patients younger than 2 years of age.

13. c. The varicella vaccine is effective in preventing or modifying disease if given within 72 hours of exposure and possibly up to 120 hours of exposure. It should not be given prior to 12 months because of passive immunity transferred maternally. The vaccine has a 96% seroconversion rate. It is 95% to 100% effective in preventing severe disease and 71% to 91% efficacious in preventing all symptoms of this disease. ACIP and Centers for Disease Control and Prevention recommend that all children receive a booster dose of varicella, scheduled with the MMR booster at 4 to 6 years, and for older children and adolescents, no sooner than 4 weeks after the initial dose.

14. b. The new human papillomavirus vaccine (HPV) is recommended in a three-dose schedule, with the second and third doses administered 2 and 6 months after the first dose. The routine vaccination with HPV is recommended for females age 11 or 12 years; the vaccination series can be started in females as young as age 9 years; a catch-up vaccination is recommended for females age 12 to 26 years who have not been fully vaccinated. A history of sexual activity is not a contraindication to vaccination.

Solution to the Clinical Case Management Problem

During the past few years, there have been both additional immunizations added to the recommended schedule by ACIP and changes in schedules and booster doses. The new rotavirus vaccine has been added to protect children from the most common cause of diarrhea resulting in morbidity, mortality, and hospitalization in the United States. After the initial vaccine was removed from the market, additional work has been done to develop this vaccine. Studies will likely show whether the ages at which it is given can be expanded since safety and efficacy outside of these age ranges has not been studied. Currently, the first dose must be given by 12 weeks (range, 6 to 12 weeks) and the third dose must be given by 32 weeks. The new human papillomavirus represents a shift in our prevention strategy of cervical dysplasia and cancer. Now recommended at age 11 or 12 years but approved for ages as young as 9 years and as old as 26 years, this vaccine will likely decrease the rates of not only cervical cancer but also lesser degrees of dysplasia that necessitate expensive and painful treatment with colposcopy, biopsy, and cryotherapy. In response to the resurgence of pertussis, and epidemiological evidence of waning immunity, the new TDaP vaccine will provide increased protection to unimmunized infants and those older than 2 months of age by increasing the herd immunity. As with the MMR booster, the addition of the varicella booster is particularly important to the small percentage of nonresponders and to the entire population as disease-acquired immunity diminishes with time. The new meningococcal vaccine will decrease this devastating disease in a broader population group; studies have shown that only a small percentage of cases are related to epidemics. New recommendations to vaccinate all children, at a younger age, with the hepatitis A vaccine have been necessary since data have shown that the disease occurs even in "low-risk" populations. Expansion of the use of the influenza vaccine to a wider population of children after deaths and hospitalizations were documented will help to control this disease among the entire population.

Epidemiological data have enabled public health authorities to follow these diseases and improve targets to control these illnesses, decreasing both the burden of disease and the cost to the individual and to society.

Summary

Figures 100-1 and 100-2 indicate the recommended ages for routine administration of currently licensed childhood vaccines, as of January 2007, for children through age 18 years. The new immunization schedules are separated into 0 to 6 years and 7 to 18 years. Figure 100-3 shows the recommended catch-up schedule for both groups. Additional information is available at www.cdc.gov/nip/recs/child-schedule.htm. Any dose not given at the recommended age should be given at any subsequent visit when indicated and feasible. Additional vaccines may be licensed and recommended during subsequent years. Licensed combination vaccines may be used whenever any components of the combination are indicated, the vaccine's other components are not contraindicated, and if approved by the Food and Drug Administration for that dose of the series. Providers should consult the respective Advisory Committee on Immunization Practices statement for detailed recommendations. Clinically significant adverse events that follow immunization should be reported to the Vaccine Adverse Event Reporting System. Providers should consult the manufacturers' package inserts for detailed recommendations.

IMMUNIZATIONS, AGES 7 TO 18 YEARS

1. Tetanus and diphtheria toxoids and acellular pertussis vaccine (TDaP): Adolescent preparation is recommended at age 11 or 12 years for those who have completed the recommended childhood DTaP/DTP vaccination series and have not received a tetanus and diphtheria toxoids vaccine (Td) booster dose. Adolescents 13 to 18 years who missed the 11- or 12-year Td/TDaP booster dose should also receive a single dose of TDaP if they have completed the recommended childhood DTP/DTaP vaccination series. Subsequent Td is recommended every 10 years.

2. Human papillomavirus vaccine (HPV): Administer the first dose of the HPV series to females at age 11 or 12 years. Administer the second dose 2 months after the first dose and the third dose 6 months after the first dose. Administer the HPV series to females at age 13 to 18 years if not previously vaccinated.

3. Meningococcal vaccine: Meningococcal conjugate vaccine (MCV4) should be given to all children at the 11- or 12-year-old visit as well as to unvaccinated adolescents at high school entry (15 years of age). Other adolescents who wish to decrease their risk for meningococcal disease may also be vaccinated. All college freshmen living in dormitories should also be vaccinated, preferably with MCV4, although meningococcal polysaccharide vaccine (MPSV4) is an acceptable alternative. Vaccination against invasive meningococcal disease is recommended for children older than 2 years of age and adolescents with terminal complement deficiencies or anatomic or functional asplenia and certain other high-risk groups; see *MMWR* 54(RR-7):1–21, 2005. Use MPSV4 for children age 2 to 10 years and MCV4 for older children, although MPSV4 is an acceptable alternative.

4. Pneumococcal polysaccharide vaccine (PPV): Administer for certain high-risk groups. See *MMWR* 46(RR-8):1–24, 1997; and *MMWR* 49(RR-9):1–35, 2000.

5. Influenza vaccine—see Figures 100-1 to 100-3.

6. Hepatitis A vaccine—see Figures 100-1 to 100-3.

7. Hepatitis B vaccine—see Figures 100-1 to 100-3.

8. Inactivated poliovirus vaccine (IPV): For children who received an all-IPV or all-OPV series, a fourth dose is not necessary if the third dose was administered at age older than 4 years.

   If both OPV and IPV were administered as part of a series, a total of four doses should be administered, regardless of the child's current age.

9. Measles, mumps, and rubella vaccine (MMR)—see Figures 100-1 to 100-3.

10. Varicella vaccine: Administer two doses of varicella vaccine to people without evidence of immunity. Administer two doses of varicella vaccine to people age older than 13 years at least 3 months apart. Do not repeat the second dose if administered more than 28 days after the first dose. Administer two doses of varicella vaccine to people age older than 13 years at least 4 weeks apart.

Recommended Immunization Schedule for Persons Aged 0–6 Years—UNITED STATES • 2008
For those who fall behind or start late, see the catch-up schedule

Vaccine ▼ Age ▶	Birth	1 month	2 months	4 months	6 months	12 months	15 months	18 months	19–23 months	2–3 years	4–6 years
Hepatitis B[1]	HepB	HepB		see footnote 1		HepB					
Rotavirus[2]			Rota	Rota	Rota						
Diphtheria, Tetanus, Pertussis[3]			DTaP	DTaP	DTaP	see footnote 3	DTaP				DTaP
Haemophilus influenzae type b[4]			Hib	Hib	Hib[4]	Hib					
Pneumococcal[5]			PCV	PCV	PCV	PCV				PPV	
Inactivated Poliovirus			IPV	IPV		IPV					IPV
Influenza[6]						Influenza (Yearly)					
Measles, Mumps, Rubella[7]						MMR					MMR
Varicella[8]						Varicella					Varicella
Hepatitis A[9]						HepA (2 doses)				HepA Series	
Meningococcal[10]										MCV4	

Range of recommended ages

Certain high-risk groups

This schedule indicates the recommended ages for routine administration of currently licensed childhood vaccines, as of December 1, 2007, for children aged 0 through 6 years. Additional information is available at **www.cdc.gov/vaccines/recs/schedules**. Any dose not administered at the recommended age should be administered at any subsequent visit, when indicated and feasible. Additional vaccines may be licensed and recommended during the year. Licensed combination vaccines may be used whenever any components of the combination are indicated and other components of the vaccine are not contraindicated and if approved by the Food and Drug Administration for that dose of the series. Providers should consult the respective Advisory Committee on Immunization Practices statement for detailed recommendations, including for **high-risk conditions: http://www.cdc.gov/vaccines/pubs/ACIP-list.htm**. Clinically significant adverse events that follow immunization should be reported to the Vaccine Adverse Event Reporting System (VAERS). Guidance about how to obtain and complete a VAERS form is available at **www.vaers.hhs.gov** or by telephone, **800-822-7967**.

1. **Hepatitis B vaccine (HepB).** *(Minimum age: birth)*
   At birth:
   • Administer monovalent HepB to all newborns prior to hospital discharge.
   • If mother is hepatitis B surface antigen (HBsAg) positive, administer HepB and 0.5 mL of hepatitis B immune globulin (HBIG) within 12 hours of birth.
   • If mother's HBsAg status is unknown, administer HepB within 12 hours of birth. Determine the HBsAg status as soon as possible and if HBsAg positive, administer HBIG (no later than age 1 week).
   • If mother is HBsAg negative, the birth dose can be delayed, in rare cases, with a provider's order and a copy of the mother's negative HBsAg laboratory report in the infant's medical record.
   After the birth dose:
   • The HepB series should be completed with either monovalent HepB or a combination vaccine containing HepB. The second dose should be administered at age 1–2 months. The final dose should be administered no earlier than age 24 weeks. Infants born to HBsAg-positive mothers should be tested for HBsAg and antibody to HBsAg after completion of at least 3 doses of a licensed HepB series, at age 9–18 months (generally at the next well-child visit).
   4-month dose:
   • It is permissible to administer 4 doses of HepB when combination vaccines are administered after the birth dose. If monovalent HepB is used for doses after the birth dose, a dose at age 4 months is not needed.

2. **Rotavirus vaccine (Rota).** *(Minimum age: 6 weeks)*
   • Administer the first dose at age 6–12 weeks.
   • Do not start the series later than age 12 weeks.
   • Administer the final dose in the series by age 32 weeks. Do not administer any dose later than age 32 weeks.
   • Data on safety and efficacy outside of these age ranges are insufficient.

3. **Diphtheria and tetanus toxoids and acellular pertussis vaccine (DTaP).** *(Minimum age: 6 weeks)*
   • The fourth dose of DTaP may be administered as early as age 12 months, provided 6 months have elapsed since the third dose.
   • Administer the final dose in the series at age 4–6 years.

4. *Haemophilus influenzae* **type b conjugate vaccine (Hib).** *(Minimum age: 6 weeks)*
   • If PRP-OMP (PedvaxHIB® or ComVax® [Merck]) is administered at ages 2 and 4 months, a dose at age 6 months is not required.
   • TriHIBit® (DTaP/Hib) combination products should not be used for primary immunization but can be used as boosters following any Hib vaccine in children age 12 months or older.

5. **Pneumococcal vaccine.** *(Minimum age: 6 weeks for pneumococcal conjugate vaccine [PCV]; 2 years for pneumococcal polysaccharide vaccine [PPV])*
   • Administer one dose of PCV to all healthy children aged 24–59 months having any incomplete schedule.
   • Administer PPV to children aged 2 years and older with underlying medical conditions.

6. **Influenza vaccine.** *(Minimum age: 6 months for trivalent inactivated influenza vaccine [TIV]; 2 years for live, attenuated influenza vaccine [LAIV])*
   • Administer annually to children aged 6–59 months and to all eligible close contacts of children aged 0–59 months.
   • Administer annually to children 5 years of age and older with certain risk factors, to other persons (including household members) in close contact with persons in groups at higher risk, and to any child whose parents request vaccination.
   • For healthy persons (those who do not have underlying medical conditions that predispose them to influenza complications) ages 2–49 years, either LAIV or TIV may be used.
   • Children receiving TIV should receive 0.25 mL if age 6–35 months or 0.5 mL if age 3 years or older.
   • Administer 2 doses (separated by 4 weeks or longer) to children younger than 9 years who are receiving influenza vaccine for the first time or who were vaccinated for the first time last season but only received one dose.

7. **Measles, mumps, and rubella vaccine (MMR).** *(Minimum age: 12 months)*
   • Administer the second dose of MMR at age 4–6 years. MMR may be administered before age 4–6 years, provided 4 weeks or more have elapsed since the first dose.

8. **Varicella vaccine.** *(Minimum age: 12 months)*
   • Administer second dose at age 4–6 years; may be administered 3 months or more after first dose.
   • Do not repeat second dose if administered 28 days or more after first dose.

9. **Hepatitis A vaccine (HepA).** *(Minimum age: 12 months)*
   • Administer to all children aged 1 year (i.e., aged 12–23 months). Administer the 2 doses in the series at least 6 months apart.
   • Children not fully vaccinated by age 2 years can be vaccinated at subsequent visits.
   • HepA is recommended for certain other groups of children, including in areas where vaccination programs target older children.

10. **Meningococcal vaccine.** *(Minimum age: 2 years for meningococcal conjugate vaccine (MCV4) and for meningococcal polysaccharide vaccine (MPSV4))*
    • Administer MCV4 to children aged 2–10 years with terminal complement deficiencies or anatomic or functional asplenia and certain other high-risk groups. MPSV4 is also acceptable.
    • Administer MCV4 to persons who received MPSV4 3 or more years previously and remain at increased risk for meningococcal disease.

The Recommended Immunization Schedules for Persons Aged 0–18 Years are approved by the Advisory Committee on Immunization Practices (www.cdc.gov/vaccines/recs/acip), the American Academy of Pediatrics (http://www.aap.org), and the American Academy of Family Physicians (http://www.aafp.org).

DEPARTMENT OF HEALTH AND HUMAN SERVICES • CENTERS FOR DISEASE CONTROL AND PREVENTION • SAFER • HEALTHIER • PEOPLE™

Figure 100-1

Recommended immunization schedule for persons age 0 to 6 years. (Available at www.cdc.gov/vaccines/recs/schedules/child-schedule.htm#printable.)

Recommended Immunization Schedule for Persons Aged 7–18 Years—UNITED STATES • 2008
For those who fall behind or start late, see the green bars and the catch-up schedule

Vaccine ▼ Age ▶	7–10 years	11–12 years	13–18 years
Diphtheria, Tetanus, Pertussis[1]	see footnote 1	Tdap	Tdap
Human Papillomavirus[2]	see footnote 2	HPV (3 doses)	HPV Series
Meningococcal[3]	MCV4	MCV4	MCV4
Pneumococcal[4]	PPV		
Influenza[5]	Influenza (Yearly)		
Hepatitis A[6]	HepA Series		
Hepatitis B[7]	HepB Series		
Inactivated Poliovirus[8]	IPV Series		
Measles, Mumps, Rubella[9]	MMR Series		
Varicella[10]	Varicella Series		

Range of recommended ages

Catch-up immunization

Certain high-risk groups

This schedule indicates the recommended ages for routine administration of currently licensed childhood vaccines, as of December 1, 2007, for children aged 7–18 years. Additional information is available at **www.cdc.gov/vaccines/recs/schedules**. Any dose not administered at the recommended age should be administered at any subsequent visit, when indicated and feasible. Additional vaccines may be licensed and recommended during the year. Licensed combination vaccines may be used whenever any components of the combination are indicated and other components of the vaccine are not contraindicated and if approved by the Food and Drug Administration for that dose of the series. Providers should consult the respective Advisory Committee on Immunization Practices statement for detailed recommendations, including for **high-risk conditions: http://www.cdc.gov/vaccines/pubs/ACIP-list.htm**. Clinically significant adverse events that follow immunization should be reported to the Vaccine Adverse Event Reporting System (VAERS). Guidance about how to obtain and complete a VAERS form is available at **www.vaers.hhs.gov** or by telephone, **800-822-7967**.

1. Tetanus and diphtheria toxoids and acellular pertussis vaccine (Tdap). *(Minimum age: 10 years for BOOSTRIX® and 11 years for ADACEL™)*
- Administer at age 11–12 years for those who have completed the recommended childhood DTP/DTaP vaccination series and have not received a tetanus and diphtheria toxoids (Td) booster dose.
- 13–18-year-olds who missed the 11–12 year Tdap or received Td only are encouraged to receive one dose of Tdap 5 years after the last Td/DTaP dose.

2. Human papillomavirus vaccine (HPV). *(Minimum age: 9 years)*
- Administer the first dose of the HPV vaccine series to females at age 11–12 years.
- Administer the second dose 2 months after the first dose and the third dose 6 months after the first dose.
- Administer the HPV vaccine series to females at age 13–18 years if not previously vaccinated.

3. Meningococcal vaccine.
- Administer MCV4 at age 11–12 years and at age 13–18 years if not previously vaccinated. MPSV4 is an acceptable alternative.
- Administer MCV4 to previously unvaccinated college freshmen living in dormitories.
- MCV4 is recommended for children aged 2–10 years with terminal complement deficiencies or anatomic or functional asplenia and certain other high-risk groups.
- Persons who received MPSV4 3 or more years previously and remain at increased risk for meningococcal disease should be vaccinated with MCV4.

4. Pneumococcal polysaccharide vaccine (PPV).
- Administer PPV to certain high-risk groups.

5. Influenza vaccine.
- Administer annually to all close contacts of children aged 0–59 months.
- Administer annually to persons with certain risk factors, health-care workers, and other persons (including household members) in close contact with persons in groups at higher risk.

- Administer 2 doses (separated by 4 weeks or longer) to children younger than 9 years who are receiving influenza vaccine for the first time or who were vaccinated for the first time last season but only received one dose.
- For healthy nonpregnant persons (those who do not have underlying medical conditions that predispose them to influenza complications) ages 2–49 years, either LAIV or TIV may be used.

6. Hepatitis A vaccine (HepA).
- Administer the 2 doses in the series at least 6 months apart.
- HepA is recommended for certain other groups of children, including in areas where vaccination programs target older children.

7. Hepatitis B vaccine (HepB).
- Administer the 3-dose series to those who were not previously vaccinated.
- A 2-dose series of Recombivax HB® is licensed for children aged 11–15 years.

8. Inactivated poliovirus vaccine (IPV).
- For children who received an all-IPV or all-oral poliovirus (OPV) series, a fourth dose is not necessary if the third dose was administered at age 4 years or older.
- If both OPV and IPV were administered as part of a series, a total of 4 doses should be administered, regardless of the child's current age.

9. Measles, mumps, and rubella vaccine (MMR).
- If not previously vaccinated, administer 2 doses of MMR during any visit, with 4 or more weeks between the doses.

10. Varicella vaccine.
- Administer 2 doses of varicella vaccine to persons younger than 13 years of age at least 3 months apart. Do not repeat the second dose if administered 28 or more days following the first dose.
- Administer 2 doses of varicella vaccine to persons aged 13 years or older at least 4 weeks apart.

The Recommended Immunization Schedules for Persons Aged 0–18 Years are approved by the Advisory Committee on Immunization Practices (www.cdc.gov/vaccines/recs/acip), the American Academy of Pediatrics (http://www.aap.org), and the American Academy of Family Physicians (http://www.aafp.org).

DEPARTMENT OF HEALTH AND HUMAN SERVICES • CENTERS FOR DISEASE CONTROL AND PREVENTION
SAFER • HEALTHIER • PEOPLE™

Figure 100-2

Recommended immunization schedule for persons age 7 to 18 years. (Available at www.cdc.gov/vaccines/recs/schedules/child-schedule.htm#printable.)

Catch-up Immunization Schedule
UNITED STATES • 2008
for Persons Aged 4 Months–18 Years Who Start Late or Who Are More Than 1 Month Behind

The table below provides catch-up schedules and minimum intervals between doses for children whose vaccinations have been delayed. A vaccine series does not need to be restarted, regardless of the time that has elapsed between doses. Use the section appropriate for the child's age.

Vaccine	Minimum Age for Dose 1	Minimum Interval Between Doses			
		Dose 1 to Dose 2	**Dose 2 to Dose 3**	**Dose 3 to Dose 4**	**Dose 4 to Dose 5**
	**CATCH-UP SCHEDULE FOR PERSONS AGED 4 MONTHS–6 YEARS**				
Hepatitis B[1]	Birth	4 weeks	8 weeks (and 16 weeks after first dose)		
Rotavirus[2]	6 wks	4 weeks	4 weeks		
Diphtheria, Tetanus, Pertussis[3]	6 wks	4 weeks	4 weeks	6 months	6 months[3]
Haemophilus influenzae type b[4]	6 wks	**4 weeks** if first dose administered at younger than 12 months of age / **8 weeks (as final dose)** if first dose administered at age 12-14 months / **No further doses needed** if first dose administered at 15 months of age or older	**4 weeks**[4] if current age is younger than 12 months / **8 weeks (as final dose)**[4] if current age is 12 months or older and second dose administered at younger than 15 months of age / **No further doses needed** if previous dose administered at age 15 months or older	**8 weeks (as final dose)** This dose only necessary for children aged 12 months–5 years who received 3 doses before age 12 months	
Pneumococcal[5]	6 wks	**4 weeks** if first dose administered at younger than 12 months of age / **8 weeks (as final dose)** if first dose administered at age 12 months or older or current age 24–59 months / **No further doses needed** for healthy children if first dose administered at age 24 months or older	**4 weeks** if current age is younger than 12 months / **8 weeks (as final dose)** if current age is 12 months or older / **No further doses needed** for healthy children if previous dose administered at age 24 months or older	**8 weeks (as final dose)** This dose only necessary for children aged 12 months–5 years who received 3 doses before age 12 months	
Inactivated Poliovirus[6]	6 wks	4 weeks	4 weeks	4 weeks[6]	
Measles, Mumps, Rubella[7]	12 mos	4 weeks			
Varicella[8]	12 mos	3 months			
Hepatitis A[9]	12 mos	6 months			
	**CATCH-UP SCHEDULE FOR PERSONS AGED 7–18 YEARS**				
Tetanus, Diphtheria/ Tetanus, Diphtheria, Pertussis[10]	7 yrs[10]	4 weeks	**4 weeks** if first dose administered at younger than 12 months of age / **6 months** if first dose administered at age 12 months or older	**6 months** if first dose administered at younger than 12 months of age	
Human Papillomavirus[11]	9 yrs	4 weeks	12 weeks (and 24 weeks after the first dose)		
Hepatitis A[9]	12 mos	6 months			
Hepatitis B[1]	Birth	4 weeks	8 weeks (and 16 weeks after first dose)		
Inactivated Poliovirus[6]	6 wks	4 weeks	4 weeks	4 weeks[6]	
Measles, Mumps, Rubella[7]	12 mos	4 weeks			
Varicella[8]	12 mos	**4 weeks** if first dose administered at age 13 years or older / **3 months** if first dose administered at younger than 13 years of age			

1. Hepatitis B vaccine (HepB).
- Administer the 3-dose series to those who were not previously vaccinated.
- A 2-dose series of Recombivax HB® is licensed for children aged 11–15 years.

2. Rotavirus vaccine (Rota).
- Do not start the series later than age 12 weeks.
- Administer the final dose in the series by age 32 weeks.
- Do not administer a dose later than age 32 weeks.
- Data on safety and efficacy outside of these age ranges are insufficient.

3. Diphtheria and tetanus toxoids and acellular pertussis vaccine (DTaP).
- The fifth dose is not necessary if the fourth dose was administered at age 4 years or older.
- DTaP is not indicated for persons aged 7 years or older.

4. *Haemophilus influenzae* type b conjugate vaccine (Hib).
- Vaccine is not generally recommended for children aged 5 years or older.
- If current age is younger than 12 months and the first 2 doses were PRP-OMP (PedvaxHIB® or ComVax® [Merck]), the third (and final) dose should be administered at age 12–15 months and at least 8 weeks after the second dose.
- If first dose was administered at age 7–11 months, administer 2 doses separated by 4 weeks plus a booster at age 12–15 months.

5. Pneumococcal conjugate vaccine (PCV).
- Administer one dose of PCV to all healthy children aged 24–59 months having any incomplete schedule.
- For children with underlying medical conditions, administer 2 doses of PCV at least 8 weeks apart if previously received less than 3 doses, or 1 dose of PCV if previously received 3 doses.

6. Inactivated poliovirus vaccine (IPV).
- For children who received an all-IPV or all-oral poliovirus (OPV) series, a fourth dose is not necessary if third dose was administered at age 4 years or older.

- If both OPV and IPV were administered as part of a series, a total of 4 doses should be administered, regardless of the child's current age.
- IPV is not routinely recommended for persons aged 18 years and older.

7. Measles, mumps, and rubella vaccine (MMR).
- The second dose of MMR is recommended routinely at age 4–6 years but may be administered earlier if desired.
- If not previously vaccinated, administer 2 doses of MMR during any visit with 4 or more weeks between the doses.

8. Varicella vaccine.
- The second dose of varicella vaccine is recommended routinely at age 4–6 years but may be administered earlier if desired.
- Do not repeat the second dose in persons younger than 13 years of age if administered 28 or more days after the first dose.

9. Hepatitis A vaccine (HepA).
- HepA is recommended for certain groups of children, including in areas where vaccination programs target older children. See *MMWR* 2006;55(No. RR-7):1–23.

10. Tetanus and diphtheria toxoids vaccine (Td) and tetanus and diphtheria toxoids and acellular pertussis vaccine (Tdap).
- Tdap should be substituted for a single dose of Td in the primary catch-up series or as a booster if age appropriate; use Td for other doses.
- A 5-year interval from the last Td dose is encouraged when Tdap is used as a booster dose. A booster (fourth) dose is needed if any of the previous doses were administered at younger than 12 months of age. Refer to ACIP recommendations for further information. See *MMWR* 2006;55(No. RR-3).

11. Human papillomavirus vaccine (HPV).
- Administer the HPV vaccine series to females at age 13–18 years if not previously vaccinated.

Figure 100-3

Catch-up immunization schedule for persons age 4 months to 18 years. (Available at www.cdc.gov/vaccines/recs/schedules/child-schedule.htm#printable.)

Suggested Reading

American Academy of Pediatrics: *2003 Red Book: Report of the Committee on Infectious Diseases*, 26th ed. Oakbrook Terrace, IL: American Academy of Pediatrics Press, 2003.

Atkinson W, Kroger A: ACIP recommendations: General recommendations on immunization. *MMWR* 55(RR15):1–48, 2006.

Centers for Disease Control and Prevention: Recommended immunization schedules for persons aged 0–18 years—United States, 2007. *MMWR* 55(51/52):1–4, 2007.

Centers for Disease Control and Prevention: National Immunization Program. Available at www.cdc.gov/nip/home-hcp.htm.

Offit PA: Addressing parents' concerns: Do vaccines cause allergic or autoimmune diseases? *Pediatrics* 111(3):654–659, 2003.

Swain G, Bower D: Office based immunization practice. In: Rakel RE, Bope ET, eds, *Conn's Current Therapy 2003*, 55th ed. Philadelphia: Elsevier, 2003.

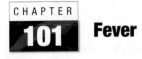

Fever

CLINICAL CASE PROBLEM 1

A 15-Month-Old Child with Persistent Fever

A 15-month-old is seen in your office for the fourth time this month with unexplained intermittent episodes of fever of 39°C. The mother has used children's ibuprofen to treat the fever and has been able to bring the temperature down to 38°C. However, the mother is now frustrated because this is her fourth visit to the office and nobody knows why her child is continuing to have these fevers. The child is not in day care and has no history of any serious illnesses, travel, or sick contacts. The child has had no symptoms of an upper respiratory infection.

On examination, the child is actively playing with his toys. He does not look ill or toxic. His rectal temperature is 39°C. The head, neck, lungs, cardiovascular, abdominal, neurologic, and musculoskeletal examination are all normal.

Your clinical judgment is that the child looks well and has no serious illness.

SELECT THE BEST ANSWER TO THE FOLLOWING QUESTIONS

1. What is your diagnosis at this time?
   a. recurrent viral infection
   b. fever without a focus
   c. infantile febrile response
   d. fever of unknown origin
   e. periodic fever, aphthous ulcers, pharyngitis, and adenopathy (PFAFA) syndrome

2. What is the most appropriate next step in the workup of this patient?

   a. obtain an immediate consultation with an infectious disease specialist
   b. start the child empirically taking antibiotics
   c. order a complete blood count (CBC) and urinalysis
   d. obtain a more detailed history
   e. obtain a chest x-ray

3. Which of the following represents the strict definition of fever of unknown origin (FUO)?
   a. fever in a child that persists for more than 1 month
   b. fever for more than 3 weeks with no diagnosis after three outpatient visits or 3 days in the hospital
   c. no diagnosis after 1 week of intelligent and intensive evaluation in the hospital
   d. b and c
   e. all of the above

4. Which of the following is the one preliminary diagnosis in this case that you should always consider?
   a. drug fever
   b. factitious fever
   c. occult bacteremia
   d. malignancy
   e. collagen vascular disease

5. The mother is very frustrated and wants to know what initial test you are going to do to determine what is going on with her son. Which of the following will you tell her?
   a. chest x-ray
   b. lumbar puncture
   c. white blood cell (WBC) count
   d. urine culture
   e. blood culture

6. What is the most common organism causing occult bacteremia in children?
   a. *Haemophilus influenza*
   b. *Mycoplasma pneumoniae*
   c. *Streptococcus pneumoniae*

d. *Salmonella*
e. *Neisseria meningitidis*

7. The most common cause(s) of recurrent fever occurring at regular intervals in a child is (are)?
   a. PFAPA
   b. Epstein–Barr virus
   c. parvovirus B19
   d. cytomegalovirus
   e. all of the above

8. What is the most common condition seen in infants with occult bacteremia?
   a. cellulitis
   b. pneumoniae
   c. otitis media
   d. pharyngitis
   e. osteomyelitis

9. Which of the following statements regarding the presumptive use of antibiotics in infants with a FUO is (are) false?
   a. presumptive use of antibiotics in infants with a FUO decreases morbidity and mortality
   b. the later the use of antibiotics, the greater the risk of morbidity and mortality
   c. presumptive use of oral antibiotics reliably prevents the risk of meningitis
   d. all of the statements are false
   e. b and c

10. In a child between the ages of 3 and 36 months, the probability of occult bacteremia is decreased if
    a. temperature is less than 39°C
    b. WBC range is between 5000 and 15,000 cells/mm³
    c. there is a negative exposure history
    d. all of the above decrease probability
    e. none of the above decrease probability

11. Recent developments in pediatric care have caused rethinking of the presumptive treatment and laboratory evaluation of the febrile child. The developments include:
    a. decrease in *H. influenza* type b infection through immunization
    b. increase in poliomyelitis due to reduced immunization levels
    c. widespread use of conjugated pneumococcal vaccine
    d. a and c
    e. all of the above

CLINICAL CASE PROBLEM 2

A 3-Year-Old with a Rash and Fever

A 3-year-old girl presents to the family health center with a fever for the past 36 hours. Maximum temperature was 40°C at 2 AM, which decreased to 38.7°F with children's ibuprofen. Her appetite and fluid intake have decreased during the past 24 hours.

Physical examination shows an ill-appearing child. Her temperature is 37.2°C. The skin has a macular–papular petechial rash on the chest and back. The remainder of the physical examination is normal.

12. Which of the following best describes your clinical impression at this time?
    a. viral syndrome
    b. meningitis
    c. sepsis
    d. b and c
    e. any of the above

13. Which laboratory testing would you order at this time?
    a. CBC
    b. blood culture
    c. urine culture
    d. lumbar puncture
    e. all of the above

14. Which of the following is the most likely organism that you need to consider in this situation?
    a. *S. pneumoniae*
    b. *H. influenzae*
    c. *N. meningitidis*
    d. *M. pneumoniae*
    e. *Listeria monocytogenes*

15. Which one of the following antibiotics would you consider in the treatment of this condition?
    a. Fortaz
    b. Rocephin
    c. Unasyn
    d. Zithromax
    e. Tequinol

16. What would you do next concerning this patient?
    a. immediate hospitalization
    b. outpatient antibiotics
    c. symptomatic treatment with analgesics and antipyretics only
    d. blood and urine cultures with outpatient follow-up in 24 hours
    e. all of the above

L. monocytogenes, and group B streptococcus account for the remaining 10%.

Clinical Case Management Problem

Describe a reasonable approach to the diagnosis and management of a fever without a focus in a 1-year-old infant.

Answers

1. d. This child has a fever of unknown origin. Most FUOs are the result of atypical presentation of common illnesses. A thorough evaluation, including history, physical examination, and selected tests, will reveal the etiology in most cases. Fever without localizing signs and symptoms is a common diagnostic dilemma for physicians caring for children younger than age 2 years. The classic definition of FUO is a fever of 38°C or higher for more than 3 weeks with no diagnosis after three outpatient visits or 3 days in the hospital.

In contrast, fever without focus is usually of acute onset and presents for less than 1 week.

PFAFA syndrome is characterized by periodic episodes of high fever (39°C) lasting 3 to 6 days and recurring every 21 days, accompanied by aphthous stomatitis, pharyngitis, and cervical adenopathy. The cause of PFAFA is unknown, although viral and autoimmune mechanisms have been postulated. This is by far the most common cause of predictable recurrent fevers with regular intervals.

2. d. The next step is to obtain a more detailed history, including the fever itself (remittent, intermittent, hectic, or sustained) and a history of exposure to infective agents such as siblings, pets, or chemicals.

3. d. See answer 1.

4. c. Fever without focus is caused by occult bacteremia until proved otherwise.

5. c. The diagnosis of FUO rarely is made with screening laboratory tests. Screening labs may direct further investigations. Suspicion of the presence of occult bacteremia depends in part on the value of the WBC. This is the most appropriate next step in the workup for infants who are 3 to 24 months of age.

6. c. The most common organism causing occult bacteremia in children is *S. pneumoniae*. This organism is responsible for approximately 65% of cases of occult bacteremia. *H. influenzae* is the second leading cause with approximately 25%. *N. meningitides,*

7. a. The other choices cause recurrent fevers at irregular intervals. PFAFA is the only one that causes recurrent fevers at regular intervals.

8. c. The most common condition in infants and children associated with occult bacteremia is otitis media. This most commonly is caused by *S. pneumoniae,* followed by *H. influenzae* type b.

S. pneumoniae also causes pneumonia and meningitis in infants and children.

9. d. The use of presumptive or prophylactic antibiotics in the prevention of morbidity or mortality associated with bacteremia is controversial. Although oral antibiotics may retard the emergence of some less serious focal bacterial disease (strep throat, otitis media, and pneumonia), they do not reliably prevent meningitis. There is no evidence that the sooner a presumptive antibiotic is used, the greater it will affect morbidity and mortality from any disease.

10. d. The probability of occult bacteremia is decreased if any of the following criteria are met: (1) temperature of less than 39°C, (2) WBC 5000 to 15,000 cells/mm^3, and (3) negative exposure history.

11. d. *H. influenzae* and pneumococcal vaccines have caused a change in the prevalence of particular diseases, especially in the 36 months and younger group. No firm changes in recommendations have occurred to date, but consideration should be given to the changing patterns of bacteremia as a result of new immunizations.

12. b. A prodromal respiratory illness or sore throat often precedes the fever, headache, stiff neck, and vomiting that characterize acute meningitis. In infants between the ages of 3 and 24 months, symptoms and signs are less predictable. There are some red flags in this presentation that should alarm the physician. There are no localizing signs for an infection. The rash is suspect because it could be secondary to septicemia.

13. e. All the above.

14. a. Although all of these organisms can cause meningitis, *S. pneumoniae* is still the leading cause in this age group.

15. b. A third-generation cephalosporin is usually added because it is highly effective against common meningeal pathogens in patients of all ages. However, in areas of high pneumococcal resistance, vancomycin with or without rifampin should be added. In newborns, ampicillin is usually added to cover *Listeria* and gentamicin may be added to expand the gram-negative coverage. These patterns of treatment are changing continually based on resistance in the community and availability of newer antibiotics. For example, Levaquin is a newer antibiotic that has a very broad range of coverage, including gram-positive/negative anaerobic and atypical organisms. The dilemma is that inappropriate or overuse of these antibiotics has also led to increased resistance within the community.

16. **a.** This child requires immediate hospitalization for a septic workup including a lumbar puncture and intravenous antibiotics. Meningitis is a very insidious disease and can be rapidly fatal if treatment is not instituted immediately.

Solution to the Clinical Case Management Problem

A reasonable approach to the diagnosis and management of fever without a focus in a 1-year-old child is as follows:

1. A proper history and physical examination are both sensitive and specific in determining the prevalence of occult bacteremia. Does the child appear ill? If no, then reassure the parent. If yes, then consider this a serious sign and continue investigation. Consider the following in an infant: quality of cry, reaction to parent stimulation, color hydration, and response (talk and smile) to social overtones.

2. Remember the risks for occult bacteremia: fever higher than 40°C, WBC <5000 cells/mm³, WBC >15,000 cells/mm³, and positive exposure history.

3. Remember the importance of repeated examinations and continuing contact with parents if fever without a focus is diagnosed and the child is allowed to go home.

4. Remember the most common organisms associated with occult bacteremia: *S. pneumoniae, H. influenzae,* group A β-hemolytic *Streptococcus,* and *N. meningitidis.*

5. Remember the most common conditions associated with occult bacteremia: otitis media, bacterial pneumonia, streptococcal pharyngitis, and meningitis. Consider the possibility of febrile convulsions if the temperature is above 40°C.

6. Remember that not all infants with fever have to be treated with antipyretics. Antipyretics do not speed the resolution of the condition. They may, in fact, hide certain symptoms.

7. Remember that symptomatic treatment (tepid sponge baths) may be just as effective as antipyretics.

8. Remember the importance of repeated reassessment of a child with fever without a focus until either the fever abates or the condition becomes overt.

9. Remember that if you are going to use an antipyretic to treat a child with a fever without a focus, the preferred agent is acetaminophen or ibuprofen.

10. Remember that blood cultures should be obtained before the increase in temperature.

Summary

See the Solution to the Clinical Case Management Problem.

Suggested Reading

Mourad O, et al: A comprehensive evidence-based approach to fever of unknown origin. *Arch Intern Med* 165(5):545–551, 2003.

Sur DK, Bukont EI: Evaluating fever of unidentifiable source in young children. *Am Fam Physician* 75:1805–1811, 2007.

Titus MO, Wright SW: Prevalence of serious bacterial infections in febrile infants with respiratory syncytial virus infection. *Pediatrics* 112(2):282–284, 2003.

CLINICAL CASE PROBLEM 1

A 6-Month-Old Infant with an Upper Respiratory Tract Infection

A 6-month-old infant is brought to your office by his mother. He has had a runny nose, cough, and a mild fever for the past 4 days. The infant was playful but occasionally fussy, and his temperature reached 39°C (102°F). He is otherwise healthy and his immunizations are up-to-date.

On physical examination, the child looks well and is afebrile. He has nasal congestion and a hyperemic pharynx. Tympanic membranes look normal. His lungs are clear and heart sounds are regular.

SELECT THE BEST ANSWER TO THE FOLLOWING QUESTIONS

1. The infant's mother is very concerned about the fever. Your recommendation to her would be
   a. treat the fever with baby aspirin if it reaches 39°C again
   b. treat the fever with elixir of acetaminophen if it reaches 39°C again
   c. treat the fever by alternating doses of acetaminophen and ibuprofen every 4 hours
   d. use only symptomatic treatment (lukewarm bath, cool clothes, and fan in the room)
   e. tell the mother that everyone has a different opinion; as far as you are concerned, she can do whatever she wants

2. What is the analgesic agent of choice in the treatment of childhood fever and mild childhood pain?
   a. elixir of naproxen
   b. elixir of hydromorphone
   c. elixir of acetaminophen
   d. children's aspirin, 75 mg
   e. elixir of acetaminophen and codeine

3. Which of the following statements most accurately reflects current practice recommendations regarding antipyretics and analgesic for fever and mild pain in children?
   a. aspirin is still the analgesic of choice in the treatment of infant and childhood pain
   b. aspirin is not contraindicated in the treatment of infant and childhood pain associated with upper respiratory infections (URIs)
   c. aspirin is a more potent analgesic than acetaminophen or ibuprofen
   d. acetaminophen is the most widely used antipyretic and mild analgesic for children
   e. ibuprofen is the preferred agent

4. Regarding the use of antihistamines in children, which of the following statements is true?
   a. cold-related nasal congestion and rhinorrhea is primarily due to histamine release
   b. antihistamines shorten the duration of upper respiratory tract illness in children
   c. antihistamine use reduces the incidence of common complications such as otitis media
   d. antihistamines have been shown to be of benefit in reducing rhinorrhea and cough in children with cold
   e. young children may develop seizures when given antihistamine doses (tablets or suppositories) that are meant for older children (on a milligram per kilogram basis)

5. Regarding the relief of nasal congestion in infants and children, which of the following statements is true?
   a. antihistamines produce excellent relief of pediatric nasal congestion
   b. intranasal and oral decongestants have been shown to relieve nasal symptoms in young children
   c. supportive treatment such as humidified air, bulb suctioning, and saline nasal drops is of no significant benefit
   d. nasal bulb suctioning done too frequently can cause nasal trauma, swelling of nasal mucosa, and greater congestion
   e. combined antihistamine and decongestant treatment has been shown to benefit young children

The child returns 3 days later with his mother. She states that despite your treatment the child has not improved. He now has significantly greater nasal congestion and is having difficulty breathing at night. She has been using an over-the-counter (OTC) cold medication and asks if she should use something stronger.

Physical examination is completely normal. You do not notice any change in the state of the nasal congestion.

6. With respect to treatment of this infant at this time, what would you tell the mother?
   a. decongestants have not been shown to reduce the duration of viral URI symptoms
   b. use nasal saline with bulb suctioning of nasal passage and humidified air instead of a decongestant
   c. reassure the mother and educate her about common cold and antihistamine–decongestant use
   d. overstimulation is a common side effect when decongestant preparations are given to children
   e. all of the above statements are true

CLINICAL CASE PROBLEM 2

A 18-Month-Old Infant with a Persistent Cough

The parent of an 18-month-old girl calls your office with a complaint that the toddler has had a persistent cough for the past 10 days. You saw the child for a routine checkup a few months ago. The cough is nonproductive, and the mother believes it is significantly interfering with the child's sleep. The child is otherwise well. She makes an appointment to see you in a couple of days and asks if you could recommend an OTC cough medication for her child.

7. Regarding the use of antitussives or expectorants in infants and children, which of the following statements is true?
   a. there is a lack of evidence that any OTC medicine is effective in treating pediatric cough
   b. centrally acting cough suppressants such as codeine and dextromethorphan are effective in treating pediatric cough
   c. dextromethorphan has been shown to significantly decrease the duration of respiratory tract infection symptoms in children
   d. use of dextromethorphan has not been related to any serious adverse reactions in children
   e. none of the above are true

CLINICAL CASE PROBLEM 3

A 13-Month-Old Infant with Nausea and Vomiting

A mother brings her 13-month-old infant to the office for assessment of vomiting and diarrhea. The child has had these symptoms for approximately 2 days. The child is otherwise active and healthy.

On physical examination, the child has dry, cracked lips, and the oral mucus membranes appear moist. There are no other abnormalities found. You diagnose the infant as having viral gastroenteritis and recommend hydration as treatment. The mother asks if you could recommend something "over-the-counter" for this illness.

8. What do you tell the mother regarding use of antiemetics and antimotility agents available OTC?
   a. antiemetics have been shown to decrease the length of viral gastroenteritis in infants
   b. use of antimotility agents such as loperamide is associated with complications such as ileus and respiratory depression
   c. viral gastroenteritis is self-limited and does not need any treatment other than prevention of dehydration
   d. b and c
   e. a, b, and c

CLINICAL CASE PROBLEM 4

An 8-Month-Old Infant with Fever, Diarrhea, and Red Cheeks

A mother brings her 8-month-old infant to your office for assessment of fever, diarrhea, and red cheeks that she attributes to teething. She was advised by her neighbor to purchase a preparation of topical benzocaine. This has not helped.

On examination, the infant has a temperature of 39°C. There are no other abnormalities.

9. Which of the following statements regarding this infant is true?
   a. the symptoms described are probably caused by teething
   b. acetaminophen is a reasonable treatment for a child who is teething
   c. teething often begins at 4 to 6 months of age and continues intermittently up to the age of 2 years
   d. b and c
   e. a, b, and c

10. In addition to the side effects of the various ingredients in OTC cough and cold preparations, which of the following are also potential hazards when these medications are given?
    a. risk of potential serious overdose, especially in children younger than 2 years of age

b. if symptoms are not controlled, parents sometimes intentionally, without intending to harm, give higher than recommended doses

c. parents are often unaware of the possible side effects

d. parents sometimes give the medications for one of the side effects—sedation

e. all of the above

Answers

1. **b.** The basic axiom relevant to this question is that "not all fever has to be treated with drugs." Fever with temperatures less than 39°C in healthy children generally does not require treatment. Temperatures above this may cause significant discomfort and may need the administration of an antipyretic. Increased body temperature is associated with decreased microbial reproduction and increased inflammatory reaction. Therefore, most evidence suggests that fever is beneficial and should be treated in selected circumstances. Febrile convulsions, which may occur in approximately 4% of children, may be of concern in a susceptible child with rapidly rising fever. Acetaminophen is the best choice. There is no evidence that alternating acetaminophen with ibuprofen is of any benefit, and it may not be safe. Symptomatic treatment such as tepid sponge bathing is helpful when used with antipyretic therapy.

2. **c.** The analgesic agent of choice in the treatment of childhood fever and mild to moderate childhood pain is acetaminophen. Hydromorphone is a strong narcotic. Naproxen is a nonsteroidal anti-inflammatory agent, and aspirin is contraindicated (see answer 3).

Acetaminophen with codeine elixir is available and may be indicated in more severe pain syndromes in childhood.

3. **d.** Acetaminophen is the most widely accepted analgesic of choice for the treatment of fever and childhood pain. Pediatric use of aspirin has decreased since the 1970s after a report of its association with Reye's syndrome. Aspirin use for fever reduction and mild pain associated with URIs is not recommended in children. Not all childhood pain needs to be treated with drugs. Many children will do just as well and feel just as well without drug use.

4. **e.** Antihistamines remain a popular therapy for cold-associated symptoms such as rhinorrhea and congestion. The mechanisms causing these in a viral URI differ from the allergy-related rhinorrhea secondary to histamine release. Antihistamines do not alleviate these symptoms to a clinically significant degree, especially in the pediatric population. They do not shorten the course of the viral illness, nor do they prevent its complications. They may produce tachycardia, blurred vision, agitation, hyperactivity, and seizures when given in toxic doses. The younger the child, the easier it is to inadvertently produce antihistamine toxicity. Treatment of a viral URI in an infant or young child should consist of reassurance and cool steam or saline nasal drops (if nasal congestion is present) and bulb syringe suctioning of nasal passages.

5. **c.** Supportive therapy with humidified air, nasal saline drops, and bulb suctioning is effective in producing relief of nasal congestion in infants and young children. These therapies are safer and less expensive than medications. Saline nasal drops may be used before suctioning. Suctioning is most likely to be helpful before feeds and sleep. However, done too frequently, suctioning may lead to nasal trauma, mucosal swelling, and greater congestion. If steam is being used in a humidifier in the child's room, it is safer to use a humidifier that emits cool steam to avoid the risk of burns. However, the use of warm steam (such as from turning on the shower in the bathroom) also produces significant symptomatic relief of nasal congestion. Steam appears to be the key in symptom resolution without any added ingredients in the water.

6. **e.** Education of parents about the lack of benefit and known risks of OTC cough and cold preparations is the key to treating irritating symptoms of the common cold. Sympathomimetics do not decrease the duration of illness. They have not been shown to be of benefit in young children, and they may cause significant side effects and toxicity even with use of topical agents. If parents insist on using these medications, then it should be negotiated to discontinue in 2 days if no benefit is observed.

7. **a.** Centrally acting cough suppressants such as dextromethorphan and codeine are not recommended for treatment of cough associated with viral illnesses. It is the most common ingredient in OTC cough medicines. As well as producing drowsiness, it has been reported to produce respiratory depression, abnormal limb movements, and coma in infants and children. As with antihistamines and decongestants, dextromethorphan has not been shown to shorten the duration of respiratory tract illness in children or adults.

Many cough preparations also contain an expectorant. The combination of a cough suppressant and an expectorant is not recommended.

Time remains the best cure for the viral URI symptoms. The use of a nasal aspirator (bulb syringe) will help to clear a young infant's nasal secretions and make feeding easier. Saline nasal drops may also be used. In infants who are irritable and feverish from viral symptoms, acetaminophen is the safest OTC drug to use.

8. **d.** Antimotility agents and antiemetics should not be used for the treatment of vomiting and diarrhea secondary to gastroenteritis in children (especially very young children). These agents have not been shown to be beneficial in the treatment of viral gastroenteritis and are associated with adverse effects. Maintenance of hydration is the mainstay in the treatment of viral gastroenteritis. In cases in which oral hydration cannot be maintained because of severe vomiting and in cases of severe dehydration, intravenous hydration may be considered.

9. **d.** Teething usually begins at 6 to 8 months of age and continues until the age of 2 years. Although often blamed on teething, there is no good evidence that fever, mood disturbances, appearance of illness, sleep disturbance, drooling, diarrhea, strong urine, red cheeks, rashes, or flushing of the face or body are associated with teething. Although topical benzocaine usually does not produce any side effects, cases of methemoglobinemia have been reported in children who have been treated with this agent.

Teething is best treated with reassurance and appropriate doses of acetaminophen.

10. **e.** All are potential hazards when OTC cold and cough medications are given to infants and children. It is very important for physicians to inquire about and educate parents on the use of all OTC medications.

Summary

1. URIs: There is no evidence that antihistamines, decongestants, cough suppressants, or expectorants are of any value in the treatment of viral URI symptoms in infants and young children. Potential toxicity is present with all of these agents.
2. Cough: Suppression of cough may be hazardous and contraindicated in many pulmonary diseases. Coughs due to URI are short-lived and treated with fluids and humidity.
3. Nausea and vomiting: Dimenhydrinate is not useful and is potentially toxic.
4. Teething: There is no evidence that rash, diarrhea, vomiting, nasal congestion, irritability, or sleeplessness are associated with teething. Benzocaine preparations should be avoided. Reassurance and judicious use of acetaminophen may be indicated.
5. Physicians need to inquire about the use of all OTC medications and need to educate parents about their effectiveness and safety.

Suggested Reading

Gunn VL, et al: Toxicity of over-the-counter cough and cold medications. *Pediatrics* 108(3):E52, 2001.

Pappas D, Owen-Hendley J: The common cold. In: Long SS, Pickering LK, Prober CG, eds, *Principles and Practice of Pediatric Infectious Diseases*, 2nd ed. Philadelphia: Churchill Livingstone, 2003.

Simasek M: Treatment of the common cold. *Am Fam Physician* 75(4):515–520, 2007.

Turner RB: Viral respiratory infections—Common cold. In: Rakel RE, Bope ET, eds, *Conn's Current Therapy 2006*, 58th ed. Philadelphia: Saunders, 2005.

Turner RB, Hayden GF: The common cold. In: Behrman RE, et al, eds, *Nelson Textbook of Pediatrics*, 17th ed. Philadelphia: Saunders, 2004.

CHAPTER 103

Diaper Rash and Other Infant Dermatitis

CLINICAL CASE PROBLEM 1

A 2-Month-Old Infant with a Rash on His Cheeks

A 2-month-old infant is brought to your office by his mother. He developed an erythematous, dry skin rash on both cheeks approximately 1 week ago. Although the rash is always present, the mother states that it seems to be worse after she feeds him.

The mother breast-fed for the first 4 weeks of life, but she returned to work 4 weeks ago and switched the baby from breast-feeding to bottle-feeding. The mother has a history of asthma, and the father has seasonal allergies.

On examination, the child appears healthy. He has an erythematous maculopapular eruption that covers his cheeks, and he appears to be developing an erythematous rash on his neck, both wrists, and both hands (Fig. 103-1). The rest of the physical examination is within normal limits.

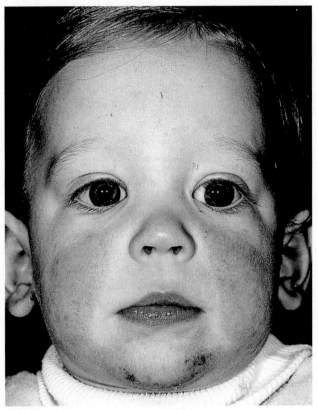

Figure 103-1

A 2-month-old infant with an erythematous maculopapular eruption covering his cheeks. (Reproduced from Habif TB: *Clinical Dermatology*, 4th ed. St. Louis, MO: Mosby, 2004, Figure 5-5, with permission.) (See Color Plate 1.)

SELECT THE BEST ANSWER TO THE FOLLOWING QUESTIONS

1. What is the most likely cause of this infant's skin rash?
   a. atopic dermatitis
   b. allergic contact dermatitis
   c. seborrheic dermatitis
   d. infectious eczematoid dermatitis
   e. none of the above

2. What is (are) the recommended initial treatment(s) of the skin rash in the infant presented?
   a. skin hydration with petroleum products
   b. local corticosteroid therapy
   c. minimizing bathing and the use of soap
   d. topical calcineurin inhibitor (Elidel)
   e. a, b, and c

3. What other conditions are not routinely associated with this condition?
   a. asthma
   b. allergic rhinitis

   c. wool sensitivity
   d. keratosis pilaris
   e. immunodeficiency

4. Which statement is false regarding the prognosis and treatment of this condition?
   a. 50% of these patients will improve by 18 months
   b. smallpox vaccine is contraindicated in these patients because of the risk of eczema herpeticum
   c. since topical corticosteroids rarely control symptoms, systemic steroids are usually required
   d. some adults continue to have localized rash
   e. up to 80% of these patients will develop allergy or allergic rhinitis symptoms

5. Which statement is not true regarding the etiology of this condition?
   a. a maternal history of allergy or asthma is the most important genetic predictor
   b. breast-feeding offers no advantage over formula-feeding in this condition

c. Eosinophilia is common in these patients

d. there is an increased production of allergen-specific T cells and some interleukins, leading to elevated IgE levels in patients with this condition

e. food allergies are important triggers in 40% of young children with this condition

CLINICAL CASE PROBLEM 2

A 3-Week-Old Infant with a Crusty Head

A grandmother brings in a 3-week-old infant with the complaint that she has "crusting" on her hair. Since it has been quite cold, the grandmother (who cares for the child) has been careful not to bathe the child too often, and she does not use shampoo. The child is bottle-feeding and has otherwise had no health problems. On examination, the infant appears healthy and interactive. Her scalp is covered with a crusty, yellowish rash with some erythema and crusting at the base of the ears and scalp (Fig. 103-2).

6. The most likely diagnosis of this rash is
   a. atopic dermatitis
   b. allergic contact dermatitis
   c. seborrheic dermatitis
   d. infectious eczematoid dermatitis
   e. none of the above

7. Recommended treatment of the rash initially is
   a. antifungal cream (e.g., clotrimazole)
   b. gentle cleansing of the scalp with a soft washcloth and baby shampoo, using oil to remove scales if needed

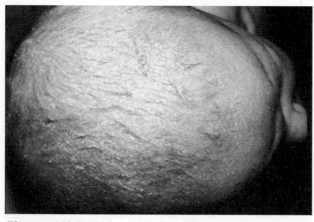

Figure 103-2

A 3-week-old infant with a crusty, yellowish rash with some erythema on her scalp. (Reproduced from Cohen BA: *Pediatric Dermatology*, 3rd ed. Philadelphia: Mosby, 2005, with permission.) (See Color Plate 2.)

c. antibiotics (preferably anti-staphylococcal antibiotics)

d. observation

e. none of the above

CLINICAL CASE PROBLEM 3

A 2-Week-Old Infant Who Looks "Too Ugly for Photos"

A 2-week-old infant, a product of a normal birth and delivery, is brought to your office because the mother says she cannot take baby photos since his skin "won't clear up." According to the mother, ever since birth the child has had small pimple-like lesions on his face and scattered over his body that come and go (Fig. 103-3). Sometimes, they get slightly erythematous, but they are not crusty. The baby is not bothered by them, but his face looks "so ugly his mother doesn't want to get his photo taken." She wants medicine to "get rid of it."

8. What is the most likely diagnosis in this infant?
   a. atopic dermatitis
   b. milia

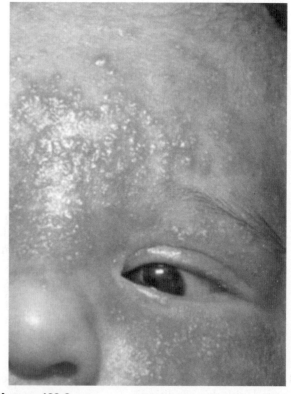

Figure 103-3

A 2-week-old infant with small pimple-like lesions on his face. (Reproduced from Cohen BA: *Pediatric Dermatology*, 3rd ed. Philadelphia: Mosby, 2005, with permission.) (See Color Plate 3.)

c. seborrheic dermatitis

d. miliaria

e. infantile acne

9. What is (are) the treatment(s) of choice for the condition described here?

   a. wet compresses

   b. topical corticosteroids

   c. topical clotrimazole

   d. reassurance

   e. a, b, and c

CLINICAL CASE PROBLEM 4

An 8-Month-Old Infant with a Long-Term Persistent Diaper Rash

An 8-month-old infant is brought to your office by his mother for assessment of a diaper rash. His mother has tried cornstarch powder, vitamin E cream, zinc oxide, and a prescribed corticosteroid cream from a different physician.

On examination, the infant has an intensely erythematous diaper dermatitis that has a scalloped border and a sharply demarcated edge. There are numerous "satellite lesions" present on the lower abdomen and thighs (Fig. 103-4).

10. What is the most likely diagnosis in this infant?

    a. atopic dermatitis

    b. allergic contact dermatitis

    c. seborrheic dermatitis

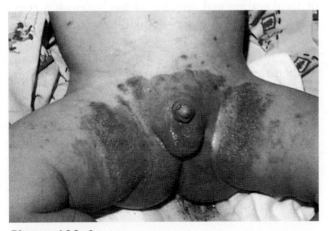

Figure 103-4

An 8-month-old infant with an intensely erythematous diaper dermatitis including a scalloped border and sharply demarcated edge. "Satellite lesions" are also present on the lower abdomen and thighs. (Reproduced from Behrman R, Kliegman R, Jenson H: Cutaneous fungal infections. In: *Nelson Textbook of Pediatrics*, 17th ed. Philadelphia: Saunders, 2004, Figure 656-5, with permission.) (See Color Plate 4.)

d. infectious eczematoid dermatitis

e. candidal diaper dermatitis

11. What is the treatment of choice for this infant's diaper rash?

    a. a topical corticosteroid

    b. a topical antibiotic

    c. a systemic antibiotic

    d. a topical antifungal agent

    e. none of the above

CLINICAL CASE PROBLEM 5

A 4-Month-Old Infant with a Diaper Rash Caused by Dirty Diapers

A 4-month-old infant is brought to your office by her mother. Her mother complains that the child has a diaper rash that is probably related to her "not changing the diapers often." The mother has five other children and was trying to save money by using fewer diapers. She admits that she waits until the diaper is soaked before changing it.

On examination, the infant has erythematous, scaly, papulovesicular diaper dermatitis with numerous bullous lesions, fissures, and erosions.

12. What is the most likely diagnosis in this infant?

    a. atopic dermatitis

    b. primary irritant contact dermatitis

    c. seborrheic dermatitis

    d. fungal dermatitis

    e. allergic contact dermatitis

13. What is (are) the treatment(s) of choice for the infant described here?

    a. zinc oxide paste or other barrier ointments

    b. topical hydrocortisone

    c. systemic antibiotics

    d. a and b

    e. a, b, and c

14. What differentiates a candidal diaper rash from irritant diaper dermatitis?

    a. irritant diaper dermatitis spares the crural folds

    b. candidal diaper rash has satellite lesions

    c. irritant diaper dermatitis involves the crural folds

    d. candidal diaper dermatitis is usually associated with fissures and erosions

    e. a and b

Answers

1. **a.** Atopic dermatitis is an inflammatory skin disease characterized by erythema, edema, pruritus, exudation, crusting, and scaling. It is often referred to as the "itch that rashes." Atopic dermatitis can be classified as infantile (up to 2 years), childhood (2 to 12 years), and adult atopic dermatitis. Infantile atopic dermatitis usually presents at 4 months of age, and 50% of cases resolve by 18 months. The areas most commonly affected include the cheeks, neck, wrists, hands, and extensor aspects of the extremities. Spread often occurs from extensor to flexor. Pruritus may lead to intense scratching and secondary infection. In older children, flexural surfaces are involved, often with xerosis and lichenification. Atopic dermatitis may be exacerbated by food allergies (in approximately 40% of cases), such as from eggs, wheat, peanuts, or cow's milk; environmental stimuli such as dust mites or animal dander; or emotional stress.

2. **e.** The treatment of atopic dermatitis begins with the avoidance of any environmental factors that precipitate the condition and also maintenance of the skin barrier. Disruption of the acid mantle of the skin by alkaline soaps is a major factor in the development and worsening of the condition. Use of non-soap alternatives (Aveeno, Cetaphil, and Dove) or pH-neutral cleaners and bathing only dirty skin areas comprise the most important maintenance therapy. In addition, emollients (e.g., petroleum products) to restore skin hydration should be applied within 3 minutes of bathing. Excessive drying of the skin should be avoided. Atopic dermatitis is best managed with local therapy. Flare-ups of the condition are treated with topical corticosteroid creams or lotions. To further prevent scratching, the fingernails should be cut short. Percutaneous absorption of corticosteroid does occur, and atrophy of the skin should be watched for. This can be avoided by using only low or moderate potency topical corticosteroids. Topical calcineurin inhibitors such as pimecrolimus (Elidel) are not approved for infants younger than 2 years of age, especially since the addition of the Food and Drug Administration black box warning for lymphomas and skin cancer, but they are used for second-line therapy in older children and are still used by some physicians in place of high-potency steroids in younger children with severe atopic dermatitis. Systemic antihistamines and nonsedating antihistamines have to be used to control pruritus, but not in infants. These can improve sleep and prevent more excoriations and secondary infections. Secondarily infected atopic dermatitis may often be managed by topical mupirocin, but occasionally it may require systemic treatment.

3. **e.** Atopic dermatitis is often associated with a family history of allergies, asthma, hay fever, or atopic dermatitis. Individuals are more sensitive to certain fibers, particularly wool. Rough fibers tend to be more irritating than smooth fibers in clothing textiles. Keratosis pilaris, which is characterized by asymptomatic horny follicular papules on the upper arms, buttocks, and thighs, is another manifestation of atopic dermatitis. Immunodeficiency (severe combined immunodeficiency, Wiskott–Aldrich syndrome, etc.) should be considered in an infant with a rash that does not resolve, but it is not typical of atopic dermatitis in general.

4. **c.** Atopic dermatitis is largely a condition of children. Nearly 60% present with symptoms as infants in the first 12 months of life, and another 25% of patients will have disease presentation by age 5 years. Of those who present in infancy, 50% will resolve by 18 months. Topical corticosteroids and treatment with skin hydration are adequate treatment for most infants and young children, but many also require treatment with topical calcineurin inhibitors (older than age 2 years) and with antihistamines. Smallpox vaccine is contraindicated due to risk of eczema herpaticum. Adults may persist in having localized rashes, and a few may have severe disease. When not treated, the condition may become very severe.

5. **b.** Breast-feeding is very important to prevent atopic dermatitis, particularly if breast-feeding is exclusive and continued until the infant is more than 6 months of age.

6. **c.** Pityriasis capita, or cradle cap—a diffuse or focal scaling and crusting of the scalp—is a common form of seborrheic dermatitis seen in infancy. Seborrheic dermatitis is most common in children during the first 3 months of life. Typically, it is a dry, scaly, erythematous, papular dermatitis that is usually nonpruritic. It may involve the face, neck, retroauricular areas, axillae, and diaper area. The dermatitis may be patchy or focal, or it may spread to involve the entire body. Although common, the etiology of seborrheic dermatitis is unclear, but it is possibly related to the proliferation of the Mallassezia species. Hormonal and genetic factors as well as alteration of essential fatty acid patterns are also thought to play a major role.

7. **b.** Generally, gentle cleaning with a soft washcloth, occasionally using baby or mineral oil to remove scales, is curative for cradle cap. If the seborrheic dermatitis extends onto the face or persists, a low-dose hydrocortisone cream may be used for a short time or selenium shampoo may be used on the scalp. Often, caretakers are afraid to shampoo the hair, causing buildup of the crust.

8. **e.** This infant has infantile acne, a benign condition that generally only presents problems of appearances and for photographs. It spontaneously resolves and does not require treatment. It should be distinguished from atopic dermatitis, seborrheic dermatitis, erythema toxicum neonatorum, and neonatal pustular melanosis. Erythema toxicum neonatorum usually appears soon after birth and lasts up to 2 weeks. It is characterized by vesicles, pustules, and papules on an erythematous halo base. Transient pustular neonatal melanosis, more common in dark-skinned infants, also has vesicles and pustules, but no erythematous base, and may have a collarette of scale. Milia are epidermal inclusion cysts and miliaria is essentially a "heat rash."

9. **d.** Reassurance that it will clear, and an understanding that no treatment is necessary, is important. None of the other treatments listed are necessary.

10. **e.** This infant has candidal diaper dermatitis, which presents as an erythematous confluent plaque formed by papules and vesiculopustules, with a scalloped border and a sharply demarcated edge. Candidal diaper dermatitis can usually be distinguished from other childhood diaper dermatoses by the presence of "satellite lesions" produced at some distance from the primary eruption. Although this child's rash is not primarily perianal, streptococcal dermatitis should be considered in the case of a chronic perianal rash. Diagnosis can be made by culture, and it responds to treatment with amoxicillin. Intertrigo, common in infants with overlapping skin and fat folds, usually responds to treatment to decrease the moisture. Primary irritant dermatitis is discussed later.

11. **d.** The treatment of choice in candidal diaper dermatitis is a topical antifungal agent. Topical miconazole, clotrimazole, or ketoconazole are commonly used. In an infant with a severe inflammatory reaction, a topical corticosteroid may be mixed 50/50 with a topical antifungal agent and applied on a regular basis for a few days to 1 week. Rather than using a high-potency steroid/antifungal combination, however, use of a low-potency steroid such as hydrocortisone with the antifungal agent is preferred because the infant is at risk for striae and local complications of steroid therapy.

12. **b.** This child has a primary irritant contact dermatitis. Irritant contact dermatitis is a reaction to friction, maceration, and prolonged contact with urine and feces. It usually presents as an erythematous, scaly dermatitis with papulovesicular or bullous lesions, fissures, and erosions. The eruption can be either patchy or confluent. The genitocrural folds are often spared.

Secondary infection with either bacteria or yeast can occur. The infant can be in considerable discomfort because of the marked inflammation that is sometimes associated with this type of diaper rash. Primary irritant diaper dermatitis should be managed by frequent changing of diapers and thorough washing of the genitalia with warm water and a mild soap. Occlusive plastic pants that promote maceration should be avoided. If cloth diapers are used, they should be changed frequently, as should disposable diapers. Drying out the skin by allowing the infant to go without diapers can be helpful but can be logistically challenging.

13. **d.** An occlusive topical agent such as zinc oxide or A&D ointment can be applied until healing occurs. Topical 1% hydrocortisone ointment is also very useful in the management of diaper dermatitis in its more severe form. Systemic antibiotics are not indicated in the treatment of primary irritant diaper dermatitis. Again, the primary treatment is frequent diaper changing or leaving the child without a diaper as much as possible until the skin heals.

14. **e.** A useful diagnostic pearl for differentiating candidal diaper rash from irritant diaper dermatitis is that candidal diaper rash tends to involve the warm, moist folds of the skin, whereas irritant diaper dermatitis tends to spare the folds, occurring mainly in the areas of greatest skin contact with urine and feces. Candidal diaper rash also tends to present with satellite lesions and will worsen with prolonged topical corticosteroid therapy.

Summary

ATOPIC DERMATITIS

1. Diagnostic clue: usually begins and is more prominent on the cheeks of infants
2. Treatment: avoidance of soaps and limited bathing frequency; use of agents to promote skin hydration; low-dose corticosteroids may be used, and in children older than 2 years, or in particularly severe cases in younger children, topical calcineurin inhibitors may be used (Elidel approved for children older than age 2 years)
3. Strong association with allergies and asthma, with 80% of patients developing these, and a strong maternal family history of these illnesses

SEBORRHEIC DERMATITIS

1. Diagnostic clue: cradle cap typically presents in early infancy
2. Treatment: gentle cleansing with soap and removal of scales with oil; low-dose corticosteroids and occasionally antifungal agents may be used if needed

CANDIDAL DERMATITIS

1. Diagnostic clue: satellite lesions around the peripheral area of the main area of dermatitis
2. Treatment: topical miconazole, topical clotrimazole, mild topical hydrocortisone mixed with a topical antifungal agent when severe inflammation is present

PRIMARY IRRITANT DERMATITIS

1. Diagnostic clue: maceration, often a history of infrequent diaper changes and prolonged exposure to urine and feces
2. Treatment: occlusive topical agent such as zinc oxide or petroleum jelly or zinc oxide applied over hydrocortisone base when severe inflammation is present; frequent diaper changes essential

Erythema toxicorum neonatorum, milia, miliaria, and transient pustular neonatal melanosis are all self-limited skin conditions of the newborn that do not require treatment.

Suggested Reading

Behrman RE, Kliegman R, Jenson H: *Nelson Textbook of Pediatrics*, 17th ed. Saunders, Philadelphia: 2004.

Boiko S: Making rash decisions in the diaper area. *Pediatr Ann* 29(1): 50–56, 2000.

Habif TB: *Clinical Dermatology: A Color Guide to Diagnosis and Therapy*, 4th ed. St. Louis, MO: Mosby, 2004.

Johns Hopkins Hospital: *Harriet Lane Handbook: A Manual for Pediatric House Officers*, 17th ed. St. Louis, MO: Mosby, 2005.

Johnson BA, Nunley JR: Treatment of seborrheic dermatitis. *Am Fam Physician* 61:2703–2710, 2713–2714, 2000.

Scheinfeld N: Diaper dermatitis: A review and brief survey of eruptions of the diaper area. *Am J Clin Dermatol* 6(5):273–281, 2005.

CHAPTER

104 Failure to Thrive and Short Stature

CLINICAL CASE PROBLEM 1

An 8-Month-Old Infant Who Appears Malnourished

An 8-month-old infant is brought to the emergency department by his mother for an assessment of an upper respiratory tract infection. He has been coughing for the past 3 days and has had a runny nose. On examination, his temperature is 37.5°C. His weight is below the 3rd percentile for his age, his length is at the 25th percentile, and his head circumference is at the 50th percentile. He appears malnourished and has thin extremities, a narrow face, prominent ribs, and wasted buttocks. He has a prominent diaper rash, unwashed skin, a skin rash that resembles the skin infection impetigo contagiosum on his face, uncut fingernails, and dirty clothing.

SELECT THE BEST ANSWER TO THE FOLLOWING QUESTIONS

1. What is the most likely diagnosis in the infant described?
   a. nonorganic failure to thrive (FTT)
   b. organic FTT
   c. child neglect
   d. a and c
   e. b and c

2. Nonorganic FTT represents what fraction of FTT?
   a. 10%
   b. 25%
   c. 50%
   d. 75%
   e. 90%

3. What is the most likely cause of this child's condition?
   a. maternal deprivation
   b. cystic fibrosis
   c. constitutionally small for age
   d. infantile autism
   e. congenital bilateral sensorineural hearing loss

4. What is (are) the procedure(s) of choice for this infant at this time?
   a. provision of a high-calorie formula; reassessment of the infant in 1 week
   b. initiation of outpatient investigations in the child to exclude serious organic disease
   c. treatment of the respiratory tract infection and instruction to the mother in correct feeding practices
   d. all of the above
   e. none of the above

5. Where is follow-up of this child best performed?
   a. in the hospital outpatient department
   b. in the hospital emergency room
   c. in the family physician's office
   d. in the home by the public health nurse
   e. in the social worker's office

6. The initial follow-up plan suggests the frequency of visits for the child to be which of the following?
   a. every month
   b. every 3 months
   c. every week
   d. every 6 weeks
   e. every 6 months

7. The environment that exists for this child should be thoroughly assessed for which of the following?
   a. child abuse or potential for child abuse
   b. spousal abuse or potential for spousal abuse
   c. level of family income
   d. inappropriate parental coping mechanisms: alcohol and drug use
   e. all of the above

CLINICAL CASE PROBLEM 2

Falling Off the Growth Curve

A 9-month-old infant comes in for a routine examination and immunizations. The infant has fallen off the previous centile line. The patient's mother has an 8th-grade education, lives on state support, and has not identified the father of the child. On questioning, the mother indicates that she has been living with her parents but has been told she must find a place of her own. She has signs of depression.

Examination shows an infant with no physical anomalies but whose weight is disproportionate to height and has fallen off the curve set in the first 9 months.

8. There is a strong relationship to this child's diagnosis and which of the following?
   a. parental education level
   b. poverty
   c. family stress
   d. markers of eating disorders
   e. none of the above

9. As assistance is provided for the mother for the depression and financial challenges, the infant will
   a. benefit from a behavioral feeding program
   b. take several years to catch up with height/weight ratio
   c. Catch up with his peers by age 1 year
   d. a and c
   e. a and b

10. Which of the following investigations should be performed in a child with FTT or a child in which short stature is unlikely to be familial in nature?
    a. complete blood count (CBC)
    b. complete urinalysis
    c. serum blood urea nitrogen (BUN) and creatinine
    d. T4 and thyroid-stimulating hormone (TSH)
    e. all of the above

CLINICAL CASE PROBLEM 3

A 13-Year-Old Female Who Is Short with a Webbed Neck

A 13-year-old female is brought to your office for assessment of her short stature. On examination, the child has a height and weight below the 5th percentile, a webbed neck, lack of breast bud development, a high-arched palate, and a low-set posterior hairline.

11. What is the most likely diagnosis in this child?
    a. Noonan's syndrome
    b. trisomy 21
    c. Turner's syndrome
    d. fragile X syndrome
    e. constitutional delay of growth

12. What is the most common cause of short stature in children?
    a. familial short stature
    b. chromosomal abnormality
    c. constitutional delay of growth
    d. hypothyroidism
    e. psychosocial dwarfism

13. Bone age can sometimes be used to differentiate certain causes of short stature in children. With respect to bone age, which of the following statements is true?
    a. bone age is normal in both familial short stature and constitutional delay of growth
    b. bone age is normal in familial short stature and delayed in constitutional delay of growth
    c. bone age is normal in constitutional delay of growth and delayed in growth hormone deficiency
    d. bone age is delayed in both familial short stature and short stature caused by hypothyroidism
    e. bone age is variable and cannot be used to differentiate familial short stature and constitutional delay

14. Psychosocial dwarfism is a situation in which poor physical growth may be associated with an unfavorable psychosocial situation. With respect to psychosocial dwarfism, which of the following statements is (are) true?
    a. sleep and eating aberrations occur in these children
    b. growth usually returns to normal when the stress is removed
    c. behavioral problems are common in these children
    d. a, b, and c are true
    e. a, b, and c are false

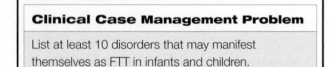

Clinical Case Management Problem

List at least 10 disorders that may manifest themselves as FTT in infants and children.

Answers

1. **d.** This child most likely has nonorganic FTT, secondary to child neglect.

2. **e.** Approximately 90% of FTT is nonorganic in origin.

3. **a.** FTT may be a result of organic causes, nonorganic causes, or both. Nonorganic causes predominate. Nonorganic FTT includes psychologic FTT (maternal deprivation), child neglect, lack of education regarding feeding, and errors in feeding. Nonorganic FTT is most often attributable to maternal deprivation (as in this case) or lack of a nurturing environment at home. Organic FTT is caused most commonly by a medical condition impairing the child's ability to take in, absorb, or metabolize adequate calories.

4. **e.** The treatment of choice at this time is to hospitalize the child and to give unlimited feedings for a minimum period of 1 week. At the same time, a careful physical examination and laboratory investigations including CBC, complete urinalysis, renal function testing, and serum TSH level can be completed. If the child lives in an inner-city neighborhood with older housing stock, a serum lead level test should also be done. The family physician should involve social services and also initiate a detailed assessment of the child's home environment. Before the child is discharged home, the home environment must be assessed and the parents of the child must be given explicit instructions in feeding practices.

5. **d.** If the child begins to gain weight rapidly and reestablish his health in the hospital (which is very likely), reassessment ideally should be done in the environment that allowed the development of the problem in the first place (at least on some occasions). This is obviously the home, and the health care professional in the best position to do this is probably the public health nurse or the community health nurse.

6. **c.** The initial follow-up supervision should be close and frequent—every week for the first 6 weeks following discharge from the hospital is reasonable.

7. **e.** Maternal neglect resulting in nonorganic FTT should not be just left at that; the reasons need to be investigated. A mother who neglects her child (a form of child abuse) is also at risk for committing other forms of child abuse. In addition, she is at greater than average risk of being abused by her husband or partner. Remember that family violence begets family violence, and in this case we already have established that a form of family violence (child abuse [neglect]) exists.

8. **c.** According to recent research, there is no clear relation between weight faltering and maternal deprivation, educational level, or markers of eating disorders.

9. **c.** Evidence indicates that infants of mothers with depression and stress are more than twice as likely to have FTT symptoms but are no different from their peers by the age of 1 year. Occasionally, infants will have developed problem eating behaviors and will benefit from behavioral intervention even as the mother is treated.

10. e. Recommended investigations in a child with FTT or a child in whom short stature is unlikely to be familial in nature should include CBC, complete urinalysis, serum BUN and creatinine, erythrocyte sedimentation rate (ESR), serum thyroxine, TSH, and bone age hand x-ray. Serum lead level, stool for ova and parasites, and liver enzymes (serum bilirubin, alanine aminotransferase, and aspartate aminotransferase) may be considered when the clinical history is suggestive.

11. c. The most likely cause of this child's short stature is Turner's syndrome. Noonan's syndrome (an autosomal dominant trait with widely variable expressivity) also has short stature and neck webbing as its most common presentation. It can be distinguished from Turner's syndrome easily, however, by its normal chromosome complement and characteristic facies including hypertelorism and ptosis. Patients with Turner's syndrome will have either a 45 XO chromosome complement or a mosaic involving loss of sex chromosomal material. Trisomy 21 will usually be recognized long before the age of 13 years. The fragile X syndrome is associated with mental retardation and macroorchidism in males.

12. a. The most common cause of short stature in children is short parents. When a short child who is growing at a normal rate and has a normal bone age is found to have a strong family history of short stature, familial short stature is the most likely cause. Other causes of short stature include constitutional delay of growth, chromosomal abnormalities, intrauterine growth restriction, chronic diseases such as renal disease or inflammatory bowel disease, hypothyroidism, adrenal hyperplasia, growth hormone deficiency or resistance, psychosocial dwarfism, and idiopathic short stature.

13. b. Bone age determination can distinguish between the two most common causes of short stature: familial short stature and constitutional delay of growth. Children with familial short stature have normal bone ages. Constitutional delay of growth, which is really a delay in reaching ultimate height and sexual maturation, presents with delayed bone age and delayed sexual maturation. Hypothyroidism and growth hormone deficiency usually present with a delayed bone age.

14. d. Inadequate growth in children may be associated with an unfavorable psychologic environment. In this situation, the child may show transiently low human growth hormone levels during periods of stress. He or she may also have behavioral, sleep, and eating disturbances. Both growth and growth hormone levels return to normal when the psychologic stressors are removed.

Solution to the Clinical Case Management Problem

Disorders that may manifest themselves as FTT in infants and children include the following: (1) emotional/ psychologic factors, (2) ventral nervous system (central nervous system [CNS]) abnormality, (3) gastrointestinal (GI) malformation (pyloric stenosis, tracheoesophageal fistula, and cleft palate) or disease (Hirschsprung's disease, gastroesophageal reflux, chronic diarrheal syndromes and malabsorption diseases, inflammatory bowel disease, liver disease, or parasites), (4) congenital or acquired heart disease (cardiac failure), (5) chronic renal disease (anomalies and renal failure), (6) chromosomal disorders (Down syndrome and Turner's syndrome), (7) chronic infection (GI system, kidney, pulmonary system, CNS, tuberculosis, human immunodeficiency virus, and hepatitis), (8) inborn error of metabolism (hypothyroidism/hyperthyroidism/hyperaldosteronism), (9) malignancies (neuroblastoma, nephroblastoma, and glioma), (10) anemias, (11) congenital low-birth-weight syndrome (fetal alcohol or drug exposure), (12) cystic fibrosis, (13) bronchopulmonary dysplasia, and (14) drug reactions.

Summary

FAILURE TO THRIVE
1. Nonorganic: psychologic FTT, maternal deprivation, child neglect, lack of education regarding feeding, and errors in feeding. Suspect family dysfunction and monitor carefully in these cases.

2. Organic FTT: See the Solution to the Clinical Case Management Problem.
3. Treatment
   a. An initial period of hospitalization is indicated in most cases. Unlimited feedings (especially to any

infant) should be given in these cases, and a complete investigation should be performed to attempt to elucidate the cause.

b. When the child goes home, careful and frequent observation is indicated, especially in the initial period. Some of these observations should take place in the environment (the home) in which the problems began (for nonorganic FTT). Weekly observation is indicated initially.

SHORT STATURE

1. Familial short stature is the most common cause.

2. Familial short stature can be differentiated from constitutional delay of growth (the second most common cause) by bone age.

3. Other causes of short stature include chromosomal abnormalities, intrauterine growth restriction, hypothyroidism, psychosocial dwarfism, Turner's syndrome, and growth hormone deficiency.

4. Investigations of a child with short stature should include CBC, complete urinalysis, serum BUN/creatinine, liver enzymes and bilirubin, ESR, serum thyroxine, TSH, and x-ray of the hands and wrist for bone age (Fig. 104-1).

Figure 104-1

Summary of diagnosis and approach to small stature. CBC, complete blood count; FTT, failure to thrive; UA, urinalysis.

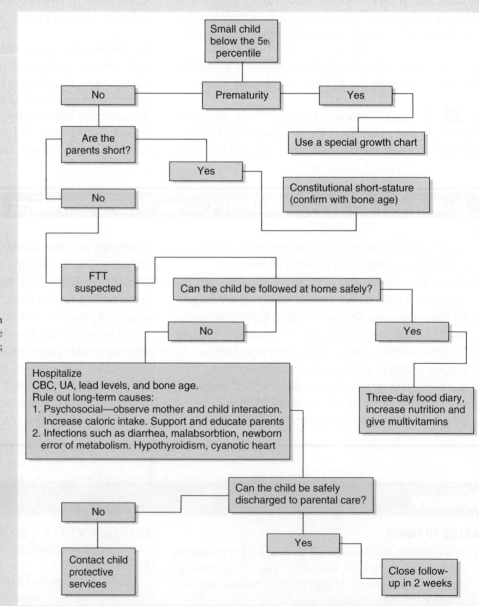

Suggested Reading

Johnson CF: Nonorganic failure to thrive. In: Behrman RE, Klegman RM, Jenson HB, eds, *Nelson Textbook of Pediatrics*, 17th ed. Philadelphia: Saunders, 2004.

Jolley CD: Failure to thrive. *Curr Problems Pediatr Adolesc Health Care* 33(6):183–206, 2003.

Krugman SD: Failure to thrive. *Am Fam Physician* 68(5):879–884, 2003.

Rudolf MC: What is the long term outcome for children who fail to thrive? A systematic review. *Arch Dis Child* 90(9):925–927, 2005.

Shah MD: Failure to thrive in children. *J Clin Gastroenterol* 35(5): 371–374, 2002.

Wright CM, Parkinson KN, Drewett RF: The influence of maternal socioeconomic and emotional factors on infant weight gain and weight faltering (failure to thrive): Data from a prospective birth cohort. *Arch Dis Child* 91(3):312–317, 2006.

CHAPTER 105 Child Abuse

CLINICAL CASE PROBLEM 1

A 2-Month-Old Infant Who Fell Off a Sofa and Fractured His Humerus

A 2-month-old infant is brought to the hospital emergency room (ER) by his mother. She says that he rolled off the sofa the previous night and injured his right arm.

On examination, the infant is crying inconsolably and has a swollen, bruised right arm. An x-ray reveals a spiral fracture of the right humerus. There are also a number of old abrasions and old bruises that appear to be in various stages of healing. The remainder of the physical examination is normal. The mother says that the child has been well since the birth of him and his twin. Neither infant has had any significant medical illnesses.

SELECT THE BEST ANSWER TO THE FOLLOWING QUESTIONS

1. Given the history, the physical examination, and the x-ray report, what should you do now?
   a. obtain an orthopedic consultation
   b. prescribe a sling for the child's arm
   c. investigate the child for possible coagulopathy
   d. suggest that the mother purchase a walker instead of laying her child on a sofa
   e. discuss the details of the incident more fully with the mother and contact the hospital social worker

2. After your initial intervention or recommendation, what is the next step you should take?
   a. ask the mother to return with the child for follow-up in 3 weeks
   b. ask the mother to return with the child for follow-up in 1 week

   c. arrange for the family physician to see the child at home the following day
   d. hospitalize the child
   e. none of the above

3. Which of the following has the lowest priority as part of this child's initial workup?
   a. obtaining a skeletal survey
   b. performing a funduscopic examination
   c. contacting the state child protection services
   d. testing for osteogenesis imperfecta
   e. obtaining a computed tomography (CT) scan of head

4. A physician should report suspected child abuse to the state agency for child protection when?
   a. only if the physician is certain that the child is being abused
   b. only if the perpetrator confesses
   c. any time the physician has a reasonable suspicion of abuse
   d. only if the child is being abused physically
   e. only if the abuse is witnessed

5. When other children reside in the home of a child who is a suspected or confirmed victim of child abuse, which of the following statements is true?
   a. evidence indicates that there is usually a single "scapegoat" and if the abused child has been identified, other children are generally safe
   b. experts recommend that contact children are at risk of abuse and medical evaluation is warranted
   c. evidence is clear that all siblings are at significant risk and confirmation of abuse of one child should immediately lead to removal of all siblings from the home until appropriate intervention has occurred
   d. abuse of other children in the home is only of concern in sexual abuse cases, so evaluation/protection of other children in the home need only occur in cases of sexual abuse
   e. evidence indicates that neglect is the only form of child abuse that is likely to be shared across multiple children and further investigation need be pursued only in cases of proven neglect

CLINICAL CASE PROBLEM 2

A Blistered 8-Month-Old Baby

An 8-month-old child is brought to the hospital ER with a large blistering burn covering both feet and ankles. There are also burns on the child's buttocks. The father states that the patient's 5-year-old brother must have turned on the hot water while they were bathing together.

6. As the ER doctor in charge, what is your next step?
   a. treat the burn and move on to the next patient: time is money!
   b. call the police and have the hospital security guards detain and restrain the father
   c. obtain a more detailed history of the child's present injury and his previous health; at the same time, immerse the child's buttocks in cold water in an attempt to minimize damage from the burn
   d. obtain a more detailed history of the child's present injury and his previous health, try to make the child comfortable with analgesics, and apply a burn dressing as soon as possible
   e. use a confrontational approach and accuse the father of concealing information and abusing the child; have your resident deal with the immediate burn injury

7. Which one of the following statements most accurately reflects the situation in a family in which there has been documented child abuse?
   a. in most cases, the child has to be permanently removed from the family and placed in a foster home
   b. rehabilitation of parents who have been involved in child abuse is almost always unsuccessful
   c. with comprehensive and intensive treatment of the entire family, 80% to 90% of families involved in child abuse or neglect can be successfully rehabilitated
   d. in most cases, child abuse will leave a permanent scar on the child's personality
   e. in a situation in which one child in a family has been abused, there is usually no increased risk to other children in the same family

8. Which of the following statements concerning child abuse in relation to spousal abuse is true?
   a. women who are abused are unlikely to abuse their children
   b. men who abuse their wives or partners are unlikely to abuse their children

   c. men who abuse their wives are much more likely to abuse their children than are men who do not abuse their wives
   d. there is no correlation between the various forms of family violence
   e. parents who abuse their children are unlikely to have come from families in which they themselves were abused or their mother was abused

9. Regarding the epidemiology of child abuse, which of the following statements is (are) true?
   a. in 1997, the National Committee for the Prevention of Child Abuse estimated that more than 3 million cases of child abuse and neglect were reported to public social service agencies in the United States
   b. approximately 1000 deaths are caused by child abuse and neglect each year in the United States
   c. each year, more than 200,000 new cases of child sexual abuse are reported in the United States
   d. it is estimated that by the age of 18 years, one of every three or four girls will be sexually assaulted and one of every six to eight boys will be sexually assaulted
   e. all of the above are true

CLINICAL CASE PROBLEM 3

An 8-Year-Old-Girl and a New Stepfather

An 8-year-old girl presents to your office with vaginal discharge, nail biting, and declining school performance. Her mother indicates that the child has always been a good student but seems to be falling behind. There has been some stress at home because the mother remarried 9 months earlier and the stepfather and his two children, ages 2 and 4 years, have become part of the family. According to the mother, the relationship between the patient and her stepfather is wonderful; she indicates that he seems to enjoy having an older child and often the two run family errands or go on outings to the zoo or library together.

10. Which aspects of the history should raise your concern about possible sexual abuse?
    a. the presence of vaginal discharge in a prepubertal girl
    b. recent change in family status with non-blood relatives in household
    c. behavioral change in patient
    d. none of the above
    e. a, b, and c

11. Sexual abuse of children includes which of the following?
    a. penetrating vaginal, anal, or oral intercourse
    b. inappropriate touching
    c. visual exposure to masturbation
    d. sexually explicit, suggestive talk or threats
    e. all of the above

12. What form of interview should be conducted to try to determine if abuse is present?
    a. one or both parents should be present at all times
    b. asking medical history, menstrual history, and sexual history helps the physician determine language and development of child
    c. ask straightforward questions at a level understood by the patient
    d. a, b, and c
    e. b and c

13. If history confirms your suspicions, what steps should be taken to collect evidence?
    a. examination under anesthesia should not be done because risk far outweighs benefit
    b. speculum exam is necessary to collect appropriate data/evidence
    c. colposcopy is recommended in order to facilitate evaluation and documentation with digital imaging
    d. exam must be done immediately upon suspicion in order to minimize loss of evidence
    e. if the last reported incident occurred more than 72 hours prior to visit, no physical exam will be necessary and history alone will be adequate

Answers

1. **e.** Such a child is almost always a victim of child abuse. Child abuse is defined as any maltreatment of children or adolescents by their parents, guardians, or other caretakers. The definition includes physical abuse, sexual abuse, physical neglect, medical neglect, emotional abuse, and emotional neglect.

The physician must be able to distinguish accidental from nonaccidental injury. Clues to nonaccidental injury in this case include the following:

A discrepant history: The explanation given by the parent does not fit the pattern and severity of the medical findings. Thus, the "baby rolling off the sofa" is a totally inadequate explanation for a fractured humerus.
A delay in seeking care: The injury occurred the previous night, but the mother waited until the next day to bring the baby to the ER.

Story inappropriate for developmental level: 2-month-old babies should not be able to coordinate rolling activity. Although all parents still should be counseled against leaving any baby unattended on a table, adult bed, or sofa, the story does not fit the developmental level of the baby.

Although the fracture must be treated, the treatment of the fracture should not be the focus of attention. An orthopedic consultation may be appropriate depending on the severity of the fracture.

It would be inappropriate to suggest the purchase of a walker at the best of times because this is associated with an increased incidence of falls and injuries, and the American Academy of Pediatrics has counseled against their use.

A coagulopathy could explain excessive bleeding with mild trauma; it could not explain the fractures in this child's case.

2. **d.** The most appropriate action at this time is to hospitalize the child. This removes the child to a safe environment and permits time for a complete evaluation. Trusting a family to follow up, especially when abuse is suspected, would be inappropriate.

3. **d.** Any infant with a suspicious injury needs a skeletal survey. This should be done in parts with multiple views instead of one anterior–posterior x-ray view (the so-called "babygram"). Suspicious lesions include multiple fractures, fractures at different stages of healing, spiral fractures, metaphyseal chip fractures (so-called "bucket handle fractures"), and posterior rib fractures. A funduscopic examination is needed to rule out retinal hemorrhages. Children with evidence of "shaken baby syndrome" (i.e., multiple fractures, retinal hemorrhages, and posterior rib fractures) require a head CT scan to rule out subdural hemorrhages. Infants have very large heads in relation to the rest of their bodies and are very susceptible to shearing and impact injuries with shaking.

Physicians are mandated reporters and are required by law to report suspected abuse to the state agency. A complete evaluation of family dynamics and a detailed history of family members (including psychiatric, substance abuse, and domestic violence history) should also be obtained. Although osteogenesis imperfecta is in the differential diagnosis of multiple fractures, it is a rare disorder and is much less likely in this case. Nonetheless, this possibility should be considered and ruled out before any other action is taken.

4. **c.** Physicians are mandated reporters of child abuse. This includes any type of child abuse. The physician is obligated by law to report any suspicion of abuse to child protection authorities. It is not the physician's duty to "prove" the abuse, although the physician must document all history and statements carefully (and sometimes take photographs) because they may be used as evidence. The physician is not liable if the investigation finds the claim of abuse to be false. Reporting is made in good faith and with good intentions whenever there is suspicion. The physician may be liable if there was clear evidence of abuse and the abuse was not reported.

5. b. Child abuse physicians perceive that contact children (others in the home in which child abuse occurs) are at risk of abuse and that medical evaluation for abuse is warranted for these children. However, there is no consensus on the extent of these evaluations.

6. d. The most appropriate next steps at this time are as follows:

1. Treat the child's burn injury: Use analgesics and apply an appropriate sterile dressing. Cold-water immersion is inappropriate and actually may extend the injury and trauma. Because of the extent of the burns and the fact that they cross joint lines (over the toes and ankles), the child should be admitted (preferably to a burn center) for observation, burn care, and possible intravenous fluids.
2. Obtain a more detailed history of the child's present injury and his previous health. This is the classic "stocking" distribution of an immersion burn. The child is held over hot water and the feet are forced into the water. When the child tries to pull up the feet, the buttocks are now the lowest point and are immersed. If the child had indeed been sitting in the bath when the hot water was turned on, the burn would be more diffuse. Regardless, an 8-month-old and a 5-year-old should never be bathing alone together.

Although it seems obvious what actually has happened here, it is important that as complete a history as possible be taken and documented for legal purposes.

7. c. With comprehensive and intensive treatment of the entire family, 80% to 90% of families involved in child abuse or neglect (excluding incest) can be rehabilitated to provide adequate and appropriate care for their children. Approximately 10% to 15% of such families can only be stabilized and will require an indefinite continuation of support services until the children in the family become independent. In only 2% or 3% of cases is termination of parental rights or continued foster care necessary (again, excluding incest).

8. c. Men who abuse their wives are more likely to abuse their children than men who do not abuse their wives. In fact, the abuse of a spouse is an absolute red flag to inquire about child abuse. It is estimated that approximately 25% to 50% of men who abuse their wives also abuse their children.

Women who are currently abused (as spouses or partners) or who have been abused in the past (as children) are also more likely to abuse their children than women who are not abused or who have not been abused (either as a spouse or as a child).

Parents who abuse their children are much more likely than not to have come from nuclear families in which abuse occurred. Most commonly, they were abused as children, although the witnessing of abuse as a child is also a common characteristic.

Thus, abuse is very much a family affair and not only moves from generation to generation at different times but also occurs among different generations at the same time. That is, it may well be that child abuse, spousal abuse, and elder abuse are occurring at the same time in the same family.

9. e. According to the National Committee to Prevent Child Abuse and the National Clearinghouse on Child Abuse Information, in 1997 almost 3.2 million cases of child abuse and neglect were reported to public social service agencies; 33% of these cases were substantiated. Neglect accounts for approximately 52% of the reports, physical abuse for approximately 24% to 26%, sexual abuse for approximately 7% to 13%, emotional maltreatment for approximately 6%, and medical neglect for approximately 3%. Each year in the United States, approximately 1000 children die as a result of fatal physical injuries from beatings or other physical trauma. It is estimated that one in every three or four girls will be sexually assaulted by the age of 18 years, and one of every six to eight boys will be sexually assaulted. It should be remembered that the actual occurrence rates are likely to be higher than these estimates because many maltreated children go unrecognized and many are reluctant to report the abuse, particularly sexual abuse.

10. e. All of the these should raise concerns.

11. e. Sexual abuse does not just include penetration and sexual intercourse. Forcing a child to watch masturbation or copulatory activity, fondling and touching a child's private areas, and using sexually explicit language with or without threats can also be sexual abuse. Internet chat rooms are a more recent area where parents need to make sure that their children are safe. Although some children inadvertently find sexually explicit chat rooms, there are also people targeting children and young adolescents under the supposed safety and anonymity of the Internet.

A few generalities follow:

1. Mothers abuse their children more often than do fathers. Approximately two-thirds of perpetrators are women, who are responsible for approximately 75% of neglect and medical neglect cases. However, men are responsible for approximately 75% of the sexual abuse cases.
2. Girls are abused more often than boys. The overall ratio is approximately 53%:46%. However, girls are subjected to sexual abuse at almost twice the rate as boys. For both sexes, 22% to 23% of the incidents of sexual abuse occur before the age of 8 years.
3. Strangers are seldom the perpetrators of child abuse. Of abusers, 77% are a parent and 11% are a close relative.
4. One parent is usually the active perpetrator, and the other parent passively accepts the abuse.

12. e. The interview should be done without the parents present, if possible, to allow the patient to answer without fear, coercion, or parental supplementation. Finding the correct level of language and the understanding level of the patient can be a challenge. Physicians who plan to interview or evaluate suspected victims should consider special training.

13. c. Timing of the physical examination depends on the last reported incident and whether symptoms are currently present. Because this child has a complaint of vaginal discharge, an exam should be done. If there are no current symptoms or the reported incident was more than 72 hours earlier, an exam can be scheduled and the recommendation is for the exam to be done with health care professionals familiar with forensic examinations. Examination under anesthesia should be considered for acutely assaulted prepubertal girls with persistent vaginal or rectal bleeding or severe abdominal pain. Culture analysis is the standard of care for children. Speculum exam is not recommended for prepubertal girls because an adequate exam can be done with proper technique and positioning.

Summary

Table 105-1 provides recommendations for approaching child abuse.

1. Prevalence

Approximately 3 million cases of abuse are reported each year in the United States; more than 1000 children die every year of injuries incurred from child abuse in the United States.

2. Definition

Child abuse can be defined as any short-term, intermediate-term, or long-term situation in a family in which a child is physically abused, sexually abused, emotionally or psychologically abused, physically neglected, emotionally neglected, or medically neglected by any other member of that family.

3. Characteristics

Child abuse occurs across all races and socioeconomic levels. Most commonly, child abuse is perpetrated by a close relative, usually the parent. Mothers abuse their children more often than fathers, girls are abused more often than boys, and one parent is usually the "active perpetrator" and the other parent is the "passive perpetrator." Strangers are rarely involved in child abuse.

Risk factors for abuse include parents raised in a harsh family environment, increasing home stressors, a decreased ability to cope with frustration or stress in a parent, a parental history of being abused, unplanned or unwanted pregnancy, socially isolated single parents, unemployment, alcohol or drug abuse, depression in a parent, a mentally impaired or physically impaired child, poverty, and unrealistic parental expectations.

4. "Red lights" for child abuse

Suspect child abuse if (a) there is a discrepant history (what is said to have happened does not match the injury pattern); (b) there is a delay in seeking care; (c) there was a recent family crisis; (d) there are unrealistic expectations put on the child by the parents; (e) there is a pattern of increasing severity of so-called accidents; (f) families are living under stressful living conditions, including overcrowding and poverty; (g) there is a real lack of a support system for the family and the family members; (h) aggressive behavior is displayed by the child; (i) you are aware of underlying psychiatric disease in either the father or the mother; or (j) there is either alcohol abuse or drug abuse in the father or the mother.

Table 105-1 | Child Abuse: Key Recommendations for Practice

Clinical Recommendation	Evidence Rating	Comments
Early childhood home visitation programs are recommended to reduce child maltreatment among high-risk families	A	Systematic review showed a 40% reduction in maltreatment episodes
All suspected cases of child abuse should be reported to child protective services	C	Legal mandate
Primary care physicians should incorporate preventive education into their practice and include abuse as part of their differential diagnosis	C	Detection at first presentation reduces morbidity and mortality
A multidisciplinary approach to evaluating, diagnosing, and treating child abuse is recommended	C	Expert opinion
A skeletal survey should be done in all children younger than 3 years with suspicious trauma	C	Based on the American Academy of Pediatrics and the American College of Radiology guidelines
Evaluation of a sexually abused child requires specialized training and experience	C	Expert opinion
There is insufficient evidence to recommend for or against routine screening of parents or guardians for abuse of children	C	U.S. Preventive Services Task Force 2004 guideline

A, consistent, good-quality patient-oriented evidence; B, inconsistent or limited-quality patient-oriented evidence; C, consensus, disease-oriented evidence, usual practice, expert opinion, or case series. Adapted from McDonald KC: Child abuse: Approach and management. *Am Fam Physician* 75:221–228, 2007.

5. Acute treatment

The acute treatment (no matter what type of child abuse is being dealt with) is hospitalization of the child. This allows time to subcategorize the type of child abuse that has occurred (often more than one type); observe the child and the child's behavior in a safe environment; investigate the child from a physical, psychological, and social perspective; obtain all details necessary to clearly understand this episode of abuse and any others that have taken place before this; and interview the parents, grandparents, and other family members.

6. Immediate and long-term treatment

The ultimate goal in a situation in which child abuse has occurred is to eventually return the child to the home. However, first it is necessary to (a) restore the child to a healthy state, (b) identify and understand the reason for the abuse, (c) provide individual and family counseling to the parents and the family, (d) treat coexisting psychiatric conditions in both parents (alcoholism, drug abuse, and depression), and (e) set up an ongoing counseling program for the individuals in the family.

7. Establish a contract with the abusing parents

"I will call if I get to a stage where I think I can no longer handle it." Remember that family violence begets family violence. Where you find one type, you will likely find another type (child abuse, spousal abuse, or elder abuse).

Suggested Reading

American Medical Association: Data on violence between intimates. Available at www.ama-assn.org/ama/pub/category/13577.html#child_maltreatment.

Campbell KA, Bogen DL, Berger RP: The other children: A survey of child abuse physicians on the medical evaluation of children living with a physically abused child. *Arch Pediatr Adolesc Med* 160:1241–1246, 2006.

Lahoti SL, McClain N, Girardet R, et al: Evaluating a child for sexual abuse. *Am Fam Physician* 63:883–892, 2001.

McDonald KC: Child abuse: Approach and management. *Am Fam Physician* 75:221–228, 2007.

Nagler J: Child abuse and neglect. *Curr Opin Pediatr* 14(2):251–254, 2002.

National Clearinghouse on Child Abuse Information. Available at www.nccanchcalib.com.

Santucci KA, Hsiao AL: Advances in clinical forensic medicine. *Curr Opin Pediatr* 15(3):304–308, 2003.

CHAPTER

106 **Common Cold**

CLINICAL CASE PROBLEM 1

A 4-Year-Old Child with a Runny Nose,
Sore Throat, and Nonproductive Cough

A 4-year-old child with a runny nose, congestion, sneezing, and a nonproductive cough comes to your office with his mother. These symptoms started 4 days ago with a sore throat that has since resolved. His appetite is mildly decreased, but he is well otherwise. He has had no fever, chills, or any other symptoms.

On examination, the child's temperature is 37.6°C. His ears are clear, and his throat is slightly hyperemic. He has grayish thick nasal discharge and the nasal mucosa appears swollen with erythematous nasal turbinates. His lung fields are clear, there is no significant cervical lymphadenopathy, and no other localizing signs are present.

The child's history is unremarkable, and he has had no significant medical illnesses. His immunizations are up to date.

SELECT THE BEST ANSWER TO THE FOLLOWING QUESTIONS

1. What is the most likely diagnosis in this child?
   a. allergic rhinitis
   b. nasal foreign body
   c. early streptococcal pharyngitis
   d. pertussis
   e. viral upper respiratory infection (URI)

2. What is the most frequent pathogen associated with this condition?
   a. *Streptococcus pneumoniae*
   b. rhinovirus
   c. parainfluenza A
   d. adenovirus
   e. respiratory syncytial virus (RSV)

3. What investigation should be done at this time?
   a. complete blood count (CBC)
   b. chest x-ray
   c. rapid strep test
   d. nasal smear
   e. nothing at this time

4. Which of the following statements regarding the common cold is true?
   a. adults are affected less than children
   b. the highest incidence of the common cold is among children of kindergarten age
   c. adults with young children at home have an increased number of colds
   d. infants with older siblings in school or day care have an increased incidence of colds
   e. all of the above are true

5. Which of the following statements regarding treatment of the condition described in this case is true?
   a. the use of antibiotics has been shown to decrease the probability of complications; their routine use is reasonable
   b. supportive care with humidified air and nasal saline drops has been shown to be beneficial in symptom relief
   c. dextromethorphan and codeine can be used to suppress cough associated with the condition
   d. zinc lozenges have been shown to be effective therapy in children
   e. antihistamine–decongestant combinations have been shown to be effective in reducing symptoms

6. Preschool children who did not attend a child care are subject to how many colds on an average yearly basis?
   a. 10 to 12
   b. 7 or 8
   c. 3 or 4
   d. 6 to 8
   e. 5 or 6

7. What is the most effective preventive measure against the common cold?
   a. megadoses of vitamin C
   b. meticulous hand washing
   c. extra sleep
   d. avoiding all contact with children and adults who have a cold
   e. pleconaril

CLINICAL CASE PROBLEM 2

A 6-Month-Old with Nasal Congestion
and Difficulty Feeding

A 6-month-old infant is brought to your office by her mother, who states that the child has been having nasal congestion for 5 days. The mother states that the child had a clear runny nose at first but now

575

the drainage is thick and yellow and she seems to be having difficulty with taking the bottle because "she just starts to snort and then spits it out." She also reports the baby has had only low-grade temperatures of less than 100.4°F. The mother tells you that the baby seems cranky but is consolable and has had difficulty sleeping because of the breathing. She is concerned because her 5-year-old child's birthday party is in 2 days and she does not want to get everyone infected. She asks you for an antibiotic.

On examination, the infant is afebrile. There is no tachypnea. The conjunctivae are slightly hyperemic but without purulent exudates. The nose is congested with erythematous mucosa and thick yellow drainage bilaterally. The ears are clear. The throat is pink, but postnasal drip is noted. The chest is without retractions and is clear to auscultation.

8. What is the diagnosis?
 a. bronchiolitis
 b. bacterial rhinosinusitis
 c. viral rhinosinusitis
 d. bacterial conjunctivitis
 e. allergic rhinitis

9. Which of the following agents is the least likely cause of the condition?
 a. RSV
 b. rhinovirus
 c. parainfluenza virus
 d. adenovirus
 e. bordetella pertussis

10. Which of the following statements about the treatment of this condition in infants is true?
 a. aspirin should be avoided
 b. medications other than acetaminophen and ibuprofen should be avoided
 c. nasal saline drops are not helpful
 d. decongestants and antihistamines are helpful
 e. expectorants have been proven to be effective

11. Which of the following is the most common bacterial complication of this condition?
 a. sinusitis
 b. pneumonia
 c. meningitis
 d. otitis media
 e. pharyngitis

12. Which of the following statements is true and is the best answer to the mother's concern?
 a. the infant is no longer infectious so there is no need to worry about spread of infection

 b. evidence does not support the use of antibiotics in URIs, and, in fact, there is an increased risk of adverse effect with their use
 c. viral shedding lasts up to 14 days, so the infant most likely will spread the infection to all those that attend her sibling's party
 d. the color of the baby's nasal discharge suggests a bacterial infection and antibiotics will be prescribed, so there should be no concern for transmission to others
 e. none of the above are true

13. Which of the following statements about complementary and alternative therapies used for the common cold is true?
 a. prophylactic use of echinacea has no impact on the frequency, severity, or duration of URIs
 b. echinacea products that use the root are better than those that use the aerial part in treatment of cold
 c. zinc has been shown to be of benefit in treating viral upper respiratory symptoms in children
 d. vitamin C prophylaxis in high doses significantly reduces symptom severity and duration of cold in the general population

---

Clinical Case Management Problem

An 8-year-old male is brought to your office with "a cold." He has had the cold for approximately 10 days, and his rhinorrhea, cough, and congestion continue. His mother tells you that she has just seen her family doctor for the same symptoms and an antibiotic was prescribed. She asks you to prescribe the same for her son. On examination, the boy has nasal congestion and a hyperemic throat. No other abnormalities are found. Discuss your approach to this patient's request.

Answers

1. e. This child most likely has the common cold or URI. It is a viral infection that typically occurs 2 or 3 day after infection. The first symptom noted is usually a scratchy throat, which resolves by the second or third day and nasal symptoms predominate. All the choices listed are conditions that may mimic a cold. Sneezing and itching are predominant symptoms in allergic rhinitis. Foreign bodies are usually associated with unilateral foul-smelling discharge. Pertussis, associated with paroxysmal or persistent cough, is unlikely because he is vaccinated. The presence of a runny nose and a cough significantly diminishes the probability of streptococcal pharyngitis.

2. **b.** The most common cause of the common cold is a rhinovirus. Rhinoviruses are responsible for approximately 30% to 40% of all cases of the common cold, especially in early fall. Rhinoviruses and corona viruses are agents primarily associated with colds. Other viruses, such as influenza, parainfluenza, RSV, adenovirus, enterovirus, and mumps and measles viruses, are responsible for colds associated with other clinical syndromes. More than 100 serospecific rhinovirus types have been established, and many viruses remain untyped.

The absence of significant fever, cervical lymphadenopathy, and exudates along with the presence of rhinorrhea and cough significantly decrease the probability of *S. pneumoniae* as a cause of this patient's symptoms.

3. **e.** Routine laboratory studies are not helpful or required for diagnosis and management of the common cold. Because the pretest probability of a streptococcal pharyngitis is very low, it is inappropriate to order a rapid antigen test for streptococcus.

4. **e.** In general, the common cold affects children significantly more frequently than adults. The highest incidence is among children of kindergarten age. Adults with young children at home have an increased number of colds, as do infants with older siblings. Often, parents notice the latter (the "second sibling syndrome") and sometimes need reassurance that their children do not have some other constitutional weakness. Children in out-of-home day cares have 50% more colds than those cared for only at home. This difference deceases as the length of time spent in day care increases; however, the incidence of illness is higher in the day care group in the first 3 years of life.

5. **b.** Treatment of the common cold focuses on relief of irritating symptoms of rhinorrhea, nasal congestion, and cough. Cold is a viral illness and antibiotics are not recommended for treatment or prevention of secondary bacterial infection such as otitis media. Use of centrally acting sympathomimetics, such as dextromethorphan and codeine, is not recommended for treating cough due to viral illness in children. They may be of some benefit in adults but may lead to serious adverse effects and dosing errors in children. Antihistamines have not been shown to alleviate these symptoms to a clinically significant degree in children or adults. Even if a slight clinical benefit exists, there are risks and adverse effects; hence, they should be used with caution. Antihistamine–decongestant combinations may be of some benefit in adults and adolescents but have not shown any benefit in young children. Parental education on the use and side effects of these medications is the key to treatment. If parents insist on using medications, then the physician should negotiate discontinuation of medication if symptoms do not improve in 2 days.

Rhinoviruses are temperature sensitive. A controlled study testing warm (30°C) humidified air against hot (45°C) humidified air to provide nasal hyperthermia for 20 to 30 minutes demonstrated a significant reduction in the severity and duration of common cold symptoms at higher temperatures. Thus, it may be that this "old-fashioned" remedy has some basis in fact. Nasal saline drops have also been found to provide relief from congestion. These have the least amount of side effects and are useful in providing some comfort.

The use of zinc lozenges for treating the common cold in children has been demonstrated to be ineffective.

6. **a.** Preschool-age children, 1 to 5 years old, who do not attend a day care are subject to seven or eight colds annually. Infants younger than 1 year average six or seven colds a year. Children in day cares or preschools have a higher incidence because they have greater exposure to the illness. Parents experience approximately four colds and teenagers approximately four or five colds a year.

7. **b.** The most effective preventive measure against the common cold is meticulous hand washing and avoidance of contact with the face or nose. There is increasing evidence that aerosol spread of the cold viruses is less important than indirect spread. Experiments suggest that cold-causing viruses can be spread by self-inoculation from deposits of virus on such surfaces as plastics to the surface of the finger and then transferred to mucous membranes of the nose and eye. This is particularly true if the inoculum is still moist.

Extra sleep and megadoses of vitamin C have not been shown to be at all effective.

It is unrealistic to suggest avoiding all contact with children and adults who have colds. Cold viruses are everywhere and will continue to be everywhere.

Placinoral is a rhinovirus capsid-function inhibitor that exhibits antiviral activity; however, the Food and Drug Administration has not approved the use of the drug based on questions regarding its safety.

8. **c.** The infant has a common cold, in this case causing mostly a rhinosinusitis. In infants, bacterial and viral rhinosinusitis are difficult to distinguish from one another. Bacterial rhinosinusitis is a possible complication of viral rhinosinusitis and should be expected if the patient has symptoms lasting more than 10 days with purulent rhinorrhea, severe illness with fever higher than 39°C, and facial pain.

The patient does not have bacterial conjunctivitis because there is no drainage from the eyes. Bronchiolitis is most often caused by RSV, which is the most common viral pathogen causing lower respiratory tract illness in infants. Tachypnea and respiratory distress including wheezing are common presentations. Other manifestations of RSV in infants can be lethargy, irritability, apneic episodes, and poor feeding.

Allergic rhinitis does not present with fever and usually is associated with pale, edematous, or violaceous turbinates.

9. e. Bordetella pertussis, mycoplasma pneumonia, and group A streptococcus all in catarrhal stage may manifest as upper respiratory infection. All the other choices include the viruses that most frequently cause the common cold.

10. b. Decongestant and antihistamine use in infants has the potential for unusual central nervous system or cardiovascular side effects, such as extreme lethargy or irritability, that far outweigh the small potential benefits. For most URIs, the best treatment is no pharmacologic treatment; however, in those with fever, antipyretics may be used. Aspirin should be avoided because of the risk of Reye's syndrome. Expectorants have not been proven to be effective for cough. Cough suppressants are also contraindicated for infants and, in fact, can cause paradoxical bronchoconstriction in some. Nasal saline drops followed by gentle bulb syringe suction can help to loosen secretions and relieve obstruction temporarily and can be particularly helpful just prior to feeding.

11. d. Otitis media is the most common bacterial complication of the common cold, occurring in

approximately 2% of patients with colds. Sinusitis, pneumonia, and pharyngitis are less common complications. Meningitis is not a typical complication of viral URIs but rarely can be caused by adenovirus in infants or patients who are immunocompromised.

12. b. There is not enough evidence of important benefits of antibiotics for the treatment of URIs. Indeed, studies have shown significant increases in adverse effects with their use.

The infant is likely still infectious. Viral shedding during a URI usually lasts 7 to 14 days and occasionally longer. Even so, most transmission is thought to be by self-inoculation by contaminated hands and some by droplet spread through sneezing; it is unlikely that the infant will spread the infection to all the guests unless parents and sibling neglect to wash their hands and inoculate most household surfaces just before the guests arrive (because viruses can live up to a few hours on plastic surfaces).

The color and thickness of nasal secretions do not help to differentiate between bacterial, viral, or allergic cause.

13. a. Echinacea for prophylaxis of URIs does not significantly decrease the frequency, severity, or duration of URIs. There is great difficulty in interpreting the research on echinacea because of the heterogeneity of the product (i.e., there is no standardization of any particular component). Regardless, it is one of the top three herbs sold in the United States. Vitamin C prophylaxis may modestly reduce the duration and severity of the common cold in the general population and may reduce the incidence of the illness in people exposed to physical and environmental stresses.

Solution to the Clinical Case Management Problem

The prescription of antibiotics for an obvious viral infection (the common cold is probably the best example) is likely the most frequent "mistake" made by family physicians. It is obviously much easier to prescribe an antibiotic for the child than to explain to the parent why one is not needed. Considering that URIs are a frequent presenting complaint to a family physician's office, this "mistake" may actually occur several times a day in an average practice. A reasonable approach to take to this patient's request may be the following:

1. Explain the viral nature of the symptoms and your certainty in coming to that conclusion regarding the patient.
2. Explain the side effects of antibiotics, including drug intolerance, drug allergy, and the possibility of creating an environment in the patient's body that promotes the growth of resistant organisms.
3. Thoroughly discuss some alternatives to antibiotic therapy that the patient may pursue for symptom relief. For children older than age 5 years, these include the use of steam, antihistamines,

decongestants, and cough suppressants. Also suggest increased rest and fluid hydration.

4. Take the opportunity to discuss how meticulous hand washing and related hygienic measures can significantly decrease spread of the common cold among family members.

5. Repeat the following age-old edict to the parent: "The symptoms will abate in a week with antibiotics and in 7 days without." (Having said that, remember that 30% of patients with common cold symptoms who had visited a physician still had a cough and a runny nose by the eighth day.)

6. Do not compromise your principles and prescribe an antibiotic when you know it is, at best, not indicated and possibly harmful. If the parent insists on an antibiotic, consider this an opportunity to discuss your philosophy of care with the patient: Have the parent consider whether he or she is comfortable with the advice you are giving. If not, you should ask the parent if he or she really wishes to continue care in your practice.

This can actually be done in a very pleasant manner. There is rarely a problem in reaching a mutually agreeable position. It comes down to a question of trust between the parent, the patient, and the physician.

Summary

1. As the most common presentation of an URI, the cold is the most common problem presenting to the family physician (Table 106-1).
2. Viral infections are the major, if not the only, cause of common colds.
3. Rhinovirus is the most common pathogen (30% to 40%); influenza, parainfluenza A, B, and C, and RSV comprise another 15%.
4. The differential diagnosis of a cold includes allergic rhinitis, vasomotor rhinitis, intranasal foreign body, and sinusitis.
5. No laboratory investigations are necessary: The combination of rhinorrhea, cough, congestion, sneezing, and a sore throat (or some reasonable combination) in the absence of significant fever, cervical nodes, or an exudate virtually rules out streptococcal pharyngitis.
6. Prevention of spread to family members is best accomplished by meticulous hygiene. Self-inoculation and direct transfer via hand-to-hand contact is more important than aerosol spread.

7. Treatment is symptomatic: steam, nasal saline, and bulb suction. Decongestants and antihistamines, which are commonly used, have no proven benefit.
8. Antibiotics have no role in the treatment of uncomplicated URI.

Table 106-1	Characteristics of Viral Colds in Adults and Young Children	
Characteristic	**Adults**	**Children <6 years**
Frequency	2–4 per year	One per month, September–April
Fever	Rare	Common during first 3 days
Nasal manifestations	Congestion	Colored nasal discharge
Duration of illness	5–7 days	14 days

Modified from Hendley JO: Epidemiology, pathogenesis, and treatment of the common cold. *Semin Pediatr Infect Dis* 9:50–55, 1998.

Suggested Reading

Ebell MH: Antihistamines for the common cold. *Am Fam Physician* 70(3):486, 2004.

Gunn VL, Taha SH, Liebelt EL, Serwint JR: Toxicity of over-the-counter cough and cold medications. *Pediatrics* 108(3):E52, 2001.

Pappas D, Owen-Hendley J: The common cold. In: Long SS, Pickering LK, Probe CG, eds, *Principles and Practice of Pediatric Infectious Diseases*, 2nd ed. Philadelphia: Saunders, 2003.

Pratter MR: Cough and the common cold: ACCP evidence-based clinical practice guidelines. *Chest* 129(1 Suppl):72S–74S, 2006.

Simasek M: Treatment of the common cold. *Am Fam Physician* 75(4):515–520, 2007.

Turner, RB: Viral respiratory infections—Common cold. In: Rakel RE, Bope ET, eds, *Conn's Current Therapy*, 58th ed. Philadelphia: Saunders, 2006.

Turner RB, Hayden GF: The common cold. In: Behrman RE, et al, eds, *Nelson Textbook of Pediatrics*, 17th ed. Philadelphia: Saunders, 2004.

Wong DM: Guidelines for the use of antibiotics in acute upper respiratory tract infections. *Am Fam Physician* 74(6):956–966, 2006.

CLINICAL CASE PROBLEM 1

A 20-Month-Old Child Who Is Febrile, Fussy, and Pulling at His Ear

A mother comes to your office with her 20-month-old son. The child has been breast-fed, and he continues to breast-feed at night, although he is slowly weaning. He usually comes only for well child checks and has rarely been in for upper respiratory infections or other illness. According to the mother, her child (who usually stays at home) went to the church nursery 2 weeks ago and since then has had some rhinorrhea. For the past 24 hours, he has been febrile, to 101°F, and has been fussy but has still been eating and playing.

On examination, the child appears mildly ill but nontoxic. He has nasal congestion and a hyperemic throat. The left tympanic membrane is normal, and the right tympanic membrane is bulging and red, with fluid detected by pneumatic otoscopy. The lungs are clear. The child's temperature is 101°F.

SELECT THE BEST ANSWER TO THE FOLLOWING QUESTIONS

1. What is the most likely diagnosis in this child?
   a. acute otitis media (AOM)
   b. otitis media without effusion
   c. chronic otitis media (COM)
   d. otitis media with effusion (OME)
   e. none of the above

2. The mother has considered echinacea and other "herbal" treatments for her child, but she tells you that she would prefer not to use antibiotics unless absolutely indicated. You tell her that
   a. because of the fever, otalgia, certain diagnosis, and the child's young age, you recommend antibiotic treatment with follow-up in 48 to 72 hours
   b. because of recent literature reviews you have done, and your understanding of her preference to avoid medications, observation is an option provided that she can bring the child for follow-up

   c. serious complications of otitis media, such as hearing loss, perforation of the tympanic membrane, subdural empyema, and brain abscess, only happen in developing countries with malnourished children
   d. avoid all analgesics for the otalgia since they can mask the severity of the infection
   e. because the child is younger than 2 years of age and has high fever, immediate myringotomy is recommended

3. If you chose to prescribe antibiotics for this child, which would be your first choice, assuming the child has no drug allergies?
   a. I would not prescribe antibiotics
   b. cefdinir (Omnicef) 7 mg/kg orally twice daily for 5 to 10 days
   c. amoxicillin 40 to 45 mg/kg orally twice daily for 10 days
   d. ceftriaxone 50 mg/kg intramuscularly (IM) for 3 days
   e. amoxicillin–clavulanate 45 mg/kg orally twice daily for 10 days

4. What are the three most common bacterial organisms in order of frequency that are responsible for the condition described here?
   a. *Streptococcus pneumoniae,* group A streptococci, *Haemophilus influenzae*
   b. *S. pneumoniae, H. influenzae, Staphylococcus aureus*
   c. *S. pneumoniae, H. influenzae, Moraxella catarrhalis*
   d. *H. influenzae, S. pneumoniae,* group A streptococci
   e. *H. influenzae, S. pneumoniae, M. catarrhalis*

5. The mother wants to know if her visit to the church nursery could have contributed to the illness. You explain
   a. her child may have contracted an upper respiratory tract viral infection in the nursery, which led to congestion of the respiratory mucosa of the nose, nasopharynx, and eustachian tube, leading to blockage of the eustachian tube, middle ear secretion accumulation, and growth of organisms
   b. her child is still breast-feeding and is more likely to contract viruses, even outside of the church nursery
   c. ear infections are unpredictable and nearly all children have them; leave the child in the nursery as often as possible
   d. none of the above are true
   e. b and c are true

6. Which of the following statements is (are) true concerning the prevalence of AOM?

a. 60% to 80% of children have at least one episode of AOM by 5 years of age, and 80% to 90% of children have at least one episode by age 8 years

b. 60% to 80% of children have at least one episode of AOM by 1 year of age, and 80% to 90% of children have at least one episode by 2 or 3 years of age

c. the highest incidence of AOM occurs between 6 and 24 months and then decreases with age, except at 5 and 6 years—the time of school entry

d. the highest incidence of AOM occurs between 24 and 48 months and then decreases with age, except at 5 and 6 years—the time of school entry

e. both b and c

CLINICAL CASE PROBLEM 2

A 24-Month-Old Female with an Upper Respiratory Tract Infection But No External Signs of an Acute Ear Infection

A 24-month-old female child presents for her well child check. She has a mild upper respiratory infection, but according to her parents she has been cheerful, eating well, and is afebrile.

On examination, you note a middle ear effusion, confirmed by pneumatic otoscopy, and the tympanic membrane is dull but not red. The rest of the examination is normal except for mild, clear rhinorrhea.

7. What is the most likely diagnosis in this child?
   a. AOM
   b. otitis media without effusion
   c. COM
   d. OME
   e. upper respiratory infection only

8. You recommend/prescribe which of the following treatments for this child?
   a. treatment with amoxicillin and follow-up in 48 to 72 hours
   b. no antibiotics, but follow-up to assess persistence or clearance of the effusion
   c. no treatment, no follow-up
   d. treatment with cefdinir, amoxicillin/clavulanate, or ceftriaxone
   e. referral to an ear, nose, and throat (ENT) surgeon for tympanostomy tubes

9. Which of the following is true with regard to this patient?
   a. steroids should be prescribed because they have been shown to decrease the duration of this condition
   b. in most cases, this condition resolves spontaneously within 3 months
   c. topical or systemic decongestants should be prescribed to improve eustachian tube function
   d. eustachian tube–middle ear inflation should be performed as soon as possible to decrease the likelihood of developing hearing loss and language delay
   e. if present for more than 3 months, bilateral myringotomy with ventilation tube placement is necessary, regardless of hearing

CLINICAL CASE PROBLEM 3

A 2-Year-Old Boy Tugging at His Ear

A 2-year-old boy presents with a 1-day history of tugging at his right ear, rhinorrhea, and a temperature of 37.9°C (100.2°F). He is not lethargic or toxic appearing, but he is irritable. On examination, the tympanic membrane is dull, but not erythematous, and has decreased mobility.

10. Which of the following would you diagnose?
    a. AOM—certain diagnosis
    b. AOM—uncertain diagnosis
    c. COM—certain diagnosis
    d. COM—uncertain diagnosis
    e. OME

11. Which of the following is an acceptable plan of treatment for this patient?
    a. provide acetaminophen for analgesia, and have the parents observe the child carefully for 48 to 72 hours; reevaluate if he does not improve
    b. prescribe amoxicillin 45 mg/kg/day orally twice daily if not penicillin allergic and follow-up in 10 to 14 days if he is improving
    c. give ceftriaxone IM 50 mg/kg in one dose
    d. both a and b are acceptable
    e. all of the above are acceptable

12. What is the most likely diagnosis in a patient with discharge from the ear present for 6 weeks and a history of multiple ear infections treated with antibiotics?
    a. AOM
    b. otitis media without effusion

c. COM with perforation
d. OME
e. otitis externa

13. How is recurrent otitis media defined?
    a. three or more episodes of AOM that occur within 6 months, or four episodes that occur within 1 year
    b. four or more episodes of AOM that occur within 6 months, or five episodes that occur within 1 year
    c. five or more episodes of AOM that occur within 6 months, or six episodes that occur within 1 year
    d. six or more episodes of AOM that occur within 6 months, or eight episodes that occur within 1 year
    e. two or more episodes of AOM that occur within 6 months, or three or more episodes that occur within 1 year

14. Which of the following statements regarding recurrent otitis media is true?
    a. recurrent bouts of AOM usually occur in the winter or early spring
    b. recurrent bouts of AOM should be managed by myringotomy and the insertion of ventilation tubes
    c. medical management appears to be less effective and is not as safe as myringotomy and tubes in children with recurrent AOM
    d. amoxicillin does not have a major role to play in the management of recurrent AOM
    e. antibiotic prophylaxis should be given for at least 6 months to 1 year

15. Which of the following is not considered important to prevent otitis media?
    a. avoid exposure to passive smoking
    b. wean by 6 months of age and switch to bottle-feeding
    c. complete vaccination, especially pneumococcal and influenza
    d. avoid pacifier use beyond 10 months
    e. avoid exposure to large numbers of children as in day care

16. Indications for use of second-line medications in the treatment of AOM include all of the following except
    a. failure to respond to first-line drugs (resistant or persistent AOM)
    b. history of lack of response to first-line drug (failure of medication on at least two occasions in the current respiratory season)

c. hypersensitivity to first-line medications
d. coexisting illness requiring a second-line medication
e. parents insist on the use of a particular medication based on what their friends have recommended

17. All of the following would be considerations for referral to an ENT specialist for placement of tympanostomy tubes except
    a. superimposed asthma and allergies placing the child at greater risk for recurrent otitis media
    b. development of advanced middle ear disease involving tympanic membrane atrophy, retraction pockets, ossicular erosion, or cholesteatoma
    c. bilateral or unilateral OME for more than 3 months with a hearing threshold of 20 dB or worse
    d. recurrent otitis media that fails medical management (prophylaxis failure two times during a 2- to 6-month period)
    e. children with craniofacial abnormalities, cleft palate, Down syndrome, and speech or language delays

18. Tympanocentesis with aspiration of middle ear fluid should be considered in all of the following patients except
    a. a child who presents with AOM and complains of tinnitus, vertigo, and hearing loss
    b. a child who develops a suppurative intracranial complication of OM
    c. an immunologically impaired patient with AOM who does not improve with antibiotic treatment
    d. a child who has extreme ear pain and appears toxic
    e. a child already taking antibiotics who develops an AOM

Clinical Case Management Problem

A father brings in his 15-month-old son who has had frequent visits for mild upper respiratory infections and both AOM and OME. He has had two episodes of AOM and on follow-up exam still has OME at 6 months. The father does not want tympanostomy tubes placed, unless needed, but is concerned that his son is not speaking as well as his older child, who is currently 5 years old, did at that age. He asks for your advice.

Answers

1. **a.** AOM is also known as acute suppurative, acute purulent, or acute bacterial otitis media. The pathophysiology is an effusion of the middle ear that becomes infected with viruses and/or bacteria. There is often a rapid onset of signs and symptoms such as fever; ear pain; a red, bulging, tympanic membrane; and fluid behind the middle ear. This child has a definitive (certain) diagnosis because he presents with fever, otalgia, a red ear, and an effusion.

2. **a.** Since this child is younger than 2 years of age and has a definitive diagnosis of AOM, antibiotics are recommended. If the child had an uncertain diagnosis, and nonsevere illness (fever < 39°C and no severe otalgia), observation would be acceptable. None of the other answers are appropriate. Myringotomy is generally reserved for immunosuppressed children or infants, or those in whom unusual organisms are suspected. Analgesics are recommended, generally acetaminophen. Complications are more common in developing countries but can still occur in developed countries.

3. **c.** The history indicates that the child has never had an episode of otitis media. Based on this information, the American Academy of Pediatrics (AAP) and American Academy of Family Physicians (AAFP) recommend amoxicillin 40 to 45 mg/kg twice daily for first-line treatment. If the child had high fever or toxicity or was unable to take oral medications, the first choice would be amoxicillin/clavulanate and ceftriaxone, respectively. The duration of treatment depends on the patient's age and other patient factors. In children older than 2 years of age without underlying medical conditions, 5 to 7 days of antibiotics is usually sufficient treatment. Younger children and those with craniofacial abnormalities, chronic or recurrent otitis media, or perforation of the tympanic membrane should be treated for 10 days. A patient who does not improve while taking amoxicillin most likely has an infection with a β-lactamase-producing organism. In this case, second-line agents including cefuroxime axetil, amoxicillin–clavulanate, and intramuscular ceftriaxone would be appropriate choices if the child did not improve.

4. **c.** The bacteriology of AOM suggests that the following bacterial organisms (in order of incidence) are responsible for most cases of AOM: (1) *S. pneumoniae*, (2) *H. influenzae*, (3) *M. catarrhalis*, (4) group A streptococci, and (5) *S. aureus* and anaerobic bacteria. The microbiology of AOM before the introduction of the heptavalent pneumococcal conjugate vaccine has been documented. The main causes are the same, but the number of cases of *S. pneumoniae* are decreasing. In contrast, since the *H. influenzae* isolates are predominately nontypable, the conjugate Hib vaccine has had little impact on *Haemophilus* AOM. Viral infections are frequently associated with AOM—most commonly respiratory syncytial virus, rhinoviruses, influenza, and adenoviruses.

5. **a.** The pathogenesis of otitis media follows a similar sequence of events in most children: An antecedent event results in congestion of the respiratory mucosa, which congests the mucosa in the eustachian tube and obstructs the narrowest portion of the tube, the isthmus. This obstruction causes negative pressure, accumulation of secretions in the middle ear, and accumulation of these secretions that serve as a nidus of infection. Breast-feeding decreases the risk of otitis media, and exposure to children in day care or, in this case, a church nursery setting increases the risk.

6. **e.** Between 60% and 80% of infants have at least one episode of AOM by 1 year of age, and 80% to 90% of children have at least one episode by 2 or 3 years. The highest incidence occurs between 6 and 24 months, and then the incidence declines with the exception of the time for school entry at 5 and 6 years. The peak age-specific attack rate occurs between 6 and 18 months of age. Day care and tobacco smoke increase risk, as does Native American ethnicity, whereas breast-feeding decreases the risk.

7. **d.** OME (serous otitis media, glue ear) is defined as the presence of a middle ear effusion in the absence of acute signs of infection. Specifically, in a child without fever, otalgia, or systemic symptoms and the presence of an effusion diagnosed by pneumatic otoscopy, tympanometry, or reflectometry, OME is diagnosed. OME may be classified as acute, subacute, and chronic based on the duration of the effusion. OME with effusions present for less than 3 weeks are acute, subacute effusions are present for 3 weeks to 3 months, and chronic effusions are those present for longer than 3 months. Treatment is generally based on the duration of the effusion and associated symptoms or risk factors.

8. **b.** OME, as in this child, is often found on a routine exam on an asymptomatic child with a mild upper respiratory infection. In this child, the length of time the effusion has been present is unknown.

If there are risk factors for learning problems or any signs of language delay, or if the child has a history of a hearing threshold of worse than 20 dB, as well as in cases in which the effusion persists for more than 3 months, a referral is warranted. Since most effusions resolve spontaneously, this child should be followed until resolution of her effusion, provided she has no signs of hearing difficulty. If it persists beyond 3 months, she should be evaluated for hearing. Antibiotics are not routinely recommended, although some physicians will give a course of antibiotics in the case of a persistent effusion despite the fact that this has not shown any long-term benefit.

9. b. OME is a middle ear effusion without signs or symptoms of acute infection. The effusion clears spontaneously by 3 months in 90% of children. Neither oral or nasal steroids nor decongestants have proved to be effective for this condition. Using the method of Politzer or the Valsalva maneuver to open the eustachian tubes has not been shown to be effective in the treatment of OME. Even if the effusion is present for more than 3 months, myringotomy and ventilation tubes are not indicated unless there is hearing loss or other findings suggesting delayed learning.

10. b. This patient has an uncertain diagnosis of AOM.

11. d. There is evidence of effusion and acute symptoms, but no evidence of inflammation. The illness is not severe because the child has only a low-grade fever and no otalgia. Observation for 48 to 72 hours or treatment with amoxicillin are acceptable plans of action.

12. c. COM is synonymous with chronic suppurative, purulent, or intractable otitis media. There is a pronounced, intractable middle ear pathologic condition with or without suppurative otorrhea. Suppurative refers to an active infection, and otorrhea refers to a discharge through a perforated tympanic membrane.

13. a. Recurrent otitis media is defined as three or more episodes of AOM that occur within 6 months or four episodes within 1 year.

14. a. Recurrent bouts of acute otitis usually occur in the winter or early spring. Such recurrent episodes can be managed to some extent with prophylactic antibiotics. Prophylaxis should not be given for more than

6 months to decrease the likelihood of colonization by resistant bacteria. Although a myringotomy and the insertion of ventilation tubes ultimately may have to be performed, it is not the first-line option. Medical management with antibiotics has been shown, in most studies, to be just as effective. Half-strength amoxicillin or sulfisoxazole is reasonable prophylactic therapy.

15. b. Breast-feeding should be encouraged because it decreases the incidence of otitis media. For those children who bottle-feed, they should be fed sitting up. Breast-feeding for at least 6 months should be strongly encouraged.

16. e. All of the answers are appropriate reasons to use second-line antibiotics for treatment (i.e., not amoxicillin). In addition, culture-proven resistance from a tympanocentesis is another indication. Certainly, parents often will know which medication their child responds to, but some may have erroneous information and their choice of antibiotics should not be the only determining factor.

17. a. Other indications for referral include refractory OM with moderate to severe symptoms after two different antibiotics; medical treatment failure due to multiple drug allergy or intolerance; at least two recurrences of otitis media within 2 or 3 months following ventilating tube extrusion with failed medical management; a history of 6 or more months of effusions out of the previous 12 months; and impending or actual complications of AOM, such as mastoiditis, lateral sinus thrombosis, meningitis, and brain abscess.

18. a. The diagnosis of AOM is made clinically based on symptoms and the appearance of the tympanic membrane; however, in certain circumstances, tympanocentesis with aspiration of the middle ear fluid may be considered to aid in diagnosis (by culture) but also in alleviating severe pain. Patients who appear toxic or who develop either suppurative intratemporal or intracranial complications should have tympanocentesis. A newborn or otherwise immunologically deficient patient who does not improve with empiric therapy may warrant tympanocentesis because unusual organisms may be involved. Similarly, a child who is taking antibiotics and develops a new AOM may also be considered for tympanocentesis to culture for resistant organisms.

Complaints of tinnitus, hearing loss, and vertigo are not uncommon, especially in older children, and do not implicate a need for tympanocentesis.

Solution to the Clinical Case Management Problem

As discussed previously, the decision for ENT referral for tympanostomy tubes is based on many factors. According to the Agency for Healthcare Research and Quality, AAP, and AAFP recommendations, since this child has had an effusion for 3 months and has evidence of possible hearing problems, you should immediately perform a hearing evaluation. If he does, in fact, have a hearing threshold worse than 20 dB, he should be referred for tympanostomy tubes. If, however, his hearing is adequate, you can consider prophylaxis with amoxicillin 20 mg/kg/day for 2 to 6 months and close follow-up. If he continues to have infections, has a persistent effusion for 12 months, or develops hearing loss, he should be referred. You should also explore other factors, such as exposure to passive smoking, day care, or other preventive actions the family can take.

Summary

AOM is the most frequent diagnosis in sick children visiting physicians' offices. By 1 year, 60% to 80% of infants will have at least one episode, and by 2 or 3 years 80% to 90% will have had an episode.

The diagnosis of otitis media requires evidence of the following:

1. Recent, usually abrupt, onset of signs and symptoms of middle ear inflammation and effusion; and
2. The presence of middle ear effusion indicated by any of the following: limited or absent mobility of the tympanic membrane, bulging of the tympanic membrane, air fluid level behind the tympanic membrane, or otorrhea; and
3. Signs or symptoms of middle ear inflammation as indicated by either distinct otalgia (pain clearly referable to the ear that affects normal activity or sleep) or distinct erythema of the tympanic membrane.

New evidenced-based guidelines from the AAP and AAFP differentiate AOM by certain and uncertain diagnosis based on the signs of inflammation. Decisions to treat with antibiotics are based on age, severity and certainty of diagnosis, as well as reliability of follow-up. Severity of diagnosis is defined by temperature of 39°C (102.2°F) or moderate to severe otalgia. Pneumatic otoscopy is recommended, occasionally with tympanometry or reflectometry, to verify the presence of a middle ear effusion. For pneumococcal-resistant or β-lactamase-producing strains of bacteria, first-line treatment is high-dose amoxicillin (90 mg/kg/day). An excellent encounter form is available at www.aafp.org/fpm/20040600/52acut.html, which incorporates the major points of the recommendations with antibiotics and their dosages.

The most common bacterial causative agents in order of frequency are *Pneumococci* (25% to 50%), *H. influenzae* (15% to 30%), and *M. catarrhalis* (3% to 20%). Risk factors for OM include bottle-feeding, exposure to day care, exposure to passive smoking, craniofacial abnormalities, and Native American ethnicity.

For AOM, otitis media with effusion, physicians should refer if children have risk factors, persistent effusions for more than 3 months, or a hearing threshold worse than 20 dB. Most effusions will clear in 3 months. Antibiotic prophylaxis, most commonly amoxicillin 20 mg/kg/day, may be used in cases of recurrent OM of more than three episodes in 6 months or four episodes in 12 months. Although severe complications of OM are not common, they may be life threatening and include mastoiditis, lateral sinus thrombosis, meningitis, brain abscess, otic hydrocephalus, and facial paralysis as well as hearing loss.

Suggested Reading

American Academy of Family Physicians, American Academy of Otolaryngology–Head and Neck Surgery, and American Academy of Pediatrics Subcommittee on Otitis Media with Effusion: Clinical practice guidelines: Otitis media with effusion. *Pediatrics* 113:1412–1429, 2004.

American Academy of Pediatrics Subcommittee on Management of Acute Otitis Media: Clinical practice guideline: Diagnosis and management of acute otitis media. *Pediatrics* 113(5):1451–1465, 2004.

Ebell M: Acute otitis media in children: Point of care guidelines. *Am Fam Physician* 69(12):2896–2898, 2004.

Glaszious PP, DelMar CB, Sanders SL, Hayem M: Antibiotics for acute otitis media in children. *Cochrane Database Syst Rev* (3): 2002.

Hendley JO: Otitis media. *N Engl J Med* 347:1169–1174, 2002.

CLINICAL CASE PROBLEM 1

An 18-Month-Old Infant with an Upper Respiratory Tract Infection

An 18-month-old is brought to the emergency department by his mother. He developed an upper respiratory tract infection 2 days ago and suddenly this evening developed a harsh, barky cough and difficulty breathing.

On examination, the child is coughing and his temperature is 38.5°C. His respiratory rate is 40 breaths/minute, and he is in some respiratory distress. The breath sounds that are heard appear to be transmitted from the upper airway. There are nasal flaring and suprasternal, infrasternal, and intercostal retractions.

SELECT THE BEST ANSWER TO THE FOLLOWING QUESTIONS

1. What is the most likely diagnosis in this child?
   a. viral pneumonia
   b. acute epiglottitis
   c. bronchiolitis
   d. croup
   e. bacterial pneumonia

2. The causative agent responsible for this child's condition is most likely which of the following?
   a. adenovirus
   b. pneumococcus
   c. parainfluenza virus
   d. *Haemophilus influenzae*
   e. respiratory syncytial virus (RSV)

3. What is the treatment of choice for moderate cases of the disorder described?
   a. racemic epinephrine
   b. aerosolized budesonide
   c. humidification
   d. dexamethasone intravenously
   e. a, b, and c

4. The presence of which symptoms would increase the likelihood of admission and intubation?
   a. stridor
   b. cyanosis
   c. tachycardia
   d. sternal retractions
   e. all of the above

5. Differentiating between viral croup and spasmodic croup can be challenging. The major differentiator is
   a. spasmodic croup is less likely to have fever
   b. viral croup is not associated with asthma
   c. spasmodic croup does not have a family history component
   d. spasmodic croup lasts much longer than viral croup
   e. viral croup is seen in much younger patients

CLINICAL CASE PROBLEM 2

A 5-Year-Old Child Who Has Been Talking Strangely and Is Anorexic

A 5-year-old child is brought to the emergency department by his mother. The mother tells you that for the past 24 hours the child has been "talking strangely" and drooling. He has had no appetite and has not been drinking.

6. Based on this history, what is the diagnosis of major concern?
   a. viral pneumonia
   b. acute epiglottitis
   c. bronchiolitis
   d. croup
   e. bacterial pneumonia

7. Since the onset of widespread vaccination with *H. influenza* type b, *H. influenzae* as a cause of epiglottitis has
   a. disappeared
   b. been replaced by *Streptococcus pneumonia* and varicella-zoster
   c. continued to be a causative organism but reduced in frequency by a factor of 1000%
   d. not changed
   e. been diagnosed only in immunocompromised patients

8. What is the diagnostic procedure that can substantiate the diagnosis you made in response to question 7 for the patient described here?
   a. white blood cell count
   b. erythrocyte sedimentation rate
   c. chest x-ray
   d. lateral x-ray of the neck
   e. computed tomography scan of the head and neck

9. What is the treatment of choice for this patient?
a. intubation and full respiratory support
b. oral ampicillin and careful observation
c. intravenous (IV) ceftriaxone
d. supplemental oxygen by mask
e. a and c

Answers

1. d. A child with croup (the most common form being acute laryngotracheobronchitis) usually has a typical upper respiratory tract infection for several days before the brassy, barking cough, inspiratory stridor, and respiratory distress become apparent. As the infection extends downward involving the bronchi and the bronchioles, respiratory difficulty increases and the expiratory phase of respiration becomes labored and prolonged.

The child often appears restless, agitated, and frightened. The child's temperature may be only slightly elevated, or it may be as high as 39°C to 40°C (102°F to 104°F).

Croup can be characterized based on the severity of symptoms. In mild croup, stridor is present with excitement only or is present at rest without signs of respiratory distress. In moderate croup, stridor occurs at rest and there is intercostal, suprasternal, or subcostal retractions. In severe croup, there is severe respiratory distress, decreased air entry, and an altered level of consciousness. Children with severe croup should be hospitalized and intubated under controlled conditions.

2. c. Most cases of croup (the most common form being acute laryngotracheobronchitis) are caused by the parainfluenza group of viruses. RSV, influenza, and adenoviruses may be implicated in some cases.

3. e. Until recently, the treatment of choice for mild to moderate cases of croup was simple humidification. However, it has been clearly established that nebulized budesonide (an inhaled glucosteroid) or oral (not IV) dexamethasone are of significant benefit in young children with mild to moderate croup. In moderate or severe cases, nebulized racemic epinephrine has been proven to be of value.

4. e. Hospitalization is indicated in children with increasing or persistent respiratory distress, fatigue, cyanosis, or dehydration.

5. a. Spasmodic croup is less likely to have fever. However, it is viral, not spasmodic, croup that is associated with development of asthma later. Spasmodic croup is more likely to have a component of family history and it lasts hours rather than the 2 to 4 days for viral croup. The age range is approximately the same for both.

6. b. This child must be suspected of having acute epiglottitis until proved otherwise. Acute epiglottitis, a potentially lethal condition, occurs in children ages 2 to 7 years and peaks at the age of 3.5 years. The incidence of this disease has decreased 10-fold due to routine immunization against *H. influenzae*. Acute epiglottitis is characterized by a fulminating course of fever, sore throat, dyspnea, rapidly progressive respiratory obstruction, and prostration. In minutes or hours, epiglottitis can lead to complete obstruction of the airway and death unless adequate treatment is administered.

Respiratory distress is the first symptom. The child may be well at bed time but awaken later in the evening with a high fever, aphonia, drooling, and moderate to severe respiratory distress with stridor. An older child or adult will often complain of a "sore throat." Severe respiratory distress may ensue within minutes or hours of the onset.

7. c. Although *H. influenza* type B was once the most common cause of epiglottitis, it continues to be a significant agent. Other organisms, such as *S. pneumonia*, *Haemophilus parainfluenzae*, varicella-zoster, and *Staphylococcus aureus*, are also causes.

8. d. On physical examination, the child is noted to have moderate to severe respiratory distress with inspiratory and, at times, expiratory stridor. There is drooling and an abundance of mucus and saliva, which also may result in rhonchi. With progression, stridor and breath sounds may become diminished as the patient tires. If this diagnosis is suspected, necessary equipment should be obtained and someone qualified to intubate the child should be summoned immediately; both the equipment and the person should accompany the patient for any diagnostic studies. The diagnosis can be made by a lateral x-ray of the neck, which will clearly show the swollen epiglottis (thumb sign).

9. e. The child's pharynx should not be examined with a tongue depressor. The diagnosis requires direct visualization by laryngoscopy with the ability to intubate immediately. The treatment of choice for a child with acute epiglottis is as follows:

1. An artificial airway must be established immediately. Untreated patients have substantial mortality even when observed in the hospital with appropriate intubation equipment nearby. Oxygen is administered.
2. IV ceftriaxone or ampicillin and chloramphenicol should be given pending culture and susceptibility reports because the condition can be caused by multiple agents.

Summary

DIFFERENTIATING BETWEEN EPIGLOTTITIS AND CROUP (Table 108-1)

Croup: The most common form is acute laryngotracheobronchitis. A harsh, barky cough in a young infant is almost pathognomonic of croup. Respiratory distress can be pronounced.

1. Causative agent: parainfluenza virus
2. Treatment: humidified oxygen, plus oral or nebulized corticosteroids; racemic epinephrine in moderate to severe cases

Acute epiglottitis: Symptoms include drooling, very sore throat, and difficulty swallowing liquids (this can be used as a diagnostic test).

1. Do not attempt visualization of the epiglottis unless prepared to intubate

2. Lateral x-ray of the neck for diagnosis (thumb sign swollen epiglottis)
3. Causative agent was *H. influenzae* (before immunization); now strep and others
4. Treatment: intubation, respiratory support, and IV ceftriaxone

Table 108-1	Characteristics of Epiglottitis and Croup	
Epiglottitis	**Croup**
Sudden onset	Gradual onset
High fever	Low-grade fever
Dysphagia present	Mild or no dysphagia
No cough	Barking, "croupy" cough
Posturing to facilitate air exchange	No particular posturing

Suggested Reading

Ewig JM: Croup. *Pediatr Ann* 31(2):125–130, 2002.
Knutson D, Aring A: Viral croup. *Am Fam Physician* 69:535–542, 2004.
Moore M, Little P: Humidified air inhalation for treating croup. *Cochrane Database Syst Rev* (3):CD002870, 2006.
Russell K, Wiebe N, Saenz A, et al: Glucocorticoids for croup. *Cochrane Database Syst Rev* (4):CD001955, 2003.

Stroud RH, Friedman NR: An update on inflammatory disorders of the pediatric airway: Epiglottitis, croup, and tracheitis. *Am J Otolaryngol* 22(4):268–275, 2001.
Wright RB, Pomerantz WJ, Luria JW: New approaches to respiratory infections in children. Bronchiolitis and croup. *Emerg Med Clin North Am* 20(1):93–114, 2002.

CHAPTER

109   Bronchiolitis and Pneumonia

CLINICAL CASE PROBLEM 1

A 4-Month-Old with Cough, Fever, and Wheezing

A 4-month-old infant presents to the emergency department with cough and fever. The infant has been sick for 3 days but worsened in severity during the past 24 hours. Past medical history is otherwise negative. He was born preterm at 35 weeks but was discharged home after 3 days. Birth weight was 7 pounds and maternal group B strep was negative. Immunizations are current.

Vital signs include a rectal temperature of 100.8°F, pulse of 120 beats/minute, blood pressure within normal limits, and a respiratory rate of 60 breaths/minute. The infant is well hydrated but ill appearing. Grunting, nasal flaring,

intracostal retractions, and increased respiratory effort are evident. Wheezing and crackles are noted on physical exam. Chest radiographs show patchy atelectasis and hyperinflation of the lungs.

SELECT THE BEST ANSWER TO THE FOLLOWING QUESTIONS

1. Which statement regarding management of this condition is true?
   a. bronchodilators provide a consistent benefit for this illness
   b. corticosteroids are routinely indicated for initial management
   c. ribavirin should not be used routinely in this condition
   d. intravenous fluids are required for infants younger than 1 year of age
   e. chest physiotherapy provides proven benefit for this condition

2. The most common cause of bronchiolitis is
   a. human metapneumovirus

b. adenovirus

c. parainfluenza

d. respiratory syncytial virus (RSV)

e. influenza

3. Which of the following statements about RSV is untrue?

a. diagnosis is most often made by clinical exam

b. infection with RSV confers life-long immunity in healthy individuals

c. 90% of children are infected with RSV within the first 2 years of life

d. the highest incidence of infection occurs between December and March

e. mortality from RSV has decreased during the past two decades

4. All of the following are associated with increased risk of severe bronchiolitis except

a. premature birth (gestational age <37 weeks)

b. bronchopulmonary dysplasia

c. cystic fibrosis

d. immunocompromised status

e. hemodynamically insignificant atrial septal defect

5. Pathologic features of acute bronchiolitis include all but

a. necrosis of respiratory epithelial cells

b. lymphocytic infiltration of the peribronchial tree

c. increased mucous clearance

d. destruction of epithelial ciliated cells

e. mucous plugging with small airway obstruction

6. In which of the following patients is palivizumab not indicated?

a. 3-month-old male born at 39 weeks of gestation with tetralogy of Fallot

b. 2-month-old female born at 28 weeks of gestation

c. 1-month-old female born at 33 weeks of gestation with no current health issues

d. 2-month-old male born at 34 weeks of gestation who is in day care and has school-aged siblings

e. 2-month-old male born at 30 weeks of gestation with bronchopulmonary dysplasia requiring oxygen therapy

7. Which of the following statements regarding antibiotic use in bronchiolitis is true?

a. use of antibiotics is recommended in all infants younger than 3 months of age

b. antibiotics likely benefit infants with severe bronchiolitis who require mechanical ventilation

c. there is an elevated risk of bacteremia in febrile children with bronchiolitis

d. numerous randomized controlled trials (RCTs) support the use of antibiotics for bronchiolitis

e. antibiotics significantly improve the clinical course of bronchiolitis

CLINICAL CASE PROBLEM 2

A 3-Year-Old with Fever, Cough, and Wheezing

A 3-year-old child is brought to the office for cough and fever. He has been sick for the past 4 days, but symptoms acutely worsened this morning. Appetite and activity levels are both decreased. Past medical history is unremarkable and immunizations are current. He lives at home with two brothers and goes to day care during the week. There are no sick contacts.

On physical examination, he has a temperature of 38.5°C, pulse of 120 beats/minute, respiratory rate of 60 breaths/minute, and normal blood pressure. He appears mildly toxic but not cyanotic. Ears, nose, and throat are unremarkable. Retractions, grunting, and accessory muscle use are noted on the lung exam. Localized rales and wheezing are noted over the right lower lung zones.

8. Which of the following interventions provides the most useful information at this time?

a. chest radiograph

b. pulse oximetry

c. complete blood count with differential

d. rapid antigen tests for influenza A and B

e. C-reactive protein level

9. Which of the following statements about childhood pneumonia is true?

a. pneumonia accounts for approximately 5% of childhood deaths worldwide

b. 1.9 million children worldwide die annually from acute respiratory tract infections

c. the majority of deaths from childhood community-acquired pneumonia (CAP) occur in Central and South America

d. human immunodeficiency virus (HIV) has a minor influence on the incidence and severity of childhood pneumonia

e. conjugated pneumococcal vaccines are ineffective in children younger than 5 years of age

10. Which of the following statements about CAP in neonates is false?
    a. group B streptococcus and gram-negative enteric bacteria are the most common pathogens
    b. infection occurs via vertical transmission
    c. nontoxic neonates may be managed as outpatients with close follow-up
    d. intravenous ampicillin plus gentamicin is recommended antibiotic therapy
    e. blood, urine, and cerebrospinal fluid should be obtained prior to beginning antibiotic therapy

11. What is the most common bacterial cause of CAP after the neonatal period?
    a. *Streptococcus pneumoniae*
    b. *Haemophilus influenzae* type B
    c. *Staphylococcus aureus*
    d. *Moraxella catarrhalis*
    e. *Mycoplasma pneumonia*

12. Which of the following signs is suggestive of hypoxemia?
    a. inability to feed
    b. altered mental status
    c. cyanosis
    d. head nodding
    e. all of the above

13. Which of the following statements is true regarding CAP in infants older than 4 months and preschool-aged children?
    a. bacterial infections are the most common cause of CAP in this age group
    b. bacterial infections most frequently occur during the winter
    c. fever, arthralgia, and cough in a school-aged child suggest pneumococcal pneumonia
    d. viral pneumonia is most frequent in the spring
    e. withholding antibiotic treatment is appropriate if a virus is suspected and close follow-up is possible

14. Which of the following statements about antibiotic therapy in CAP is true?
    a. antibiotic therapy should be continued for a total of 5 days
    b. follow-up of patients treated as outpatients is required within 1 week
    c. a transition to oral antibiotics is appropriate after 48 hours of intravenous antibiotics
    d. the choice of antibiotics for children with CAP is generally made on an empiric basis
    e. a patient with a negative antibody assay for pneumococcus is not at risk for strep infection and should be treated solely with macrolides

Answers

1. **c.** Inhaled ribavirin is an antiviral medication used to treat bronchiolitis. Some studies document improvement in the respiratory score and decreased hospital length of stay with ribavirin. Indications for its use are controversial. It may be considered for treatment of patients predisposed to developing severe RSV-related morbidity because of underlying health problems.

Bronchodilator use is also controversial. Current recommendations do not support routine bronchodilator use in the treatment of bronchiolitis. A Cochrane review examined eight RCTs on inhaled bronchodilator therapy in bronchiolitis ($N = 394$). One in four children who were treated with bronchodilators showed transient improvement, although it was of unclear significance. Both albuterol/salbutamol and epinephrine are available options. Although a recent Cochrane review found insufficient evidence to support epinephrine use, it was believed to be favorable to salbutamol. Little supporting evidence exists from RCTs, but clinical practice suggests that a nebulized bronchodilator trial is appropriate in select infants. When good clinical response is noted, therapy is continued.

Corticosteroid treatment is also not routinely recommended, although almost 60% of admitted infants receive these medications. A Cochrane review of glucocorticoid use in acute bronchiolitis did not show a benefit.

Infants with mild disease may not require intravenous fluids. If feeding is not compromised and the respiratory rate is below 60 to 70 breaths/minute, a trial of oral feeds is appropriate. Infants with cough, retractions, or nasal flaring may be at increased risk for aspiration. Intravenous fluids are appropriate in this subset of patients until respiratory status improves.

Chest physiotherapy is not routinely recommended in the treatment of bronchiolitis. A Cochrane review of three RCTs did not show benefit for either vibration or percussion physiotherapy, although nasal suctioning provides some temporary benefits.

2. **d.** Respiratory syncytial virus is the most common agent in bronchiolitis. Other viruses that cause bronchiolitis are adenoviruses, influenza, parainfluenza, and human metapneumovirus. Less common agents include *M. pneumonia*, which occurs sporadically.

3. **b.** Infection with RSV does not confer immunity, and reinfection with RSV is common. Ninety percent of children are exposed to RSV by 2 years of age. The diagnosis is made clinically. Late winter and early spring are the most common seasons for RSV

infection. Mortality from RSV in the United States decreased from 4500 annual deaths in 1985 to 390 deaths in 1999.

4. **e.** Several factors are associated with an increased severity of RSV infection. Delivery at less than 37 weeks of gestational age and age younger than 12 weeks are both associated with more severe infections. Young infants may develop apnea and require more intensive surveillance than older children. Immunocompromised status, chronic lung disease, and hemodynamically significant congenital heart disease are also associated with higher risk of disease progression and mortality.

5. **c.** Pathologic changes in acute bronchiolitis include necrosis of the respiratory epithelium, destruction of respiratory ciliated cells, and peribronchial lymphocytic infiltration. This leads to increased mucous production, bronchial wall edema, and impaired clearance of small airways. Mucous clearance is impaired rather than increased in bronchiolitis.

6. **c.** Certain infants and children should be offered prophylactic vaccination with palivizumab. Injections (15 mg/kg/dose) are given monthly beginning in November or December. Infants younger than 24 months of age and children with chronic lung disease requiring treatment with supplemental oxygen, bronchodilators, diuretics, or corticosteroids should receive prophylaxis. The presence of hemodynamically significant congenital heart disease, serious pulmonary disease, or immune dysfunction also mandates immunization. Premature infants without underlying heart or lung disease may require immunization depending on the gestational age at birth. Table 109-1 details recommendations for palivizumab administration based on gestational age/prematurity. Infants younger than 28 weeks of gestation who will be less than 12 months of age at the beginning of RSV season should be immunized. Infants 32 to 35 weeks of gestational age need to be immunized if they have additional risk factors (Table 109-2).

7. **b.** Few RCTs examine antibiotic use in bronchiolitis. No studies demonstrate improvement in symptoms, fever, radiographic findings, or clinical course in bronchiolitis patients who receive antibiotics. The risk of bacteremia in febrile children with bronchiolitis is quite low (0.2%). Current recommendations do not support routine antibiotic use, although more research is needed. Severely ill children who require mechanical ventilation or intensive care unit admission are at higher risk for bacterial coinfection and may benefit from antibiotic therapy.

Table 109-1	Indications for Respiratory Syncytial Virus(RSV) Prophylaxis	
Patient Group	**Patient Age at Beginning of RSV Season**
Chronic lung disease/ bronchopulmonary dysplasia requiring any of the following therapies within 6 mo of RSV season	≤2 yr
Supplemental oxygen	
Diuretics	
Corticosteroids	
Bronchodilators	
Hemodynamically significant congenital cardiac disease	≤2 yr
Immune compromise (except prematurity)	≤2 yr
Prematurity without chronic heart or lung issues	
≤28 weeks' gestational age	≤12 mo
28– 32 weeks' gestational age	≤6 mo
32–35 weeks' gestational age	≤6 mo with two additional risk factors

Table 109-2	Respiratory Synctial Virus Risk Factors
School-age siblings
Day care attendance
Environmental pollution exposure
Severe neuromuscular disease
Family history of asthma
Multiple gestation delivery (i.e., twins and triplets)
Low birth weight (<2500 g)
Congenital lung abnormalities
Crowded living conditions

8. **b.** The presentation is consistent with CAP. In most cases, isolation of the infectious agent is not critical and treatment proceeds empirically. Oxygen saturation with pulse oximetry provides important data regarding hypoxia. Complete blood count, C-reactive protein, and erythrocyte sedimentation rate do not distinguish viral from bacterial infections and are not routinely indicated. Testing for influenza A and B is appropriate in certain scenarios, but it is less useful than pulse oximetry. Chest radiographs do not distinguish between bacterial and viral CAP as definitively as once believed. Lobar consolidation and interstitial infiltrates are identified in viral, bacterial, and combination infections, limiting the generalizability of findings. Radiographs are indicated when CAP is unresponsive to therapy or of prolonged course, the clinical picture is uncertain, or abscess/pleural effusion is suspected.

9. b. Pneumonia accounts for a large percentage of pediatric disease worldwide. It is responsible for approximately 20% of childhood deaths, mostly in underdeveloped countries. Half of the 1.9 million annual deaths from childhood respiratory infections occur in Africa. CAP in African children accounts for 30% to 40% of hospital admissions and 15% to 28% of deaths in children. The HIV epidemic has greatly worsened the incidence, severity, and outcomes for childhood CAP in developing nations.

A conjugate, heptavalent pneumoccocal vaccine is available in the United States. The vaccine provides immunity against the seven most common serotypes of *S. pneumoniae* in children. The vaccine is immunogenic, safe, and effective in children immunized as early as 6 weeks of age. Initial outcomes demonstrate a decrease in the incidence of invasive disease and a decrease in pneumococcal pneumonia, especially in children younger than 2 years of age. The polysaccharide pneumococcal vaccine is used in adults but is ineffective in children younger than 5 years of age.

10. c. Group B streptococcus and gram-negative enteric bacteria (*Escherichia coli*) are the most common pathogens encountered in neonates from birth to 20 days of age. Other common causes include *Listeria monocytogenes*, with group D streptococci, *H. influenzae*, and *Ureaplasma urealyticum* seen less commonly. Transmission is usually vertical. Infants younger than 3 weeks with respiratory findings should be admitted to the hospital and cultures of blood, urine, and cerebrospinal fluid obtained. Antibiotic selection is generally intravenous or intramuscular ampicillin and gentamicin with or without cefotaxime.

11. a. *Streptococcus pneumoniae* is the most common bacterial etiology of CAP past the neonatal period. *Hemophilus*, *S. aureus*, and *Moraxella* are less common

bacterial causes. Both mycoplasma and chlamydia pneumonia are common atypical causes of CAP in older children.

12. e. No single sign reliably predicts hypoxia. Since sensitivity is low for most signs, a combination of signs must be used. Respiratory rate greater than 60 breaths per minute, altered mental status, and feeding difficulties all suggest hypoxemia. Head nodding and cyanosis are highly specific for hypoxia.

13. e. In children between 4 months and 5 years of age, viruses are the most common cause of CAP. RSV is the most common agent. Infections occur more often in fall and winter. Associated symptoms include rhinorrhea, sore throat, and diarrhea. If a viral etiology is suspected and follow-up is guaranteed, antibiotics do not have to be given.

Pneumococci are the most common bacterial cause of CAP in this age group. Symptoms usually begin abruptly with high fever and productive cough. Bacterial CAP occurs without regard to season. Children with headache, gastrointestinal complaints, arthralgia, and cough are most likely to have *Mycoplasma* infections.

14. d. Determining the etiology of CAP is difficult in children; antibiotics are usually selected empirically. The duration of therapy is 7 to 10 days in uncomplicated CAP. For outpatient management of CAP, follow-up is indicated within 1 to 3 days after diagnosis. In children who fail to respond appropriately to therapy, evaluation for empyema, abscess, or nonsusceptible organisms should be undertaken.

Rapid antigen tests are available for adenovirus, parainfluenza strains 1 through 3, influenza A and B, and RSV. Nasopharyngeal washings are used to determine the cause of CAP. Pneumococcal antigen and antibody assays are not sensitive enough to diagnose *S. pneumoniae* infection. Immune complex detection may be a useful test in children younger than 2 years old and is currently in development.

Summary

Bronchiolitis is a viral lower respiratory tract infection that is common during the first 2 years of life. RSV is the most common infectious agent, although influenza, adenovirus, parainfluenza, and human metapneumovirus also cause bronchiolitis. RSV is most common during the winter and early spring. Most children are exposed by age 2 years. Reinfection with RSV is common because infection does not confer immunity.

Pathophysiologic features of bronchiolitis include inflammation, edema, and necrosis of the epithelial linings of the small airways. Increased mucous production and bronchospasm are seen in conjunction with wheeze, cough, accessory muscle use, tachypnea, and rhinorrhea.

Evidence-based treatment for bronchiolitis is detailed in the clinical practice guidelines from the American Academy of Pediatrics. Indications for use of the antiviral ribavirin are controversial. Some studies document improvement in respiratory score and decreased hospital length of stay. Inhaled ribavirin may be considered when severe RSV disease is present in patients with health conditions that predispose them to increased risk from this infection.

The effectiveness of bronchodilator use (i.e., epinephrine, albuterol, and salbutamol) is also not well understood. A Cochrane review examined eight RCTs of bronchodilator use ($N = 394$). Twenty-five percent of treated patients had transient improvement, although it was of unclear significance. Another Cochrane review also found insufficient evidence to support epinephrine use. Current recommendations do not support routine use of bronchodilators in bronchiolitis. Clinical practice suggests that a nebulized bronchodilator trial is appropriate in select infants. When good clinical response is noted, bronchodilators are a reasonable intervention.

Although 60% of admitted infants receive corticosteroids, routine glucocorticoid use is not recommended because a Cochrane review did not show a benefit for steroids given in acute bronchiolitis.

Infants with mild disease may not need intravenous fluids. If feeding is not compromised and the respiratory rate is below 60 to 70 breaths/minute, a trial of oral feeds is appropriate. Infants with retractions, nasal flaring, or coughing may be at increased risk of aspiration. Intravenous fluids are appropriate in this subset of patients until the condition improves.

Chest physiotherapy is also not routinely recommended in treatment of bronchiolitis. A Cochrane review of three RCTs did not show benefit for either vibration or percussion physiotherapy, although nasal suctioning provides some temporary benefits.

Few RCTs have examined the use of antibiotics in bronchiolitis. No studies demonstrate an improvement in symptoms, fever, radiographic findings, or clinical course in patients with bronchiolitis who receive antibiotics. The risk of bacteremia in children with bronchiolitis and concomitant fever is quite low (0.2%). Children with severe illness who require mechanical ventilation or intensive care unit admission are at higher risk for bacterial coinfection and may benefit from antibiotic therapy. Current recommendations do not support routine antibiotic use, although more research is needed.

Palivizumab is a prophylactic immunization indicated for certain infants at high risk for RSV disease (see Tables 109-1 and 109-2). The recommended dose is 15 mg/kg of weight; injections are given in five monthly doses beginning in November or December. Infants and children with lung disease requiring medical therapy, hemodynamically significant congenital heart disease, and immunosuppression should be immunized. Prematurity is also an indication in certain cases.

Behavioral intervention helps prevent the spread of RSV. Sanitation and hand washing are important because RSV secretions are highly contagious. Passive smoking increases the risk of having RSV infection. Pulmonary function in infants of mothers who smoke during or after pregnancy is significantly decreased. Breast-feeding has a protective effect; a meta-analysis showed a threefold greater risk for hospitalization in non-breast-fed infants with lower respiratory tract infection.

CAP is one of the most common serious infections in children. The incidence is 34 to 40 cases per 1000 in the United States and Europe. Disease burden is significantly higher in developing regions such as Africa. Infectious causes of CAP are numerous but often specific to certain ages (Table 109-3).

Diagnosis of CAP is strongly suggested when fever and cyanosis are found in conjunction with more than one of the following: cough, nasal flaring, retractions, rales, tachypnea, and diminished breath sounds. Younger children are noted to have tachypnea, nasal flaring, and fever, whereas older children often have rales, tactile fremitus, pleural rub, and bronchial breath sounds.

Although isolation of the causative agent is generally not necessary in routine CAP, sputum cultures can be obtained in those with severe illness. Adequate sputum for gram stain and culture has more than 25 leukocytes and less than 25 squamous epithelial cells per low power field. Pulse oximetry is recommended in children with respiratory distress. Complete blood counts, erythrocyte sedimentation rates, and C-reactive protein do not distinguish viral from bacterial causes and are not routinely indicated. Although radiographic findings of consolidation have traditionally been ascribed to pneumococcal infection and interstitial infiltrates to viral CAP, the studies may not differentiate between illness type as well as previously thought. Chest radiographs are most useful in children with prolonged illness, atypical presentation/symptoms, worsening infection, or when pulmonary effusion or abscess is suspected.

Treatment of CAP is based on the child's age and clinical picture. If bacterial CAP is suspected, antibiotics should be started promptly. Table 109-3 lists recommended regimens based on age. Infants from birth to 20 days of age, febrile infants from 3 weeks to 3 months of age, and children who appear toxic generally should be hospitalized. Antibiotics are prescribed for a total of 7 to 10 days. Follow-up radiographs are not indicated unless the clinical condition does not improve.

Vaccines that reduce the incidence of CAP include *H. influenza* type B and influenza. Use of the conjugated vaccine against the seven most active strains of *S. pneumoniae* has resulted in a decreased incidence of invasive streptococcal disease in the United States.

Table 109-3 | Etiology and Medication Recommendations for Community-Acquired Pneumonia in Childhood

Age	Common Causes, Bacterial	Common Causes, Viral	Inpatient or Outpatient Management	Recommended Medications
Birth to 20 days	*E. coli*, group B strep, *Listeria*	Cytomegalovirus, herpes simplex (uncommon)	Admit	IV or IM ampicillin plus gentamicin with or without IV cefotaxime
3 wk to 3 mo	*Chlamydia trachomatis*, *S. pneumoniae*	Adenovirus, influenza, parainfluenza, RSV	Admit if hypoxic or febrile	If outpatient, oral azithromycin or erythromycin If admitted, IV erythromycin; add IV cefotaxime or IV cefuroxime
4 mo to 5 yr	*Chlamydia pneumoniae*, *Mycoplasma*, *S. pneumoniae*	Adenovirus, influenza, parainfluenza, rhinovirus, RSV	Outpatient management	Outpatient: amoxicillin or amoxicillin–clavulanate; azithromycin, erythromycin Inpatient: IV cefotaxime or cefuroxime For pneumococcal infection: ampicillin
5 yr to adolescence	*C. pneumoniae*, *M. pneumoniae*, *S. pneumoniae*	Adenovirus, Epstein–Barr, influenza, parainfluenza, rhinovirus, RSV, varicella (less common)	Outpatient management	Outpatient: oral azithromycin, clarithromycin, or erythromycin Inpatient: IV cefuroxime plus erythromycin For pneumococcal infection: IV ampicillin

Adapted from data in Ostapchuk M, Roberts D, Haddy R: Community-acquired pneumonia in infants and children. *Am Fam Physician* 70: 899–908, 2004.

Suggested Reading

American Academy of Pediatrics Subcommittee on Diagnosis and Management of Bronchiolitis: Diagnosis and management of bronchiolitis. *Pediatrics* 118:1774–1793, 2006.

Ayieko P, English M:In children aged 2–59 months with pneumonia, which clinical signs best predict hypoxemia? *J Tropical Pediatr* 52(5):307–310, 2006.

Ostapchuk M, Roberts D, Haddy R: Community-acquired pneumonia in infants and children. *Am Fam Physician* 70:899–908, 2004.

Perrotta C, Ortiz Z, Roque M: Chest physiotherapy for acute bronchiolitis in pediatric patients between 0 and 24 months old. *Cochrane Database Syst Rev* (7):CD004873, 2007.

Spurling GK, Fonseka K, Doust J, et al: Antibiotics for bronchiolitis in children. *Cochrane Database Syst Rev* (1):CD005189, 2007.

Zar H, Madhi S: Childhood pneumonia—Progress and challenges. *S Afr Med J* 96:890–900, 2006.

CHAPTER 110 · Childhood Asthma

CLINICAL CASE PROBLEM 1

My Child Is Usually Healthy, but He Wheezes Sometimes

A 2-year-old African American male presents for his well child checkup. His parents tell you that he has been doing well, but he has had episodes of wheezing four times during the past year. He is the product of an uncomplicated pregnancy and delivery, but he was hospitalized at age 6 months for bronchiolitis. Both parents have a history of allergies, and his father has asthma. His mother smoked during pregnancy but quit smoking last year. The child was never breast-fed.

SELECT THE BEST ANSWER TO THE FOLLOWING QUESTIONS

1. Which of the following is true concerning this child?
   a. you cannot diagnose this child with asthma because he is too young
   b. children who have four or more episodes of wheezing and a clinical picture consistent with asthma should be diagnosed and treated according to current guidelines once other causes of wheezing have been excluded
   c. since his mother quit smoking, this child is at no increased risk for asthma
   d. since he had bronchiolitis at 6 months, he cannot be diagnosed with asthma
   e. African Americans have much less severe asthma than other races, so this child does not need to be diagnosed with asthma now

2. Which of the following differential diagnoses should you exclude in this child?
   a. foreign body
   b. viral bronchiolitis
   c. heart disease
   d. vocal cord dysfunction
   e. all of the above

3. Which of the following is true concerning treatment of this child?
   a. there are virtually no studies using inhaled corticosteroids in children of this age
   b. inhaled corticosteroids should not routinely be used in children younger than 5 years of age due to growth retardation
   c. because of recurrent episodes of wheezing, with a strong family history, this child should be treated with inhaled corticosteroids
   d. levalbuterol is far superior to albuterol in this age group and should be used
   e. rescue medication should be avoided in children in this age group

4. In discussing treatment plans with the parents, they ask about various medications used in asthma therapy. Which of the following medications has been shown to be most effective in the treatment of asthma in children and should be used at first-line treatment if maintenance therapy is begun?
   a. leukotriene inhibitor
   b. nedocromil
   c. long-acting β_2-agonist inhaler or nebulizer
   d. inhaled corticosteroids as an inhaler or nebulizer
   e. none of the above

5. Which of the following statements is false concerning asthma in children?
   a. 50% to 80% of children with asthma develop symptoms before 5 years of age
   b. atopic dermatitis and rhinitis not related to viral infections during the first year are both strongly related to the development of asthma, and atopy is the strongest predictor that wheezing will progress to asthma
   c. many young children have elevated immunoglobulin E (IgE) levels from 9 months of age
   d. perinatal exposure to tobacco smoke is associated with the onset of asthma
   e. wheezing and cough are usually worse in the midday, after lunch, related to increased reflux

6. Which of the following is included in the diagnosis of asthma in children?
   a. symptoms of episodic airflow obstruction
   b. at least partially reversible airflow obstruction
   c. wheezing with allergic rhinitis
   d. a, b, and c
   e. a and b

CLINICAL CASE PROBLEM 2

7-Year-Old with Rhinitis and Chest Tightness

A 7-year-old female presents to your office with a history of 1 week of gradually increasing chest tightness and mild dyspnea. She has had nasal drainage and a nighttime cough. Her mother states that she has had no fever and has been going to school. Her medical history is significant for only one previous episode of wheezing for which she was treated with an antibiotic and an inhaler. Her family history is significant for an older brother with asthma. Her father is a smoker.

On examination, she has a temperature of 99.9°F, blood pressure of 90/50 mmHg, respiratory rate of 20 breaths/minute, and pulse of 100 beats/minute. She appears in no distress but is audibly wheezing. She has mild nasal turbinate swelling, postnasal drainage, and diffuse expiratory wheezes. After a nebulizer treatment with albuterol, she feels much better, and her lungs are completely clear.

7. Which of the following do you advise the patient and her parent?
   a. she may or may not have asthma, but she has symptoms of airway reactivity; you prescribe an albuterol inhaler with a spacer device and advise that her father must stop smoking immediately or ensure she is not exposed to any cigarette smoke
   b. she definitely has asthma; you prescribe an albuterol inhaler, a short course of prednisone, and an inhaled corticosteroid
   c. she has acute bronchitis and should respond well to an antibiotic alone
   d. she needs to follow-up with you in a short period of time to determine if further treatment is necessary and should call immediately if she is worsening
   e. a and d

The child does not keep her follow-up appointment, although when your nurse calls to check, her mother states that she is completely well. Four months later, she comes in for a visit because she is having a nighttime cough. After a complete history, you find that she has continued to have chest tightness and dyspnea several days a week, especially after running in gym class, and two or three nights each month she cannot sleep well due to coughing. She has no fever, rhinorhea, or other symptoms. She finished her inhaler a month ago, after which her symptoms increased.

8. She has a completely normal physical exam and her peak flow is 90% predicted. Which of the following diagnoses and treatments are correct?

a. diagnose her with asthmatic bronchitis; treat her with an antibiotic and a course of oral steroids
b. diagnose her with mild intermittent asthma; renew her albuterol inhaler
c. diagnose her with mild persistent asthma; renew her albuterol inhaler, begin an inhaled corticosteroid inhaler, and instruct her in asthma management
d. diagnose her with exercise-induced asthma only; renew her albuterol inhaler and instruct her in management of exercise-induced asthma
e. diagnose her with moderate persistent asthma; renew her albuterol inhaler, begin a steroid inhaler and leukotriene inhibitor or nedocromil, and instruct her in asthma management

9. The patient returns for regular follow-up but she continues to have symptoms that require her to use the rescue medication four or five times a week. She now has daily symptoms and coughs more than one night a week. Which of the following would be appropriate to recommend?
   a. review triggers and try to eliminate them
   b. continue her dose of inhaled corticosteroid at the recommended dose and add a long-acting β-agonist
   c. add a leukotriene inhibitor or nedocromil if needed
   d. a, b, and c
   e. continue with the same treatment but increase her inhaled steroid because long-acting β-agonists are too dangerous

10. While discussing elimination of triggers with the child and her parents, you mention all of the following as possible triggers. Which of these is most commonly implicated in causing exacerbations, and possibly even influencing the development of asthma in populations as a whole?
    a. dust mites and tobacco smoke
    b. cockroach antigens
    c. animal dander
    d. outdoor pollutants
    e. violence

11. Disease severity in asthma is not determined by which of the following?
    a. nighttime symptoms and their frequency
    b. pulmonary function measures
    c. use of rescue medications
    d. physical symptoms, including chest tightness and dyspnea, and their frequency
    e. the presence of nasal eosinophils

short course of oral steroids. When he returns in 3 days, he has already improved dramatically and has a normal physical exam. You spend additional time with the patient and his grandmother, and you have your nurse spend time reviewing an action plan as well. Which of the following is true concerning monitoring of asthma in children?
a. written action plans are a waste of time and provide no benefit
b. peak expiratory flow monitoring has shown the greatest statistical benefit in management of asthma
c. although some studies are inconclusive, a written action plan has been shown to improve asthma management and outcomes
d. written action plans only work in families with educated parents
e. compliance is rarely a problem in pediatric asthma since parents are generally concerned about their children

15. Written action plans for asthma patients should include all of the following except
a. peak flow monitoring instructions, with green, yellow, and red zones indicating normal, decreasing, or emergency peak flow zones, respectively
b. instructions on self-adjusting allergy immunotherapy based on symptoms
c. management of the environment (avoidance of triggers)
d. management of maintenance medications and medications for exacerbations

16. Based on the history of this patient, which medicine do you recommend for maintenance?
a. inhaled corticosteroid with a long-acting β_2-agonist
b. short-acting β_2-agonist only
c. nasal steroids only
d. no treatment, only follow-up
e. leukotriene modifier only

17. Which of the following facts is (are) true concerning asthma?
a. the incidence in the United States is increasing
b. more than 10% of children younger than age 18 years in the United States have been diagnosed with asthma
c. it is found more often in children with a personal or family history of atopy
d. a and c
e. all of the above

CLINICAL CASE PROBLEM 3

Lost Continuity with Revolving Homes

A 13-year-old male presents to your office, brought by his grandmother. He has been treated by you for allergic rhinitis in the spring, when the pollen count was increased, and now it is winter. He has been living with his mother but spends summers with his father. Because of his living arrangements, his medical care has been inconsistent. According to the child and his grandmother, he was diagnosed with asthma at age 8 years. He has had one or two exacerbations a year that have required an emergency room visit. He was hospitalized 3 days for "pneumonia and asthma" at age 10 years. He has been prescribed a variety of medications, but he tells you that he left his inhaler at his father's house and currently he does not have any medications. He seems to understand very little about asthma.

The patient complains of "a little" fever, nasal congestion, and intermittent wheezing. He tells you that he has taken a bottle of over-the-counter cough syrup in the past 3 days because he coughs so much at night. Vital signs are normal. Physical examination is normal except for nasal congestion without sinus tenderness and scattered expiratory wheezes with no rales, rhonchi, or eegophony.

12. Which of the following statements is true?
a. this child likely has an acute exacerbation of asthma due to viral infection, superimposed on untreated mild or moderate persistent asthma
b. this child likely has severe persistent asthma
c. this child likely has pneumonia
d. this child likely has acute sinusitis
e. this child likely has cystic fibrosis

13. The grandmother tells you that the other doctors told her the child would "outgrow" his asthma. You explain to her that the following pathologic change(s) is(are) found in the airways of patients with asthma, with or without symptoms:
a. airway remodeling
b. airway smooth muscle hypertrophy
c. airway epithelial cell destruction
d. airway decreased submucosal vascularity
e. a, b, and c

14. You check an influenza swab, which is negative, and treat the child with inhaled albuterol with a spacer, an inhaled corticosteroid, and a

18. All of the following statements concerning treatment of asthma in children have level A (highest level, randomized controlled trials) evidence except
    a. a spacer with a meter-dose inhaler is as effective as a nebulizer either for treatment of an acute exacerbation of asthma or for maintenance therapy
    b. sublingual immunotherapy is as effective as traditional immunotherapy (injections)
    c. oral corticosteroids should be administered within 45 minutes, or as quickly as possible, during an acute exacerbation of asthma to decrease hospitalizations and emergency room stay
    d. moderate doses of inhaled corticosteroids are recommended as first-line treatment in children with mild or moderate persistent asthma because they are more effective in improving symptoms and lung function in children than leukotriene inhibitors, inhaled long-acting β_2-agonists, and inhaled nedocromil
    e. physicians should consider adding inhaled ipratropium bromide (Atrovent) with inhaled β_2-agonist particularly in the setting of a more severe asthma exacerbation

19. Which of the following statements concerning use of oral corticosteroids in children with asthma is true?
    a. a regular, low-dose oral corticosteroid (e.g., prednisone) has less effect on growth rate and bone mass than short bursts of steroids
    b. oral corticosteroids and inhaled or nebulized corticosteroids are equally effective in the acute asthma exacerbation
    c. repeated short courses of oral corticosteroids at 1 mg/kg/day to treat acute exacerbations of asthma have not shown any effect on adrenal function, bone mineralization, or bone metabolism
    d. intravenous corticosteroids are more effective than oral corticosteroids in children with an intact gastrointestinal tract who can take oral medications
    e. oral corticosteroids given early in the acute flare-up of asthma have no impact on the rate of hospitalization

20. Goals of asthma therapy (according to recent recommendations) include all of the following except
    a. minimal or no chronic symptoms day or night
    b. minimal use of any medications
    c. minimal or no exacerbations
    d. no limitations on activities; no school missed
    e. minimal use of short-acting inhaled β_2-agonists

21. Which of the following statements is correct, according to the most recent guidelines for asthma management?
    a. the stepwise approach is intended to replace the clinical decision making required to meet individual patient needs so that if a patient has a bad outcome, the physician can legally defend him- or herself
    b. there are exact guidelines on management of asthma in infants
    c. gain control as quickly as possible (a course of short systemic corticosteroids may be required) and then step down to the least medication necessary to maintain control
    d. advise consultation with an asthma specialist for all patients with mild persistent asthma
    e. if control of asthma symptoms is not maintained, never step up. Once diagnosed as one "class" of asthma, a patient is always in that class

---

Clinical Case Management Problem

An 8-year-old female who is your patient and whom you have diagnosed with moderate persistent asthma recently has been coming in more frequently with chest tightness and nighttime cough. You are not sure if the child and parents are compliant with the medication, and you are very sure they are not compliant with avoidance measures. In addition to possibly adding medications, what can you do to improve this child's quality of life?

Answers

1. **b.** Failure to diagnose young children with asthma, despite the presence of four episodes of wheezing, may lead to increased hospitalizations and complications and deprive the child of disease-modifying therapy. Bronchiolitis, especially respiratory syncytial virus, is associated with an increased risk of later asthma, as is a family history of allergy or atopy. Smoking during pregnancy is associated with an increased risk of asthma, and breast-feeding decreases risk. African Americans have a higher risk for fatal asthma attacks and more severe asthma.

2. **e.** In the infant and child, it is important to exclude other possible causes of wheezing, especially since pulmonary function tests cannot be easily performed. Foreign body, viral bronchiolitis, heart disease, vocal cord dysfunction, enlarged lymph nodes, tumor,

allergic sinusitis, and cystic fibrosis should also be considered. Because the child in this case has had four episodes of wheezing and no signs of other illnesses, these conditions are unlikely.

3. c. This child should be treated with inhaled corticosteroids. Since most young children cannot use an inhaler, inhaled budenoside (Pulmicort) in a nebulizer twice a day is often preferred. As with all asthma patients, identifying triggers, patient education, and close monitoring are important. Levalbuterol has not been found superior to albuterol in children, and it is much more costly. Rescue medication (most commonly albuterol) should be used as needed. Long-term studies have not shown adrenal or growth suppression with inhaled corticosteroids in children. The National Asthma and Education Prevention Program (NAEPP) examined studies using inhaled corticosteroids early in the course of asthma to attempt to decrease the progression of the disease. Initial studies in children established the safety and effectiveness of inhaled steroids in children but were inconclusive in establishing that inhaled steroids changed the disease progression.

4. d. Studies have confirmed that inhaled corticosteroids are the preferred medication for maintenance therapy in the management of childhood asthma. NAEPP recommendations clearly reflect this. Other therapies, such as nasal steroids, leukotriene inhibitors, nedocromil, long-acting β-agonists, or theophyline, are added to the inhaled corticosteroids and should not be used as first-line therapy. In children younger than age 5 years, leukotriene inhibitors and cromolyn remain alternatives, but inhaled corticosteroids are associated with improved lung function, decreased emergency room visits, and decreased hospitalizations in all age groups.

5. e. A child who presents with wheezing, chest tightness, and cough that are worse in the late evening or early morning hours, particularly with a history of atopy, rhinitis not related to viral infections, family history of allergy and/or asthma, and perinatal exposure to tobacco smoke, likely has asthma. In young children, pulmonary function tests are difficult, but serum IgE levels are generally elevated from 9 months of age.

6. e. The definition of asthma, adapted from NAEPP, includes the following: Episodic symptoms of airflow obstruction, symptoms of at least partially reversible airflow obstruction, and alternative diagnosis excluded. Wheezing with allergic rhinitis may be associated with asthma but is not in the definition.

7. e. Although you suspect asthma, this child also has tobacco exposure and an acute upper respiratory infection. Her symptoms may be from the bronchial reactivity due to acute bronchitis. Treatment with an antibiotic has not been shown to benefit patients with or without asthma unless sinusitis or pneumonia is likely. In this child with no toxicity, no sinus tenderness, and no fever, that is unlikely. At this visit, treatment of her wheezing with a bronchodilator, without addition of steroids, is appropriate. If her symptoms persist, or she is not clearing, further workup for pneumonia or consideration of oral steroids or antibiotics might be appropriate. Most important, the parents must understand the importance of stopping her exposure to cigarette smoke, a known trigger for asthma, and the importance of close follow-up to determine if she does indeed have asthma.

8. c. Now the patient has symptoms that, according to the NAEPP definition, place her in the category of mild persistent asthma. At this time, she should be placed on an inhaled steroid with a rescue medication (albuterol), instructed in asthma self-management, and followed closely.

9. d. Now this child is classified as having moderate persistent asthma. The child is using her rescue medication more than twice a week, which indicates she does not have adequate treatment for her asthma. Reassessing her forced expiratory volume in 1 second (FEV_1) and close monitoring of peak flow are important. Emphasizing again the need for no cigarette exposure is very important. Treatment options will include adding a long-acting β-agonist, adding a leukotriene modifier, adding nasal steroids (particularly in patients with prominent allergic rhinitis), and avoiding triggers. Increasing the dose to high-dose inhaled corticosteroids is no longer recommended in children. If triggers seem prominent, consideration should be given for allergy testing to determine which allergens should be avoided. Although the child does have a component of exercise-induced asthma, this is also best treated with inhaled steroids. Lung function, hospitalization rates, and emergency room visits are much improved in children on a combination of inhaled steroids with a long-acting β-agonist. Due to the recent findings of increased mortality with long-acting β-agonists, even with inhaled corticosteroids, these medications are only recommended for mild persistent asthma and worse, not for mild intermittent asthma.

10. a. Although all of the choices may trigger asthma in some children, dust mites and tobacco smoke have been implicated most often and may play a role in even causing asthma. Cockroach antigens, animal dander (especially cats), molds, and outdoor pollutants cause exacerbation in many children as well. Violence is believed to increase asthma due to a stress-related increase in production of inflammatory mediators.

11. e. All of the choices are in the NAEPP stepwise approach to treatment for asthma except the presence of nasal eosinophils (Table 110-1).

12. a. This child has a history consistent with a diagnosis of asthma—likely mild or moderate persistent asthma. His social situation is common in the pediatric population, making control of his asthma even more difficult. With the increase in symptoms of wheezing most recently, he has an acute exacerbation that must be treated first. Although he does not have definite signs of pneumonia or sinusitis, some clinicians would give antibiotics in a case such as this, particularly if x-rays are not done to exclude other diagnosis. Because it is winter, a flue screen should be considered, depending on exposure history.

13. e. Airway remodeling has a major role in the pathogenesis of asthma. Prolonged inflammation leads to permanent structural changes, despite the fact that asthma is generally a "reversible" disease. Pathologic changes include smooth muscle hypertrophy, epithelial cell destruction, increased submucosal vascularity, and angiogenesis. Adolescence may mark an improvement in asthma symptoms, but some patients worsen.

14. c. Written action plans tell patients how to adjust their medications, manage their environment, and manage routine and exacerbation of symptoms with or without peak flow monitoring. NAEPP recommends written action plans and peak flow monitoring even though some studies are inconclusive. Peak flow monitoring, in particular, has not been statistically shown to improve outcomes, but studies vary in their quality, and NAEPP still recommends its use. A Cochrane review of patients who used asthma management plans showed decrease hospitalizations and emergency room visits and improved lung function.

15. b. Using peak flow monitoring is useful to help patients (or parents) identify when they need to increase medication, begin rescue medication for an exacerbation, or see a physician.

Table 110-1	Stepwise Approach for Managing Children with Asthma			
	Step 1: Mild Intermittent	**Step 2: Mild Persistent**	**Step 3: Moderate Persistent**	**Step 4: Severe Persistent**
Symptoms	Daytime: Symptoms no more than twice a week	Daytime: Symptoms more than twice weekly but no more than once daily	Daytime: Daily symptoms	Daytime: Continuous symptoms
Exacerbations	Brief exacerbations	Exacerbations may affect activity	Exacerbations affect activity, occur twice a week and may last for days	Frequent exacerbations
Nocturnal symptoms	Nocturnal symptoms no more than twice a month	Nocturnal symptoms more than twice a month	Nocturnal symptoms more than twice weekly	Frequent nocturnal symptoms
FEV_1 and peak flow	FEV_1 and peak flow <80%	FEV_1 and peak flow <80% predicted	FEV_1 or peak flow <60–80% predicted	FEV_1 and peak flow <60% predicted
Variability of peak flow	Peak flow variability <20%	Peak flow variability 20–30%	Peak flow variability >30%	Peak flow variability >30%
Treatment	No daily medication Short-acting rescue bronchodilator	Short-acting rescue bronchodilator with daily controller inhaled corticosteroid	Short-acting rescue bronchodilator with daily controller inhaled corticosteroid and long-acting β_2-agonist	Short-acting rescue bronchodilator with daily controller inhaled corticosteroid and long-acting β_2-agonist and oral steroids if needed

Adapted from the National Heart, Lung, and Blood Institute. Available at www.nhlbi.nih.gov/guidelines/asthma.

16. **a.** With his history of recurrent episodes and hospitalization, this child likely has moderate persistent asthma and he should be on an inhaled corticosteroid with a long-acting β_2-agonist. Addition of nasal steroids and leukotriene modifiers would be appropriate if this is not adequate. Short-acting β_2-agonists should be prescribed for rescue medication, and their use should be monitored closely.

17. **d.** Asthma is on the rise in the United States. Currently, more than 5% (not 10%) of children in the United States—nearly 5 million children—have asthma.

18. **b.** Although sublingual immunotherapy is being used, it has not been compared with injection immunotherapy and has not been shown to improve lung function and symptoms in the treatment of asthma.

19. **c.** Chronic use of oral corticosteroids has, of course, multiple long-term side effects, including growth suppression, adrenal suppression, and decreased bone mineralization. Repeated short courses of oral steroids, however, have not shown any of these negative effects. Although inhaled and nebulized corticosteroids are excellent for maintenance, oral corticosteroids are superior, and equally effective compared to intravenous corticosteroids, in an acute attack.

20. **b.** The goal of therapy is to use adequate medication to control symptoms while producing minimal or no adverse effects from the medication(s).

21. **c.** The stepwise approach for managing asthma is intended to assist, not replace, the clinical decision-making process. The patient is assigned to the most severe step in which any feature occurs. Treatment is reviewed every 1 to 6 months; a gradual stepwise reduction in treatment may be possible. If control is not maintained, then consider a step up after reviewing the patient's adherence, medication technique, and environmental control. Gain control as quickly as possible and then step down to the least medication necessary to maintain control. Minimize use of short-acting inhaled β_2-agonists to less than one canister a month. Provide parent education on management of asthma and control of environmental factors that make asthma worse. Consultation with an asthma specialist is recommended for patients with moderate or severe persistent asthma.

Solution to the Clinical Case Management Problem

It is sometimes very difficult to assess the compliance of a pediatric patient's asthma therapy, particularly if the parents seem uninterested. Expert Panel Report number 2 of the NAEPP lists the four components of asthma management as measurement of assessment and monitoring, control of factors contributing to asthma severity, pharmacologic therapy, and patient education to facilitate partnership in asthma care.

In this case, since you suspect lack of compliance with avoidance measures and medication use, patient and parent education will be the most important focus. Checking her spirometry in comparison to previous visits, reviewing her peak flow monitor records (if she has kept them), and examining the number of refills of rescue medication and maintenance medication are all essential. Patient education should begin with the diagnosis and should be done by not only the physician but also the entire health care team. Basic facts about asthma, the role of medications, recognition and treatment of exacerbations, peak flow monitoring, and environmental modifications should be taught. A child of this age can be involved in the education as well, and asthma camps are available in some areas. Helping the parents to understand that management of asthma will improve their quality of life as well (fewer visits to the emergency department and physician) may help to motivate change. Having the parents explain the action plan after it is presented, to ensure they understand the plan, is essential. The child should demonstrate use of the inhaler with a spacer device and use of the peak flow monitor in the office. At each visit, the physician should review possible triggers and try to elucidate if the child is worsening due to noncompliance of her inhaled corticosteroid and other medication or if she has a new pet or other new exposure. Some physicians have asthma support groups or scheduled days for special asthma programs in their clinics.

Summary

The incidence of asthma in children in the United States has increased 160% since 1980. The disease currently affects nearly 5 million children in the United States. NAEPP has helped clinicians to standardize treatment based on the latest evidence available.

Asthma is a chronic inflammatory disorder of the airways in which mast cells, eosinophils, T lymphocytes, neutrophils, epithelial cells, and other cellular elements play a role. Reversibility of airway obstruction, either spontaneously or with treatment, is the hallmark of asthma.

The diagnosis of asthma in children is primarily clinical, with treatment based on severity of the asthma. The key features of asthma are bronchial hyperreactivity and airway reversibility. Other causes of wheezing must be ruled out prior to the diagnosis of asthma, particularly in younger children, in whom spirometry is difficult. Differential diagnosis includes bronchitis, bronchiolitis, foreign body, cystic fibrosis, gastroesophageal reflux disease, tumor, etc. An improvement of more than 12% in FEV_1 or peak flow after treatment with a bronchodilator or corticosteroids confirms the diagnosis.

Symptoms characteristic of asthma include wheezing, chest tightness, breathlessness, and cough (particularly at night). In children, atopy and allergic disease are strongly related to asthma. Physical findings are prolonged expiratory phase, use of accessory muscles of respiration, wheezing, tachypnea, and intercostals retractions.

For children of all ages, inhaled corticosteroids are the drug of choice, although nedocromil and leukotriene inhibitors may be considered in children younger than age 5 years and as supplemental therapy in all children. Multiple studies have shown no long-term growth suppression in even young children on inhaled corticosteroids; however, they have shown a marked decrease in emergency room visits, hospitalization, exacerbation, and death.

In addition to pharmacologic treatment of asthma, identification and avoidance of triggers are particularly important in children. Most children have an allergic component, and adequate treatment of allergic rhinitis with nasal corticosteroids, avoidance of allergens, leukotriene inhibitors, and immunotherapy all improve asthma outcomes.

NAEPP and recent research emphasize that a self-management plan and a thorough education plan is critical for improving clinical outcomes in asthmatics. A stepwise approach for management is used with a quick relief plan for exacerbations as well as a step up and step down plan to monitor patients based on their classification severity and clinical features for daily therapy.

Suggested Reading

Courtney A, McCarter D, Pollart S: Childhood asthma: Treatment update. *Am Fam Physician* 71(10):1959–1968, 2005.

Mintz M: Asthma update. Part I: Diagnosis, monitoring, and prevention of disease progression. *Am Fam Physician* 70(5):893–898, 2004.

Mintz M: Asthma update. Part II: Medical management. *Am Fam Physician* 70(6):1061–1066, 2004.

National Asthma Education and Prevention Program: *Guidelines for the Diagnosis and Management of Asthma: Expert Panel Report 2*, NIH publication No. 97-4051. Bethesda, MD: U.S. Department of Health and Human Services, Public Health Service, National Institutes of Health, National Heart, Lung, and Blood Institute, 1997.

National Asthma Education and Prevention Program: *Expert Panel Report: Guidelines for the Diagnosis and Management of Asthma: Update on Selected Topics—2002*, NIH publication No. 02–5074. Bethesda, MD: U.S. Department of Health and Human Services, Public Health Service, National Institutes of Health, National Heart, Lung, and Blood Institute, 2003.

National Institutes of Health, Heart, Lung, and Blood Institute: *Practical Guide for the Diagnosis and Management of Asthma, Based on Expert Panel Report 2*. Bethesda, MD: National Institutes of Health, 2003, pp. 1–60.

111 Allergic Rhinitis

CLINICAL CASE PROBLEM 1

A 6-Year-Old Male with a Perennial Cold

A 6-year-old male is brought to your office by his grandmother, who states that he has had a "stuffy, runny nose for what seems forever." The grandmother states that the child started to have a runny nose 9 or 10 months ago associated with congestion and occasionally "fits of sneezing." He has not had any fever, cough, wheezing, headache, or ear pain. Over-the-counter oral "cold medicines" have helped somewhat.

On further questioning, you find out that the child lives with his parents in a fully carpeted home. He also received a puppy for his birthday a few months ago. The only significant past medical history is of some mild eczema. The mother has a history of asthma as a child.

On examination, there is bilateral clear rhinorrhea and obvious turbinate swelling with a pale blue mucosa. The child is mouth breathing and several times during the examination is noted to rub his nose upward with the palm of his hand. Some cobblestoning is noted on the posterior pharynx. The chest examination is negative.

SELECT THE BEST ANSWER TO YHE FOLLOWING QUESTIONS

1. What is the most likely diagnosis in this child?
   a. infectious rhinitis
   b. vasomotor rhinitis
   c. seasonal allergic rhinitis
   d. perennial allergic rhinitis
   e. rhinitis medicamentosa

2. The most common complication(s) associated with this condition is (are)
   a. epistaxis
   b. sinusitis and otitis media
   c. nasal polyps
   d. all of the above
   e. none of the above

3. Elevation of which of the following immunoglobulins is associated with this condition?
   a. immunoglobulin A (IgA)
   b. IgE
   c. IgG
   d. IgM
   e. no immunoglobulin is associated with the condition

4. What type of allergen is this condition most often associated with?
   a. house dust mites, animal dander, and molds
   b. pollen, especially from grasses, trees, and weeds
   c. cigarette smoke
   d. nonspecific environmental pollutants
   e. all of the above

5. Which of the following physical signs associated with the condition described here is found most commonly in children and not adults?
   a. "shiners"
   b. nasal crease
   c. mouth breathing
   d. the "salute sign"
   e. posterior pharyngeal wall lymphoid hyperplasia

6. Which of the following is the most common predisposing factor to the condition described here?
   a. family history
   b. smoke exposure
   c. chronic use
   d. asthma
   e. eczema

CLINICAL CASE PROBLEM 2

Too Many Colds Lasting Too Long

A father who owns a landscaping business brings his 3-year-old daughter to your office with a complaint of 6 weeks of runny nose, congestion, sneezing, and cough. He further notes that the child seems to have long colds especially during spring, early summer, and, occasionally, late summer. The child also had an episode of difficulty breathing a few days ago for which they visited a local emergency room and were given an inhaler.

7. What do you think this child has?
   a. asthma
   b. seasonal allergic rhinitis
   c. gastroesophageal reflux
   d. common cold
   e. rhinitis medicamentosa

8. What is the first step in treatment that you would recommend to these patients?
   a. immunotherapy
   b. turbinectomy

c. refer to an allergist
d. dietary restrictions
e. environmental control measures and allergen avoidance

9. What is the most effective pharmacologic treatment for the condition described here?
   a. intranasal cromolyn sodium
   b. intranasal corticosteroids
   c. antihistamines
   d. oral or topical decongestants
   e. leukotriene receptor antagonists

10. Which of the following therapies for allergic rhinitis has the fewest side effects?
    a. immunotherapy
    b. intranasal cromolyn sodium
    c. intranasal corticosteroids
    d. antihistamines
    e. leukotriene receptor antagonists

11. The mother of the child calls your office and requests "blood work" to confirm the diagnosis before she starts the child on the medications you recommended. You call back and tell her which of the following?
    a. laboratory testing is not essential for diagnosis or initiation of treatment
    b. radioallergosorbent testing (RAST) will be ordered
    c. she should not call the office again
    d. the child should be tested for food allergies
    e. you will order nasal smear, complete blood count (CBC), and serum IgE levels

12. 12. Which of the following is not a physiologically based treatment for allergic rhinitis?
    a. leukotriene receptor antagonist
    b. oral corticosteroids
    c. anticholinergics
    d. guaifenesin
    e. antihistamines

13. Which of the following systemic diseases is not associated with rhinitis?
    a. hypertension
    b. sarcoidosis
    c. Wegener's granulomatosis
    d. hypothyroidism
    e. amyloidosis

14. All of the following statements about immunotherapy are true except
    a. approximately 80% to 85% of patients will have significant long-lasting relief with continued therapy

b. it should not be initiated during pregnancy
c. anaphylaxis is rare
d. skin testing must be done prior to initiation
e. it is more effective for allergens of perennial rhinitis than for allergens of seasonal rhinitis

15. In patients with significant allergic rhinitis, quality of life is
    a. as debilitating as that of patients with moderate to severe reactive airway disease
    b. compromised as a result of decreased restful sleep
    c. not impaired in any way
    d. a and b
    e. a, b, and c

16. Which of the following statements about vasomotor rhinitis is false?
    a. nasal smears lack eosinophils
    b. the predominant feature is congestion and rhinorrhea, not sneezing and itching
    c. symptoms are associated with changes in temperature or humidity
    d. it is common in children
    e. hot or spicy foods can elicit symptoms

Clinical Case Management Problem

Define and describe rhinitis medicamentosa.

Answers

1. d. The child has allergic rhinitis with no seasonal pattern and seems to have perennial symptoms. There is no fever, purulent rhinorrhea, fetid breath, headache, or ear pain to suggest an infection. Allergic rhinitis is the sixth leading type of chronic disease in the United States and the most common nasal problem.

Symptoms of allergic rhinitis include intermittent nasal congestion; rhinorrhea; sneezing; watery eyes; and pruritus of the nose, palate, pharynx, ears, and eyes. Nasal congestion is more severe at night, causing mouth breathing, snoring, interference with sleep, tiredness, and irritability.

Physical signs include clear nasal secretions; edematous, boggy, bluish mucus membranes; and swollen turbinates. Exam might also reveal abnormalities of facial development, dental malocclusion, the "allergic gape" (continuous open mouth breathing), the "allergic shiners" (dark circles under the eyes), and the transverse nasal crease.

2. d. Sinusitis and otitis media are common complications of untreated allergic rhinitis caused by inflammation and obstruction of the sinus ostia and eustachian tube. Nasal polyps are a rare complication of allergic rhinitis and occur less in children than adults. However, they are a feature of cystic fibrosis. Epistaxis can occur with severe acute allergic rhinitis. Approximately 60% of patients with allergic rhinitis have asthma, and even those who do not may exhibit bronchial hyperresponsiveness.

3. b. The exposure to an allergen of an atopic host results in IgE production and infiltration of the nasal mucosa by inflammatory cells. Re-exposure to the allergen leads to bridging of IgE to the mast cells, resulting in initiation of "early phase reaction" characterized by degranulation of mast cells and release of inflammatory mediators such as histamine. "Late phase reaction" starts 6 to 8 hours after exposure, with secretion of eosinophil-derived mediators and damage to nasal epithelium. Repeated intranasal introduction of allergens causes "priming," a brisk response to a reduced provocation dose.

4. a. Perennial allergic rhinitis is most often associated with indoor allergens: house dust mites, animal dander, and molds. Cat and dog allergies are of major importance in the United States. Cockroaches and feathers can also be causes. Rare causes include cigarette smoke and nonspecific environmental pollutants.

5. d. All of the listed physical findings are found in patients with allergies; however, one is most likely to actually visualize the upward motion of nose rubbing (the salute) in children and not adults. Chronic nose rubbing and wrinkling of the nose is theorized to cause the horizontal nasal crease that is commonly seen at the junction of the bridge of the nose with the bulbous tip of the nose. Posterior pharyngeal wall lymphoid hyperplasia is also commonly known as "cobblestoning."

6. a. Family history is the most common predisposing factor to allergic rhinitis. Greater risk exists if more than one parent is atopic.

7. b. Seasonal allergic rhinitis (also known as hay fever or pollinosis) is caused by outdoor inhaled allergens, including tree, grass, and weed pollens. In temperate climates, airborne pollen responsible for seasonal allergic rhinitis appears in distinct phases. Gastroesophageal reflux disease can cause reflex bronchospasm, but this is unlikely the case here. Rhinitis medicamentosa is rebound nasal congestion with overuse of nasal decongestants.

8. e. The first and most important step in the treatment would be avoidance of known allergens and nonspecific or initial triggers. Identification and elimination is easiest for feathers, cockroaches, and dust mites. Use of allergen-proof mattress and pillow covers and removal of carpets are helpful steps, as is washing bed linens in hot water. Dehumidification is beneficial because mites thrive in high humidity. Most patients with pets are not willing to remove the pet from the household; however, not allowing the pet in the bedroom helps considerably. HEPA filters in bedrooms may be beneficial.

Pollen is the most difficult to avoid. Patients and parents need to be educated to avoid the outdoors during highest pollen count days, which is often not possible because of the patient's activities. Washing and changing clothes upon coming indoors during high pollen season is recommended. Another intervention is to keep windows closed and use air conditioning. If windows need to be opened, then daytime is better than night because many pollen counts such as mold and trees are highest at night. Window filters or filtering fans could be used as an alternative. Turbinectomy is an extreme measure taken when all other therapies have failed. Dietary restrictions do not help because allergic rhinitis is not triggered by food. Referral to an allergist may be considered for allergy testing in patients with severe symptoms that are unresponsive to conventional treatment and adherence to lifestyle changes or when the diagnosis is in question.

9. b. Intranasal corticosteroids (INCs) are by far the most efficacious agents for allergic rhinitis approved for use in children as young as 2 years of age. Intranasal cromolyn is most effective as a preventive medication when initiated before the onset of pollination. No clinically significant adverse effects are associated with this medication, making it attractive for use in children. It is less efficacious than INCs, however, and regular use—four times per day—is required for clinical effectiveness, thus reducing compliance. Antihistamines are useful for rhinorrhea and pruritus; however, they do not relieve congestion. Nonsedating forms, such as loratadine, ceterizine, and fexofenadine, are better choices because studies have shown that older antihistamines can cause psychomotor or cognitive impairment even without sedation. Topical decongestants can be used only for 3 to 5 days; if used longer, they can cause rebound congestion. Oral decongestants can be used with antihistamines but can cause hyperactivity and insomnia. They should be used with caution in patients with hypertension, thyroid disease, diabetes, and enlarged prostates. Leukotriene antagonists have similar efficacy to antihistamines but work better in combination with them.

10. b. Intranasal cromolyn sodium has almost no side effects other than possible local irritation and sneezing. The problems with this therapy are that it is not very efficacious and it is prophylactic, so it should be started prior to onset of symptoms and needs to be used four to six times daily. Thus, compliance is an issue. Antihistamines can cause sedation and interfere with school or work function. Immunotherapy can cause local reactions and, more important, anaphylaxis. Intranasal steroids can cause local irritation and bleeding and, rarely, septal perforation. Topical steroids do have some systemic absorption; however, in recommended doses they do not cause hypothalamic–pituitary axis suppression. Some studies do show minor effects on growth, so for children the lowest effective dose for the shortest amount of time necessary is recommended. Leukotriene receptor antagonists can cause influenza-like symptoms.

11. **a.** Laboratory studies are not always necessary, especially in patients with a clear-cut seasonal pattern and classic history. Food allergens do not trigger allergic rhinitis, so testing for this is not required. If the history is confusing, nasal smears can be done. Eosinophils in the smear indicate allergy. Eosinophilia in a CBC may suggest allergic rhinitis. Serum IgE values are not routinely recommended to test for atopy; however, an elevated value supports the diagnosis. Diagnostic tests such as RAST are helpful to confirm diagnosis and to determine specific triggers, and they may be appropriate in patients with severe symptoms not responsive to traditional treatment or with uncertain diagnosis.

12. **d.** Guaifenesin is an expectorant and is not indicated for the treatment of allergic rhinitis. Leukotriene antagonists inhibit the immune cascade, which can potentially cause allergic symptoms, and have been discussed previously. Oral corticosteroids are not routinely recommended but can be used for severe, acute disease for a short term as potent anti-inflammatory agents. Anticholinergics and topical ipratropium bromide are effective in treating the watery rhinorrhea of allergies. Antihistamines also help with pruritus.

13. **a.** Although antihypertensive agents such as reserpine can cause rhinorrhea, hypertension is not associated with allergic rhinitis. The other systemic diseases can be associated with rhinitis.

14. **e.** Immunotherapy is indicated in patients who do not have adequate relief from pharmacologic treatment, who cannot tolerate the medications, or in whom the pharmacologic treatments are contraindicated for other medical reasons. Immunotherapy has been proved to be effective for seasonal-type allergens such as grass, ragweed, and trees. Its efficacy in controlling dust and mold-related symptoms is not clear. There is no absolute recommendation for duration of therapy, but most believe that with 3 to 5 years of adequate symptom control, immunotherapy can be stopped, and that 65% of these patients will have continued long-lasting relief. If a patient does not show any improvement after 1 year of immunotherapy, it should be discontinued. All of the other statements about immunotherapy are true.

15. **d.** Allergic rhinitis can cause significant morbidity. It can be associated with other disorders, such as asthma, otitis media, eustachian dysfunction, sinusitis, atopic dermatitis, and allergic conjunctivitis. This can contribute to learning disabilities, sleep disorder, and daytime fatigue leading to compromised daily activity level and impaired school performance.

16. **d.** Vasomotor rhinitis is rarely seen in children. This disorder is poorly understood and is theoretically the result of an imbalance of the autonomic nervous system control of mucosal vasculature and mucous glands in which symptoms mimic allergic rhinitis but no allergic cause is found on testing.

Solution to the Clinical Case Management Problem

Rhinitis medicamentosa is the term used to describe the chronic nasal congestion that results as a rebound effect of prolonged or excessive use of topical nasal decongestant nose drops that work by vasoconstriction. The rebound swelling is caused by interstitial edema, not vasodilation. Therefore, topical decongestants should not be used for more than 5 days. Similar consequences can result from chronic topical use of other vasoconstrictors, such as cocaine. On examination, the nasal mucosa appears beefy red and swollen and may show areas of punctate bleeding. Diagnosis depends on history, physical exam, and positive response to nasal steroid treatment, which is required to wean off the offending medication.

Summary

Classification: Causes of seasonal allergic rhinitis (also known as hay fever or seasonal pollinosis) include tree, weed, and grass pollen; mold spores are a less likely cause. Seasonal allergic rhinitis is temporally related to seasons with high pollen counts and is variable by geographic location.

Perennial allergic rhinitis: Symptoms present at least 9 months out of the year; causes include dust mites, animal dander, feathers, mold, and cockroaches.

Frequency distribution: Approximately 20% seasonal, 40% perennial, and 40% mixed.

Etiology: Prolonged exposure to allergens is associated with allergen-specific IgE production leading to a cascade of events on re-exposure resulting in symptoms of allergic rhinitis.

Symptoms: Symptoms include nasal congestion; rhinorrhea; nasal and palatal pruritus; sneezing; nasal discharge; eye redness, itching, and tearing; and irritability and fatigue.

Signs

1. Allergic shiners: dark, puffy lower eyelids from venous stasis caused by impaired blood flow through inflamed, edematous nasal mucous membranes
2. Allergic salute: rubbing nose with palm of hand in an upward motion, usually only seen in children; this gives rise to nasal crease, a horizontal skin fold over the bridge of nose
3. Dennis–Morgan lines: extra skin folds on the lower eyelids secondary to recurrent conjunctival edema
4. Pale, blue, boggy nasal turbinates and mucous membranes
5. Postnasal drainage
6. Cobblestoning (lymphoid hyperplasia) of posterior pharyngeal wall
7. Allergic gape: continuous mouth breathing

Diagnosis: The diagnosis is made by clinical history and physical exam, nasal smear with eosinophils, RAST or enzyme-linked immunosorbent assay testing, and skin allergy testing.

Associated disorders: These include chronic sinusitis, otitis media (acute and chronic), adenoid and tonsillar hypertrophy associated with obstructive sleep apnea, asthma, and atopic dermatitis.

Differential diagnosis: This includes eosinophilic nonallergic rhinitis, infectious rhinitis, vasomotor rhinitis, rhinitis medicamentosa, and systemic diseases (sarcoidosis, Wegener's granulomatosis, amyloidosis, and hypothyroidism).

Treatment: This involves the avoidance of allergen as much as is feasible. Inhaled corticosteroids are most effective and first-line therapy, and they are approved for children as young as 2 years of age. Nonsedating antihistamine and leukotriene receptor antagonists (not any more efficacious than antihistamines alone, but better response when added to antihistamines) can also be used. Mast cell stabilizers can be useful in some symptom relief; use decongestants sparingly. Immunotherapy can be considered in children older than age 5 years.

Suggested Reading

Behrman RE, Kliegman RM, Jenson HB, eds: *Nelson Textbook of Pediatrics*, 17th ed. Philadelphia: Saunders, 2004.

Lai L, Casale TB, Stokes J: Pediatric allergic rhinitis: Treatment. *Immunol Allergy Clin North Am* 25:283–299, 2005.

Mahr T, Sheth K: Update on allergic rhinitis. *Pediatr Rev* 26:284–289, 2005.

Milgrom H, Leung D: Allergic rhinitis. In: Behrman RE, Kliegman RM, Jenson HB, eds, *Nelson Textbook of Pediatrics*, 17th ed. Philadelphia: Saunders, 2004.

Passalacqua G, Durham S: Allergic rhinitis and its impact on asthma update: Allergen immunotherapy. *J Allergy Clin Immunol* 119(4):881–891, 2007.

Quillen D, Feller D: Diagnosing rhinitis: Allergic vs. nonallergic. *Am Fam Physician* 73: 1583–1590, 2006.

Wheeler P, Wheeler S: Vasomotor rhinitis. *Am Fam Physician* 72(6):1057–1062, 2005.

c. there is dermatomal distribution of the lesions
d. diagnosis is usually made on clinical findings
e. these lesions are not seen in immunocompromised patients

CLINICAL CASE PROBLEM 1

A 3-Year-Old with a Rash and Fever

A 3-year-old comes to your office with fatigue and irritability and a low-grade fever that he has had for 3 days. The father relates to you that the child attends day care, where a virus is "going around." The father used acetaminophen, which has helped to decrease irritability; although the child's appetite is suppressed, he is still taking in a good amount of fluids.

On physical examination, the child does not look ill. His temperature is 38°C. His skin examination shows scattered small vesicles on an erythematous base. The rash was seen first on the face and seems to be spreading to the trunk.

SELECT THE BEST ANSWER TO THE FOLLOWING QUESTIONS

1. What is the most likely diagnosis in this child at this time?
   a. rubella (German measles)
   b. adenoviral exanthem
   c. varicella-zoster
   d. mumps
   e. rubeola

2. What is the most outstanding feature of this illness?
   a. constitutional symptoms
   b. the appearance of a rash at the same time as the temperature falls
   c. the description of the lesion as a "dew drop on a rose petal"
   d. recurrence of the rash in adulthood
   e. benign nature of this infection

3. What is the causative agent of this infection?
   a. human parvovirus
   b. adenovirus
   c. rhinovirus
   d. human herpesvirus
   e. Epstein–Barr virus

4. This infection can occur in adulthood. Which of the following is a unique feature in this recurrence?
   a. incidence varies with gender and race
   b. there is no long-term sequelae with the recurrence

5. What is the current recommendation for the treatment and prevention of this condition?
   a. no antibiotics, no vaccinations
   b. no antibiotics, an antiviral agent to prevent complications
   c. no antibiotics, one vaccination in childhood
   d. antibiotics, no vaccinations in childhood
   e. no antiviral, no antibiotics, two vaccinations in childhood

6. The father is concerned about his 5-year-old child contracting the disease. What will you tell him?
   a. there is no cause for concern
   b. the child will get herpes zoster infection
   c. the child is exposed and will get severe varicella infection
   d. all of the above
   e. none of the above

7. What is (are) a complication(s) associated with varicella infection?
   a. scarring
   b. secondary bacterial infection with staphylococcus and streptococcus
   c. pneumonia
   d. encephalitis and cerebellar ataxia
   e. all of the above

CLINICAL CASE PROBLEM 2

A 5-Year-Old with Cough, Coryza, and Conjunctivitis

A 5-year-old whose family believes that immunizations can cause autism is brought to the office with a 3-day history of fever, nonproductive cough, coryza, and conjunctivitis. This morning, a rash appeared on his forehead and behind the ears, and it appears to be spreading to his upper arms and chest.

On physical examination, you note a fine maculopapular rash over the face that appears to be spreading to the back and thighs.

8. What is the most likely diagnosis in this patient?
   a. roseola infantum
   b. scarlet fever
   c. meningococcemia
   d. rubeola
   e. rubella

9. What are the hallmark signs and symptoms of this infection?
   a. Koplik's spots
   b. coalescing erythematous maculopapular rash
   c. suboccipital and postauricular lymph node enlargement
   d. conjunctivitis
   e. all of the above

10. Which of the following is a relatively common complication of this infection?
    a. encephalomyelitis
    b. myocarditis
    c. pneumonia
    d. thrombocytopenic purpura
    e. keratoconjunctivitis

11. What treatment recommendations will you make to the father?
    a. amoxicillin
    b. erythromycin
    c. supportive care
    d. vitamin A
    e. ribavirin

12. What is the recommended immunization schedule for the prevention of this infection?
    a. four doses at 2, 4, and 6 months with a booster at 15 months
    b. three doses at 2, 4, and 6 months
    c. two doses at 12 to 15 months and 4 to 6 years
    d. three doses at 0, 1, and, 6 months
    e. two doses at 1 year and 15 months

13. What would be the recommendations for the exposed members of the family?
    a. none
    b. administration of immunoglobulin and measles vaccine
    c. immunoglobulin only
    d. measles vaccine
    e. vitamin A

CLINICAL CASE PROBLEM 3

A 4-Year-Old with a Bright Red Rash on Both Cheeks

A 4-year-old is brought to the office by his mother. The child has had a low-grade fever, headache, and a sore throat for the past week. Four days ago, he suddenly developed a bright red rash on his cheeks, which during the past 2 days has spread to the trunk, arms, and legs.

On physical examination, the child has erythema of the cheeks and a maculopapular rash with central clearing on the trunk spreading to the extremities. There are no other significant findings.

14. What is the most likely diagnosis in this child?
    a. rubella
    b. scarlet fever
    c. human herpesvirus 6
    d. erythema infectiosum
    e. measles

15. What is the causative agent of this infection?
    a. herpesvirus 6
    b. human papillomavirus
    c. rhinovirus
    d. human parvovirus B19
    e. adenovirus

16. What are the cardinal features of this infection?
    a. circumoral pallor and sandpaper-like appearance of the trunk
    b. fine pustular appearance and a bright red macular–papular rash with central clearing
    c. erythematous cheeks with a lacy reticular pattern
    d. coalesced lesions in various stages (vesicles, bullae, and papules)
    e. none of the above

17. The mother asks you what she can do about the slap-cheeked appearance. People are staring at her as though she has been abusing her child.
    a. tell her to tell them to stop staring; it's none of their business
    b. tell her to give the child acetaminophen every 4 to 6 hours
    c. tell her to wash the face repeatedly with cold water
    d. advise her to keep the child out of the sun
    e. tell her that if it does not clear in 3 to 5 days, you will give her an antibiotic cream

18. The mother then tells you that she is 4 months pregnant and asks whether she should be worried about anything. What do you tell her?
    a. there is no cause for concern; this is a self-limiting illness
    b. there is a small chance for fetal demise or congenital defects
    c. tell her you are too busy and ask her why she doesn't just look it up on the Internet like everyone else
    d. all of the above
    e. none of the above

MATCHING QUESTIONS

Eleven disease-producing pathogens or disease entities are listed, and 11 disease-defining characteristics are listed after. Match each disease-producing pathogen or disease entity to its defining characteristic.

19. Herpes varicella
20. Herpes simplex
21. Coxsackievirus
22. Kawasaki disease
23. Adenovirus
24. Lyme disease
25. Parainfluenza virus
26. Tinea versicolor
27. Tinea corporis
28. Pityriasis rosea
29. Molluscum contagiosum

a. Discrete, dome-shaped papules
b. Herald patch
c. Erythema chronicum migrans
d. Hand-foot-and-mouth disease
e. Acute gingivostomatitis
f. Ringworm
g. Primary cause of conjunctivitis
h. Primary cause of infectious croup
i. Hyperpigmented or hypopigmented lesions
j. Coronary vasculitis
k. "Crops of lesions": vesicles

Answers

1. c. This is a classic presentation of chickenpox (varicella-zoster). A prodrome of low-grade fever and general malaise usually precedes the defining rash by 1 or 2 days. The rash begins as scattered red macules seen first on the face and trunk progressing to the classic lesion of small vesicles with erythematous bases. The lesions spread centrifugally to involve all skin surfaces and possibly mucous membranes (lips and vulva). Lesions at different stages of development are found simultaneously. They are pruritic, and scratching may lead to excoriations and superficial skin infections and scarring. Treatment is symptomatic.

2. c. The classic description of the lesion is a "dew drop on a rose petal," corresponding to a clear vesicle on an erythematous base.

3. d. Varicella-zoster virus (VZV) is a neurotropic human herpesvirus. The herpesviruses are a large group of double-stranded DNA viruses that also includes oral and genital herpes (herpes simplex virus types 1 and 2), Epstein–Barr virus, and cytomegalovirus.

4. c. Herpes zoster (shingles) is caused by reactivation of latent VZV. Therefore, shingles is uncommon in childhood and has no seasonal variation. It is seen primarily in the elderly or in the immunocompromised, especially those with human immunodeficiency virus or lymphoreticular malignancies. When the virus is reactivated from its latent state in the dorsal root ganglia, inflammatory changes occur in the sensory root ganglia and in the skin of the associated dermatome. The clinical presentation is that of an erythematous vesicular rash associated with pain before, during, and after the rash in a dermatomal distribution.

5. e. Antibiotics are not recommended. Antiviral therapy with acyclovir is not recommended routinely in the treatment of uncomplicated chickenpox in an otherwise healthy child because of marginal benefit, cost of therapy, and low risk of complications. The Centers for Disease Control and Prevention recommends the first dose of varicella vaccine at 12 to 15 months of age and a newly recommended second dose administered at 4 to 6 years of age.

6. e. Varicella has a transmission rate of 65% to 86% to susceptible household contacts. Patients are contagious from 24 to 48 hours before onset of rash until all vesicles are crusted (3 to 7 days from onset). Incidence has declined considerably secondary to vaccination. "Breakthrough varicella" may occur in immunized children but is usually very mild. Herpes zoster is very rare in children younger than 10 years of age unless infected in utero or in the first year of life.

7. e. Complications are rare in immunocompetent patients. The most common complication is scarring and skin superinfection with staphylococcus and streptococcus. Other complications mentioned are rare. Central nervous system complications are highest among patients younger than 5 years or older than 20 years of age.

8. d. The diagnosis is apparent from the characteristic clinical presentation. The rash must be distinguished from all other conditions mentioned as well as from those resulting from echovirus, coxsackievirus, and adenovirus; infectious mononucleosis; toxoplasmosis; rickettsial diseases; Kawasaki disease; serum sickness; and drug rashes.

9. e. Major symptoms of measles are Koplik's spots, a coalescing erythematous maculopapular rash, suboccipital and postauricular lymph node enlargement, and conjunctivitis. Rubeola (measles) has an incubation period of 8 to 12 days from exposure to onset of symptoms. The prodromal phase includes fever, nonspecific upper respiratory symptom and signs (i.e., cough, coryza, conjunctivitis, and a low- to moderate-grade fever), followed by an exanthematous phase. Koplik's spots (1-mm, bluish-white lesions on an erythematous base) can be seen only during the first few days of symptoms. They usually appear on the buccal mucosa opposite the lower molars and quickly coalesce into larger lesions. The temperature in rubeola increases as the rash appears. Erythematous maculopapular rash, which blanches, starts at the hairline and spreads to the forehead, face, neck, trunk, and extremities, including the palms and soles. The rash begins to disappear in approximately 3 days in the same manner (from head down). Fine desquamation may occur during healing. The total duration of the rash is approximately 7 days.

10. c. The more common complications are bronchopneumonia and otitis media. Encephalitis, myocarditis, thrombocytopenic purpura, and keratoconjunctivitis giant cell pneumonia are much less common; however, all are possible. Subacute sclerosing panencephalitis can occur as a complication of measles many years after the acute episode but is now extremely rare in the United States.

11. c. There is no specific therapy. Treatment is entirely supportive. Antipyretics (acetaminophen or ibuprofen) for fever, bed rest, and adequate fluid intake are advised. Bacterial complications (e.g., otitis media) may need to be treated with antibiotics.

12. c. The recommended immunization schedule for measles is two doses at 12 to 15 months and 4 to 6 years. Experts agree that there is no association between autism and measles–mumps–rubella vaccination.

13. b. Measles vaccination is recommended for susceptible household contacts within less than 72 hours of exposure. For prolonged exposure (more than 72 hours), immunoglobulin (IG), along with measles vaccine, is indicated. IG can prevent disease if given within 6 days of exposure. It is recommended for individuals with significant exposure to a patient with measles, particularly those at risk of complications (e.g., household members, children younger than 1 year of age, pregnant women, and immunocompromised individuals). Immunocompetent household contacts do not need IG if they have received at least one dose of measles vaccine at age 12 months or older.

14. d. See answer 17.

15. d. See answer 17.

16. c. See answer 17.

17. d. Erythema infectiosum is caused by human parvovirus B19. It occurs mostly during spring months; localized outbreaks among children and adolescents are common. The infection begins as a low-grade fever and produces a three-stage rash. In the first stage, a bright red "slapped-cheek" rash appears on the cheeks and forehead with circumoral pallor. During the second stage, rash spreads distally to the trunk and extremities with a lacy reticular appearance as it resolves. The third stage is highly variable, with rash recurring for up to several weeks. Recurrences after exercise, application of heat, or emotional distress are not uncommon. Constitutional symptoms include headache, pharyngitis, myalgias, arthritis, gastrointestinal upset, and coryza. The illness usually lasts 5 to 10 days. The rash may last from a few days to several weeks. It is frequently pruritic. Treatment is symptomatic.

18. b. Primary infection with human parvovirus B19 in pregnant women is associated with nonimmune fetal hydrops and fetal demise. The reported frequency after exposure ranges from 5% to 15%. Therefore, the mother should try to avoid contagion.

19. k. The viral agent is herpes varicella (chickenpox). Disease-defining characteristics are crops of small, red papules that develop into oval vesicles on an erythematous base.

20. e. The viral agent is herpes simplex virus. The disease-defining characteristic is acute herpetic gingivostomatitis, which is the most common cause of stomatitis in children ages 1 to 3 years.

21. d. The viral agent is coxsackievirus A16. Disease-defining characteristics are hand-foot-and-mouth disease and an enteroviral exanthem–enanthem with the distribution portrayed by the name.

22. j. The disease entity is Kawasaki disease. The disease-defining characteristic is coronary vasculitis, also known as mucocutaneous lymph node syndrome or infantile polyarteritis. Cardiac involvement is the most important manifestation of Kawasaki disease (10% to 40% of children within the first 2 weeks of illness). The causal agent is unknown.

23. g. The viral agent is adenovirus. The disease-defining characteristic is adenovirus, the most common cause of conjunctivitis.

24. c. The disease entity is Lyme disease. The disease-defining characteristic is erythema chronicum migrans, which begins as an erythematous macule or papule at the site of a tick bite. The causative organism is *Borrelia burgdorferi*, which develops into an expanding erythematous annular lesion with central clearing and often reaches a diameter of 16 cm.

25. h. The viral agent is parainfluenza virus. The disease-defining characteristic is that it is the most common cause of infectious croup.

26. i. The disease entity is tinea versicolor. The disease-defining characteristic is hypopigmented or hyperpigmented macules covered with a fine scale. Lesions begin in a perifollicular location, enlarge, and form confluent patches, most commonly on the neck, upper chest, back, and upper arms. The causative organism is dimorphic yeast (*Pityrosporon orbiculare* [*Malassezia furfur*]).

27. f. The disease entity is tinea corporis. The disease-defining characteristic is ringworm, the common name for a group of disorders known as dermatophytoses. The three principal genera responsible for dermato-phyte infections are Trichophyton, Microsporum, and Epidermophyton. A classical lesion begins as a dry, mildly erythematous, elevated, scaly papule or plaque and spreads centrifugally as it clears centrally to form the characteristic annular lesion responsible for the designation ringworm.

28. b. The disease entity is pityriasis rosea. The disease-defining characteristic is the herald patch, a solitary, round, or oval lesion that may occur anywhere on the body and is often but not always identifiable by its large size. The herald patch usually precedes the generalized maculopapular eruption of oval or round lesions that crop. The rash can assume a characteristic Christmas-tree appearance on the back.

29. a. The disease entity is molluscum contagiosum. The disease-defining characteristic describes a disorder characterized by discrete, dome-shaped papules varying in size from 1 to 5 mm. Typically, these lesions have a central umbilication from which a cheesy material can be expressed. The papules may occur anywhere on the body, but the face, eyelids, neck, axillae, and thighs are sites of predilection. The causative agent is a DNA virus, the largest member of the poxvirus group.

Summary

The summary is limited to a discussion of what are termed the "big five" viral exanthems in children because most other conditions are discussed in the chapter.

1. Roseola infantum (exanthema subitum): erythematous maculopapular rash (Figs. 112-1 and 112-2)
   a. HHV-6 and HHV-7 infection
   b. 95% in children younger than age 3 years; peak incidence at 6 to 15 months of age
   c. High fever (37.9°C to 40°C [101°F to 106°F]) followed by the appearance of rash within 12 to 24 hour after fever resolution
2. Erythema infectiosum (fifth disease): hallmark of erythema infectiosum is the characteristic rash, which occurs in three stages (Fig. 112-3)
   a. Initial stage: erythematous facial flushing or "slapped cheek" appearance
   b. Second stage: lacy reticular rash spreading concurrently to trunk and proximal extremities
   c. Third stage: rash resolves spontaneously without desquamation; can recur with exposure to sun, heat, stress, and exercise
3. Rubella: rash similar to that of mild rubeola or scarlet fever
   a. Most characteristic sign is retro auricular, posterior cervical, and postoccipital lymphadenopathy
   b. Mild constitutional symptoms

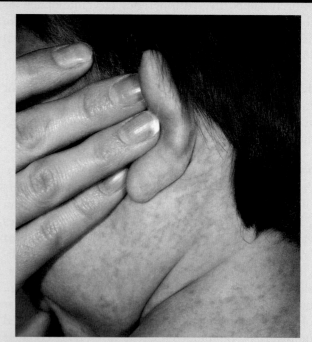

Figure 112-1

Roseola: Numerous pale pink, almond-shaped macules. (Reprinted with permission from Habif TP: *Clinical Dermatology*, 4th ed. St. Louis: Mosby, 2004.) (See Color Plate 5.)

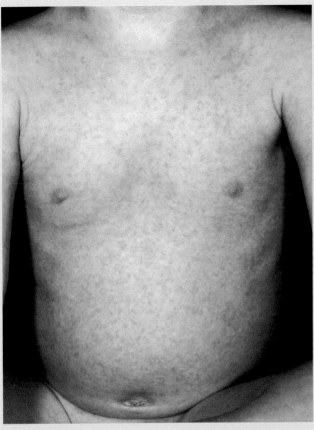

Figure 112-2

Roseola: Pale pink macules may appear first on the neck. (Reprinted with permission from Habif TP: *Clinical Dermatology*, 4th ed. St. Louis: Mosby, 2004.) (See Color Plate 6.)

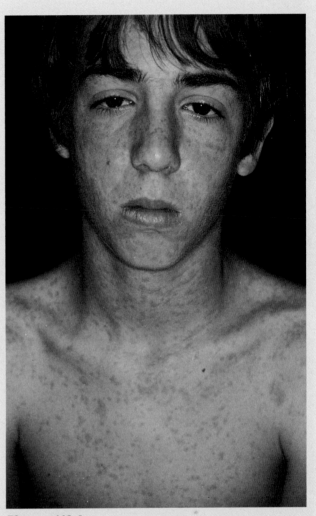

Figure 112-4

Measles. Early eruptive stage with involvement of the face and trunk. Eruption has become confluent on the face. (Reprinted with permission from Habif TP: *Clinical Dermatology*, 4th ed. St. Louis: Mosby, 2004.) (See Color Plate 8.)

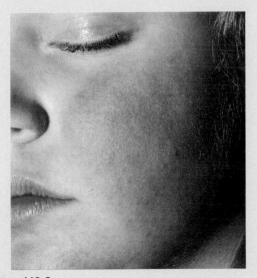

Figure 112-3

Erythema infectiosum. Facial erythema "slapped cheek." The red plaque covers the cheek and spares the nasolabial fold and the circumoral region. (Reprinted with permission from Habif TP: *Clinical Dermatology*, 4th ed. St. Louis: Mosby, 2004.) (See Color Plate 7.)

4. Measles (rubeola): maculopapular rash erupting successively over the neck and face, trunk, arms, and legs, accompanied by a high fever (Fig. 112-4)
   a. Three clinical stages: an incubation stage, a prodromal stage with an enanthem (Koplik's spots, pathognomonic), and a final stage with a maculopapular rash accompanied by high fever
   b. Prodromal symptoms include three Cs: cough, coryza, and conjunctivitis
   c. Lymph nodes at the angle of the jaw and in the posterior cervical region usually enlarged
   d. Severity of the disease directly related to the extent and confluence of the rash; mnemonic is cc-CPK: cough, coryza, conjunctivitis, photophobia, Koplik's spots
5. Scarlet fever: upper respiratory tract infection associated with a characteristic rash, caused by group A β-hemolytic streptococcus (Figs. 112-5 to 112-7)

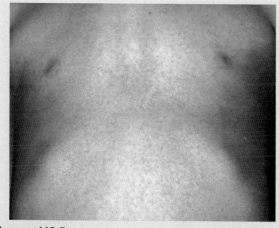

Figure 112-5

Scarlet fever: Early eruptive stage on the trunk showing numerous pinpoint red papules. (Reprinted with permission from Habif TP: *Clinical Dermatology*, 4th ed. St. Louis: Mosby, 2004.) (See Color Plate 9.)

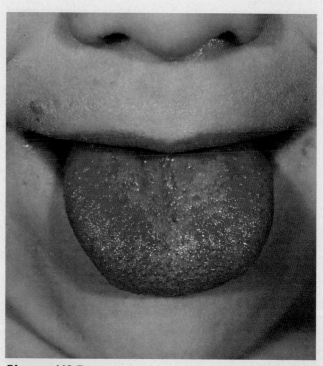

Figure 112-7

Scarlet fever: "Strawberry tongue." (Reprinted with permission from Habif TP: *Clinical Dermatology*, 4th ed. St. Louis: Mosby, 2004.) (See Color Plate 11.)

a. Presents as fever, chills, headache, vomiting, and pharyngitis
b. Diffuse, finely papular, erythematous eruption producing a bright red discoloration of the skin, which blanches on pressure and has the texture of coarse sandpaper
c. Circumoral pallor common
d. Penicillin V is drug of choice

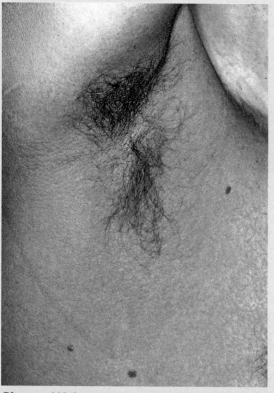

Figure 112-6

Scarlet fever: Fully evolved eruption. Numerous papules giving a sandpaper-like texture to the skin. (Reprinted with permission from Habif TP: *Clinical Dermatology*, 4th ed. St. Louis: Mosby, 2004.) (See Color Plate 10.)

Suggested Reading

Behrman RE, Kliegman RM, Jenson HB, eds: *Nelson Textbook of Pediatrics*, 17th ed. Philadelphia: Saunders, 2004.
Habif TP: *Clinical Dermatology*, 4th ed. St. Louis: Mosby, 2004.

COLOR PLATES

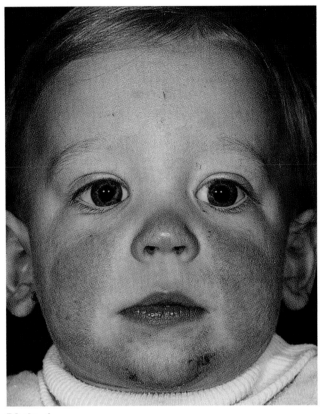

Plate 1

A 2-month-old infant with an erythematous maculopapular eruption covering his cheeks. (Reproduced from Habif TB: *Clinical Dermatology*, 4th ed. St. Louis, MO: Mosby, 2004, Figure 5-5, with permission.) (See Fig. 103-1.)

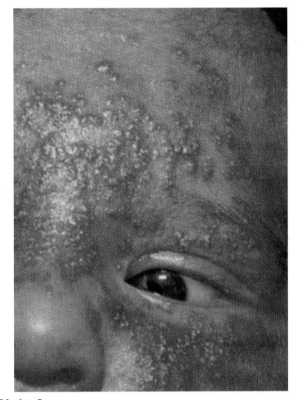

Plate 3

A 2-week-old infant with small pimple-like lesions on his face. (Reproduced from Cohen BA: *Pediatric Dermatology*, 3rd ed. Philadelphia: Mosby, 2005, with permission.) (See Fig. 103-3.)

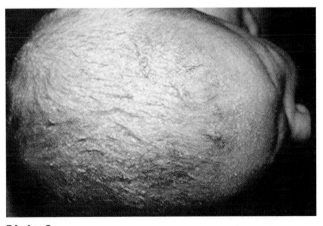

Plate 2

A 3-week-old infant with a crusty, yellowish rash with some erythema on her scalp. (Reproduced from Cohen BA: *Pediatric Dermatology*, 3rd ed. Philadelphia: Mosby, 2005, with permission.) (See Fig. 103-2.)

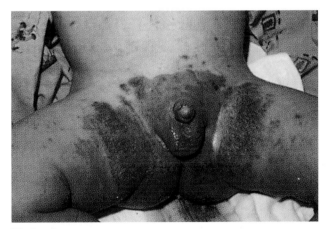

Plate 4

An 8-month-old infant with an intensely erythematous diaper dermatitis including a scalloped border and sharply demarcated edge. "Satellite lesions" are also present on the lower abdomen and thighs. (Reproduced from Behrman R, Kliegman R, Jenson H: Cutaneous fungal infections. In: *Nelson Textbook of Pediatrics*, 17th ed. Philadelphia: Saunders, 2004, Figure 656-5, with permission.) (See Fig. 103-4.)

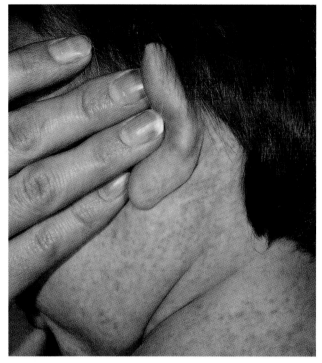

Plate 5

Roseola: Numerous pale pink, almond-shaped macules. (Reprinted with permission from Habif TP: *Clinical Dermatology*, 4th ed. St. Louis: Mosby, 2004.) (See Fig. 112-1.)

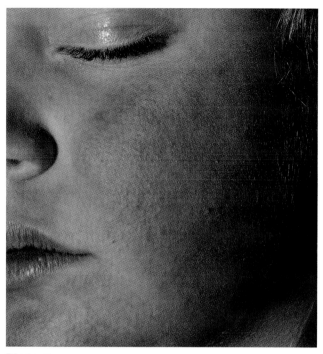

Plate 7

Erythema infectiosum. Facial erythema "slapped cheek." The red plaque covers the cheek and spares the nasolabial fold and the circumoral region. (Reprinted with permission from Habif TP: *Clinical Dermatology*, 4th ed. St. Louis: Mosby, 2004.) (See Fig. 112-3.)

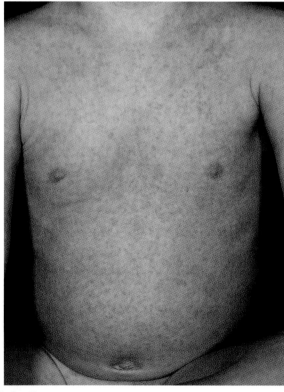

Plate 6

Roseola: Pale pink macules may appear first on the neck. (Reprinted with permission from Habif TP: *Clinical Dermatology*, 4th ed. St. Louis: Mosby, 2004.) (See Fig. 112-2.)

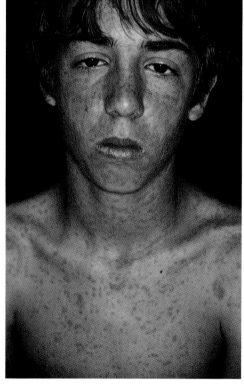

Plate 8

Measles. Early eruptive stage with involvement of the face and trunk. Eruption has become confluent on the face. (Reprinted with permission from Habif TP: *Clinical Dermatology*, 4th ed. St. Louis: Mosby, 2004.) (See Fig. 112-4.)

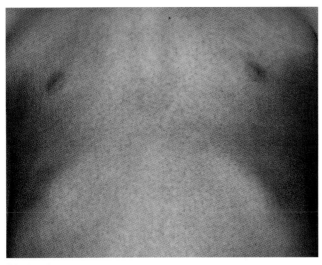

Plate 9

Scarlet fever: Early eruptive stage on the trunk showing numerous pinpoint red papules. (Reprinted with permission from Habif TP: *Clinical Dermatology*, 4th ed. St. Louis: Mosby, 2004.) (See Fig. 112-5.)

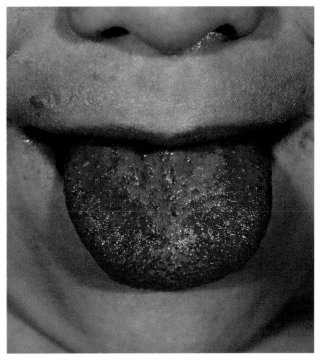

Plate 11

Scarlet fever: "Strawberry tongue." (Reprinted with permission from Habif TP: *Clinical Dermatology*, 4th ed. St. Louis: Mosby, 2004.) (See Fig. 112-7.)

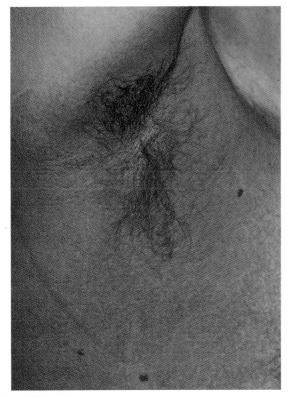

Plate 10

Scarlet fever: Fully evolved eruption. Numerous papules giving a sandpaper-like texture to the skin. (Reprinted with permission from Habif TP: *Clinical Dermatology*, 4th ed. St. Louis: Mosby, 2004.) (See Fig. 112-6.)

Cardiac Murmurs

CLINICAL CASE PROBLEM 1

A 3-Year-Old Child with a Cardiac Murmur

A 3-year-old child is brought to your office by his mother for a periodic health examination. The child has been well and has no history of significant medical illness. He has reached all of his developmental milestones.

On physical examination, the child is in the 50th percentile for weight and height. His blood pressure is 90/70 mmHg. He has a grade II/VI short ejection systolic murmur heard maximally along the left sternal edge from the midsternum to the lower end of the sternum. There is no radiation of the murmur to either the neck or the back. There is a musical quality to the sound and no associated thrill with this murmur. The child's pulse is 84 beats/minute and regular. The femoral artery pulses are normal and are not delayed. The rest of the physical examination is normal.

SELECT THE BEST ANSWER TO THE FOLLOWING QUESTIONS

1. Which of the following statements best reflect(s) the character of this heart murmur?
   a. the location of the heart murmur (mid to low sternum) increases the probability of this murmur being pathologic
   b. systolic timing of the heart murmur increases the probability of this murmur being pathologic
   c. grade of the murmur (II/VI rather than I/VI) increases the probability of this murmur being pathologic
   d. musical quality of the sound and no thrill associated
   e. all of the above

2. This murmur is best referred to as which of the following?
   a. Gibson's murmur
   b. Austin Flint murmur
   c. Still's murmur
   d. Carey Coombs murmur
   e. Graham Steell murmur

3. Which of the following signs or symptoms is not associated with "innocent" cardiac murmurs?
   a. low frequency
   b. an associated thrill
   c. short ejection systolic in timing
   d. grade I or grade II in audibility
   e. a and b

4. The intensity of the murmur is increased by which of the following?
   a. anemic states
   b. exercise
   c. febrile illness
   d. anxiety or excitement
   e. all of the above

5. At this time, what should you do?
   a. call the pediatric cardiologist immediately
   b. tell the child's mother that the child has a heart murmur but "not to worry…it probably isn't anything important"
   c. tell the mother that all heart murmurs need to be taken very seriously; therefore, it is probably best to have the pediatric cardiologist do "every test he can"
   d. tell the mother that the heart sound you hear (a very soft murmur) is very common and occurs in at least half of all children
   e. tell her nothing; there is no need to cause her unnecessary worry

6. At this time, which of the following investigations should be performed on the child?
   a. a chest x-ray
   b. an electrocardiogram (ECG)
   c. an echocardiogram
   d. none of the above
   e. a, b, and c

CLINICAL CASE PROBLEM 2

A 2-Week-Old Infant with a Harsh Grade III/VI Pansystolic Heart Murmur

A 2-week-old infant is brought to your office by his mother for a checkup and establishment of care. They have just moved into the area and you have not seen the baby before. The mother states that the baby was born at term and she had a normal pregnancy.

On examination, the infant has a grade III/VI harsh pansystolic heart murmur heard along the lower left sternal edge. There is no radiation of the murmur. The heart rate is 82 beats/minute and regular. There is no thrill. The blood pressure is 80/60 mmHg. No other abnormalities are found on examination. The infant is in the 50th percentile for height and weight.

7. What is the most likely cardiac diagnosis in this infant?
   a. innocent cardiac murmur
   b. tetralogy of Fallot
   c. pulmonary atresia
   d. ventricular septal defect (VSD)
   e. coarctation of the aorta

8. At this time, the infant should
   a. have immediate surgery
   b. be managed with digoxin and diuretics
   c. be managed with digoxin, diuretics, and an angiotensin-converting enzyme inhibitor
   d. have an immediate cardiac catheterization performed followed by surgical closure within 3 months
   e. none of the above

9. What preventive health practices should be followed for the infant described here?
   a. prophylaxis against bacterial endocarditis if dental work is to be done
   b. cardiac catheterizations every 3 months until resolution
   c. echocardiograms every 3 months until resolution
   d. a and c
   e. none of the above

10. What is the prevalence of cardiac murmurs in childhood?
    a. 50%
    b. 60%
    c. 70%
    d. 80%
    e. 90%

11. What is the most common pathologic cardiac murmur in childhood?
    a. atrial septal defect (ASD)
    b. tetralogy of Fallot
    c. VSD
    d. transposition of the great arteries
    e. aortic stenosis

12. Which of the following is (are) a common innocent cardiac murmur(s) in childhood?
    a. pulmonary flow murmur of newborn (systolic)
    b. venous hum of late infancy and early childhood

    c. Still's aortic vibratory systolic murmur
    d. pulmonary ejection systolic murmur of adolescence and childhood
    e. all of the above

CLINICAL CASE PROBLEM 3

A Baby with Abnormal Facies and a Murmur

A mother brings her child in for a 2-month visit. She gives a history of no prenatal care and a normal vaginal delivery. The baby has received no medical care since discharge. The infant has a large, protruding tongue; short palpebral fissures; and epicanthal folds. He has a simian palmar crease and a large space between the first and second toes. On cardiac examination, you note a harsh III/VI systolic murmur on the left sternal border.

13. Your leading cardiac diagnosis is
    a. Still's murmur
    b. VSD
    c. teratology of Fallot
    d. endocardial cushion defect
    e. hypoplastic left heart

CLINICAL CASE PROBLEM 4

Heart Murmur in a Term Infant

You are asked to evaluate a term infant in the delivery room. He was born a few minutes earlier by spontaneous vaginal delivery with Apgar scores of 9 and 9. The mother had good prenatal care and a normal pregnancy. No significant family history is noted. On physical examination, the infant appears alert and is active and crying. Acrocyanosis is noted on extremities. A grade II/VI soft, systolic murmur is audible at the left upper sternal border. Otherwise, the exam is completely normal.

14. What would you do about the murmur at this time?
    a. order an ECG and chest x-ray
    b. order an echocardiogram
    c. get a cardiology consultation
    d. perform a second detailed physical exam at 24 hours
    e. all newborns have transient murmurs; it will go away eventually

Answers

1. e. This murmur has all the characteristics of an innocent classic vibratory murmur of childhood. It is a low-frequency vibratory, "twanging string," groaning, squeaking, or musical murmur located at the mid to low sternal border. It is systolic in timing and has no associated thrill. Most important, the child appears healthy, with normal growth and development. The grading of murmurs is from I to VI. Grade I is very faintly auscultated with the stethoscope. Grade II can be heard more clearly. Grade III is a loud murmur with no associated thrill. Grade IV is also loud, with a palpable thrill. Grade V can be heard with the stethoscope tilted off of the patient's chest, and grade VI can be heard without a stethoscope. Location, quality, and timing (systole or diastole) are critical characteristics of a murmur.

2. c. This murmur, which is described as "vibratory" or "musical" in nature, is known as Still's murmur. Still's murmur is safely diagnosed clinically, and laboratory studies add nothing to its assessment. However, any murmur associated with failure to thrive, no matter how innocent sounding, should prompt further investigation. All others are diastolic murmurs.

3. b. A palpable thrill is always pathologic and demands a further workup. A murmur associated with thrill increases the grading of the murmur to a grade IV. A murmur is likely pathological if the patient is symptomatic or physical exam reveals cyanosis, abnormal pulse, abnormal heart sounds, diastolic murmur, or systolic murmur grade III or more associated with thrill and abnormal ECG or chest x-ray.

4. e. Other characteristics of an innocent cardiac murmur (e.g., a Still's murmur) include the following: It is low in frequency and localized, and it is seldom greater than grade II/VI in intensity. Still's murmur is best heard with the bell of the stethoscope in a supine position. Anxiety, febrile illness, anemic states, and exercise increase the intensity. The murmur may disappear briefly with a maximum Valsalva maneuver.

5. d. In explaining heart murmurs to parents, not just what you say but also how you say it is very important. It is important to be reassuring in your tone and inform the mother that more than 80% of children have innocent murmurs of one type or another sometime during childhood, usually beginning at approximately age 3 or 4 years. Make sure that you provide an opportunity for the mother to ask any questions that she may have.

It is extremely unwise not to tell the parents when you detect a heart murmur in a young child. Sooner or later, someone is going to hear it and mention it. At that time, it will come back to haunt you. It is far better to tell the parent(s) that a heart murmur exists but that you are confident that it is innocent. If you are not positive, an elective referral to a pediatric cardiologist would be reasonable.

6. d. Still's murmur is safely diagnosed clinically, and laboratory and diagnostic imaging studies add nothing to its assessment. It may be confused with VSD. A VSD murmur is usually harsh, grade II–III/VI accompanied by a palpable thrill.

7. d. This infant most likely has a small VSD. Most commonly, the murmur is detected at 2 to 6 weeks of age when the infant returns for the initial checkup after hospital discharge. The typical heart murmur associated with a VSD is harsh, pansystolic, and best heard at the lower left sternal edge. Even as the VSD becomes smaller, it maintains its regurgitant characteristic of starting off with the first heart sound (holosystolic timing). As a VSD closes and becomes smaller, the murmur can actually become louder until the VSD is closed. Infants with small VSDs are well developed and acyanotic. Infants with large VSDs may have poor weight gain or show signs of congestive heart failure (CHF) before 2 or 3 months of age.

8. e. Watchful expectation should be pursued. The prognosis is excellent, and the defect will likely close spontaneously. As the VSD becomes smaller, the murmur becomes shorter and maintains its regurgitant characteristics (i.e., it starts off with the first heart sound). Spontaneous closure occurs in 30% to 40% of cases, even more frequently in small defects. Pediatric cardiology referral is appropriate for serial examinations and echocardiograms. Infants with large VSD who develop CHF and growth retardation should be treated first with digoxin and diuretics. If this fails, then surgical intervention is necessary within the first 6 months of life.

9. a. The only prophylaxis that needs to be followed in this child is protection with antibiotic therapy (penicillin, amoxicillin, or erythromycin for patients allergic to penicillin) before any dental procedure or any other procedure that would increase the probability of bacterial endocarditis. This obviously can be discontinued when the defect closes. Serial echocardiograms are indicated. Different cardiologists have different recommendations for the frequency of examination, but every 6 to 12 months is the range, not every 3 months. Cardiac catheterization is not indicated for this lesion.

10. d. More than 80% of children have innocent murmurs of one type or another sometime during childhood, usually beginning at approximately age 3 or 4 years. Half of full-term newborn infants have systolic murmurs sometime during the first week of life. The vast majority of these murmurs are innocent in nature and do not reflect any cardiac pathologic condition.

11. c. The most common pathologic cardiac murmur in childhood is VSD. With a VSD, the cardiac murmur is often not present at birth but is first heard at the 2- to 4-week well baby checkup. As discussed previously, the most common outcome of this congenital heart defect is spontaneous closure. In some cases, however, surgical closure is indicated. The most uncommon scenario is the development of congestive cardiac failure secondary to VSD.

The relative frequencies of pathologic cardiac murmurs in childhood are as follows: VSD, 38%; ASD, 18%; pulmonary valve stenosis, 13%; pulmonary artery stenosis, 7%; aortic valve stenosis, 4%; patent ductus arteriosis (PDA), 4%; mitral valve prolapse, 4%; and all others, 11%.

12. e. The common functional or common innocent murmurs of infancy and childhood include the following: (1) pulmonary flow murmur of newborn (systolic), (2) venous hum of late infancy and early childhood, (3) Still's aortic vibratory systolic murmur, and (4) pulmonary ejection systolic murmur of late adolescence and childhood.

13. d. This infant has the characteristic stigmata of Down syndrome, or trisomy 21. At least 50% of infants with Down syndrome have some type of congenital heart disease. Endocardial cushion defect or atrioventricular canal is the most common lesion in this population, followed by VSD. Congestive heart failure can develop in these infants. Most infants with congenital heart disease and trisomy 21 should be identified on prenatal screening. Care must be taken in patients with no prenatal care and little medical follow-up. Any newborn identified with the features of trisomy 21 should have a screening echocardiogram.

14. d. This is the transient systolic murmur of PDA. It is audible at the upper left sternal border and in the left infraclavicular area on the first day, and it usually disappears soon thereafter. As in older infants and children, not all heart murmurs in neonates are pathologic. More than 50% of term-born infants are found to have innocent systolic murmurs at some time during the first week of life. The prevalence is even higher in premature infants. The incidence of structural congenital heart disease is estimated to be less than 1% of all live births. The infant should have a detailed exam at 24 hours and again prior to discharge before any further decisions are made. Acrocyanosis, a normal phenomenon, should also be distinguished from central cyanosis.

Summary

Murmurs are common in the pediatric population, and the role of the primary care physician is to differentiate the common innocent murmur from the more pathologic ones.

1. Prevalence of murmurs
   a. More than 50% of infants and 80% of children usually beginning at approximately age 3 or 4 years have some type of innocent murmur.
   b. Innocent/pathologic: 10/1.
2. Epidemiology: Experienced clinical assessment is just as sensitive and specific as echocardiography and more sensitive and specific than electrocardiography. Any concern or doubt on the part of the primary care physician should warrant referral to a pediatric cardiologist. Evaluation begins with a pointed history and a systematic physical examination, including careful palpation of pulses and cardiac impulses, assessment of skin color, and complete cardiac examination.
3. Innocent murmurs: These are almost exclusively ejection systolic, generally soft, never associated with a palpable thrill, and subject to variation with changes in the patient's position.
   a. Still's murmur (most common)
   b. Venous hum (second most common)
   c. Pulmonary flow murmur: most common in newborn infants
   d. Neonatal pulmonary artery branch murmur
4. Pathologic murmurs: Clinical features include grade III or louder intensity, pansystolic timing, a harsh quality, location of maximum intensity at the left upper sternal border, and the presence of abnormal S2 or an early to midsystolic click.
   a. VSD (most common)
   b. ASD (second most common)
   c. Pulmonary valve stenosis

5. The following are clinical signs and symptoms that are reassuring for the family physician during evaluation of a childhood cardiac murmur:
   a. No evidence of failure to thrive
   b. No symptoms (shortness of breath, blue lips, lethargy, and having to stop and rest while playing) or signs (cyanosis, diastolic murmur, parasternal heave, thrill, loud murmur greater than II/VI, and pansystolic murmur) to suggest pathologic murmur
   c. Murmur accentuated by sitting forward
   d. Murmur accentuated by exercise or increased heart rate resulting from another cause
   e. Murmur accentuated by fever, anxiety, restlessness, or crying, suggests an innocent murmur
   f. No radiation
   g. Located lower (rather than higher) along the left sternal edge
   h. Not associated with other characteristics of abnormal murmurs, including sweating while eating, clubbing, associated anomalies or abnormal facies, edema, and arrhythmias

Suggested Reading

Frommelt MA: Differential diagnosis and approach to a heart murmur in term infants. *Pediatr Clin North Am* 51:1023–1032, 2004.

Johns Hopkins Hospital: *The Harriet Lane Handbook: A Manual for Pediatric House Officers*, 17th ed. St. Louis: Mosby, 2005.

Park MK: *Pediatric Cardiology for Practitioners*, 4th ed. St. Louis: Mosby, 2002.

Pelech AN: The physiology of cardiac auscultation. *Pediatr Clin North Am* 51(6):1515–1535, 2004.

CHAPTER 114

Vomiting and Diarrhea

CLINICAL CASE PROBLEM 1

An 18-Month-Old Infant with Diarrhea

A mother brings her 15-month-old son who has diarrhea to your office for evaluation. The child has been having on average approximately seven loose stools per day for the past 4 days. The stool is watery without any mucus or blood. He also vomited several times during the first 2 days but now it appears to be subsiding. He has been drinking fluids but has not had much appetite for food. For the past 2 days, he has been running a "low-grade fever" and appears to have some abdominal discomfort. He attends a local day care, where some of the children have had similar symptoms.

On physical examination, the child is active without any fever. He has dry, cracked lips with moist oral mucosa. The ears, throat, lungs, and abdomen are normal. There are no abdominal masses and no palpable tenderness.

SELECT THE BEST ANSWER TO THE FOLLOWING QUESTIONS

1. What is the most likely cause of this toddler's symptoms?
   a. astrovirus
   b. rotavirus
   c. coxsackievirus
   d. norovirus
   e. *Shigella*

2. What is the treatment of choice in this infant at this time?
   a. admission to the hospital for intravenous (IV) therapy
   b. observation in the hospital and oral rehydration therapy
   c. treatment at home with fluids including fruit juices and noncarbonated beverages
   d. treatment at home with an oral rehydrating solution
   e. none of the above

3. Investigations at this time should include which of the following?
   a. complete blood count
   b. fecal smear
   c. microscopic examination of stool for ova and parasite
   d. enzyme immunoassay
   e. nothing at this time

4. Which of the following statements regarding diarrhea caused by the agent identified in response to question 1 is true?
   a. upper respiratory tract symptoms frequently precede the gastrointestinal symptoms

b. worldwide, this organism is estimated to cause more than 125 million cases of diarrhea annually in children younger than 5 years of age

c. it is seen most commonly in summer months

d. frequent complications include meningitis and osteomyelitis

e. a and b

5. Which of the following statements about the treatment of the condition described here is true?
   a. rehydration can be accomplished in most patients via the oral route
   b. clear liquids such as flat soda, fruit juice, and sports drinks, are appropriate for rehydration of young children
   c. BRAT (bananas, rice, applesauce, and toast) diet has been shown to be superior to a regular diet
   d. oral rehydration is not indicated in moderate dehydration
   e. prolonged (>12 hours) administration of exclusive clear liquids or dilute formula is clinically beneficial

6. Which of the following represents the composition of an ideal rehydrating solution for moderate dehydration?
   a. 45 mM Na$^+$, 20 mM K$^+$, 70 mM Cl$^-$, 100 mM citrate, and 110 mM glucose
   b. 50 mM Na$^+$, 30 mM K$^+$, 80 mM Cl$^-$, 10 mM citrate, and 100 mM glucose
   c. 90 mM Na$^+$, 20 mM K$^+$, 80 mM Cl$^-$, 10 mM citrate, and 111 mM glucose
   d. 90 mM Na$^+$, 30 mM K$^+$, 80 mM Cl$^-$, 20 mM citrate, and 111 mM glucose
   e. 90 mM Na$^+$, 30 mM K$^+$, 80 mM Cl$^-$, 20 mM citrate, and 100 mM glucose

7. Which of the following statements regarding the prevention of the infection caused by the agent identified in response to question 1 is true?
   a. RotaShield is the only vaccine approved in the United States for prevention of rotavirus gastroenteritis (vomiting and diarrhea)
   b. RotaTeq is the only vaccine approved in the United States for prevention of rotavirus gastroenteritis
   c. there is no approved vaccine in the United States for prevention of rotavirus gastroenteritis
   d. vaccination has not been shown to be of benefit in prevention of rotavirus gastroenteritis
   e. none of the above

8. What is the most common bacterial cause of diarrhea in children?

   a. *Salmonella*
   b. *Shigella*
   c. *Campylobacter*
   d. *Escherichia coli*
   e. *Enterococcus*

9. Which of the following infectious agents may produce bloody diarrhea in infants and children?
   a. *Shigella*
   b. *Salmonella*
   c. enteroinvasive *E. coli*
   d. *Enterococcus*
   e. a, b, and c
   f. all of the above

10. Which of the following statements about enterohemorrhagic *E. coli* O157:H7 is false?
    a. infection is transmitted by undercooked ground beef, unpasteurized milk, and other vehicles contaminated with bovine feces
    b. outbreaks have been linked to contaminated apple cider, raw vegetables, and drinking water
    c. person-to-person transmission is uncommon in outbreaks
    d. the dose necessary to cause infection is low
    e. hemolytic uremic syndrome is a serious complication of infection

11. Which of the following is (are) a common cause(s) of antibiotic-associated diarrhea in infants and children?
    a. ampicillin
    b. clindamycin
    c. amoxicillin
    d. cephalosporins
    e. all of the above

CLINICAL CASE PROBLEM 2

A 23-Month-Old Infant with Sunken Eyeballs and Doughy Skin

An 23-month-old infant is brought to the emergency department by his mother. He has had diarrhea and vomiting for the past 3 days and appears to be at least 15% dehydrated. His eyeballs are sunken, and his skin is doughy. The child has no satisfactory veins in which to place an IV line.

12. What should you do now?
    a. attempt oral rehydration therapy
    b. perform a venous cutdown in the ankle
    c. begin an interosseous infusion

d. begin a subcutaneous infusion

e. any one of the above

13. Which of the following investigations should not be performed on any child who has ongoing diarrhea and severe dehydration?
    a. urine-specific gravity
    b. stool evaluation for blood
    c. stool evaluation for fecal leukocytes
    d. stool cultures
    e. serum electrolytes

CLINICAL CASE PROBLEM 3

A 3-Year-Old Male with Diarrhea Who Had Been Camping

A mother comes to your office with her 3-year-old boy who has developed severe crampy diarrhea and mild fever. The family has just returned from a camping trip in the Rocky Mountains; the child became sick on the third day. He was apparently drinking water from a local stream.

14. What is the most likely diagnosis in this patient?
    a. viral gastroenteritis
    b. *Shigella* gastroenteritis
    c. *Salmonella* gastroenteritis
    d. giardiasis
    e. amebiasis

15. Which of the following pediatric infections often presents with diarrhea as the initial symptoms?
    a. acute appendicitis
    b. otitis media
    c. urinary tract infections
    d. pneumonia
    e. all of the above

16. Which of the following is the most common cause of acute abdominal pain in children?
    a. constipation
    b. intussusception
    c. volvulus
    d. gastroenteritis
    e. mesenteric lymphadenitis

17. All of the following factors are associated with an increased risk of gastroenteritis except
    a. day care attendance
    b. travel to an endemic area
    c. exposure to unsanitary conditions
    d. age older than 5 years
    e. ingestion of contaminated food or water

Clinical Case Management Problem

Discuss the most common cause of childhood death from gastroenteritis (worldwide). Comment on community health aspects of this condition.

Answers

1. **b.** The most common cause of childhood gastroenteritis is rotavirus. Symptoms of rotavirus infection include low-grade fever, anorexia, nausea, vomiting, diarrhea, and abdominal cramps. Dehydration may occur. The disease typically runs its course in 4 to 10 days. Astroviruses are the second most important agent of viral gastroenteritis in young children, followed by enteric adenoviruses and calciviruses, such as Norwalk agents and noroviruses. Caliciviruses are small, 27- to 35-nm, viruses that are the most common cause of gastroenteritis outbreaks in older children and adults.

2. **d.** Because this child does not appear to be significantly dehydrated, hospitalization is not required. The treatment of choice is home oral rehydration therapy. Fruit juices (undiluted) and commercial beverages are not recommended because of high osmolarity and the danger of hypernatremia or exacerbation of stool losses.

3. **e.** Investigations do not need to be performed routinely in children with signs and symptoms of acute gastroenteritis. Testing for a specific etiologic agent such as those for rotavirus, ova, parasites, or bacteria is only marginally helpful and not recommended. Serum electrolytes are useful in children with severe dehydration requiring IV hydration. Gross or occult blood in stool should raise suspicion of pathogens such as *Shigella* or *Campylobacter*, although hemorrhagic *E. coli* mentioned previously, is the most common agent. It is responsible for more than 50% of cases of Large numbers of leukocytes in fecal smear may indicate inflammatory bacterial process. In the absence of white blood cells or blood, stool cultures have a very low yield. Most noninflammatory diarrhea is self-limited, and confirming etiologic agents does not alter clinical management. The mainstay of treatment is oral rehydration therapy.

4. **e.** Viruses are the most common cause of wintertime diarrhea in infants. Rotavirus presents as acute diarrhea in children and accounts for 20% to 60% of hospitalization for children with diarrhea worldwide. The other viral causes are listed in answer 1. The majority of infants and children who develop rotavirus develop an upper respiratory tract infection preceding

the gastrointestinal symptoms. The respiratory tract symptoms include rhinorrhea, cough, pharyngeal erythema, and otitis media. Dehydration is the most common complication. Meningitis and osteomyelitis are infrequent complications that can occur with bacterial causes of gastroenteritis, such as *Shigella*, *Salmonella*, and *E. coli*.

5. a. Rehydration can be accomplished in most patients via the oral route. Oral rehydration therapy seems to be a preferred treatment option for patients with moderate dehydration from gastroenteritis. Modern rehydration solutions containing appropriate quantities of sodium and glucose promote optimal absorption of fluid from the intestine. Other clear liquids such as flat soda, fruit juice, and sports drinks are inappropriate for rehydration of young children with significant stool loss. Prolonged (>12 hours) administration of exclusive clear liquids or dilute formula is without clinical benefit and actually prolongs the duration of diarrhea. Hypocaloric diets low in protein and fat such as BRAT have not been shown to be superior to a regular diet.

6. c. Oral rehydration therapy effectively resolves most cases of pediatric gastroenteritis. The World Health Organization recommended standard for oral rehydration therapy is 90 mM Na+, 20 mM K+, 80 mM Cl-, 10 mM citrate, and 111 mM glucose.

Among the common oral rehydration solutions used, Rehydralyte has the closest composition to the World Health Organization's recommended formula. Pedialyte is less ideal because it contains only 45 mEq/L of sodium instead of 90 mEq/L. Although these solutions are best suited as maintenance solutions, they can satisfactorily rehydrate children who are mildly or moderately dehydrated.

Clear liquids should not be given to infants with diarrhea because they have a low sodium content, a low potassium content, and a high carbohydrate content. Examples of clear liquids include apple juice, carbonated beverages, and sports beverages.

7. b. RotaTeq is the only vaccine approved in the United States for prevention of rotavirus gastroenteritis (vomiting and diarrhea). The Centers for Disease Control and Prevention recommendation is for infants to receive three doses of the oral vaccine at 2, 4, and 6 months of age. Children should receive the first dose of the vaccine by 12 weeks of age and should receive all doses of the vaccine by 32 weeks of age. There are insufficient data on safety and efficacy outside of these age ranges. RotaShield, another rotavirus vaccine, was withdrawn from the market in 1999 after it was found to be associated with intussusception.

8. c. The most common cause of bacterial gastroenteritis in both children and adults is *Campylobacter jejuni*.

Campylobacter gastroenteritis typically begins with fever and malaise, followed by nausea, vomiting, diarrhea, fever, and abdominal pain. The diarrhea is often profuse and may contain blood. The illness is self-limited, lasting less than 1 week in 60% of cases. Recurrences and chronic symptoms can occur, especially in infants.

Symptoms caused by *C. jejuni* usually occur as a result of endotoxin production. Invasive strains also occur and produce disease. *Campylobacter* is treated effectively with erythromycin, although the infection is usually self-limiting and clears up when left untreated.

9. e. *Salmonella* gastroenteritis begins with watery diarrhea and is accompanied by fever and nausea. As with *Campylobacter*, *Salmonella* produces disease both by mucosal invasion and by endotoxin production, and the diarrhea may be bloody. Most cases of *Salmonella* gastroenteritis do not require antibiotic therapy.

Shigella gastroenteritis begins with watery diarrhea, high fever, and malaise; this is usually followed in 24 hours by tenesmus and frank dysentery. Mucosal invasion with frank ulceration and hemorrhage often occur. Dehydration is common. *Shigella* gastroenteritis should be treated with trimethoprim–sulfamethoxazole.

E. coli gastroenteritis may occur as an enteropathic, enterohemorrhagic, enterotoxigenic, or enteroinvasive infection. Enteropathic *E. coli* usually produces a mild self-limited illness. Enterohemorrhagic *E. coli* produces diarrhea that is initially watery and later becomes bloody. Enterotoxigenic *E. coli* is the most common cause of traveler's diarrhea. Enteroinvasive *E. coli* invades the mucosa and produces a dysentery-like illness with bloody stool.

In infants and children, *Yersinia enterocolitica* may produce acute and chronic gastroenteritis and mesenteric lymphadenitis. Occasionally, mesenteric lymphadenitis is extremely difficult to distinguish from acute appendicitis. Diarrhea, fever, and crampy abdominal pain are the most common presenting symptoms. Treatment is symptomatic only; antibiotic therapy is unnecessary.

Enterococcus is not a cause of bacterial gastroenteritis in children.

10. c. *E. coli* O157:H7 infections in the United States have become more common. Outbreaks have been linked to contaminated water, apple cider, salami, yogurt, undercooked beef, and raw vegetables. Person-to-person transmission is high during outbreaks, and the infectious dose is low (approximately 100 organisms). Enterohemorrhagic *E. coli* infection can progress to hemolytic uremic syndrome (especially O157:H7).

Enteropathic *E. coli* infection is seen primarily in infants. Enterotoxigenic *E. coli* infection is usually brief and self-limited. This is the most common cause of traveler's diarrhea.

11. e. Diarrhea is one of the most common complications associated with antibiotic therapy. The most common cause of antibiotic-associated diarrhea is ampicillin. Amoxicillin, ampicillin, other penicillins (including β-lactamase-stable agents), cephalosporins (second and third generation), and clindamycin are some of the agents most frequently associated with antibiotic-associated diarrhea. These are common and generally self-limiting. Most cases resolve on discontinuation of the drug. However, occasionally a pseudomembranous colitis may develop because of an overgrowth of *Clostridium difficile* or release of its toxin. The prognosis of severe *C. difficile*-induced pseudomembranous colitis cases is poor, with a 20% to 30% fatality rate and a 10% to 20% relapse rate. Treatment of severe cases consists of oral vancomycin or metronidazole.

12. c. In a young infant or child who presents with severe dehydration, it is often very difficult to establish good IV access. A skull vein is a possibility, but even that is difficult. An excellent alternative is an interosseous infusion (usually placed in the tibia). A large bore needle is used after local anesthesia has been infiltrated around the bone. This allows easy access and affords an excellent alternative to venous access.

13. d. The investigations that should be performed on all children who have ongoing diarrhea include urine-specific gravity, stool analysis for blood, and stool analysis for fecal leukocytes. A urine-specific gravity of less than 1.015 suggests adequate hydration.

If a patient presents with bloody diarrhea, high fever, persistent symptoms, tenesmus, or a history of foreign travel, a stool culture and examination of the stool for ova and parasites should be performed. Routine stool culture, however, is not cost-effective.

Other investigations that should be considered in a toxic child include complete blood count, serum electrolytes, and serum osmolality.

14. d. Gastroenteritis that begins while camping in the Rocky Mountains most likely is caused by giardiasis. Giardiasis needs a very low "organism load" to produce a very painful gastroenteritis. Giardiasis is the most common parasitic cause of gastroenteritis; however, parasitic infections in total account for less than 10% of all cases of gastroenteritis. The recommended treatment is metronidazole and rehydration.

15. e. Many nonenteric infections may produce diarrhea as the first and most prominent symptom. These include otitis media, urinary tract infection, acute appendicitis (from inflammation extending to involve the ureter on the right side of the body), lower lobe pneumonia, and mesenteric lymphadenitis (*Y. enterocolitica*).

16. d. The most common medical cause of abdominal pain in children is gastroenteritis. The most common surgical cause is appendicitis. Intussusception and volvulus are not common; however, intussusception is the most common cause of bowel obstruction in childhood. Patients will often have emesis and bloody stool, but only approximately 50% will have the characteristic "currant-jelly" stool. Although constipation is common, it does not most commonly present as acute abdominal pain. Mesenteric lymphadenitis often presents similar to appendicitis and can be caused by *Y. enterocolitica* and pseudotuberculosis and *G. lamblia*.

17. d. Factors that increase susceptibility to infection with enteropathogens include young age, immune deficiency, measles, malnutrition, travel to an endemic area, lack of breast-feeding, exposure to unsanitary conditions, ingestion of contaminated food or water, level of maternal education, and attendance at a child care center.

Solution to the Clinical Case Management Problem

The most common cause of gastroenteritis-produced death in infants and children worldwide is cholera. Cholera is both endemic and epidemic, and both have a seasonal pattern. Contaminated water is the major source of infectivity and transmission, and cholera becomes an epidemic when crowded conditions such as refugee camps are established.

The responsible organism is *Vibrio cholerae*. The resulting illness is sudden in onset and produces severe rice-water diarrhea and severe dehydration that can quickly lead to death. Most cases can be treated effectively by oral rehydration with a balanced electrolyte solution.

Summary

1. Prevalence: During the first 3 years of life, the average child experiences one to three episodes of diarrhea per year.
2. Viral gastroenteritis: Viruses are the most common agents causing diarrheal illnesses in the United States.
   a. Rotavirus is the most common cause (50%). It is most common in winter months, spreading via a fecal–oral route. It typically begins with mild to moderate fever and vomiting, followed by frequent watery stools. Dehydration and electrolyte disturbance are the most common sequelae.
   b. Other viral agents producing gastroenteritis include (i) Norwalk agent (parvovirus), (ii) coxsackievirus, (iii) echovirus, (iv) adenovirus, (v) calicivirus, and (vi) astrovirus.
3. Bacterial gastroenteritis accounts for 2% to 10% of cases of diarrhea.
   a. *Campylobacter jejuni* is the most common bacterial cause.
   b. Other bacterial agents include *Salmonella*, *Shigella*, *Yersinia*, and *E. coli*.
4. Parasitic gastroenteritis: Giardiasis ("beaver fever") is the most common, followed by *Campylobacter*.

Entamoeba histolytica is a common cause of diarrhea and dysentery in developing countries.

5. Diagnosis: Routine laboratory testing is not necessary in most children. Children who are severely dehydrated or who have failed oral replacement therapy should be evaluated by having a complete urinalysis performed, including urine-specific gravity, and a stool examination for blood and fecal leukocytes. Specific gravity of 1.015 or less suggests adequate hydration.

   If bloody diarrhea, persistent symptoms, fever, tenesmus, or recent foreign travel are present, a stool culture for ova and parasites should be done. In mild and self-limiting diarrhea, a stool culture is not cost-effective.

6. Treatment: Most children can be managed by oral rehydration therapy using a solution containing 90 mM Na^+, 20 mM K^+, 80 mM Cl^-, 10 mM citrate, and 111 mM glucose. Resumption of a normal diet for age results in a more rapid recovery. Breast-feeding should be continued.

   Antibiotic therapy should be initiated for *Shigella* (trimethoprim–sulfamethoxazole) and *C. jejuni* (erythromycin).

7. Prevention remains the most vital measure in managing diarrheal disease.

Suggested Reading

Behrman RE, Kliegman RM, Jenson HB, eds: *Nelson Textbook of Pediatrics*, 17th ed. Philadelphia: Saunders, 2004.

Bellemare S: Oral versus intravenous rehydration of moderately dehydrated children: A randomized, controlled trial. *J Pediatr* 147(1):125–126, 2005.

Dennehy PH: Acute diarrheal disease in children: Epidemiology, prevention, and treatment. *Infect Dis Clin North Am* 19(3):585–602, 2005.

Leung A, Sigalet D: Acute abdominal pain in children. *Am Fam Physician* 67:2321–2326, 2003.

Pickering L, Snyder J: Gastroenteritis. In: Behrman RE, Kliegman RM, Jenson HB, eds, *Nelson Textbook of Pediatrics*, 17th ed. Philadelphia: Saunders, 2004.

CHAPTER

115 Recurrent Abdominal Pain

CLINICAL CASE PROBLEM 1

A 13-Year-Old Female with Recurrent Abdominal Pain

A 13-year-old female is brought to your office with a history of recurring abdominal pain. She has had episodes of abdominal pain at least once or twice a week for the past 3 months. These episodes last approximately 6 to 8 hours. You have seen her for the same problem on many occasions. The following were done previously and all results were normal: complete blood count (CBC); erythrocyte sedimentation rate (ESR); urinalysis; stool for ova and parasites; an ultrasound of the kidneys, ureter, and bladder; and an abdominal plain film. The pain is described as umbilical in location with a quality described as a "dull ache." She rates the pain at a baseline quantity of 6/10, with increases to 8/10 and decreases to 4/10. It is not associated with any food intake, and it is not associated with any diarrhea or constipation. Her mother says that she has been missing school because of the pain.

On physical examination, the girl is in no apparent distress. Her vital signs, height, and weight are normal for her age. On abdominal exam there is slight tenderness in the area of the periumbilical region. There is no hepatosplenomegaly and no other masses.

SELECT THE BEST ANSWER TO THE FOLLOWING QUESTIONS

1. What is the most likely diagnosis in this patient?
   a. recurrent abdominal pain (RAP) syndrome
   b. lactose intolerance
   c. Crohn's disease
   d. mesenteric lymphadenitis
   e. chronic appendicitis

2. What is the prevalence of this condition in children?
   a. 1%
   b. 5%
   c. 15%
   d. 20%
   e. 25%

3. Regarding the physiologic basis for the pain that occurs in the condition described here, which of the following statements is (are) true?
   a. the pain can be conceptualized as a disorder that provokes pain pathways
   b. the pain can be conceptualized as an alteration in the patient's threshold to pain
   c. there is evidence that an abnormality in the autonomic nervous system is involved in this condition
   d. there is evidence that intestinal motility can be affected along with the occurrence of hyperalgesia
   e. all of the above statements are true

4. Which of the following statements regarding school attendance and the condition described is true?
   a. there is no association between school attendance and the condition described
   b. school phobia (reluctance to attend school) may be an important contributing factor in many cases of this condition
   c. children with this condition usually achieve higher marks than their counterparts without this condition
   d. there is no association between stressful events at school and this condition
   e. none of the above statements are true

5. Which of the following should be considered "red flags" in the history of RAP syndrome?
   a. localization of the pain away from the umbilicus
   b. constitutional symptoms, such as recurrent fever and loss of appetite or energy
   c. pain not associated with change in bowel habits, particularly diarrhea, constipation, or nocturnal bowel movements
   d. RAP occurring in a child older than 5 years of age
   e. a and b

6. The mother of the patient is extremely anxious and wants to know if the investigations need to be repeated at this time. You tell her which of the following?
   a. a CBC, ESR, and urinalysis will be repeated
   b. no further testing needs to be done
   c. kidneys, ureter, and bladder (KUB) x-ray needs to be done
   d. abdominal ultrasound needs to be done
   e. the next step will be to perform an upper gastrointestinal endoscopy (EGD) to "rule out all possibilities"

7. Which of the following is the treatment of choice for the condition described?
   a. muscle relaxants
   b. tricyclic antidepressants
   c. narcotic analgesics
   d. nonsteroidal anti-inflammatory drugs
   e. none of the above

Clinical Case Management Problem

List nine frequent causes of acute abdominal pain for each of the following: (1) infancy (<2 years), (2) preschool (2 to 5 years), (3) school age (5 to 10 years), and (4) adolescence (11 to 15 years).

Answers

1. **a.** The most likely diagnosis in this patient is RAP syndrome. RAP in children is defined as episodes of pain occurring at least monthly for 3 consecutive months with a severity that interrupts routine functioning. The signs and symptoms of RAP syndrome are marked by their lack of specificity. The crucial separation of organic from nonorganic pain can be based on a few important findings, including the specificity and consistency of the pain and the relationship of the pain to meals and movement. The patient with nonspecific RAP tends to look well; to have pain that is inconsistent in relationship to meals and to movement; and to be free of the occurrence of additional symptoms such as nausea, vomiting, or dysuria. Early investigators found an organic cause

for RAP in 5% to 10% of children. With advancement in medical technology, the percentage of patients with unexplained pain is decreasing.

Lactose intolerance is often confused with RAP syndrome in childhood and with irritable bowel syndrome in adults. In fact, these two syndromes can coexist. Lactose intolerance is usually associated with flatus and diarrhea. Crohn's disease and mesenteric lymphadenitis are usually associated with systemic symptoms. The lack of systemic symptoms in this patient is strong evidence against these diagnoses. Chronic appendicitis, if it exists, is more likely to be associated with pain in the right lower quadrant and with nausea and vomiting.

2. c. RAP affects approximately 15% of middle and high school students. Approximately 10% of students who experience abdominal pain seek medical evaluation. The likelihood of seeking medical attention is proportional to the severity and frequency of abdominal pain and its impact on school attendance. RAP affects males and females equally until age 9 years. After that, the incidence in females increased such that between 9 and 12 years, the female-to-male ratio is 1.5:1. The overall incidence appears to peak at 10 to 12 years. RAP is rare among children younger than 5 years of age, and an organic cause must be considered even more carefully in this age group.

3. e. There are many theories related to RAP syndrome in children. Pain in children is conceptualized as a disorder that provokes pain pathways or an alteration in the patient's threshold to pain. A widely held plausible explanation in these cases is some abnormality in the functioning of the autonomic nervous system. This is thought to result in altered intestinal motility and the occurrence of hyperalgesia and altered secretory pathways.

There are some clear warning signs and symptoms that should raise the likelihood of underlying organic disease. Complaint of localizing pain, pain associated with change in bowel habits, repeated vomiting, altered vital signs, anorexia or weakness, and RAP syndrome occurring in a child younger than age 4 years should be investigated vigorously. Constitutional signs of weight loss, growth restriction or cessation, organomegaly and localized tenderness, hernias, or swelling similarly should be pursued.

4. b. School phobia (reluctance to attend school) may be an important contributing factor in many cases of RAP syndrome in childhood. There is a significant association between stressful events at school and RAP syndrome. Children with this condition, on average, achieve lower grades than their cohorts without this condition. This actually may be more associated with diminished school attendance than anything else. There is a significant association between stressful events at school and exacerbations of this condition.

5. e. The most powerful diagnostic tools for the problem of RAP in childhood are a thorough history and physical examination. A correct diagnosis can usually be suspected following a good history and physical examination. Red flags on the history of RAP syndrome are localization of the pain away from the umbilicus; pain associated with change in bowel habits, particularly diarrhea, constipation, or nocturnal bowel movements; pain associated with night wakening; repetitive emesis, especially if bilious; constitutional symptoms such as recurrent fever; loss of appetite or energy; and RAP occurring in a child younger than 4 years of age.

6. b. This child has already had numerous investigations. It is pointless to repeat them unless her condition is markedly different from previous episodes. The possible mechanisms associated with abdominal pain are so numerous and poorly understood that the investigation and treatment of these cases of RAP in childhood test not only the physician's scientific acumen but also his or her skill in the practice of the art of medicine. The "rule out all possibilities" approach can lead to a spiral of investigations that simply reinforces the impression that some hidden cause has been overlooked and must be unmasked, even when the clinician is convinced of the functional nature of the pain. In only 10% of cases of RAP syndrome is an organic cause found. Therefore, in most cases, investigations can be limited to a CBC, urinalysis, stool specimen for occult blood, white cells, culture, and ova and parasite examination. A flat plate of the abdomen can define significant constipation if this is suspected by history or examination, and abdominal ultrasonography may be of use for diagnosing renal, gynecologic, or cystic etiologies. An EGD is not indicated at this time.

7. e. Treatment for RAP syndrome in childhood should not be based on pharmacotherapy, especially pharmacotherapy that may do more harm than good. The first and admittedly most challenging task is to explain the concept of functional abdominal pain to the parents. Many parents will assume that pain that has a "nonphysical" origin implies imagined or contrived pain—that the child is "faking it." The most convincing method of divesting the parents of this notion is to compare the abdominal pain with headache in adults. Most adults have occasional headaches, and although the cause is rarely associated with any abnormal physical findings or investigations, the pain is undoubtedly real and not imagined. The parents need to maintain a sympathetic attitude that acknowledges the pain but encourages continued activities and school attendance to the greatest degree possible. Young children are highly suggestible, and parents should refrain from questioning the child about the pain if the child is not complaining.

The role of increased dietary fiber in alleviating the pain is unclear; however, the diets of many children are lacking in fiber, and a trial of increasing fiber by dietary modification seems a prudent strategy that will do no harm. Laxatives and, occasionally, enemas may be beneficial when there is evidence of retained stool or suspicion of constipation. The impulse to commence a trial of empiric medication to provide symptomatic relief should be resisted.

Solution to the Clinical Case Management Problem

Nine frequent causes of acute abdominal pain in infancy, preschool, school age, and adolescence are listed in the table.

Additional causes for all ages include mesenteric lymphadenitis, tumor, pneumonia, constipation, sickling syndrome, cystic fibrosis, diabetes mellitus, and celiac disease (Table 115-1).

Table 115-1 Frequent Causes of Acute Abdominal Pain

Infancy	Preschool	School Age	Adolescence
Colic	Gastroenteritis	Gastroenteritis	Gastroenteritis
Gastroenteritis	Urinary tract infection	Urinary tract infection	Urinary tract infection
Milk intolerance	Trauma	Appendicitis	Appendicitis
Intussusception	Intussusception/constipation	Recurrent abdominal pain syndrome	Pelvic inflammatory disease/dysmenorrhea
Urinary tract infection	Henoch–Schönlein purpura/ sickle cell disease	Inflammatory bowel disease	Inflammatory bowel disease
Trauma/abuse	Appendicitis	Ingestions	Peptic ulcer disease
Volvulus/intestinal anomaly (Meckel's)	Hemolytic uremic syndrome	Gonadal torsion	Ingestion
Incarcerated hernia	Lead and other ingestions	Lactose intolerance	Gonadal torsion
Other	Ketoacidosis	Wilms' tumor	Pregnancy

Summary

1. Definition: Episodes of abdominal pain occurring at least monthly for 3 months that interrupts routine functioning.
2. Prevalence in school-age children (4 to 16 years) is approximately 10%, equally affecting both sexes. Peak incidence is at age 9 years.
3. The diagnosis of RAP syndrome can be made from the following:
   a. History and physical examination
   b. CBC, urinalysis, ESR, stool for ova and parasites, occult blood, KUB x-ray, and abdominal ultrasound
   c. The absence of symptoms of organic etiology: age younger than 5 years, fever, weight loss, joint symptoms, abnormal growth, localized away from the umbilicus, wake the patient from sleep, vomiting, diarrhea, and blood in the stool
4. Do not overinvestigate or overtreat patients with RAP in childhood. The vast majority of cases (85% to 90%) are nonorganic in origin.
5. Treatment should be supportive and should consist of reestablishing a healthy lifestyle, eating a well-balanced diet, exercising daily, and avoiding stress (especially at school).
6. There is a strong association between school phobia (school avoidance) and RAP syndrome. Take a careful history of school performance, school fears, and general feelings about attending school.

Suggested Reading

Leung AK, Sigalet D: Acute abdominal pain in children. *Am Fam Physician* 67(11):2321–2326, 2003.

Subcommittee on Chronic Abdominal Pain: Chronic abdominal pain in children. *Pediatrics* 115(3): e370–e381, 2005.

Thiessen PN: Recurrent abdominal pain. *Pediatr Rev* 23(2):39–46, 2002.

Weydert JA: Systematic review of treatments for recurrent abdominal pain. *Pediatrics* 11(1):e1–e11, 2003.

Wyllie R: Recurrent abdominal pain of childhood. In: Behrman RE, Kliegman RM, Jenson HB, eds, *Nelson Textbook of Pediatrics*, 17th ed. Philadelphia: Saunders, 2004.

Zeiter DK: Recurrent abdominal pain in children. *Pediatr Clin North Am* 49(1):53–71, 2002.

CHAPTER 116 Enuresis

CLINICAL CASE PROBLEM 1

Bed-wetting in a 6-Year-Old

A mother and her 6-year-old son come to the office with a concern that he continues to have nighttime wetting several times a week. He is the second child of three. He is in the first grade and struggling with his performance. He has had no medical problems, no history of developmental delay, and was the product of a normal uncomplicated pregnancy and delivery. Since the birth of the third child, his behavior has been poor. The examination of other body systems is normal. He does not have laboratory evidence of a urinary tract infection.

SELECT THE BEST ANSWER TO THE FOLLOWING QUESTIONS

1. What is the most likely diagnosis in this child?
   a. school phobia
   b. nocturnal enuresis
   c. small bladder syndrome
   d. masked childhood depression
   e. none of the above

2. A child is defined as enuretic if he or she has not attained full bladder control by what age?
   a. 3 years
   b. 4 years
   c. 5 years
   d. 6 years
   e. 8 years

3. With respect to this condition, which of the following statements is true?
   a. at age 5 years, less than 5% of children have this condition
   b. there is no relationship to family history

   c. the condition is significantly more common in boys
   d. the condition usually implies significant psychopathology in the child
   e. bladder capacity is usually less in these children

4. Which of the following investigations is most important in a child with enuresis?
   a. urinalysis
   b. urine culture
   c. complete blood count (CBC)
   d. complete cystometric evaluation
   e. intravenous pyelography (IVP)

5. Which of the following should be used in the treatment of this patient?
   a. imipramine
   b. desmopressin
   c. oxybutynin
   d. biofeedback
   e. all of the above

CLINICAL CASE PROBLEM 2

Family Upheaval Due to Bed-wetting

A mother brings her 8-year-old son to the office seeking treatment for his diagnosis of bed-wetting or nocturnal enuresis. Her husband works long hours. The mother is employed outside the home. The stress of wet beds multiple times per week is causing significant family disruption due to additional work created by the wet linens; anger by the father, who believes his son should be able to control the problem; and social withdrawal by the son, who is embarrassed by the problem.

6. Classical conditioning using an alarm system that wakens the child when wetting starts is one consideration. Which of the following statements is true?
   a. since the effect is virtually immediate, it offers a good solution in this case
   b. it requires no effort on the part of the parents, so it is a good solution for this family

c. it is the most commonly prescribed intervention, so there are many satisfied patients to vouch for the process

d. it can be arduous for the child because it disrupts the sleep cycle

e. none of the above

7. Which of the following statements is (are) true regarding the use of bedwetting alarms?

    a. for resolution of bedwetting, the alarm may need to be used for 15 weeks

    b. the treatment dropout rate is up to 30%

    c. the alarm should not be used in children younger than age 5 years

    d. a and c

    e. a, b, and c

8. Which of the following should not be used in the treatment of this condition?

    a. punishing the child

    b. limiting or eliminating liquids after dinner

    c. providing the child with a feeling of inferiority for having the problem

    d. all of the above

    e. a and c

9. Which of the following is the drug of choice in the pharmacologic treatment of this disorder?

    a. oxybutynin chloride

    b. imipramine

    c. diazepam

    d. desmopressin

    e. most pharmacologic therapies have been shown to be no more effective than placebo

10. Clearly, this child has psychological issues, as demonstrated by his social withdrawal and strained relationships with his family. Which of the following statements is (are) true regarding his psychological status?

    a. it is likely that his psychological problems are the cause of his enuresis

    b. most psychological problems related to enuresis are the result of the bedwetting and not the cause of the bedwetting

    c. enuresis is often symptom substitution for other neurotic or emotional symptoms

    d. commonly associated psychological symptoms are low self-esteem and high anxiety

    e. b and d

Answers

1. **b.** Nocturnal enuresis is defined as involuntary urination in sleep without urological or neurological causes after the age of 5 years at which time bladder control would normally be expected. He does not meet the criteria for school phobia and there is no information that suggests a diagnosis of masked depression. There is no such condition as small bladder syndrome.

2. **c.** Enuresis is usually defined as the involuntary discharge of urine after the age at which bladder control usually should have been established (age 5 years). As just classified, this child has nocturnal enuresis (only at night).

3. **c.** The prevalence of enuresis decreases with increasing age. Thus, 82% of 2-year-old children, 49% of 3-year-old children, 26% of 4-year-old children, and 15% to 25% of 5-year-old children still wet beds on a regular basis. Enuresis is definitely more common in children when one or both parents were enuretic as children. It is significantly more common in boys than girls. The psychological issues seem to be the result of the enuresis rather than the cause. Bladder capacity is usually the same in children with and without enuresis, although functional capacity may be less in those with enuresis.

4. **a.** The only mandatory laboratory evaluation for children with enuresis is a urinalysis. The following are all important abnormalities that may be associated with enuresis: the presence of white blood cells in the urine as a result of a urinary tract infection, low urinary specific gravity as a result of diabetes insipidus, proteinuria, hematuria as a result of renal disease, and glucosuria as a result of diabetes mellitus. Urine culture, CBC, IVP, and cystometric evaluation should be performed only if specific indications suggest the need. Posterior urethral valves (especially in boys) may be associated with enuresis.

5. **e.** Pharmacological therapy is directed at alleviating the symptoms of nocturnal enuresis rather than curing the condition. Imipramine has been noted to have a response rate of 20% to 36%. Desmopressin has a wide range of efficacy from 10% to 86%. Oxybutynin increases functional bladder capacity, but in double-blind, placebo-controlled studies had no advantage over placebo. Biofeedback has an immediate success rate of 80%, but the long-term success rate is 60%.

6. **d.** It can be difficult for the child because nocturnal enuresis is believed to be primarily a sleep disturbance, so further disturbing sleep is problematic. The treatment requires work, inconvenience, and dedication to the treatment process and may take 2 or 3 months to have an effect; thus, families may lose patience and the stress may have a negative effect on the conditioning.

7. e. For resolution of bedwetting, the alarm may need to be used for 15 weeks. The treatment dropout rate is up to 30% and the alarm should not be used in children younger than age 5 years.

8. e. Because there is usually no identifiable cause of enuresis and the disorder tends to remit spontaneously even if not treated, treatment should be conservative. The following methods are approved for the treatment of enuresis:

1. Appropriate toilet training (scheduled voiding times especially in the evening; wake up to urinate in the middle of the night).
2. Behavior modification (bell or buzzer) and pad: These treatments are the most successful in achieving cure. The alarm should not be used in children younger than age 5 years and may require up to 15 weeks to achieve continence. There is a 10% to 30% dropout rate. Possible predictors of a poor response include an unstable or chaotic family situation, behavioral deviance in the child, high parental anxiety level, and low parental education level.
3. Positive reinforcement system that charts the child's progress: Although all of the approved methods are effective and should be used together, it appears that the most effective behavior-modification method is the buzzer or bell and pad system.

9. e. The evidence-based literature has moved from recommending desmopressin instead of imipramine to suggesting that there is not sufficient evidence to recommend one or the other; both seem to have little or no carryover after discontinuing treatment. The evidence comparing the two head to head is unreliable or conflicting in two small trials, and most trials are not large enough to reasonably assess the side effects. In the small randomized controlled trials, there were no instances of serious events or death with either treatment, although adverse events were much more frequently reported for imipramine-treated children.

10. e. Enuresis often causes psychological problems, such as low self-esteem and anxiety, and can create family dysfunction. Most evidence suggests that there is no occurrence of symptom substitution and that children do not show an increase in behavior or psychological problems except for their response to the bedwetting.

Summary

1. Prevalence: 7% to 20% at the age when bladder control should have been fully achieved (i.e., after age 5 years)
2. Classification of subtypes of enuresis is based on whether the child has ever achieved bladder control:
   a. Primary enuresis: Child has never been dry.
   b. Secondary enuresis: Child has been dry for a period but becomes enuretic later.
3. Classification based on period when child does not have bladder control:
   a. Nocturnal enuresis: Enuresis at night only.
   b. Diurnal enuresis: Enuresis during the day only.
   c. Nocturnal and diurnal enuresis: Enuresis during both day and night.
4. Pathophysiology: Immaturity on the part of the autonomic nervous system that controls the bladder in the vast majority of cases. Infrequently, enuresis is associated with organic problems, such as congenital urinary tract system abnormality or urinary tract infection. Only 20% of children with enuresis have a psychodevelopmental disorder (lower intelligence quotient or behavioral disorder). Secondary enuresis is often associated with a stressful environmental event.
5. Investigations: Urinalysis is the only mandatory investigation for nocturnal enuresis. If enuresis also occurs in the daytime or if urinary flow is small or interrupted, a renal ultrasound and a careful neurologic examination (including inspection of the sacral area for structural abnormalities) are indicated.
6. Treatment: Because the pathophysiology of enuresis is not completely clear, the therapeutic approach is still based on empirical data. Therapy is aimed at alleviating the symptoms of nocturnal enuresis rather than at curing the condition.
   a. Imipramine is no longer recommended for the treatment of enuresis in most children due to the potential for complications. Desmopressin is useful in achieving dry nights but patients often revert to pretreatment levels when the medication is discontinued.
   b. A behavior-modification program is the treatment of choice, including buzzer/bell and pad, positive reinforcement, charting progress to increase confidence and self-esteem, urinating before bedtime, avoiding liquids after the evening meal, and avoiding psychological trauma through blame or belittling the child.

Suggested Reading

Golbin AZ: Nocturnal enuresis: A disorder of sleep. In: Golbin AZ, Kravitz HM, Keith LG, eds, *Sleep Psychiatry*. New York: Taylor & Francis, 2004.

Sulkes SB, Dosa NP: Developmental and behavioral pediatrics: Enuresis. In: Behrman RE, Kliegman RM, eds, *Nelson Essentials of Pediatrics*, 4th ed. Philadelphia: Saunders, 2002.

Thiedke CC: Nocturnal enuresis. *Am Fam Physician* 67:1499–1506, 1509–1510, 2003.

Lymphoma and Leukemia

c. chronic myelogenous leukemia
d. Hodgkin's disease
e. non-Hodgkin's lymphoma

CLINICAL CASE PROBLEM 1

A 14-Year-Old Male with a Mediastinal Mass

A 14-year-old male is brought into the office by his parents. For the past 2 weeks, he has been very tired and has felt short of breath. The mother tells you that she thinks he has been losing weight. On physical examination, the child is alert and in no distress; vital signs are normal, but he has lost 8 pounds since his last visit 6 months ago. The lungs are clear bilaterally, and the heart examination is normal. You palpate an enlarged supraclavicular node. Chest radiography reveals a large mediastinal mass.

SELECT THE BEST ANSWER TO THE FOLLOWING QUESTIONS

1. What is the most likely diagnosis?
   a. acute streptococcal pneumonia
   b. mycoplasma pneumonia
   c. mononucleosis
   d. Hodgkin's disease
   e. tuberculosis

2. Which of the following is commonly associated with non-Hodgkin's lymphoma?
   a. intussusception in a child older than age 5 years
   b. intraabdominal mass
   c. superior vena cava obstruction
   d. airway obstruction
   e. all of the above

3. The presence of Reed–Sternberg cells in tissue is diagnostic of which disease?
   a. Hodgkin's disease
   b. lymphoblastic lymphoma
   c. Burkitt's lymphoma
   d. large cell lymphoma
   e. non-Hodgkin's disease

4. The most common malignancy in childhood is which of the following?
   a. acute lymphoblastic leukemia (ALL)
   b. acute myeloid leukemia (AML)

CLINICAL CASE PROBLEM 2

"My Little Is All Bruised Up"

A 3-year-old female presents for her well child visit. The physician notes pallor and bruising. On physical examination, the vital signs are normal but there is a generalized lymphadenopathy and hepatosplenomegaly. A complete blood count (CBC) reveals a white blood cell (WBC) count of 33,000/mm^3 and a platelet count of 81,000/mm^3. The peripheral blood smear shows blasts, and the lactate dehydrogenase activity is elevated. CBC shows blasts as well as hypochromic red blood cells.

5. The most common leukemia among children is which of the following?
   a. acute myelogenous leukemia
   b. acute lymphocytic leukemia
   c. chronic myelogenous leukemia (CML)
   d. chronic lymphocytic leukemia (CLL)
   e. equal numbers of AML and ALL

6. Most cases of ALL are diagnosed between the ages of which of the following ranges?
   a. birth and 2 years
   b. 2 and 3 years
   c. 12 and 15 years
   d. 8 and 12 years
   e. 5 and 15 years

7. Which ethnic group has the highest frequency of ALL?
   a. white
   b. Hispanic
   c. African American
   d. Asian
   e. no ethnic variation

8. Which of the statements regarding the disease described in here is true?
   a. the peak age of onset is 12 years
   b. at the time of diagnosis, most patients have a thrombocytosis
   c. a CBC with differential is the most useful initial test
   d. a chest x-ray is the most useful initial test
   e. none of the above

9. Which of the following increases the risk of a child developing AML?
a. previous exposure to benzene
b. previous exposure to ionizing radiation
c. neurofibromatosis
d. a and c
e. a, b, and c

Answers

1. d. There are two types of lymphomas: Hodgkin's disease and non-Hodgkin's lymphoma. Hodgkin's disease is the more common type of lymphoma.

Nonspecific signs and symptoms observed in children with lymphoma include malaise, fever, painless adenopathy, headache, nausea, vomiting, weight loss, abdominal pain, intussusception, intermittent obstruction, diarrhea, pruritus, swelling of the face and neck, cough, and shortness of breath with no history of reactive airway disease.

Hodgkin's disease commonly presents with painless cervical adenopathy. Early lymph node biopsy should be considered if there is no identifiable infection in the region drained by an enlarged node, a node is greater than 2 cm, there is supraclavicular adenopathy or an abnormal chest x-ray, or a lymph node is increasing in size after 2 weeks or does not resolve after 4 to 8 weeks.

When Hodgkin's disease is suspected, a chest x-ray should be ordered. Half of all patients will have either mediastinal adenopathy or an anterior mediastinal mass. The blood count is usually normal, and acute phase reactants such as the erythrocyte sedimentation rate are often elevated.

2. e. The onset of symptoms is more rapid in non-Hodgkin's lymphoma than Hodgkin's disease. Shortness of breath and abdominal symptoms such as intussusception, obstruction, and abdominal mass are more common in non-Hodgkin's lymphoma.

Non-Hodgkin's lymphoma is divided into three groups: lymphoblastic, small noncleaved cell, and large cell. The presentation of non-Hodgkin's lymphoma depends on the cell type. Lymphoblastic lymphoma commonly presents with symptoms of airway obstruction or superior vena cava obstruction. This is the result of mediastinal disease. Small noncleaved cell lymphomas and large cell lymphomas often present with signs or symptoms related to abdominal disease.

3. a. The presence of Reed–Sternberg cells in tissue is diagnostic of Hodgkin's disease. These cells are large and multinucleated, and they have abundant cytoplasm.

4. a. ALL is the most common malignancy of childhood. It accounts for approximately 25% of all cancer diagnosis in children younger than age 15 years.

5. b. AML is the most common leukemia in adults, but it is less common in children. Seventy-three percent of childhood leukemia is acute lymphocytic leukemia. CML is very rare in children, occurring in approximately 2% of childhood leukemia cases. CLL is also unusual in children.

6. b. The peak incidence for ALL is 2 and 3 years of age.

7. b. Hispanics have a frequency of 43 per 1 million. The frequency for whites is 30 to 40 per 1 million, and that for African Americans is approximately one-third the rate of whites.

8. c. The most useful initial test to perform in patients suspected of having ALL is a CBC with differential. In most cases, there will be an increase or decrease in at least one or two cell types. The WBC count may be decreased, normal, or elevated, and the differential will show a neutropenia. Blasts may be seen on the peripheral smear. Most patients with ALL will have a decreased hemoglobin and platelet count at the time of diagnosis. The diagnosis of ALL is confirmed by a bone marrow examination showing more than 25% lymphoblasts. A chest radiograph should be obtained to search for a possible mediastinal mass. With combination chemotherapy, the prognosis of ALL is very good.

9. e. A less common type of leukemia seen in children is AML. Risk factors for AML include exposure to ionizing radiation or benzene, previous treatment with cytotoxic chemotherapeutic agents, and certain congenital syndromes such as neurofibromatosis. Most patients will have no identifiable risk factors. The incidence of AML is bimodal and peaks at the ages of 2 and 16 years. Leukemia during the first 4 weeks of life is most often AML.

Children with AML may present with fever, pallor, weight loss, or fatigue. In some cases, sepsis or bleeding may be the initial presentation of AML. A CBC will show anemia, thrombocytopenia, and an elevated or low WBC count. Bone marrow aspirate will show more than 30% myeloblasts.

Summary

Lymphoma
HODGKIN'S DISEASE

1. It is the most common type of lymphoma (incidence approximately 5.5 to 12.1 cases per 100,000).
2. Bimodal incidence is late teen/young adult and mid-50s.
3. Presentation: It commonly presents with painless cervical adenopathy; may have splenomegaly or enlargement of other immune tissue, fever, weight loss, fatigue, or night sweats.
4. If diagnosis is suspected, a chest radiograph should be obtained to search for mediastinal adenopathy or anterior mediastinal mass.
5. Reed–Sternberg cells are diagnostic of Hodgkin's disease. Viral DNA has been found in Reed–Sternberg cells. Epstein–Barr virus has been implicated in approximately 50% of all cases of Hodgkin's lymphoma in the United States.
6. Treatment involves multiagent chemotherapy and, in some cases, radiation therapy. Patients with lower stage disease have more than a 90% survival rate; those with a higher stage disease have more than a 70% survival rate.

NON-HODGKIN'S LYMPHOMA

Slightly less common than pediatric Hodgkin's.
1. Groups
   a. Lymphoblastic
   b. Small noncleaved cell
   c. Large cell
2. It has a more rapid onset of symptoms than in Hodgkin's disease.
3. Shortness of breath, intussusception, bowel obstruction, and abdominal mass are more common in non-Hodgkin's lymphoma than in Hodgkin's disease.
4. The presentation of non-Hodgkin's lymphoma depends on cell type.
   a. Lymphoblastic lymphoma commonly presents with airway obstruction of superior vena cava obstruction.
   b. Small noncleaved cell and large cell lymphomas commonly present with signs and symptoms related to abdominal disease.
5. Treatment is based on multiagent chemotherapy based on the histologic subtype. Since the late 1960s, treatment has progressed rapidly. Rather than an inevitable death sentence, the current cure rate is approximately 65% to 90%.

Leukemia
CLASSIFICATION

1. Myelogenous—proliferation of WBCs, red blood cells with or without platelet precursors
2. Lymphocytic—proliferation of bone marrow precursors of lymphocytes

ALL

1. Most common malignancy of childhood, accounting for approximately 23% of all childhood malignancies. There are approximately 2000 to 2500 new cases per year or 30 to 40 per 1 million.
   a. Hispanic incidence is 43 per 1 million.
   b. It is three times more common in white than in African American children.
2. Peak incidence is 2 and 3 years of age.
3. Common presentation includes (a) intermittent fevers; (b) bone pain; (c) cutaneous or mucosal bleeding; (d) petechiae, purpura; (e) pallor; (f) lymphadenopathy; (g) hepatosplenomegaly; (h) swelling of the face; (i) testicular enlargement; and (j) subcutaneous nodules (leukemia cutis).
4. CBC with differential: (a) WBCs increased, decreased, or normal; (b) neutropenia; (c) anemia; and (d) thrombocytopenia.
5. Bone marrow shows a large number of leukemic blasts.
6. Obtain chest radiograph to search for mediastinal widening or mass.
7. Treatment is chemotherapy based. Although it was a death sentence a few decades ago, there is currently a 95% remission rate and 75% to 95% of patients are disease free at 5 years.

AML

1. It is less common than ALL. Overall, it accounts for approximately 20% of childhood leukemias.
2. The peak incidence is at 2 and 16 years of age. Because the incidence of ALL starts later and decreases more rapidly, AML accounts for a larger fraction of cases in children younger than 2 years and older than 5 years.
3. Leukemia during the first 4 weeks of life is most often AML and accounts for approximately 50% by adolescence.
4. Risk factors include (a) previous exposure to benzene, ionizing radiation, or cytotoxic chemotherapeutic agents and (b) certain congenital syndromes, such as neurofibromatosis, Noonan syndrome, Fanconi anemia, and Down syndrome.
5. Common presentation includes (a) fever, (b) pallor, (c) weight loss, (d) fatigue, (e) cutaneous or mucosal bleeding, and (f) menorrhagia.
6. CBC with differential: (a) anemia, (b) thrombocytopenia, and (c) elevated or low WBCs.
7. Bone marrow aspirate shows more than 30% myeloblasts.
8. Treatment is intensive chemotherapy. Overall cure rate is approximately 50%. (Children with Down syndrome do best with less intensive treatment.)

Suggested Reading

Albano EA, Stork LC, Greffe BS, et al: Neoplastic disease. In: Hay WW, Jr, Hayward AR, Levin MJ, Sondheimer JM, eds, *Current Pediatric Diagnosis & Treatment.* New York: Lange/McGraw–Hill, 2003.

Brown VI: Acute lymphoblastic leukemia. In: Schwartz MW, ed., *The 5-Minute Pediatric Consult.* Philadelphia: Lippincott Williams & Wilkins, 2003.

Gajra A, Vajpayee N, Grethlein S: B-cell lymphoma. Emedicine, March 2007.

Habermann TM: Improving outcomes in patients with lymphoma. Continuing medical education activity. *Medscape,* 2007.

Kang T, Shankar SM: Acute myeloid leukemia. In: Schwartz MW, ed., *The 5-Minute Pediatric Consult.* Philadelphia: Lippincott Williams & Wilkins, 2003.

Mester B, Nieters A, Deeg E, et al: Occupation and malignant lymphoma: A population based case control study in Germany. *Occup Environ Med* 63(1):17–26, 2006.

Reaman GH: Pediatric oncology: Current views and outcomes. *Pediatr Clin North Am* 49(6):1305–1318, 2002.

Schöllkopf C, Smedby KE, Hjalgrim H, et al: Cigarette smoking and risk of non-Hodgkin's lymphoma—A population-based case–control study. *Cancer Epidemiol Biomarkers Prev* 14(7):1791–1796, 2005.

Velez MC: Lymphomas. *Pediatr Rev* 24(11):380–386, 2003.

CHAPTER

118   Sickle Cell Disease

CLINICAL CASE PROBLEM 1

A 10-Year-Old Male with Diffuse Musculoskeletal Pain

Parents bring their 10-year-old son to the office, reporting that he has had several episodes of abdominal, arm, leg, and back pain during the past 2 weeks, each lasting 1 to 5 hours, with the last one prompting emergency room care. At that time, he was treated with narcotic analgesics and intravenous fluids. He was referred to you for follow-up and primary care. He was diagnosed with sickle cell anemia as an infant and has received pneumococcal vaccine, but he is not on any chronic medications.

SELECT THE BEST ANSWER TO THE FOLLOWING QUESTIONS

1. What is the pathophysiology of sickle cell anemia?
   a. replacement of normal hemoglobin A by hemoglobin C
   b. replacement of normal hemoglobin A by hemoglobin F
   c. substitution of glutamic acid by valine in the sixth position of the beta chain of hemoglobin A
   d. substitution of glutamic acid by lysine in the sixth position of the beta chain of hemoglobin A
   e. a and c

2. What is the most likely type of crisis just experienced by this patient?
   a. aplastic crisis
   b. hemolytic crisis
   c. neutropenic crisis
   d. sequestration crisis
   e. vasoocclusive crisis

3. In vasoocclusion, which of the following contribute(s) to the crisis?
   a. activated vascular endothelium
   b. hypocoagulability
   c. altered nitric oxide metabolism
   d. a and c
   e. all of the above

4. What is (are) the long-term complication(s) of this type of crisis?
   a. autoinfarction of the spleen
   b. liver failure secondary to infarction
   c. papillary necrosis with secondary renal complications
   d. transient ischemic attacks
   e. all of the above

5. In which of the following ethnic groups does sickle cell anemia not occur?
   a. African American
   b. Italian
   c. Saudi Arabian
   d. Northwest European
   e. Greek

6. Which of the following vaccinations should the patient receive?
   a. 23-valent pneumococcal vaccine
   b. 7-valent pneumococcal conjugate vaccine
   c. annual influenza vaccine
   d. meningococcal vaccine
   e. all of the above

CLINICAL CASE PROBLEM 2

Headache in a Child of Middle Eastern Descent

A recently immigrated family from the Middle East comes to the office with their 3-year-old daughter, who has been complaining of a prolonged headache that parents thought was due to the stress of the move. On examination, vital signs are normal and there are no focal changes. On history, the mother reports that her brother (the patient's uncle) has sickle cell trait. However, the patient has not been screened for hemoglobinopathies. You recommend that this child should be screened due to family history, newly effective preventative measures, and the opportunity for early intervention.

7. In children, which of the following is (are) the possible acute complication(s) of this condition?
   a. cerebrovascular accident
   b. splenic sequestration
   c. multiple organ failure syndrome
   d. acute chest syndrome
   e. all of the above

8. In children, chronic manifestations of sickle cell anemia include which of the following?
   a. proliferative retinopathy
   b. pulmonary hypertension
   c. avascular necrosis
   d. cholelithiasis
   e. all of the above

9. Appropriate prevention interventions/evaluations to consider include which of the following?
   a. evaluation of transcranial blood flow
   b. hydroxyurea until age 4 years
   c. antibiotics prophylaxis
   d. a and c
   e. b and c

Clinical Case Management Problem

An 8-year-old with sickle cell disease presents to the emergency room with fever, chest pain, cough, and trouble breathing. She was in the emergency department for a pain crisis 2½ days ago. She has recently had an upper respiratory infection and suddenly felt much worse. Describe the diagnosis, treatment, and prognosis for this patient.

Answers

1. **c.** Replacement of normal hemoglobin A by hemoglobin S is caused by substitution of glutamic acid by valine in the sixth position of the beta chain of hemoglobin A.

2. **e.** This patient most likely presents with a vaso-occlusive crisis caused by obstruction of the microcirculation by sickled red blood cells (RBCs) and ischemia. A hemolytic crisis usually presents with sudden onset of anemia secondary to the sequestration of RBCs in the spleen. Aplasia can be a result of a hemotologic crisis usually precipitated by folic acid deficiency or parvovirus infection. A neutropenic crisis is not a term usually used for sickle cell crises, with most sickle cell patients presenting with leukocytosis. A sequestration crisis is another term for a hemolytic crisis.

3. **d.** The vasoocclusion of the disease once thought to involve only the polymerization of hemoglobin S is now known to include leukocytes, activated vascular endothelium, altered nitric oxide metabolism, hypercoagulability, and ischemia–reperfusion injury.

4. **e.** All of the organs listed can be damaged by the occlusion of their blood flow by sickled cells.

5. **d.** The sickle cell disorder occurs most often in those of African descent but also has a high frequency in Mediterranean, Caribbean, South and Central American, Arab, and East Indian populations.

6. **e.** All of the usual childhood immunizations should be provided as well as the influenza vaccine due to decreased immunity secondary to potential functional asplenia. The 7-valent pneumococcal vaccine decreases the incidence of invasive pneumococcal infection in children younger than age 2 years, but since children with sickle cell remain susceptible to life-threatening pneumococcal infections, they should receive the 23-valent if they are 2 years old or older.

7. **c.** Acute complications of this disease include acute chest syndrome. It is the second most common reason for hospitalization of patients with sickle cell anemia after painful crisis. It is the most common cause of death in sickle cell patients. Triggers include infection, fat embolism, and hypoventilation secondary to bone infarct in ribs, sternum, or thoracic vertebrae. Acute sequestration can cause acute anemia. Multiple organ failure syndrome involves the acute development of severe dysfunction in at least two of three major organs during a painful episode.
   Up to 30% of individuals with hemoglobin SS suffer a stroke, and recurrence is not unusual.

8. **e.** The prevalence of pulmonary hypertension in adults may be as high as 30%, although children can be affected as well. Proliferative retinopathy is seen secondary to microvascular occlusion and ischemia. Avascular necrosis of the femoral head is very common

in patients with sickle cell disease and can lead to significant disability. Cholelithiasis results from high bilirubin levels from constant hemolysis.

9. **d.** Evaluation of transcranial blood flow by specialized transcranial Doppler ultrasound is recommended for asymptomatic children. If transcranial blood flow velocity is 200 cm/second or more, the patient is at high risk of stroke and is a candidate for chronic transfusion. Daily antibiotic prophylaxis for infants and children consists of penicillin V potassium starting by 2 months of age. The prophylaxis can be stopped safely at 5 years of age for patients without a history of invasive pneumococcal infection or splenectomy. Hydroxyurea should be considered for older adolescents and adults but not children.

Solution to the Clinical Case Management Problem

Survival is improved with aggressive treatment, so a high index of suspicion should be maintained. Symptoms include new-onset chest pain, fever, wheezing, dyspnea or tachypnea, cough, and hypoxemia. Chest radiograph shows a new pulmonary infiltrate. Diagnostics include blood and sputum culture, pulse oximetry, daily CBC and serum chemistries, arterial blood gas measurements for changes in O_2 saturations, and pre- and posttransfusion hemoglobin S concentration (hemoglobin electrophoresis).

Treatment includes the following:

Prompt consultation with a pulmonologist or hematologist
Supplemental oxygen for Po_2 below 80 mmHg or oxygen saturation below 95%

Incentive spirometry while awake
Broad-spectrum antibiotic therapy (include coverage for atypical organisms)
Fluid management with careful intake and output management
Bronchodilator therapy if needed
Aggressive pain management with respiratory monitoring
Transfusion therapy for hypoxemia or clinical deterioration

Regarding the prognosis, 30% of patients with hemoglobin SS disease will have one episode of acute chest syndrome and half of those will have recurrent episodes. It can lead to adult respiratory distress syndrome. It is the most common cause of death in sickle cell patients.

Summary

1. Population at greatest risk: African Americans—1 in 12 (8%) carry the sickle cell trait. That is, they are heterozygous (HbA/HbS) for sickle cell. Those who are homozygous (HbS/HbS) have sickle cell disease.
2. Diagnosis
   a. Blood smear: red blood cells sickle and hemolyze
   b. Hemoglobin electrophoresis
3. Clinical manifestations
   a. Hemolytic anemia: Severe hemolytic anemia with hematocrit values varying between 18% and 30%. The mean red blood cell survival is between 10 and 15 days.
   b. Acute pain crises and chronic organ damage: The morbidity and mortality are primarily a result of recurrent vasoocclusive phenomena causing damage through microinfarcts that produce the painful crisis and macroinfarcts that produce organ damage.

   c. Pulmonary function restriction: Impairment of pulmonary function is common. Resting arterial PO_2 is reduced in part because of the intrapulmonary arterial–venous shunting. Because HbS/Hbs red blood cells have decreased oxygen affinity, arterial blood is significantly undersaturated.
   d. Congestive cardiac failure: HbS/Hbs homozygotes frequently develop overt congestive heart failure (CHF). The pathophysiology of this CHF is associated with the severe chronic anemia and hypoxemia (high-output cardiac failure).
   e. Cerebrovascular accidents (CVAs): The primary causes of a CVA are cerebral thrombosis or subarachnoid hemorrhage. Hemiplegia is encountered more frequently than coma, convulsions, or visual disturbances.
   f. Ophthalmologic complications: These include retinal infarcts, peripheral vessel disease, arteriovenous

anomalies, vitreous hemorrhage, proliferative retinopathy, and retinal detachment.

g. Genitourinary complications: Patients develop significant and prolonged painless hematuria as a result of papillary infarcts. The amount of blood loss can be so significant that iron deficiency develops. Longer surviving patients with HbS/Hbs disease develop progressive renal failure. Boys and young men with sickle cell disease occasionally develop priapism.

h. Hepatobiliary complications: Patients can be icteric because of the hemolytic anemia discussed previously. The hyperbilirubinemia that is associated with sickle cell disease is nonconjugated hyperbilirubinemia. Patients with sickle cell disease are also at increased risk of gallstone formation.

i. Skeletal complications: The skeletal complications include expansion of the red marrow, bony infarcts, and avascular necrosis of joints in hip and shoulder. The biconcave, or "fishmouth," vertebrae are virtually pathognomonic for sickle cell disease. The hand–foot syndrome is a painful swelling of the hand or foot caused by infarction of the bone marrow in metacarpal or metatarsal bones and phalanges.

j. Skin disease: Chronic skin ulcers often occur in the lower extremities.

k. Splenic sequestration: The spleen becomes enlarged as a result of the rapid sequestration of sickled blood. The acute anemia that results may be rapidly fatal and should be treated with emergency blood transfusions.

l. Aplastic crises: The previously mentioned aplastic crises, which usually occur when a child is recovering from an infection, are caused by human parvovirus B19. Profound anemia occurs, and blood transfusions are necessary to treat it.

4. Treatment

a. Treatment and, when possible, prevention of complications (recurrent CVAs) may be prevented by starting the child on a chronic transfusion program.

b. Nutritional supplements: Folic acid 1 mg/day.

c. Immunizations or vaccines: *Haemophilus influenzae* B, pneumococcal vaccine, and all other routine vaccinations recommended for other children, as summarized in Chapter 100.

d. Prophylactic antibiotics: Penicillin V 125 mg twice daily up to age 3 years, then 250 mg twice daily up to age 5 years.

e. Pain control for acute pain crises and other painful events: Intravenous fluids and analgesics as needed; do not be afraid to use narcotic analgesics.

f. Painless hematuria: Aminocaproic acid.

g. Transfusion: Indicated for symptomatic episodes of acute anemia, severe symptomatic episodes of acute anemia, severe symptomatic chronic anemia, prevention of recurrent strokes in children, acute chest syndromes with hypoxia, and surgery with general anesthesia.

h. Hydroxyurea: Indicated for adolescents or adults with frequent episodes of pain, a history of the acute chest syndrome, other severe vasoocclusive complications, or severe symptomatic anemia.

i. Transplantation: Bone marrow (stem cell) transplantation has been successful; this should be considered in children and adolescents younger than age 16 years who have severe complications and an HLA-matched donor is available.

Suggested Reading

Hulbert ML, Scothorn DJ, Panepinto JA, et al: The pathophysiology, prevention, and treatment of stroke in sickle cell disease. *Curr Opin Hematol* 14(3):191–197, 2007.

Mehta SR, Afenyi-Annan A, Byrns PJ, Lottenberg R: Opportunities to improve outcomes in sickle cell disease. *Am Fam Physician* 74(2):303–310, 2006.

Melton CS, Haynes J: Sickle acute lung injury: Role of prevention and early aggressive intervention strategies on outcome. *Clin Chest Medicine* 27:487–502, 2006.

National Institutes of Health: *The Management of Sickle Cell Disease*, publication No. 02–2117, 4th ed. Bethesda, MD: National Institutes of Health, 2002.

Quinn CT, Miller ST: Risk factors and prediction of outcomes in children and adolescents who have sickle cell anemia. *Hematol Oncol Clin North Am* 18:1339–1354, 2004.

Wang WC, Morales KH, Scher CD, et al: Effect of long-term transfusion on growth in children with sickle cell anemia: Results of the Stop Trial. *J Pediatr* 147(2):244–247, 2005.

119 Physical Activity and Nutrition

CLINICAL CASE PROBLEM 1

A 12 Year-Old Boy Who Is Overweight

A mother comes into your clinic with her 12-year-old son. She is concerned that he might be overweight and wants some advice on weight-loss programs. The patient has been healthy with no medical problems. On examination, he is in the 70th percentile for height and more than 97th percentile for weight.

SELECT THE BEST ANSWER TO THE FOLLOWING QUESTIONS

1. Questions that you want to ask this mother include which of the following?
   a. how much time does the patient spend watching television and playing video games?
   b. how much physical activity does the patient receive at home and how much physical education at school?
   c. what type of snacks does he eat and how frequently?
   d. how much juice and soda does he consume?
   e. all of the above

2. Barriers to effective interventions designed to encourage a healthy diet include all of the following except
   a. parents purchasing high-calorie snacks
   b. cognitive developmental stage of the child and ability to understand cause and long-term effects
   c. perceived lack of time
   d. expense of fast foods compared to foods cooked at home
   e. plenitude and availability of inexpensive fast food, junk food, and soda

3. According to recent statistics, which of the following is true about overweight and obese children in the United States?
   a. interventions to decrease obesity are showing positive results
   b. parents' exercise and eating habits do not matter as long as they teach their children what is correct
   c. schools have adopted recommendations to increase exercise and require all children to participate in sports activities through their senior year in high school
   d. the group with the highest percentage of overweight children among different ethnic groups is non-Hispanic black girls
   e. there is no relation between obesity in childhood and adolescence and obesity in adulthood

4. Strength training in children
   a. has been shown to be beneficial when provided in a supervised environment
   b. has no proven benefit in increasing fitness or helping with weight loss
   c. actually can cause children to gain significant amounts of weight
   d. endangers growth plates and increases risk of injuries
   e. should focus on heavy weights and few repetitions

5. Effective nutritional interventions for obese children include which of the following?
   a. allowing the child/adolescent to choose food at the grocery store
   b. very low-carbohydrate/high-fat diets
   c. increasing consumption of fruit drinks
   d. eating while watching television
   e. adding more fruits and vegetables to the diet while eliminating sodas and juices

6. Which of the following statements is false?
   a. peak bone mass is achieved in childhood and adolescence
   b. the extent and duration of breast-feeding have been found to be inversely associated with risk of obesity in later childhood
   c. early menarche is clearly associated with the degree of overweight, with a twofold increase in rate of early menarche associated with a high body mass index (BMI)
   d. maternal obesity, low cognitive stimulation in the home, and low socioeconomic status all predict development of obesity
   e. obesity in adulthood has a higher correlation with obesity in younger children than with obesity in adolescence

7. During the past three decades, the rate of obesity has
   a. more than doubled for preschool children ages 2 to 5 years and adolescents ages 12 to 19 years and more than tripled for children ages 6 to 11 years
   b. increased slightly for preschool children and 6- to 11-year-olds but decreased in 12- to 19-year-olds due to anorexia nervosa and bulimia

c. been slowly increasing in all groups
d. been the same
e. none of the above are true

A School with a Large Overweight Student Population

You are hired by the school board as a consultant for the district to assist them in making changes to improve the obesity epidemic in the area. As a result of national and local campaigns, the parents and teachers have recognized that many children are overweight and obese, but they are not sure what to do. You review the height and weight data for the children and find that 25% of the children are over the 97th percentile for weight. You decide to investigate what is being done in other areas and what recommendations you can make to change this worrisome trend.

8. You make all of the following recommendations to the school board except
   a. school lunches should have two vegetables and/or fruits, not including fruit juices
   b. yearly height, weight, and BMI measurements and calculations should be done on all students, with the information provided to the parents
   c. snack bars, vending machines, and before- and after-school snack programs must eliminate soft drinks and energy-dense, high-calorie snacks and replace them with vegetables and fruits
   d. all students must be in regular, structured physical education classes for 30 minutes a day
   e. parents should not be allowed to use any school facilities after school hours because these facilities should be preserved for the children only

9. As you research the physical education programs in your school and others throughout the country, you find that the following is a true statement:
   a. all of the physical education period is dedicated to physical activity
   b. physical education classes have decreased dramatically in frequency and duration throughout the country
   c. daily physical education classes in school have no association with physical activity as adults
   d. recess periods are equivalent to structured physical education periods
   e. school physical education programs meet the current recommendations for physical activity in children

10. In educating the board and parents, you tell them that the results of increasing physical activity in children include all of the following except
    a. increased fitness levels
    b. decreased risk of obesity and some chronic diseases, such as diabetes mellitus and heart disease
    c. increased skills in teamwork, leadership, and socialization
    d. decreased anxiety and stress
    e. worsening academic performance as a result of time spent exercising

11. Some members of the community argue with you that they cannot afford to pay for more athletic programs and physical education teachers. You explain that the long-term costs of childhood obesity include which of the following?
    a. increased incidence of endocrine problems, especially type 2 diabetes mellitus
    b. increased orthopedic problems, such as slipped capital femoral epiphysis and genu varum
    c. increased urinary tract infections
    d. increased problems in cardiovascular health (hypercholesterolemia and dyslipidemia, hypertension)
    e. increased mental health problems (depression and low self-esteem)

12. In parent–teacher conferences, which of the following statements could you use in informing the parents?
    a. television commercials have no influence on food choices made by children/adolescents
    b. since most families eat their evening meal at home, eating out minimally affects a child's nutrition
    c. eat and exercise how you would like your children to do so—they learn by example more than by lecture
    d. since children generally will choose a healthier meal with a greater percentage of fruits and vegetables over a high-fat meal, let your child choose the menu
    e. the amount of time children spend in front of a television or computer screen is not important, as long as they do not eat the wrong foods

13. You ask the school nurse to help you calculate the BMI of the students. Which statement about BMI is false?
    a. BMI is the ratio of weight in kilograms to the square of height in meters
    b. BMI is used to define overweight and obesity because it correlates well with more accurate

measures of body fat and with obesity-related comorbid conditions
c. BMI between the 85th and 95th percentiles for age and sex is considered at risk of overweight
d. BMI can overestimate obesity in children because they are shorter; it is more accurate in adults
e. BMI at or higher than the 95th percentile is considered overweight or obese

Answers

1. e. Obesity is increasing at epidemic proportions in the United States and other industrialized countries, especially among children and adolescents. All of the choices listed are important in evaluating an obese child. Television and video games have been associated with childhood and adolescent obesity. The amount of physical activity and physical education at school are important factors in weight maintenance and general health. High-fat snacks and juice and soda consumption are important culprits in childhood and adolescent obesity. Sometimes, requesting the mother or patient keep a food diary will help in obtaining an accurate picture of true intake.

2. d. Parents are generally responsible for food shopping. If the parents want their children to eat healthy food, then they cannot buy junk food and not expect the children to want it. The cognitive developmental stage of children is also important to institute changes in behavior. Children and early adolescents have more difficulty understanding the importance of long-term effects on health. Perceived lack of time is a major barrier to behavioral changes. In this modern age, children's schedules are packed like never before. Fast food seems a convenient option for many families without time or resources to cook healthier meals. Soda and junk food are usually cheaper and more available than fruits and vegetables. The relatively cheap cost of fast food—as well as chips, sweets, and high-calorie snacks—compared to that of fresh fruits and vegetables is a barrier. Nutritional recommendations should be met with the basic food groups. Parents who need further help in constructing healthy diets for themselves and their children can benefit by consulting a trained nutritionist.

3. d. Efforts to decrease obesity among children and adolescents have not been effective. In fact, the numbers are even more alarming than in previous years, with adolescent non-Hispanic black females having higher than a 25% incidence of overweight and obesity. Parental behavior and modeling does affect children, and overweight children become overweight adults. Recommended interventions, including a minimum of 30 minutes per day of structured exercise and changes in school cafeteria food, are often not followed due to financial, time, or societal issues.

4. a. Strength training in children has been shown to be beneficial in increasing fitness and in helping to lose weight. Muscle burns more calories at baseline than fat, so building muscles can actually help burn calories. Muscle weighs more than fat, so as muscle mass grows, body weight can actually increase slightly, but when this occurs it is negligible and is offset by the health benefits. When children learn strength training in a supervised environment with good technique, there is very low risk for injury and no risk to growth plates. Strength training in children should emphasize low weights and more repetitions.

5. e. Few children eat the recommended five or six servings of fruits and vegetables a day. Replacing high-calorie and minimally nutritious sodas and juices with these improves the intake of micro- and macronutrients while decreasing empty calories. Children can participate in shopping at the grocery store for healthy food, but left to their own devices they will generally choose high-fat snacks over fruits and vegetables. Fad diets popular with adults, such as very low-carbohydrate/high-fat and very low-fat diets, have not been studied in children and are therefore not recommended. General nutritional guidelines from the U.S. Department of Agriculture recommend that fat intake be approximately 30% of total calories for the day. An obese child or adolescent should have less fat in the diet than this recommendation but should continue to eat a well-balanced diet. Fruit drinks are a hidden source of calories. Many parents believe that fruit drinks must be healthy for their children. They also taste good, and children enjoy drinking them. However, many fruit drinks contain only approximately 5% to 10% of actual fruit juice. Even 100% fruit juice is high in calories and low in fiber and other nutrients essential to a healthy diet. School-age children and adolescents should not drink much more than 10 to 12 ounces of juice per day. Eating while watching television has been shown to increase food intake. Television commercials also feature high-fat foods that make children want fast food and junk food instead of healthier choices.

6. e. Obesity in adolescence is a higher predictor of obesity in adulthood than that in younger children. The extent and duration of breast-feeding are inversely associated with risk of obesity, whereas early menarche, high-risk behaviors, low cognitive stimulation in the home, maternal obesity, low socioeconomic status, and the absence of family meals are associated with increased obesity risk. Television viewing of more than

4 hours a day is associated with a significant increase in BMI compared to that of children who watch less than 2 hours. Peak bone mass is achieved in childhood/adolescence and is improved by increased calcium intake at that time. Soft drinks and smoking cigarettes both have adverse effects on bone mineralization. Weight-bearing physical activity and strength training increase bone density and decrease the risk of osteoporosis and stress fractures.

7. a. The prevalence of obesity in children, as well as adults, is now epidemic. More than 6 million children in the United States are considered obese. During the past three decades, these numbers have more than doubled for preschool children ages 2 to 5 years and adolescents ages 12 to 19 years and more than tripled for children ages 6 to 11 years. Although anorexia and bulimia are health concerns in adolescents, they do not affect the epidemic of obesity.

8. e. Choices a through d have been recommended in the recent Institute of Medicine (IOM) report, as well as by others, to improve health and decrease obesity in children. Many children do not receive regular checkups, but measurement of height, weight, and BMI calculation will help the child and parents to detect developing obesity. Since the behavior of the parents affects that of the children, IOM recommends that schools allow after-hours use of the recreational facilities by families. Since obesity has a multifactoral cause, addressing it at the school, family, and societal levels is essential.

9. b. School physical education programs do not even come close to meeting the current recommendations for physical activity in children. Current recommendations advocate 30 to 60 minutes of moderate to vigorous physical activity a day at least 5 days per week. Physical education in schools is shaped by state law. In recent years, with increasing demand for students' time and decreasing availability of qualified teachers, physical education programs have suffered. Many schools have physical education classes one to three times per week. Very few schools have daily classes. Some schools try to use open recess periods to meet requirements. Some children are active during free recess periods, but many are not, choosing to stand and socialize or read. Even in dedicated physical education classes, more than half of the allotted time can be wasted with changing and showering. Physical education programs need to be supported in schools to help children meet current recommendations for physical activity.

10. e. Physical activity in children has many benefits. Children can achieve increased fitness levels, increased strength, and decreased risk of obesity and related health problems such as insulin resistance. Children who participate in physical activity and team sports are found to have improved skills in teamwork, leadership, confidence, and socialization. Anxiety and stress are decreased, and depression is improved. In one study, adolescents who engaged in regular physical activity were statistically less likely to have thoughts of suicide. Academic performance has actually been found to be improved by participation in regular physical activity. Some researchers believe that students who play sports have to budget their time more efficiently and are more disciplined and organized. Some also believe that participating in regular physical activity provides increased energy and a sense of well-being that allows greater concentration.

11. c. Long-term costs of childhood obesity are frightening. Obesity is associated with significant health problems including cardiovascular health, the endocrine system, mental health, orthopedic complications, pulmonary (asthma and obstructive sleep apnea), gastrointestinal complications, and the probability of obesity persisting into adulthood (80% at adolescence). The potential future health costs associated with pediatric obesity prompted the Surgeon General to predict that preventable morbidity and mortality associated with the obesity epidemic could exceed that of cigarette smoking.

12. c. Television commercials constantly advertise fast food; when children are overwhelmed by so many messages, combined with the convenience and cheapness of fast food, they generally will choose fast food and soda. Children should have five servings of fruits and vegetables per day, and only 10 to 12 ounces of fruit drink per day, as discussed previously. During the past three decades, tremendous societal changes have occurred so that many families do not have a parent at home to prepare the evening meal. Many families frequently eat at restaurants, where food may have more fat, sodium, and less nutritious content (especially fast food). Children learn by example. Obese parents have more obese children, so parents should be encouraged to model a healthy lifestyle to their children. Even with a nutritious diet, if children spend significant time in front of television and computer screens they will not get adequate physical exercise and will still suffer from being overweight. Parents should limit screen viewing to 1 or 2 hours a day.

13. d. BMI is not less accurate in children than in adults. The pediatric growth charts for the U.S. population now include BMI for age and gender so that BMI can be tracked longitudinally.

Summary

According to an IOM report, reversing the rapid increase in obesity among children and adolescents in the United States will require a multipronged approach as comprehensive as the national antismoking campaign. Efforts will have to be combined by schools, families, communities, industry, and government.

The prevalence of overweight children and obesity has dramatically increased in the United States, and it is now the major public health concern among children. Since the 1970s, the prevalence of overweight children ages 2 to 5 years has doubled, and it has tripled for school-aged children. Although Healthy People 2010 indicated overweight and obesity as one of the 10 top public health indicators and set a target prevalence of 5%, there has been little success in reaching the target. The National Health and Nutrition Examination Survey (NHANES) monitors the nutritional status of the population. The most recent NHANES data (2003 and 2004) showed that the prevalence of overweight for children ages 6 to 11 years and 12 to 19 years was 18.8% and 17.4% respectively. The number of overweight children has increased in all age groups, but the prevalence rate was slightly higher among adolescent non-Hispanic white boys (19.1%) than among non-Hispanic black boys (18.5%) and Mexican-American boys (18.3%). Among girls, the racial disparity was even greater, with non-Hispanic black girls having the highest prevalence of overweight (25.4%) compared to non-Hispanic white (15.4%) and Mexican-American (14.1%) girls.

Obesity is directly related to many chronic health problems, most notably type 2 diabetes but also asthma, sleep apnea, depression, and cardiovascular disease.

The U.S. Preventive Services Task Force found insufficient evidence for the effectiveness of counseling and other preventive interventions and insufficient evidence to recommend for or against routine screening for overweight in children and adolescents as a means to prevent adverse health outcomes. Until further research is done, the American Academy of Pediatrics and IOM recommend monitoring BMI in children, encouraging parents to provide healthy food choices, promoting physical activity, and, most important, modeling good food choices and exercise. Downloadable growth and BMI charts are available from the Centers for Disease Control and Prevention at www.cdc.gov/nchs.

The CDC recommends 30 to 60 minutes of moderate to vigorous physical activity per day at least 5 days per week in all children. In adolescents, participation in regular physical activity has been associated with decreased smoking; decreased drug use; increased fruit and vegetable consumption; decreased risk of pregnancy and sexually transmitted diseases; decreased anxiety, stress, and depression; decreased illicit drug use; increased seat belt use; increased academic performance, and other positive health-related behaviors. There are many perceived and real barriers to adequate physical activity, including bad weather, lack of time and access to facilities or equipment, lack of safety, and lack of energy. Attempts must be made to further characterize and eliminate these barriers. Physical education classes are currently inadequate to meet the physical activity recommendations for children and adolescents. Increased availability of exercise opportunities and facilities increases activity. Use of school facilities after-hours, particularly in communities with few exercise areas, has been encouraged by many experts. Strength training in a well-supervised environment is beneficial for children in terms of overall fitness and strength. Peak bone mass is achieved in adolescence. Calcium intake and physical activity during this time can help determine later bone mineral density and the risk of future osteoporosis and stress fractures.

Adequate nutrition and a healthy diet are also critical in childhood and adolescence. Parents must model good eating behavior and make good food purchases. Despite the convenience and inexpensive price tag of many fast-food meals, parents must make the added effort to find and prepare well-balanced and healthy meals, providing plenty of fresh fruits and vegetables and less than 30% of total calories as fat. Fruit juice is often an unrecognized culprit in childhood obesity and is not a substitute for fresh fruits.

Suggested Reading

American Academy of Pediatrics Committee on Nutrition: Policy statement: Prevention of pediatric overweight and obesity. *Pediatrics* 112(2):424–428, 2003.

Centers for Disease Control and Prevention: *Healthy People 2010.* Available at www.cdc.gov.

Goran MI, Ball DC, Cruz ML: Obesity and risk of type 2 diabetes and cardiovascular disease in children and adolescents. *J Clin Endocrinol Metab* 88(4):1417–1427, 2003.

Hill JC, Smith PC, Meadows SE: What are the most effective interventions to reduce childhood obesity? *J Fam Pract* 51(10):891, 2002.

Koplan J, Liverman CT, Kraak VA: *Preventing Childhood Obesity: Health in the Balance.* Washington, DC: National Academies Press, 2005. Available at http://books.nap.edu/catalog/11015. html.

Sothern MS, Gordon ST: Prevention of obesity in young children: A critical challenge for medical professionals. *Clin Pediatr* 42(2):101–111, 2003.

U.S. Preventive Services Task Force: Screening and interventions for overweight in children and adolescents: Recommendation statement. *Pediatrics* 116(1):205–209, 2005.

The Limping Child

CLINICAL CASE PROBLEM 1

An 18-Month-Old with Pain while Walking

An 18-month-old male is brought in by his parents because for the past week he has cried whenever they put him down to walk. They deny any injury.

SELECT THE BEST ANSWER TO THE FOLLOWING QUESTIONS

1. The differential diagnosis of limp in this young child includes which of the following?
   a. urinary tract infection
   b. septic arthritis of the hip
   c. fracture
   d. puncture wound of the foot
   e. all of the above

2. Foot problems in young children include which of the following?
   a. puncture
   b. avascular necrosis of navicular head or infarction of second metatarsal
   c. stress fracture
   d. ingrown toenails
   e. all of the above

CLINICAL CASE PROBLEM 2

A 5-Year-Old with Fever, Fatigue, and Pain in Leg

A 5-year-old has fever and fatigue and refuses to bear weight on the right leg. You suspect septic arthritis.

3. Which laboratory findings would you expect to find?
   a. elevated C-reactive protein
   b. normal erythrocyte sedimentation rate
   c. low peripheral white blood cell count
   d. high glucose in joint fluid
   e. significantly low platelet count

4. What other conditions should you consider in this child?
   a. compound fracture
   b. viral synovitis
   c. Legg–Calve–Perthes disease
   d. osteomyelitis
   e. b and d

CLINICAL CASE PROBLEM 3

A 12-Year-Old with a Limp and Thigh Pain

A 12-year-old develops a limp and complains of right thigh pain.

5. What conditions should be included in the differential diagnosis?
   a. transient synovitis
   b. slipped femoral capital epiphysis
   c. fracture
   d. gonococcal arthritis
   e. all of the above

6. Osgood–Schlatter disease is
   a. found in young children but not teenagers
   b. a condition affecting the patellar tendon insertion into the tibial tubercle
   c. best treated with surgery
   d. viral in origin
   e. treated surgically

7. Which diagnostic modality is correctly paired with the condition it best assesses?
   a. ultrasound of the hip: osteomyelitis
   b. plain x-ray: Legg–Calve–Perthes disease
   c. history and physical examination: Osgood–Schlatter disease
   d. magnetic resonance imaging (MRI): bone tumor
   e. all of the above

CLINICAL CASE PROBLEM 4

A 9-Year-Old Male with Leg Pain

A 9-year-old male comes to your office with his mother. He complains of a recurrent (nightly) pain in both legs. The pain is so severe that it wakes him from sleep. It is described as a "deep pain." The pain is bilateral and usually is gone by morning. There is no associated fever, chills, limp, or other symptoms. There is no pain during the day.

His history has been excellent. He has had no significant medical illnesses. On examination, the child has no limp and no leg length discrepancy.

8. What is the most likely diagnosis in this child?
   a. slipped capital femoral epiphysis (SCFE)
   b. Legg–Calve–Perthes disease
   c. osteogenic sarcoma
   d. Ewing's sarcoma
   e. "growing pains"

9. What is the preferred treatment for this condition?
   a. surgical fixation
   b. bracing or traction
   c. amputation
   d. radiotherapy followed by chemotherapy
   e. none of the above

10. Regarding limb pain in children, which of the following statements is (are) true?
    a. limb pain is a common presenting complaint in children
    b. there is significant association between limb pain, headache, and abdominal pain
    c. there is frequently an association between limb pain in children and pain of other types in family members
    d. there is frequently an emotional component to limb pain in children
    e. all of the above are true

11. The following criteria describe which of the following childhood orthopedic conditions listed: (1) The condition occurs as a result of acute trauma or in a more subtle manner over time; (2) the typical patient is a somewhat overweight and sedentary teenage boy; (3) pain is located either in the groin or on the medial side of the knee; (4) the hip is held in abduction and external rotation, and there is marked limitation of internal rotation; and (5) diagnosis is made by x-ray.
    Which of the following is most likely?
    a. SCFE
    b. Legg–Calve–Perthes disease
    c. osteogenic sarcoma
    d. Ewing's sarcoma
    e. "growing pains"

12. What is the preferred treatment for the condition described in question 11?
    a. surgical fixation
    b. bracing or traction
    c. amputation

d. radiotherapy followed by chemotherapy
e. none of the above

Answers

1. **e.** Causes of limp in young children include puncture wounds, sprain, bruise, synovitis, and fracture. As many as 20% of young children with a limp have an unsuspected fracture. Spiral fractures of the distal one-third of the tibia can be unsuspected and the result of a minor injury. Other common fractures in children include torus fractures from impaction injuries and greenstick fractures from direct trauma.

2. **e.** Any of these conditions can occur in a young child and should be considered during evaluation of limp or refusal to walk.

3. **a.** Septic arthritis is characterized by refusal to bear weight; fever; and elevation in white blood cell count, C-reactive protein, and erythrocyte sedimentation rate. Ultrasound can aid in diagnosis and in guiding joint aspiration. Fluid aspirated from joints suspected of infection should be sent for the following laboratory studies: cell count and differential, glucose, culture and sensitivity, Gram's stain, and crystal examination. Glucose levels in infected joint fluid are usually low.

4. **e.** In the 4- to 10-year old range, fracture, puncture, sprain, bruising, viral synovitis, septic arthritis, osteomyelitis, Legg–Calve–Perthes disease, tumor, and juvenile rheumatoid arthritis should be in the differential diagnosis. However, Legg–Calve–Perthes disease does not usually present with fever and fatigue, but instead with a painful limp. Compound fracture presents with bone protruding from the skin and should not present as a difficult differential diagnosis.

5. **e.** Transient synovitis should be part of the differential diagnosis for limp in children of all ages. All of these conditions should be considered in older children with limp. Gonococcal arthritis can be contracted even at this young age. Thigh pain can be the chief complaint even when the pathology is in the hip or knee; referred pain and nonspecific complaints are common in children.

6. **b.** Osgood–Schlatter disease is a common cause of knee pain in adolescent athletes. Pain and tenderness occur just below the knee and can be bilateral. The quadriceps inserts into the patellar tendon, and this tendon inserts into the tibial tubercle. As the

quadricep muscle develops, with growth and strength the tendon insertion is stressed and becomes inflamed. Treatment is rest and ice; the condition usually resolves when the growth spurt is over.

7. e. In addition, detection of stress fractures can be aided by three-phase bone scan.

8. e. This child has typical "growing pains" or idiopathic limb pain.

Growing pains occur in 15% to 30% of otherwise normal children. They consist of deep pain often in the lower limbs that can be severe enough to wake the child from sleep. The pains occur intermittently, are always bilateral, are poorly localized, and are usually completely gone in the morning. The pains can sometimes be aggravated by heavy exercise during the day, but day pain is never a regular characteristic of growing pains. They can be improved by nonpharmacologic therapies such as heat, massage, and physiotherapy. There is no limp or apparent disability, and the cause is unknown.

There is often a psychological component to growing pains. There seems to be a relation between limb pain, abdominal pain, and headaches in children and an inherited or environmentally determined link between siblings with pain and parents with pain.

9. e. Treatment consists of reassuring the family about the benign, self-limited course of the condition. Systematic treatment such as heat and an analgesic can be provided. Although avoidance of activities that aggravate the condition should be advised, this must be balanced against the positive benefits of maintaining some type of exercise program. Inform the family that if clinical features change, the child should be brought back to the office for reevaluation.

10. e. Limb pain is a common presenting complaint in primary care practice. It is estimated to account for 5% to 10% of pediatric visits.

With limb pain in childhood, there is frequently an emotional component. There is a relation between growing pains and headache and abdominal pain in children with these symptoms, who often come from "pain-prone" families. The parents often have had pain as children that sometimes persisted into adulthood. In up to 33% of cases, this "childhood pain syndrome" persists.

11. a. SCFE is most likely. Physiologically, SCFE occurs before the epiphyseal plate closes and usually at a time before and during the maximal pubertal growth spurt (13 to 15 years old in males and 11 to 13 years old in females). This condition is the most common adolescent hip disorder. Obesity is present in 80% of children with this disorder. It is more common in males. In nearly 50% of cases, both hips will ultimately be affected.

12. a. An SCFE is an orthopedic emergency. Immediate hospitalization and operative fixation is indicated. Stabilization of the SCFE is essential if acute or gradual slipping is to be prevented. In severe chronic (and poorly aligned) SCFE, osteotomies are required to realign and stabilize the capital femoral epiphysis. Prompt intervention is also required to minimize avascular necrosis of the femoral head as a result of slippage.

Summary

1. Limp is defined as abnormal gait due to pain

Pain can be referred, and children are not always accurate at pointing to the source or site of pain. A detailed history and physical examination are required, including analysis of gait, but x-rays may or may not be needed.

A child with a limp is a common presentation in family medicine. History and physical examination are critical. A careful observation of gait and preferred position of the affected leg will aid in diagnosis. Frequent follow-up is often critical to reassure that a condition is benign. The most important distinction to make is the difference between urgent and nonurgent conditions. Urgent conditions often require consultation with a specialist and/or hospitalization for treatment. Patients with nonurgent conditions can be reassured, treated with conservative measures, and followed closely.

If there is no history of trauma, plain films are usually normal; however, plain x-ray is all that is needed to diagnose slipped femoral capital epiphysis. Ultrasound detects transient synovitis, and plain x-ray is not needed in this case. Ultrasound can also detect osteomyelitis and Legg–Calve–Perthes disease. Bone scans and joint aspiration are also sometimes needed. Aspiration is needed in the case of fever, elevated C-reactive protein, elevated erythrocyte sedimentation rate, refusal to bear weight, and high white blood cell count. These factors are suggestive of septic arthritis. Bone scan can be helpful in younger children.

Bone scan can be helpful when the child limps but physical examination is nonfocal. Bone scan can help identify Legg–Calve–Perthes disease. Radiation exposure is high enough in computed tomography (CT) scanning to limit its use, except in preoperative studies for known fracture and when searching for stress fracture in osteopenic children with normal MRI.

MRI is helpful in detecting stress fracture, early Legg–Calve–Perthes disease, and osteomyelitis—especially in differentiating osteomyelitis from bone infarct.

If the exam is nonfocal in a child age 0 to 5 years, x-ray of the pelvis and lower extremities is appropriate and has minimal radiation exposure. Three-phase bone scan and MRI of pelvis/lower extremity can be very helpful, whereas ultrasound of hip and spine x-rays are less appropriate. If the physical examination is focal but septic arthritis is not suspected in these young children, plain x-ray of the suspected site is most appropriate, and bone scan and MRI can also be helpful. Ultrasound and CT are less helpful. When septic arthritis is suspected, plain x-ray and ultrasound (most useful when the suspected site is the hip) have the highest efficacy.

In the newborn, ultrasound can detect developmental dysplasia of the hip. Bone scan detects occult fracture, osteomyelitis, and Legg–Calve–Perthes disease. MRI is best for bone tumors and soft tissue problems.

Blood cultures should be obtained when septic arthritis or osteomyelitis is suspected. Joint fluid should be sent for cell count, differential, glucose, culture and Gram stain, and crystal examination.

Toddlers with foot problems should be evaluated for avascular necrosis of the navicular head and second metatarsal infarction. Stress fractures can occur in these young children; ingrown toenails can cause limp. Infection after puncture wound should be evaluated for osteomyelitis; *Pseudomonas aeruginosa* should be suspected.

2. Common causes of childhood limp by urgency

a. Urgent: (i) toxic or transient synovitis, (ii) septic arthritis, (iii) osteomyelitis, (iv) Legg–Calve–Perthes disease, (v) slipped capital femoral epiphysis, and (vi) malignancies (uncommon)

b. Nonurgent: (i) growing pains, (ii) school phobias, (iii) Osgood–Schlatter disease, (iv) osteochondritis dissecans (consultation strongly suggested), (v) chondromalacia patellae, and (vi) other patellofemoral disorders or syndromes

3. Common causes of limp by age are shown in the following table

0–4 years	4–10 years	10–18 years
Hip dysplasia	Fracture	Slipped capital
Fracture	Puncture wound	femoral epiphysis*
Puncture	Strain/sprain/	Fracture
Sprain/strain/	bruising	Sprain/strain/bruise
bruising	Viral synovitis*	Osgood–Schlatters
Septic arthritis	Septic arthritis	Bone tumor
Viral synovitis*	Osteomyelitis	Osteomyelitis
Bone tumor	Legg–Calve–	
	Perthes disease*	
	Bone tumor	
	Juvenile	
	rheumatoid	
	arthritis	

* Most common cause(s) in the age group.

Suggested Reading

Beach CB, Ficke JR: The limping child. *eMedicine*: 2007. Available at www.emedicine.com/orthoped/topic412.htm.

Fordham L, Gunderman R, Blatt ER, et al; Expert Panel on Pediatric Imaging: *Limping child—Ages 0-5 years*. Reston, VA: American College of Radiology, 2007. Available at www.guidelines.gov.

Leet, AI, Skaggs, DL: Evaluation of the acutely limping child. *Am Fam Physician* 61:1011–1018, 2000.

CHAPTER
121 **Foot and Leg Deformities**

CLINICAL CASE PROBLEM 1

An Anxious Mother with a 3-Month-Old Infant with Crooked Feet

A 3-month-old infant is brought to your office by his mother. She states that he has "crooked feet." She has been told by her friend that he will "need a number of casts to correct this." On examination, the infant's feet are everted. The heel position as viewed from behind with his feet dorsiflexed is valgus. No other abnormalities are found. The mother's pregnancy was unremarkable. The birth weight of the infant was 10 pounds, 8 ounces.

SELECT THE BEST ANSWER TO THE FOLLOWING QUESTIONS

1. What is the most likely diagnosis in this infant?
   a. congenital calcaneovalgus
   b. metatarsus valgus
   c. metatarsus varus
   d. talipes equinovarus
   e. clubfoot

2. What is the treatment of choice in this child?
   a. serial casts
   b. bilateral osteotomies
   c. Denis–Browne splints
   d. immediate referral to an orthopedic surgeon
   e. reassurance and foot exercises

CLINICAL CASE PROBLEM 2

A 4-Week-Old Infant with "Toeing In"

A mother brings her 4-week-old infant to the office for assessment of her child's "toeing in." She states that another physician has told her that this probably will require "serial casts" to correct. On physical examination, both feet deviate medially. The feet dorsiflex easily, and the heels are in a neutral position. The lateral borders of the feet are convex.

3. What is the most likely diagnosis in this patient?
   a. calcaneovalgus
   b. metatarsus varus
   c. metatarsus valgus
   d. talipes equinovarus
   e. clubfoot

4. What is the most likely predisposing factor to the diagnosis described in this case?
   a. abnormality at the embryo stage of development
   b. hereditary susceptibility to the condition
   c. position of the fetus in utero
   d. abnormality in the shape of the maternal uterus
   e. abnormality in the formation of the fetal legs and feet

5. What is the treatment of choice for the majority of patients with the condition described in this case?
   a. serial casts
   b. bilateral osteotomies
   c. Denis–Browne splints
   d. immediate referral to an orthopedic surgeon
   e. reassurance and foot exercises

CLINICAL CASE PROBLEM 3

A 15-Month-Old with "Bowlegs"

Parents bring their 15-month-old infant into your office for an assessment of "his bowlegs." They note that the child has been "bowlegged" since he began to walk 3 months ago. On examination, the toddler's feet point inward and his knees point straight ahead.

6. On the basis of the information provided, what is the most likely diagnosis?
   a. internal tibial torsion
   b. internal femoral torsion
   c. metatarsus varus
   d. fixed tibia varum
   e. calcaneovalgus

7. What is the treatment of choice for the child described in this case?
   a. serial casts
   b. bilateral osteotomies
   c. Denis–Browne splints
   d. immediate referral to an orthopedic surgeon
   e. reassurance and leg exercises

CLINICAL CASE PROBLEM 4

An 18-Month-Old with Twisted Legs

A mother comes to your office with her 18-month-old infant. She tells you that her child appears to have "both legs twisted inward from the hips."

You examine the child and confirm that the mother's impression appears to be correct. The anterior aspect of the patellae is directed medially, and the hip internal rotation is greater than external rotation.

8. What is the most likely diagnosis in this patient?
   a. internal tibial torsion
   b. excessive femoral anteversion
   c. flexible flatfeet
   d. metatarsus adductus
   e. metatarsus varus

9. What is the most common cause of intoeing in children older than age 3 years?
   a. internal tibial torsion
   b. excessive femoral anteversion
   c. metatarsus adductus
   d. metatarsus varus
   e. none of the above

10. What is the initial treatment of choice for the condition described in this case?
    a. serial casts
    b. bilateral osteotomies
    c. Denis–Browne splints
    d. immediate referral to an orthopedic surgeon
    e. watchful waiting

11. What is the most common method of measuring the degree of the condition described in this case?
    a. computed tomography scan of the lower leg
    b. ultrasonography of the lower leg
    c. biplanar radiography of the lower leg
    d. magnetic resonance imaging scan of the lower leg
    e. none of the above

CLINICAL CASE PROBLEM 5

A 6-Month-Old with Crooked Feet

A mother brings her 6-month-old infant to your office for assessment. She tells you that her child's feet are "completely crooked" and that there is no way she can correct it. On examination, you are unable to dorsiflex either foot. You notice that the heels are in the varus position (medial deviation) and the sole is kidney shaped when viewed from the bottom.

12. What is the most likely diagnosis in this infant?
    a. talipes equinovarus
    b. metatarsus adductus
    c. internal tibial torsion

d. excessive femoral anteversion
e. none of the above

13. Which of the following treatments may be indicated for correction of the condition described in this case?
    a. posterior medial release of the heel cords
    b. serial casts
    c. reassurance and foot exercises
    d. a and b
    e. a, b, and c

14. Which of the following may be associated with the condition described in this case?
    a. congenital dislocation of the hip
    b. spina bifida
    c. myotonic dystrophy
    d. a and b
    e. a, b, and c

CLINICAL CASE PROBLEM 6

A 21-Month-Old Child with Flat Feet

A mother comes to your office with her 21-month-old infant. She tells you that he "slaps his feet when he walks." Her father-in-law has informed her that he has "flat feet" and instructed her to "be sure the doctor does something about it." On examination, you observe the child walking. There certainly does seem to be a difference between the contour of the foot when weight-bearing compared to when not weight-bearing. Otherwise, the examination is normal.

15. Assuming that the abnormalities in this child's feet involve arch support and ligamentous laxity, what is the most likely diagnosis?
    a. muscular dystrophy
    b. cerebral palsy
    c. flexible flatfeet
    d. osteochondrosis
    e. obesity

16. What is the most common difference between weight-bearing and non-weight-bearing in this condition?
    a. difference in the "heel lift"
    b. difference in "toe lift"
    c. difference in foot varus
    d. difference in foot valgus
    e. difference in sag versus nonsag weight-bearing

17. Which of the following coexisting conditions is (are) associated with this condition?

a. muscular dystrophy
b. cerebral palsy
c. congenital heel cord tightness
d. a and c
e. a, b, and c

18. What is the treatment of choice for the primary condition described in this case?
a. corrective orthopedic shoes
b. orthotic inserts
c. flexible, well-fitted soft shoes
d. specially designed shoes
e. none of the above; normal activity

Answers

1. a. The most likely diagnosis is congenital calcaneovalgus.

2. e. The calcaneovalgus foot is a common neonatal foot deformity. It is the result of positional confinement in utero. The foot has a banana-shaped sole (lateral deviation); dorsiflexes quite easily because of a stretched, abnormally long heel cord; and has a heel that deviates laterally. Prognosis is excellent; most cases improve spontaneously and rapidly. Parents who are uncomfortable with the prescription of observation alone should be encouraged to exercise the child's foot at each diaper change by stretching the ligaments and stretching the dorsal tendons.

Only in the rare instance that the foot remains severely deformed should corrective casts be applied. If the calcaneovalgus foot can be only partially corrected, a flexible flatfoot results. This calcaneovalgus foot must be differentiated from a congenital vertical talus (congenital convex pes valgus), which is associated with neurologic disorders such as spina bifida or arthrogyrposis in approximately 50% of cases. The vertical talus foot has a "rocker-bottom" appearance with a tight heel cord, and it often requires surgery.

3. b. This child has metatarsus adductus and metatarsus varus. They are used synonymously in practice, although they describe slightly different variations in the forefoot. In both cases, the sole is kidney bean shaped (medial deviation), and the foot is easily dorsiflexed.

4. c. Metatarsus adductus varus may be either bilateral or unilateral; it is probably secondary to in utero positioning and confinement. Two conditions associated with metatarsus are muscular torticollis and congenital hip dysplasia.

5. e. Metatarsus adductus usually improves spontaneously; this applies to at least 85% of cases. The severity of the metatarsus adductus, determined from the examination, should be documented. Severity is classified as follows: Category A is mild/flexible, category B is moderate/fixed, and category C is severe/rigid. The vast majority of cases fall into the mild/flexible group (category A). The parents can be taught to stretch the child's foot by firmly holding and stabilizing the heel and stretching the forefoot laterally, holding it to a count of five. The exercise can be performed five times at each diaper change. Category B metatarsus adductus may need to be treated by serial casting. Category C metatarsus adductus may need corrective surgery.

6. a. Internal tibial torsion is a normal finding in newborns. The mean tibial torsion at maturity is 15 to 20 degrees. At birth, the mean tibial torsion is 5 degrees—that is, 10 to 15 degrees inward compared with that of adults. Internal tibial torsion usually presents at walking age, and affected children have an inward foot progression angle. When the child walks, it can be observed that the kneecaps point forward but the foot points inward. Internal tibial torsion is thus a physiologic bowing of the lower extremities produced by the external rotation of the femur and internal rotation of the tibia.

7. e. The natural history of internal tibial torsion is spontaneous resolution in more than 95% of children. Internal tibial torsion usually resolves by 7 or 8 years of age, at which time the rotator conformation of the bones is largely established. Reassurance and leg exercises are the treatment of choice for the management of internal tibial torsion.

8. b. The most likely diagnosis is excessive femoral anteversion.

9. b. The most common cause of intoeing in children older than age 3 years is excessive femoral anteversion. The femoral neck is normally anteverted 10 degrees to 15 degrees with respect to the axis of the femoral condyles in the knee of adults. The femoral neck is more anteverted in children. In one large study, the average degree of anteversion of the femur in children between the ages of 3 months and 12 months was 39 degrees, and it was 31 degrees in 1- and 2-year-old children.

10. e. The treatment of choice in children with excessive femoral anteversion is "watchful waiting." In 90% to 95% of children, the degree of anteversion will decrease progressively to a level that is both within the normal range and acceptable to the parents.

11. **c.** A number of techniques have been devised to accurately measure the degree of femoral anteversion. The most commonly used techniques involve biplanar radiography. In children in whom excessive femoral anteversion is the cause of their intoeing, the typical clinical finding is that the child is observed to walk with his or her patellae and feet pointing inward. The clinical diagnosis is made by having the child lie prone or supine with the hips extended and externally rotating the hip. In children with excess femoral anteversion, most of the arc of rotation of the hip will be inward.

12. **a.** This child has talipes equinovarus (clubfoot). When a child develops clubfoot, you notice the following: (1) the inability to dorsiflex the clubfoot (heel equines), (2) the presence of heel varus (medial deviation), and (3) a sole that is kidney shaped (forefoot and midfoot adductus). Mild cases of clubfoot can be attributed to deformation caused by intrauterine compression, whereas more severe, fixed cases are usually secondary to underlying anatomic abnormalities such as an abnormal talus.

13. **d.** Treatment options for talipes equinovarus include corrective serial casts and posterior medial release of the heel cords. The proportion of children requiring corrective surgery varies from 75% if full anatomic, radiographic, and clinical correction is attempted to less than 50% if mild radiographic and clinical deformity is accepted.

14. **e.** Accompanying deformities with talipes equinovarus include congenital dislocation of the hip, spina bifida, moronic dystrophy, and arthrogryposis.

15. **c.** This child has flexible flatfeet. The flexible flatfoot is extremely common, with an incidence ranging from 7% to 22%.

16. **e.** The condition is often hidden by normal adipose tissue and usually becomes noticeable after a child begins to stand. The most common cause of the flexible flatfoot is ligamentous laxity, which allows the foot to sag with weight-bearing. Children often present with accompanying hyperextension of fingers, elbows, and knees and a family history of flatfeet and ligamentous laxity. A child with flexible flatfeet secondary to ligamentous laxity can form a good arch when asked to stand on tiptoe. The heel rolls into a varus position (medial deviation) on tiptoe, and good strength of the ankle and foot muscles is assured. When the child walks, the difference that can be seen immediately is that when the child is not bearing weight there is an arch. When the child is bearing weight, there is no arch.

17. **e.** Although flexible flatfeet are usually not associated with any secondary conditions (i.e., primary flexible flatfeet), it must be recognized that flexible flatfeet can be secondary to muscular dystrophy, mild cerebral palsy, or congenital tightness of the heel cords.

18. **e.** Although many treatments have been advocated for flatfeet (corrective shoes, custom orthotics, corrective inserts, and flexible flatfoot wear), none have been shown to be better than "no treatment" or "watchful expectation."

Summary

1. Prevalence of foot and leg deformities: common (up to 10% of infants)
2. Foot deformities in infants and children
   a. Congenital calcaneovalgus foot: very common neonatal foot deformity. It results from the fetal position in utero. The foot has a banana-shaped sole (lateral deviation) and dorsiflexes quite easily because of a stretched, abnormally long heel cord and a heel that deviates laterally. No intervention is beneficial.
   b. Metatarsus adductus (metatarsus varus): most common congenital foot deformity. The sole is kidney bean shaped (medial deviation), and the foot is easily dorsiflexed. Treatment consists of foot exercises and watchful waiting.
   c. Talipes equinovarus (clubfoot): characterized by the inability to dorsiflex the foot, the presence of a heel varus (medial deviation), and a sole that is kidney bean shaped when viewed from the bottom.

The tarsal navicular position is abnormal. A tight heel cord is exceedingly common. Many cases are caused by intrauterine position. Treatment with either serial casts or surgical posterior medial heel cord releases is required.
3. Other causes of intoeing in young children
   a. Internal tibial torsion: The entire foot points inward and the patella points straight ahead. Treatment consists of normal activity.
   b. Excessive femoral anteversion: The entire leg turns in so that both the patella and the foot are facing medially (medial femoral torsion or increased anteversion of the hips). Treatment consists of normal activity.
4. Flexible flatfeet: When the foot is not bearing weight, the arch of the foot is preserved. When the child is bearing weight, the arch of the foot is not preserved. Treatment consists of normal activity.

5. Assessment of any child with foot or leg deformity requires a thorough pregnancy and birth history, taking care to elicit any history of complications, including oligohydramnios. Physical examination must include observation of the child during normal activity. A thorough examination of the musculoskeletal system should include observation of foot varus versus foot valgus and also the flexibility of varus or valgus deformity. A neurologic examination is also essential. Parent education materials should be tailored to literacy level; extended family should also be considered, and additional information may be needed at multiple literacy levels. Parents should be given information about the importance of adequate exercise, and they should be discouraged from limiting the child's normal activities if the diagnosis is one that does not require intervention. Close follow-up, possibly more frequently than the usual well child visit schedule, and, if needed, consultation with a pediatric orthopedist should be pursued.

Suggested Reading

Behrman R, Kliegman RM, Jenson HB, eds: *Nelson Textbook of Pediatrics*, 17th ed. Philadelphia: Saunders, 2004.

Göksan SB, Bursali A, Bilgili F, et al: Ponseti technique for the correction of idiopathic clubfeet presenting up to 1 year of age. A preliminary study in children with untreated or complex deformities. *Arch Orthop Trauma Surg* 126:15–21, 2006.

Hoffinger SA: Evaluation and management of pediatric foot deformities. *Pediatr Clin North Am* 43(5):1091–1111, 1996.

Sass P, Hassan G: Lower extremity abnormalities in children. *Am Fam Physician* 68:461–468, 2003.

Wall EJ: Practical primary pediatric orthopedics. *Nurs Clin North Am* 35:95–113, 2000.

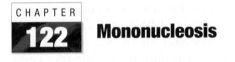

CHAPTER **122** **Mononucleosis**

CLINICAL CASE PROBLEM 1

Pharyngitis and Heptosplenomegaly

A 16-year-old previously healthy female is brought to your office for an urgent care visit. She complains of a severe sore throat for the past 3 days. Yesterday, she developed a fever to 102°F and noted pus on her tonsils. Her mother kept her home from school and she "has just been lying around." She has a diagnosis of mild persistent asthma but stopped using her inhalers 2 months ago. The patient says that she really "only used the inhalers before she played lacrosse anyway." She denies previous hospitalizations or surgery. Her immunizations are current.

On examination, her temperature is 101.5°F, oxygen saturation is 99%, and pulse is 80 beats/minute. Greenish pharyngeal exudate and significant lymphadenopathy are noted in the posterior cervical and auricular areas. Neurologic exam is nonfocal; Brudinsky and Kernig signs are negative. Heart is regular rate and rhythm and no expiratory wheeze is present. She has a small, palpable mass in the left upper quadrant of the abdomen. The liver is 1 cm below the costal margin and mildly tender.

SELECT THE BEST ANSWER TO THE FOLLOWING QUESTIONS

1. At this point, which of the following is least likely in the differential diagnosis?
   a. hepatitis A
   b. group A β-hemolytic strep
   c. infectious mononucleosis (IM)
   d. acute asthma exacerbation
   e. gonococcal pharyngitis

2. Which of the following historical questions is least pertinent at this time?
   a. has she had a recent diphtheria–tetanus–acellular pertussis (DTaP) booster?
   b. is the patient sexually active?
   c. has she been exposed to anyone with strep throat?
   d. has she had any gastrointestinal symptoms or recent foreign travel?
   e. does she have stridor or problems breathing because of the sore throat?

On further questioning, the patient states that she recently returned from a music camp in Vermont. With her mother out of the room, she denies that she has had sexual intercourse but admits to "messing around" with one of the male campers. She has no history of recurrent strep pharyngitis, nor is anyone in her immediate family ill. She denies jaundice or diarrhea.

3. All of the following tests are reasonable at this time except
   a. gonococcal swab of the pharynx

b. rapid test for group A β-hemolytic strep
c. Western blot for human immunodeficiency virus (HIV)
d. heterophile antibody test (monospot)
e. hepatitis panel

4. A heterophile antibody test is ordered and the result is negative. Which of the following statements is false?
a. these tests are available in either latex agglutination or solid-phase immunoassay types
b. the test is less sensitive in patients younger than age 12 years
c. the patient is unlikely to have IM because of the high sensitivity of the test
d. the test is less accurate in the first weeks of illness
e. the heterophile antibody response is due to immunoglobulin M (IgM)

5. Additional lab results are available, including a negative rapid strep test. A complete blood count with differential is done. Which of the following differential profiles is most predictive of IM?
a. the presence of greater than 50% lymphocytes
b. greater than 50% lymphocytes combined with less than 10% atypical lymphocytes
c. less than 10% atypical lymphocytes
d. a lymphocyte to white blood cell count ratio greater than 0.35
e. the presence of greater than 40% neutrophils

6. IM is sometimes strongly suspected by history and physical, but heterophile antibody testing is negative. Which serologic pattern best supports a diagnosis of acute IM?
a. a negative Epstein–Barr nuclear antigen (EBNA)
b. a positive anti-EBNA and a negative viral capsid antigen (VCA) IgM
c. elevated antibody levels against VCA IgG and VCA IgM
d. low level of VCA IgG and a negative test for VCA IgM
e. negative VCA tests for both IgG and IgM

7. Transmission routes for infectious mononucleosis include all of the following except:
a. feces
b. blood
c. solid organs
d. saliva
e. genital secretions

8. Which of the following statements about Epstein–Barr virus (EBV) is true?

a. EBV replicates primarily in T lymphocytes
b. intermittent excretion of EBV occurs for 6 months after initial infection
c. EBV is a betaherpes virus
d. EBV is the most common cause of IM
e. EBV is communicable for 30 to 45 days

9. Which of the following statements about EBV is correct?
a. humans are the only source of EBV
b. mononucleosis tends to occur most frequently in late winter and early spring
c. viral particles are viable in oral secretions for several hours outside the body
d. endemic infections are uncommon in group settings of young adults (i.e., boarding school and the military)
e. a and c

10. Which of the following demographic statements about EBV is true?
a. EBV infection in developing countries most often affects the 15- to 25-year old age group
b. the majority of children in industrialized countries are exposed to EBV by the age of 2 years
c. high socioeconomic status is associated with EBV seropositivity during the adolescent years
d. EBV has four distinct subtypes
e. Dual infection with types 1 and 2 occurs mostly in individuals infected with HIV

CLINICAL CASE PROBLEM 2

Pharyngitis, Fever, and Lymphadenopathy

During your shift in the emergency department, an 18-year-old male is brought in by his girlfriend. He appears acutely ill. He is febrile (temperature, 102.7°F), blood pressure is 80/40 mmHg, and pulse is 130 beats/minute. On initial examination, he is in respiratory distress with an oxygen saturation of 88%. His oropharynx shows exudative obstructive tonsilar hypertrophy. Severe lymphadenopathy is noted in the posterior auricular chain.

According to his girlfriend, the patient had a sore throat that worsened during the past 2 or 3 days. She states that he is generally in good health. He has no medical issues, has never had surgery, and takes no medications. He is allergic to penicillin, which was discovered 2 days ago when he got a prescription for penicillin VK to treat a tooth abscess. He developed a generalized rash but did not have breathing problems or angioedema. His dentist was concerned because the patient had previously taken penicillin without incident. The patient recently returned home from college for summer vacation.

11. At this point, what is the most important action to take?
    a. conduct a thorough physical exam
    b. order both rapid strep and heterophile antibody tests
    c. emergently give subcutaneous epinephrine, solumedrol, and benadryl to manage acute penicillin anaphylaxis
    d. make definitive plans for airway management and obtain an emergent ear, nose, and throat consultation
    e. order a cross-table neck radiograph to assess the risk of impending airway compromise

12. Flexible laryngoscopy shows diffuse swelling of the palatal and pharyngeal wall, supraglottis, and epiglottis. He is successfully intubated, sedated, and placed on 100% oxygen. Heterophile antibody testing obtained after intubation is positive. Which of the following interventions is indicated at this time?
    a. intravenous acyclovir
    b. intravenous corticosteroids
    c. acetaminophen
    d. intravenous ranitidine
    e. intravenous gancyclovir

13. In patients without life-threatening IM complications, which of the following statements about steroid use is false?
    a. several trials demonstrate that steroids provide initial relief of sore throat at 12 hours, but that the benefit does not last longer than 2 to 4 days
    b. there is currently not enough evidence to recommend steroid treatment for symptom control in uncomplicated IM
    c. the effectiveness of steroid treatment for post-IM fatigue is uncertain
    d. patients with acute IM who receive corticosteroids are less likely to be admitted, less likely to develop complications, and have shorter hospitalizations than those who do not receive steroids
    e. factors associated with steroid use include more than one physician encounter, inpatient admission, and otolaryngology consultation

14. Central nervous system complications from EBV include all of the following except

    a. transverse myelitis
    b. optic neuritis
    c. encephalitis
    d. seizures
    e. cranial nerve palsies

15. EBV is associated with several other disorders, including all but the following:
    a. nasopharyngeal carcinoma
    b. Burkitt's lymphoma
    c. Hodgkin's disease
    d. non-Hodgkin's disease
    e. chronic fatigue syndrome

16. Which of the following statements about IM is true?
    a. patients with IM are unlikely to have splenomegaly
    b. the risk of splenic rupture is 1%
    c. most ruptures occur between the weeks 4 and 6 of infection
    d. physical exam is superior to ultrasound for diagnosing splenomegaly
    e. splenic rupture may occur nontraumatically

17. What is the best advice for the athlete who wishes to return to play after having mononucleosis?
    a. patients should avoid athletics for a minimum of 3 or 4 weeks
    b. patients should not participate in athletics until they are asymptomatic
    c. avoidance of athletics is recommended until the patient is asymptomatic and a minimum of 3 or 4 weeks has passed
    d. an ultrasound to rule out splenomegaly is necessary before a patient can return to play
    e. participating in noncontact sports creates no risk for splenic rupture

Answers

1. **d.** The patient has a history of mild persistent asthma but has not used inhalers in the past several months. She has never been hospitalized nor intubated for an exacerbation. From the history, her asthma more closely fits an exercise-induced pattern. With normal vital signs and no acute pulmonary findings, acute asthma exacerbation is an unlikely cause of her symptoms.

2. **a.** Since immunizations are current, the likelihood of diphtheria is low. A booster dose of DTaP is required between age 12 and 15 years. Infections with *Corynebacterium diphtheriae* have a 2- to 4-week incubation period. This infection generally presents

with pharyngitis and cervical lymphadenopathy. A distinctive exudative grayish-white membrane extending to the soft palate is characteristic of this infection. Serosanguinous nasal drainage is also common.

3. **c.** Although acute HIV seroconversion can cause sore throat, fatigue, and low-grade fever, it is an unlikely diagnosis given the patient's negative history for sexual intercourse. If the veracity of the history is in question, the appropriate screening test is an enzyme-linked immunosorbent assay. Western blot is used to confirm a positive screening test for HIV. Gonococcal pharyngitis causes severe sore throat, fever, and characteristic greenish pharyngeal exudate. A pharyngeal swab is indicated in patients at risk for gonorrhea via receptive oral sex. Because both IM and group A β-hemolytic strep share symptoms of exudate, lymphadenopathy, and palatine petechiae, a rapid strep swab and monospot are indicated. Hepatitis A is associated with symptoms of fatigue, recent travel, and malaise.

4. **c.** The heterophile antibody test reacts to IgM and becomes positive during the first 2 weeks of infection. The false-negative rate approaches 25% during the initial week, decreases to 5% to 10% during the second week, and is approximately 5% during the third week. The test is particularly poor at detecting IM in children younger than age 4 years. Paul–Bunnell latex agglutination and solid-phase immunoassays have largely replaced earlier tests that detected antibodies by agglutination of sheep and horse red blood cells. Because the patient has been sick for only 3 days, the result may be a false negative.

5. **d.** Hoagland's criteria for IM mandate at least 10% atypical lymphocytes and at least 50% lymphocytes in addition to fever, lymphadenopathy, and pharyngitis confirmed by serologic testing. Although specific, the criteria frequently miss patients who actually have IM. A recently published retrospective pilot study compared lymphocyte and white blood counts with the monospot test for the diagnosis of acute IM. A lymphocyte to white blood cell (L:WCC) ratio of greater than 0.35 was 100% specific and 90% sensitive for detecting IM. This measurement may be useful to distinguish bacterial tonsillitis from IM, permitting more judicious use of heterophile antibody testing.

6. **c.** Antibody testing for VCA and anti-EBNA is performed when heterophile testing is negative but clinical presentation suggests IM. VCA IgG antibodies are high during initial infection. Levels then decrease and persist for life. VCA IgM antibodies indicate acute infection of recent onset. VCA IgM levels dissipate

over time. Anti-EBNA becomes positive several weeks to months after infection. Negative VCA for both IgG and IgM suggests infection from a source other than IM. The IgG spike during early infection and the presence of IgM antibodies indicate acute IM.

7. **a.** EBV infection is usually subclinical. The virus establishes a persistent infection in lymphocytes and is then excreted in low levels in saliva. EBV is also transmitted through blood and solid organs. Patients with recently confirmed EBV or with an infection clinically resembling EBV should be counseled not to donate blood or organs. EBV viral particles are found in both female and male genital secretions, although this is not considered a major route of transmission. EBV is not transmitted via feces.

8. **d.** Intermittent excretion of EBV occurs in affected individuals throughout their lifetime. It is unknown how long a person may transmit the infection once he or she is infected. Although replication primarily occurs in β-lymphocytes, epithelial cells in the pharynx and parotid duct may also sustain EBV growth. EBV is a gammaherpes virus of the genus *Lymphocryptovirus* and is the most common cause of IM.

9. **e.** Mononucleosis has no seasonal predilection. Humans are the sole source of EBV. Spread is usually by close personal contact (i.e., saliva). The virus lives in secretions for several hours outside the body. EBV transmission by blood transfusion is less common, but it is a concern in organ transplantation. The incubation period is a lengthy 30 to 50 days. Outbreaks in institutional settings with groups of young people are common.

10. **e.** EBV seroconversion occurs in two waves. The first peak occurs from ages 2 to 4 years, and a second peak occurs at approximately age 15 years. Demographic factors influence when infection is most likely to occur. In nonindustrialized countries, most children are exposed to EBV by the age of 2 years. Seroconversion is shifted toward older age groups in industrialized societies. High socioeconomic status increases the probability of EBV seronegativity in late adolescence.

EBV subtypes are identified as type 1 and type 2 (also A and B). Type 1 is more prevalent worldwide. Type 2 is more often found in Africa and is less common in heterosexual men. Concomitant infection with types 1 and 2 is associated with HIV seropositivity.

11. **d.** Planning for definitive airway management is critical. The working diagnosis indicates IM. Although significant airway compromise is rare, it occurs in 1% to 3.5% of cases. Intubation using fiberoptic laryngoscopy is indicated secondary to the patient's airway compromise. If intubation attempts are unsuccessful, personnel capable of performing a tracheostomy may become necessary. Although completing the physical exam and ordering confirmatory blood work is important, the compromised airway takes precedence. Choices c and e are not indicated. Since penicillins cause a morbilliform rash in patients with IM, it is unlikely that the patient has a true penicillin allergy.

12. b. Corticosteroids for IM are indicated only in patients with impending airway compromise, hemophagocytic syndrome, hemolytic anemia, massive splenomegaly, or myocarditis. Options include intravenous dexamethasone 0.5 mg/kg or equivalent doses of methylprednisolone given every 8 hours for at least 24 to 48 hours. Acetaminophen is appropriate for fever control but is less urgent than steroids. Neither acyclovir nor valacyclovir show consistent clinical benefit, although they may be useful in patients with EBV-induced lymphoproliferative problems after organ transplantation. Ranitidine shows no benefit for treating IM.

13. d. No apparent increases or decreases in admission rates, length of hospitalization, or complications are found between patients with IM who are given steroids and those who are treated conservatively. Although steroids provide relief of sore throat symptoms in the first 12 hours, the benefit is not seen after 2 to 4 days. One trial demonstrated that steroids may improve fatigue after 1 month, but it combined steroids with valacylovir. Patients who have more contact with the health care system, specialty consultation, or admission are more likely to be treated with steroids. There is not enough evidence to recommend use of steroids for symptom control in uncomplicated IM.

14. d. EBV infection causes several neurologic complications, including Guillain–Barré syndrome, transverse myelitis, meningitis, encephalitis, optic neuritis, and cranial nerve palsies.

15. e. EBV is linked with several lymphoproliferative abnormalities of the B and T lymphocytes. Burkitt's lymphoma is a B lymphocyte tumor primarily found in central Africa. Nasopharyngeal carcinoma is seen most often in Southeast Asia. Both Hodgkin's and non-Hodgkin's lymphomas are linked to EBV. Immunocompromised people and organ transplant recipients are at higher risk, especially in the case of liver and heart transplantation. Approximately 10% of patients with IM develop postinfection fatigue, although an association between EBV and chronic fatigue syndrome is uncertain.

16. e. Some degree of splenomegaly is likely present in IM. Most patients do not have evidence of splenomegaly on physical exam. Although ultrasound is more sensitive in detecting splenomegaly, routine ultrasound is not indicated. The risk of splenic rupture is 0.1%, with the majority of cases occurring during the first 3 weeks. Rupture often occurs via nontraumatic mechanisms.

17. c. The current literature recommends that participation in athletics should be restricted until the patient is asymptomatic and at least 3 or 4 weeks have elapsed. Longer time frames of 6 weeks to several months have been suggested by some experts. Although ultrasound is better than clinical exam for detecting splenomegaly, the number needed to treat, the cost, and the fact that the risk of rupture decreases after 1 month make this option impractical. Since nearly half of splenic ruptures are atraumatic in etiology, noncontact sports are also not recommended.

Summary

Infectious mononucleosis is a common infection in adolescents and young adults in industrialized societies. IM is most often caused by exposure to EBV, a gammaherpes-type virus. The infection is often subclinical in young children, with EBV establishing a persistent presence in the β-lymphocytes. Low-level viral excretion continues throughout life. Exposure to EBV is generally from close contact, usually saliva, although EBV is identified in genital secretions of males and females and in blood and solid transplanted organs. There are two peaks of exposure: the first from 2 to 4 years and the second at approximately 15 years. In nonindustrialized countries, the majority of children are exposed to EBV by 2 years of age. In adolescents in socioeconomically privileged Western cultures, seronegativity into young adulthood is not uncommon.

Symptoms of IM include sore throat, lymphadenopathy, tonsilar enlargement, and fever. Palatal petechiea, hepatosplenomegaly, and exudative pharyngitis are common. The spectrum of disease is broad, ranging from subclinical infection to fulminate death. The incubation period is 30 to 50 days. The differential diagnosis of IM includes group A β-hemolytic strep pharyngitis, acute cytomegalovirus, HIV, toxoplasmosis, and hepatitis.

Several diagnostic tests are available to diagnose IM. The initial test is generally the heterophile antibody test (monospot) in latex agglutination or solid-phase immunoassay form. The heterophile antibody response occurs due to the presence of IgM. Although relatively specific, the test has a false-negative rate as high as 25% during the first week of infection and 5% to 10% in the second week. Complete blood counts with greater than 50% lymphocytes and 10% atypical lymphocytes also strongly suggest IM. An L:WCC ratio of greater than 0.35 may also distinguish IM from bacterial pharyngitis. In cases in which clinical suspicion is high but the heterophile antibody is negative, serologic antibody tests are necessary.

The most commonly performed test is VCA antibodies. IgM antibodies develop during acute infection and disappear over several months: IgG has an initial peak with acute infection and then persists for life. EBNA antibodies develop several weeks to months after initial infection. Early antigen occurs early in the course of EBV. Since many patients with IM are coinfected with group A strep infections, a rapid strep test is also prudent.

The main therapy for IM is supportive care. In mild cases, hydration, acetaminophen, throat lozenges, and nonsteroidal anti-inflammatories may be all that is necessary. Severe cases often require hospitalization and respiratory support. The role of steroids in mild IM is unclear. Although some improvement in sore throat is noted by 12 hours in those who are treated with steroids, the benefit is lost by 2 to 4 days. Since steroids have a risk of adverse effects, they are not recommended at this time for symptom control in mild IM. In cases in which the patient is at risk for impending airway obstruction, massive splenomegaly, hemophagocytosis, or myocarditis, intravenous dexamethasone or an equivalent steroid are generally given for 24 to 48 hours. Oral steroids are then given for 7 days with subsequent tapering. Approximately 10% of patients develop fatigue-type symptoms, although a relationship with chronic fatigue syndrome has not been clearly delineated.

Possible complications of EBV include meningitis, cranial nerve palsies, interstitial nephritis, myocarditis, and thrombocytopenia. The most feared complication is splenic rupture, which occurs in 0.1% of cases. Risk is greatest in the first 3 or 4 weeks postinfection. Many ruptures are nontraumatic in origin. Therefore, patients should not participate in noncontact sports until they are asymptomatic and at least 3 or 4 weeks have passed ("C" level recommendation). Patients are encouraged to advance to normal activity levels as tolerated; enforced bed rest has not been demonstrated to improve outcomes.

EBV is associated with several notable diseases, including Burkitt's lymphoma, nasopharyngeal carcinoma, Hodgkin's and non-Hodgkin's lymphomas, and other epithelial neoplasms. An EBV vaccine that targets gp350, a viral receptor protein, is currently in phase II clinical trials.

Suggested Reading

Candy B, Hotopf M: Steroids for symptom control in infectious mononucleosis. *Cochrane Database Syst Rev* (3):CD004402, 2006.

Crawford DH, Macsween KF, Higgins CD: A cohort study among university students: Identification of risk factors for Epstein–Barr virus seroconversion and infectious mononucleosis. *Clin Infect Dis* 43:276–282, 2006.

Ebell M: Epstein–Barr virus infectious mononucleosis. *Am Fam Physician* 70(7):1279–1287, 2004.

Pickering LK, ed: *Red Book: 2006 Report of the Committee on Infectious Diseases*, 27th ed., Section 3. Elk Grove Village, IL: American Academy of Pediatrics, 2006.

Wolf DM, Friedrichs I, Toma AG: Lymphocyte–white blood cell count ratio: A quickly available screening tool to differentiate acute purulent tonsillitis from glandular fever. *Arch Otolaryngol Head Neck Surg* 13:61–64, 2007.

Adolescent Development

CLINICAL CASE PROBLEM 1

13-Year-Old Comes for a Sports Physical

A 13-year-old comes to the office for a sports physical. According to his mom, he used to see a pediatrician, but he believes he is too old for that now. This is his initial visit to the family health center.

On taking the history, you notice that he seldom makes eye contact and appears anxious, more than usual for a child his age. The physical exam is benign, including a complete neurological and musculoskeletal exam.

SELECT THE BEST ANSWER TO THE FOLLOWING QUESTIONS

1. Regarding the patient described, you should do which of the following?
   a. ask the parent if she has any concerns about his growth and development
   b. refer the patient to a psychologist
   c. attempt to identify an underlying agenda
   d. consult a school counselor
   e. all of the above

2. To facilitate further discussion with this patient at this time, you should say?
   a. you are in good health, so I'll see you next year
   b. we need to schedule you for some routine blood work
   c. why don't you ask your mom if she has any questions
   d. I get the feeling that there is something on your mind that you would like to talk about.... I'm listening
   e. I am too busy today, but why don't you make a follow-up appointment with your guidance counselor

3. During this first visit, which of the following issues should be addressed?
   a. body image
   b. home environment
   c. education
   d. sex, drugs, and alcohol
   e. all of the above

4. In the United States, the leading cause of death among people age 15 to 24 years is which of the following?
   a. homicide
   b. suicide
   c. accidents
   d. human immunodeficiency virus (HIV) infection
   e. cancer

5. Which psychiatric disorder is least common in adolescents?
   a. depression
   b. anxiety
   c. schizophrenia
   d. adjustment disorder
   e. antisocial personality disorder

6. Children in midadolescence are concerned primarily with which of the following?
   a. strong emphasis on the new peer group
   b. struggle with sense of identity
   c. realization that parents are not perfect and identification of their faults
   d. movement toward independence
   e. a and d

7. What major factor(s) is (are) most important to ensure healthy development of the adolescent?
   a. encouragement toward independence
   b. the establishment of boundaries
   c. teaching of discipline
   d. a prolonged supportive environment
   e. a and d

8. Risk factors for alcohol and drug use in the adolescent include all of the following except
   a. divorce or separation of parents
   b. poor school performance
   c. sexual promiscuity
   d. peer group
   e. socioeconomic status

9. Regarding visits to family physicians by adolescents, which of the following is (are) true?
   a. adolescents make regular visits to the doctor
   b. 25% of adolescents have chronic conditions necessitating a visit to the doctor
   c. adolescents are open about asking questions regarding sexual issues
   d. a and c
   e. none of the above

10. What is the second leading cause of death among people age 15 to 24 years in the United States?
    a. motor vehicle accidents

b. suicide
c. homicide
d. cancer
e. acquired immune deficiency syndrome

CLINICAL CASE PROBLEM 2

A Young Driver with Health Problems

A 16-year-old comes to the office for a follow-up of an emergency department visit following a minor motor vehicle accident in which she was a front seat passenger. She has some facial lacerations that are healing and a bruised knee from hitting the dashboard. She is accompanied by her mother.

11. In following up the motor vehicle accident, you should ask which questions?
    a. were you wearing a seat belt?
    b. how many people were in the car?
    c. were you or the driver drinking?
    d. all of the above
    e. none of the above

12. In following up the answer to question 11, it is a reasonable time to talk with the patient and her mother about limitations on teen driving that increase the safety of beginning drivers. These include
    a. limit on the number of teens in the car
    b. learner must remain crash/conviction free
    c. limitation on nighttime driving
    d. all occupants must wear safety belts
    e. all of the above

13. During the history and evaluation, you note that the patient is significantly underweight. Thus, you make a point during the examination to do a full oral exam and note some etching and abrasion of the front teeth. You are concerned that this patient is showing signs of which of the following?
    a. anorexia
    b. bulimia
    c. vitamin K deficiency
    d. dental caries
    e. oral thrush

14. While you are talking to the mother, the patient asks the nurse if she can return to see you without her mother. Your nurse answers how?
    a. because the patient is underage, parental permission is necessary, so the parent would have

to come along or provide written permission to see the patient
    b. because you have treated her for some time, you can see her without parental consent and just bill the insurance
    c. if the problem is about reproductive issues, you can see her without parental consent
    d. since the patient is not emancipated, you cannot see her without parental consent for any purpose
    e. a and c

Clinical Case Management Problem

Describe the preventive medicine strategies that should be incorporated into an office visit in which an adolescent comes to his or her physician for acute episodic care.

Answers

1. **c.** This adolescent is obviously very anxious about something. The physical examination may be the perfect opportunity to have the parent leave so that you can have a discussion in private and attempt to identify why he is so anxious. There is a high probability the patient may have some issues that he may disclose to you.

2. **d.** At this time, you should attempt, if possible, to identify exactly what the patient's agenda may be. An appropriate opener would be "I get the feeling that there is something you would like to talk about... I'm listening." More direct questions would be about school, friends, peers, sexual orientation, drugs, alcohol, and so on. A good way to approach these issues would be to state, "I know that a lot of people your age are starting to have sex or use drugs and alcohol. Are you aware of anyone in your school that may be doing this?" This is a nonthreatening way of approaching a sensitive topic.

3. **e.** Body image, home environment, education, and sex, drugs, and alcohol are all topics that may be important to find out about the adolescent.

4. **c.** The leading cause of death among people age 15 to 24 years is accidents.

5. **c.** Schizophrenia is the least likely mental illness in adolescents. The peak incidence is usually age 18 to 25 years. The other conditions are much more prevalent in the adolescent population.

6. **e.** Although there is a continuum of development, there are three identified phases of adolescent development. In early adolescence, there is a preoccupation with bodily changes. Early adolescents often feel uncertain about their appearance, and their interests are directed toward themselves. This is a period marked by high levels of physical activity and mood swings.

In midadolescence, the major concern is independence. The peer group dominates social life, and risk behaviors become more prevalent. This is a time of heightened sexual curiosity and exploration.

In late adolescence, there is greater emotional stability with the establishment of a firmer self-identity. There is goal-directed behavior and more adult-type thinking, with an acceptance of social and cultural institutions. The adolescent begins to act like an adult, thinking about the future and weighing the risks, benefits, and consequences of life decisions.

7. **e.** Experts believe that the key ingredient to ensure healthy adolescent development is a prolonged supportive environment with graded steps toward autonomy. Healthy development is encouraged by a process of mutual positive engagement between the adolescent, various adults, and peers. Youth groups and other social organizations (e.g., Boy Scouts) can have a very positive impact toward the development of an independent, mature adolescent.

8. **e.** Divorce or separation of parents, poor school performance, sexual promiscuity, and peer group pressure are all risk factors for alcohol and substance abuse. Socioeconomic status is not.

9. **e.** Acute episodic care is the most frequent reason adolescents visit physicians' offices. These visits most frequently involve respiratory tract infections, skin conditions, genitourinary concerns, musculoskeletal injuries, or psychological disorders.

Among adolescents, 10% have chronic medical conditions (diabetes, asthma, epilepsy, irritable bowel disorder, etc.) necessitating regular visits.

School and sports physicals are the only other times when adolescents will make a regular visit to the physician's office. Therefore, it is incumbent for physicians to attempt to discuss a healthy lifestyle during any of these visits.

10. **c.** It is a poor commentary on social conditions in the United States, but homicide is the second leading cause of death among young people age 15 to 24 years.

11. **d.** One in four drivers age 15 to 20 years who are killed in crashes was intoxicated. More than one in three drivers questioned admit to riding in an automobile with an intoxicated driver. A significant number of teens admit to not wearing safety belts. Having multiple teens in the car increases the risk of accidents.

12. **e.** Graduated licensing has demonstrated a reduction in automobile accidents. It allows young drivers to gain driving experience under controlled circumstances. Usually, there are levels such as learner, intermediate, and full driver. Driver permits are linked to the following: zero tolerance for alcohol use, nighttime driving limitations, limits on teen passengers, all occupants must wear seat belts, and the permit holder must remain crash and conviction free to maintain the permit.

13. **b.** Due to the peer pressures of adolescence and the normal progress toward self-identity, teen years are a time during which females in particular tend to think they are overweight. Although a number of eating disorders should be considered, the binge/purge behavior is high on your list due to the damage to the front teeth caused by repeated exposure to gastric acids. Oral thrush causes white plaque, and dental caries are usually discoloration or cavitation as opposed to enamel damage. Anorexia can cause the weight problem but is less likely to cause the dental signs.

14. **e.** Generally, parental consent is required unless an underage patient is emancipated or it is an emergency in which awaiting consent would endanger the patient. However, in almost every jurisdiction, teens are entitled to medical privacy when they seek reproductive health care, including contraceptives, prenatal care, pregnancy and delivery services, HIV testing, and diagnosis and treatment of sexually transmitted diseases. In most jurisdictions, the only reproductive procedure underage patients cannot green-light is sterilization.

Solution to the Clinical Case Management Problem

Universal: Adolescence is a period when at least one health maintenance examination should be carried out. Episodic care visits are an ideal time to carry out these health screenings and assessments. A mnemonic useful in screening adolescents is SAFE TIMES:

S = Sexuality issues

A = Affect (depression) and abuse (drugs)

F = Family (function and medical history)

E = Examination (sensitive and appropriate)

T = Timing of development (body image)

I = Immunizations

M = Minerals (nutritional issues)

E = Education, employment (school and work issues)

S = Safety (vehicle)

Summary

The following are five recognized psychosocial issues that teens deal with during their adolescent years:

1. Establishing an identity

This is one of the most important tasks of adolescents.

Teens begin to integrate the opinions of influential others (e.g., parents, other caring adults, and friends) into their own likes and dislikes.

People with secure identities know where they fit (or where they do not want to fit) in their world.

2. Establishing autonomy

Establishing autonomy during the teen years means becoming an independent and self-governing person within relationships.

Autonomous teens have gained the ability to make and follow through with their own decisions, live by their own set of principles of right and wrong, and have become less emotionally dependent on parents.

Autonomy is a necessary achievement if a teen is to become self-sufficient in society.

3. Establishing intimacy

Many equate intimacy with sex, which of course it is not.

Intimacy is usually first learned within the context of same-sex friendships and then utilized in romantic relationships.

Intimacy refers to close relationships in which people are open, honest, caring, and trusting.

4. Becoming comfortable with one's sexuality

Teen years mark the first time that young people are both physically mature enough to reproduce and cognitively advanced enough to think about it.

More than half of most high school students report being sexually active.

Many experts agree that the mixed messages teens receive about sexuality contribute to problems such as teen pregnancy and sexually transmitted diseases.

5. Achievement

Society tends to foster and value attitudes of competition and success.

Because of cognitive advances, teens begin to see the relationship between their current abilities and plans and their future vocational aspirations.

Suggested Reading

Culbertson JL: Childhood and adolescent psychologic development. *Pediatr Clin North Am* 50(4):741–764, vii, 2003.

Goran MI: Obesity and risk of type 2 diabetes and cardiovascular disease in children and adolescents. *J Clin Endocrinol Metab* 88(4):1417–1427, 2003.

National Safety Council: Young drivers. Available at http://www.nsc.org/resources/Factsheets/road/young_drivers.aspx.

Towey K, Fleming M: *Healthy Youth 2010: Supporting the 21 Critical Adolescent Objectives.* Chicago: American Medical Association, 2001.

Weiss GG: Reduce liability risk when treating young patients. *Medical Economics* February 1, 2008.

Windle M, Windle RC: Adolescent tobacco, alcohol, and drug use: Current findings. *Adolesc Med* 10(1):153–163, 1999.

CHAPTER 124 Adolescent Safety

CLINICAL CASE PROBLEM 1

Routine Examinations as Safety Updates

RJ is a 15-year-old male brought to the office for a well adolescent physical by his father. He has no current health issues and takes no medications. After his father leaves the room, RJ denies sexual activity and alcohol, tobacco, or drug use. Both RJ and his father are concerned because a student at the high school was arrested for threatening another student with a gun. RJ's father admits to having several rifles in the home for hunting. He is concerned about gun safety because of the events at school. In addition, RJ is quite happy that he will soon obtain his driver's license. His father asks whether driver education at school will decrease his son's chances of having an accident.

SELECT THE BEST ANSWER TO THE FOLLOWING QUESTIONS

1. What is the leading cause of injury and all-cause mortality in adolescents?
   a. drowning
   b. firearm violence
   c. motor vehicle accidents
   d. suicide
   e. fires

2. Which of the following age groups has the highest crash rate per miles driven?
   a. 16-year-olds
   b. 17- to 19-year-olds
   c. 20- to 24-year-olds
   d. 25- to 29-year-olds
   e. 30- to 69-year-olds

3. Which of the following is least strongly associated with adolescent driver accidents and injuries?
   a. risk-taking behaviors
   b. nighttime driving
   c. marijuana use
   d. attention-deficit/hyperactivity disorder (ADHD)
   e. truancy

4. Which of the following interventions does not reduce crash and injury rates among new teenaged drivers?
   a. limit on nighttime driving (curfews)
   b. mandatory school drivers education courses
   c. requirements that drivers remain crash free before receiving a regular driver's license
   d. staging licensure into a three-step learner's permit, intermediate stage, and regular driver's license
   e. restrictions on the number of passengers during the intermediate stage

5. What is the second leading cause of death in adolescents age 15 to 19 years?
   a. drowning
   b. suicide
   c. firearms
   d. all-terrain vehicle accidents
   e. alcohol

6. Exposure to direct or indirect gun violence is associated with all of the following except
   a. withdrawal from family and friends
   b. substance use
   c. aggressive or delinquent behavior
   d. ADHD
   e. future involvement in violence

7. Which of the following statements regarding adolescent firearm violence is correct?
   a. gun ownership is not an independent risk for homicide in the home
   b. suicide risk in homes with firearms is no higher than in homes without firearms
   c. safe storage practices include storing ammunition with the firearm in a locked location
   d. parents are more receptive to gun safety counseling when it is provided by their child's physician
   e. physician counseling about firearm issues such as purchasing guns, disposing of guns, or buying safety locks is effective in changing patients' attitudes about firearm safety

CLINICAL CASE PROBLEM 2

"Could My Daughter Be on Drugs?"

SL is a 14-year-old female who is brought to the office for "problems." Her mother accompanies her and has concerns that her daughter is performing poorly in school and "hanging out with the wrong crowd." She recently quit the tennis team and is more solitary at home. Her mother found a pack of cigarettes when she was cleaning her daughter's room. She wants her daughter tested for drug use.

8. Which of the following is not a cause of false-positive urine drug screening in adolescents?
   a. cooking alcohol
   b. dextromethorphan
   c. poppy seeds
   d. pseudoephedrine
   e. none of the above

9. Which of the following substances is detectable on routine urine drug screening?
   a. 3,4-methylenedioxymethamphetamine (Ecstasy)
   b. oxycodone
   c. nitrous oxide
   d. tetrahydrocannabinol
   e. none of the above

10. How long is one-time use of marijuana detectable on a routine drug screen?
    a. less than 1 day
    b. 1 to 3 days
    c. 1 week
    d. 1 month
    e. 4 to 6 weeks

11. Which of the following policies is the greatest deterrent to teenage smoking?
    a. taxation of cigarettes
    b. antismoking campaigns
    c. access controls to obtaining tobacco (i.e., age restrictions)
    d. public smoking bans
    e. bans on tobacco advertising

SL is brought back for a follow-up visit. Her urine drug screen and alcohol level are both negative. When you speak with SL when her mother is out of the room, she confides that she is being bullied by several girls at school. She has been threatened and made fun of by this group. She is afraid to tell her mother and teachers, and she has dealt with the situation by avoiding social and athletic events at school.

12. What percentage of young adolescents experience some type of bullying behavior in the United States?
    a. 5%
    b. 10%
    c. 25%
    d. 50%
    e. 75%

13. Which of the following statements about peer bullying is correct?
    a. it is not intended to harm or be aggressive
    b. it occurs within interpersonal relationships and is used to create a power imbalance

c. it usually occurs as a one-time event
d. indirect bullying employs verbal attacks by teen boys
e. direct bullying includes verbal and/or physical attacks

14. Which of the following statements regarding bullying behavior is true?
    a. adolescents who are bullied have increased risk for violent behavior as adults
    b. comprehensive school-based interventions for reducing bullying consistently decrease the incidence of this behavior
    c. being an adolescent bully is not associated with later criminal behavior
    d. family characteristics of low cohesion and parental involvement are not linked with the likelihood of bullying
    e. single-parent family structure is not related to greater bullying among adolescents

Answers

1. c. Motor vehicle accidents are the leading cause of death for 16- to 20-year-olds. Two-thirds of adolescents who die in crashes are male. Of those killed, the majority (63%) are driving. A total of 5500 teenagers die annually, 450,000 are injured, and 27,000 of those injured require hospitalization as a result of motor vehicle accidents.

2. a. Adolescent drivers represent 6% of total drivers and account for 14% of fatal accidents. In terms of total crashes per 1 million miles driven, 16- to 19-year-olds have a crash rate twice that of 20- to 24-year-olds, three times that of 25- to 29-year-olds, and four times that of the 30- to 69-year-old age group. Younger drivers are at increased risk. Crash rates for 16-year-old drivers are significantly higher than for 17-year-olds (35 crashes verses 20 crashes per 1 million miles).

3. e. Multiple factors contribute to the increased rates of teenage driver injury and mortality. Risk taking is common in adolescents, although inexperience with driving certainly also plays a role. Driving with teenage passengers significantly increases the risk of a crash. Sixteen- and 17-year-olds have a 40% increased risk of accident when one friend is in the car. With three or more teenage passengers, the risk increases fourfold. Driving with a male teenage passenger results in faster speed and riskier driving than when a female is in the car. Curfews for night driving often prohibit driving after midnight, but 58% of fatal crashes occur between 9 PM and midnight. Marijuana use is seen with 6% to 25% of drivers involved in severe injury crashes. Teenagers diagnosed with ADHD are two to four times more likely to be injured in motor vehicle accidents. Truancy per se is not directly linked with accidents, although it likely has an indirect effect.

4. **b.** The majority of states have graduated driver licensing (GDL) laws. GDL consists of three stages: the learner's permit, an intermediate stage, and the regular driver's license. A recent Cochrane review of 12 GDL programs found a 31% decrease in overall crashes in 16-year-old drivers in the first year. Although evidence shows that GDL is effective in reducing crashes, the magnitude of effect is unknown. Three other provisions of GDL thought to reduce crashes are limits on night driving, requirements to stay crash free, and restrictions on the number of passengers in the car. Traditional driver education courses provide relatively little behind-the-wheel instruction. Several literature reviews show that courses are not effective in reducing crashes and may allow for earlier licensure of younger at-risk drivers.

5. **c.** Firearm-related deaths rank second only to motor vehicle accidents in injuries to 15- to 19-year-olds. Firearm mortality is higher than death from any disease category in this age group. In 2002, 2474 individuals age 15 to 19 years were killed by firearms, and 11,014 were seen in emergency departments for nonfatal injuries.

6. **d.** Firearm violence is linked with serious psychological sequelae both in communities in which violence is common and through media coverage of gun violence. Negative effects on child development include withdrawal, aggressive/delinquent behavior, substance use disorders, mental illness, poor school performance, and future violent behavior.

7. **d.** Ownership of a gun is a known risk factor for homicide in the home. Firearms in the home are associated with a threefold increased risk of homicide, usually by a family member or acquaintance. Suicide is five times higher in homes with guns. Safe storage methods include keeping guns unloaded and locked up, ideally separate from any ammunition. Counseling on gun safety by a parent's physician does not demonstrate a significant effect on changing habits. Parents may be more receptive to counseling from their child's physician.

8. **a.** Alcohol used for cooking does not cause a false-positive alcohol screen. Ingesting large amounts of poppy seeds can result in a false-positive screen for opioids. Confirmatory tests may incorrectly indicate cocaine or morphine use. Dextromethorphan and pseudoephedrine are common ingredients in cold relief products. Dextromethorphan cross-reacts with phencyclidine hydrochloride assays but not opioid assays. Pseudoephedrine can cross-react with an amphetamine screen.

9. **d.** Tetrahydrocannabinol (marijuana) is detectable on conventional urine drug screens. Inhaled nitrous oxide is detectable in blood or urine for a short period after exposure only when specific processing is done. Ecstasy is not routinely detected in most drug screens. Specially ordered tests can identify the substance in urine. Oxycodone is a semisynthetic opioid that is not tested on a routine urine screen. Its presence is only detectable by tests that must be specifically requested from the laboratory.

10. **b.** Urine drug screening for marijuana after one-time use remains positive for 1 to 3 days. Marijuana is highly lipophilic, and prolonged use concentrates marijuana metabolites in the body's fat stores. In regular users, cannabis is detected for 4 to 6 weeks on a urine drug test. Secondhand marijuana exposure does not cause false-positive urine drug screens.

11. **a.** Tobacco control policies directed at adolescents include various restrictive laws, public smoking bans, and advertising regulations. Taxation policies are the most effective deterrent to keep teens from either starting or continuing smoking. Price increases in tobacco products impact teen smokers to a greater degree than adults. For each 10% increase in price per pack, an estimated 15% fewer cigarettes may be consumed by adolescents.

12. **e.** Three-fourths of adolescents experience some type of bullying. Name calling, rumors, and public ridicule are common vehicles. One-third of this group experience more serious coercion or unwanted physical contact. Bullying behavior peaks in early adolescence and tapers off in later years.

13. **e.** Bullying, harassment, and victimization are all terms used to describe aggressive peer relationships. Bullying refers to behavior that is aggressive and intended to harm another. It occurs repetitively over time where power imbalances exist between individuals. Direct bullying involves overt verbal or physical assaults, whereas indirect bullying uses ignoring or gossiping behaviors that involve third parties. Direct bullying occurs more frequently with boys, whereas girls are more apt to employ indirect methods.

14. **a.** Bullying has long-term consequences, including increased violent behavior in adulthood in both bullies and those who are bullied. Former bullies have a fourfold increase in criminal behavior at age 24 years. Family dynamics of low parental involvement, poor warmth, minimal family cohesion, and single-parent homes are all linked with an increase in bullying behavior. It is uncertain whether school-based interventions to reduce bullying have a significant effect.

Summary

Adolescent safety is an important topic to discuss during routine periodic health exams. Automobile accidents are the leading cause of death in 16- to 20-year-olds. The majority of deaths occur in males, although tens of thousands of teens require hospitalization annually due to injuries sustained in automobile crashes.

Adolescents account for 14% of fatal crashes despite the fact that they make up only 6% of total drivers. The crash rate for 16-year-old drivers is substantially higher than that of older teenagers. Factors contributing to this increased risk are manifold. Risk taking in adolescents, combined with inexperience, is likely a major factor. Other risks include driving with teenage passengers, especially males; drug and alcohol use; and driving at night. Graduated driver licensing laws are used in the majority of states in an attempt to decrease mortality rates in this age group. Requirements for licensure are staged and consist of the learner's permit followed by an intermediate stage and, lastly, a regular driver's license. Whether GDL programs decrease mortality is not completely understood. Curfews for night driving, limiting teen passengers in the car, and revoking licenses of teenagers who wreck are also legislated with GDL. School-based driver education courses may inadvertently allow for licensure of younger at-risk drivers.

Firearm-related deaths are the second leading cause of injuries in 15- to 19-year-olds. Gun violence takes a severe psychological toll both in communities in which it is rampant and from media coverage of firearm violence. Effects on adolescent development include substance use disorders, mental illness, poor school performance, withdrawal, delinquent behavior, and future violent tendencies. A gun in the home is a known risk for homicide. Safe storage entails keeping the gun locked up and unloaded. Ammunition should be stored separately from the firearm. Although counseling by the parent's physician does not change attitudes regarding gun safety, counseling by the child's physician may.

Urine drug testing and screening for alcohol use are increasingly used in the school setting to detect substance use in adolescents. Providers ordering drug screening should be aware of what the standard screens can and cannot detect. Ecstasy, oxycodone, and nitrous oxide are drugs of choice in many adolescents, and specialized testing is needed to screen for them. Several substances and drugs cross-react with the standard drug panels and cause false-positive results. Gas chromatography is required for confirmation with any positive urine drug screen.

Bullying affects 75% of adolescents. This type of behavior peaks in early adolescence and gradually tapers off. It involves behavior that is repetitive, aggressive, and designed to harm another person. Home situations characterized by minimal parental involvement, single-parent homes, and poor family cohesion are often associated with adolescents who bully. Direct bullying involves overt physical or verbal assault, whereas indirect bullying uses third-party gossip and innuendo to disrupt social relationships. Both bullies and their victims have long-term sequelae, including lower self-esteem and future violent tendencies. Whether school programs on bullying prevention are effective is not clear.

Suggested Reading

Committee on Injury, Violence, and Poison Prevention and Commitee on Adolescence: The teen driver. *Pediatrics* 188:2570–2581, 2006.

Ding A: Curbing adolescent smoking: A review of the effectiveness of various policies. *Yale J Biology Med* 78:37–44, 2005.

Duke N, Resnick M, Borowsky I: Adolescent firearm violence: Position paper of the Society for Adolescent Medicine. *J Adolesc Health* 37:171–174, 2005.

Eisenberg M, Aalsma M: Bullying and peer victimization: Position paper of the Society for Adolescent Medicine. *J Adolesc Health* 36:88–91, 2005.

Hartling L, Wiebe N, Russell K, et al: Graduated driver licensing for reducing motor vehicle crashes among young drivers. *Cochrane Database Syst Rev* (1):CD003300, 2007.

Levy S, Harris S, Sherritt L, et al: Drug testing of adolescents in ambulatory medicine. *Arch Pediatr Adolesc Med* 160:146–150, 2006.

GERIATRIC MEDICINE

CHAPTER

125 Functional Assessment of the Elderly

CLINICAL CASE PROBLEM 1

A Worrisome Visit

John was concerned when he visited his mother. His father had died 3 months ago from congestive heart failure at the age of 82 years. Although he thought his mother was doing well, based on what he saw, he was quite concerned. He and his family live 220 miles away in another state, he has no siblings, and his ability to visit his mother is limited at best. He had been calling her twice a week and she reassured him that everything was fine and she was getting along pretty well. He knew she had a severe case of arthritis of the hands and knees but was unaware how this had affected her ability to function independently. When he visited with his two children, he was amazed at how much weight she had lost in the past 3 months and the amount of spoiled food in the refrigerator. The home was unkempt and she appeared to be wearing clothes that were soiled and not ironed.

He sat down with his mother to discuss this issue, and she admitted that her abilities to care for herself had declined throughout the years and her husband had assisted her in many of her activities of daily living. She was ashamed of the state of her home and her son asked why they had not told him of their needs: "Dad and I did not want to worry you and your family," was her reply. Together, they looked to provide some assistance for her. They contacted her primary physician, who referred them to a geriatric center for a comprehensive evaluation.

This included evaluation for physical, cognitive, and social concerns. Although she denied depression, with the loss of her husband, her inability to care for herself, and the declining function, depression was certainly a concern and a support system needed to be in place.

How could a comprehensive geriatric assessment assist John's mother with her current needs?

SELECT THE BEST ANSWER TO THE FOLLOWING QUESTIONS

1. What percentage of those older than age 65 years in the United States have one or more chronic conditions?
   a. 84%
   b. 70%
   c. 53%
   d. 28%
   e. 10%

2. What is the most common chronic condition?
   a. arthritis
   b. heart disease
   c. hypertension
   d. diabetes
   e. chronic obstructive pulmonary disease

3. Older men exhibit a higher percentage of limitations at all ages than do older women.
   a. true
   b. false

4. Activities of daily living include all the following except
   a. bathing
   b. dressing
   c. toileting
   d. handling finances
   e. feeding

5. Abnormalities of gait include which of the following?
   a. path deviation
   b. diminished height and length of step
   c. difficulty turning
   d. trips, slips, and near fall
   e. all of the above

6. The "timed get up and go" test should be completed in how many seconds to be considered a normal examination?
   a. less than 10 seconds
   b. less than 15 seconds
   c. less than 20 seconds
   d. less than 25 seconds
   e. less than 30 seconds

7. Poor nutritional assessment may be manifested by which of the following?
   a. A body mass index of less than 20 kg/m²
   b. unintentional weight loss of more than 10 pounds in 6 months
   c. visual inspection
   d. none of the above
   e. all of the above

8. Significant impairment in vision can be confirmed by the use of a Snellen chart if the patient is unable to read greater than 20/40.
   a. true
   b. false

9. Hearing loss in the elderly can lead to which of the following associations?
   a. depression
   b. social isolation
   c. dissatisfaction with living
   d. all of the above
   e. none of the above

10. After the age of 65 years, the prevalence of cognitive decline doubles every 5 years, and it approaches 40% to 50% by the age of 90 years.
    a. true
    b. false

11. The Mini-Cog is an assessment instrument consisting of:
    a. clock drawing test
    b. three-item recall
    c. Mini-Mental State Examination
    d. a and b

12. Hearing loss in the elderly is usually
    a. unilateral and in the high-frequency range
    b. unilateral and in the low-frequency range
    c. bilateral and in the high-frequency range
    d. bilateral and in the low-frequency range

13. A comprehensive geriatric assessment is most successful if the geriatric team maintains control of the patient.
    a. true
    b. false

14. Risk factors for adult drivers include which of the following?
    a. poor visual acuity (less than 20/40)
    b. dementia (especially with visual–spatial problems)
    c. impaired neck and trunk rotation
    d. poor motor coordination and speed of movement
    e. all of the above

Answers

1. **a.** In the United States in 2000, 84% of people aged 65 years or older had one or more chronic conditions. Hypertension is the most common, followed by arthritic conditions, heart disease, chronic obstructive pulmonary disease, cancer, sinusitis, and diabetes. Other common conditions include ulcers, strokes, and kidney disease. Although 80% of the elderly report two or more chronic diseases, only 36% report being in poor health.

2. **c.** See answer 1.

3. **b.** False. Older women exhibit a higher percentage of limitations than do men. In the United States, the majority of people younger than age 85 years report no difficulty in activities of daily living or instrumental activities of daily living. Differences between racial and ethnic groups exist as well. Among those age 70 years or older, black Americans are 1.5 times as likely as white Americans to be unable to perform one or more activities of daily living. When older people need assistance with functioning, they rely first on their family.

4. **d.** Functional status refers to a person's ability to perform tasks that are required for living. These tasks are referred to as activities of daily living and include bathing, dressing, feeding, toileting, grooming, and ambulating. Instrumental activities of daily living include handling finances, shopping, food preparation, housekeeping, laundry, independent traveling, and taking their own medications. Scales are then utilized to determine the level of a patient's function and his or her ability to live independently.

5. e. Gait disorders are common in older adults and are a predictor of functional decline. The disturbance in gait is usually multifactorial and a full assessment should consider a number of different causes. Because gait disturbances are commonly associated with falls and disability in older adults, proper evaluation is essential.

6. a. The "timed get up and go" test consists of the following tasks: rising from a chair, walking 10 feet, turning around, returning to the chair, turning, and sitting back down in the chair. The ability to accomplish this sequence of maneuvers in less than10 seconds shows that the patient has intact mobility. Those who take 20 seconds or longer require further evaluation for either physical or cognitive decline.

7. e. Poor nutrition in older individuals may reflect concurrent medical illnesses, depression, dementia, inability to shop or cook, inability to feed oneself, or financial hardship.

8. a. True. Many elderly patients are unaware of their visual deficits. Visual impairment from cataracts, glaucoma, macular degeneration, and abnormalities of accommodation worsen with ageing and often result in decreased vision. Asking about difficulty with driving, watching television, or reading may help identify underlying problems that were previously left undiagnosed. When using a Snellen chart, the inability to read greater than 20/40 is the criteria for visual impairment.

9. d. The importance of adequate hearing screening is essential in evaluating elderly patients. The risk of social isolation, depression, and a lack of appreciation for living directly impact the quality of life and in many cases can be corrected. This initial assessment can be done by asking questions first and then using a handheld Audioscope for testing purposes. The inability to hear a 40-db tone at 1000 or 2000 Hz in both ears or at either of these frequencies in one ear is considered abnormal and should be evaluated further. Always check for cerumen impaction in each patient as a possible cause for hearing loss.

10. a. True. The prevalence of dementia is 40% to 50% at age 90 years. Because most patients with dementia do not realize the extent of their disease, it is important for practitioners to question both the patient and a close family member or friend if memory loss is considered. A brief cognitive screen is important, and this may include the Folstein Mini Mental Status Exam. A test score of less than 24 on the Folstein would be consistent with an underlying dementia and should be investigated. This test will assess orientation, registration, attention and calculation, recall, language skills, and visual–spatial skills. Because loss of short-term memory is typically the first sign of dementia, the three-item recall in 1 minute test should be performed.

11. d. The clock drawing test is combined with the three-item recall to form the Mini-Cog assessment. The clock drawing test is valuable because it assesses executive function and visual–spatial skills, and the three-item recall in 1 minute may indicate impaired short-term memory, typically the first sign of dementia.

12. c. Bilateral high-frequency loss is most common.

13. a. True. Comprehensive geriatric assessment is intended to determine a patient's medical, psychosocial, and functional capabilities and limitations. The main goal is to develop an overall plan for treatment and long-term follow-up. It requires a highly trained team and is expensive and time-consuming. Success generally requires the geriatric team to take over the direct care of the patient. The greatest success in terms of improving function, reducing nursing home placement, and reducing hospital readmissions occurs in a patient-centered geriatric unit that is staffed by highly trained professionals.

14. e. Although the absolute number of crashes involving older drivers is low, the number of crashes per mile driven and the likelihood of serious injury or death are higher than for any age group other than 16- to 24-year-olds. Medications and alcohol may also contribute significantly to impaired driving skills. It is therefore essential that this function be screened for in each individual.

Suggested Readings

American Geriatrics Society: *Geriatric Review Syllabus, A Core Curriculum in Geriatric Medicine*, 6th ed. New York: American Geriatrics Society, 2006, pp. 4–5, 46–47, 92–93, 199.

American Geriatrics Society: *Geriatrics at Your Fingertips, 2006–2007*. New York: American Geriatrics Society, 2006, pp. 215–217.

Cohen HJ, Feussner JR, Weinberger M, et al: A controlled trial of inpatient and outpatient geriatric evaluation and management. *N Engl J Med* 346(12):905–912, 2002.

Gill TM, Kurland B: The burden and patterns of disability in activities of daily living among community living older persons. *J Gerontol Biol Sci Med Sci* 58:70–75, 2003.

126 Polypharmacy and Drug Reactions in the Elderly

CLINICAL CASE PROBLEM 1

A 75-Year-Old Female with a Bagful of Pills

A 75-year-old female comes to your office for the first time with her daughter. Her daughter describes her mother as having undergone "a marked personality change." Apparently, her elderly mother began seeing "pink rats coming out of the wall" and she began "hearing and seeing people from outer space" floating down into her field of vision.

The patient's daughter brings in her mother's medications in a bag. She describes a visit to her mother's previous physician 1 week ago. At that time, the doctor prescribed a number of medications, including pills for her blood pressure, pills for her heart, pills for her arthritis, pills for her stomach, pills for her anxiety, pills for her depression, and pills for her insomnia.

On further questioning, the daughter states that her mother had been fairly well before the physician visit but had (unfortunately) mentioned "a few minor ailments." In response to the patient's complaints, the physician prescribed hydrochlorothiazide, propranolol, nifedipine, digoxin, ibuprofen, cimetidine, Maalox, amitriptyline, and triazolam.

You are well aware of the fact that medications in the elderly can often produce significant side effects. You suspect that there is a connection between the pink rats, the space men, and the pills.

On examination, the patient is agitated and confused. Her blood pressure is 100/70 mmHg, and her pulse is 54 beats/minute and regular. She has a bruise on her head from a fall 3 days ago. Examination of the cardiovascular system reveals a normal S1 and S2 with a grade VI systolic murmur heard along the left sternal edge. There are no other abnormalities.

SELECT THE BEST ANSWER TO THE FOLLOWING QUESTIONS

1. Which of the following statements regarding this patient's acute medical problem is true?
   a. this patient's problem is unlikely to be related to her medications
   b. this patient's presentation is unusual following the initiation of medications in the elderly
   c. this patient's problem is unlikely to lead to hospitalization
   d. this patient's problem is likely to be transient
   e. none of the above statements are true

2. Which of the following statements regarding the use of drugs in the elderly is true?
   a. elderly patients should be treated the same way as younger patients with respect to drug initiation
   b. elderly patients generally need the same dose of medications as younger patients
   c. psychotropic drugs are unlikely to produce significant side effects in elderly patients
   d. elderly patients on multiple medications should be reassessed on a yearly basis
   e. none of the above statements are true

3. Regarding elderly patients in chronic care facilities, which of the following statements regarding medication use is (are) true?
   a. elderly patients in chronic care facilities are usually on fewer medications than elderly patients living on their own
   b. elderly patients in chronic care facilities are usually on between 8 and 13 different medications at any one time
   c. elderly patients in chronic care facilities are likely to experience iatrogenic side effects from medications at one time or another
   d. b and c are true
   e. a, b, and c are true

CLINICAL CASE PROBLEM 2

An 85-Year-Old Female Patient with a Dangerously High Blood Pressure

An 85-year-old female patient of yours was placed on a combination of hydrochlorothiazide and clonidine because of a "dangerously high" blood pressure of 150/95 mmHg. When you hear this story, you are concerned about possible adverse side effects. Your worst fear comes true when you find yourself attending her in the emergency department with a serious adverse event you believe is directly related to the medications on which she was placed.

4. Which of the following specialists will you call to manage this adverse event?
   a. a rheumatologist

b. a general surgeon or a general internist

c. a gerontologist

d. an orthopedic surgeon

e. a psychiatrist

5. The patient becomes acutely short of breath. The adverse effect that you feared has now led to a complication. What is that complication?

a. deep venous thrombosis (DVT) leading to a pulmonary embolus

b. splenic infarct

c. cerebrovascular accident

d. aplastic anemia

e. drug-induced psychosis

6. What is the most likely medication causing the pink rats and the people from outer space in the patient described in Clinical Case Problem 1?

a. propranolol

b. hydrochlorothiazide

c. ibuprofen

d. cimetidine

e. digoxin

7. Consider the possibility that the adverse event and its complication just described did not occur. Considering the rapid introduction of multiple medications that took place on the visit to the other physician, what would be the most appropriate course of action at this time?

a. discontinue the digoxin

b. discontinue the hydrochlorothiazide

c. discontinue the propranolol

d. discontinue the triazolam

e. discontinue all medications, observe in a geriatric day hospital environment, and reevaluate the patient continuously for the first few weeks

8. Of the drug combinations listed, which is the most likely to result in a drug–drug interaction in the elderly?

a. cimetidine and propranolol

b. digoxin and hydrochlorothiazide

c. ibuprofen and captopril

d. triazolam and amitriptyline

e. haloperidol

9. What is the most common potentially serious side effect of tricyclic antidepressants in elderly patients?

a. dry mouth

b. constipation

c. bladder spasm

d. orthostatic hypotension

e. sedation

10. Which of the following combinations of pharmacologic agents is most commonly associated with adverse drug reactions (ADRs) in the elderly?

a. cardiovascular drugs, psychotropics, and antibiotics

b. cardiovascular drugs, psychotropics, and analgesics

c. gastrointestinal drugs, psychotropics, and analgesics

d. gastrointestinal drugs, psychotropics, and antibiotics

11. Which of the following pharmacologic parameters may be associated with ADRs in the elderly?

a. altered free serum concentration of drug

b. altered volume of distribution

c. altered renal drug clearance

d. altered tissue sensitivity of the drug

e. all of the above

12. Which of the following is (are) an example(s) of ADRs in the elderly?

a. drug side effects

b. drug toxicity

c. drug–disease interaction

d. drug–drug interaction

e. all of the above

13. Some pharmacologic agents are excreted virtually unchanged by the kidneys. The dosages of these drugs must be carefully titrated in any elderly patient with renal impairment or potential renal impairment. Drugs in this category include which of the following?

a. cimetidine

b. gentamicin

c. lithium

d. all of the above

e. none of the above

14. Regarding antipsychotic drug therapy in the elderly, which of the following statements is (are) true?

a. antipsychotic drugs are often prescribed for behavior that chronic care staff find objectionable

b. tardive dyskinesia is a frequent side effect of antipsychotic drug use in the elderly

c. antipsychotic drugs are prescribed much more frequently in institutionalized patients than in noninstitutionalized patients

d. all of the above statements are true

e. none of the above statements are true

15. Underprescribed medications in older adults may include which of the following?
   a. angiotensin-converting enzyme inhibitors for heart failure
   b. beta blockers for heart failure and following a myocardial infarction
   c. warfarin for atrial fibrillation
   d. aspirin within 24 hours of an acute myocardial infarction
   e. all of the above

Clinical Case Management Problem

List 10 rules that will minimize ADRs in the elderly.

Answers

1. e. This patient's problem can be characterized in the following manner: (1) It is likely to be related to the bagful of medications on which she was started; (2) it is very common following the initiation of medication in the elderly, especially multiple medications; (3) it is very unlikely to be transient unless some or all of the medications are discontinued; and (4) it will commonly lead to hospitalization.

It is believed that up to 20% of hospitalizations, and perhaps significantly more in the elderly, are a result of iatrogenic disease. Iatrogenic disease is almost always associated with multiple medication use.

2. e. The following are some helpful guidelines on the initiation of drugs in the elderly:

1. Drug initiation in the elderly should be done cautiously. The general rule should be to start very low and go very slow.
2. The elderly patient usually needs a considerably lower dose of drug than does the young adult. This is, of course, especially true of drugs that are renally excreted. The general rule on drug initiation in elderly patients is "no more than 50% of the usual adult dose; no more than one drug at a time. Increases not any more quickly than once a week."
3. Psychotropic drugs should be used with special caution. Psychotropic medications are frequently misused in the elderly and dosing should be monitored closely.
4. All elderly patients should have a formal drug review performed at least every 3 months. At that time, all drugs and the drug doses should be seriously considered for reduction or discontinuation, especially if the elderly patient has symptoms that suggest an ADR to one or more of the drugs that he or she is taking.

3. d. Patients in chronic care facilities have the following characteristics with respect to medication use:

1. They are usually on multiple medications. The average number of medications used by the institutionalized elderly is 8 per day. Standard orders may increase this to 13 medications per day.
2. The most usual scenario is that medications are always added but never subtracted. Thus, the number simply continues to increase.
3. Iatrogenic side effects from medication use in chronic care facilities are extremely common. Considering the number of medications that these residents are taking, they are actually far more likely to experience at least one ADR per year than not.
4. In comparison to senior citizens living on their own in the community, the number of medications used by institutional-based elderly patients is greater.

4. d. The combination of hydrochlorothiazide and clonidine is likely to produce significant orthostatic hypotension in the elderly patient. The most "adverse effect of the adverse effect" is a fall in the elderly leading to a fracture of the neck of the femur. Thus, the specialist that you most likely will call is an orthopedic surgeon.

5. a. The most serious complication from a hip fracture is immobility leading to DVT. The development of a DVT is, of course, directly correlated with a subsequent pulmonary embolus.

The mortality of elders in the first year following a hip fracture is approximately 25%. Prevention is the best treatment.

Prevention is best accomplished by significantly limiting the number of medications an elder patient is on, especially medications that tend to produce orthostatic hypotension. It should be noted that sedative hypnotics increase the risk for hip fractures considerably.

6. a. The most common medication-induced cause of hallucinations in elderly patients is propranolol. Many elderly patients who are started on propranolol develop visual or auditory hallucinations. Unfortunately, many of these patients are then started on antipsychotic medications to treat the hallucinations rather than evaluating their medication list.

7. e. The most reasonable course of action at this time is to stop everything and start again. The rapid introduction of the nine medications listed was a recipe for disaster. In an attempt to counteract the disaster, this logically should take place in the supervised setting of at least a geriatric day hospital. Many geriatric assessment units do exactly that when an elder is admitted for the assessment of any medical problem. With elders who have been on multiple medications for long periods of time, the safest place to accomplish this is in the hospital under close observation. Of elderly hospital admissions, 10% to 17% are a result of inappropriate medication use. Use these hospitalizations to properly assess medications and to develop appropriate treatment plans.

8. b. Patients who develop ADRs are more likely to be taking six or more drugs than those who do not develop an ADR. The most commonly identified combination likely to result in a drug–drug interaction is digoxin with a diuretic. In this case, the ADR most likely to be produced is hypokalemia. The hypokalemia produced will often lead to digoxin toxicity in the susceptible elder. These combinations are considered secondary drug reactions, which require at least two drugs to cause an interaction.

9. d. All of the side effects listed are common side effects of tricyclic antidepressant medications. The side effects that are caused by an anticholinergic mechanism include dry mouth, blurred vision, constipation, bladder spasm and urinary retention, and sedation.

The orthostatic hypotension is caused by an α-adrenergic blockade and is potentially the most serious due to the association described previously between the following series of events: (1) orthostatic hypotension, (2) falls in the elder, (3) fractured neck of the femur, (4) DVT, and (5) pulmonary embolism.

Excess morbidity and mortality are associated with events 3, 4, and 5 in the chain. In addition, always follow cardiac status when using digoxin, evaluating for bradycardia and dysrhythmias.

10. b. The three most common drug classes associated with ADRs in the elderly are cardiovascular drugs, psychotropic drugs, and analgesics (especially nonsteroidal anti-inflammatory drugs [NSAIDs]). Unfortunately, many of the drugs used in the treatment of geriatric patients are prescribed for symptoms related to the effects and the diseases of aging and not necessarily for a specific acute disease where function can be restored. This results, of course, in the elder being on the particular agent for a longer period.

11. e. Many physiologic and social variables increase the incidence of ADRs in elderly patients. They include the number of drugs, compliance, absorption of drug, concentration of free drug in the serum, volume of distribution, tissue sensitivity, metabolic clearance, renal drug clearance, general homeostasis, and concentration of serum albumin.

12. e. An ADR is defined as any unintended or undesired effect of a drug in a patient. This may include abnormal laboratory values, patient symptoms, and signs on physical examination.

ADRs can be divided into side effects (dry mouth from tricyclic antidepressants and hypokalemia from diuretics), drug toxicity (daytime sedation from hypnotics, diarrhea from laxatives, and syncope from antihypertensive agents), drug–disease interaction (benzodiazepine and drugs with anticholinergic properties may affect the cognitive function in Alzheimer's patients), drug–drug interaction (digoxin and diuretics), and secondary effects (haloperidol causing drug-induced parkinsonism).

13. d. The kidney is the major source of elimination of many commonly prescribed drugs. Drugs that undergo extensive renal clearance and that are therefore likely to accumulate in the elderly include digoxin, gentamicin and other aminoglycosides, lithium, cimetidine, cotrimoxazole, disopyramide, nadolol, procainamide, and sulfonamides. Remember that NSAIDs may increase renal toxicity, especially in high-risk patients.

14. d. Psychotropic drugs are commonly prescribed for geriatric patients. Indications for the use of these drugs are not well established. In nursing home situations, psychotropic drugs are often prescribed for behaviors that staff members find objectionable (i.e., for the benefit of the staff, not the patient); the patient may, in fact, remain on this (these) drug(s) for long periods. The institutionalized elderly are 10 times more likely to receive antipsychotic agents as age-matched noninstitutionalized controls.

15. e. All of the named medications and situations are true. Other medications include HMG-CoA reductase inhibitors for primary prevention, gastroprotective agents for patients at high risk for NSAID-induced gastrointestinal bleeding, and narcotic analgesics for pain control.

Double-blind, randomized controlled trials have not established the efficacy of antipsychotic drug use in Alzheimer's disease. Tardive dyskinesia, rigidity, and excessive sedation are frequent side effects of antipsychotic drug use. In many states, the use of psychotropic medication must be well documented with specific goals for behavior. The use of chemical restraints through the use of psychotropic medications is not justified.

It should be noted that the use of newer antipsychotic agents, such as risperidone (Risperdal), olanzapine (Zyprexa), and quetiapine (Seroqual), has been shown to be effective in the treatment of psychotic behavior and neurobehavioral manifestations in patients with severe Alzheimer's disease.

Solution to the Clinical Case Management Problem

The following is a good set of rules for prescribing medication in geriatric patients:

1. Recognize that there is no drug to treat senescence.
2. Recognize that mere prolongation of life is not a valid reason for using medications that decrease the quality of life.
3. Make sure that the effects of treatment outweigh the risks.
4. Establish a priority order for treatment.
5. Keep the number of drugs administered concurrently to a minimum.
6. Know your patient well. Consider renal and hepatic impairment. Consider what else (including over-the-counter medications) is being taken and who else is prescribing drugs.
7. Always begin with nonpharmacologic therapy first, if possible.
8. If you decide to prescribe a drug, know it well. Consider using a few drugs often rather than many drugs infrequently.
9. Select the dose carefully: Start very low and go very slow.
10. Anticipate and minimize ADRs by considering side effect profiles.
11. Determine whether or not the patient needs help using the medication.
12. Educate the patient and family.
13. Continually reevaluate whether or not your patient needs a specific drug.
14. Perform a drug review every 3 months on every elder on more than one medication.
15. Use medication diaries: Have patients bring in all medications and over-the-counter and herbal medications used.
16. Check serum levels when indicated.
17. Destroy old medications.
18. Use medication cards.

Summary

1. Prevalence: Drug reactions are common, especially in institutionalized elderly, who are on an average of 13 medications. ADRs are at least twice as common in elderly patients as in younger patients.
2. Types of ADRs: (a) side effects, (b) drug toxicity, (c) drug–disease interaction, (d) drug–drug interaction
3. Most common drugs associated with ADRs: (a) cardiovascular drugs, (b) psychotropic drugs, (c) analgesics
4. Set of reasonable rules: Follow the set of rules listed in the Clinical Case Management Solution
5. Categories of ADRs
   a. Primary ADR (one drug with one side reaction): (i) Cimetidine causes psychosis and (ii) propranolol induces depression.
   b. Secondary ADR (requires at least two drugs to cause an interaction): Erythromycin and theophylline used together are toxic.
   c. Drug withdrawal syndromes: (i) Beta blocker withdrawal leads to angina and (ii) addictive drugs cause withdrawal syndromes (benzodiazepines).
   d. Tertiary ADR: Benzodiazepines result in a higher incidence of falls.
6. Physician factors implicated in ADRs
   a. The physician gives a high-risk drug to a vulnerable host (NSAID for a patient with peptic ulcer disease).
   b. The physician gives a highly interactive drug to a pharmacologically vulnerable patient (i.e., captopril given to a patient on a potassium-sparing agent).
   c. The physician prescribes an inappropriate drug to treat an unrecognized drug side effect (i.e., antidepressant given to treat beta blocker depression).
7. Automatic or standard drug orders in intensive care unit, chronic care unit, or chronic care facilities should be reviewed on a regular basis.
8. Ensure appropriate follow-up.
9. Obtain a complete drug history.
10. Avoid prescribing before a diagnosis is made.
11. Review medications regularly and before adding a new medication.
12. Know the actions, adverse effects, and toxicity of the medications you prescribe.
13. Start at a low dose and titrate according to tolerability and response.
14. Attempt to maximize dose before switching to another.
15. Avoid using one drug to treat the side effects of another.

Suggested Reading

American Geriatric Society: *Geriatric Review Syllabus, A Core Curriculum in Geriatric Medicine*, 6th ed. Chicago: American Geriatric Society, 2006, pp. 72–79.

Goulding MR: Inappropriate medication prescribing for elderly ambulatory patients. *Arch Intern Med* 164(3):305–312, 2004.

Pham CB, Dickman RL: Minimizing adverse drug events in the elderly. *Am Fam Physician* 76:1837–1844, 2007.

CHAPTER
127 The Propensity and Consequences of Falls among the Elderly

CLINICAL CASE PROBLEM 1

An 81-Year-Old Female Who Is Repeatedly Falling

An 81-year-old female is brought to your office by her daughter. The elderly mother has been falling repeatedly for at least 3 months. The falling has been getting progressively worse, and the patient's daughter is very concerned about the possibility of her mother "breaking her hip."

On examination, the patient is a frail, elderly female in no acute distress. She appears somewhat depressed, but her Mini-Mental Status Examination score is 27. The patient's blood pressure is 180/75 mmHg. Her pulse is 84 beats/minute and irregular. No other abnormalities are found.

SELECT THE BEST ANSWER TO THE FOLLOWING QUESTIONS

1. What is the prevalence of falls among community-based elderly patients between the ages of 70 and 75 years?
   a. 5% per year
   b. 10% per year
   c. 20% per year
   d. 30% per year
   e. 50% per year

2. Which of the following statements regarding falls in the elderly is (are) true?
   a. the prevalence of falling in the elderly increases with advancing age
   b. elderly patients who are physically active may be at greater risk of falling than those who are not
   c. approximately 55% of elderly patients who fall once will fall again
   d. falling in the elderly may not necessarily be a marker of functional decline
   e. all of the above statements are true

3. Which of the following is the most feared morbid outcome of falling among elderly patients?
   a. fracture of the hip
   b. fracture of the radius
   c. subdural hematoma
   d. epidural hematoma
   e. cervical fracture

4. Potential reversible causes of falling in the elderly include which of the following?
   a. medications
   b. postprandial hypotension
   c. alcohol use
   d. urinary urgency
   e. all of the above

5. Which of the following are predisposing risk factors for falls in the elderly?
   a. visual impairment
   b. cerebrovascular accidents
   c. Alzheimer's disease
   d. normal pressure hydrocephalus
   e. all of the above

6. Regarding the incidence of falling and medication use in the elderly, which of the following statements is (are) true?
   a. multiple drug use is associated with an increased incidence of falling in the elderly
   b. the higher the drug dosage, the greater the probability of falling
   c. drug interactions are a major contributing factor to an increased incidence of falling in the elderly
   d. a and b
   e. a, b, and c

7. Falling in the elderly is most commonly associated with which of the following pathophysiologic factors?
   a. orthostatic hypotension
   b. decreased left ventricular output
   c. decreased cerebral circulation
   d. increased left ventricular output
   e. none of the above

8. Which of the following medications is most likely to lead to a serious fall in an elderly patient?
   a. amitriptyline
   b. hydrochlorothiazide
   c. enalapril
   d. nifedipine
   e. fluoxetine

9. What is the prevalence of falling among institutionalized elderly patients?
   a. 50% per year
   b. 40% per year
   c. 30% per year
   d. 20% per year
   e. 10% per year

10. Which of the following statements regarding the use of restraints in elderly patients as a means to prevent falls is (are) true?
    a. restraints have been shown to reduce the incidence of falling in the elderly
    b. no study has ever shown a decrease in falls with restraint use in the elderly
    c. potential complications of restraint use in the elderly include strangulation, vascular damage, and neurologic damage
    d. a and c
    e. b and c

11. What percentage of elderly patients are not able to get up after a fall?
    a. 10%
    b. 20%
    c. 30%
    d. 40%
    e. 50%

12. Various risk factors consistently identified from multiple cohort studies include which of the following?
    a. age
    b. cognitive impairment
    c. female gender
    d. past history of a fall
    e. all of the above

13. Preventive measures for fall should include which of the following?
    a. strength and balance programs
    b. educational programs
    c. medication reviews
    d. environmental modifications
    e. all of the above
    f. none of the above

Clinical Case Management Problem

Describe the preventive measures that may result in a reduction in falls in the elderly.

Answers

1. **d.** According to several community-based surveys, approximately 30% of people older than the age of 65 years experience falls each year in situations in which there are no overwhelming intrinsic causes (e.g., syncope).

2. **e.** Approximately 55% of elders who fall have multiple falling episodes. The likelihood of falling increases with age. As illustrated by this very high prevalence of 30% among community-based people, falling is not just confined to the frail elderly; healthy elderly patients fall as well during ordinary daily activities. This suggests that falling is not merely a marker of functional decline in the elderly. Although the elder we picture as falling is the frail elder with multiple medical problems, it may well be the case that falling is more prevalent among the more healthy elders who are more, not less, physically active.

3. **a.** The most feared outcome of falls in the elderly is a fracture of the hip. This is especially common among elderly women who have significant osteoporosis.

   The escalating cost of health care has resulted in increased expectations and demands concerning cost-effective health care. Hip fracture results in the death of at least 12,000 elderly Americans per year. In elderly females with hip fractures, the mortality is approximately 20% in the first year.

4. **e.** Potential reversible causes of falling include medication, alcohol, postprandial hypotension (30 to 60 minutes after a meal), urinary urgency, insomnia, peripheral edema, and environmental factors.

5. **e.** Vision, hearing, vestibular function, and proprioception are the major sensory modalities related to stability. Thus, declines in vision, hearing, imbalance leading to vertigo and dizziness, peripheral neuropathies, and cervical degenerative disease are the most common causes of falls in elderly patients.

   Other associated diseases or conditions associated with falls in the elderly include cerebrovascular accidents, Parkinson's disease, normal-pressure hydrocephalus, dementia (Alzheimer's disease), severe osteoarthritis or rheumatoid arthritis, and medications causing orthostatic hypotension.

6. **e.** Iatrogenic disease is a major cause of falls in the elderly. This iatrogenic disease, which is almost completely related to medication use, is a serious problem in elders. As discussed previously, the average number of medications per elder (especially in the institutionalized setting) is between 8 and 13. Elderly patients on benzodiazepines have an increased risk of falling. Multiple drugs, increased drug dosage, and drug–drug interactions are all reasons for orthostatic hypotension (an alpha-blockade phenomenon) and sedation (the two most common predisposing pathophysiologic mechanisms associated with falling in the elderly).

7. **a.** Decreased left ventricular output, most closely associated with congestive heart failure, may also play a prominent role in some cases of falling, but orthostatic hypotension is the most common cause.

8. **a.** Amitriptyline, hydrochlorothiazide, enalapril, and nifedipine may all be associated with falling in the elderly. Enalapril and hydrochlorothiazide are more likely to be associated with falling when given concomitantly. In addition, the first-dose hypotensive effect of an angiotensin-converting enzyme (ACE) inhibitor should be remembered; that is, it is much safer to give the first dose of an ACE inhibitor to an elder in your office, where this possible side effect can be monitored.

Of the four medications listed, however, the most prominent predisposing to falls in the elderly is amitriptyline, a tricyclic antidepressant. Amitriptyline predisposes to falls by a combination of two mechanisms: its anticholinergic mechanism and its alpha-blockade mechanism. This drug should be used judiciously in the elderly. Starting very low and going very slowly will minimize falling as a result of drug use in elderly patients.

9. **a.** More than half of ambulatory nursing home patients fall each year. The estimated annual incidence is 1600 falls per 1000 beds. The higher frequency of falling among institutionalized elderly patients results both from the greater frailty of these patients compared to community-based elderly patients and from the greater reliability of reporting in an institutional setting.

10. **e.** No study has confirmed or suggested that the risk of falling in the elderly is lessened because of the use of restraining devices. On the other hand, restraining devices have been shown to result in significant morbidity and mortality from strangulation, neurologic damage, and vascular damage. In some countries (e.g., the United Kingdom), restraints are almost forbidden. In the United States, the situation appears to be the opposite. In some institutions, they are used routinely. Restraints have other side effects, including anxiety, anger, agitation, and paranoia.

11. **e.** Of the elderly who fall, only 50% are able to get up. Thus, experiencing what is referred to as the "long lie," is associated with lasting declines in functional status.

12. **e.** Additional risk factors include lower extremity weakness, gait problems, foot disorders, poor balance, psychotropic medications, arthritis, hypovitamin D, and Parkinson's disease.

13. **e.** Also included in studies was tai chi, which proved to be effective; withdrawal of psychotropic medications; and cardiac pacing for high-risk individuals.

Solution to the Clinical Case Management Problem

A preventive program for minimizing falls in the elderly should include the following:

1. Identification of intrinsic risk factors
   a. A thorough clinical evaluation aimed at identifying all contributing risk factors for falling is the first, most important step. Directly observing balance and gait has proven to be effective in identifying residents at risk for falling.
   b. A careful review of all situations may identify problem situations to be avoided in the future.
   c. A complete medication review with elimination of all unnecessary medications and a decrease in the dose of all others will minimize falls.

2. Environmental prevention
   a. General environmental measures include ensuring adequate lighting without glare; having dry, nonslippery floors that are free of obstacles and contamination; having high, firm chairs; and having raised toilet seats.
   b. Restraints should be used only when there appears to be no other alternative. Restraints should not take the place of close supervision and attention to the risk factors discussed previously. Alternatives to restraints, including wedges in chairs for maintenance of position and organized walking and grid barriers for prevention of wandering, may afford the necessary protection.

Summary

1. Prevalence: 30% per year in community-based elders and 50% per year in institutionalized elders
2. Major complication: fracture of the femur and resulting morbidity and mortality from surgery, deep venous thrombosis, and pulmonary embolus
3. Major predisposing conditions precipitating major complications
   a. Vision, hearing, vestibular function, and proprioception impairments
   b. Other conditions associated with increased risk: Alzheimer's disease, Parkinson's disease, and iatrogenic disease (mainly medication use, including the psychotropic agents and the cardiovascular agents—the agents with the greatest probability of producing sedation and other anticholinergic side effects and alpha-blockade side effects [orthostatic hypotension])
   c. 1 or 2 (above) associated with significant osteoporosis increases the risk
4. Elder populations at greatest risk
   a. Active elderly patients who are at increased risk because of significant activity levels in whom even a minor impairment may be enough to cause significant problems
   b. The "frail elderly" who have concomitant chronic medical conditions
   c. The institutionalized elderly
   d. This list may, in fact, include most elders
5. Prevention
   a. Prevent the development of osteoporosis in postmenopausal women whenever possible (estrogens, calcitonin, calcium, and biphosphonates).
   b. Carefully examine identifying intrinsic risk factors and environmental protection methods in helping to prevent falls.
   c. Medications
      i. Provide a medication review to every elder every 3 months.
      ii. Keep the number of medications to a minimum.
      iii. In starting medications, start very low and go very slow.
      iv. To minimize falls, minimize adverse drug reactions.

Suggested Reading

American Geriatric Society: *Geriatric Review Syllabus, A Core Curriculum in Geriatric Medicine*, 6th ed. Chicago: American Geriatric Society, 2006, pp. 201–209.

Gillespie LD, Gillespie WJ, Robertson MC, et al: Intervention for preventing falls in elderly people. *Cochrane Database Syst Rev* (3):CD000340, 2001.

Rao SS: Preventing falls in the elderly. *Am Fam Physician* 71(1):81–88, 2005.

Weinstock M, Neides D: *Residents Guide to Ambulatory Care*, 3rd ed.. Columbus, OH: Anadem, 2002, pp. 105–106.

Urinary Incontinence in the Elderly

CLINICAL CASE PROBLEM 1

An 88-Year-Old Institutionalized Female with Urinary Incontinence

An 88-year-old female patient who you care for and who resides in a chronic care facility is having increasing difficulties with "bedwetting." She is embarrassed to talk about this, but the nurses inform you that it is a problem and is getting progressively worse.

On your last weekly visit, the charge nurse requested permission from you to insert an indwelling urinary catheter. At that time, the patient had been incontinent continuously for 6 days. The charge nurse clearly tells you, "I haven't got enough staff to keep changing sheets 10 times a day. Please do something."

SELECT THE BEST ANSWER TO THE FOLLOWING QUESTIONS

1. At this time, what should your instructions to the charge nurse be?
   a. insert the indwelling catheter; call me if there are any more problems
   b. begin intermittent 4-hour catheterization to avoid the necessity of inserting an indwelling catheter
   c. wait and see what happens over the next couple of weeks

d. order some routine blood work to attempt to determine the cause of the problem

e. clearly indicate that you will begin investigation of this problem now; ask the charge nurse, in return, to attempt to manage the current situation for only a short time longer

2. Regarding urinary incontinence in the elderly, which of the following statements is false?
   a. 50% of elderly patients in nursing homes have established urinary incontinence
   b. 15% to 30% of elderly patients in a community setting have developed urinary incontinence
   c. women are twice as likely as men to have urinary incontinence
   d. humiliation and embarrassment are significant life problems for the patient with urinary incontinence
   e. none of the above statements are false

3. What is the most common type of urinary incontinence in elderly patients?
   a. urge incontinence
   b. stress incontinence
   c. complex incontinence
   d. overflow incontinence
   e. functional incontinence

4. Which of the following statements regarding incontinence in the elderly is (are) true?
   a. stress incontinence is usually manifested by loss of small amounts of urine as intraabdominal pressure increases
   b. overflow incontinence occurs through bladder distention
   c. prostatic obstruction is a common cause of overflow incontinence
   d. functional incontinence is characterized by an involuntary loss of urine despite normal bladder and urethral functioning
   e. all of the above statements are true

5. Which of the following is (are) a contributing factor(s) to urinary incontinence in the elderly?
   a. loss of the ability of the elderly to concentrate urine
   b. decreased bladder capacity
   c. decreased urethral closing pressure
   d. decreased mobility
   e. all of the above

6. Which of the following classes of drugs has not been implicated in the pathogenesis of urinary incontinence in the elderly?
   a. thiazide diuretics

   b. neuroleptics
   c. sedatives
   d. antibiotics
   e. hypnotics

7. Which of the following nonpharmacologic treatments may be effective in the management of urinary incontinence in the elderly?
   a. Kegel exercises
   b. biofeedback
   c. behavioral toilet training
   d. clean intermittent catheterization
   e. all of the above

8. Which of the following cause(s) acute (reversible) urinary incontinence in the elderly?
   a. delirium
   b. restricted mobility
   c. infection
   d. drugs
   e. all of the above

9. Anticholinergic and narcotic drugs are most commonly associated with which of the following types of urinary incontinence?
   a. urge incontinence
   b. stress incontinence
   c. overflow incontinence
   d. complex incontinence
   e. functional incontinence

10. Which of the following components of the diagnostic evaluation of urinary incontinence is not necessary in every elderly patient with the disorder?
    a. complete history
    b. focused physical examination
    c. renal ultrasound
    d. complete urinalysis
    e. postvoiding residual (PVR) urine determination

11. PVR urine is considered definitely abnormal when it exceeds which of the following?
    a. any amount is abnormal
    b. 100 mL
    c. 75 mL
    d. 50 mL
    e. 10 mL

12. What is (are) the drug(s) of choice for the pharmacologic management of stress incontinence?
    a. supplemental estrogen
    b. α-adrenergic agonists
    c. cholinergic agents
    d. a and b
    e. all of the above

13. Which of the following types of urinary incontinence is most amenable to surgical intervention?
    a. urge incontinence
    b. stress incontinence
    c. overflow incontinence
    d. complex incontinence
    e. functional incontinence

14. Which of the following are indications for the use of a chronic indwelling catheter in elderly patients with incontinence?
    a. urinary retention causing persistent overflow incontinence
    b. chronic skin wounds or pressure ulcers that can be contaminated by incontinent urine
    c. terminally ill or severely impaired elderly patients for whom bed and clothing changes are uncomfortable
    d. urinary retention that cannot be controlled medically or surgically
    e. none of the above statements are true
    f. a, b, c, and d

15. Alzheimer's disease, Parkinson's disease, and cerebrovascular disease are usually associated with which of the following types of urinary incontinence?
    a. urge incontinence
    b. stress incontinence
    c. overflow incontinence
    d. complex incontinence
    e. functional incontinence

16. Behavioral training for urge incontinence includes which of the following?
    a. patient should stand still or sit down and not race quickly to the bathroom
    b. patient should contract his or her pelvic muscle
    c. patient should concentrate on making the urge decrease
    d. when urge is under control, the patient should walk slowly to the bathroom
    e. a, b, and c
    f. a, b, c, and d

17. An abnormal PVR detected by catheter insertion or ultrasound may be caused by which of the following conditions?
    a. detrusor muscle weakness
    b. neuropathy
    c. fecal impaction
    d. medications
    e. all of the above

18. Mental status testing is not an important part of the workup for urinary incontinence.
    a. true
    b. false

19. A mixed urinary incontinence usually consists of what forms of incontinence?
    a. urge and overflow incontinence
    b. urge and stress incontinence
    c. stress and functional incontinence
    d. overflow and functional incontinence

Clinical Case Management Problem

List the patient-dependent (4) and caregiver-dependent (2) behaviorally oriented training procedures that may be beneficial in the management of urinary incontinence in the elderly.

Answers

1. **e.** In an elderly patient who has just become incontinent, it is inappropriate to insert a Foley catheter or do anything else until you have established the cause. The pathophysiology of urinary incontinence in the elderly population is complex, even among patients with dementia. Elderly patients deserve the same intensive investigation of the cause of incontinence as you would perform in a younger individual.

2. **e.** Fifty percent of elderly patients in nursing homes have urinary incontinence. Of elderly patients in the community, 15% to 30% have urinary incontinence. Women are twice as likely as men to develop urinary incontinence. Humiliation and embarrassment are important consequences of urinary incontinence in elderly patients. This embarrassment leads to social isolation and subsequent anxiety and depression. Incontinence is the second leading cause of admission of elderly patients to long-term care facilities. In the United States, it is estimated that the total health care costs associated with urinary incontinence are more than $26 billion per year.

   Physical consequences, such as predisposition to skin irritations and subsequent skin ulcers and infections, are major problems.

3. **a.** The most common type of urinary incontinence in the elderly population is urge incontinence. Urge incontinence (also known as detrusor hyperreflexia) is

characterized by leakage of urine caused by strong and sudden sensations of bladder urgency. Patients with urge incontinence may also experience frequency, urgency, and nocturia. Urge incontinence is also called unstable bladder, uninhibited bladder, and hyperreflexic bladder. Many conditions may predispose to urge incontinence, including cerebrovascular accidents, Parkinson's disease, Alzheimer's disease, spinal cord injury or tumor, multiple sclerosis, prostatic hypertrophy, and interstitial cystitis. Urge incontinence may also be present in patients in whom no neurologic or genitourinary abnormality is present.

4. e. Stress incontinence (urethral incompetence) is characterized by loss of small amounts of urine secondary to increases in intraabdominal pressure. Stress incontinence is most commonly associated with pelvic floor weakening through childbirth, obesity, injury, menopause and aging, and sphincter damage.

Overflow incontinence occurs with bladder overdistention. Overdistention results in a constant leakage of small amounts of urine or "dribbling," a physiologic situation in which the intracystic pressure exceeds the intraurethral resistance. Bladder overdistention is usually caused by an enlarged prostate, urethral stricture, or fecal impaction. A hypotonic bladder secondary to diabetes mellitus, syphilis, spinal cord compression, or anticholinergic medications may also result in overflow incontinence.

Complex incontinence refers to incontinence that has both urge and stress components.

Functional incontinence refers to involuntary loss of urine despite normal bladder and urethral functioning. This is most commonly seen with severe dementia and closed head injuries. There is an inability or unwillingness to toilet because of physical, cognitive, psychologic, or environmental factors.

5. e. Many factors are associated with the development and maintenance of urinary incontinence in the elderly. These include a loss of the ability of the kidney to concentrate urine, a decreased bladder capacity, decreased urethral closing pressure following menopause, decreased mobility, decreased vision, depression, secondary inattention to bladder cues, and an inadequate environmental setting.

The importance of drugs in the causation of elderly incontinence is discussed in answer 6.

6. d. Drug use is a common cause of incontinence in the elderly. The major drugs implicated as a cause of urinary incontinence in the elderly and the pathology involved are summarized in Table 128-1.

Table 128-1	Drugs Causing Urinary Incontinence in the Elderly
Drug Class	**Pathology**
Diuretics	Polyuria, frequency, urgency
Anticholinergics	Urinary retention, overflow incontinence, impaction
Antidepressants	Anticholinergic actions, sedation
Antipsychotics	Anticholinergic actions, sedation, rigidity, immobility
Sedative hypnotics	Sedation, delirium, immobility, muscle relaxation
Narcotic analgesics	Urinary retention, fecal impaction, sedation, delirium
α-Adrenergic	Urethral relaxation blockers Urinary retention agonists
β-Adrenergic	Urinary retention blockers
Calcium channel blocker	Urinary retention
Alcohol	Polyuria, frequency, urgency, sedation, delirium, immobility

7. e. Nonpharmacologic treatments are both available and useful in the treatment of all forms of urinary incontinence in the elderly. The treatments include the following:

1. Stress incontinence: (a) pelvic muscle (Kegel) exercises, (b) biofeedback, (c) behavioral therapies (prompted voiding, habit training, and scheduled toileting), and (d) transcutaneous electrical nerve stimulation (TENS)
2. Urge incontinence: (a) biofeedback, (b) behavioral therapies (as previously listed), and (c) TENS
3. Overflow incontinence: (a) intermittent catheterization and (b) indwelling catheterization (use only for chronic urinary retention, nonhealing pressure ulcers in incontinent patients, and when required to promote comfort)
4. Functional incontinence: (a) behavioral therapies (as previously listed), (b) environmental manipulations, (c) incontinence undergarments and pads, (d) external collection devices, (e) indwelling catheters (if necessary), and (f) TENS

In the past, TENS has been used successfully to treat chronic pain syndromes. An exciting new development provides another opportunity to avoid both surgery and pharmacologic agents in the treatment of incontinence. The use of a pessary TENS unit has been shown to be effective for stress incontinence and urge incontinence. More trials need to be carried out before definitive conclusions can be made, but initial results are promising.

8. e. Causes of acute and reversible forms of urinary incontinence are provided by the DRIP pneumonic:

Delirium
Restricted mobility, retention
Infection (urinary tract), inflammation (urethritis or atrophic vaginitis), impaction (fecal)
Polyuria (diabetes mellitus, diabetes insipidus, congestive heart failure, and venous insufficiency), pharmaceuticals

9. c. Urinary retention with overflow incontinence must be considered when any patient who was previously completely continent suddenly becomes incontinent. The causes include immobility, anticholinergic drugs, narcotic analgesic drugs, calcium channel blockers, beta blockers, fecal impaction, and spinal cord compression resulting from metastatic cancer.

10. c. The evaluation of urinary incontinence in the elderly should be undertaken with the same precision and care as evaluation and investigation of other urinary problems in younger patients.

All elderly patients who present with urinary incontinence should have the following procedures performed: (1) a complete history, (2) a complete medication review (ideally, every elderly patient on more than one drug should have this done every 3 months), (3) an age-specific focused physical examination (U.S. Preventive Services Task Force recommendation), (4) a complete urinalysis, (5) a urine culture, and (6) a PVR urine determination.

A renal ultrasound needs to be done only if problems such as urinary obstruction (a renal tumor), uremia, or the inability of the kidneys to concentrate urine are suspected.

11. b. A PVR urine should be performed on every elderly patient with incontinence to exclude significant degrees of urinary retention. Neither the history nor the physical examination is sensitive or specific enough for this purpose in elderly patients. The PVR urine can be done either by itself as a simple one-test procedure or in conjunction with other simple urodynamic investigations.

To maximize the accuracy of PVR urine, the measurement should be performed within a few minutes of voiding. A PVR volume of 100 mL or less in the absence of straining reflects adequate bladder emptying in elderly patients. If more than 100 mL, it suggests detrusor weakness, neuropathy, outlet obstruction, or detrusor hyperactivity with impaired contractility.

12. d. The ideal combination of pharmacologic agents for certain patients with stress incontinence involves supplemental estrogen and an α-adrenergic agonist.

For patients with stress incontinence, pharmacologic management is appropriate if the following criteria are met: (1) The patient is motivated, (2) the degree of stress incontinence is "mild to moderate," (3) there is no major associated anatomical abnormality (e.g., a large cystocele), and (4) the patient does not have any contraindications to the use of these drugs.

Pharmacologic treatment of stress incontinence is as efficacious as, but not more efficacious than, nonpharmacologic treatment. Approximately 75% of patients improve with each. Combining the two modalities improves the efficacy of treatment.

Supplemental estrogen has not been found, by itself, to be as effective as when used in combination with an α-adrenergic agonist. If either oral or vaginal estrogen is used for a prolonged period of time (more than a few months), then cyclic progesterone should be added to protect the endometrium. A combination of oral Premarin (0.3 mg/day) and oral pseudoephedrine (Sudafed) 30 to 60 mg twice daily would be a good starting point for pharmacologic treatment of stress incontinence.

13. b. The type of incontinence that is most amenable to surgical intervention is stress incontinence. The indication for surgery in stress incontinence is continued significant bothersome leakage that occurs after attempts at nonsurgical treatment and patients who, along with their stress incontinence, also have a significant degree of pelvic prolapse.

The second most amenable subtype of incontinence that may be significantly improved with surgery is outflow obstruction caused by prostatic hypertrophy or prostatic carcinoma in men. With benign prostatic hypertrophy, it would be prudent to reduce the size of the prostate and decrease obstruction by use of a 5-α-reductase inhibitor or an α-adrenergic blocker (doxazosin, terazosin, or prazosin) before contemplating surgery.

14. f. The indications for chronic indwelling catheter use include the following:

1. Urinary retention that is (a) causing persistent overflow incontinence, (b) causing symptomatic infections, (c) producing renal dysfunction, (d) unable to be corrected surgically or medically, and (e) not practically managed with intermittent catheterization
2. Skin wounds, pressure sores, or irritations that are being contaminated by incontinent urine
3. Care of terminally ill or severely impaired patients for whom bed and clothing changes are uncomfortable or disruptive
4. Preference of patient or caregiver when a patient has failed to respond to more specific treatments

15. a. Central nervous system disorders, such as cerebrovascular accidents (stroke), dementia, Parkinson's disease, and suprasacral spinal cord injury, are associated with detrusor motor or sensory instability resulting in urge incontinence.

16. **f.** All described are part of behavioral training.

17. **e.** All conditions listed can cause abnormal PVR.

18. **b.** False. Mental status testing is very important in evaluating a patient for urinary incontinence. Remembering to go to the bathroom, to toilet oneself, and finding the bathroom can be very confusing for a patient with dementia. As a result, they may have a higher incidence of incontinence. In addition, the ability to functionally go to the bathroom and use the facilities and adjust clothing may also be impaired.

19. **b.** Although this combination is more common in females with mixed incontinence, it may also occur in men with an enlarged prostate gland.

Solution to the Clinical Case Management Problem

Following are examples of behaviorally oriented training procedures for urinary incontinence:

1. Patient-dependent procedures: (a) pelvic muscle (Kegel) exercises, (b) biofeedback, (c) behavioral training, and (c) bladder retraining

2. Caregiver-dependent procedures: (a) scheduled toileting or prompted voiding and (b) habit training

Summary

1. Definition: the involuntary loss of urine in sufficient amount or frequency to be a social or health problem
2. Subtypes of urinary incontinence: acute (reversible) versus persistent urinary incontinence
3. Acute (reversible) urinary incontinence: DRIP mnemonic: **d**elirium; **r**estricted mobility, retention; **i**nfection, inflammation, impaction; **p**olyuria, pharmaceuticals
4. Persistent urinary incontinence
   a. Stress: Involuntary loss of urine (usually small amounts) with increases in intraabdominal pressure (e.g., cough, laugh, or exercise). Common causes include weakness and laxity of pelvic floor musculature and bladder outlet or urethral sphincter weakness.
   b. Urge: Leakage of urine (often larger volumes, but variable) because of inability to delay voiding after sensation or bladder fullness is perceived; also known as detrusor hyperreflexia. Common causes include detrusor motor or sensory instability, isolated or associated with one or more of the following: cystitis, urethritis, tumors, stones, diverticula, or outflow obstruction; also central nervous system disorders such as stroke, dementia, Parkinson's disease, and suprasacral spinal cord injury.
   c. Overflow: Leakage of urine (usually small amounts) resulting from mechanical forces on an overdistended bladder or from other effects of urinary retention on either bladder or sphincter function. Common causes include anatomic obstruction by prostate, stricture, and cystocele; hypotonic bladder associated with diabetes mellitus or a spinal cord injury; neurogenic (detrusor–sphincter dyssynergy) associated with multiple sclerosis; or supraspinal cord lesions.
   d. Functional: Urinary leakage associated with the inability to toilet because of impairment of cognitive or physical functioning, psychologic unwillingness, or environmental barriers. Common causes include severe dementia and other neurologic disorders or psychologic factors such as depression, regression, anger, and hostility.
5. Prevalence of urinary incontinence in the elderly is as follows: (a) institutionalized elderly, 50%; (b) elderly patients living in the community, 5% to 15%.
6. Investigations: The basic investigations for all elderly patients with urinary incontinence are (a) complete history, (b) complete physical examination, (c) complete medication review (every 3 months), (d) complete urinalysis, (e) urine for culture and sensitivity, and (f) PVR urine determination.
7. Primary treatments for different types of geriatric urinary incontinence
   a. Stress incontinence: (1) pelvic muscle (Kegel) exercises; (2) α-adrenergic agonists; (3) supplemental

estrogen (oral or vaginal); (4) biofeedback, behavioral training; (5) surgical bladder neck suspension; and (6) periurethral injections

b. Urge incontinence: (1) bladder relaxants, (2) estrogen (if vaginal atrophy is present), (3) behavioral procedures (biofeedback and behavioral therapy), and (4) surgical removal of obstructing or other irritating pathologic lesions

c. Overflow incontinence: (1) surgical removal of obstruction, (2) intermittent catheterization (if practical), and (3) indwelling catheterization

d. Functional incontinence: (1) behavioral therapies (prompted voiding, habit training, or scheduled toileting), (2) environmental manipulations, (3) incontinence undergarments and pads, (4) external collection devices, (5) bladder relaxants (select patients), and (6) indwelling catheters (select patients)

Suggested Reading

American Geriatric Society: *Geriatric Review Syllabus, A Core Curriculum in Geriatric Medicine*, 6th ed. Chicago: American Geriatric Society, 2006, pp. 189–194.

Dmochowski R, Staskin D: Mixed incontinence: Definitions, outcomes, and interventions. *Curr Opin Urol* 15(6):374–379, 2005.

Hashim H, Abrams P: Overactive bladder: An update. *Curr Opin Urol* 17(4):231–236, 2007.

Nygaard IE, Kreder KJ: Pharmacologic therapy of lower urinary tract dysfunction. *Clin Obstet Gynecol* 47(1):83–92, 2004.

Teunissen TA, de Jonge A, van Weel C, Lagro-Janssen AL: Treating urinary incontinence in the elderly—Conservative therapies that work: A systematic review. *J Fam Practice* 53(1):25–30, 32, 2004.

CHAPTER

129   Prostate Disease

CLINICAL CASE PROBLEM 1

A 75-Year-Old Male with Nocturia, Hesitancy, and a Slow Urinary Flow

A 75-year-old male comes to your office with a 6-month history of nocturia, hesitancy, a slow flow of urine, and terminal dribbling. The symptoms have been progressing. Otherwise, he is well and has had no significant medical illnesses.

On examination, his abdomen is normal. He has an enlarged prostate gland, which is smooth in contour and firm and has no nodules or irregularities.

SELECT THE BEST ANSWER TO THE FOLLOWING QUESTIONS

1. What is the most likely diagnosis in this patient?
   a. benign prostatic hypertrophy (BPH)
   b. carcinoma of the bladder
   c. prostatic carcinoma
   d. urethral stricture
   e. chronic prostatitis

2. Which of the following symptoms is (are) associated with the condition described in this case?
   a. dysuria
   b. daytime frequency
   c. incomplete voiding
   d. urgency
   e. all of the above

3. Which of the following pharmacologic treatments may be indicated in the treatment of the condition described in this case?
   a. finasteride
   b. prazosin
   c. terazosin
   d. a, b, and c
   e. none of the above

4. Before the medical or surgical treatment of the condition described here, which of the following should be performed?
   a. digital rectal examination
   b. transrectal ultrasound
   c. computed tomography (CT) scan of the pelvis
   d. a and b
   e. all of the above

5. Which of the following surgical procedures is the treatment of choice for severe cases of the condition described here?
   a. transurethral resection of the prostate (TURP)

b. open prostatectomy
c. transurethral incision of the prostate
d. hyperthermia of the prostate
e. balloon dilatation of the prostate

CLINICAL CASE PROBLEM 2

A 58-Year-Old Male with Hesitancy of the Urinary Stream and Bone Pain

A 58-year-old male comes to your office with a 3-month history of gradually worsening hesitancy of urinary stream, urgency, nocturia, and terminal dribbling. He also complains of lumbar and pelvic bone pain present for the past 3 weeks.

On physical examination, the prostate is enlarged and very hard. There is some tenderness over the pelvic ischium on the left side and at the fourth and fifth lumbar vertebrae.

6. Which of the following statements regarding this patient's condition is false?
   a. the most likely diagnosis is prostatic carcinoma
   b. radiotherapy is the most probable first line of therapy in the management of this patient
   c. this patient most likely has metastatic disease
   d. the evaluation of this patient should include a bone scan
   e. combination chemotherapy may be indicated for the treatment of this condition

7. Which of the following statements regarding carcinoma of the prostate is (are) true?
   a. prostatic cancer is a major public health problem in men
   b. prostatic cancer is now the most prevalent cancer in men
   c. bone is the most common site of metastatic disease
   d. all of the above statements are true
   e. none of the above statements are true

8. Which of the following is (are) a risk factor(s) for the disease described in the patient in this case?
   a. increased age
   b. African American men
   c. positive family history for the disease
   d. dietary fat intake
   e. all of the above

9. Which of the following statements is true regarding screening for this disorder?
   a. routine digital rectal examination (DGE) in men after the age of 55 years is recommended

b. routine use of prostate-specific antigen analysis (PSA) in men after the age of 55 years is recommended
c. routine combined use of PSA and DGE in men after the age of 55 years is recommended
d. routine combined use of PSA and DGE in men after the age of 65 years is recommended
e. there is insufficient evidence to recommend routine screening of men for prostate cancer at any age

10. Which of the following is the treatment of choice for stage A-1 of this disease in an 81-year-old male?
    a. radiation therapy
    b. radical prostatectomy
    c. hormone therapy
    d. combination chemotherapy
    e. none of the above

11. What is the most common symptom with which a male with prostatic cancer presents?
    a. a feeling of "hardness" in the rectal area
    b. obstructive voiding symptoms
    c. anorexia
    d. weight loss
    e. bone pain

CLINICAL CASE PROBLEM 3

A 24-Year-Old Male with Fever, Suprapubic Discomfort, and Inhibited Urinary Voiding

A 24-year-old male comes to your office with a 2-day history of fever, chills, perineal and suprapubic discomfort, dysuria, and inhibited urinary voiding.

On physical examination, the lower abdomen is tender. A digital rectal examination reveals a swollen, boggy, and tender prostate. Examination of the urine reveals pus cells and bacterial rods. The man has no history of similar symptoms.

12. What is the most likely diagnosis in this patient?
    a. acute prostatitis
    b. acute cystitis
    c. chronic prostatitis
    d. acute perineal pain syndrome
    e. acute nongonococcal urethritis

13. What is the most likely organism responsible for the condition described in this case?
    a. *Escherichia coli*
    b. *Pseudomonas*

c. *Proteus*
d. *Serratia*
e. *Chlamydia trachomatis*

14. What is the pharmacologic agent of choice for the condition described in this case?
a. trimethoprim–sulfamethoxazole (TMP-SMX)
b. erythromycin
c. ampicillin
d. tetracycline
e. gentamicin

Clinical Case Management Problem

Describe the therapeutic mechanism and the therapeutic effects of the drug finasteride for the treatment of BPH.

Answers

1. a. The most likely diagnosis in this patient is BPH. Hyperplasia of the prostate causes increased outflow resistance.

2. e. The symptoms of BPH are described as either obstructive or irritative. Obstructive symptoms are attributed to the mechanical obstruction of the prostatic urethra by the hyperplastic tissue and include the following: (1) hesitancy, (2) weakening of the urinary stream, (3) intermittent urinary stream, (4) feeling of residual urine (incomplete bladder emptying), (5) urinary retention, and (6) postmicturition urinary dribbling.

Irritative symptoms are attributed to involuntary contractions of the vesical detrusor muscle (detrusor instability) and are associated with obstruction in approximately 50% of patients with prostatism. These symptoms include (1) nocturia, (2) daytime frequency, (3) urgency, (4) urge incontinence, and (5) dysuria.

Differential diagnosis includes carcinoma of the prostate, neuropathic bladder, chronic prostatitis, and urethral stricture.

3. d. The pharmacologic treatment of BPH is directed toward relaxation of the prostatic smooth muscle fibers through inhibition of α-adrenergic receptors and toward regression of the hyperplastic tissue by hormonal suppression.

The growth of BPH depends on the presence of the androgenic hormone testosterone and its derivative dihydrotestosterone (via conversion by the enzyme 5-α reductase). The strategy of antiandrogenic therapy in BPH is to interfere with dihydrotestosterone production. Many antiandrogenic drugs have been tried, but the most promising is the 5-α reductase inhibitor finasteride. Finasteride (Proscar) 5 mg/day results in a 20% reduction in prostatic size and a modest improvement of the urine and symptom score. It also has a low incidence of adverse effects. Finasteride significantly decreases the PSA level, and detection of cancer of the prostate becomes difficult. Finasteride treatment should be considered in patients with moderate symptoms of prostatism. If the patient improves and side effects are minimal, continuation of therapy under careful urologic control is appropriate.

The tone of prostatic smooth muscle is mediated by α_1-adrenoreceptor stimulation. Selective or nonselective antagonists relax the smooth muscle, resulting in a diminution of urethral resistance, improvement of urine flow, and a significant improvement in symptoms. The results of double-blind, randomized controlled trials have demonstrated the short-term efficacy of selective α_1-blockade. Selective α_1-blocking drugs, such as terazosin (Hytrin), doxazosin (Cardura), and prazosin (Minipress), represent an option for patients with moderate symptoms. The long-term efficacy remains to be established.

4. d. The following should be performed before any medical or surgical intervention for BPH: (1) a history with use of a validated screening tool such as the International Prostate Symptom Scale, (2) a focused physical examination, and (3) a DRE. Other studies in evidence-based reviews have been deemed unnecessary. Ultrasound (transrectal or abdominal), determination of postvoiding residual urine, routine urinalysis and culture, electrolytes (especially urea and creatinine), PSA levels, and cystoscopy are sometimes performed when complications are present.

5. a. In general, TURP remains both safe and efficacious and is the "gold standard" against which all other treatments, both medical and surgical, must be measured. More than 80% of patients experience subjective improvement, including a significant improvement in urine flow rate. Approximately 15%, however, report no benefit 1 year after surgery. Complications of surgery can be significant, with many patients left with chronic incontinence and/or impotence.

Other surgical treatment options include so-called minimally invasive procedures. Those undergoing investigation include transurethral laser-induced prostatectomy, transurethral balloon dilatation of the prostate, laser ablation, high-intensity ultrasound thermotherapy, microwave thermotherapy, electrovaporization, and radiofrequency vaporization.

6. **b.** This patient most likely has a prostatic carcinoma with osseous bone metastases. Evaluation of this patient should include a PSA level, a bone scan, plain x-rays of the pelvis and lumbar areas, and a CT scan of the pelvis. The patient should receive hormonal therapy if these investigations confirm stage D carcinoma of the prostate (pelvic lymph node metastases or distant metastases). Although radiotherapy for stage D cancer is not entirely ruled out, it is not a first-line option.

7. **d.** Prostate cancer represents the most common tumor among men in the United States. The most important risk factor for cancer of the prostate is age; the disease prevalence increases almost exponentially after age 50 years. The true prevalence is unknown, but estimates can be obtained from autopsy series or from a series of patients undergoing TURP. These series suggest that the prevalence of the disease is approximately 30% in men age 60 to 69 years and approximately 67% in men age 80 to 89 years. It approaches 100% in men older than 90 years of age. The incidence among various populations is similar in autopsy samples, but the clinical incidence varies considerably. This suggests that environmental/dietary differences among various cultural groups may be important determinants of the rate of cancer growth. It has been reported that cancerous growth is promoted by a high-fat diet, including the omega-3 α-linolenic acid and, surprisingly, also by high calcium intake. Conversely, growth has been reported to be inhibited by aspirin, a diet rich in fish (a rich source of longer chain omega-3 fatty acids), whole grains, lycopene and β-carotene (antioxidants), cruciferous vegetables, and vitamin D. Apparently, diet plays a role, but most of these studies are preliminary in nature and the results need to be investigated further by well-executed, evidence-based studies.

A July 2003 study reported that finasteride reduced the risk of prostate cancer by 25%, but unfortunately patients who did develop cancer while taking finasteride had a more aggressive form of the disease; there were also sexual side effects, including reduced libido, decreased ejaculate volume, and erectile dysfunction.

The most common site of prostatic metastases is bone.

8. **e.** As mentioned in answer 7, increasing age is the most important risk factor for carcinoma of the prostate. Other risk factors include African American race, dietary fat intake, positive family history for carcinoma of the prostate, and possible exposure to certain chemicals (herbicides and pesticides). Certain occupations, such as farming and work in the industrial chemical industry, seem to present an especially high risk.

9. **e.** Although the combined use of DGE and PSA has increased the accuracy of prostate cancer diagnosis, routine screening is not recommended primarily because many cancers remain asymptomatic; it is also feared that prostate screening programs may result in unnecessary biopsy and the resultant cost and risk of complications in some men who, if left alone, would have suffered no symptoms for the rest of their lives. In addition, even after DGE and PSA analysis, the diagnosis is uncertain. The result of the digital examination is subjective, and BPH and other benign conditions will increase PSA values into the "gray" risk zone of 4 to 10 ng/mL, causing false-positive results, which again will trigger further studies. However, treatment of BPH with finasteride reduces PSA values and causes false-negative results. Rather than routine screening, it is recommended that testing be done on high-risk subjects on an individual basis at the physician's discretion.

Regular PSA analyses on high-risk subjects performed on a yearly or biyearly basis that show a rapid increase in PSA values are extremely suspicious, even if the value stays below 4 ng/mL. Also, the validity of an elevated PSA value can be further checked by a "free PSA test," a measure of unbound PSA. A free PSA value of 25% or greater means the risk of cancer is low, even if the total PSA value is higher than 4 ng/mL, whereas a free value of less than 10% means the risk is very high. However, again there is a zone of uncertainty between 10% and 25%, making biopsy inevitable in such cases.

10. **e.** Multiple treatment options exist for localized prostate cancer. Studies of the natural history of untreated stages A and B disease attest to the slow progression of these lesions, with disease-specific survival rates in excess of 85% at 10 years. For this reason, a watch-and-wait policy for older patients and those with significant other comorbid conditions is a reasonable option. For younger patients with a long life expectancy (more than 10 years), treatment for cure can be accomplished with radical prostatectomy, external beam radiotherapy, or interstitial radiotherapy in which the radiation source is placed close to the tumor. Radical proctectomy is the classical approach in which the prostate is removed from the urethra. Provided the tumor is still contained within the prostate, there is essentially no chance of remission or metastasis, and modern surgical techniques have greatly reduced the risk of nerve damage that can result in long-term urinary incontinence and impotency. External beam radiotherapy produces equivalent results and avoids the trauma of surgery and hospitalization, but it does require daily doses for 4 to 6 weeks and can cause fatigue and irritation. Moreover, it has a non-inconsequential chance of producing impotence. Interstitial radiotherapy involves implantation of radioactive "seeds," which are permitted to slowly destroy the prostate tissue. Although it has gained in popularity during the past decade, the jury is still out concerning effectiveness and potential side effects.

11. b. The diagnosis of prostate cancer is usually a serendipitous finding. Signs and symptoms of the disease are usually encountered only at an advanced stage. These signs and symptoms include anorexia, bone pain, neurologic deficits, obstructive voiding symptoms, and weight loss. Of these, the most common initial presenting symptom is obstruction to voiding.

12. a. This patient's symptoms are classic for acute bacterial prostatitis. They include both systemic symptoms (fever and chills) and local urinary symptoms

such as perineal and suprapubic discomfort, dysuria, and inhibited urinary voiding.

The DRE that reveals a swollen, tender, and boggy prostate is probably the most sensitive and specific diagnostic test for prostatitis. When performing the rectal examination in a patient with systemic symptoms, it is imperative that the prostate gland not be massaged; this may release a significant number of bacteria into the bloodstream. Only when systemic symptoms are absent can the prostate gland be safely massaged to obtain a prostatic specimen for culture.

13. a. The two bacteria responsible for most cases of bacterial prostatitis are *E. coli* and *Klebsiella*. Nonbacterial prostatitis is most often caused by *C. trachomatis* or *Ureaplasma urealyticum*.

14. a. The drugs of choice for the treatment of acute prostatitis are TMP-SMX, norfloxacin, and ciprofloxacin. Antibiotic treatment should continue for at least 4 weeks.

Solution to the Clinical Case Management Problem

The medical treatment of BPH has been revolutionized. The growth of BPH depends on the presence of the androgenic hormone testosterone and its derivative dihydrotestosterone (via conversion by the enzyme 5-α reductase). The strategy of antiandrogenic therapy in BPH is to interfere with dihydrotestosterone production.

As mentioned in answer 3, finasteride results in an approximately 20% reduction in prostatic size and a modest improvement in the flow rate of urine and symptom score, and it has a very low rate of adverse

effects. The main adverse effects are a decrease in libido and/or erectile dysfunction. Finasteride also significantly decreases the serum PSA level and thus reduces the ability to screen for carcinoma of the prostate.

The treatment of BPH with finasteride should be considered in patients with moderate symptoms of prostatism. If the patient improves while taking the drug and does not experience significant side effects, continuation of therapy under careful physician supervision is reasonable.

Summary

BPH

1. Symptoms: both obstructive symptoms (hesitancy, weak stream, intermittent urinary stream, feeling of incomplete emptying, urinary retention, and terminal dribbling) and irritative symptoms (nocturia, daytime frequency, urgency, urge incontinence, and dysuria).
2. Investigations: history with validated symptom scoring tool, physical examination, and rectal examination. Other studies, such as urinalysis, culture, transrectal ultrasound, residual urine, electrolytes, blood urea nitrogen, creatinine, serum PSA, and cystoscopy, are often performed but have not been shown to change

treatment decisions or outcomes in evidence-based reviews.
3. Treatment: pharmacologic treatment—5-α reductase inhibitor (finasteride), α-receptor blocker (prazosin and terazosin); surgical treatment—TURP; minimally invasive procedures under investigation and may mitigate complications of TURP

CARCINOMA OF THE PROSTATE

1. Prevalence: Carcinoma of the prostate is the most prevalent malignancy in men and the second leading cause of death from cancer.

2. Symptoms and signs: Symptoms and signs are the same as those of BPH, except abnormalities are found on examination of the prostate.

3. Treatment: Multiple treatment trials are under way, and effective treatment strategies are a matter of debate. Consider all options with the patient, including watchful waiting, because all therapies have their advantages and disadvantages. One set of recommendations is as follows: (a) stages A and B-1 (younger than age 65 years), prostatectomy or radiation; (b) stages A and B-1 (older than age 65 years), watchful waiting; (c) stages B and C, radiotherapy; (d) stage D asymptomatic, await the onset of symptoms or hormone therapy; and stage D symptomatic, hormone therapy (orchiectomy, antiandrogens, luteinizing hormone, releasing hormone analogues). Combination chemotherapy can be used in hormone-resistant cases.

PROSTATITIS

1. Acute bacterial prostatitis
   a. Symptoms: fever, chills, perineal and suprapubic discomfort, dysuria, and inhibited urinary voiding
   b. Treatment: Septra, norfloxacin, and ciprofloxacin
   c. Organisms: *E. coli/Klebsiella. Chlamydia trachomatis* is thought to be the major cause of nonbacterial prostatitis.

2. Chronic prostatitis
   a. Symptoms: Either asymptomatic or symptoms are less prominent than in acute bacterial prostatitis.
   b. Investigation: Perform a three-part urine culture (third after prostatic massage).
   c. Treatment: Effective treatment is poor. Consider the same drugs as those used to treat acute bacterial prostatitis.

Suggested Reading

Batstone GR, Doble A: Chronic prostatitis. *Curr Opin Urol* 13(1):23–29, 2003.

Harris R, Lohr KN: Screening for prostate cancer: An update of the evidence for the U.S. Preventive Services Task Force. *Ann Intern Med* 137(11):917–929, 2002.

Katz A, Katz A: The top 13: What family physicians should know about prostate cancer. *Can Fam Physician* 54(2):198–203, 2008.

Wilt TJ, N'Dow J: Benign prostatic hyperplasia. Part 1: Diagnosis. *BMJ* 336(7636):146–149, 2008.

Wilt TJ, N'Dow J: Benign prostatic hyperplasia. Part 2: Management. *BMJ* 336(7637):206–210, 2008.

CHAPTER

130 Pressure Ulcers

CLINICAL CASE PROBLEM 1

An 80-Year-Old Female Nursing Home Resident with a Pressure Ulcer

You are called to a nursing home to see an 80-year-old female with a fever of 40°C. The patient is disoriented and confused. The nursing home staff has had difficulty treating her pressure ulcers, especially one on her sacrum.

On physical examination, the patient's blood pressure is 110/80 mmHg, and her pulse is 72 beats/minute and regular. There is a 10 × 5 cm pressure ulcer on her sacrum. Also, there is a purulent, foul-smelling discharge coming from that ulcer.

SELECT THE BEST ANSWER TO THE FOLLOWING QUESTIONS

1. Which of the following diseases or conditions is (are) a risk factor(s) for the development of pressure ulcers?
   a. immobility
   b. dementia
   c. Parkinson's disease
   d. congestive heart failure
   e. a, b, and c
   f. a, b, c, and d

2. Which of the following nutritional or physiologic variables increase(s) the risk of pressure ulcers?
   a. hypoalbuminemia
   b. moist skin
   c. increased pressure
   d. a and b
   e. a, b, and c

3. Regarding the pathophysiology of pressure ulcers, which of the following factors has (have) been implicated in their cause?
   a. the pressure of the body weight
   b. shearing forces
   c. friction
   d. moisture
   e. a, b, and d
   f. a, b, c, and d

4. Which of the following statements concerning the prevention and cause of pressure ulcers is false?
   a. pressure ulcers are impossible to prevent in immobilized elderly patients
   b. good nutrition in the elderly will help prevent pressure ulcers
   c. anemia in the elderly patient predisposes to the formation of pressure ulcers
   d. incontinence in the elderly increases the risk of pressure ulcers by a factor of five
   e. patients who sit for long periods are just as likely to develop pressure ulcers as bedridden patients

5. Concerning the patient described in this case, how long would it take the large ulcer to develop from a small, untreated ulcer?
   a. 28 days
   b. 21 to 28 days
   c. 14 to 20 days
   d. 7 to 10 days
   e. 1 or 2 days

6. Which of the following anatomic sites is the least common site for the development of a pressure ulcer?
   a. ischial tuberosity
   b. lateral malleolus
   c. medial malleolus
   d. sacrum
   e. greater trochanter

7. With respect to pathophysiology, which of the following factors contributes to the formation of pressure ulcers?
   a. blood and lymphatic vessel obstruction
   b. plasma leakage into the interstitial space
   c. hemorrhage
   d. bacterial deposition at the site of the pressure-induced injury
   e. muscle cell death
   f. all of the above

8. Which of the following statements concerning pressure ulcers and mortality in elderly patients is (are) true?
   a. there appears to be no increase in mortality among elderly individuals who develop pressure ulcers
   b. failure of a pressure ulcer to heal or improve has not been associated with a higher death rate in institutionalized elderly
   c. in-hospital death rates for patients with pressure ulcers range from 23% to 36%
   d. all of the above statements are true
   e. none of the above statements are true

9. Patients at high risk for the development of pressure ulcers should be repositioned how frequently?
   a. every 2 hours
   b. every 4 hours
   c. every 6 hours
   d. every 8 hours
   e. every 12 hours

10. Which of the following descriptions best illustrate(s) the nature of bacteria usually found in an infected pressure ulcer?
    a. gram-positive aerobic cocci alone
    b. gram-negative aerobic rods alone
    c. anaerobic bacteria alone
    d. a and c
    e. a, b, and c

11. What are the best initial antibiotic treatments for an infected pressure ulcer?
    a. tetracycline and gentamicin
    b. clindamycin and gentamicin
    c. cephalexin and doxycycline
    d. penicillin and gentamicin
    e. trimethoprim–sulfamethoxazole

12. What is the most common and serious complication of pressure ulcers in elderly patients?
    a. anemia
    b. hypoproteinemia
    c. infection
    d. contracture
    e. bone resorption

13. Bacterial sepsis leading to septic shock in pressure ulcers is most closely associated with which of the following bacteria?
    a. *Bacteroides fragilis*
    b. *Pseudomonas aeruginosa*
    c. *Proteus mirabilis*
    d. *Staphylococcus aureus*
    e. *Providencia* spp.

A 78-Year-Old Immobilized Male with a 1-cm Area of Erythema and Bruising on His Heel

A 78-year-old immobilized male is seen with a 1-cm area of erythema and bruising on his left heel.

14. Which of the following is the most important aspect of the treatment of this pressure ulcer at this time?
    a. application of a full-thickness skin graft
    b. extensive debridement of the area and cleansing with an iodine-based solution
    c. application of a foam pad to protect the heel from further damage
    d. application of microscopic beaded dextran to the lesion
    e. elevation of the left leg by 30 degrees

15. Which of the following statements concerning the use of pressure-reducing devices in the prevention and treatment of pressure ulcers is true?
    a. with the proper use of pressure-reducing devices, all pressure ulcers can be prevented
    b. there is consensus regarding the pressure-reducing devices of first choice
    c. sheepskin can be considered a pressure-reducing device of first choice
    d. there appears to be little difference between the products indicated for the prevention and treatment of pressure ulcers
    e. none of the above are true

16. Which of the following factors has (have) been associated with a more favorable outcome in the prevention and treatment of pressure ulcers?
    a. educational programs for health professionals
    b. educational programs for families and caregivers
    c. multidisciplinary health care
    d. b and c
    e. a, b, and c

17. Concerning local wound care in superficial pressure ulcers, which of the following is (are) acceptable for cleaning the ulcer and disinfecting the ulcer?
    a. povidone–iodine
    b. hydrogen peroxide
    c. hypochlorite solutions
    d. all of the above
    e. none of the above

18. Which of the following pressure-reducing devices should not be used for the prevention and treatment of pressure ulcers?
    a. an air-fluidized bed
    b. a sheepskin mattress
    c. a conventional foam pad
    d. an air mattress
    e. a water mattress

19. The debridement of moist, exudative wounds originating from the formation of pressure ulcers may be augmented by the use of which of the following?
    a. hydrophilic polymers
    b. enzymatic agents
    c. acetic acid
    d. a and b
    e. all of the above

20. Which of the following statements concerning the use of occlusive dressings for treating pressure ulcers is (are) true?
    a. hydrocolloid dressings and transparent films improve the healing rate of superficial pressure ulcers
    b. hydrocolloid has proven to be effective in treating deep pressure ulcers as well as superficial pressure ulcers
    c. hydrocolloid dressings and transparent films may remain in place for several days
    d. a and c
    e. all of the above statements are true

21. Proper skin care in patients to prevent pressure ulcers includes which of the following?
    a. therapeutic massage of high-risk areas
    b. avoiding perspiration, wound drainage, urine, and feces
    c. use of disposable undergarments
    d. b and c
    e. all of the above

22. Methods of debridement utilized to remove necrotic devitalized tissue include which of the following?
    a. mechanical
    b. enzymatic
    c. autolyte
    d. surgical
    e. all of the above

23. Transparent film occlusive dressing should be utilized for what stage of pressure ulcers?
    a. stage I
    b. stage II
    c. stage III
    d. stage IV
    e. all of the above

Clinical Case Management Problem

Pressure ulcers can be classified into four stages dependent on the degree of thickness of penetration of the epidermis and deeper tissues. Because the therapy varies depending on the stage of the ulcer, it is important to understand the difference between the four stages. Provide the definitions of stages I, II, III, and IV pressure ulcers.

Answers

1. **f.** See answer 2.

2. **e.** Risk factors for pressure ulcers include the following:

1. Any disease process leading to immobility and limited activity levels, such as a spinal cord injury, dementia, Parkinson's disease, severe congestive heart failure, and chronic obstructive pulmonary disease. This can cause unrelieved pressure that results in damage of underlying tissue.
2. Other factors include urinary incontinence (moisture) and nutritional factors such as a decreased lymphocyte count, hypoalbuminemia, inadequate dietary intake, decreased body weight, and a depleted triceps skinfold thickness. Poor nutrition status may be secondary to immobility, poor financial status, isolation, and poor dentition.
3. Potential risk factors identified in prospective studies include moist skin, increased body temperature, decreased blood pressure, older age, and an altered level of consciousness. Cardiovascular disease, strokes, diabetes, fractures, bed or wheelchair confinement, impaired level of consciousness, and hypotension are all independently associated with pressure ulcers.

3. **f.** The pathophysiology of pressure ulcers includes the interaction of all of the following:

1. Pressure: Contact pressures of 60 to 70 mmHg for 1 or 2 hours lead to degeneration of muscle fibers. Repeated exposures to pressure will cause skin necrosis because of decreased oxygen tension, vessel leakage, and lack of nutrients. Pressure is considered the most significant risk factor for developing pressure ulcers.
2. Shearing forces: Shearing forces are tangential forces that are exerted when a person is seated or when the head of the bed is elevated and the person

slides toward the floor or foot of the bed. Shearing forces disrupt subcutaneous vessels and cause ischemia and subsequent necrosis.
3. Friction: Friction has been shown to cause intraepidermal blisters. When unroofed, these lesions result in superficial erosions. This kind of injury can occur when a patient is pulled across a sheet or when the patient has repetitive movements that expose a bony prominence to such frictional forces.
4. Moisture: Intermediate degrees of moisture increase the amount of friction produced by the rubbing interface, whereas extremes of moisture or dryness decrease the frictional forces between the two surfaces rubbing against each other. Moisture macerates skin tissue, predisposing the skin to breakdown.

4. **a.** Pressure ulcers are not impossible to prevent in immobilized elderly patients. It is true that it is difficult to prevent all pressure ulcers, but many of those that do develop in immobilized elderly patients are, in fact, preventable.

Good nutrition in elderly patients will help prevent pressure ulcers.

Anemia and incontinence are predisposing factors to the development of pressure ulcers.

Elderly patients who sit for long periods of time are just as likely to develop pressure ulcers as bedridden patients.

5. **e.** Erythema may progress to ulceration quickly. A small ulcer can progress to a large ulcer within 24 to 48 hours. The progression is caused by local edema or infection, with the former being the most important factor. As in the patient described in Clinical Case Problem 1, severe infection can lead to septicemia, which must be recognized and treated with appropriate systemic antibiotic therapy.

6. **c.** The most common sites for pressure ulcers to develop are (1) the sacrum, (2) the trochanters, (3) the heels, (4) the lateral malleoli, and (5) the buttocks over the ischium.

The least common site of those listed for the formation of pressure ulcers is the medial malleoli.

7. **f.** The ultimate chain of pathophysiologic events involved in the formation of pressure ulcers is as follows: (1) Ischemia is associated with the occlusion of blood and lymphatic vessels; (2) as plasma leaks into the interstitium, diffusing substances increase between the cellular elements of skin and blood vessels; (3) ultimately, hemorrhage occurs and leads to erythema of the skin that is unable to be blanched; (4) bacteria are

deposited at sites of pressure-induced injury and set up a deep suppurative process; and (5) the accumulation of edema fluid, blood, inflammatory cells, toxic wastes, and bacteria ultimately and progressively leads to the death of muscle, subcutaneous tissue, and epidermal tissue.

The damage caused by shearing forces is probably mediated by pressure-induced ischemia in deep tissues as well as by direct mechanical injury to the subcutaneous tissue.

8. c. Increased death rates have been consistently observed in elderly patients who develop pressure ulcers. In addition, failure of an ulcer to heal or improve has been associated with a higher rate of death in nursing home residents. In-hospital death rates for patients with pressure ulcers range from 23% to 36%. Most of these deaths are in debilitated patients; in many cases, it is difficult to separate what contribution the actual pressure ulcer makes to the process. The development of a pressure sore quadruples the risk of death for institutionalized patients.

9. a. Data support the recommendation that high-risk patients should be repositioned every 2 hours to prevent pressure ulcers from forming and to minimize the size, thickness, and infectivity rate of pressure ulcers that have already formed.

10. e. Infected pressure ulcers are usually associated with *P. aeruginosa*, *Providencia* spp., *Proteus* spp., *S. aureus*, and anaerobic bacteria (particularly *B. fragilis*). The best combination of antibiotics, therefore, is one that will treat gram-positive aerobic cocci (present in 39% of isolates), gram-negative aerobic rods, and anaerobic bacteria.

11. b. One realizes the risk of using a powerful agent such as gentamicin in a debilitated elder; however, the elder who is debilitated most likely by that time has acquired a serious bacteremia/septicemia. Check creatinine clearance and adjust the gentamicin dose accordingly.

12. c. Sepsis is the most common and most serious complication of pressure ulcers in elderly patients. Contraction and bone resorption are also complications of pressure ulcers.

Anemia and hypoproteinemia are risk factors for the formation of pressure ulcers.

13. a. With respect to infection, bacteremia, septicemia, and death, (1) most infected pressure ulcers are polymicrobial; (2) most infected polymicrobial pressure ulcers have *B. fragilis* as one of the major

organisms involved; and (3) infected pressure ulcers also lead to other infectious complications, such as bacterial cellulitis, osteomyelitis, and septic arthritis.

14. c. The short time interval between the formation of a small area of erythema and a true pressure ulcer has already been described.

The most important therapy at this time is to try to protect the patient's heel from progressing to any further stage of damage. This is best done by using a foam pad or other piece of protective apparatus.

15. b. Regarding the formation of pressure ulcers, the prevention of pressure ulcers, and the pressure-reducing devices available, the following facts have emerged:

1. Despite nurses' best efforts, the use of proper positioning alone is not sufficient to prevent all pressure ulcers. Even with pressure-reducing devices, this is not always possible.
2. The use of water mattresses or alternating air mattresses decreased the incidence of pressure ulcers by 50% compared with conventional hospital mattresses.
3. Although sheepskin products are very popular, it has been demonstrated that sheepskins and 2-inch convoluted foam pad products do not have the capability to sufficiently decrease pressure to eliminate the risk of cutaneous injury.
4. The following have been demonstrated to have superior efficacy in preventing pressure ulcers: a foam mattress, a static air mattress, an alternating air mattress, and a gel or water mattress. In addition, the use of air-fluidized and low-air-loss beds is recommended (especially for stage III and stage IV ulcers).

16. e. Several studies have demonstrated a significant decrease in pressure ulcer incidence after an educational program and a multidisciplinary team approach to the problem of pressure ulcers. Such educational programs should be directed at all levels of health care professionals, patients, family, and caregivers.

17. e. Topical antiseptics, such as hypochlorite solutions, povidone–iodine, acetic acid iodophor, and hydrogen peroxide, should be avoided in cleaning and debriding a pressure ulcer because of the potential of these compounds to inhibit wound healing. The preferred alternative is normal saline.

18. b. A sheepskin mattress should not be used for the prevention and treatment of pressure ulcers. See the critique in answer 15 for further details.

19. **d.** The debridement of moist, exudative wounds may be augmented by using hydrophilic polymers such as dextranomer. Enzymatic agents such as collagenase, fibrinolysin, deoxyribonuclease, streptokinase, and streptodornase may be helpful in aiding debridement.

20. **d.** Once an ulcer is clean and granulation or epithelialization begins to occur, a moist wound environment should be maintained without disturbing the healing tissue. Superficial lesions heal by migration of epithelial cells from the borders of an ulcer; deep lesions heal as granulation tissue fills the base of the wound. Controlled studies have shown that the use of occlusive dressing such as transparent films and hydrocolloid dressings improves healing of stage II pressure ulcers. These dressings remain in place for several days and allow a layer of serous exudate to form underneath the dressing. This facilitates the further migration of epithelial cells. Although these dressings have not been shown to improve the effective healing rate of deep ulcers, they do reduce the nursing time needed for treatment.

Clean stage III and clean stage IV ulcers should be dressed with a gauze dressing kept moistened with normal saline. Moist dressings should be kept off surrounding skin to avoid macerating normal tissues. Unless there are symptoms or signs of infection, these dressings can stay in place for several days.

21. **d.** Therapeutic massage of high-risk areas is not recommended. It was believed that this would enhance circulation, but postmortem biopsies found degenerated tissue in the areas massaged.

22. **e.** Enzymatic debridement is a topical debridement using an agent to dissolve necrotic areas. Autolytic debridement uses synthetic dressings to allow devitalized tissue to self-digest from the enzymes found in the ulcer fluids. Surgical debridement uses scalpels, forceps, and scissors to debride wounds.

23. **a.** Transparent film should be utilized primarily for stage I ulcers. Although it may also be used for early stage II ulcers, these are usually treated with a foam island.

Solution to the Clinical Case Management Problem

The classification of pressure ulcers in elderly patients is as follows:

1. Stage I pressure ulcers present as erythema of intact skin that is unable to be blanched.
2. Stage II pressure ulcers involve partial-thickness skin loss involving the epidermis or the dermis.

3. Stage III pressure ulcers extend from the subcutaneous tissues to the deep fascia and typically show undermining.
4. Stage IV pressure ulcers involve muscle or bone. Full-thickness injury is often manifested by eschar, frequently involving muscle and bone, but cannot be staged until the eschar is removed.

Summary

TERMINOLOGY

1. The term pressure ulcer is preferred at this time.
2. Previous terms included the following:
   a. Decubitus ulcers
   b. Bedsores
   c. Pressure sores

PREVALENCE

1. The prevalence of pressure ulcers among patients in acute care hospitals ranges from 1% to 10%, and it ranges from 15% to 25% in long-term care facilities.
2. Among patients expected to be hospitalized and confined to bed or chair for at least 1 week, the prevalence of stage II and greater pressure ulcers is as high as 28%.

3. The prevalence of pressure ulcers in nursing homes is similar to that reported in acute care hospitals. As many as 20% to 33% of patients admitted to nursing homes have stage II or greater pressure ulcers. Less than 20% of pressure ulcers develop in the nursing home and in the home care setting; more than 60% develop in the acute care setting.
4. Pressure ulcers affect 3 million people annually, at a cost of more than $5 billion per year.

COMPLICATIONS

1. Sepsis is the most serious complication of pressure ulcers.
2. Other complications include local infections, cellulitis, and osteomyelitis. In addition, infected pressure

ulcers may be deeply undermined and lead to osteomyelitis or penetrate into the abdominal cavity and cause peritonitis. Infected pressure ulcers lead to nosocomial reservoirs for antibiotic-resistant bacteria.

3. Pressure ulcer infections have the following characteristics:
   a. They are polymicrobial.
   b. Gram-positive anaerobic cocci, gram-negative anaerobic rods, and aerobic bacteria are the most common organisms found.
   c. Specific organisms commonly found include: *P. aeruginosa*, *Providencia* spp., *Proteus* spp., *S. aureus*, and *B. fragilis*.

MORTALITY

1. Failure of a pressure ulcer to heal is associated with a higher rate of death in nursing home residents.
2. In-hospital death rates for patients with pressure ulcers range from 23% to 36%. Most of these deaths involve patients with severe underlying disease.

RISK FACTORS

1. Disease processes leading to immobility or reduced activity
2. Spinal cord injury
3. Dementias
4. Parkinson's disease
5. Congestive cardiac failure
6. Incontinence
7. Nutritional factors: inadequate intake of protein, vitamins, minerals, calcium, or calories leading to cachexia, hypoalbuminemia, decreased body weight, and decreased triceps skinfold thickness

PATHOPHYSIOLOGY

Four factors have been implicated in the pathogenesis of pressure ulcers: (1) pressure, (2) shearing forces, (3) friction, and (4) moisture.

PATHOPHYSIOLOGIC SERIES OF EVENTS IN PRESSURE ULCER FORMATION

1. Pressure on tissues overlying bone prominence
2. Ischemia produced by occlusion of blood vessels and lymphatic vessels
3. Endothelial cell swelling and vessel leak
4. Plasma leakage into the interstitium
5. Increased distance between cellular elements of skin and blood vessels
6. Hemorrhage
7. Erythema of the skin that is unable to be blanched
8. Continued accumulation of edema fluid, blood, inflammatory cells, toxic wastes, and bacteria
9. Death of muscle, subcutaneous tissue, and epidermal skin

PREVENTION OF PRESSURE ULCERS

1. Formal risk assessment: A formal "risk assessment" for the development of pressure ulcers should be done on all patients.
2. Frequent repositioning
   a. Patients at highest risk should be repositioned every 2 hours.
   b. Lower risk patients should be repositioned two to four times a day.
3. Technique of repositioning: Repositioning should be performed so that a person at risk is repositioned without pressure on vulnerable bony prominences. Most of these sites are avoided by positioning patients with the back at a 30-degree angle to the support surface, alternatively from the right to the left sides and to the supine position.
4. Pressure-reducing devices
   a. Although sheepskins and 2-inch convoluted foam pads are popular, they do not have the capability to sufficiently decrease pressure to eliminate risk of cutaneous injury.
   b. Preferred devices include static air mattresses, alternating air mattresses, gel mattresses, and water mattresses.
   c. Lifting devices or bed linen movement (not bed linen drag) will minimize friction and shear-induced injuries during transfers and position changes.

EDUCATION

1. There is a significant decrease in pressure ulcer incidence after an educational program and a multidisciplinary team approach to the problem of pressure ulcers is implemented.
2. Educational interventions should be targeted to all levels of health care providers, patients, families, and caregivers.

ASSESSMENT OF PATIENTS WITH PRESSURE ULCERS

1. Appropriate assessment and treatment of underlying diseases and conditions that have put the person at risk for developing pressure ulcers
2. Nutritional assessment particularly important
3. Assessment of associated infections (as previously discussed)

TREATMENT OF PRESSURE ULCERS

1. Systemic treatment
   a. Vitamin C: The patient should take 500 mg twice daily (84% reduction in pressure ulcer surface area in patients taking this vitamin).
   b. Drug combination of choice: clindamycin and gentamicin; monitor and watch renal function carefully while the patient is on gentamicin.
   c. Air-fluidized bed therapy is a major improvement over the conventional bed.

2. Local wound care
   a. Normal saline is the agent of choice for cleaning and for gentile debridement. Avoid povidone–iodine, hypochlorite, mild acetic acid, and hydrogen peroxide.
   b. Surgical debridement is augmented with wet-to-dry dressings using normal saline.
   c. The debridement of moist, exudative lesions is facilitated by using hydrophilic polymers. Enzymatic agents should be used only until the ulcer bed becomes clean.
   d. Once clean and granulation or epithelialization begins to occur, a moist wound environment should be maintained. Occlusive dressings and hydrocolloid dressings improve healing rates for stage II ulcers. Stage III and stage IV ulcers should be dressed with a gauze soaked in normal saline.
   e. Surgical therapies should be used to remove necrotic tissue that cannot be removed any other way and that if not removed will cause septicemia and death. Surgical flaps (a more elective procedure) should be carefully considered, especially on debilitated, cachectic patients. Rule out osteomyelitis if clinically suspected.

Suggested Reading

American Geriatric Society: *Geriatric Review Syllabus, A Core Curriculum in Geriatric Medicine*, 6th ed. Chicago: American Geriatric Society, 2006, pp. 259–268.

Graumlich JF, Blough LS, McLaughlin RG, et al: Healing pressure ulcers with collagen or hydrocolloid: A randomized, controlled trial. *J Am Geriatr Soc* 51:147–154, 2003.

Keast DH, Parslow N, Houghton PE, et al: Best practice recommendations for the prevention and treatment of pressure ulcers: Update 2006. *Adv Skin Wound Care* 20(8):447–462, 2007.

Langemo D, Anderson J, Hanson D, et al: Nutritional considerations in wound care. *Adv Skin Wound Care* 19(6):297–298, 300, 303, 2006.

Niezgoda JA, Mendez-Eastman S: The effective management of pressure ulcers. *Adv Skin Wound Care* 19(suppl 1):3–15, 2006.

---

131 Constipation in the Elderly

CLINICAL CASE PROBLEM 1

A 78-Year-Old Female with Constipation

A 78-year-old female comes to your office with a 5-year history of "constipation." The patient, who has had significant difficulties with ischemic heart disease, is currently on atenolol and verapamil.

On examination, the patient's blood pressure is 180/95 mmHg. Her pulse is 72 beats/minute and regular. Upon examination, the head and neck, the lungs, the cardiovascular system, and the abdomen are all normal. Digital rectal examination (DRE) reveals impacted stool.

SELECT THE BEST ANSWER TO THE FOLLOWING QUESTIONS

1. Constipation is best defined as which of the following?
   a. only one bowel movement in 3 days
   b. only two bowel movements in 10 days
   c. only three bowel movements in 7 days
   d. only four bowel movements in 7 days
   e. none of the above

2. What is the most accurate elderly patient definition of constipation?
   a. anything less than one bowel movement per day
   b. any defecation difficulty
   c. anything less than two bowel movements per day
   d. any straining at stool
   e. any of the above: constipation to the elderly means almost anything vaguely associated with bowel movements

3. Which of the following is (are) associated with constipation in the elderly?
   a. impaired general health status
   b. increased medication use
   c. decreased level of exercise
   d. all of the above
   e. none of the above

4. Which of the following drug classes is (are) associated with constipation?
   a. tricyclic antidepressants
   b. anticholinergic agents
   c. calcium channel blockers
   d. all of the above
   e. none of the above

5. Concerning the history and physical examination of elderly patients with constipation, which of the following should be performed?
   a. DRE
   b. complete medication review
   c. functional inquiry of the gastrointestinal (GI) system
   d. a and b
   e. all of the above

6. Which of the following is (are) a complication(s) associated with constipation in the elderly?
   a. fecal impaction
   b. diarrhea
   c. anal fissures
   d. sigmoid volvulus
   e. a and c
   f. all of the above

7. Which of the following is not a recommended treatment for constipation in the elderly?
   a. a bowel training regime
   b. an exercise program
   c. chronic laxative use
   d. a high-fiber diet
   e. an above average consumption of fluids

8. Which of the following drugs is most closely associated with constipation in the elderly?
   a. hydrochlorothiazide
   b. verapamil
   c. atenolol
   d. acetaminophen
   e. fluoxetine

9. Constipation in the elderly is most closely associated with which of the following?
   a. fecal impaction
   b. diarrhea
   c. crampy back pain
   d. a and c
   e. all of the above

10. What is the self-reported percentage incidence of constipation in elderly Americans?
   a. 10%
   b. 20%
   c. 30%
   d. 40%
   e. 50%

11. What is the laxative group most closely associated with long-term side effects in the elderly?
   a. stimulant laxatives
   b. hyperosmolar laxatives
   c. saline laxatives
   d. emollient laxatives
   e. stool softeners

CLINICAL CASE PROBLEM 2

An 86-Year-Old Male with Stage IV Carcinoma of the Prostate

An 86-year-old male with stage IV carcinoma of the prostate comes to your office seeking "pain relief." He has bony metastatic disease and his pain was well controlled on a combination of diclofenac and morphine sulfate. With the morphine, his pain decreased from 9/10 to 2/10. However, 5 days after morphine was started he began to experience more severe pain. You decide to increase the morphine dose and see him in a week. He returns after that week with worse pain than before; it is now 13/10. You increase the morphine dose even further and ask him to return in another week. He returns a week later doubled over in pain that he describes as 15/10.

12. At this time, what would you do?
   a. switch the patient to hydromorphone
   b. switch the patient to methadone
   c. switch the patient to fentanyl (patch)
   d. switch the patient to oxycodone
   e. none of the above

13. At this time, your physical examination maneuver of choice for the patient is which of the following?
   a. none; you do not believe in the sensitivity, specificity, and positive predictive value of physical examination techniques anymore
   b. palpation of the abdomen
   c. percussion of the abdomen
   d. auscultation of the abdomen for bowel sounds
   e. none of the above

14. At this time, which of the following is the investigation of choice for this patient?
   a. magnetic resonance imaging scan
   b. repeat bone scan
   c. computed tomography scan of the pelvis
   d. serum calcium level to "look for that ever-elusive entity, hypercalcemia"
   e. none of the above

15. What is the most common cause of abdominal pain in the elderly?
   a. angiodysplasia
   b. diverticulitis
   c. spastic colon of the elderly syndrome
   d. the aging gut syndrome
   e. none of the above

Clinical Case Management Problem

Name the drug in each of the drug classes listed that is most commonly responsible for constipation in the elderly: (1) antihypertensive agent, (2) antianginal agent, (3) medical diagnostic agent, (4) antacid, (5) nutritional supplement, (6) analgesic, (7) antipsychotic, (8) antidepressant, (9) anticholinergic, and (10) inexpensive osteoporotic therapy agent.

Answers

1. e. Constipation is usually medically defined as fewer than three bowel movements per week. It is a major problem for elderly patients in developed countries. This is substantiated by the increase in the use of laxative therapies. Approximately 30% of patients older than age 65 years are regular laxative users. Constipation refers to infrequent, incomplete, or painful evacuation of stool.

2. e. Physicians tend to define constipation on the basis of the frequency of stooling and the consistency of stooling. To the elder, on the other hand, constipation can mean almost anything, including any difficulties in defecation such as straining at stool, anything less frequent than one or two bowel movements per day that are completely normal in every way (shape, caliber, diameter, length, and color), and anything else vaguely related to the bowel movement. The point is, you must ask the elder what he or she means by constipation. It is almost a guarantee that the patient's definition will not match yours.

Again, it is important to realize that there is a significant discrepancy between what physicians define as constipation in the elderly and what the elderly define as constipation. For many elderly patients, the daily bowel movement is a significant mark of health.

3. d. The factors that appear to be associated with constipation in the elderly include an impaired general health status, an increased number of medications other than laxatives, diminished mobility, and diminished physical activity.

The true effect of diet on bowel habits is unclear. There is epidemiologic evidence from developed countries that greater amounts of crude dietary fiber are associated with a lesser prevalence of various GI disorders, including diverticular disease, colorectal cancer, and constipation. However, there may be intervening variables that account for some of this difference.

4. d. A significant number of drug classes are associated with constipation, especially constipation in the elderly. These include (1) antacids (aluminum hydroxide and calcium carbonate), (2) anticholinergic agents (trihexyphenidyl), (3) antidepressants (tricyclic antidepressants and lithium carbonate), (4) antihypertensive–antiarrhythmics (calcium channel blockers [especially verapamil] and diuretics), (5) metals (bismuth, iron, and heavy metals), (6) narcotic analgesics (any narcotic analgesic, but especially codeine and opiates), (7) nonsteroidal anti-inflammatory drugs (all may produce constipation in the elderly), (8) sympathomimetics (pseudoephedrine), (9) antipsychotics, and (10) anti-parkinsonian drugs.

5. e. When an elderly patient complains of constipation, a careful history is the most important aspect of the evaluation. Sometimes all that is required is reassurance from the physician that there is a broad range of normal bowel frequency.

Symptoms of disorders that impair the motility of the large bowel should be sought. These general medical conditions include hypothyroidism, hyperparathyroidism, scleroderma, Parkinson's disease, cerebrovascular accidents, and diabetes mellitus.

Localized colorectal diseases, such as tumors or other constricting lesions that may cause constipation, are often accompanied by other symptoms. Thus, the history must include questions concerning abdominal pain, weight loss, and bleeding per rectum. In idiopathic, dietary, and drug-related constipation, there are usually no symptoms other than constipation, although a complaint of an abdominal bloating sensation is common with severe constipation.

A DRE is a sensitive screening tool in detecting anal lesions, although fissures and hemorrhoids, unless they are thrombosed or large, are found more reliably on anoscopy. Anoscopy should be performed routinely in constipated elderly patients. DRE of the anal canal and rectum is useful in assessing the tone of the internal anal sphincter and also the strength of the external sphincter and the puborectalis muscle.

The amount and the consistency of stool felt in the rectum may, in fact, indicate what type of constipation is present. Patients with a failure of the defecation mechanism tend to have much stool in the rectal vault, whereas those patients with colonic atony or irritable bowel syndrome have little or no stool in the rectum between defecations.

6. f. Although for most elderly patients constipation is just a minor annoyance, for some elders it is much more than that. The elders who are most susceptible to constipation are those who are institutionalized or bedridden.

Complications of constipation in the elderly include the following:

1. Fecal impaction is heralded by crampy, lower abdominal and lower back pain.
2. Stercoral ulcers are common in the patient who is bedridden. They are caused by pressure necrosis of the rectal or sigmoid mucosa due to a fecal mass. In some cases, the ulcer may present as rectal bleeding.
3. Anal fissures may result from excessive straining at stool and the subsequent complications that develop, including tears and passive congestion of the tissues near the dentate line. The problem is enhanced by the irritating effect of hard stools and toilet paper. Intraabdominal pressures of up to 300 mmHg are generated during straining. Excessive straining at stool may cause prolapse of the anal mucosa, venous distention, and internal hemorrhoids.
4. Megacolon in the elderly is almost always idiopathic. Chronic use of cathartics over a period of years may lead to an acquired degeneration of the colonic myenteric plexus and subsequent megacolon. Bacterial overgrowth may occur and further complicate matters.
5. Volvulus, especially of the sigmoid colon, occurs most commonly in institutionalized, bed-bound, elderly patients and carries a high mortality rate.
6. There is evidence that chronic constipation is a risk factor for the development of carcinoma of the colon, particularly in women. This might be related to increased exposure time of susceptible mucosa to potentially carcinogenic substances.

7. c. The treatment of constipation is primarily nonpharmacologic. In large part, it involves inducing the patient to adopt a "healthier lifestyle." This includes a bowel training regime (a schedule of regular times for attempting defecation); regular exercise (bedridden patients are at great risk of constipation and often respond poorly to treatment); dietary adjustment to increase the amount of fiber in the diet; and an increased consumption of liquids, particularly water. Some foods that are exceptionally high in fiber include 100% bran cereal, beans (baked, kidney, lima, and navy), canned peas, raspberries, and broccoli.

It is not recommended that a regular or chronic laxative regime be part of a routine prophylactic and treatment protocol for constipation.

8. b. The drug that is most closely associated with the development of constipation in the elderly is verapamil.

Verapamil is a calcium channel blocker commonly used to treat hypertension. Constipation develops in approximately 16% of patients who take verapamil for any length of time, and this percentage may be significantly higher in the elderly, especially in institutionalized and bedridden patients. The development of constipation-related complications previously discussed may follow.

Constipation may also occur as a side effect of the use of hydrochlorothiazide, atenolol, or fluoxetine, but it does not appear to be a major side effect with these drugs (see answer 4).

9. e. Constipation is often associated with fecal impaction; diarrhea; and crampy, lower abdominal and lower back pain.

Fecal impaction is the result of prolonged exposure of accumulated stool to the absorptive forces of the colon and rectum. The stool may become rocklike in consistency in the rectum (70%), in the sigmoid colon (20%), and in the distal colon (10%).

Symptoms of crampy, lower abdominal and lower back pain are common. Diarrhea may paradoxically follow the constipation, which leads to the impaction (watery material making its way around the impacted mass of stool). The impaction can sometimes be evacuated by the patient after the oral administration of polyethylene glycol (GoLYTELY), but manual disimpaction is usually required.

10. c. A survey in the United States of community-dwelling people older than age 65 years found that 30% of men and 29% of women considered themselves constipated. In the month preceding the survey, 24% of the men and 20% of the women had used laxatives.

11. a. The laxative group used to treat constipation can be divided into six major categories:

Bulk-forming laxatives: Bulk-forming laxatives include the various fiber-containing preparations and are thought to act in two major ways. They are hydrophilic and tend to increase the stool mass and soften the stool consistency. They are the safest laxatives and are generally well tolerated by elderly patients when introduced gradually.

Emollient laxatives: Emollients, or stool softeners, include mineral oil and the newer docusate salts such as dioctyl sodium sulfosuccinate (Colace). Mineral oil is generally not recommended because safer, more effective agents are available. The newer agents lower surface tension, allowing water to enter the stool more readily. They are generally well tolerated and may be particularly useful in bed-bound elderly patients who are at risk for fecal impaction.

Saline laxatives: Saline laxatives and enemas are salts of magnesium and sodium. Those in most common use are oral milk of magnesia, oral magnesium citrate, and sodium phosphate (Fleet's enema). All of these agents function as hyperosmolar agents and cause net secretion of fluid into the colon. Colonic motility is increased by these agents via release of the hormone cholecystokinin. Chronic use of magnesium-containing saline laxatives in elderly patients may contribute to hypermagnesemia (especially when there is associated impaired renal function). The phosphate-containing preparations may also induce hypocalcemia when high doses are used. The phosphate-containing enemas may cause damage to the rectum; this may occur via the nozzle part of the instrument or via a direct toxic effect exerted by the hypertonic saline on the rectal mucosa.

Hyperosmotic laxatives: Hyperosmolar laxatives such as lactulose draw water into the gut lumen by an osmotic action. Lactulose is an indigestible agent that is metabolized by bacteria to hydrogen and organic acids. This causes acidification of the colon, which, in addition to its osmotic effect, may alter electrolyte transport and colonic mobility.

Stimulant laxatives: Stimulant laxatives include the anthraquinone derivatives cascara, senna, and aloe; phenolphthalein; and bisacodyl (Dulcolax) tablets. Complications of the stimulant laxatives include melanosis coli from the anthraquinone group and Stevens–Johnson syndrome, dermatitis, and photosensitivity reactions from the phenolphthalein group. Although bisacodyl tablets are probably safer than the rest of the stimulant laxatives, all of the agents can cause electrolyte imbalance and precipitate hypokalemia, fluid and salt overload, and diarrhea. Thus, the stimulant laxatives are the laxatives most closely associated with long-term side effects.

Lavage laxatives: Lavage laxatives are the newest group of laxatives. They include the agents GoLYTELY and COLyte. They work by stimulating neither secretion nor motility but by passing unimpeded through the GI tract. They are the most commonly used agents for bowel preparation before flexible sigmoidoscopy and colonoscopy.

12. e. In this patient, the increasing and different abdominal pain was caused by constipation. This patient had actually not had a bowel movement for 9 days. Thus, the increasing severe abdominal pain (caused by increasing doses of morphine) completely overshadowed his previous pain (the pain caused by metastatic bone disease). Therefore, switching to another painkiller is not a logical response.

13. e. The physical examination maneuver of choice in this patient is a DRE to confirm impacted stool.

14. e. The investigation of choice is an x-ray of the kidneys, ureter, and bladder to confirm stool throughout the colon.

15. e. Remember, constipation is the most common cause of abdominal pain in the elderly.

This patient's problem was treated by manual disimpaction, tap water enemas, and lactulose. To reduce the possibility of severe constipation, you should treat patients who you start on narcotic analgesics by following these two rules: (1) Start a bowel regimen at the same time as you start the narcotic, and (2) maintain the bowel regimen for as long as you maintain the patient on the narcotic.

Solution to the Clinical Case Management Problem

The drug classes and their most common offenders are listed in the following table:

Drug Class	Most Common Offender
Antihypertensive	Verapamil
Antianginal agents	Verapamil
Medical diagnostic agent	Barium sulfate
Antacids	Aluminum hydroxide
Nutritional supplement	Iron
Narcotic analgesics	Codeine
Antipsychotics	Thioridazine
Antidepressants	Amitriptyline
Anticholinergics	Trihexyphenidyl
Osteoporosis therapy	Calcium carbonate (TUMS)

Summary

1. Prevalence
The reported prevalence of constipation in the elderly is 30%.

2. Definition
Constipation is usually defined as fewer than three bowel movements per week.

3. Causes
The causes of constipation include declined or impaired general health status in the elderly, increasing number of medications (verapamil), and diminished mobility and physical activity.

4. Diagnosis and investigation
The patient's complete medical history is the most important part of the evaluation (remember to include complete functional inquiry of the GI tract). DRE is the most important part of the physical examination; anoscopy should accompany DRE. DRE and anoscopy may detect fissures, fistulas, strictures, carcinoma, or hemorrhoids.

5. Complications
The complications of constipation in the elderly include the following: (a) fecal impaction, crampy abdominal and back pain, and overflow diarrhea; (b) stercoral ulcers; (c) anal fissures and anal fistulas; (d) hemorrhoids (internal and external); (e) megacolon; (f) sigmoid volvulus; and (g) risk factor for carcinoma of the colon.

6. Treatment
a. Nonpharmacologic: (i) bowel training; (ii) exercise; (iii) high-fiber diet, up to 20 to 25 g/day; and (iv) increased fluid intake, at least 1500 mL/day.
b. Pharmacologic (laxatives): (i) bulk laxatives (recommended: psyllium, methylcellulose, and polycarbophil), (ii) emollient laxatives (mineral oil is not recommended, but Colace is recommended), (iii) saline laxatives and enemas (not recommended on long-term basis), (iv) hyperosmolar laxatives (recommended: milk of magnesia, magnesium citrate, lactulose, sorbitol, glycerin, and polyethylene glycol), (v) stimulant laxatives (not recommended: castor oil, Dulcolax, aloe, cascara, and senna), (vi) use saline or tap water enemas two times per week, and (vii) oil retention enema for refractory constipation only.

7. Rules summary
a. Always ask yourself the question, "Why is the patient constipated?" Constipation is not part of the normal aging process.
b. Cancer is a common diagnosis in elderly patients. Most elderly patients with cancer will eventually require a narcotic analgesic. When that time comes, always start a constipation-correcting bowel regime at the same time.

Suggested Reading

American Geriatric Society: *Geriatric Review Syllabus, A Core Curriculum in Geriatric Medicine,* 6th ed. Chicago: American Geriatric Society, 2006, pp. 394–395.

Bleser S, Brunton S, Carmichael B, et al: Management of chronic constipation: Recommendations from a consensus panel. *J Fam Practice* 54(8):691–698, 2005.
Leung FW: Etiologic factors of chronic constipation: Review of the scientific evidence. *Digestive Dis Sci* 52(2):313–316, 2007.

132 Pneumonia and Other Common Infectious Diseases of the Elderly

CLINICAL CASE PROBLEM 1

An 81-Year-Old Male Who Lives by Himself and Has Increasing Confusion and Shortness of Breath

A previously healthy 81-year-old male is brought to the emergency department by his daughter. He lives by himself. He was well until 3 days ago. At that time, he became somewhat confused and began wandering aimlessly around the house and muttering incoherently. For the past 3 days, he has had both nausea and anorexia. In addition, he became short of breath last night.

On physical examination, his temperature is 100.8°F, and his blood pressure is 100/70 mmHg. His pulse is 96 beats/minute and regular. His respiratory rate is 28 breaths/minute and his respirations appear slightly labored. On auscultation of his lung fields, there are a few rales bilaterally but no other abnormalities. His white blood cell (WBC) count is 11,000/mm³. His chest x-ray reveals right lower lobe consolidation. His P_{O_2} is 65 mmHg and his P_{CO_2} is 40 mmHg.

SELECT THE BEST ANSWER TO THE FOLLOWING QUESTIONS

1. What is the most likely diagnosis in this patient?
   a. bacterial pneumonia
   b. viral pneumonia
   c. fungal pneumonia
   d. aspiration pneumonia
   e. obstructive pneumonia

2. What is the most likely pathogen in this patient's pneumonia?
   a. *Klebsiella pneumoniae*
   b. *Haemophilus influenzae*
   c. influenza type B
   d. *Escherichia coli*
   e. *Streptococcus pneumoniae*

CLINICAL CASE PROBLEM 2

An 84-Year-Old Female Who Is Currently Residing in a Long-Term Care Facility and Has Increasing Confusion and Shortness of Breath

A presentation with almost identical symptoms and signs as those of the patient in Clinical Case Problem 1 occurs in an 84-year-old female who is currently residing in a long-term care facility and who has many chronic medical conditions. Compare her presentation to the presentation of the patient described in Clinical Case Problem 1.

3. Which of the following statements is (are) true?
   a. the prognosis is likely to be similar in both individuals
   b. the responsible organism is likely to be the same
   c. the treatment is likely to be the same
   d. all of the above statements are true
   e. none of the above statements are true

4. What is the treatment of choice for the patient described in Clinical Case Problem 1?
   a. amoxicillin
   b. erythromycin
   c. gentamicin
   d. ceftriaxone
   e. amphotericin B

5. Which of the following is (are) a risk factor(s) for the development of urinary tract infections in elderly patients?
   a. advanced age
   b. decreased bladder emptying
   c. prostatic hypertrophy
   d. decreased host defense mechanisms
   e. all of the above

6. What is the most common pathogen in urinary tract infections in noncatheterized elderly patients?
   a. *Serratia* sp.
   b. *Proteus mirabilis*
   c. *Klebsiella* sp.
   d. *E. coli*
   e. *Pseudomonas aeruginosa*

CLINICAL CASE PROBLEM 3

An 81-Year-Old Female with Dysuria, Frequency, Urgency, and Incontinence

An 81-year-old female comes to your office with a 5-day history of dysuria, frequency, urgency, and incontinence. She has no other symptoms, including no costovertebral angle (CVA) tenderness. The patient lives at home by herself and has had no major medical problems.

On examination, her temperature is 101°F. Her blood pressure is 150/80 mmHg, and her pulse is 84 beats/minute and regular. No other abnormalities are found.

7. Which of the following statements concerning this patient is (are) true?
   a. the most likely diagnosis is acute bacterial cystitis
   b. the most likely organism is *P. aeruginosa*
   c. amoxicillin is a reasonable first-choice antibiotic
   d. this patient should be treated for 14 days
   e. all of the above statements are true

8. If this patient were a male with relapsing infections, you would consider chronic prostatitis as a cause. Concerning chronic prostatitis in elderly patients, which of the following statements is (are) true?
   a. chronic prostatitis is the most common cause of relapsing urinary tract infections in elderly males
   b. prostatic massage is not helpful in establishing a diagnosis
   c. *Klebsiella* is the most common pathogen in this condition
   d. with prolonged therapy, relapse becomes unlikely
   e. all of the above statements are true

CLINICAL CASE PROBLEM 4

A 75-Year-Old Female with Fever, Chills, Confusion, Dysuria, and Diarrhea

A 75-year-old female comes to your office with a 2-day history of fever, chills, confusion, dysuria, and diarrhea. There are no other symptoms, including no back pain.

On examination, the patient's temperature is 100.5°F. Her blood pressure is 120/75 mmHg, and her pulse is 96 beats/minute and regular. There is no demonstrable CVA tenderness.

9. What is the most likely diagnosis in this patient?
   a. acute bacterial cystitis
   b. viral gastroenteritis
   c. acute pyelonephritis
   d. bacterial gastroenteritis
   e. none of the above

10. Regarding the use of antibiotics in elderly patients with indwelling catheters, which of the following statements is (are) true?
    a. indwelling urinary catheters are the leading cause of nosocomial infections
    b. indwelling urinary catheters are the most common predisposing factor in hospital-acquired, fatal, gram-negative sepsis
    c. by the time a urinary catheter has been in place for 2 weeks, 50% of catheterized patients have significant bacteriuria
    d. all of the above statements are true
    e. none of the above statements are true

11. What is the leading cause of death from infection in hospitalized elderly patients?
    a. bacterial pneumonia
    b. urinary tract infection
    c. pressure ulcers
    d. diverticulitis
    e. septic arthritis

12. What is the leading cause of death from infection in institutionalized elderly patients?
    a. bacterial pneumonia
    b. urinary tract infection
    c. pressure ulcers
    d. diverticulitis
    e. septic arthritis

13. What is the leading cause of death from infection in elderly individuals living in the community?
    a. bacterial pneumonia
    b. urinary tract infection
    c. pressure ulcers
    d. diverticulitis
    e. septic arthritis

14. In considering acute appendicitis in elderly patients, which of the following statements is (are) true?
    a. the presenting signs and symptoms are similar to those of younger patients
    b. gangrene of the appendix is uncommon
    c. morbidity and mortality are much higher than in younger patients
    d. all of the above statements are true
    e. none of the above statements are true

15. Which of the following statements concerning fever in elderly patients is (are) true?
    a. fever in elderly patients is more likely to be the result of a serious pathologic condition than in younger patients

b. compared to younger patients, older adults often fail to show a temperature elevation despite having a serious infectious disease
c. in elderly patients with fever of undetermined origin (FUO), a localized infection (e.g., an abscess) is often found
d. all of the above statements are true
e. none of the above statements are true

Clinical Case Management Problem

Consider the following functional states or levels of care in elderly patients and the following primary considerations in infectious or inflammatory disease. In order of frequency, what are the three most common primary infectious diseases in each of the following groups?

1. Independent healthy elderly individuals living in the community
2. Hospitalized elderly patients
3. Nursing home or institutionalized elderly residents

Answers

1. **a.** The most likely diagnosis in this patient is a bacterial pneumonia. The presentation of bacterial pneumonia in elderly patients is usually much more subtle and nonspecific than in younger patients. As illustrated in this case presentation, confusion is a very common early sign. Other nonspecific early signs include disorientation and a change (decrease) in the elder's interest level. A fall is often part of the presenting symptoms and signs of elder infectious illness, possibly resulting from dehydration associated with infectious processes.

Findings on physical examination are also nonspecific. The patient may be afebrile. Signs of consolidation are often absent. Rales are common but not specific. An increased respiratory rate (as in this patient) may precede other signs and symptoms. Pleuritic chest pain, dyspnea, productive cough, chills, and rigors are not always present in the elderly.

The specificity of laboratory abnormalities found in elders with bacterial pneumonia is low. An increased WBC count (less than 10,000 mm³) is commonly found, but as well as being nonspecific, the WBC count also suffers from low sensitivity. Hypoxemia is a common finding. In elderly patients with bacterial pneumonia, the correlation between clinical findings and radiologic findings is poor. Up to 50% have a normal WBC count, but 95% have a left shift. An infiltrate in chest x-ray may not show up until the patient is properly hydrated.

2. **e.** The most likely pathogen associated with community-acquired pneumonia is *S. pneumoniae*. *H. influenzae*, *K. pneumoniae*, and gram-negative bacilli are much less common unless there is associated chronic obstructive pulmonary disease or an immune-compromising condition. Expected organisms for community-acquired pneumonia include strep pneumonia, respiratory viruses, *H. influenzae*, gram negative bacteria, *Moraxella catarrhalis*, legionella, tuberculosis, and endemic fungi (listed in order of frequency of occurrence).

In summary, the difference between younger adults and older adults with regard to community-acquired bacterial pneumonia is that *S. pneumoniae* is the responsible organism in 60% to 80% of younger patients but only 40% to 60% of elderly patients.

3. **b.** The most important differences between the two presentations are as follows:
1. The patient presented in Clinical Case Problem 1 resides in the community, whereas the patient presented in Clinical Case Problem 2 resides in a long-term care facility.
2. The patient presented in Clinical Case Problem 1 is otherwise healthy and has no significant medical problems, whereas the patient presented in Clinical Case Problem 2 has many other chronic health problems.
3. The organism found in the patient in Clinical Case Problem 1 is likely to be the most common cause of bacterial community-acquired pneumonia. The most likely organism to be found in the patient in Clinical Case Problem 2 is still *S. pneumoniae*, but other candidates should be considered, such as *H. influenzae*, *K. pneumoniae*, or other gram-negative organisms.
4. Because it is more likely to find gram-negative organisms in the patient in Clinical Case Problem 2, the treatments may be different.
5. The virulence of the organism in the patient in Clinical Case Problem 2 is likely to be significantly greater than the virulence of the organism in the patient in Clinical Case Problem 1. Thus, the prognosis in the patient in Clinical Case Problem 2 is significantly less favorable than that of the patient in Clinical Case Problem 1.

4. **d.** The treatment of choice for a community-acquired bacterial pneumonia in an elderly patient is an agent that is active against *S. pneumoniae*, *H. influenzae*, *Mycoplasma pneumoniae*, *Chlamydia pneumoniae*, and *Legionella* spp. The current recommendation from the Infectious Disease Society of America is a β-lactam and β-lactamase combination or advanced cepahalosporin (ceftriaxone and cefotaxime) with or without a macrolide such as erythromycin, azithromycin, or clarithromycin. An alternative would be one of the quinolones, such as levofloxacin, sparfloxacin, or gatifloxacin.

5. **e.** Urinary tract infections in the elderly are second only to respiratory tract infections as causes of febrile illness in patients older than age 65 years. The risk factors for urinary tract infections in the elderly include the following: (1) advanced age (the older the patient, the greater the risk, which appears to be immune-system dependent); (2) decreased functional ability resulting from cerebral vascular accidents, dementia, neurologic deficits, functional ability, and other chronic underlying illness; (3) decreased bladder emptying resulting from neurogenic bladder, bladder-outlet obstruction (e.g., prostatic hypertrophy), and drugs with anticholinergic side effects; (4) nosocomial spread of organisms, spread from hospitalized patients with asymptomatic bacteriuria and the use of indwelling urinary catheters; and (5) physiologic changes such as decreased vaginal glycogen and increased vaginal pH in women and decreased prostatic secretions and increased prostatic calculi in men.

6. **d.** The most common organism responsible for urinary tract infections in elderly patients who do not have indwelling urinary catheters is *E. coli*. Other gram-negative organisms responsible include *Klebsiella*, *Enterococcus*, *Pseudomonas*, and *Proteus mirabilis*. However, in the absence of a complication (e.g., an indwelling catheter), *E. coli* still predominates. The difference between younger adults and older adults with respect to the cause of uncomplicated urinary tract infections is that although *E. coli* is the most common agent in both younger adults and older patients, the percentage of infections caused by *E. coli* is lower in older patients; that is, in older patients with an acute uncomplicated urinary tract infection there is an increased chance of an infection caused by *Klebsiella*, *Enterococcus*, *Proteus mirabilis*, or *Pseudomonas*.

7. **a.** Regarding Clinical Case Problem 3, the following facts can be stated:
1. This appears to be an uncomplicated urinary tract infection.

2. The most likely infecting organism is *E. coli*, but *Klebsiella*, *Proteus mirabilis*, and *Pseudomonas aeruginosa* must also be considered.
3. The most likely diagnosis is acute bacterial cystitis, which is confirmed when there are no signs or symptoms of upper urinary tract infection and the bacterial count is greater than 100,000 organisms per milliliter of urine. The most common symptoms encountered in acute bacterial cystitis are lower abdominal or pelvic pain, dysuria, increased frequency of urination, and recent episodes of urinary incontinence.
4. The first-line drug in this case would be a fluorquinolone because of trimethoprim–sulfamethoxazole (TMP-SMX) resistance of 10% to 20%. A cephalosporin or amoxicillin/clavulanic acid (especially if enterococcal infection is suspected) would also be a reasonable choice as first-line therapy. Although treatment with single-dose therapy is reasonable for younger adults, it cannot be recommended for the elderly.

8. **a.** Chronic bacterial prostatitis is the most common cause of relapsing urinary tract infection in elderly males. Acute bacterial prostatitis is much more common in younger males and chronic bacterial prostatitis is much more common in older patients. The diagnosis of chronic bacterial prostatitis is established by culturing prostatic secretions obtained by prostatic massage. The most common causative organism is *E. coli*, and *K. pneumoniae*, *Proteus*, and *Enterococcus* are other organisms associated with the condition. The preferred antibiotic treatment is a quinolone antibiotic such as ciprofloxacin or levofloxacin (quinolones may be more effective than TMP-SMX and must be given for 12 weeks). Relapses are common, even with prolonged therapy. This condition may be ameliorated by transurethral resection of the prostate.

9. **c.** The patient in Clinical Case Problem 4 has acute pyelonephritis. Elderly patients who develop a syndrome of fever, chills, and irritating voiding symptoms likely have acute pyelonephritis despite the absence of CVA tenderness. In fact, not more than half of elders who develop pyelonephritis have the back pain and CVA tenderness that is classic in younger patients with the disease. Some elders do not even have fever. Geriatric patients often also have gastrointestinal symptoms such as diarrhea or pulmonary symptoms with upper urinary tract infections. This infection must be suspected in elderly patients who are immunocompromised and incapacitated (hospitalized patients and long-term care facility patients).

The probability of septicemia/generalized sepsis is greatly increased in elderly patients who develop urinary tract infections. Bacteremia is much more common in elderly patients who develop pyelonephritis, and the urinary tract is the source of bacteremia in more than one-third of elders admitted to the hospital with generalized sepsis. Thus, blood cultures are mandatory before initiating treatment. From sepsis follows septic shock in up to 20% of elders with acute pyelonephritis. As with lower urinary tract infections, the most common organisms involved are *E. coli*, *Klebsiella*, *Proteus*, and *Pseudomonas*.

For elderly patients, the best initial antibiotic choice for suspected pyelonephritis is a fluorquinonolone because of excellent bioavailability and increased resistance to TMP-SMX.

10. d. By 2 weeks, 50% of catheterized patients have significant bacteriuria, and after 1 month virtually all patients do.

Indwelling urinary catheters are a leading cause of nosocomial infection and one of the most common predisposing factors in hospital-acquired, gram-negative sepsis. Patients who have asymptomatic bacteriuria should not be treated with antibiotics. This applies to catheterized patients as well.

11. b. In the hospitalized elder, the most common cause of morbidity and mortality is septicemia from a urinary tract infection.

12. a. Elderly patients living in long-term care facilities are susceptible to bacterial pneumonia, which is the most common cause of death from an infective source.

13. a. The leading infective causes of morbidity and mortality in elderly patients vary depending on location of the elder's habitation.

The most common cause of death from an infective source is bacterial pneumonia in elderly patients living in the community as well as those living in long-term care facilities. This serves to illustrate the importance of preventive services designated for this age group. The U.S. Task Force on the Periodic Health Examination recommends the following: (1) All individuals older than age 65 years should receive annual influenza vaccinations, and (2) all individuals older than age 65 years should receive the Pneumovax vaccination. (Consider revaccination every 6 or 7 years.)

Although bacterial pneumonia is discussed as the primary cause of morbidity and mortality, it must be understood that viral pneumonia frequently predates bacterial pneumonia (i.e., influenza produces a viral pneumonia that leads to a secondary bacterial pneumonia).

14. c. Acute appendicitis is primarily a disease of younger patients in their second or third decade of life. However, it also occurs with increasing frequency in males older than age 80 years. The mortality in this age group is 10%. As with other abdominal infections such as acute cholecystitis, the increased severity of disease is largely caused by the atypical presentation of the signs and symptoms of acute inflammation (or, more appropriately, the lack of signs and symptoms of acute inflammation). Instead of the classic time sequence of periumbilical pain; anorexia, nausea, and vomiting; and movement of the pain to the right lower quadrant seen in younger patients, the elderly male with acute appendicitis usually has a prolonged period of vague abdominal discomfort.

There may be mild nausea and anorexia, but vomiting is unusual. As localized peritonitis develops, pain may appear in the right lower quadrant. Rebound tenderness and abdominal guarding, which are very common in younger adults, are uncommon in the elderly.

Perforation of the appendix is much more common in the elderly because of the narrowing of the lumen and the atherosclerotic changes in the artery supplying the appendix. In elderly patients, approximately 70% of cases of acute appendicitis rupture compared with 20% in younger patients.

In summary, critical differences between younger adults and older adults with appendicitis are that the elderly have atypical symptoms, a high rate of perforation, and a high mortality rate (10%).

15. d. In children and in young and middle-aged adults, fever is often the result of a relatively benign disease. Such is not the case with the elderly. The rapid development of an elevated body temperature in an older adult is almost invariably the result of a serious infection such as pneumonia, urinary tract infection, or an intraabdominal abscess. Although the presence of fever in an older adult usually indicates a serious infection or other serious disease process (e.g., neoplasia and connective tissue disorders), elderly patients are two or three times as likely to demonstrate a lack of febrile response to the presence of serious disease.

In older adults who have FUO, the probability of a localized infection such as an abscess is high. In summary, elders with a fever usually have a serious rather than a benign disease process occurring. Always be aggressive in evaluating elders with fever.

Solution to the Clinical Case Management Problem

Primary considerations in infectious diseases in the elderly depending on the habitation status of the elder are as follows:

1. The three primary types of infection for elders living in a community setting are (a) bacterial pneumonia; (b) urinary tract infections; and (c) intraabdominal infections, including cholecystitis, diverticulitis, and appendicitis.
2. The three primary types of infection for hospitalized elders are (a) urinary tract infections, (b) bacterial

pneumonia (gram negative, anaerobes, gram positive, and fungi), and (c) surgical wound infections.
3. The three primary types of infection for nursing home or other institutionalized elders are (a) bacterial pneumonia (*S. pneumoniae*, gram negative, *Staphylococcus aureus*, anaerobes, *H. influenzae*, group B streptococcus, and chlamydia), (b) urinary tract infections, and (c) decubitus ulcers.

Suggested Reading

American Geriatric Society: *Geriatric Review Syllabus, A Core Curriculum in Geriatric Medicine*, 6th ed. Chicago: American Geriatric Society, 2006, pp. 332–338, 429.

Furman CD, Rayner AV, Pelcher-Tobin E: Pneumonia in residents of long term care facilities. *Am Fam Physician* 70:1495–1500, 2004.

Lutfiyya MN, Henley E, Chang LF, Reyburn SW: Diagnosis and treatment of community-acquired pneumonia. *Am Fam Physician* 73(3):442–450, 2006.

Ramakrishnan K, Scheid DC: Diagnosis and management of acute pyelonephritis in adults. *Am Fam Physician* 71(5):933–942, 2005.

CHAPTER

133 Polymyalgia Rheumatica and Temporal Arteritis

CLINICAL CASE PROBLEM 1

An 82-Year-Old Female with Aching and Stiffness in the Shoulder and Hip Girdles

An 82-year-old female comes to your office with "stiffness" and "aching" in the shoulders and hips present for the past 3 months. The onset was quite abrupt. The stiffness and aching are bilateral in both upper and lower limbs. The symptoms are especially severe in the morning. The patient says that it is difficult to get out of a chair and difficult to move her arms above her head.

The patient also mentions significant malaise and fatigue and has experienced a 20-pound weight loss. She mentions a mild fever and also a feeling of "depression."

On examination, the patient's blood pressure and pulse are normal. Although the patient describes "significant weakness," there are no objective findings.

SELECT THE BEST ANSWER TO THE FOLLOWING QUESTIONS

1. What is the most likely diagnosis in this patient?
   a. osteoarthritis
   b. rheumatoid arthritis (RA)
   c. polymyalgia rheumatica (PMR)
   d. polymyositis
   e. acute degenerative arthritis

2. Which of the following disorders is most closely associated with the geriatric population?
   a. PMR
   b. osteoarthritis
   c. RA
   d. degenerative arthritis
   e. polymyositis

3. Which of the following statements regarding the condition described is (are) true?
   a. the cause of the disease is unknown
   b. this disease is most likely autoimmune in origin
   c. the overall prevalence of this condition is approximately 17 out of 100,000 patients
   d. family aggregation of this disorder has been described
   e. all of the above statements are true

4. Which of the following statements regarding this condition is (are) true?
   a. there are no significant complications or related disorders of concern
   b. hypothyroidism, hyperthyroidism, and hyperparathyroidism are part of the differential diagnosis
   c. systemic lupus erythematosus must be considered a potential diagnostic possibility
   d. b and c
   e. a, b, and c

5. What is (are) the major difference(s) between PMR and polymyositis?
   a. marked proximal muscle weakness in polymyositis
   b. marked proximal muscle tenderness in polymyositis
   c. elevated muscle enzymes such as creatine kinase (CK) in polymyositis
   d. a and b
   e. a, b, and c

6. Which of the following is the investigation of choice in PMR?
   a. muscle CK
   b. erythrocyte sedimentation rate (ESR)
   c. antinuclear antibody titer
   d. rheumatoid factor titer
   e. computed tomography scan of the shoulders and hip girdle

7. Which of the following is (are) a manifestation(s) of giant cell arteritis (GCA), also known as temporal arteritis?
   a. jaw claudication
   b. headaches
   c. amaurosis fugax
   d. scalp tenderness
   e. all of the above

8. Of the symptoms and signs listed in question 7, which is (are) the most worrisome
   a. jaw claudication
   b. headaches
   c. amaurosis fugax
   d. scalp tenderness
   e. all of the symptoms are equally worrisome

9. The symptom(s) and sign(s) identified in question 8 as most worrisome can lead to which of the following (greatly feared) complications of GCA?
   a. permanent hemiplegia
   b. permanent bilateral and complete sensorineural hearing loss
   c. permanent monocular or binocular total blindness
   d. permanent bilateral and complete sensorineural and conductive hearing losses
   e. permanent quadriplegia

10. What is the treatment of choice for both PMR and GCA?
    a. intravenous (IV) pulsed steroids
    b. oral prednisone: 20 mg/day for PMR and 60 mg/day for GCA
    c. oral methotrexate
    d. cyclosporine IV every third day for 4 weeks
    e. IV dihydroergotamine

11. What is the pathophysiologic cause of temporal arteritis?
    a. inflammation of the middle meningeal artery
    b. inflammation of the temporal artery
    c. inflammation of the common carotid artery
    d. inflammation of the internal carotid artery
    e. inflammation of the external carotid artery

12. Complications of long-term steroid use in the elderly include which of the following?
    a. diabetes mellitus
    b. glaucoma
    c. accelerated cataracts
    d. skin atrophy
    e. all of the above

13. The incidence of aneurysm formation in patients with a history of GCA is
    a. 5%
    b. 10%
    c. 15%
    d. 20%
    e. none of the above

Clinical Case Management Problem

An 82-year-old female comes to your office with a history of shoulder girdle pain and hip pain progressing to involve other joints of the upper and lower extremities. Provide a differential diagnosis for this patient's pain.

Answers

1. **C.** The diagnosis in this patient is PMR. This is an important diagnosis to make in the elderly.

2. **a.** Of all the musculoskeletal conditions, PMR is most closely identified with the geriatric population.

PMR is a diagnosis that is often missed, a diagnosis in which vague symptoms are present, and a diagnosis that is often characterized by the patient's seeing multiple doctors without being correctly diagnosed.

PMR is characterized by aching and stiffness in the shoulder and hip girdles. Profound morning stiffness is especially suggestive of this disorder and should be specifically sought out. The diagnosis of PMR is seldom seen before the age of 50 years; its mean age of onset is 70 years. The onset may be either abrupt or gradual. The stiffness that is present in the hips and the shoulders may become generalized, involving the neck and knees and even extending into the wrists and fingers.

There are also prominent constitutional symptoms, including malaise, weight loss, low-grade fever, and depression.

3. **e.** The cause of PMR is unknown, although an autoimmune process appears to be related to the condition. The overall prevalence of PMR is 17/100,000 people. In addition, family aggregation is common.

4. **d.** The differential diagnosis of PMR in the elderly includes hypothyroidism, hyperthyroidism, hyperparathyroidism, systemic lupus erythematosus, RA, osteoarthritis or degenerative arthritis, and polymyositis.

The most important complication of concern in PMR is its association with GCA.

5. **e.** The differences between PMR and polymyositis on clinical examination are as follows: (1) There is marked weakness associated with proximal muscle pain in polymyositis, (2) there is marked muscle tenderness associated with the proximal muscle pain in polymyositis, and (3) laboratory examination reveals elevated muscle enzymes only in polymyositis.

6. **b.** Both PMR and GCA are characterized by elevations in ESR. Elevations to levels greater than 100 mm/hour may be seen in either disease; elevations to levels greater than 50 mm/hour are almost universal. C-reactive protein may also be elevated and should be checked if GCA is suspected. Combinations of ESR and C-reactive protein elevations are 97% specific for GCA compared to ESR alone.

7. **e.** Manifestations of temporal arteritis include headache, scalp tenderness, visual symptoms, jaw claudication, constitutional symptoms (fever, weight loss, anorexia, and fatigue), polymyalgia symptoms (aching and stiffness of the trunk and proximal muscle groups), cough, and amaurosis fugax.

8. **c.** Of the symptoms listed in answer 7, the most worrisome is amaurosis fugax. Amaurosis fugax, defined as brief visual loss, is related to ischemia of the posterior ciliary branch of the ophthalmic artery and can lead to blindness if not treated quickly.

9. **c.** The transient visual loss of amaurosis fugax may foretell by days, weeks, or sometimes even months the most dreaded complication, permanent monocular or binocular blindness. If any ocular involvement is present, IV methylprednisolone should be initiated immediately to try to prevent blindness.

10. **b.** Oral prednisone is the treatment of choice for both PMR and GCA. The dosage is as follows: (1) PMR: 20 mg/day by mouth for 4 weeks with gradual reduction thereafter but maintained for at least 1 year; and (2) temporal arteritis: 60 mg/day by mouth for 4 weeks with gradual reduction beginning at 4 weeks but with maintenance therapy for 1 or 2 years. Dosage should be adjusted by monitoring the ESR.

11. **b.** From a pathologic standpoint, the cause of temporal arteritis is inflammation of the temporal artery. From a local anatomic standpoint, this results in temporal headache (generally unilateral and accompanied by temporal artery swelling and tenderness). Temporal artery biopsy is the definitive diagnostic procedure for GCA and should include a segment at least 2 cm long. Because of the potential for ocular involvement, treatment should be started immediately, even if biopsy cannot be done within 1 week. It is believed that with treatment the characteristic pathology of GCA may be present for up to 2 weeks, but do not wait for the biopsy results.

12. **e.** Long-term use of steroids in the elderly may result in many adverse side effects that need to be followed. These may include muscle atrophy, diabetes mellitus, hypertension, glaucoma, skin atrophy, and accelerated cataracts.

13. **b.** The incidence of aneurysm formation in those with a history of GCA is approximately 10%, with thoracic and abdominal aneurysm discovery at 5.9 and 2.5 years, respectively. As a result of these findings, patients should be evaluated yearly for the formation of aneurysm if they have had GCA.

Solution to the Clinical Case Management Problem

The differential diagnosis includes the following:

1. Nonmusculoskeletal problems: hypothyroidism, hyperthyroidism, and hyperparathyroidism
2. Musculoskeletal problems: systemic lupus erythematosus, RA, osteoarthritis or degenerative arthritis, PMR, and polymyositis
3. Other important systemic conditions: metastatic bone cancer and multiple myeloma

Summary

PMR

1. Epidemiology: Of all the musculoskeletal conditions, none is so closely identified with the geriatric population as PMR.
2. Prevalence: A prevalence rate of 17/100,000 people older than age 50 years has been established (average age, approximately 70 years old).
3. Symptoms: Symptoms include either sudden onset or gradual onset of pain (usually bilateral).
   a. Initial manifestations: Pain, aching, and stiffness in the shoulder girdle and hip girdle; profound morning stiffness; and patients may complain of fatigue, malaise, weight loss, and depression.
   b. Progression: Pain, aching, and stiffness progress to other joints in the upper and lower extremities.
   c. Clue: The patient tells you that suddenly he or she can no longer get out of bed in the morning.
4. Diagnosis: Elevated ESR (almost always greater than 50 mm/hour; frequently greater than 100 mm/hour). Other findings may be a normocytic normochromic anemia, elevated platelet count, and increased C-reactive protein. Liver enzymes, especially alkaline phosphatase, are increased in one-third of patients. Muscle enzymes are normal.
5. Complication: Temporal arteritis with eventual blindness is the major complication.
6. Treatment: Prednisone, 20 mg/day for 1 month and taper; maintain for 1 year. Response can be seen in 1 or 2 days.
7. Differential diagnosis: See the Solution to the Clinical Case Management Problem.

TEMPORAL ARTERITIS

1. Presenting signs and symptoms
   a. Pain, aching, and stiffness in the shoulder and hip girdles, as previously described.
   b. Additional systemic signs and symptoms of inflammation include the following: (i) fever (high spiking), (ii) weight loss, (iii) malaise, (iv) jaw claudication, (v) transient visual complaints leading to blindness if left untreated, (vi) extremity claudication, and (vii) aortic aneurysm.
   c. Significant local signs and symptoms are (i) temporal headache (unilateral), (ii) temporal artery swelling and tenderness (but not always tender), and (iii) significant neurologic symptoms (see answers 7 to 9).
2. Diagnosis
   a. ESR (as mentioned previously).
   b. Temporal artery biopsy: If you suspect temporal arteritis, do not wait for a surgeon to perform a biopsy. Treat the condition with prednisone immediately. Of patients with PMR, 10% to 15% may develop GCA, and 40% to 60% of patients with GCA will have PMR.
3. Complications: Permanent monocular or binocular blindness are major complications.
4. Treatment: Treatment is high-dose prednisone, 40 mg/day for 4 weeks; taper slowly and maintain for 1 or 2 years. Other dosing may include 1 to 1.5 mg/kg/day for 4 weeks. If symptoms are ocular, use IV methylprednisolone immediately.

Suggested Reading

American Geriatric Society: *Geriatric Review Syllabus, A Core Curriculum in Geriatric Medicine*, 6th ed. Chicago: American Geriatric Society, 2006, pp. 439–440.

Unwin B, Williams CM, Gilliland W: Polymyalgia rheumatica and giant cell arteritis. *Am Fam Physician* 74(9):1547–1554, 2006.

Weyand CM, Goronzy JJ: Giant-cell arteritis and polymyalgia rheumatica. *Ann Intern Med* 139(6):505–515, 2003.

CHAPTER 134

Hypertension Management in the Elderly

An 80-Year-Old Male with Hypertension

An 80-year-old white male, previously healthy, comes to your office for a periodic health examination. He was last seen by a physician 20 years ago. His blood pressure is recorded as 185/95 mmHg.

A complete history reveals no other cardiovascular risk factors. A complete physical examination reveals no evidence of end organ damage or secondary causes of hypertension.

Basic laboratory investigations, including a complete blood count, urinalysis, electrolytes, serum calcium, fasting blood sugar, plasma cholesterol, uric acid, and an electrocardiogram, are all normal.

The patient is on a fixed income and is trying to keep up with payments for his wife's nursing home care.

SELECT THE BEST ANSWER TO THE FOLLOWING QUESTIONS

1. Based on the information given, what would you do now?
   a. begin therapy with a thiazide diuretic
   b. begin therapy with a calcium channel blocker
   c. begin therapy with an angiotensin-converting enzyme (ACE) inhibitor
   d. begin therapy with a beta blocker
   e. none of the above

Following further investigation and two more visits, appropriate therapy is prescribed for the patient, and he returns in 1 month for follow-up care. His blood pressure remains elevated at 185/92 mmHg. A visit 1 week later yields the same blood pressure reading.

You also discuss nonpharmacologic treatment with him, and it appears obvious to you that he is not prepared to alter his "hamburgers and chips" diet. He also states that exercise would kill him.

2. What would you do now?
   a. prescribe a thiazide diuretic
   b. prescribe a calcium channel blocker
   c. prescribe a beta blocker
   d. prescribe an ACE inhibitor
   e. prescribe a vasodilator

Appropriate therapy is prescribed for the patient, and he returns in 1 month for follow-up care. His blood pressure is now 170/90 mmHg and his serum potassium level has decreased from 4 to 3 mEq/L.

3. At this time, what would you do?
   a. substitute an ACE inhibitor for the present medication
   b. substitute a calcium channel blocker for the present medication
   c. substitute a beta blocker for the present medication
   d. substitute a vasodilator for the present medication
   e. review the type and dose of the drug class being prescribed

The patient has the necessary intervention made. When he returns next month for follow-up care, his blood pressure is 175/90 mmHg.

4. At this time, what would you do?
   a. add an ACE inhibitor
   b. add a calcium channel blocker
   c. add a beta blocker
   d. add a vasodilator
   e. maximize the dose of a beta blocker

5. Which of the following statements regarding the treatment of hypertension in the elderly is (are) true?
   a. isolated systolic hypertension in the elderly should not be treated
   b. the benefits of treating elderly hypertensive patients have not been established
   c. no change in morbidity or mortality has been demonstrated for elderly patients treated with antihypertensives
   d. elderly patients treated for hypertension are likely to benefit only from a reduction in cerebrovascular morbidity and mortality, not cardiac morbidity or mortality
   e. none of the above are true

6. Regarding the epidemiologic importance of elevations in systolic versus diastolic blood pressure in elderly patients, which of the following statements is true?
   a. elevation of systolic blood pressure is not as important as elevation of diastolic blood pressure
   b. elevation of systolic blood pressure, although important, does not correlate well with cardiovascular morbidity and mortality

c. elevations of systolic and diastolic blood pressure are equally important
d. elevated systolic blood pressure is a greater risk for subsequent cardiovascular morbidity and mortality than diastolic blood pressure
e. the relative importance of elevations in systolic blood pressure in terms of cardiovascular morbidity and mortality is unclear

7. With respect to morbidity and mortality and treatment of systolic hypertension in the elderly, which of the following epidemiologic categories show(s) a significant decrease (compared to placebo) when systolic blood pressure is treated?
a. total stroke morbidity
b. total stroke mortality
c. total coronary artery mortality
d. a and b
e. a, b, and c
f. none of the above

8. Which of the following drug combinations should be avoided in elderly hypertensive patients?
a. hydrochlorothiazide (HCT)/amiloride and enalapril
b. HCT/amiloride and nifedipine
c. HCT/amiloride and atenolol
d. HCT/amiloride and hydralazine
e. HCT/amiloride and reserpine

9. In a long-term care setting, blood pressure readings tend to be higher during what time of day?
a. before breakfast
b. before lunch
c. after dinner
d. before bedtime

10. Postprandial hypotension in long-term care facilities is often associated with which of the following?
a. falls
b. syncopal episodes
c. stroke
d. overall mortality
e. all of the above

11. The auscatory gap may lead to an underestimation of which form of blood pressure?
a. diastolic blood pressure
b. systolic blood pressure
c. both
d. neither

CLINICAL CASE PROBLEM 2

A 75-Year-Old African American Male with Angina Pectoris

A 75-year-old African American male with angina pectoris is found, on physical examination, to have a blood pressure of 170/100 mmHg. His angina is controlled on isosorbide dinitrate, 30 mg four times per day. His blood pressure reading is repeated on several occasions and remains unchanged.

12. At this time, what is the most reasonable treatment for this patient's blood pressure?
a. a calcium channel blocker
b. a beta blocker
c. a thiazide diuretic
d. an ACE inhibitor
e. a and/or c

CLINICAL CASE PROBLEM 3

A Hypertensive 72-Year-Old White Female with a Previous Myocardial Infarction and Mild Congestive Heart Failure

A 72-year-old white female with a previous myocardial infarction (MI) and mild congestive heart failure (CHF) (controlled with furosemide 40 mg four times per day) comes to your office for a routine assessment. She is found to have a blood pressure of 190/100 mmHg. This reading is repeated on two occasions.

13. What would be the most appropriate treatment for her hypertension?
a. an ACE inhibitor
b. a calcium channel blocker
c. a beta blocker
d. a thiazide diuretic
e. none of the above

CLINICAL CASE PROBLEM 4

A Hypertensive 72-Year-Old White Male with Diabetes

A 72-year-old white male with a 20-year history of non-insulin-dependent diabetes mellitus is found to have a blood pressure of 170/105 mmHg. He has no history of angina pectoris or other significant vascular disease. He had never been diagnosed as hypertensive.

His blood pressure is repeated on two additional occasions and the readings remain the same. Laboratory evaluation reveals microalbuminuria.

14. At this time, what would be the most appropriate treatment for this patient's blood pressure?
    a. a thiazide diuretic
    b. a beta blocker
    c. a calcium channel blocker
    d. an ACE inhibitor
    e. a vasodilator

15. What is the recommended dosage of HCT for the treatment of hypertension in the elderly?
    a. 12.5 to 25 mg
    b. 25 to 50 mg
    c. 50 to 75 mg
    d. 75 to 100 mg
    e. whatever you want

Clinical Case Management Problem

An 80-year-old African-American male with systolic hypertension (210/85 mmHg) is a new patient to your practice. He says he has been healthy all of his life. From three consecutive readings you determine that the patient is truly hypertensive. Discuss your approach to this patient with respect to education and counseling regarding his hypertension. Include lifestyle advice, medication advice, and other pertinent advice that you consider important.

Answers

1. **e.** Although this patient has a systolic blood pressure of 185 mmHg, you should consider that this is only one reading and it cannot be assumed to represent his "true blood pressure." Even if you were able to make the diagnosis of hypertension at this time, you would still want to begin with nonpharmacologic therapy.

This patient should have his blood pressure rechecked on two other occasions before the diagnosis of hypertension is made. If there is a concern, then it would be reasonable to utilize ambulatory monitoring at home and have the patient report back to you if certain parameters are not met. This requires an accurate and well-calibrated blood pressure cuff.

2. **a.** Studies have clearly demonstrated the importance of treating systolic hypertension in the elderly. In fact, it should be treated with the same rigor and aggressiveness as diastolic hypertension.

Because of the patient's fixed income and the proven efficacy of thiazide diuretics in reducing morbidity and mortality from cardiovascular disease, a low-dose (12.5 to 25 mg) thiazide diuretic would be the agent of choice. It would be reasonable to follow recommendations and start with 12.5 mg/day. Thiazide diuretic has proven to decrease morbidity and mortality. Chlorthalidone has also been extensively studied and would be an alternative at 12.5 mg/day.

3. **e.** At this time, the most reasonable alternative would be to review both the dose and the drug class.

On the positive side, this patient's systolic blood pressure has dropped (from 185 to 170 mmHg). On the negative side, his potassium has also dropped (from 4 to 3 mEq/L). This is a significant drop and puts this patient into the danger zone for hypokalemia—the level at which dysrhythmias begin to be a serious concern.

4. **c.** The most appropriate strategy at this time would be to add a beta blocker. Remember, the initial goal will be to reduce the systolic blood pressure to 160 mmHg and then eventually to 140 mmHg over a period of months. The most reasonable strategy in this case would likely be to reduce the dose of the thiazide diuretic to an absolute minimum (12.5 mg) if started at 25 mg/day and add a beta blocker (e.g., atenolol). This combination of drugs (thiazide and beta blocker) was selected because of recommendations made in the Seventh Report of the Joint National Committee on Prevention, Detection, Evaluation, and Treatment of High Blood Pressure (JNC-VII), which documented the reduction in cardiovascular morbidity and mortality induced by thiazides and beta blockers. A cardioselective beta blocker should be used in the elderly especially if there is a history of MI or ischemic heart disease. Cardioselective beta blockers also result in fewer side effects than nonselective beta blockers.

Potassium supplementation should also be considered.

5. **e.** There is ample evidence to show that antihypertensive therapy prevents cerebrovascular accidents, congestive cardiac failure, and other blood pressure-related complications. The Systolic Hypertension in the Elderly Program showed a reduction in MI and other coronary events in older patients with moderate to severe ischemic heart disease. Other more recent studies confirm this finding.

6. c. The most important advance in the treatment of hypertension in the elderly is the clear and unequivocal recognition that systolic hypertension is as important as diastolic hypertension as a risk factor for cardiovascular morbidity and mortality and should be aggressively treated. The goal of systolic blood pressure reduction is a reading not exceeding 160 mmHg. The ideal control would be a systolic blood pressure less than 140 mmHg.

7. e. See answer 5.

8. a. Of the choices provided, the drug combination that should clearly be avoided in elderly patients is HCT/amiloride and enalapril. Both amiloride and enalapril are potassium-sparing drugs. In an elderly patient with decreased renal function, this can lead to profound and rapid hyperkalemia with subsequent complications.

9. c. In a long-term care facility, approximately one-third to two-thirds of the residents have hypertension. Inaccuracies result from measurement errors and from temporal variability, particularly in relation to meals.

10. e. Because of the increase in side effects associated with the elderly, you must consider many factors when treating this patient. Does the side effect of treatment medications have such a negative consequence on the patient's quality of life that it is not worth treating with medication? For example, is there a significant increase in the number of falls or syncopal episodes? If so, treatment may be more detrimental than not treating.

11. b. The auscatory gap is found in patients with systolic hypertension and is usually an indication of arterial stiffness. To determine systolic blood pressure more accurately, palpation will avoid this problem.

12. e. See the Solution to the Clinical Case Management Problem.

13. a. Considering that this elderly female has CHF as well as hypertension, the treatment of choice is an ACE inhibitor. ACE inhibitors reduce both preload and afterload in hypertensive patients and thus are the drug class of choice for the management of CHF. ACE inhibitors have minimal side effects, primarily cough with enalapril and taste disturbances with captopril. For patients with left ventricular hypertrophy, an ACE inhibitor, a combination of hydralazine and isosorbide dinitrate, beta blockers, or spironolactone have been shown to decrease mortality. Patients started on an ACE inhibitor should have their blood pressure checked in 1 week and serum creatinine in 1 month.

14. d. Patients with diabetes mellitus and resulting renal impairment or microalbuminuria should definitely be treated with ACE inhibitors as the drug class of choice. There is evidence that ACE inhibitors can be "renal protective agents" in patients with diabetes mellitus and can even be indicated as a prophylactic measure. Additional studies have shown that patients with microalbuminuria can also respond to angiotensin receptor blockers.

15. a. The recommended, or "correct," dose of HCT or other thiazide diuretic is the lowest dose that effectively controls the blood pressure and at the same time minimizes all of the metabolic side effects associated with thiazide diuretics.

Solution to the Clinical Case Management Problem

Provide advice for an 80-year-old African-American male with documented systolic hypertension:

1. Review the patient's diet with him. Attempt to have the patient's spouse present (if available) while discussing this.
2. Encourage the patient to adopt the general recommendations of the American Heart Association's type I diet. This includes no more than 300 mg of cholesterol per day, no more than 30% of calories from fat, and no more than 10% of calories from saturated fat.
3. Encourage the patient to begin a "gentle" aerobic exercise program. The most reasonable exercise for a man of this age would be a walking program.
4. Advise the patient to decrease his alcohol intake to no more than two drinks per day.
5. Encourage the patient to stop smoking (cutting down might be more reasonable) if he is a smoker.
6. Start "nonpharmacologic maneuvers" along with treatment.

Summary

1. The most important point is that systolic hypertension in the elderly (and in the young as well) is as important as diastolic hypertension.
2. Diagnosis of hypertension in the elderly: New criteria established by JNC-VII (see answer 4).
3. Treatment of hypertension in the elderly reduces cerebrovascular morbidity, cerebrovascular mortality, cardiovascular morbidity, and cardiovascular mortality.
4. A substantial proportion of patients with mild or moderate hypertension can be controlled with a single agent, and in most this control will be maintained in the long term.
5. Assessment of cardiac risk factors: Smoking, dyslipidemia, and diabetes are important in the elderly.
6. Assessment of end organ damage: Left ventricular hypertrophy, coronary artery disease, CHF, stroke or transient ischemic attacks, renal disease, peripheral arterial disease, and retinopathy are important and often require treatment.
7. Consider renal artery stenosis if hypertension is sudden in onset, if there is a sudden rise in blood pressure, or if blood pressure is elevated with three medications. Workup would include listening for a bruit, renography, and aortogram.
8. Conditions requiring emergent lowering of blood pressure include hypertensive encephalopathy, intracranial hemorrhage, unstable angina, acute MI, acute left ventricular failure with pulmonary edema, and dissecting aortic aneurysm.

Suggested Reading

American Geriatric Society: *Geriatric Review Syllabus, A Core Curriculum in Geriatric Medicine*, 6th ed. Chicago: American Geriatric Society, 2006, pp. 361–368.

Asmar R: Benefits of blood pressure reduction in elderly patients. *J Hypertens Suppl* 21(6):S25–S30, 2003.

Chobanian AV, Bakris GL, Black, HR, et al: The seventh report of the Joint National Committee on Prevention, Detection, Evaluation, and Treatment of High Blood Pressure (JNC-7). *JAMA* 289(19):2560–2571, 2003.

Franco V, Oparil S, Carretero OA: Hypertensive therapy: Part I. *Circulation* 109(24):2953–2958, 2004.

Staessen JA, Richart T, Birkenhager WH: Less atherosclerosis and lower blood pressure for a meaningful life perspective with more brain. *Hypertension* 49(3):389–400, 2007.

CHAPTER

135 Cerebrovascular Accidents

CLINICAL CASE PROBLEM 1

A 67-Year-Old Male with a Sudden-Onset Left-Sided Hemiplegia, Dysphagia, and a "Visual Problem"

A 67-year-old male is brought to the emergency department by ambulance after the gradual onset of the following: inability to move his right leg, followed by his right arm; speech impairment; and a "visual problem."

On examination, the patient has a flaccid paralysis of the muscles of the right leg and the muscles (excluding the deltoid) of the right arm, a homonymous hemianopia, and dysphagia. In addition, he "does not recognize" that he is paralyzed, nor can he turn his eyes toward the right side. His deep tendon reflexes are hyperreflexive on the right side. His right great toe is upgoing.

It is now 6 hours since the symptoms began. It appears from talking to his wife that his symptoms are "still changing."

SELECT THE BEST ANSWER TO THE FOLLOWING QUESTIONS

1. What is the most likely diagnosis at this time?
   a. transient ischemic attack (TIA)
   b. completed stroke
   c. stroke-in-evolution
   d. subarachnoid hemorrhage
   e. complicated migraine

2. The location of symptoms correlates the site of the lesion to which of the following?
   a. left middle cerebral artery
   b. right middle cerebral artery
   c. left anterior cerebral artery
   d. right anterior cerebral artery
   e. left posterior cerebral artery

3. What is the most likely pathophysiologic process involved in this patient at this time?
   a. thrombotic stroke
   b. embolic stroke
   c. hemorrhagic stroke
   d. lacunar stroke
   e. subarachnoid hemorrhage

4. What is the most common pathophysiologic process in patients who have suffered a cerebrovascular accident (CVA)?
   a. thrombotic stroke
   b. embolic stroke
   c. hemorrhagic stroke
   d. lacunar stroke
   e. subarachnoid hemorrhage

5. In which of the following conditions would you most likely find an embolic phenomenon as the pathophysiology of a CVA?
   a. hypertension
   b. atrial fibrillation
   c. ventricular fibrillation
   d. a young woman on the oral contraceptive pill
   e. b and d

6. What is the number one risk factor for CVAs?
   a. cigarette smoking
   b. hypertension
   c. hypercholesterolemia
   d. hypertriglyceridemia
   e. hypothyroidism

7. Lacunar strokes (lacunar infarcts) are most closely associated with which of the following?
   a. thrombosis
   b. embolization
   c. hypertension
   d. subarachnoid bleeding
   e. cerebral infarction

CLINICAL CASE PROBLEM 2

A 47-Year-Old Patient with Mental Status Impairment, Foot Drop, and Left-Sided Hemiplegia and Numbness

A 47-year-old patient develops the following symptoms and signs: impaired mental status including confusion, amnesia, perseveration, and personality changes; foot drop; apraxia on the affected side; left-sided hemiplegia; and left-sided numbness (both muscle power and sensation retained to some degree in left upper extremity).

8. This patient most likely has had a CVA affecting which of the following arteries?
   a. right middle cerebral artery
   b. posterior cerebral artery
   c. vertebral–basilar artery
   d. right anterior cerebral artery
   e. posterior/inferior cerebellar artery

CLINICAL CASE PROBLEM 3

A 77-Year-Old Female with Nystagmus, Homonymous Hemianopia, and Facial Numbness Weakness

A 77-year-old female presents to the emergency department with the following signs/symptoms: dysarthria and dysphagia, vertigo, nausea, syncope, memory loss and disorientation, and ataxic gait.

On physical examination, the patient has nystagmus, homonymous hemianopia, numbness in the area of the 12th cranial nerve, and facial weakness. You suspect a CVA.

9. Which of the following arteries is most likely to be involved?
   a. middle cerebral artery
   b. posterior cerebral artery
   c. vertebral–basilar artery
   d. anterior cerebral artery
   e. posterior inferior cerebellar artery

10. There are many sources of potential emboli that may cause a CVA. The most common source of cerebral emboli is which of the following?
    a. carotid arteries
    b. aortic arch
    c. heart
    d. vertebral–basilar arteries
    e. middle cerebral artery

11. The role of computed tomography (CT) scanning within the first 24 hours of a stroke includes which of the following?
    a. to exclude hemorrhages
    b. to exclude tumors
    c. to exclude abscesses
    d. to diagnose stroke
    e. a, b, and c

12. The use of anticoagulation is clearly effective in preventing recurrent cardioembolic strokes from atrial fibrillation, a recent myocardial infarction, valvular disease, or a patent foramen ovale. Contraindications to the use of anticoagulation include which of the following?
    a. hemorrhage on CT scan
    b. large cerebral infarctions
    c. evidence of bacterial endocarditis
    d. a and b
    e. all of the above

13. A TIA is most closely associated with which of the following?
    a. amaurosis fugax
    b. subarachnoid hemorrhage
    c. lacunar hemorrhage
    d. intracranial aneurysm
    e. fusiform aneurysm

14. A ruptured berry aneurysm is usually located in which of the following?
    a. anterior cerebral artery distribution
    b. posterior cerebral artery distribution
    c. circle of Willis
    d. middle cerebral artery distribution
    e. none of the above

15. A patient is suspected of having a cerebral infarction. If you had the opportunity to order only one investigation, what investigation would that be?
    a. a regular angiogram of the cerebral circulation
    b. a CT scan of the brain without contrast
    c. a magnetic resonance imaging (MRI) angiogram of the brain
    d. a digital subtraction angiogram of the brain
    e. an immediate lumbar puncture

16. Which of the following is not a risk factor for the development of a CVA?
    a. diabetes mellitus type 1
    b. diabetes mellitus type 2
    c. African American race
    d. cigarette smoking
    e. diabetes insipidus

17. The incidence of stroke in the United States during the past 15 years has done which of the following?
    a. increased significantly
    b. increased slightly
    c. decreased significantly
    d. decreased slightly
    e. nobody really knows for sure

CLINICAL CASE PROBLEM 4

A 42-Year-Old White Male with a "Curtain Coming down" over His Eyes

A 42-year-old white male presents to your office with a complaint of decreased vision that, with further questioning, is described as "a curtain coming down over my eyes." The patient's past medical history included hypertension and hyperlipidemia, and he recently admitted to extensive use of cocaine. He denies intravenous drug use, vertigo, diplopia, ataxia, or an abnormal heart rate.

18. If you had the choice of one test to help determine the etiology of his symptoms, what would that be?
    a. ultrasound of the carotid arteries
    b. CT scan of the brain
    c. MRI scan of the brain
    d. fluorescein angiography of the fundi
    e. lumbar puncture

19. Which of the following statements regarding carotid endarterectomy (CEA) is (are) true?
    a. CEA is indicated in the presence of a completed stroke
    b. CEA is indicated in the presence of a complete arterial occlusion
    c. randomized, controlled trials have established the benefit of CEA over standard medical therapy for the treatment of carotid artery stenosis
    d. CEA has been established as the treatment of choice in patients with a documented TIA and a tightly stenotic lesion greater than 70%
    e. nobody really knows for sure

20. In a patient with an asymptomatic carotid bruit, for whom evaluation reveals a high-grade stenosis, recommended treatment would include:
    a. watchful waiting
    b. anticoagulation therapy with aspirin or ticlopidine
    c. CEA
    d. CEA and aspirin
    e. none of the above

21. In the diagnostic workup of a patient with a TIA, a lumbar puncture should be utilized when?
    a. in all diagnostic workups
    b. only when meningitis is suspected
    c. in any patient considered to have a subarachnoid hemorrhage when a CT scan is not diagnostic
    d. there are no clinical indications for a lumbar puncture in the workup of a patient with a TIA or CVA

22. Among the following, which is (are) the preferred diagnostic test(s) for evaluating patients with a cardiac embolic phenomenon?
a. transthoracic echocardiography
b. transesophageal echocardiography
c. magnetic resonance angiography
d. all of the above
e. none of the above

23. The main indication for the use of magnetic resonance angiography is which of the following?
a. to diagnose an acute stroke
b. to evaluate for coronary artery stenosis
c. if considering emergent thrombolytic therapy to reverse stroke progression
d. all of the above
e. none of the above

24. The first-line choice in prophylaxis of pulmonary embolus in patients who have had an acute ischemic stroke is which of the following?
a. acetylsalicylic acid (ASA)
b. clopidogrel (Plavix)
c. ticlopidine
d. enoxaparin
e. warfarin

Clinical Case Management Problem

Define the following terms: (1) transient ischemic attack, (2) stroke-in-evolution, and (3) completed stroke.

Answers

1. **c.** At this time, the most likely diagnosis is stroke-in-evolution. The typical development of thrombotic stroke causes a clinical syndrome known as stroke-in-evolution. An intermittent or slow progression over hours to days is characteristic of stroke-in-evolution or slow hemorrhage.

Also referred to as a progressing stroke, the exact etiology must be defined, although ischemic stroke is most common.

2. **a.** The symptoms that this patient is currently experiencing suggest a lesion of the left middle cerebral artery. The signs/symptoms of middle cerebral artery occlusion are (1) dysphagia (left hemisphere involvement), dyslexia, and dysgraphia; (2) contralateral hemiparesis or hemiplegia; (3) contralateral hemisensory disturbances; (4) rapid deterioration in consciousness from confusion to coma; (5) homonymous hemianopsia; (6) denial of or lack of recognition of a paralyzed extremity; (7) eyes deviated to the side of the lesion; and (8) global aphasia if dominant hemisphere is involved.

3. **a.** Because of the slow and continuing progression of the central nervous system symptomatology, this is much more characteristic of a thrombotic stroke rather than an embolic or hemorrhagic stroke.

4. **a.** The pathophysiology of stroke in order of frequency (from most common to least common) is (1) thrombotic stroke, (2) embolic stroke, (3) hemorrhagic stroke, (4) lacunar stroke (lacunar infarct), and (5) subarachnoid hemorrhage.

5. **b.** An embolic stroke involves fragments that break from a thrombus formed outside the brain in the heart, aorta, common carotid, or thorax. Emboli infrequently arise from the ascending aorta or the common carotid artery. The embolus usually involves small vessels and obstructs at a bifurcation or other point of narrowing, thus enabling ischemia to develop and extend. An embolus may completely occlude the lumen of the vessel, or it may remain in place or break into fragments and move up the vessel. The most common source of emboli is the heart.

Conditions associated with the onset of an embolic stroke include (1) atrial fibrillation; (2) myocardial infarction; (3) endocarditis; (4) rheumatic heart disease; (5) valvular prostheses; (6) atrial septal defect; (7) disorders of the aorta; (8) disorders of the carotids; (9) disorders of the vertebral–basilar system; and (10) other embolic phenomena, such as air, fat, and tumor.

6. **b.** CVAs or strokes remain the third-leading cause of death in the United States. The most important risk factor for stroke is hypertension. The decrease in the incidence of stroke is largely due to the successful, aggressive, and ideal treatment of hypertension in the United States. The risk of stroke is three times higher in those with hypertension and is twice as high in those with isolated systolic hypertension.

Other factors that are important in the etiology of stroke include (1) age (the older the patient, the greater the risk), (2) other heart disease (valvular, conductive, infective, and atherosclerotic), (3) cigarette smoking, (4) diabetes mellitus (type 1 and type 2), (5) the oral contraceptive pill when combined with smoking and older age, (6) race (African Americans are more prone than white Americans), (7) family history (of lipid disorders or cardiovascular diseases in general), and (8) sex (strokes are more common in females than in males).

7. **c.** Lacunar strokes (lacunar infarcts) are infarcts smaller than 1 mm in size and involve the small perforating arteries predominately in the basal ganglia, pons, cerebellum, internal capsule, and, less commonly, deep cerebral white matter. Lacunar infarcts are primarily associated with hypertension. Because of the subcortical location and small area of infarction, these strokes may have pure motor and sensory deficits, ipsilateral ataxia, and dysarthria. They may appear on CT scan as small hypodense areas. Prognosis and recovery are usually good.

8. **d.** This patient most likely has a lesion in the territory of the right anterior cerebral artery. Signs and symptoms of a CVA in the territory of the anterior cerebral artery include (1) mental status impairments including confusion, amnesia, perseveration, personality changes (flat affect and apathy), and cognitive changes (short attention span, slowness, and deterioration of intellectual function); (2) urinary continence (long duration); (3) contralateral hemiparesis or hemiplegia; (4) sensory impairments (contralateral); (5) foot and leg deficits (more frequent than arm deficits) and contralateral leg/foot paralysis; (6) apraxia on affected side; (7) expressive aphasia (for left hemisphere only); (8) deviation of the eyes and head toward the affected side; (9) abulia (lack of initiative); and (10) gait dysfunction.

9. **c.** This patient has had a CVA involving the vertebral–basilar system. The signs and symptoms of vertebral–basilar stroke are (1) dysarthria and dysphagia; (2) vertigo, nausea, and vomiting; (3) disorientation; (4) ataxic gait (ipsilateral cerebellar ataxia); (5) visual symptoms (double vision and blurred vision); (6) dysphagia; (7) ocular signs (nystagmus, conjugate gaze paralysis, and ophthalmoplegia); (8) akinetic mutism (locked-in syndrome when basilar artery occlusion occurs); (9) numbness of lips and face; (10) facial weakness, alternating motor paresis; and (11) drop attacks, syncope (Doppler studies can detect vertebrobasilar embolic sources).

10. **c.** The most common source of cerebral emboli is from the heart.

11. **e.** Ischemic stroke changes usually will not show up on a CT scan or MRI within the first 24 hours. Therefore, the role of CT scanning is to rule out structural abnormalities such as hemorrhages, tumors, or abscesses.

12. **d.** Bacterial endocarditis would not be considered a contradiction to anticoagulation therapy, but it would be considered a precaution with those bleeding tendencies and uncontrolled hypertension. Contradiction in the case would be a patient who has a large stroke, a hemorrhagic stroke, or severe thrombocytopenia.

13. **a.** A TIA probably represents thrombotic particles causing an intermittent blockage of circulation or spasm. Amaurosis fugax, which is described by patients as "a curtain coming down in front of my eyes—a blackout," is really a TIA of the ophthalmic artery. This is associated primarily with the carotid circulation and may also present with contralateral weakness of the face, arm, legs, or numbness. In the situation of a patient with a noncardioembolic stroke or TIA, the use of ASA (325 mg), low-dose subcutaneous heparin, or both is indicated. Consider statins and ramipril as well. A complete workup, including CT scanning and carotid Doppler imaging, is warranted to search for treatable causes of TIA.

14. **c.** Intracranial aneurysms may result from arteriosclerosis, congenital abnormality, trauma, inflammation, or infection. Cocaine has been linked to aneurysm formation. The size may vary from 2 mm to 2 or 3 cm. Most aneurysms are located at bifurcations in or near the circle of Willis, particularly on the anterior or posterior communicating arteries. Aneurysm may be single, but in 20% of cases more than one aneurysm is present. The peak incidence occurs between age 35 and 60 years. Berry aneurysms are also known as saccular aneurysms. Berry aneurysms make up the majority of subarachnoid bleeds (51%).

15. **b.** The diagnostic test of choice for a cerebral infarction is a CT scan of the head. A CT scan of the brain without contrast would allow you to exclude a cerebral hemorrhage. A CT scan is preferable to an MRI in the acute stages because it is quicker, and an MRI will not easily detect bleeding during the first 48 hours.

16. **e.** The risk factors for CVAs include (1) hypertension (the most important risk factor), including isolated systolic hypertension; (2) hypercholesterolemia; (3) hypertriglyceridemia (because it has been found to be an independent risk factor for vascular disease); (4) African American race (probably due to increased risk of hypertension); (5) obesity (also related to increased risk of hypertension); (6) sedentary lifestyle related to obesity, which is related to hypertension; (7) cigarette smoking; (8) women in their later reproductive years (age 37 to 45 years) who are heavy cigarette smokers and on the oral contraceptive pill; (9) family history of CVAs; (10) family history of hyperlipidemia; (11) age older than 65 years; (12) diabetes mellitus types 1 and 2; and (13) hypothyroidism (related to hyperlipidemia).

Diabetes insipidus has nothing to do with CVA (with the possible exception of Sheenan's syndrome, postpartum pituitary necrosis).

17. **c.** Estimates vary widely. However, the incidence of stroke in the United States has declined dramatically in the past 15 years due in large part to the relative success of the treatment of hypertension. Note, however, that the incidence increases almost 20-fold with age (from 2.1 per 1000 people age 45 to 54 years to 4.5 per 1000 people age 65 to 74 years and 9.3 per 1000 people age 75 to 84 years). The incidence for women is 25% to 30% lower than that for men in the same age groups, but it surpasses that of men for people older than age 85 years.

18. **a.** This patient has had a TIA. Amaurosis fugax and his cocaine use may have contributed to this TIA. Cocaine probably caused an intense vasospasm; it is an intensely powerful vasoconstrictor—much more powerful than either angiotensin II or thromboxane. This patient needs an ultrasound of his carotid arteries, and he needs it soon. Treatment will be based on etiology, and a workup and consultation should be conducted quickly.

19. **d.** There has been a great deal of research on carotid endarterectomies (CEAs) (when to do/when not to do). Studies have demonstrated that a CEA reduces the risk of subsequent stroke in patients who have had TIAs with a high-grade stenosis. If an ulcerated plaque is present in the presence of moderate stenosis, the risk of stroke increases, and patients benefit from CEA. Based on recommendations from the North American Symptomatic Carotid Endarterectomy Trial, the optimal treatment for symptomatic carotid artery disease if the stenosis is more than 70% is CEA, provided the patient has few comorbidities and the institution performs a large number of procedures.

Further research is being conducted on the use of CEA for patients with carotid artery lesions between 30% and 70% and on patients with asymptomatic bruits with moderate stenotic lesions. These investigations may result in a recommendation to perform CEAs in such patients.

The current treatment recommendations for carotid stenosis include the following: (1) prior TIA or stroke with a stenosis of more than 70% (CEA is superior to medical management); (2) prior TIA or stroke with a stenosis of 50% to 60%, CEA or medical management with serial carotid Doppler to identify developing plaques; (3) prior TIA or stroke with stenosis of less than 50%, medical management (CEA of no benefit); (4) asymptomatic patient with stenosis of more than 80%, CEA should be considered; and (5) asymptomatic with less than 80% stenosis should consider medical management in the elderly population. Medical management includes blood pressure control, lipid control, and antiplatelet therapy.

20. **d.** Carotid artery studies report that in asymptomatic patients with a high-grade carotid artery stenosis, a CEA in combination with aspirin therapy and risk factor reduction lowers the relative risk of stroke compared to medical therapy alone.

21. **c.** A lumbar puncture should be done in any patient considered to have a subarachnoid hemorrhage when a CT scan is not diagnostic. It should be performed in patients suspected of having infective endocarditis, meningitis, or inflammatory vasculitis, searching for the presence of cerebrospinal fluid leukocytosis.

22. **a.** Transesophageal echocardiography is preferred for the evaluation of cardiogenic emboli.

23. **c.** Magnetic resonance angiography is indicated if one is considering emergent thrombolytic therapy to reverse stroke progression. Treatment must be initiated within 3 hours of onset of symptoms, and therapy doubles the chances of a favorable outcome at 3 months. The benefits must be weighed against the increased risk of intracranial hemorrhage in the elderly population.

24. **d.** Venous thromboembolism is a common complication following acute ischemic stroke. Enoxaparin is preferable to unfractionated heparin for the prevention of venous thromboembolism following acute ischemic stroke.

Solution to the Clinical Case Management Problem

1. Transient ischemic attack: A disturbance of the cerebrovascular system in which neurologic symptoms both appear and then disappear within 24 hours.
2. Stroke-in-evolution: The typical course of a thrombotic stroke. This is also known as a progressive stroke. It is best defined as an intermittent progression of a neurologic deficit over hours to days.
3. Completed stroke: A CVA that has reached its maximum destructiveness in producing neurologic deficits, although cerebral edema may not have reached its maximum.

Summary

1. Incidence: There has been a very significant decrease during the past 15 years because of better control of hypertension.

2. Pathologic classification (in order of frequency): (a) thrombotic stroke, (b) embolic stroke, (c) hemorrhagic stroke, (d) lacunar stroke, and (e) subarachnoid hemorrhage.

3. Risk factors for CVA: (a) Hypertension is the most important risk factor, (b) there is no longer any such entity as mild hypertension, and (c) see also answer 17.

4. Classification of CVAs: See the Solution to the Clinical Case Management Problem.

   It is important to evaluate and workup for TIAs. Research on the benefits of CEA and aspirin/antiplatelet therapy in preventing future TIAs or strokes is reviewed in answers 13 and 19.

5. Signs/symptoms: See details on arteries in answers 2, 8, 9, and 12.

6. Investigations/treatment: These include (a) history; (b) physical exam; (c) MRI angio or CT; (d) if not hemorrhagic and if not a completed stroke, consider heparin followed by warfarin; if it is already complete, do not follow this approach; (e) cerebral edema may become a major problem and corticosteroid therapy may be required; (f) unless contraindicated, all patients with TIAs, history of stroke, and risk factors for stroke (major) should be on aspirin prophylaxis; and (g) rehabilitation (aggressive, early, and forceful).

7. Concomitant conditions: Depression is the most important coexisting or concomitant condition. Remember that this applies to both the patient and the patient's caregiver.

8. The biopsychosocial model of illness: Few diseases are as devastating to a patient and a patient's family as stroke. Often, the person who gets lost in the ordeal is the spouse. Please remember the spouse.

9. Prevention
   a. TREAT hypertension aggressively.
   b. Treat obesity and sedentary lifestyle aggressively.
   c. Stop smoking.
   d. Remember, an aspirin a day keeps the neurologist away.

   e. Ramipril, an angiotensin-converting enzyme inhibitor, provides an early and powerful reduction in risk of stroke regardless of patient type or initial blood pressure.

   f. Statins reduce average risk of stroke by 25%. However, this reduction varies by risk stratification: There will be one fewer stroke in every 2778 low-risk patient using statins versus one fewer stroke in every 617 high-risk patient (those with preexisting cardiovascular disease).

10. Acute ischemic stroke: Blood pressure should never be lowered too quickly. In extreme cases (systolic >220 mmHg), gradual reduction to 180 mmHg should be undertaken. Intravascular volume should be maintained, and in some cases cerebral edema should be controlled with mannitol. For patients with a cerebellar infarction, neurosurgical consultation should be sought because of the risk of brain stem compression.

    Thrombolysis: For patients with ischemic deficits of less than 3 hours' duration, with no hemorrhage on CT scanning, thrombolysis with recombinant tissue plasminogen activator may be helpful. It is important to weigh the risk:benefit ratio in the elderly to lower the risk of hemorrhagic stroke associated with thrombolysis.

    Anticoagulation: Heparin is generally used when atherogenic vascular stenosis or occlusion is suspected (crescendo symptoms, unstable TIA, or posterior circulation involvement). Give for 2 to 5 days with PTT at two times normal.

    Catheter-based interventions: These are under study for acute ischemic stroke at large centers. Whether these will prove beneficial compared with standard thrombolytic therapy remains to be determined. Access to such services within appropriate time windows of opportunity will be an issue for a large part of the population if these methods prove effective.

11. Venous thromboembolism is a common complication following acute ischemic stroke. Enoxaparin is preferable to unfractionated heparin for the prevention of venous thromboembolism following acute ischemic stroke.

Suggested Reading

American Geriatric Society: *Geriatric Review Syllabus, A Core Curriculum in Geriatric Medicine*, 6th ed. Chicago: American Geriatric Society, 2006, pp. 458–461.

Bosch J, Yusuf S, Pogue J, et al: Use of ramipril in preventing stroke: Double blind randomised trial. *BMJ* 324:1–5, 2002.

Briel M, Studer M, Glass TR, et al: Effects of statins on stroke prevention in patients with and without coronary heart disease: A meta-analysis of randomized controlled trials. *Am J Med* 117:596–606, 2004.

Dickerson LM, Carek PJ, Quattelbaum RG: Prevention of recurrent ischemic stroke. *Am Fam Physician* 76:382–389, 2007.

Lees KR, Dawson J: Advances in emerging therapies 2006. *Stroke* 38(2):219–221, 2007.

Reuben D, Herr K, Pacala J, et al: *Geriatrics at Your Fingertips: 2006–2007*, 8th ed. New York: The American Geriatrics Society, 2006, pp. 137–138.

Sherman DG, Albers GW, Bladin C, et al: The efficacy and safety of enoxaparin versus unfractionated heparin for the prevention of venous thromboembolism after acute ischaemic stroke (PREVAIL Study): An open-label randomised comparison. *Lancet* 369: 1347–1355, 2007.

CHAPTER

136 Depression in the Elderly

CLINICAL CASE PROBLEM 1

*An 85-Year-Old Female Nursing Home
Resident Who Simply "Stares into Space"
and Cries Almost All the Time*

You are called to see an 85-year-old patient who moved into a nursing home 9 months ago. Previously, she was living on her own and had managed by herself since the death of her husband 6 years ago. During the past year, she has become increasingly disabled with congestive heart failure and osteoarthritis. During the past 9 months, the patient has lost 15 pounds, has not been hungry, has lost interest in all of her social activities, and has been crying almost every day. You are aware that before moving into the nursing home she was quite active.

Her mental status examination is difficult. She does, however, describe her mood as being worse in the morning. According to the staff, her short-term memory is impaired. She is currently taking furosemide and enalapril for her congestive heart failure and acetaminophen for the pain associated with osteoarthritis.

SELECT THE BEST ANSWER TO THE FOLLOWING QUESTIONS

1. What is the most likely diagnosis in this patient?
   a. major depressive illness
   b. Alzheimer's disease
   c. multi-infarct dementia
   d. hypothyroidism
   e. none of the above

2. Regarding the diagnosis of the patient described, which of the following statements is false?
   a. this condition occurs less often in older patients than in younger patients
   b. elderly patients are less likely to recover from this illness than young adults
   c. this condition is more common among institutionalized elders than elders living at home
   d. this condition may be related to physical illness
   e. this condition may be related to the move into the nursing home

3. Which of the following investigations and/or assessments should be performed in the patient described?
   a. medication review
   b. complete blood count (CBC)
   c. serum thyroid-stimulating hormone (TSH) level
   d. all of the above
   e. none of the above

4. Which of the following antidepressants is considered an agent of first choice for the treatment of depression in the elderly?
   a. imipramine
   b. nortriptyline
   c. desipramine
   d. amitriptyline
   e. fluoxetine

5. Which of the following antidepressants specifically blocks serotonin reuptake?
   a. imipramine
   b. desipramine
   c. nortriptyline
   d. amitriptyline
   e. fluoxetine

6. You decide to treat the patient with fluoxetine (Prozac). In a patient of this age, at what daily dosage would you start her?
   a. 5 mg
   b. 25 mg
   c. 50 mg
   d. 75 mg
   e. 100 mg

7. Regarding the treatment for the condition described, which of the following statements is (are) true?
   a. electroconvulsive therapy (ECT) is unlikely to be of any benefit in the treatment of this condition
   b. socialization, music therapy, and pet therapy have no role to play in the treatment of this condition
   c. cognitive and behavioral therapy may significantly improve this condition
   d. all of the above statements are true
   e. none of the above statements are true

8. Which of the following features is most commonly associated with this diagnosis in geriatric patients?
   a. acute mania
   b. hypomania
   c. extreme anxiety
   d. psychomotor agitation or retardation
   e. hypersomnia

9. The signs and symptoms of the condition described include all except which of the following?
   a. impaired concentration
   b. guilt
   c. hopelessness
   d. suicidal ideation
   e. violent or aggressive behavior

10. The length of time recommended for the pharmacologic treatment of this condition with the drug selected is at least
    a. 1 month
    b. 3 months
    c. 6 months
    d. 12 months
    e. 18 months

11. An elderly institutionalized patient is put on nortriptyline. The dose is increased up to 100 mg but no improvement is noted. You decide to substitute fluoxetine. Which of the following side effects might you anticipate with the use of fluoxetine?
    a. constipation
    b. blurred vision
    c. urinary retention
    d. dry mouth
    e. agitation

12. If the side effect selected in question 11 occurred, which of the following courses of action would be the most reasonable?
    a. increase the dose of the drug
    b. decrease the dose of the drug
    c. stop the drug
    d. elect ECT as your next option
    e. c and d

13. The prevalence of depression in elderly patients in a primary care clinic is approximately
    a. 6% to 10%
    b. 10% to 15%
    c. 20% to 25%
    d. 30% to 35%

14. Characteristics of depression in the elderly that differ from those of younger patients include which of the following?
    a. more somatic complaints
    b. report depressed mood less frequently
    c. report feeling guilty less frequently
    d. all of the above
    e. none of the above

15. Serotonin syndrome, which may lead to delirium and hyperthermia, is associated with the use of selective serotonin reuptake inhibitors (SSRIs) and what other medication(s)?
    a. monoamine oxidase inhibitors
    b. meperidine
    c. tricyclic antidepressants
    d. all of the above
    e. a and b

16. On the Geriatric Depression Scale, a score of what value is considered positive for depression?
    a. less than 5
    b. 5 to 15
    c. 20 to 25
    d. 25 to 30

17. According to the *Diagnostic and Statistical Manual of Mental Disorders*, 4th edition (*DSM-IV*) criteria for depression, a patient must have five or more symptoms for more than 2 weeks to be diagnosed with depression. These five symptoms must include which of the following?
    a. depressed mood
    b. weight loss
    c. loss of interest or pleasure
    d. a and c
    e. b and c

Clinical Case Management Problem

Part A: Discuss the differential diagnosis of depressive symptoms in the elderly.

Part B: List the three most common physical illnesses that present or manifest depression in the elderly.

Part C: Name the most common drug associated with depression in the elderly.

Part D: Name the most common drug class associated with depression as a psychoactive substance use disorder.

Answers

1. **a.** This patient has a major depressive illness. A mnemonic that is very helpful for diagnosing depression is **A SIG: E CAPS:**

   Affect: at least a 2-week period of a depressed mood or a depressed affect

   Sleep disturbance (hyposomnia, insomnia, and hypersomnia)

Interest (lack of interest in life)
Guilt or hopelessness
Energy level (decreased) or fatigue
Concentration decreased
Appetite disturbance (decreased or increased with or without weight gain or weight loss)
Psychomotor retardation or agitation
Suicidal ideation

Major depressive illness is diagnosed when there are four of eight criteria present and there is at least a 2-week period of a depressed mood or depressed affect. Despite these criteria, depression in elderly patients is more likely to occur with weight loss and less likely to occur with feelings of worthlessness and guilt. Elderly patients are no more likely than people in midlife to report cognitive problems, although they do have more difficulties with cognition during an episode of depression.

2. b. Elderly patients are just as likely to recover from a major depressive illness as are younger adults. Major depression is less prevalent among those age 65 years or older than in younger groups. However, suicide is not; it continues to increase in elderly patients at an alarming rate.

The prevalence of major depression in elderly patients in the community is between 1% and 2%. In long-term chronic care facilities, the prevalence of major depressive illness may be as high as 10% to 20%. The majority of depressed elderly patients, however, do not fit the *DSM-IV* criteria but, rather, have depressive symptoms that are associated with an adjustment reaction (as in this patient, who has just had to leave her own home) or that are associated with significant physical illness (as this patient also demonstrates).

3. d. The elderly patient with depressive symptoms should have the following evaluations: a complete history, a complete physical examination, and a complete medication review (both prescribed and over-the-counter medications). Some of the most common pharmacologic agents that contribute to depression include antihypertensive agents, such as propranolol and methyldopa, and cimetidine and sedative hypnotic drugs. In addition to the complete history and physical examination, the elderly patient should also have the following laboratory investigations: CBC, vitamin B_{12}, serum folate level, serum TSH, chest x-ray, electrocardiogram (ECG), complete urinalysis, and serum electrolytes.

4. e. SSRIs should be considered medications of choice for depression in the elderly. This is especially

true for patients with medical problems such as heart conduction defects, ischemic heart disease, prostatic hyperplasia, or uncontrolled glaucoma. Consider venlafaxine (Effexor), mirtazapine (Remeran), and bupropion (Welbutrin and Zyban) as second-line medications and nortriptyline or desipramine as third line.

5. e. The group of antidepressant agents known as SSRIs includes fluoxetine (Prozac), fluvoxamine (Luvox), sertraline (Zoloft), and paroxetine (Paxil). These drugs are considered first choice for the treatment of depression in the elderly. They offer some significant theoretic advantages in that the common tricyclic antidepressant side effects, such as dry mouth, blurred vision, tachycardia, constipation (anticholinergic), orthostatic hypotension (α-adrenergic blockade), and weight gain, may be averted by their use. They do not increase the cardiac risk caused by blockade of impulse conduction through the atrioventricular node.

6. a. The patient described in this case, an 80-year-old female, should be started on as low a dose of an SSRI as possible. A dose of 5 mg of fluoxetine would be an ideal starting dose. This dose could be increased slowly as needed to a maximum of 80 mg/day.

7. c. Elderly patients with depressive illness may be significantly improved with cognitive or behavioral psychotherapy. Attempts at increased socialization (especially in chronic care facilities) including music therapy, pet therapy, and other therapies that serve to redirect the attention of the elderly patient appear to be effective in the treatment of depression in the elderly.

ECT may be the only effective therapy for severe depression in elderly patients, especially in patients with psychotic depression. ECT is well tolerated in geriatric patients. Indications include severe depression when a rapid response is necessary and when depression is resistant to drug therapy; it is also indicated for patients unable to tolerate antidepressants or who have psychotic depression, severe catatonia, or depression with Parkinson's disease. Contraindications to ECT include an intracranial mass, recent myocardial infarction, or a recent cardiovascular accident.

8. d. Although acute mania, hypomania, extreme anxiety, and hypersomnia may all be associated with depression in elderly patients, by far the most common symptom of those listed in elderly patients is psychomotor agitation or retardation. Psychomotor agitation is the more common presentation of the two.

9. **e.** The diagnostic symptoms of depressive illness were discussed in answer 1. They do not include violent or aggressive behavior. If violent or aggressive behavior is found in a patient who has an underlying depression, there is likely another major diagnosis that would explain the symptom. In an elder, the most common diagnosis in this case would be Alzheimer's disease.

10. **c.** Geriatric patients should be treated with antidepressants for at least 6 months. After 6 months, if the patient is improved, the drug can be tapered and eventually discontinued.

11. **e.** The side effects of blurred vision, dry mouth, urinary retention, and constipation are all anticholinergic side effects that do not occur with the new SSRIs. Agitation, however, is a side effect that

may be anticipated with these drugs, especially with fluoxetine.

12. **e.** The most reasonable course of action would be to discontinue the drug and to use ECT. Two failed drug courses (with drugs of different classes) would be a reasonable indication for the use of ECT.

13. **a.** This prevalence increases in nursing home settings to approximately 12% to 20%.

14. **d.** If an elderly patient does not admit to feelings of sadness, then ask about interest or lack of interest in activities (anhedonia). If the patient is anhedonic, he or she is most likely depressed.

15. **e.** Both MAOIs and meperidine can cause serotonin syndrome.

16. **b.** The Geriatric Depression Scale is based on 15 questions. A score of 5 or higher is indicative of depression.

17. **a.** Depressed mood must be present.

Solution to the Clinical Case Management Problem

Part A
The differential diagnosis of depressive symptoms in the elderly is lengthy. It includes four major categories: mood disorders, adjustment disorders, psychoactive substance use disorders, and somatoform disorders.

1. Mood disorders: (a) major depression (single episode or recurrent); (b) dysthymia (or depressive neurosis); (c) bipolar affective disorder, depressed; and (d) depressive disorder not otherwise specified (atypical depression with mild biogenic depression)
2. Adjustment disorders: (a) primary degenerative dementia with associated depression; (b) organic mood disorder, depressed; (c) secondary to physical illness (hypothyroidism, carcinoma of the pancreas, stroke, and Parkinson's disease); and (d) secondary to pharmacologic agents (methyldopa and propranolol)
3. Psychoactive substance use disorders: (a) alcohol use or dependence and (b) sedative, hypnotic, or anxiolytic abuse or dependence

4. Somatoform disorders: hypochondriasis and somatization disorder

Part B
The three most common physical illnesses that present or manifest depression in the elderly are hypothyroidism, carcinoma of the pancreas, and cerebrovascular accident (stroke).

Part C
The most common drug associated with depression in the elderly is propranolol.

Part D
The most common drug class associated with depression is the psychoactive substance use class. This drug class includes all of the sedative–hypnotics. Sedatives and hypnotics are vastly overused in the elderly; this appears to be especially true in institutionalized elderly patients. It is much easier for nursing home staff to prescribe a sedative or hypnotic or both than to recognize and help an elder adjust to altered sleep patterns.

Summary

1. Diagnosis: Follow *DSM-IV* criteria, but recognize that the elderly are more likely to experience weight loss and cognitive problems and less likely to experience feelings of guilt and hopelessness.

2. Recognize that depression is often an adjustment reaction to life stress, environment change (especially having to leave home), and the realization of the effects of aging.

3. Prevalence: Depression prevalence is 1% or 2% in community environment and 10% to 20% in an institutional environment. Some studies suggest a much higher prevalence of 50% in an institutional environment.

4. Differential diagnosis includes mood disorders, adjustment disorders, organic mental disorders, psychoactive substance use, and somatoform disorders.

5. Investigations include Mini-Mental Status Examination; complete medication review; and laboratory evaluation including CBC, electrolytes, TSH, vitamin B_{12}, serum folate, ECG, and chest x-ray.

6. Treatment strategies
   a. Nonpharmacologic strategies include the following: (i) relaxation techniques and mind-occupying techniques such as frequent visitors, pet therapy, and music therapy; and (ii) cognitive, supportive, and behavioral psychotherapy.
   b. Pharmacologic strategies include the following: (i) Drugs of first choice are SSRIs; (ii) drugs of second choice are venlafaxine, mirtazapine, and buproprion; (iii) drugs of third choice are MAOIs; and (iv) if two drug classes fail, ECT should be considered. ECT has much more of a role to play in geriatric depression than it does in depression associated with younger patients. Before performing ECT, do a chest x-ray, ECG, serum electrolytes, and cardiac exam (may need stress test and electroencephalogram if indicated).

   Most important, depression in the elderly must not be treated with pharmacologic agents only; instead, treatment should include an equal contribution from nonpharmacologic treatments and pharmacologic agents.

Suggested Reading

American Geriatric Society: *Geriatric Review Syllabus, A Core Curriculum in Geriatric Medicine*, 6th ed. Chicago: American Geriatric Society, 2006, pp. 269–279.

Birrer RB, Vemuri SP: Depression in later life: A diagnostic and therapeutic challenge. *Am Fam Physician* 69(10):2375–2382, 2004.
Skultety KM, Zeiss A: The treatment of depression in older adults in the primary care setting: An evidence-based review. *Health Psychol* 25(6):665–674, 2006.

CHAPTER

137 Dementia and Delirium

CLINICAL CASE PROBLEM 1

A 78-Year-Old Female with Increasing Confusion, Impairment of Memory, and Inability to Look after Herself

A 78-year-old female is brought to your office by her daughter. The patient lives alone in an apartment, and her daughter is concerned about her ability to carry on living independently. Her daughter tells you that her mother began having difficulty with her memory 2 years ago, and since that time she has deteriorated in a slow, steady manner.

However, she is not totally incapacitated. She is able to perform some of the activities of daily living, including dressing and bathing. When she cooks for herself, however, she often leaves burners on, and when she drives the car she often gets lost. She has had four motor vehicle accidents in the past 3 months. Her daughter became alarmed when she learned that her mother had gone to the bank and withdrawn the entire contents of her $80,000 savings account to "give to her new boyfriend." She had asked for the entire amount in $1 bills and argued with the bank teller upon learning that this was impossible.

The daughter states that her mother's memory and confusion have been getting worse. Her personality has changed; her kind and caring mother now displays periods of both agitation and aggression.

On examination, the patient's Mini-Mental Status Examination (MMSE) is 15/30. Her blood pressure is 170/95 mmHg, and her pulse is 84 beats/minute and irregular. There is a grade II/VI systolic heart murmur heard along the left sternal edge. Examination of the respiratory system is normal. Examination of the abdomen is normal. Digital rectal examination reveals some hard stool. A detailed neurologic and musculoskeletal examination cannot be carried out because the patient could not follow instructions.

SELECT THE BEST ANSWER TO THE FOLLOWING QUESTIONS

1. Based on this history, what is the most likely diagnosis in this patient?
   a. Alzheimer's disease
   b. vascular dementia
   c. major depressive disorder
   d. hypothyroidism
   e. mixed dementia

2. At this time, what would you do?
   a. order an appropriate cost-effective laboratory investigation
   b. arrange for the patient to be admitted to a chronic care facility and placate the daughter
   c. prescribe diazepam for the daughter and haloperidol for the patient
   d. refer the patient for immediate consultation with a geriatrician
   e. begin a trial of a tricyclic antidepressant

3. Which of the following diseases is the most common treatable disease confused with Alzheimer's disease in elderly patients?
   a. hypothyroidism
   b. vascular dementia
   c. congestive heart failure
   d. major depressive disorder
   e. normal pressure hydrocephalus

4. Which of the following statements regarding Alzheimer's disease is true?
   a. Alzheimer's disease is present to some degree in all people older than 80 years
   b. Alzheimer's disease is a rapidly progressive dementia
   c. Alzheimer's disease is easy to differentiate from other dementias
   d. Alzheimer's disease is a pathologic diagnosis
   e. Alzheimer's disease usually has a sudden onset

5. In contrast to dementia, patients with depression often:
   a. complain about their cognitive deficits
   b. deny that their cognitive deficits exist
   c. try to conceal their cognitive deficits
   d. try to answer questions even if they do not know the answers
   e. perform consistently on tasks of equal difficulty

6. In contrast to dementia, the cognitive impairment associated with depression often
   a. comes on more slowly
   b. comes on more rapidly
   c. is less of an impairment
   d. is not improved with the administration of an antidepressant
   e. none of the above are true

7. Diagnostic criteria for delirium include which of the following?
   a. disturbed consciousness
   b. cognitive change
   c. rapid onset and fluctuating course
   d. evidence of a causal physical condition
   e. all of the above

8. A cost-effective workup of 2 years of slowly progressive confusion in an elderly, otherwise well patient does not include which of the following?
   a. a complete blood count (CBC)
   b. an electrolyte profile
   c. a plasma glucose level
   d. a computed tomography (CT) scan of the head
   e. all of the above investigations are cost-effective

9. After a complete dementia workup, you are unsure whether or not a patient has Alzheimer's disease or a major depressive disorder. At this time, what would you do?
   a. reexamine the patient in 3 months
   b. suggest a trial of electroconvulsive therapy
   c. arrange for the patient to be admitted to a nursing home and begin supportive psychotherapy
   d. prescribe a trial of an antidepressant
   e. none of the above

10. Which of the following is (are) an important aspect(s) of dementia management?
    a. maintenance of a daily routine
    b. making the environment safe
    c. assessment of family support
    d. minimization of external stimuli
    e. all of the above

11. Elderly patients frequently develop "acute confusional states." Acute confusional states are also known as which of the following?
    a. dementia
    b. delusional states
    c. delirium
    d. pseudodementia
    e. pseudodelirium

12. What is the most common cause of dementia in the elderly?
    a. drug-induced dementia
    b. Lewy body dementia
    c. pseudodementia
    d. Alzheimer's disease
    e. Vascular dementia

13. What is the most common symptom and finding in patients with Alzheimer's disease?
    a. a progressive decline in intellectual function
    b. memory loss
    c. impairment in judgment
    d. impairment in problem solving
    e. impaired orientation

14. What is the most important risk factor for a patient acquiring Alzheimer's disease?
    a. history of head injury
    b. history of thyroid disease
    d. family history of dementia
    e. history of psychiatric disease

15. Characteristics of Lewy body dementia include which of the following?
    a. gradual onset
    b. fluctuating symptoms
    c. symptoms of parkinsonism
    d. gradual onset but faster than that of Alzheimer's disease
    e. all of the above
    f. a, b, and c

16. What is (are) the histologic criteria for diagnosing Alzheimer's disease postmortem?
    a. senile plaques
    b. neuronal loss
    c. neurofibrillary tangles (NFTs)
    d. a and c
    e. all of the above

17. What pharmaceutical agent(s) represent(s) the best choice for treatment of Alzheimer's disease?
    a. tacrine (Cognex)
    b. donepezil (Aricept)
    c. galantamine (Reminyl)
    d. rivastigmine (Exelon)
    e. b, c, and d

18. The main predisposing factors for delirium include which of the following?
    a. age older than 65 years
    b. brain damage
    c. chronic cerebral disease
    d. b and c
    e. a, b, and c

19. The best documented hypothesis for delirium suggests which of the following?
    a. serotonin deficiency
    b. norepinephrine deficiency
    c. acetylcholine deficiency
    d. dopamine deficiency
    e. catecholamine imbalance

20. What is the most important investigation for patients suspected of having delirium?
    a. CT scan of the head
    b. magnetic resonance imaging scan of the head
    c. electroencephalogram
    d. positron emission tomography scan
    e. CBC

21. Characteristics of mild cognitive impairment include which of the following?
    a. a report by the patient (or informant) of memory loss
    b. mild abnormal memory performance for age (typically MMSE score of 24 to 28)
    c. normal general cognition
    d. normal activities or daily living
    e. all of the above

22. The use of memantine in the treatment of Alzheimer's disease is indicated for which of the following?
    a. early onset senile dementia Alzheimer's type (SDAT)
    b. mild cognitive impairment
    c. moderate cognitive impairment
    d. severe SDAT
    e. c and d

23. Two risk factors for Alzheimer's disease are age and family history. For late-onset SDAT, which apolipoprotein E (ApoE) gene on chromosome 19 is most likely to result in the disease?
    a. ApoE-2
    b. ApoE-3
    c. ApoE-4
    d. none of the above

Clinical Case Management Problem

Part A: Using the mnemonic DEMENTIA and selecting at least one cause (but in some cases many causes) for each letter, construct a complete differential diagnosis of confusion in the elderly.

Part B: List and briefly describe the distinct disorders that are part of the differential diagnosis of delirium.

Answers

1. **a.** The most likely diagnosis is Alzheimer's disease. The slow, insidious course of the decline is much more characteristic of Alzheimer's disease than of any other dementive process.

Multi-infarct dementia, in contrast, tends to produce a stepwise decline, with each step (or each decline) being temporally related to a small infarct.

Major depressive disorder tends to come on rather abruptly. This is discussed in detail in Chapter 136 and with specific relevance to the geriatric patient in answers 5 and 6. Hypothyroidism must always be considered as a reversible cause of dementia, but in this case this is an unlikely cause of the symptoms.

Dementia is characterized by evidence of short-term and long-term memory impairment with impaired abstract thinking, impaired judgment, disturbances of higher cortical thinking, and personality changes. In Alzheimer's disease, short-term memory is impaired before long-term memory; consequently, patients present with repetitive thoughts or questions, forgetting daily events or people they have know for years. It is not uncommon for the "house" this patient mentioned to be the one she lived in as a child.

2. **a.** Alzheimer's disease is a diagnosis of exclusion. Before a patient is labeled as having Alzheimer's disease, a complete history, a complete physical examination, and a cost-effective laboratory evaluation need to be performed. It is inappropriate to arrange care in a chronic care facility and to treat patients (even with an antidepressant) until a dementia workup has been done.

An appropriate cost-effective workup of dementia includes a complete history, a complete physical examination (including a neuropsychiatric evaluation), a CBC, a blood glucose, serum electrolytes, serum calcium, serum creatinine, and serum thyroid-stimulating hormone. Other tests should be done only if there is a specific indication (e.g., vitamin B_{12} and folate if macrocytosis is present). A CT or MRI should be considered if the onset of dementia is before the age of 65 years, symptoms have occurred for less than 2 years, there is evidence of focal or asymmetrical neurological deficits, the clinical picture indicates normal pressure hydrocephalus, or there is a recent history of fall or other head trauma. If a patient has a history of cancer or is on anticoagulation therapy, then neuroimaging should also be considered.

3. **d.** The most common treatable disease confused with Alzheimer's disease in elderly patients is depression. It has been estimated that up to 15% of patients who are labeled with Alzheimer's disease actually have a major depressive disorder. Many more patients with Alzheimer's disease have depression as a clinical feature of the disease. Depression, whether the primary diagnosis or a diagnosis secondary to Alzheimer's disease, will respond to pharmacotherapy and psychotherapy.

4. **d.** Alzheimer's disease is a pathologic diagnosis. The prevalence of Alzheimer's disease increases with age to approximately 30% in patients older than age 80 years. It is certainly not present in all patients of any age.

The clinical progression of Alzheimer's disease is usually slow and insidious, not rapidly progressive. It is an acquired decline in memory and at the least one other cognitive function (language, visual spatial, and executive) sufficient to affect daily life in an alert person.

It is not easy to differentiate Alzheimer's disease from other conditions or other entities. Because of the slow and insidious onset of the disease, it often goes unnoticed by both friends and family.

5. **a.** In contrast to patients with dementia, depressed patients often complain about their cognitive deficits.

6. **b.** Also in contrast to dementia, the cognitive impairment associated with depression usually comes on rapidly. It is apparent that something is wrong. Other features that suggest depression include the following: (1) a personal or family history of psychiatric illness (especially major depressive disorder), bipolar affective disorder, and alcoholism; (2) depressive symptoms preceding cognitive changes (depressed mood, loss of interest or pleasure in activities, weight loss or gain, difficulty sleeping, etc.); (3) feelings of hopelessness, guilt, and worthlessness; and (4) a poor affect on psychologic testing.

7. **e.** The *Diagnostic and Statistical Manual of Mental Disorders*, 4th edition (*DSM-IV*), criteria for the diagnosis of delirium include the following (this scheme is expanded in the Solution to the Clinical Case Management Problem): (1) a disturbed level of consciousness, such as a decreased attention span or lack of environmental awareness; (2) cognitive change, such as a memory deficit, disorientation, or language disturbance, possibly also including visual illusions or hallucination; (3) rapid onset within hours or days with a fluctuating course; and (4) evidence of a causal physical condition.

8. **d.** See answer 2.

9. **d.** A cautious trial of an antidepressant can be both a diagnostic test and a therapeutic trial because (1) it can often be difficult to differentiate a dementia from a depression; (2) a dementia may have, as part of its symptomatology, depressive symptoms; and (3) depression is reversible, whereas dementia is not.

Selective serotonin reuptake inhibitors are the most commonly used agents for the geriatric patient. They are considered the first-line choice for older patients, especially patients with heart conduction defects or ischemic disease, prostatic hyperplasia, or uncontrolled glaucoma. Second-line choices include buproprion, mirtazapine, or venlafaxine. Third-line choices include nortriptyline or desipramine. These can be used for severe melancholic depression.

In an elderly patient, you want to (1) maximize the benefit from the antidepressant without producing an adverse drug reaction; (2) start low and go slow; and (3) select an agent that has low anticholinergic, α-adrenergic, and antihistaminic side effects.

10. e. The management of dementia in the elderly involves both behavioral methods and pharmacologic methods. Regarding behavioral management, the following four principles apply to all elderly patients with a dementia-like syndrome:

1. External stimuli (especially external stimuli that may confuse, worry, or upset the elder) should be kept to a minimum.
2. A daily routine that does not vary by any significant degree should be established and maintained.
3. The environmental safety of the particular residence or facility should be maximized. This includes attention to the maximization of lighting in the home or facility, the minimization of significant noise or distractions, the installation of handrails in hallways and rooms and at bathtub edges, and the minimization of stairs in the living accommodations of the patient.
4. Support the elder's family and offer respite care where and when needed.

11. c. Delirium is often referred to as an acute confusional state (see answer 9).

12. d. The most common cause of dementia in the elderly is Alzheimer's disease, which represents approximately two-thirds of all dementing syndromes. Vascular dementia represents 15% to 25 % and Lewy body dementia is thought to represent approximately the same. The wording is important in this question. Drugs do not cause dementia; they cause delirium. The other choice, pseudodementia, is really a misnomer. Pseudodementia really represents depression that has been incorrectly diagnosed as an irreversible dementia.

13. b. Memory loss is the most common presenting feature of Alzheimer's disease, but a personality change

or an impairment in the ability to perform intellectual tasks such as calculations may herald the onset.

The five major clinical manifestations of Alzheimer's disease are as follows:

1. Memory loss: Initially, the memory loss is a loss for recent events only and is associated with an inability to learn new information. Recall of past events and previously acquired information becomes impaired at a somewhat later stage. Memory loss is the most common presenting feature of Alzheimer's disease.
2. Language impairment: Language impairment is also common among patients with Alzheimer's disease. The term *anomia*, or "word-finding difficulty," often begins with the onset of dementia. This feature usually progresses to a transcortical, sensory-like aphasia. Severe language disturbance is a poor prognostic feature of Alzheimer's disease.
3. Visuospatial disturbance: Patients with Alzheimer's disease are often characterized by a difficulty in getting around the neighborhood or house. Practical examples of visuospatial disturbances in patients with Alzheimer's disease include difficulty following directions and getting lost in a familiar place or in familiar surroundings.
4. Loss of interest in activities: The loss of interest in activities such as personal habits or community affairs parallels the intellectual decline previously discussed. This may be Alzheimer's disease first and an accompanying depression second or a primary depression manifesting itself as Alzheimer's disease.
5. Delusions and hallucinations: Delusions and hallucinations are prevalent in patients with Alzheimer's disease and tend to indicate a poor prognosis.

14. d. A family history of Alzheimer's disease is an important risk in acquiring Alzheimer's disease, especially at a younger age. Advanced age is also a risk factor, with more than 30% of those older than 85 years developing some degree of Alzheimer's disease.

15. e. The characteristics of Lewy body dementia include a gradual onset but faster than that of Alzheimer's disease, memory impairment, visuospatial impairment, hallucinations, fluctuating symptoms, parkinsonism, normal laboratory tests, and possible global atrophy.

16. d. Alzheimer's disease really is a pathologic diagnosis. The National Institute on Aging's diagnostic criteria for this disease are as follows:

The quantity of senile plaques (age-specific): Senile plaques are microscopic lesions composed of a significant percentage of amyloid.

The quantity of NFTs (age-specific): NFTs, initially described in 1907, are neuronal cytoplasmic collections of tangled filaments present in abundance in the neocortex, hippocampus, amygdala, basal forebrain, substantia nigra, locus ceruleus, and other brain stem nuclei.

Although these are the two criteria on which the diagnosis of Alzheimer's disease is based, the following is a complete list of all of the microscopic lesions seen in the brain of a patient with Alzheimer's disease: (1) neuritic plaques, (2) NFTs, (3) amyloid degeneration, and (4) neuronal loss.

Most patients with Alzheimer's disease have a slight reduction in total brain weight, with the majority ranging from 900 to 1100 g. Mild to moderate cerebral atrophy is often present.

17. e. The primary treatment for Alzheimer's patients includes the use of the cholinesterase inhibitors donepezil, galantamine, and exelon. Patients with a diagnosis of mild or moderate Alzheimer's disease should receive these medications, which will increase the level of acetylcholine in the brain. Only 25% of patients taking cholinesterase inhibitors show improvement, but 80% have a less rapid decline. Benefits include cognition, mood, behavioral symptoms, and daily function. Because of hepatic toxicity, tacrine would not be considered as first-line treatment.

18. e. Delirium (acute confusional state) is caused by one or more organic factors that bring about widespread cerebral dysfunction. The factors associated with delirium can be divided into the following subcategories:

Predisposing factors: (a) older than age 65 years, (b) brain damage, and (c) chronic cerebral disease (e.g., Alzheimer's disease)
Facilitating factors: (a) psychologic stress, (b) sleep loss or sleep deprivation, and (c) sensory deprivation or sensory overload
Precipitating (organic) causal factors: (a) primary cerebral diseases; (b) systemic diseases affecting the brain secondarily, such as metabolic encephalopathies, neoplasms, infections, cardiovascular diseases, and collagen vascular diseases; (c) intoxication with exogenous substances, such as medical drugs, recreational drugs, and poisons of plant, animal, or industrial origin; and (d) withdrawal from substances of abuse, such as alcohol and sedative–hypnotic drugs

One of the most common causes of delirium in the elderly is intoxication with anticholinergic drugs, such as tricyclic antidepressants given in doses that would be appropriate for a younger adult but not for a frail elderly patient.

The following are other common causes: (1) congestive cardiac failure, (2) pneumonia, (3) urinary tract infection, (4) cancer, (5) uremia, (6) hypokalemia, (7) dehydration, (8) hyponatremia, (9) epilepsy, and (10) cerebral infarction (right hemisphere).

Risk factors for delirium in hospitalized elderly patients include the following: (1) urinary tract infections, (2) low serum albumin levels, (3) elevated white blood cell count, (4) proteinuria, (5) prior cognitive impairment, (6) limb fracture on admission, (7) symptomatic infective disease, (8) neuroleptic drugs, (9) narcotic drugs, and (10) anticholinergic drugs.

19. c. The best documented hypothesis for delirium in the elderly suggests that the syndrome results from a widespread imbalance of neurotransmitters. It is postulated that there is a reduction in brain metabolism that results in diminished cortical function. Impairment of cerebral oxidative metabolism results in reduced synthesis of neurotransmitters, especially acetylcholine, whose relative deficiency in the brain is a common denominator in metabolic–toxic encephalopathies. Hypoxia and hypoglycemia impair acetylcholine metabolism and bring about changes in mental function. The inhibition of acetylcholine metabolism may be caused by calcium-dependent release of the neurotransmitter. Thus, the cholinergic deficit is currently the most convincing pathogenic hypothesis of delirium. Numerous experimental studies have shown that the syndrome can be readily induced by anticholinergic agents.

20. e. As discussed in answer 19, delirium is associated with many different abnormalities. One of the most important factors to rule out in the elderly is an underlying infection. Therefore, a CBC would be required. It is a low-cost test that helps rule out infection, a common reversible cause of delirium in the elderly.

21. e. All of the choices, although not meeting the criteria for dementia, are consistent with mild cognitive impairment. Screening tests for patients with dementia include the MMSE, Blessed Information Memory Concentration test (IMC). Coupled with neuropsychological testing, these tests often provide the needed information for the diagnosis of dementia. The interpretation of scores depends on the person's age and education. An MMSE score of 24 or less, or an IMC score of more than 8 (maximum score, 33; minimum score, 0) may be an indication of an underlying dementia. Patients with mild cognitive impairment have significant problems with memory, with deficits in other cognitive domains. Approximately 12% proceed to dementia each year, so they should be followed every 6 to 12 months with cognitive testing.

22. e. Mematine (Namenda) is Food and Drug Administration approved for moderate to severe stages of Alzheimer's disease. The recommended initial dose is 5 mg/day, which can then be titrated up at 5 mg/week if needed to a dose of 10 mg twice a day. The most common side effects are constipation, dizziness, and headache. Memantine has been used safely with other anticholinesterase inhibitors, but additional research in this area is under way.

23. c. Approximately 3% of the population has the ApoE 4/4 genotype and 20% has the 3/4 genotype. The ApoE-4 allele increases the risk of developing SDAT and decreases the age of onset.

Solution to the Clinical Case Management Problem

Part A

The following is an all-inclusive mnemonic on confusion in the elderly. This includes both reversible causes and nonreversible causes. The mnemonic is DEMENTIA.

D = **D**rug intoxication (especially anticholinergic agents) but includes alcohol abuse

E = **E**yes and ears (especially cataracts, diabetes mellitus, and sensory neural hearing loss)
Environment (A new environment is a common trigger for acute confusional state.)

M= **M**etabolic, including (1) hyponatremia, (2) hypokalemia, (3) hyperkalemia, (4) hypercalcemia, (5) elevated blood urea nitrogen, (6) elevated serum creatinine, and (7) elevated gamma-glutamyl transferase

E = **E**motional, including (1) major depressive disorder, (2) bipolar affective disorder, (3) schizoaffective disorder, (4) chronic schizophrenia, (5) pseudodementia (depression masking as dementia), and (6) adverse drug reaction (propranolol causes depression)
Endocrine including (1) hypothyroidism, (2) hyperthyroidism, (3) hyperglycemia, and (4) hypoglycemia

N = **N**eoplasms, including (1) benign neoplasms (rare), (2) malignancies (breast cancer, lung cancer, colon cancer, prostate cancer, lymphomas, and multiple myeloma)
Neurologic (1) normal pressure hydrocephalus, (2) Parkinson's disease, and (3) Huntington's disease

T = **T**rauma: Chronic subdural hematoma is most common. Burr holes can be life saving in a rural center if recognized.

I = **I**nfections (in order of frequency as a cause of delirium in three groups of elderly patients)
  1. Infections predominating in hospitalized patients with delirium: urinary tract infection, bacterial pneumonia, and surgical wound infections

  2. Infections predominating in nursing home patients who develop delirium: bacterial pneumonia, urinary tract infection, and pressure ulcer
  3. Independent, previously healthy individuals living in the community: bacterial pneumonia, urinary tract infection, intraabdominal infections (appendicitis and diverticulitis), and infective endocarditis
Inflammatory
  1. New-onset/recurrent inflammatory bowel disease (ulcerative colitis or regional enteritis)
  2. Collagen vascular disorders, including rheumatoid arthritis and systemic lupus erythematosis
  3. Musculoskeletal system: (1) polymyalgia rheumatica (if not treated properly, this can lead to serious consequences such as blindness) and (2) polymyositis/dermatomyositis
  4. Pericarditis
  5. Pleuritis
  6. Biliary colic
  7. Renal colic
  8. Chronic pancreatitis

A = **A**nemia: (1) iron-deficiency anemia, (2) anemia of chronic disease, (3) and macrocytic anemia (vitamin B_{12} or folate deficiency)
Atherosclerotic vascular disease or cardiovascular disease: (1) myocardial infarction, (2) pulmonary embolism, (3) cerebrovascular accident (stroke), and (4) congestive cardiac failure
Alzheimer's and other dementias: (1) Alzheimer's disease, (2) multi-infarct dementia, (3) Parkinson's disease, and (4) Huntington's disease

Part B

The distinct disorders that are part of the complex termed delirium include the following:
  1. Global disorder of cognition: This constitutes one of the essential features of delirium. In this sense, *global* refers to the main cognitive functions, including the following: (1) memory, (2) thinking,

(3) perception, (4) information acquisition, (5) information processing, (6) information retention, (7) information retrieval, and (8) utilization of information. These cognitive deficits and abnormalities constitute an essential diagnostic feature of delirium.

2. Global disorder of attention: Disturbances of the major aspects of attention are invariably present. Alertness (vigilance)—that is, readiness to respond to sensory stimuli—and the ability to mobilize, shift, sustain, and direct attention at will are always disturbed to some extent.

3. Reduced level of consciousness: This implies a diminished awareness of oneself and one's surroundings to respond to sensory inputs in a selective and sustained manner and to be able to relate the incoming information to previously acquired knowledge.

4. Disordered sleep–wake cycle: Disorganization of the sleep–wake cycle is one of the essential features of delirium. Wakefulness is abnormally increased and the patient sleeps little or not at all or it is reduced during the day but excessive during the night.

5. Disorder of psychomotor behavior: A disturbance of both verbal and nonverbal psychomotor activity is the last essential feature of delirium. A delirious patient can be predominantly either hyperactive or hypoactive. Some patients shift unpredictably from abnormally increased psychomotor activity to lethargy and vice versa.

Summary

The answer to Part A of the Clinical Case Management Problem (the mnemonic for confusion in the elderly) serves as the summary for this chapter.

Suggested Reading

American Geriatric Society: *Geriatric Review Syllabus, A Core Curriculum in Geriatric Medicine*, 6th ed. Chicago: American Geriatric Society, 2006, pp. 222–247.

Kawas C: Early Alzheimer's disease. *N Engl J Med* 349:1056–1063, 2003.

Kelley BJ, Petersen RC: Alzheimer's disease and mild cognitive impairment. *Neurol Clin* 25(3):577–609, 2007.

Moraga AV, Rodriguez-Pascual C: Accurate diagnosis of delirium in elderly patients. *Curr Opin Psychiatry* 20(3):262–267, 2007.

Rayner AV, O'Brien JG, Shoenbachler B: Behavior disorders of dementia: Recognition and treatment. *Am Fam Physician* 73(4):647–652, 2006.

CHAPTER 138 Parkinson's Disease

CLINICAL CASE PROBLEM 1

A 75-Year-Old Male with a Slow, Shuffling Gait, Tremors, and Depression

A 75-year-old male is brought to your office by his wife. She states that he has just been "staring into space" for the past 2 months. He has been unable to move around the house without falling over. Also, his movements appear to be very slow. According to his wife, he has been very depressed, is drooling, has difficulty swallowing, and is losing weight.

On examination, the patient has a slow, shuffling gait and walks in a "stooped-over" position. His blood pressure (lying) is 140/90 mmHg. His standing blood pressure is 100/70 mmHg. He has marked rigidity of his upper extremities. He also has a tremor that appears to be present only at rest.

SELECT THE BEST ANSWER TO THE FOLLOWING QUESTIONS

1. What is the most likely diagnosis in this patient?
   a. Alzheimer's disease
   b. major depressive disorder with psychomotor retardation

c. degenerative orthostatic hypotension
d. Parkinson's disease
e. multiple sclerosis

2. What is the most common presenting symptom in this disorder?
a. orthostatic hypotension
b. depression
c. gait disturbance
d. tremor
e. rigidity

3. Where is the lesion associated with the described disorder located?
a. caudate nucleus
b. substantia nigra
c. hypothalamus
d. putamen
e. globus pallidus

4. The disorder described is associated with a central nervous system neurotransmitter deficiency. What is that neurotransmitter?
a. acetylcholine
b. serotonin
c. γ-aminobutyric acid
d. dopamine
e. norepinephrine

5. Many drugs are associated with side effects that mimic some of the symptoms of the described disorder. Which of the following drugs would not produce these symptoms?
a. diazepam
b. haloperidol
c. chlorpromazine
d. perphenazine
e. reserpine

6. Which of the following statements regarding the condition described is false?
a. there is marked heterogeneity in disease presentation
b. there are at least two major subgroups of this disorder
c. patients who have marked postural instability have a better prognosis than those who have a tremor
d. personality changes commonly appear in the course of this disorder
e. significant depression and dementia appear in one-third to one-half of patients with this condition

7. What is (are) the drug(s) of choice for mild cases of the condition described (mild meaning that the main or only symptom is tremor)?
a. amantadine
b. trihexyphenidyl
c. levodopa
d. carbidopa
e. selegiline (Deprenyl)
f. a or b

8. If the symptoms progress to the point at which another agent is needed, dose-limiting side effects develop from the drugs being used, or the drugs being used begin to lose their effectiveness, what is the next step in the treatment of the disorder described?
a. selegiline
b. trihexyphenidyl
c. amantadine
d. all of the above
e. none of the above

9. Which of the following drugs may be indicated in the treatment of the disorder described?
a. bromocriptine
b. pergolide
c. amitriptyline
d. all of the above
e. none of the above

10. Which of the following symptoms is not characteristic of this disorder?
a. unilateral onset of tremor
b. unilateral onset of bradykinesia
c. impaired balance
d. muscle rigidity
e. psychomotor agitation

11. Which of the following statements regarding levodopa is false?
a. levodopa in combination with carbidopa remain the primary drugs for the treatment of most patients with the condition described
b. levodopa is unlikely to lose its effectiveness over time
c. levodopa is likely to produce an "on–off" phenomenon during treatment
d. nausea is a frequent side effect of levodopa
e. centrally mediated dyskinesia, hallucinations, dystonia, and motor fluctuations are common in levodopa-treated patients

12. Which of the following conditions is most closely associated with the condition described?
   a. major depressive disorder
   b. cerebrovascular disease
   c. epilepsy
   d. schizophrenia
   e. schizoaffective disorder

13. Which of the following statements regarding benign essential tremor is (are) true?
   a. benign essential tremor is often familial
   b. a nodding head and tremulousness of speech are often observed with benign essential tremor
   c. benign essential tremor is a resting tremor rather than an action tremor
   d. a and b
   e. all of the above statements are true

14. Benign essential tremor is frequently treated with which of the following agents?
   a. propranolol
   b. alcohol
   c. atenolol
   d. all of the above
   e. none of the above

15. What illicit drug produces symptoms closely resembling the symptoms of the condition described?
   a. a meperidine analog (MPTP)
   b. crack cocaine
   c. lysergic acid diethylamide
   d. apomorphine
   e. diamorphine (heroin)

16. Anticholinergic agents are sometimes helpful in treating tremor and drooling in patients with Parkinson's disease. Some common side effects associated with them (trihexyphenidyl and benztropine) include which of the following?
   a. constipation
   b. urinary retention
   c. hallucinations
   d. memory impairment
   e. all of the above

17. By 5 years, what percentage of patients with Parkinson's disease develop dyskinesias from the use of levodopa?
   a. 5%
   b. 10%
   c. 20%
   d. 50%

18. True or false: Deep brain stimulation (DBS) results in decreased dyskinesias, rigidity, tremors, and fluctuations.
   a. True
   b. False

19. The surgical procedure(s) useful for refractory tremor includes
   a. thalamic DBS
   b. pallidal stimulation
   c. a and b
   d. Neither a nor b

Clinical Case Management Problem

Discuss the therapeutic choices available to treat the condition described in the patient presented in Clinical Case Problem 1. Describe a logical approach to instituting these therapeutic choices in any patient with this disorder.

Answers

1. d. This patient has Parkinson's disease. The most common presenting symptoms in Parkinson's disease include tremor, bradykinesia, rigidity, impaired postural reflexes, gait disturbance, autonomic dysfunction (causing orthostatic hypotension), and depression. A "masked facies" expression is typical of the disease.

Other presenting symptoms can be constipation, vague aches and pains, paresthesias, decreased smell sensation, vestibular symptoms, pedal edema, fatigue, and weight loss.

The other choices listed in this question do not explain the constellation of presenting symptoms.

2. d. The most common presenting symptom in Parkinson's disease is a resting tremor. This symptom is seen in 70% of patients with the disease. It may initially be confined to one hand, but it usually extends to involve all limbs.

3. b. The principal pathologic feature in Parkinson's disease is degeneration of the substantia nigra. Degenerative changes are also found in other brain stem nuclei.

4. d. Parkinson's disease is associated with a depletion of dopamine in the substantia nigrostriatal pathway system.

5. **a.** Parkinsonian-like side effects are common side effects of the neuroleptic drug class. This drug class includes chlorpromazine, haloperidol, and perphenazine. In addition, the prokinetic agent metoclopramide can also produce this side effect.

Reserpine, an older antihypertensive agent, may also produce these extrapyramidal symptoms. This is relevant because many elderly individuals who were started on reserpine are still taking it. Diazepam does not produce any such side effects.

6. **c.** There is marked heterogeneity in Parkinson's disease. There are at least two major subtypes of Parkinson's disease. In one group, the symptom of tremor is the most predominant clinical symptom. In the second group, postural instability and gait difficulty (PIGD) are the predominant symptoms. There is some overlap, but most patients fit into only one subgroup. Patients with tremor-predominant Parkinson's disease have slower progression of disease and have fewer problems with bradykinesia. They are also less likely to develop significant mental symptoms.

Personality changes usually occur in the early stages, and patients often become withdrawn, apathetic, and dependent on their spouses. Significant depression occurs in half of patients, and dementia occurs in one-third of patients. As mentioned previously, these personality and mental changes are more common in patients who present with the PIGD subtype of Parkinson's disease.

7. **e.** Research from three studies has supported the use of selegiline (Deprenyl) early in the course of the disease to delay the onset of the disability and the need for initiation of levodopa therapy. The combination of levodopa and carbidopa is effective and is still considered for primary treatment, but their use should be delayed as long as possible because of their side effect profile and the eventual development of tolerance to these medications.

8. **e.** The next step in the pharmacologic treatment of Parkinson's disease is the combination of levodopa and carbidopa. Levodopa is a precursor of dopamine synthesis in the substantia nigra. The drug is usually administered in combination with carbidopa, which is a decarboxylase inhibitor. Obviously, treatment must be individualized: A general rule to follow is to start low and go slow. Sinemet is most helpful for bradykinesia.

9. **d.** Bromocriptine and pergolide are dopaminergic agonists that can be useful for sudden episodes of hesitancy or immobility, which parkinsonian patients describe as "freezing." This can be an intermittent event or a regular event. The freezing often occurs when parkinsonian patients begin to walk or they pass through a structure such as a doorway. Dyskinesias and other types of involuntary movements are also treated by these drugs. Newer dopaminergic agents include pramipexole and ropinirole.

10. **e.** The unilateral onset of tremor or bradykinesia is common in patients with Parkinson's disease. Muscle rigidity and impaired balance are other important symptoms. Psychomotor agitation (although one of the characteristic symptoms of major depressive disorder) is rare. Instead, patients with Parkinson's disease have psychomotor retardation.

11. **b.** Levodopa does lose its effectiveness over time in the treatment of Parkinson's disease. That is the reason why, in patients who have mild symptoms, it is best to begin therapy with selegiline (Deprenyl).

Levodopa does exhibit a marked "on–off" phenomenon during treatment of Parkinson's disease. This is characterized by periods of "drug working" and "drug not working." Pramipexole may be used with Sinemet to reduce these fluctuations. Catechol-*O*-methyltransferases, such as tolcapone (100 mg) or entacapone (200 mg), with each Sinemet dose may enhance the benefits of levodopa therapy.

Side effects of levodopa include nausea and vomiting, dystonias, hallucinations, dyskinesias, and motor fluctuations. Hallucinations become the most common side effect, limiting the titration of carbidopa–levodopa.

12. **a.** Depression is a common problem in patients with Parkinson's disease. The association between depression and Parkinson's disease generally follows this pathway: When depression occurs, the symptoms of Parkinson's disease become worse; the patient then believes that his or her disease has progressed quickly. This leads to a cycle that is difficult to break.

13. **d.** Benign essential tremor is the major differential diagnostic possibility when considering tremor. Benign essential tremor is familial. Typical features include generalized tremulousness, including tremulousness of speech, and a "head-nodding" motion. In contradistinction to the tremor of Parkinson's disease, benign essential tremor is an action tremor.

14. **d.** The agents of choice for treating benign essential tremor are propranolol (long acting) and primidone.

15. **a.** The illicitly made MPTP produces symptoms that are Parkinson-like in presentation. This agent appears to act as a poison on the substantia nigra. Also, the symptoms appear to be irreversible, and the individual is left with a lifetime disability.

16. **e.** All listed are common side effect.

17. **d.** Within 5 years, 50% of patients using levodopa will develop dyskinesias.

18. **a.** DBS has been used successfully in many patients.

19. **c.** Lesioning of the pallidum is sometimes successful in the treatment of contralateral dyskinesias. Thalamic stimulation of the ventral intermediate nucleus has been successful in treating the contralateral tremor.

Solution to the Clinical Case Management Problem

A reasonable therapeutic approach to the treatment of Parkinson's disease is as follows:

1. Patients with minor symptoms (not significantly impairing function): (a) no pharmacologic treatment, (b) selegiline (Deprenyl), (c) anticholinergic medications (trihexyphenidyl and benztropine; use with caution in the elderly), and (d) amantadine

2. Patients with moderate symptoms: Levodopa–carbidopa (Sinemet) is the drug of choice. Levodopa is a precursor of dopamine; carbidopa is a decarboxylase inhibitor. Although selegiline is not considered the drug of first choice, its use will increase if current research continues to support the idea that it decreases the rate of progression of Parkinson's disease or delays the use of Sinemet.

3. Patients with moderate to severe symptoms (or patients in whom the effect of levodopa has worn off): (a) selegiline (a monoamine oxidase [MAO] B inhibitor) in patients with a significant depressive component because of the MAO activity, and (b) bromocriptine and pergolide (dopamine agonists) in patients in whom dyskinesias and other involuntary movements are prominent

4. Patients with Parkinson's disease with significant depression: amitriptyline or another tricyclic antidepressant with or without anticholinergic properties (balance the benefits of the anticholinergic properties of amitriptyline against the risk of increased orthostatic disturbance and imbalance)

Summary

1. Epidemiology: After stroke and Alzheimer's disease, Parkinson's disease is the most commonly encountered neurologic disorder in the elderly population.
2. Pathologic condition: Depigmentation of the substantia nigra, which results in a decrease in brain synthesis of dopamine.
3. Major symptoms include (a) resting tremor, (b) bradykinesia, (c) rigidity, (d) impaired postural reflexes, (e) gait disturbance, (f) autonomic dysfunction, and (g) depression.
4. Major subtypes
   a. Parkinson's disease (group A): This group exhibits tremor (resting) as the major symptom and sign.
   b. Parkinson's disease (group B): This group exhibits PIGD as the major symptom. Progression of the disease is usually more rapid in this group;

neurobehavioral changes are also more common in this group.
5. Treatment: See the Solution to the Clinical Case Management Problem.
6. Other related disease entity: Benign essential tremor is an action tremor (as opposed to the resting tremor of Parkinson's disease). It is most often seen in the extremities and is sometimes associated with head nodding and tremulousness of speech. It is familial. The drug treatment of this entity includes a beta blocker, primidone, or alcohol (in moderation).
7. In refractory cases, unilateral pallidotomy may be effective in relieving signs of Parkinson's disease on the contralateral side. Deep brain stimulation of the globus pallidas or subthalamic nucleus has a lower morbidity than pallidotomy and appears to improve clinical status.

Suggested Reading

American Geriatric Society: *Geriatric Review Syllabus, A Core Curriculum in Geriatric Medicine*, 6th ed. Chicago: American Geriatric Society, 2006, pp. 462–464.

Bonuccelli U, Del Dotto P: New pharmacologic horizons in the treatment of Parkinson disease. *Neurology* 67(7 Suppl 2):S30–S38, 2006.

Frucht SJ: Parkinson disease: An update. *Neurologist* 10(4):185–194, 2004.

Hauser RA, Zesiewicz TA: Advances in the pharmacologic management of early Parkinson disease. *Neurologist* 13(3):126–132, 2007.

Roa SS, Hofmann LA, Shakil A: Parkinson disease: Diagnosis and management. *Am Fam Physician* 74(12):2046–2054, 2006.

CHAPTER

139 Elder Abuse

CLINICAL CASE PROBLEM 1

A 72-Year-Old Female with a Sore Right Shoulder and Multiple Bruises

A daughter brings her 72-year-old mother to the emergency department for assessment. The mother has Alzheimer's disease, and although she is able to communicate, she will not answer without looking at her daughter first. The daughter tells you that her mother has had Alzheimer's disease for 5 years and has been living with her for the majority of that time, and that she is always hurting herself despite attempts to help her. Her mother lies there, tears in her eyes, and seems frightened.

The daughter tells you that her mother fell on her right shoulder approximately 3 hours ago. As you look at the patient, you notice a large bruise in the area of the head of the right humerus.

On examination, there are multiple bruises on her arms, legs, and abdomen. The head of the humerus is tender. The resident who is with you tells you that he "has things pretty well squared away." He has made the diagnosis of a rare inherited bleeding disorder on the basis of (as the nurse who is caring for the patient says) "goodness knows what."

You decide that you are not satisfied with this diagnosis and need to investigate further. Meanwhile, the patient is complaining of pain and holding her shoulder. You order an x-ray of the shoulder and diagnose a fractured head of the humerus.

SELECT THE BEST ANSWER TO THE FOLLOWING QUESTIONS

1. At this time, what should you do?
   a. treat the patient's pain, provide a collar and cuff, and discharge the patient with her daughter
   b. treat the patient's pain, provide a collar and cuff for the patient, and advise the patient about safe environments
   c. treat the patient's pain and contact an orthopedic surgeon who you are sure will wish to manage this fracture with internal fixation
   d. order a complete blood count, International Normalized Ratio, and all other laboratory tests associated with intrinsic defects of the hematological and clotting system
   e. none of the above

2. What is the prevalence of elder abuse in the U.S. population?
   a. 4%
   b. 2%
   c. 10%
   d. 8%
   e. 15%

3. Regarding screening for the condition described here, which of the following statements is (are) true?
   a. screening for the condition described here is recommended by the American Medical Association
   b. it is recommended that physicians incorporate routine questions related to the condition in Clinical Case Problem 1 into their daily practice
   c. direct, concrete action should be taken when a situation is identified that confirms the diagnosis described in Clinical Case Problem 1

d. all of the above statements are true

e. none of the above statements are true

4. When comparing the prevalence of this condition in the community setting with the prevalence of the same condition in long-term care institutions, which of the following statements is (are) true?

   a. the prevalence of this condition is much higher in institutionalized elderly patients compared to elders in the community setting

   b. the institutionalized elderly patient is at greater risk of this condition because of his or her physical or psychological status

   c. one of the reasons for the high prevalence of this condition in the institutionalized elderly is lack of staff training and/or institutional understaffing

   d. all of the above statements are true

   e. none of the above statements are true

5. There are various forms of this condition. Which of the following would be placed in that category of forms?

   a. a physical form

   b. a psychological form

   c. a financial form

   d. a neglect form

   e. all of the above

6. Which of the following is (are) associated with the condition described?

   a. excessive use of restraints

   b. pushing

   c. grabbing

   d. yelling

   e. all of the above

7. What is the most common manifestation of the condition described in this case?

   a. excessive use of restraints

   b. pushing

   c. grabbing

   d. yelling

   e. slapping or hitting

8. Which of the following is not a risk factor for the condition described?

   a. unsatisfactory living arrangements

   b. low educational level of staff

   c. physical or emotional dependence on the caregiver

   d. living apart from the victim

   e. older than age 75 years

9. Which of the following is false regarding the condition described?

   a. abusive events tend to be one-time-only events

   b. abusive events tend to escalate in the same manner in which spousal abuse escalates

   c. the situation rarely resolves spontaneously

   d. many victims refuse help

   e. serious illness, crisis, admission to an institution, or even death are all long-term sequelae of this condition

10. With respect to research priorities and the condition described, which of the following is (are) true?

    a. there should be a determination of the cause of the condition in different ethnic and cultural groups in North America

    b. there should be a comprehensive assessment of the prevalence of this condition in North American long-term care institutions

    c. valid, reliable tools should be developed for use in settings such as primary care institutions, hospital emergency departments, and long-term care institutions

    d. all of the above

    e. a and c only

11. In which of the following settings is the incidence of the condition described likely to be highest based on screening history and physical examination?

    a. family physician's office

    b. local emergency department

    c. referral-based specialist's office

    d. any of the above

    e. none of the above

12. When evaluating a patient who you believe may have been abused, what characteristics should you look for?

    a. a disparity in the histories between the patient and the abuser

    b. a delay in treatment

    c. explanations that are vague and not realistic

    d. laboratory findings inconsistent with history provided

    e. all of the above

Clinical Case Management Problem

Discuss a comprehensive plan to manage elder abuse in your community.

Answers

1. e. This patient is much more likely to have injuries inflicted as a result of abuse rather than to have a rare inherited clotting disorder or anything else.

Obviously, the patient's pain and her fractured arm have to be treated. This is not, however, the end of the treatment.

Elder abuse is extremely common and is a condition that will not be diagnosed unless it is included in a differential diagnosis and considered in all situations in which it may occur. In this case, a consult to social services is essential. With the history of physical injury, it would seem that the wisest course of action at this time is removal of the patient to a safe environment.

2. a. The prevalence of elder abuse in the United States is estimated at 4%. This represents 700,000 to 1.2 million cases per year in those older than age 65 years. In many cases, this abuse is long term, repeated, or both. In one study, 58% of elderly patients had suffered previous incidents of abuse.

Some studies have estimated the prevalence of elder abuse to be much higher than 4%; 10% appears to be a more realistic figure.

3. d. When a situation arises that confirms elder abuse, direct action should be taken to rectify, improve, or resolve the situation.

The American Medical Association recommends that physicians screen for elder abuse in their practices and that they incorporate routine questions related to elder abuse and neglect when seeing elderly patients. For example, the physician may ask, "Is there any violence in your family that you want to tell me about?" "Has anyone tried to hurt or harm you?" "Are you afraid of anyone living in your home?" "Are you receiving enough care at home?" or "Did anyone take anything from you or force you to do anything that you did not want to do?"

4. d. The prevalence of elder abuse is much higher in institutionalized elderly patients than in elderly patients who live in the community. In one study of nursing home staff, 36% had witnessed physical abuse of residents in the preceding year.

5. e. The simplest definition of elder abuse is "any act of commission or omission that results in harm to an elderly person."

Elder abuse is distinguished from other crimes against elderly people by the perpetrator's occupying a position of trust. The following definition of elder abuse and neglect is proposed:

1. Physical abuse: assault, rough handling, sexual abuse, or the withholding of physical necessities such as food or other items of personal, hygienic, or medical care
2. Psychosocial abuse: verbal assault, social isolation, lack of affection, or denial of the person's participation in decisions affecting his or her life
3. Financial abuse: the misuse of money or property, including fraud or use of funds for purposes contrary to the needs, interests, or desires of the elderly person
4. Neglect: In active neglect, the caregiver consciously fails to meet the needs of the elderly person; in passive neglect, the caregiver does not intend to injure the dependent person. Neglect can lead to any of the three types of abuse.

6. e. Other categories of abuse have been proposed, such as violation of rights and medical abuse (inappropriate treatment, excessive use of restraints, and withholding of treatment). Abuse may be intentional or unintentional.

7. a. As mentioned previously, 36% of institutionalized elderly have been abused. In this study, the most common forms of abuse were excessive use of restraints (witnessed in the study by 21% of staff); pushing, grabbing, shoving, or pinching (17%); and slapping or hitting (15%).

Psychological abuse was observed by 81% of the staff; 70% had witnessed a staff member yelling at a patient in anger, 50% had seen someone insulting or swearing at a patient, and 23% had seen a patient isolated inappropriately.

8. d. Living apart from the victim is not a risk factor for elder abuse. The risk factors for elder abuse are as follows:

Situational factors:
1. Community situational factors: (a) isolation, (b) lack of money, (c) lack of community resources for additional care, and (d) unsatisfactory living arrangements
2. Institutions: (a) shortage of beds, (b) surplus of patients, (c) low staff-to-patient ratio, (d) low staff compensation, and (e) staff burnout

Characteristics of the victim: (1) physical or emotional dependence on caregiver, (2) lack of close family ties, (3) history of family violence, (4) age older than 75 years, and (5) recent deterioration in health

Characteristics of the perpetrator: (1) stress caused by financial, marital, or occupational factors; (2) deterioration in health; (3) bereavement;

(4) substance abuse; (5) psychopathologic illness; (6) related to victim; (7) living with victim; and (8) long duration of care for victim (mean, 9.5 years)

9. **a.** Elder abuse rarely resolves spontaneously; it tends to escalate in the same way as spousal abuse. Abusive events tend to be repeated and will almost always continue unless there is a major change in the environment. Such an environmental change may not occur because in 25% to 75% of cases, victims or their families refuse help. This may subsequently result in serious illness, crisis, admission to an institution, or even death.

10. **d.** The research priorities for elder abuse include (1) a determination of the causes of this condition in different ethnic and cultural groups in the United States and Canada; (2) a determination of the prevalence of abuse in American and Canadian institutions; (3) the development of valid and reliable assessment tools for use in settings such as primary care offices, hospital emergency departments, and long-term care institutions; and (4) an evaluation of the effectiveness of interventions on the prevalence of this condition.

11. **b.** The highest incidence is likely to occur at the local emergency department facility. The reason is that elders are most likely to come to the emergency department at the time of, or soon after, an event of abuse. This does not imply that screening should not occur at the other facilities; it should occur in all health care settings all of the time.

12. **e.** Additional presentations may include (1) a patient who is functionally impaired coming to the emergency room or office without his or her primary caregiver and (2) frequent visits to the emergency room for patients with chronic diseases despite a plan for medical care and adequate resources.

Solution to the Clinical Case Management Problem

A comprehensive plan to manage elder abuse should include recognition of the condition, comprehensive treatment of the condition, and a significant education component aimed at increasing public awareness of (1) the magnitude of the problem, (2) the signs and symptoms of elder abuse, and (3) the treatment options available.

The actual components of the management of elder abuse include the following:

1. Detection and risk assessment: (a) documentation of the type of abuse, the frequency and severity of abuse, the danger to the victim, and the perpetrator's intent and level of stress; (b) involvement of other health care professionals (social worker, visiting nurse, and geriatric assessment team); (c) documentation of the injuries (take photographs if possible); and (d) assessment of the victim's overall health status, the victim's functional status, and the victim's social and financial status.
2. Assessment of decision-making capacity of the victim: Assess the cognitive state and the emotional state of the victim.
3. Measures to take if the victim is competent: (a) Provide information to the victim; (b) in providing information, outline the choices or possible choices that the victim has, such as temporary relocation, home support, community agencies, and criminal charges; and (c) support the victim's decision.
4. Measures to take if the victim is not competent: (a) Separate the victim and the perpetrator; (b) relocate the victim; (c) arrange advocacy services for the victim; (d) inform a protective service agency; (e) reduce caregiver stress; (f) treat all medical disorders; (g) minimize or simplify medications; (h) seek agencies to provide respite care, support for house cleaning, personal care, and transportation; and (i) provide support groups for primary caregivers.
5. Key questions to guide intervention: (a) How safe is the patient if he or she is sent home? (b) What services or resources are available to help a stressed family? (c) Does the elderly person need to be removed to a safe environment? and (d) Does the situation need an unbiased advocate to monitor the care and finances for this patient?

Always perform an in-depth evaluation and interview when possible, and carefully document physical and psychological findings. Report suspected cases to adult protective services.

Summary

See the Solution to the Clinical Case Management Problem.

Suggested Reading

American Geriatric Society: *Geriatric Review Syllabus, A Core Curriculum in Geriatric Medicine*, 6th ed. Chicago: American Geriatric Society, 2006, pp. 86–91, 508–509.

Fulmer T, Guadagno L, Dyer CB, et al: Progress in elder abuse screening and assessment instruments. *J Am Geriatr Soc* 52(2):297–304, 2004.

Geroff AJ, Olshaker JS: Elder abuse. *Emergency Med Clin North Am* 24(2):491–505, ix, 2006.

Gnanadesigan N, Fung CH: Quality indicators for screening and prevention in vulnerable elders. *J Am Geriatr Soc* 55(Suppl 2):S417–S423, 2007.

CHAPTER 140

Emergency Treatment of Abdominal Pain in the Elderly

CLINICAL CASE PROBLEM 1

An 84-Year-Old Male with Abdominal Pain

An 84-year-old male presents with a 6-hour history of severe abdominal pain. The pain is described as follows: quality, dull, aching; quantity, severe, baseline 9/10, range 8 to 10/10; location, epigastric, radiating through to the back and flank; and chronology, began suddenly after dinner 6 hours ago. Aggravating factor is movement and relieving factor is rest; provocative maneuver is deep palpation to abdomen. He has had no previous episodes like this, no history of similar pain, and no previous significant history of angina pectoris. Associated manifestations are "faintness and dizziness" along with nausea.

On examination, the patient's blood pressure is 86/56 mmHg, and his pulse is 106 beats/minute and regular. His respiratory rate is 16 breaths/minute. He is breathing normally. Examination of the abdomen reveals no distention and normal bowel sounds. However, there is marked central abdominal tenderness to palpation.

SELECT THE BEST ANSWER TO THE FOLLOWING QUESTIONS

1. What is the major differential diagnosis in this patient's case?
   a. ruptured aortic aneurysm
   b. intestinal ischemia or infarction
   c. perforated viscus
   d. splenic infarction
   e. all of the above

2. Given the history and physical examination findings, which of the following diagnostic possibilities is most likely?
   a. ruptured aortic aneurysm
   b. intestinal ischemia or infarction
   c. perforated viscus
   d. splenic infarction
   e. myocardial infarction

3. The diagnosis of the condition described can best be confirmed by which of the following?
   a. ultrasonography
   b. computed tomography (CT) scan of the abdomen
   c. magnetic resonance imaging scans of the abdomen
   d. 12-lead electrocardiogram (ECG)
   e. laparotomy

4. What is the most important diagnostic clue that leads you to arrive at the diagnosis?
   a. the patient's hypotension
   b. the location of the abdominal pain
   c. hypotension with back and flank pain
   d. the periumbilical tenderness
   e. none of the above

5. What is the most critical early intervention that must take place in this patient?
   a. placement of an endotracheal tube
   b. establishment of intravenous (IV) access for fluid and blood replacement
   c. abdominal paracentesis
   d. administration of a thrombolytic agent
   e. establishment of an arterial line

6. In which of the following conditions do pharmacotherapy and the adverse effects of same (i.e.,
iatrogenic disease) play the greatest role?
   a. ruptured aortic aneurysm
   b. intestinal ischemia or infarction
   c. peptic ulcer perforation
   d. splenic infarction
   e. diverticulitis

7. Which drug is most often closely associated with
peptic ulcer perforation?
   a. ibuprofen
   b. piroxicam
   c. naproxen
   d. aspirin
   e. celecoxib

8. What is the treatment of choice for this patient?
   a. monitoring in the intensive care unit, thrombolytic therapy, aspirin, beta blockers, and antiarrhythmic therapy
   b. laparotomy—oversew perforation
   c. laparotomy—removal of ischemic bowel
   d. laparotomy—surgical repair of aortic aneurysm
   e. laparotomy and splenectomy

9. Which of the following statements is (are) true
regarding ruptured aortic aneurysm?
   a. more than 80% of abdominal aortic aneurysms
are asymptomatic when first diagnosed
   b. the diagnosis is often missed because physicians do not consider it
   c. most abdominal aortic aneurysms are atherosclerotic in nature
   d. all of the above are true
   e. none of the above are true

10. What is the key to reducing morbidity and mortality in the condition described?
   a. enhanced tertiary prevention
   b. enhanced secondary prevention
   c. regular yearly checkups
   d. early diagnosis and intervention
   e. early administration of thrombolytic agents

Clinical Case Management Problem

Provide the differential diagnosis for acute
abdominal pain in the elderly as an emergency room
presentation.

Answers

1. e. The differential diagnosis of abdominal pain in
the elderly is extensive. In this case, the sudden onset
of the pain and the severity of the pain strongly suggest an acute abdomen. At the top of the list would be
ruptured aortic aneurysm, perforated viscus, intestinal
ischemia or infarction, a perforated diverticulum, and
pancreatitis.

2. a. Given the history and physical findings, the
most likely diagnosis is ruptured aortic aneurysm.
The clue to ruptured aortic aneurysm in this case is
the hypotension and location of pain. The signs and
symptoms suggest at least a leaking aneurysm.

3. b. The working diagnosis can best be confirmed
by the performance of a CT scan of the abdomen.
Ultrasound and CT are both close to 100% accurate
in diagnosing an abdominal aortic aneurysm. The
CT scan is subject to less technical and interpretation
errors than an ultrasound. The CT scan also better
detects retroperitoneal hemorrhage associated with an
aneurysm rupture.

4. c. See answer 2.

5. b. Remember the ABCs. Because this patient
is breathing normally, the next most important step
is circulation. You should immediately place either a
central venous pressure line or two large bore IV lines
(two lines of at least No. 16 gauge).

6. c. See answer 7.

7. d. Iatrogenic disease (in the form of a nonsteroidal anti-inflammatory drug [NSAID] prescription) is
closely associated with perforated peptic ulcer. Many
thousands of Americans die each year from perforated
and bleeding peptic ulcers caused by the prescription of
NSAIDs.
   The NSAID that causes more peptic ulcers and is
associated with more perforated peptic ulcers than any
other agent (on a prevalence/administration rate basis)
is acetylsalicylic acid (aspirin). The risk appears to be
dose related.

8. d. The treatment of choice in this patient is
removal of the segment of the aorta affected by the
aneurysm and replacement with a graft.

9. d. More than 80% of aortic aneurysms are asymptomatic when first diagnosed. The diagnosis is often
missed because the possibility is not considered.

Most aortic aneurysms are atherosclerotic in nature and result from a generalized atherosclerotic process.

10. d. The key to reducing morbidity and mortality from aortic aneurysm is early diagnosis and intervention. Although routine screening for aortic aneurysms in the elderly is not recommended by the U.S. Preventive Services Task Force on the periodic health examination, it is wise to consider this on a risk factor basis in the patients you see. High-risk patients and patients with symptoms that even vaguely suggest aortic aneurysm probably should be evaluated by both physical examination and ultrasound.

Solution to the Clinical Case Management Problem

The following is a differential diagnosis of abdominal pain in the elderly as an emergency room presentation:

1. Nonabdominal-related causes: (a) myocardial infarction, (b) pneumonia, and (c) pericarditis
2. Abdominal-related causes: (a) constipation (major cause), (b) diverticulitis, (c) cholecystitis/ cholelithiasis, (d) peptic ulcer disease/gastritis, (e) pancreatitis, (f) appendicitis, (g) bowel obstruction (large bowel and small bowel), (h) inflammatory bowel disease, (i) carcinoma (stomach, pancreas, and colon), (j) ruptured aortic aneurysm, (k) intestinal ischemia or infarction, and (l) urinary tract sepsis

Summary

1. Diagnosis
   a. Life-threatening causes of abdominal pain may present with few findings in the elderly.
   b. The elderly are less likely to have rebound or guarding because of decreased abdominal musculature.
   c. In general, compared to younger patients, abdominal pain in the elderly often has a vague presentation and higher rates of serious disease.
   d. Constipation is the most common cause of abdominal pain in the elderly.
   e. When elderly patients present to the emergency room with sudden onset of abdominal pain, think of the following: (i) nonabdominal causes: myocardial infarction; (ii) abdominal causes: see the Solution to the Clinical Case Management Problem.

2. Investigations: basic investigations in an elderly patient with abdominal pain: CBC; electrolytes; amylase; lipase; liver function tests; ECG; kidney, ureter, and bladder x-ray; urinalysis; ultrasonography; and CT scan
3. Treatment
   a. Treat the cause.
   b. Remember ABCs in acutely ill elderly patients.
   c. Remember that elderly patients present quite differently from younger patients—they often lack the classic signs and symptoms of any acute abdominal condition.
   d. A major error with regard to acutely ill elderly patients seen in community or rural hospitals is the failure to transfer to a tertiary care center soon enough.

Suggested Reading

Ferri FF: *Ferri's Clinical Advisor*. St. Louis: Mosby, 2005, pp. 907–909.
Kasper DL, Braunwald E, Fauci AS, et al, eds: *Harrison's Principles of Medicine*. New York: McGraw–Hill, 2005, pp. 82–84.

McPhee SJ, Papadakis MA, Tierney LM, eds: *Current Medical Treatment*, 46th ed. New York: McGraw–Hill, 2007, pp. 621–629, 714–715.

BEHAVIORAL HEALTH

Depressive Disorders

CLINICAL CASE PROBLEM 1

*A 28-Year-Old Male Who Just Is
Not Himself*

A 28-year-old male comes to the office with this wife because he has been "feeling tired" during the past 4 months. He says he always feels "run down" but also notes that he does not sleep well. He says he is able to fall asleep when he goes to bed at approximately 10 PM, but he wakes up routinely at 3 AM and is unable to get back to sleep.

He notes that he often has trouble with focus and concentration, and he lacks the energy to finish his tasks at home. He used to be more active but has recently stopped playing softball with his league on Wednesday nights because he says he is "just not interested in going out anymore." His wife says he seems on edge. "He has a short fuse … it seems like even the smallest things set him off," she says. His appetite has decreased and you note a 10-pound weight loss since his last visit 6 months ago. He denies fever, chills, nausea, vomiting, or night sweats. He has no other medical problems and denies any other medication except for a "megavitamin" he hoped would help him feel more energetic. His physical examination is completely normal.

SELECT THE BEST ANSWER TO THE FOLLOWING QUESTIONS

1. What is the most likely diagnosis in this patient?
   a. adjustment disorder with depressed mood
   b. generalized anxiety disorder
   c. major depressive disorder (MDD)
   d. mood disorder caused by a general medical condition
   e. dysthymic disorder

2. What class of drugs is most often used in the disorder described?
   a. selective serotonin reuptake inhibitors (SSRIs)
   b. tricyclic antidepressants (TCAs)
   c. monoamine oxidase inhibitors (MAOIs)
   d. benzodiazepines
   e. lithium carbonate

3. Which of the following types of psychotherapy is generally considered most effective in the illness previously described?
   a. psychoanalytic psychotherapy
   b. supportive psychotherapy
   c. psychodynamic psychotherapy
   d. cognitive–behavioral psychotherapy (CBT)
   e. all of the above

4. Which of the following is least likely to induce withdrawal symptoms if abruptly discontinued?
   a. fluoxetine (Prozac)
   b. sertraline (Zoloft)
   c. citalopram (Celexa)
   d. paroxetine (Paxil)
   e. being from the same class of medications, all of the above present an equal risk of inducing withdrawal symptoms

CLINICAL CASE PROBLEM 2

*A 39-Year-Old Male Who Is Sad All
the Time*

A 39-year-old male comes to your office with a 3-year history of "feeling down." He states that he feels "depressed most of the time," although there are periods when he feels better. He is "always tired," admits to trouble concentrating at work, and says this is starting to affect his job performance at work. He has had no other symptoms. His health is otherwise good. He is not taking any medications.

5. This patient most likely suffers from which of the following?
   a. adjustment disorder
   b. dysthymic disorder
   c. MDD
   d. mood disorder caused by a general medical condition
   e. none of the above

6. What is the treatment of choice for this patient?
   a. relaxation therapy
   b. pharmacologic antidepressants
   c. CBT
   d. exercise
   e. b, c, and d

CLINICAL CASE PROBLEM 3

A 35-Year-Old Female Who Is Distressed at Work

A 35-year-old female comes to your office with a 3-month history of feeling "depressed." She feels "extremely distressed at work" and tells you that she is "burned out." You discover that she moved into a managerial position at work 4 months ago and is having a great deal of difficulty (interpersonal conflict) with two of her employees.

The patient has no history of psychiatric illness. She has no other symptoms. She is not taking any medications.

7. What is the most likely diagnosis in this patient?
   a. adjustment disorder with depressed mood
   b. dysthymic disorder
   c. MDD
   d. mood disorder caused by a general medical condition
   e. burnout

8. What is the treatment of choice for this patient?
   a. a TCA
   b. an SSRI
   c. supportive psychotherapy
   d. a and c
   e. b and c

CLINICAL CASE PROBLEM 4

A 45-Year-Old Hard-Driving Male

A 45-year-old male who is a "hard-driving" executive comes to your office with a 4-month history of feelings of sadness, irritability, loss of appetite, inability to concentrate, and a significantly decreased ability to function in his job. He tells you that he is "completely burned out."

When you question him, he tells you that he has been "using anything and everything possible to try to relax." He has missed a number of days of work recently because he "hasn't felt up to it." He also complains of increasing stomach pains and headaches during the past 2 months.

9. From the history given, what is the most likely diagnosis in this patient?
   a. MDD
   b. dysthymic disorder
   c. mood disorder caused by a general medical condition
   d. substance-induced mood disorder
   e. adjustment disorder with depressed mood

10. What is the treatment of choice for this?
    a. an SSRI
    b. a TCA
    c. an MAOI
    d. lithium carbonate
    e. none of the above

CLINICAL CASE PROBLEM 5

A 33-Year-Old Woman Who Has Lost Interest in Life

A 33-year-old woman presents to your office complaining of fatigue and decreased interest in "the things that used to make me happy." She is sleeping less and eating less, and she says that she is forcing herself to eat "because I know I have to eat something." She had been looking forward to the winter snow and had promised to help build snowmen with her two young sons. Instead, she finds herself spending less time with them as she retreats to her room. Her husband says, "It seems like this happens every year! I'm beginning to think she just doesn't like the winter."

11. On the basis of the information given, which of the following conditions is the most likely possibility in this patient?
    a. generalized anxiety disorder
    b. substance-induced mood disorder

c. adjustment disorder with depressed mood
d. MDD with a seasonal pattern
e. dysthymia disorder

12. What is the first-line treatment for this patient?
    a. an SSRI
    b. a TCA
    c. an MAOI
    d. lithium carbonate
    e. none of the above

13. As physicians, we need to inform our patients that depression is a disease like any other; it often affects body chemistry, just as diseases such as hypothyroidism, hyperthyroidism, and diabetes mellitus do. Which of the following hypotheses support(s) this argument?
    a. loss of the normal feedback mechanism inhibiting adrenocorticotropic hormone
    b. the lack of normal suppression of blood cortisol following the administration of dexamethasone
    c. the generalized decrease in noradrenergic function in patients who are depressed
    d. a and b
    e. all of the above

14. Which of the following neurotransmitters appears to be the most important mediator of depressive illness in humans?
    a. norepinephrine
    b. acetylcholine
    c. dopamine
    d. serotonin
    e. tryptophan

CLINICAL CASE PROBLEM 6

After a Myocardial Infarction

A 62-year-old male is in your office to follow-up a recent myocardial infarction requiring hospitalization and bypass surgery. During the visit, his wife tells you her husband "just doesn't seem like himself" and goes on to describe symptoms consistent with depression.

15. Which of the following is true?
    a. people who are depressed and who have pre-existing cardiovascular disease have a 3.5 times greater risk of death than patients who are not depressed
    b. there is no evidence demonstrating a connection between cardiovascular disease and depression
    c. the use of SSRI medication can exacerbate cardiovascular disease

d. TCAs are first-line treatment in patients who have undergone coronary artery bypass and who present with depression

16. A thorough patient interview is most important in evaluating patients who are depressed. In a patient with depression, which of the following questions is the most important and urgent question to ask?
    a. Is there a family history of psychiatric disorders?
    b. Is there a personal history of previous episodes of depression?
    c. Have you had any thoughts of suicide?
    d. Have you had hallucinations?
    e. Have you experienced any delusion?

Clinical Case Management Problem

Discuss a strategy for the pharmacologic management of major depressive disorder.

Answers

1. **c.** The diagnosis in this patient is MDD. This is based on the presence for at least 2 weeks of a distinct change in mood (sadness or lack of pleasure) accompanied by changes in appetite and activities, including decreased energy, psychomotor agitation or retardation, decreased appetite for food or sex, weight loss, changes in sleep–wake cycles, and depressive rumination or thoughts of suicide. Adjustment disorder with depressed mood is not diagnosed when symptoms are severe enough to be considered MDD.

Generalized anxiety disorder is characterized by excessive worry and nervousness about many problems. Mood disorders caused by general medical conditions are initiated and maintained by physiologic problems.

Dysthymic disorder is characterized by a depressed mood that persists for more than 2 years without the other features of MDD.

The criteria for MDD according to the *Diagnostic and Statistical Manual of Mental Disorders*, 4th edition (*DSM-IV*) are as follows:

1. The presence of five or more of the following symptoms during the same 2-week period. These must represent a change from previous functioning. At least one of those two symptoms must be either a or b from the following list:
    a. Depressed mood most of the day, nearly every day, as indicated by either subjective report (e.g., feeling sad or empty) or observation made by others (e.g., appears tearful)

b. Markedly diminished interest or pleasure in all or almost all activities most of the day, nearly every day (as indicated by either subjective account or observation made by others)

c. Significant weight loss when not dieting or weight gain (e.g., a change of more than 5% of body weight in a month) or a decrease or increase in appetite nearly every day

d. Insomnia or hypersomnia nearly every day

e. Psychomotor agitation or retardation nearly every day (observable by others and not merely subjective feelings of restlessness or being slowed down)

f. Fatigue or loss of energy nearly every day

g. Feelings of worthlessness or excessive or inappropriate guilt (which may be delusional) nearly every day (not merely self-reproach or guilt about being sick)

h. Diminished ability to think or concentrate or indecisiveness nearly every day (either by subjective account or observed by others)

i. Recurrent thoughts of death (not just fear of dying), recurrent suicidal ideation without a specific plan, a suicide attempt, or a specific plan for committing suicide

2. The symptoms do not meet the criteria for a mixed episode (manic depression).

3. The symptoms cause clinically significant distress or impairment in social, occupational, or other important areas of functioning.

4. The symptoms are not caused by direct physiologic effects (e.g., drug abuse or a medication) or a general medical condition.

5. The symptoms are not accounted for by bereavement (after the loss of a loved one); the symptoms persist for longer than 2 months or are characterized by a marked functional impairment, morbid preoccupation with worthlessness, suicidal ideation, psychotic symptoms, or psychomotor retardation.

A mnemonic for MDD is SIG-EM-CAPS. A diagnosis is made if a patient has five of the nine following symptoms, which must include energy/fatigue or mood:

Sleep (hypersomnia or insomnia)
Interest (lack of interest in life in general)
Guilt or hopelessness
Energy/fatigue
Mood (depressed, sadness)
Concentration (lack of)
Appetite (increased or decreased; weight loss or weight gain)
Psychomotor (retardation or agitation)
Suicidal ideation

The other choices in this question are discussed in various other answers in this chapter.

2. **a.** The pharmacologic treatment for patients with MDD is most often a member of the class of drugs known as SSRIs. The agents in this class include fluoxetine (Prozac), sertraline (Zoloft), paroxetine (Paxil), fluvoxamine (Luvox), and citalopram (Celexa) or escitalopram (Lexapro). These agents have significantly fewer side effects than older antidepressants. Major side effects may include gastrointestinal distress, decreased libido and inhibited orgasm, tremor, insomnia, somnolence, dry mouth, and a small amount of weight gain.

The SSRIs act exactly as they are named: They block the reuptake of serotonin in the brain. Mixed reuptake inhibitors (norepinephrine, 5-HT, and dopamine) are sometimes used instead of SSRIs and include bupropion (Wellbutrin), venlafaxine (Effexor), nefazodone (Serzone), and mirtazapine (Remeron). TCAs are used less commonly because they exhibit more anticholinergic side effects, including dry mouth, urinary retention, constipation, and blurred vision. They are more sedating than most SSRIs and mixed reuptake inhibitors. Other serious side effects may include orthostatic hypotension (an alpha-blockade side effect) and cardiac conduction abnormalities (an increased risk for patients with second-degree and third-degree heart block or right or left bundle branch block from a quinidine-like action). However, in select cases, the sedative action of TCAs may be beneficial in the treatment of a patient who is depressed.

Antidepressants all have comparable efficacy overall, but individual patients may respond to some antidepressants and not others. A family history of a positive response to a specific antidepressant may be helpful in determining which new antidepressant may be effective, but it is impossible to predict with certainty which antidepressant will be effective for a particular patient; therefore, a trial of two or more antidepressants is sometimes necessary. A patient should be switched to a different antidepressant if he or she does not respond after 6 weeks of treatment or if side effects are intolerable. If sexual side effects occur with use of an SSRI, then bupropion, an antidepressant with minimal sexual side effects (decreased libido), is often substituted.

Antidepressants exert multiple effects on central and autonomic nervous system pathways, at least partially by presynaptic blockade of norepinephrine or serotonin reuptake. MAOIs such as phenelzine or tranylcypromine may be effective in the treatment of patients resistant to MDD. The most common side effects of this class of drugs are dizziness, orthostatic hypotension, sexual dysfunction, insomnia, and daytime sleepiness. The greatest risk with MAOIs is the occurrence of hypertensive crises, which may be induced by the consumption of large amounts of certain foods (i.e., aged cheese and red wine) or drugs containing sympathetic stimulant activity. MAOIs are rarely prescribed in a primary care setting because side effects and significant interactions with a multitude of other medications are common.

Pharmacologic treatment of MDD is effective in approximately 70% to 75% of cases. Electroconvulsive therapy (ECT) may be useful for individuals who do not respond to antidepressants, have contraindications to antidepressants, or are in immediate danger of committing suicide. Unlike antidepressants, which often require 4 to 6 weeks to have a full effect, ECT is effective almost immediately. Although there are no absolute contraindications to its use, ECT should be prescribed only by a psychiatrist; an appropriate referral is necessary.

3. d. Most studies suggest that CBT is an effective treatment for depression. CBT helps patients change the way they interpret events and encourages a greater sense of optimism and empowerment. This method of brief psychotherapy was developed during the past two decades by Aaron T. Beck. It is used primarily for the treatment of mild to moderate depression and for patients with low self-esteem. It is a form of behavioral therapy that aims to directly remove symptoms rather than resolving underlying conflicts such as is attempted in psychodynamic psychotherapies. Cognitive behavioral therapists view the patient's conscious thoughts as central to production. The cornerstone of treatment is the belief that how patients think informs how they feel. If negative thoughts can be adjusted, the negative feelings and low mood can be improved. Both the content of thoughts and the thought processes are seen as distorted in people with such symptoms. Therapy is directed at identifying and altering these cognitive distortions.

4. a. SSRI discontinuation syndrome can present with a range of symptoms, including anxiety, agitation, gastrointestinal distress, myalgias, or a sensation of "electrical shocks" through the arms and legs. The chance of this occurring is directly related to the half-life of a given SSRI. Fluoxetine is the least likely of the drugs to produce a discontinuation syndrome on abrupt cessation of use due to its long half-life (up to 7 days). On the other hand, paroxetine has the shortest half-life (21 hours) and therefore is most likely to cause symptoms. The other SSRIs listed, sertraline and citalopram, have intermediate half-lives and have an intermediate likelihood of precipitating discontinuation symptoms.

5. b. This patient has a dysthymic disorder. Dysthymic disorder is defined as a depressive syndrome in which the patient is bothered all or most of the time by depressive symptoms. The diagnosis of dysthymic disorder is best made by following the "Rule of 2's": two of the nine symptoms required for a diagnosis of major depressive disorder are present, for at least 2 years, without interruption of symptoms for longer than 2 months. Although the symptoms of dysthymic disorder are chronic and certainly impair occupational and/or social function, they are not of sufficient severity to warrant a diagnosis of major depressive episode.

Adjustment disorder is generally more time limited and related to a specific stressor. Mood disorders caused by general medical conditions have specific physiologic causes.

6. e. Because of the long history, this patient probably should be treated with a combination approach of exercise, psychotherapy, and pharmacotherapy.

Medications used for this disorder are as described previously, although agents with more side effects should be avoided. Generally, if medications are used, the lowest effective dose is used, treatment is continued for 6 months, and the patient is reevaluated periodically afterward. Exercise has been shown to be effective in the treatment of this disorder and should be strongly encouraged. Psychotherapy (CBT as described previously) is an important component of the treatment of this condition and has been shown to reduce recurrences. Importantly, a dysthymic disorder that evolves into major depressive disorder, known as "double depression," can often be difficult to treat and often requires a combination of medication and therapy.

Relaxation therapy is more appropriate for treatment of anxiety than for depression.

7. a. This patient has an adjustment disorder with depressed mood, which is defined as a reaction to some identifiable psychosocial stressor(s) that occurs within 3 months of the onset of the depressed mood. As with any other psychiatric disorder, there is a clear impairment of occupational or social functioning. The severity of the depression is not sufficient to warrant a diagnosis of MDD. Treatment of individuals with adjustment disorder includes counseling about stress management and brief psychotherapy, and medications are rarely used.

Dysthymic disorder is characterized by 2 or more years of chronically depressed mood. Mood disorder caused by a general medical condition is caused by a known pathologic process.

Substance-induced mood disorder is directly caused by a particular substance, commonly alcohol or psychostimulants. Substance-induced mood disorder should be considered in individuals with depressive symptoms, especially those who may be under psychologic stress and using inappropriate coping mechanisms, such as the use of alcohol or drugs.

8. c. The treatment of choice for adjustment disorder is brief psychotherapy consisting of counseling and stress management. If the stressful situation cannot be changed, cognitive restructuring, relaxation and other stress management techniques, and exercise are useful for improving the ability to cope with stress. The physician should suggest specific coping strategies, with specific goals and objectives negotiated with the patient.

9. d. This patient most likely has a substance-induced mood disorder. The "tip-offs" to this diagnosis are as follows: (1) symptoms and signs of depression, (2) a self-described "burnout syndrome", (3) the missing of a number of days of work recently, and (4) the clue of "I am using anything and everything to try to relax."

The sequence of events that likely took place in this patient is as follows. The drive to keep going faster and faster "to stay on the treadmill" eventually led to a depressive disorder and occupational burnout. This was followed by inappropriate "coping mechanisms," including the use of alcohol and/or drugs to keep going. Eventually, he reached a point at which he was unable to function because of depression, "burnout syndrome," and the number of days missed at work. Therefore, his work suffered.

10. e. The steps that should be pursued in this patient's case are as follows: (1) Ask the patient about alcohol intake (specific amounts, specific times, and total intake); (2) administer an alcohol abuse questionnaire; (3) involve the patient's family, if possible; (4) if a diagnosis of substance-induced mood disorder is confirmed, get the patient's cooperation for initiating treatment; and (5) include an ongoing recovery program, possibly following detoxification. Individual, group, and family psychotherapy is often helpful.

Referral to a 12-step program such as Alcoholics Anonymous is extremely useful for both rehabilitation and relapse prevention.

11. d. This patient most likely has MDD with a seasonal pattern (or seasonal affective disorder). Patients meet the criteria for MDD but symptoms only occur during certain seasons and often remit with the transition to the next season. The most common seasons of the year for patients to experience symptoms are fall and winter, with cessation of symptoms during spring and summer. Typical symptoms include loss of interest in activities, sleep disturbances, and loss of libido. Once the pattern is identified, the treatment can include prophylactic treatment with SSRI medication in order to prevent the onset of disabling mood symptoms. Seasonal affective disorder can often be treated with light therapy (with exposure to the eye, not the skin), which appears to have a low risk of adverse effects. Light therapy is more effective if administered in the morning, and studies are beginning to show that light therapy can be as effective as SSRI medication.

The psychiatric differential diagnosis in this patient would include adjustment disorder with depressed mood, but this is less likely with the repeated pattern temporally related to the change of seasons.

12. a. Although both TCA and MAOI classes of antidepressants are often helpful in depression, the SSRI class is associated with less morbidity, and drugs in this class are generally considered first-line treatment.

13. e. Depression is associated with significant chemical and morphologic changes in the brain. When patients understand this, it helps to decrease the stigma of the diagnosis and decrease feelings of shame and inadequacy.

14. d. The following physiologic abnormalities have been described in MDD: (1) a "neurotransmitter imbalance" that appears to be caused by a relative deficiency of the neurotransmitter serotonin (the new SSRIs add confirming evidence to this hypothesis); (2) patients with MDD have hyperactivity of the hypothalamic–pituitary–adrenal axis, which results in elevated plasma cortisol levels and nonsuppression of cortisol following a dexamethasone suppression test; (3) a blunting of the normally expected increase in plasma growth hormone induced by α_2-adrenergic receptor agonists; and (4) a blunting of serotonin-mediated increase in plasma prolactin.

15. a. Approximately 65% of patients with acute myocardial infarction report experiencing symptoms of depression. Major depression is present in 15% to 22% of these patients. Depression is an independent risk factor in the development of and mortality associated with cardiovascular disease in otherwise healthy people. People who are depressed and who have pre-existing cardiovascular disease have a 3.5 times greater risk of death than patients who are not depressed and have cardiovascular disease. Physicians should assess patients for depression with any cardiovascular disease.

SSRIs are the first-line treatment in this case. TCAs are associated with cardiac arrhythmias, which are also an increased risk in the weeks after a patient has sustained a myocardial infarction.

16. **C.** The most important question to ask a patient who presents with signs and symptoms of depression is whether he or she has contemplated suicide. The following questions are useful in exploring suicidality:

1. "You seem so terribly unhappy. Have you had any thoughts about hurting yourself?"
2. "If you have, have you thought of the means by which you would do it? Have you considered a specific plan for ending your life? Under what circumstances would you carry it out?"

3. "What would it take to stop you (from killing yourself)?"
4. "Do you feel that your situation is hopeless?"

The overall mortality from suicide in individuals with MDD is 15%. Symptoms that place a patient who is depressed at higher risk for suicide are a practical and lethal plan with feelings of hopelessness. Patients must be directly asked about suicidal ideations, and steps must be taken to protect those at high risk. Such steps include making a treatment contract, mobilizing support systems, providing close observation, ensuring immediate availability of a clinician, or placing the patient in the hospital if necessary. Suicidal risk is an acute, not a chronic, problem and has to be handled as a crisis.

Solution to the Clinical Case Management Problem

A strategy for the pharmacologic management of MDD is as follows: (1) Identify and treat causes unrelated to MDD (e.g., hypothyroidism or substance abuse); (2) use single-agent pharmacotherapy as the first step; (3) if there is no satisfactory response after 4 to 6 weeks and an increase of the dose does not improve the patient's condition, or if the patient cannot tolerate the first drug, switch to a different drug that minimizes the troublesome side effects or

is from a different chemical class; and (4) if trials of two or three antidepressants are ineffective, refer to a psychiatrist for possible augmentation or other intense treatments.

A psychiatrist may elect to use ECT if several antidepressant trials in addition to nonpharmacologic treatment options have been ineffective, if there are contraindications to the use of antidepressants, or if there is a high risk of immediate suicide.

Summary

PREVALENCE
1. MDD
   a. Lifetime prevalence: 3.5% to 5.8% of the population
   b. Gender difference: more common in women than in men
   c. Age: occurs in children, adolescents, adults, and the elderly.
2. Dysthymia
   a. Lifetime prevalence: 2.1% to 4.7%
   b. Gender difference: more common in women than in men
3. Prevalence for depression in medical settings has been reported to be as high as 15%.

DIFFERENTIAL DIAGNOSIS
As described in the *DSM-IV* criteria: (1) MDD, (2) dysthymia, (3) depression caused by a general medical condition, (4) adjustment disorder with depressed mood, (5) substance-induced mood disorder, (6) manic episodes with irritable mood, and (7) mixed episodes (depression and hypomania)

DISTINGUISHING MDD FROM DYSTHYMIA
In addition to depressed mood, there are significant changes in appetite and activities, such as sleep disturbance, weight loss, severe fatigue or lack of energy, and suicidal rumination. Dysthymia is perhaps best described as "a chronic ongoing depressed mood" that lasts years rather than weeks or months.

SUBCLASSIFICATIONS OF MDD
Once a diagnosis of depression has been made, the clinician should characterize the syndrome further, if possible, into the following categories:
1. Unipolar versus bipolar
   a. MDD is unipolar.
   b. Affective disorder is bipolar.
2. Melancholic versus nonmelancholic: 40% to 60% of all hospitalizations are for melancholic depression. Symptoms include anhedonia, excessive or inappropriate guilt, early morning waking, anorexia, psychomotor

disturbance, and diurnal variation in mood. The patient who is depressed and melancholy may appear frantic, fearful, agitated, or withdrawn.

3. Psychotic versus nonpsychotic: Psychotic depressions are not rare. Studies suggest that approximately 10% to 25% of patients hospitalized for major depression have a psychotic depression. Often, patients with a psychotic depression will endorse "mood congruent" symptoms such as auditory hallucinations characterized by a voice telling them they are worthless or "no good." These are also known as "self-deprecating" auditory hallucinations.

4. Atypical depression: Atypical depression denotes symptoms that include hypersomnia instead of insomnia, hyperphagia (sometimes as a carbohydrate craving) rather than anorexia, reactivity (mood changes with environmental circumstances), and a long-standing pattern of interpersonal rejection sensitivity. It is much more common in women. Patients with atypical depression are frequently reported to have an anxious or irritable mood rather than dysphoria. They may also describe "leaden paralysis," which is the sensation that their limbs are extremely heavy and making it difficult to move.

5. Masked depression: Masked depression is similar to atypical depression. Instead of overt depression, the depression is expressed as many psychosomatic signs and symptoms.

TREATMENT

1. Follow the guidelines provided in the Solution to the Clinical Case Management Problem.
2. Consider the SSRIs as the drugs of first choice unless specific contraindications to their use are present.
3. Treat for at least 4 weeks before you consider the therapy you are using to be a therapeutic failure.
4. MDD should be treated with a combination of pharmacotherapy, psychotherapy, and exercise.

5. MDD is a recurrent disease: At 1 year following the start of therapy, 33% will be free of the disease, 33% will have had a relapse, and 33% will still be depressed. Using psychotherapy along with pharmacologic treatment significantly reduces the rate of relapse.

Three-phase approach to the treatment of depression:

1. Acute treatment phase, phase 1: time, 6 to 12 weeks. The goal of this phase of therapy is the remission of symptoms of depression.
2. Continuation treatment, phase 2: time, 4 to 9 months. The goal of this phase of therapy is to prevent a relapse of the depressive symptoms.
3. Maintenance treatment, phase 3: time, patient dependent, perhaps lifetime. The goal of this phase of therapy is to treat patients who have had three or more episodes of depression. Prevention of recurrence is the treatment goal.

Too often, medication is tapered or discontinued soon after symptoms have been brought under control; this greatly increases the patient's risk of relapse. There is no justification for lowering the effective dose of an antidepressant drug during maintenance treatment. Once the patient is asymptomatic for at least 6 months following a depressive episode, recovery from the episode is declared.

The termination of therapy must be accompanied by patient education. The key concern is the likelihood of a recurrent episode. If this is the patient's first bout of depression that needed to be treated, the recurrence rate is approximately 50%. If there have been previous episodes of depression or a family history of depression exists, the probability of a recurrence is increased significantly. The patient must be made aware of the symptoms that indicate another episode and needs to know that subsequent attacks can be treated effectively, especially if therapy is initiated early in the disease.

Suggested Reading

American Psychiatric Association: *Diagnostic and Statistical Manual of Mental Disorders*, 4th ed text revision. Washington, DC: American Psychiatric Association, 2000.

Gilbody SM, Whitty P, Grimshaw J, Thomas R: Educational and organizational interventions to improve the management of depression in primary care: A systematic review. *JAMA* 289(23): 3145–3151, 2003.

Mann JJ: The medical management of depression. *N Engl J Med* 353(17):1819–1834, 2005.

Nease DE Jr, Maloin JM: Depression screening: A practical strategy. *J Fam Pract* 52(2):118–124, 2003.

Rupke SJ, Blecke D, Renfrow M: Cognitive therapy for depression. *Am Fam Physician* 73(1):83–86, 2006.

Sutherland JE, Sutherland SJ, Hoehns JD: Achieving the best outcome in treatment of depression. *J Fam Pract* 52(3):201–209, 2003.

SELECT THE BEST ANSWER TO THE FOLLOWING QUESTIONS

CLINICAL CASE PROBLEM 1

A 42-Year-Old Computer Science Professor Who Has Just Been Anointed by God as the New Head of the Computer Age

A 42-year-old computer technician is brought to the emergency room by his wife, who complains that for the past 4 weeks her husband has become increasingly irritable, angry, and suspicious. She states, "His personality has completely changed"; "He has not slept for 6 nights and has been found by the local police using his laptop under a lamppost to work on his computer programs."

He has become preoccupied with the belief that God has anointed him as the "new leader of the computer age." Fearing that his ideas will be stolen by INTERPOL, the CIA, the state police, and the "Red Coated Mounties" from Canada, he has constructed an elaborate mathematic code that allows only him and his appointed prophets to understand the programs. He quite proudly states that "Albert Einstein wouldn't have a chance at this. It's even too clever for him!"

His wife further states that the patient has been depressed on and off throughout his life and has been taking "all kinds of junk" for the depression, none of which helped at any time. However, she claims that the patient has never had a substance abuse problem of any kind. She describes her husband's family as "a bunch of nuts." She continues to tell you that, for instance, his mother calls him at 3 o'clock almost every morning (often while he is busy getting his equipment and extension cords set up outside, rooting through the garage, knocking everything over, and waking up the entire neighborhood) just to tell him that she is thinking of him. His father has a history of numerous psychiatric hospitalizations for "weird behavior" and has received several courses of shock therapy.

During the interview, the patient volunteers little information, is extremely agitated, and paces the floor muttering, "There is no time for this ... my mission is clear!"

1. Based on the history given, what condition best describes the behavior exhibited in this patient?
   a. acute hypomania
   b. acute mania
   c. acute anxiety
   d. dementia
   e. delirium

2. Based on the patient's personal history, the condition applied in question 1, and the family history described, this is most likely a part of a condition known as which of the following?
   a. bipolar disorder
   b. alcohol intoxication
   c. major depressive disorder (MDD)
   d. schizoid personality disorder
   e. schizophrenia

3. The *Diagnostic and Statistical Manual of Mental Disorders*, 4th edition (*DSM-IV*), further subclassifies this into which of the following?
   a. schizophrenia: catatonic type
   b. schizophrenia: paranoid type
   c. bipolar I disorder
   d. bipolar II disorder
   e. atypical insanity

4. At this time, what would you do?
   a. prescribe diazepam and tell his wife that you will review the situation
   b. prescribe lithium carbonate on an outpatient basis and see the patient in 3 months
   c. prescribe fluphenazine on an outpatient basis and see the patient in 1 week
   d. prescribe a tricyclic antidepressant (TCA) on an outpatient basis and see the patient in 1 week
   e. none of the above

5. The wife of the patient calls you at your office and asks, "Doctor, what are the chances that my son will develop the same diagnosis?" What will you tell her regarding her son's relative risk of developing the disorder described compared with someone without a first-degree relative with the disease?
   a. half as much
   b. equal to
   c. 24 times as much
   d. twice as much
   e. 3.5 times as much

6. Which of the following is a symptom of lithium toxicity?
   a. weight gain
   b. psoriatic rash
   c. agranulocytosis
   d. tremor
   e. polyuria

7. Which of the following medications would not be used in patients with this disorder who are refractory to lithium carbonate?
   a. carbamazepine
   b. lamotrigine
   c. divalproex
   d. gabapentin
   e. risperidone

8. Which of the following neurotransmitters is (are) implicated most clearly in the cause of the acute manic or acute hypomanic episodes in bipolar disorder?
   a. norepinephrine
   b. dopamine
   c. serotonin
   d. a and b
   e. all of the above

9. What is the role of the family physician in the diagnosis and treatment of the condition described?
   a. family physicians routinely diagnose and treat this condition without the help of a psychiatrist
   b. family physicians are not involved in the diagnosis and treatment of this condition
   c. family physicians are in a unique position to diagnose this disease early because often a longitudinal relationship with the patient and the family exists
   d. family physicians are often involved during the maintenance phase of treatment
   e. c and d

CLINICAL CASE PROBLEM 2

A 34-Year-Old Woman with Ups and Downs

A 34-year-old woman comes to your office feeling "a little depressed" and you note that she feels sad but does not meet the definition of a current major depressive episode. As your visit continues, she also admits to feeling "really great" sometimes. She describes periods of elated mood, mildly decreased sleep with continued energy, and increased goal-directed behavior that last 2 or 3 days but never more. The symptoms are episodic but do not interfere with her work or social life.

10. Which diagnosis best characterizes this patient's presentation?
    a. cyclothymic disorder
    b. MDD
    c. bipolar disorder, type I
    d. bipolar disorder, type II
    e. generalized anxiety disorder

11. What is the pharmacologic treatment of choice for this patient's disorder?
    a. a serotonin reuptake inhibitor (SSRI)
    b. a TCA
    c. a monoamine oxidase inhibitor
    d. divalproex
    e. lithium carbonate

CLINICAL CASE PROBLEM 3

A 45-Year-Old Male Recently Treated for Depression

A 45-year-old patient you have recently diagnosed and started treating for major depression leaves a message for you saying, "I feel like I am going crazy!" He says he has not slept for days, is having racing thoughts, and is starting one project after another without finishing anything.

12. What is a likely diagnosis in this patient?
    a. medication-induced mania
    b. chronic paranoid schizophrenia
    c. generalized anxiety disorder
    d. impulsive neurotic syndrome
    e. delusional disorder

13. Which other conditions can cause mood swings?
    a. thyroid disorders
    b. adrenal disorders
    c. neurologic disorders
    d. substance abuse disorders
    e. all of the above

Clinical Case Management Problem

Describe the basic diagnostic features of bipolar disorder: manic episode and hypomanic episode.

Answers

1. **b.** The most likely diagnosis in this patient at this time is acute mania. Mania is defined as a distinct period of abnormally and persistently elevated, expansive, or

irritable mood. It may include inflated self-esteem or grandiosity, decreased need for sleep, loquaciousness, flight of ideas, distractibility, increase in goal-directed activity, activities such as unrestrained buying sprees, sexual indiscretions, and foolish business investments. These symptoms cause a marked impairment in occupational functioning.

The basic difference between mania and hypomania is that in mania there are often psychotic symptoms and a more severe impairment in normal functioning (social, occupational, etc.). In addition, the mood disturbance is more severe.

With no history of substance abuse problems, memory impairment, or general medical conditions, delirium and dementia are not likely. A diagnosis of acute anxiety does not account for many of the presenting symptoms.

2. a. This episode of acute mania is part of a bipolar disorder. For a diagnosis of bipolar disorder, at least one episode of mania or hypomania has to have occurred. This patient has a history that is very suggestive of previous episodes of major depression, which provides further evidence for a diagnosis of bipolar disorder.

His mother may also have bipolar disorder, indicated by her frequent phone calls at 3 AM. Furthermore, his father has a significant psychiatric history, and although we cannot be sure of a specific diagnosis, his treatment with electroconvulsive therapy may support a potential derangement in mood.

3. c. The *DSM-IV* subdivides bipolar disorder into two types: bipolar I and bipolar II. Bipolar I disorder identifies a patient who has had at least one true manic episode. A history of depression or hypomania may also be present in the patient with bipolar I disorder, but neither of these conditions is essential for the diagnosis. Patients with bipolar II disorder have a history of hypomania and major depressive episodes but no history of mania.

4. e. Outpatient therapy is usually not possible or safe for patients with acute mania. The treatment of choice at this time is admission to a psychiatric hospital and treatment with an antipsychotic agent such as risperidone, haloperidol, or olanzapine until the psychotic symptoms subside. He should be on a mood stabilizer at the same time. Lithium carbonate remains the drug of choice for long-term treatment of the majority of patients with bipolar disorder. It is effective treatment for acute mania and prevents relapses of both manic and depressive episodes in bipolar disorder; hence, once the diagnosis has been made, it should continue to be used prophylactically. It has also been shown to lessen suicidal thoughts and behavior

in patients with bipolar disorder. In the treatment of acute mania, it may be 10 to 14 days before the full therapeutic effect of lithium is felt. Lithium carbonate is not metabolized and therefore does not accumulate active metabolic products. However, because the therapeutic window is very narrow (0.6 to 1.2 mEq/L), blood level monitoring is necessary to determine appropriate dosing and blood levels should be drawn 10 to 12 hours after the last dose has been given.

Patients with bipolar disorder who do not respond to lithium carbonate or in whom lithium is contraindicated should be treated with anticonvulsant medications (carbamazepine or divalproex acid). Blood level monitoring is necessary for these agents as well. These anticonvulsants are almost as effective as lithium carbonate in the treatment of bipolar disorder. Approximately 30% of patients with bipolar disorder will not respond to lithium and will have to be treated with other agents.

Benzodiazepines may occasionally be useful for the treatment of severe agitation during a manic episode; however, agents such as lorazepam or clonazepam are preferred.

5. c. First-degree relatives of patients with bipolar illness are reported to be at least 24 times more likely to develop bipolar illness than relatives of control subjects. The genetic evidence is very strong for bipolar disorder. The incidence of bipolar illness and MDD is much higher in first-degree relatives of patients with bipolar illness than in the general population. However, first-degree relatives of patients with MDD only have an increase in the incidence of unipolar depression.

6. d. Although lithium is highly effective in the treatment of bipolar disorder, it is important be recognize symptoms associated with its use. Tremor is an indication of lithium toxicity. Other signs of toxicity include diarrhea, vomiting, ataxia, and restlessness. Weight gain, hypothyroidism, polyuria, and exacerbation of psoriasis can occur at therapeutic lithium levels. Agranulocytosis is not associated with lithium use.

7. d. As mentioned previously, the anticonvulsant agents carbamazepine, divalproex, and lamotrigine are useful in the treatment of bipolar disorder if lithium is contraindicated or not helpful. Atypical antipsychotics such as risperidone also have a place in maintenance therapy. Gabapentin has no role in the acute or chronic treatment of bipolar disorder because no studies support its efficacy in this regard.

8. d. The most relevant pharmacologic information relating to theories of acute mania and acute hypomania is the consistent finding that direct or indirect norepinephrine and dopamine agonists (those drugs that stimulate the noradrenergic and dopaminergic receptors or increase concentrations of these neurotransmitters in the brain) can precipitate mania or hypomania in patients with underlying bipolar illness. Stimulants such as amphetamines and cocaine can induce maniclike syndromes in patients who do not appear to have an underlying vulnerability to develop a bipolar disorder. This suggests an association of mania or hypomania with hyperadrenergic or hyperdopaminergic states.

9. **e.** During the acute manic phase described previously, patients need to be hospitalized and seen by a psychiatrist. The family physician will refer a patient with this condition until he or she is stabilized. During the maintenance phase of treatment, family physicians often resume the care of these patients, including obtaining appropriate drug levels and other blood tests. Family physicians are in a unique position to diagnose the onset of the disease because they often have longitudinal relationships with the entire family; early diagnosis and treatment of this disorder can prevent serious family and occupational disruptions. When patients have become stabilized with appropriate medication, they are often able to lead creative, productive, and satisfying lives with little impairment of social or professional functioning.

10. **a.** This patient is describing cyclothymic disorder. Cyclothymic disorder is best conceptualized as a less severe form of bipolar illness. The data indicate that approximately 30% of individuals with cyclothymia have a positive family history for bipolar illness. By definition, cyclothymic disorder is a chronic mood disturbance of at least 2 years' duration and involving numerous hypomanic and mild

depressive episodes that do not meet the diagnostic criteria for mania or major depression, do not interfere with social or occupational function, but have no periods of euthymic mood for more than 2 months. Patients with bipolar II disorder have a history of hypomania and also meet the criteria for major depressive episodes.

11. **e.** As with bipolar disorder, the treatment of choice is lithium carbonate.

12. **a.** Depression can be treated with the use of SSRI medication such as fluoxetine, but if used alone this class of medication can trigger a manic episode in some patients. Taking a thorough history of mood symptoms must include direct questioning about any history of manic or hypomanic symptoms in patients presenting with depressive symptoms. Often, a presentation of unipolar depression underlies an undiagnosed bipolar diathesis.

13. **e.** Many other conditions can cause mood swings. Abuse of substances such as amphetamines and cocaine can be diagnosed by obtaining a drug screen. Thyroid disorders can cause mood swings and are diagnosed by an appropriate physical examination and blood tests. Adrenal disorders such as Addison's disease or Cushing's syndrome, vitamin B_{12} deficiency, and neurologic disorders such as multiple sclerosis, brain tumors, epilepsy, or encephalitis can mimic bipolar disorder. Certain infections affecting brain function, especially acquired immune deficiency syndrome, can cause mental states resembling bipolar disorder. A number of medications, including corticosteroids and certain drugs used to treat anxiety, can also cause mood swings and need to be discontinued or their dose needs to be adjusted if these symptoms occur.

Solution to the Clinical Case Management Problem

Key features of bipolar disorder are as follows:

Manic Episode

1. A manic episode is a distinct period of abnormally and persistently elevated, expansive, or irritable mood lasting at least 1 week and of sufficient severity to cause marked impairment in social or occupational functioning.

2. During this period, at least three of the following symptoms are also present: (a) grandiosity, (b) decreased need for sleep, (c) hyperverbal or pressured speech, (d) flight of ideas or racing

thoughts, (e) distractibility, (f) increase in goal-directed activity or psychomotor agitation, and (g) excessive involvement in pleasurable activities that have a high potential for painful consequences.

3. There is no evidence of a physical or substance-induced cause or the presence of another major mental disorder to account for the patient's symptoms.

Key Features of Hypomanic Episodes

1. During hypomanic episodes, there is a distinctly sustained elevated, expansive, or irritable mood

lasting for at least 4 days that is clearly different from the individual's nondepressed mood but does not cause marked impairment in social or occupational functioning such as in acute mania.

2. During the mood disturbance, at least three of the following symptoms are also present to a significant degree: (a) inflated self-esteem or grandiosity, (b) decreased need for sleep, (c) more talkative than usual, (d) flight of ideas or racing thoughts, (e) distractibility, (f) increase in goal-directed activity or psychomotor agitation, and (g) excessive involvement in pleasurable activities that have a high potential for painful consequences.

3. The episode is not physical or substance induced.

Summary

PREVALENCE

1. The prevalence of bipolar disorders varies from 0.7% to 1.6% (lifetime).
2. The prevalence is greater in women than in men.
3. In general medical settings (settings that select for patients with emotional distress and physical illness), the lifetime prevalence rate is probably between 5% and 10%.

CLASSIFICATION OF BIPOLAR DISORDERS

1. Bipolar disorder I: a patient with bipolar disorder who has had at least one episode of true mania.
2. Bipolar disorder II: a patient with bipolar disorder who has not had at least one episode of true mania.
3. Cyclothymic disorder: a less severe form of bipolar disorder.

HERITABILITY OF BIPOLAR DISORDER

1. First-degree relatives of patients with bipolar affective disorder are at least 24 times more likely to develop bipolar illness than relatives of control subjects.
2. The incidence of both bipolar illness and MDD is much higher in first-degree relatives of patients with bipolar illness than in the general population.

DIAGNOSTIC CRITERIA

1. See diagnostic criteria for acute mania and acute hypomania in the Clinical Case Management Problem.

2. The other mood component of bipolar disorder is depression, which is discussed in Chapter 141.

CYCLOTHYMIC DISORDER

1. Cyclothymic disorder is defined as a less severe form of bipolar disorder. By definition, it is a chronic mood disturbance of at least 2 years' duration and involves numerous hypomanic and mild depressive episodes. These episodes do not meet the diagnostic criteria for bipolar disorder or MDD.
2. In cyclothymic disorder, there are no periods of euthymia longer than 2 months' duration.

TREATMENT

1. Acute treatment: (a) Hospitalization is required for acute mania with psychosis, (b) antipsychotic agents (olanzapine, clozapine, risperidone, and haloperidol) should be used when psychosis is present, and (c) benzodiazepines (lorazepam and clonazepam) may be useful for severe agitation during mania.
2. Maintenance and prevention of relapse: (a) Lithium carbonate is the agent of first choice (usual dosage is 900 to 1200 mg/day), (b) anticonvulsive agents (carbamazepine or divalproex) are useful when lithium is ineffective or contraindicated, and (c) other anticonvulsants such as lamotrigine may be used when the previously mentioned agents are ineffective when used alone or in combination.

Suggested Reading

American Psychiatric Association: *Diagnostic and Statistical Manual of Mental Disorders*, 4th ed, text revision. Washington, DC: American Psychiatric Association, 2000.

Glick ID, Suppes T, DeBattista C, et al: Psychopharmacologic treatment strategies for depression, bipolar disorder, and schizophrenia. *Ann Intern Med* 134(1): 47–60, 2001.

Goodnick PJ: Bipolar depression: A review of randomised clinical trials. *Expert Opin Pharmacother* 8(1):13–21, 2007.

Kaplan HI, Sadock BJ, eds: *Kaplan and Sadock's Synopsis of Psychiatry: Behavioral Sciences/Clinical Psychiatry*, 8th ed. Baltimore: Williams & Wilkins, 1998.

Tomb DA: *Psychiatry*, 6th ed. Baltimore: Williams & Wilkins, 1999.

CLINICAL CASE PROBLEM 1

A 27-Year-Old Female with Restlessness and Chronic Worry

A 27-year-old female comes to your office expressing concern about a number of bothersome issues. She says things were going "pretty well" until a few months ago when she started feeling restless and on edge. She notes feeling tired and run down and "constantly stressed out." She also describes problems falling asleep as she lies awake worrying about all of the things she needs to get done: "But even though I'm worrying about all of the things I need to get done, I have such a hard time concentrating that I can't even start in my to-do list!" She is seeking help now because this problem with focus and concentration is affecting her job performance and threatening her relationship with her long-term boyfriend.

At this point in the interview, she becomes very tense and tells you, "You know, doctor, this is really getting out of control; I feel I can't function anymore."

On physical examination, the patient's blood pressure is 130/70 mmHg, and her pulse is 94 beats/minute and regular. Her thyroid gland is within normal limits and nontender. Her cardiac examination reveals no abnormalities outside the tachycardia. Her neurologic examination is normal. The remainder of the physical examination is normal.

SELECT THE BEST ANSWER TO THE FOLLOWING QUESTIONS

1. What is the most likely diagnosis in this patient?
   a. panic disorder
   b. major depressive disorder
   c. generalized anxiety disorder (GAD)
   d. hyperthyroidism
   e. hypochondriasis

2. Of patients with the disorder described, what percentage have at least one other similar psychiatric disorder at some time in their life?
   a. 10%
   b. 30%
   c. 50%
   d. 80%
   e. no data are available

3. All of the following are true regarding anxiety seen in the primary care setting except
   a. it is the most common psychiatric illness seen by family physicians
   b. it is associated with high utilization of medical services
   c. patients often present with somatic complaints
   d. anxiety can be a normal part of other medical issues, such as asthma and cardiac pathology
   e. it is often associated with other psychiatric conditions, such as depression

4. Which of the following symptoms is generally not characteristic of the disorder described?
   a. awakening with apprehension and unrealistic concern regarding future misfortune
   b. worry out of proportion to the likelihood or impact of feared events
   c. a 6-month or longer course of anxiety and associated symptoms
   d. association of the anxiety described with depression
   e. anxiety exclusively focused on health concerns

5. Which of the following statements regarding the disorder described is (are) true?
   a. this disorder may develop between attacks in panic disorder
   b. the symptoms of this disorder are often present in episodes of depression
   c. medical conditions that produce the major symptom associated with this disorder must be excluded
   d. the disorder is accompanied by symptoms of motor tension, autonomic hyperactivity, hypervigilance, and scanning
   e. all of the above are true

6. What is the psychotherapy of choice in this disorder?
   a. cognitive–behavioral therapy (CBT)
   b. hypnosis
   c. supportive psychotherapy
   d. psychoanalytic psychotherapy
   e. none of the above

7. Which of the following pharmacologic agents is not recommended in the treatment of this disorder?
   a. venlafaxine
   b. buspirone
   c. benzodiazepines

d. selective serotonin reuptake inhibitors (SSRIs)
e. Clozaril

8. Which of the following benzodiazepines has the shortest half-life?
   a. diazepam (Valium)
   b. chlordiazepoxide (Librium)
   c. clorazepate (Tranxene)
   d. alprazolam (Xanax)
   e. clonazepam (Klonopin)

9. This disorder is more common in which of the following?
   a. elderly white males
   b. school-age children
   c. married people
   d. those of higher socioeconomic status
   e. young to middle-aged females

10. Which of the following statements is (are) true regarding this disorder?
    a. this disorder displays autosomal-dominant genetic transmission
    b. the mechanism of symptom development in this disorder may relate to a conditioned response to a stimulus that the individual has come to associate with danger
    c. a relation between the onset of this disorder and the cumulative effects of stressful life events is possible
    d. b and c
    e. a, b, and c

CLINICAL CASE PROBLEM 2

A 22-Year-Old Law Student Unable to Answer Questions in Class

A 22-year-old law student comes to your office in a state of anxiety. He is taking a law class in which 50% of the class grade is based on class participation. Although he knows the material well, he is unable to answer the questions when posed to him by the professor. He now has gone through 2 months of the 6-month class and has not been able to answer one of the 14 questions that the professor has asked him in class.

The professor asked him to make an appointment for a "little chat" the other day. At that time, he was told that he would (in the professor's words) "fail the class" unless he began to participate.

The student describes himself as a loner. He tells you that he has always been shy, but this is the first time the shyness has really threatened to have a major impact on him. His family history is significant for what he terms "this shyness." His mother has the same characteristics, but for her it does not seem to be causing the kind of life difficulties that it is causing him.

His mental status examination is essentially normal.

11. What is the most likely diagnosis in this patient?
    a. panic disorder with agoraphobia
    b. panic disorder without agoraphobia
    c. panic disorder with social phobia
    d. social phobia
    e. specific phobia

12. Which of the following is not a characteristic of the disorder described?
    a. persistent fear of humiliation
    b. exaggerated fear of humiliation
    c. embarrassment in social situations
    d. high levels of distress in particular situations
    e. fear of crowds or fear of closed-in spaces

13. Which of the following personality disorders is this disorder likely to be confused with?
    a. avoidant personality
    b. borderline personality
    c. histrionic personality
    d. obsessive–compulsive personality
    e. shy personality not otherwise specified

14. The neurochemical basis of the disorder described has been associated with which of the following neurotransmitters?
    a. epinephrine
    b. norepinephrine
    c. serotonin
    d. a and b
    e. a, b, and c

15. Which of the following pharmacologic agents is used most commonly to treat this disorder?
    a. benzodiazepines
    b. monoamine oxidase inhibitors (MAOIs)
    c. tricyclic antidepressants
    d. newer antipsychotic medications
    e. beta blockers

16. With respect to this disorder, which of the following psychotherapies is most effective?
    a. CBT
    b. brief psychodynamic therapy
    c. psychoanalysis
    d. biofeedback
    e. all of the above

CLINICAL CASE PROBLEM 3

An Anxious Young Man

A lab technician calls to tell you that a 22-year-old male you have sent for a blood draw is very anxious. He says he is terrified of having his blood drawn and almost faints at the sight of the needle.

17. Which of the following disorders is the most likely diagnosis?
    a. panic disorder
    b. social phobia
    c. GAD
    d. specific phobia
    e. obsessive–compulsive disorder

Clinical Case Management Problem

List four groups of symptoms that may manifest in the presentation of anxiety.

Answers

1. c. This patient has GAD, which is defined as unrealistic or excessive worry about several life events or activities for a period of at least 6 months during which the person has been bothered more days than not by these concerns. In addition, the following six symptoms are present: muscle tension, restlessness or feeling keyed up or on edge, easy fatigability, difficulty concentrating or a sensation of the "mind going blank" because of anxiety, trouble falling or staying asleep, and irritability. Finally, the anxiety, worry, or physical symptoms significantly interfere with the person's normal routine or usual activities, or they cause marked distress.

2. d. At least 80% of patients with GAD have had at least one other anxiety disorder in their lifetime.

3. a. The most common psychiatric illness seen by family physicians is major depression. Anxiety is associated with high utilization of medical services, and patients often present with somatic complaints. Acute anxiety can be a normal part of other medical issues, such as asthma and cardiac pathology. The most common psychiatric comorbidity with anxiety is major depression.

4. e. GAD is characterized by awakening with apprehension and concern regarding future misfortune, worry out of proportion to the likelihood or impact of feared events, a duration of 6 months or more of anxiety or associated symptoms, and an association with depressed moods.

GAD is usually not associated exclusively with health concerns. When health concerns become the focus of worry, a diagnosis of hypochondriasis or another somatoform disorder becomes more likely.

5. e. Generalized persistent anxiety may develop between attacks in panic disorder. GAD symptoms are often present during episodes of depression. As with panic disorder, medical conditions that may produce anxiety symptoms must be excluded (see answer 3).

GAD is characterized by chronic anxiety about life circumstances accompanied by symptoms of motor tension, autonomic hyperactivity, hypervigilance, and scanning.

6. a. CBT is often effective in the treatment of GAD. Cognitive therapy challenges the distortions in patients' thinking that trigger and heighten their anxiety. This technique can be combined with relaxation training, including deep breathing and progressive muscle relaxation. Biofeedback and imagery are also useful to achieve systematic desensitization. Because relaxation and anxiety are mutually exclusive, these techniques help patients to achieve relief from their symptoms. Although cognitive therapy alone may alleviate GAD symptoms, the combination of cognitive and other behavioral techniques is more effective than cognitive therapy alone.

7. e. SSRIs, especially paroxetine, are often used in the pharmacologic treatment of GAD. Venlafaxine, a mixed serotonin–norepinephrine reuptake inhibitor, can be used for short- and long-term treatment. Although commonly used, benzodiazepines have mostly short-term benefits. Longer acting agents are preferred over short-acting benzodiazepines, but their use should be limited, if possible, because withdrawal symptoms, dependency, and impaired performance are frequent. Buspirone, a nonbenzodiazepine anxiolytic, and other agents such as tricyclic antidepressants are used as well. Clozapine is an antipsychotic agent used in the treatment of patients with schizophrenia. It has no role in the treatment of GAD.

8. d. Alprazolam has the shortest half-life at 6 to 12 hours; clonazepam has a half-life of 25 hours; and diazepam, clorazepate, and chlordiazepoxide all have half-lives of up to 50 hours.

9. **e.** GAD is slightly more common in young and middle-aged females, ethnic minorities, those not currently married, and those of lower socioeconomic status.

10. **d.** Behavioral theories consider GAD, like panic disorder, to be a conditioned response to a stimulus that the individual has come to associate with danger. There is indeed some suggestion that the onset of GAD may be related to the cumulative effects of several stressful life events that have not been properly processed. There is no convincing evidence of a specific form of genetic transmission of GAD.

11. **d.** This patient has a social phobia, which is characterized by a marked and persistent fear of one or more social or performance situations in which the person is exposed to unfamiliar people or to possible scrutiny by others. These patients fear that they may act in a manner that will be humiliating or embarrassing. Examples include (as in this patient) not being able to talk when asked to speak in public, choking on food when eating in front of others, being unable to urinate in a public lavatory, hand trembling when writing in the presence of others, and saying foolish things or not being able to answer questions (as in this patient) in social situations.

In addition, exposure to the feared social situation almost invariably provokes anxiety. The individual realizes that his or her behavior is abnormal and unreasonable. The feared social or performance situation is either avoided or endured with intense anxiety. The avoidance, anxious participation, or distress in the feared social or performance situation interfere significantly with the person's normal occupational, academic, or social functioning and relationships with others.

12. **e.** Fear of crowds, in which escape may not be possible, is known as agoraphobia. Fear of closed spaces is known as claustrophobia. All the other choices correctly describe symptoms of social phobia.

13. **a.** Avoidant personality disorder has many symptoms in common with social phobia and may be very difficult to differentiate. The core feature of avoidant personality is an excessive discomfort or fear in intimate and social relationships that results in pathologic avoidance as a means of self-protection. Like patients with social phobia, these patients fear humiliation and rejection. However, patients with social phobia tend to have more specific fears with regard to social performances rather than close relationships.

14. **e.** Symptoms reported by patients with social phobia in phobic situations suggest heightened autonomic arousal. When placed in a phobic situation, social phobics experience significant increases in heart rate that are highly correlated with self-perceived physiologic arousal (in contrast to claustrophobics, who experience less heart rate increase and negative correlations between perceived and actual physiologic arousal). Stressful public speaking situations result in two- or threefold increases in plasma epinephrine levels. Increases in norepinephrine are also seen.

Until recently, epinephrine and norepinephrine were the only neurotransmitters associated with the neurochemical basis of this disorder. However, now that the new SSRI agents have been shown to be effective in socially phobic situations, serotonin is also likely to be involved. In this case, it would seem that patients with social phobia would demonstrate a relative deficiency of serotonin-mediated activity rather than an excess, as seen with epinephrine and norepinephrine.

15. **e.** Beta blockers (e.g., atenolol and propranolol) are commonly used to treat circumscribed forms of social phobia, such as fears of public speaking or performances.

Generalized social phobia is often less responsive to pharmacologic interventions. Although SSRIs are considered the drug class of choice, MAOIs, specifically phenelzine (45 to 90 mg/day), buspirone, and benzodiazepines, have been reported to occasionally be effective.

16. **a.** CBT is particularly effective for treating social phobia. The treatment consists of desensitization through graduated exposure to social situations, modifying cognitive distortions, psychoeducation, and relaxation training.

17. **d.** The most likely diagnosis in this patient is specific phobia, with a blood injection injury subtype. This is the only specific phobia with a clear genetic link, and it is commonly seen in the primary care setting. Specific phobias involve intense fear and avoidance of specific objects or situations. The individual recognizes the fear and avoidance as excessive, and the symptoms result in occupational or social impairment. Other common specific phobias include certain animals, heights, flying, closed spaces, crossing bridges, darkness, and blood. Benzodiazepines can be used to decrease acute anxiety, although CBT with exposure and desensitization to the feared stimulus is often required to fully extinguish the symptoms in the long term.

Solution to the Clinical Case Management Problem

1. Physical symptoms related to autonomic arousal, such as tachycardia, tachypnea, diaphoresis, diarrhea, and lightheadedness
2. Affective symptoms that may include increased irritability or may be experienced as "sheer terror"
3. Behavioral symptoms such as avoidance of anxiety-provoking stimuli
4. Cognitive symptoms such as worry, apprehension, or inability to concentrate and focus

Summary

GAD

1. Epidemiology: The lifetime prevalence of GAD is 5.1%.
2. Differential diagnoses include the following: (1) panic disorder; (2) somatoform disorder; (3) hypochondriasis; (4) substance abuse, including caffeine and diet pills; (5) depression (with secondary anxiety); (6) hyperthyroidism; and (7) other organic disorders (less likely).
3. Symptoms: GAD is characterized by chronic excessive anxiety concerning life circumstances accompanied by symptoms of motor tension, autonomic hyperactivity, vigilance, and scanning. These symptoms of anxiety, worry, or physical signs significantly interfere with the person's normal routine of usual activities and cause marked distress.
4. Treatment
   a. Nonpharmacologic treatment options combine behavioral interventions including (i) CBT that challenges distortions in thinking and uses positive affirmations; (ii) relaxation training, including abdominal breathing, and progressive muscle relaxation techniques; (iii) systematic desensitization using imagery and/or biofeedback; and (iv) assertiveness training.
   b. Pharmacologic treatment options include the following: (i) SSRIs, (ii) tricyclic antidepressants, (iii) venlafaxine, (iv) benzodiazepines, and (v) buspirone.

SOCIAL PHOBIA

1. Epidemiology: The estimated 6-month prevalence of social phobia is 1.2% to 2.2%.
2. Definition: Social phobia is a persistent and overwhelming fear of one or more social or performance situations in which the individual is exposed to unfamiliar people or to possible scrutiny by others. Fear of speaking in public, hand trembling, and answering questions are examples. The fear is one of not being able to perform the particular activity and of being humiliated in public because of this. It produces both embarrassment and high levels of distress.

   The individual either avoids the situation or endures it with intense anxiety. The individual also realizes that the fear is unreasonable but is powerless to do anything about it. In addition, the individual experiences occupational, social, or academic impairment with normal life activities and goals.
3. Symptoms: The individual experiences not only intense anxiety and fear but also symptoms of autonomic hyperactivity, such as blushing, trembling, tachycardia, and elevated blood pressure.
4. Neurochemistry: There is probable increased noradrenergic and adrenergic activity related to autonomic hyperarousal. Serotonin systems may also be involved, given the therapeutic effects of SSRIs in this disorder.
5. Treatment
   a. Nonpharmacologic: CBTs (including relaxation training, systematic desensitization, flooding, and cognitive reframing) are most effective for decreasing symptoms of hyperarousal.
   b. Pharmacologic: The drug class of choice is the SSRIs. Other drug classes of benefit are MAOIs (particularly phenelzine) and beta blockers (particularly atenolol and propranolol).
6. Concomitant disorders: One-third of patients with social phobia report a history of MDD.

Suggested Reading

American Psychiatric Association: *Diagnostic and Statistical Manual of Mental Disorders*, 4th ed, text revision. Washington, DC: American Psychiatric Association, 2000.

Culpepper L: Generalized anxiety disorder in primary care: Emerging issues in management and treatment. *J Clin Psychiatry* 63(Suppl 8):35–42, 2002.

House A, Stark D: Anxiety in medical patients. *BMJ* 325(7357): 207–209, 2002.

Kaplan HI, Sadock BJ: Anxiety disorders. In: Kaplan HI, Sadock BJ, eds, *Kaplan and Sadock's Synopsis of Psychiatry: Behavioral Sciences/Clinical Psychiatry*, 8th ed. Baltimore: Williams & Wilkins, 1998.

Shaner R: *Psychiatry*. Baltimore: Williams & Wilkins, 1997.

Tomb DA: *Psychiatry*, 6th ed. Baltimore: Williams & Wilkins, 1999.

Tonks A: Treating generalised anxiety disorder. *BMJ* 326(7391): 700–702, 2003.

Post-traumatic Stress Disorder

CLINICAL CASE PROBLEM 1

A 23-Year-Old Male Who Is a Returning War Veteran

A 23-year-old male is brought to your office by his wife, who states that for the past 2 months her husband has been anxious and withdrawn. He returned from active duty in the Middle East approximately 3 months ago, where he had been involved in combat for long periods of time and had witnessed the loss of life of people to whom he had been close. His wife tells you that "things have been pretty tough since he came back." Her husband has been sleeping poorly and is having nightmares "that bring it all back" with increasing frequency. He has been "on edge" and, on more than one occasion, has fallen to his knees at loud sounds such as the backfire of a car. The patient says only that he feels unhappy and "numb" but does not want to talk about "what went on over there." He says, "I just want to put it behind me."

SELECT THE BEST ANSWER TO THE FOLLOWING QUESTIONS

1. What is the most likely diagnosis in this patient?
   a. primary insomnia
   b. adjustment disorder with anxious mood
   c. major depressive disorder
   d. borderline personality disorder
   e. post-traumatic stress disorder (PTSD)

2. Characteristics of this disorder include which of the following?
   a. recurrent and intrusive recollections of disturbing events
   b. efforts to avoid thinking about what has happened in the past
   c. irritability or outbursts of anger
   d. a and b
   e. a, b, and c

3. Regarding the treatment of the disorder described in this case, which of the following statements is (are) true?
   a. treatment relies on a combination of nonpharmacologic and pharmacologic approaches
   b. nonpharmacologic treatment centers on desensitization that lowers anxiety from the conditioned stimulus
   c. tricyclic antidepressants (TCAs) have been used with some success in the treatment of this disorder
   d. monoamine oxidase inhibitors (MAOIs) have been used with some success in the treatment of this disorder
   e. all of the above statements are true

4. Which of the following drugs has the most potential for abuse in the treatment of the disorder described in this case?
   a. lithium carbonate
   b. phenelzine
   c. fluoxetine
   d. alprazolam
   e. desipramine

5. Which of the following medications generally would be considered the best choice for treatment of this disorder?
   a. sertraline
   b. phenelzine
   c. lithium carbonate
   d. alprazolam
   e. desipramine

6. Which of the following medications has been shown to be effective at decreasing nightmares associated with PTSD?
   a. hydrochlorothiazide
   b. prazosin
   c. lithium carbonate
   d. alprazolam
   e. desipramine

CLINICAL CASE PROBLEM 2

After Sexual Assault

A 27-year-old woman is diagnosed with PTSD following a violent assault. One year after the event, her initial symptoms seem to improve but she begins to feel more depressed and starts drinking alcohol excessively.

7. Which of the following is the most common comorbid psychiatric condition in women with PTSD?
   a. depression
   b. substance abuse
   c. generalized anxiety disorder
   d. delusional disorder
   e. brief psychotic disorder

Answers

1. **e.** The most likely diagnosis in this patient is PTSD. The essential features of this disorder involve the presence of intrusive recollections, emotional numbing and avoidance, difficulty sleeping, and anxiety, all occurring after a single event or chronic exposure to traumatic experiences that cause feelings of danger, helplessness, and horror.

2. **e.** Five major criteria for the diagnosis of PTSD are listed in the *Diagnostic and Statistical Manual of Mental Disorders*, 4th edition, text revision: (1) experiencing or witnessing an event that involves death, threat to life, or serious injury to self or others that was experienced with intense fear, helplessness, or horror; (2) a traumatic event that is persistently experienced in ways such as recurrent and intrusive distressing recollections, dreams, feelings, or thoughts that the event is recurring; psychological distress at exposure to symbolic events of that time, and physiologic reactivity on exposure to cues of that event; (3) persistent avoidance of stimuli associated with the trauma or numbing of general responsiveness, including efforts to avoid thoughts or feelings of the event; efforts to avoid activities, situations, or people associated with the event; inability to recall some aspect of the event (psychological amnesia); feelings of detachment or distance from others; diminished ability to have "affective feelings"; and a sense of a foreshortened future; (4) persistent symptoms of increased arousal (this is very common in war veterans) indicated by difficulty falling or staying asleep, irritability or outbursts of anger, difficulty concentrating, hypervigilance, and exaggerated startle response; and (5) marked distress or significant impairment in social or occupational functioning caused by the disturbance. Symptoms must exist for at least 1 month.

3. **e.** As is the case with other anxiety disorders, treatment for PTSD is often best accomplished with a combination of pharmacologic and nonpharmacologic therapies. Selective serotonin reuptake inhibitors (SSRIs), including sertraline, are often used as medications of first choice for treating PTSD. However, many other medications have been used, and there are few controlled trials confirming the superiority of one class of drugs over another in the treatment of this disorder. Phenelzine (an MAOI) and imipramine (a TCA) have been used often. Other drugs that have shown some efficacy include clonidine, propranolol, lithium, and buspirone.

4. **d.** Alprazolam and other benzodiazepines are relatively contraindicated in this patient because of their increased potential for substance abuse and dependence in patients with PTSD. Benzodiazepines have been used immediately after the traumatic event to help with sleep and functioning and the ability to process the event. However, the use of benzodiazepines may produce an increased incidence of PTSD if used early in treatment and can lead to worsening of PTSD symptoms after benzodiazepine withdrawal. There are also concerns about addictive potential in individuals with comorbid substance use disorders, which constitutes a large percentage of patients with PTSD.

5. **a.** PTSD is best treated with the initiation of an SSRI medication. Although many medications in this class are often used, only sertraline and paroxetine are approved by the Food and Drug Administration for use. As discussed previously, new research indicates that the early use of benzodiazepines may confer some early anxiolysis, but it may also exacerbate the symptoms of PTSD with long-term use and because of this should not be continued more than 2 weeks after a traumatic event. Because of the increased addictive potential of benzodiazepines in patients with PTSD, the use of shorter acting benzodiazepines such as alprazolam, which may confer additional addictive risk, should be avoided. This initial pharmacologic treatment should be supplemented by supportive/expressive psychotherapy (crisis counseling and/or support groups). Long-term management of PTSD requires a more complex treatment, including drugs and cognitive–behavioral therapy (CBT). Drugs used to reduce anxiety symptoms of intrusion and/or avoidance behavior include tricyclics such as imipramine, desipramine, or amitriptyline; MAOIs such as phenelzine; and SSRIs such as fluoxetine or sertraline. Trazodone, a sedating antidepressant, is often used to treat insomnia.

CBT (including relaxation training, systematic desensitization, flooding, and cognitive reframing) is effective for decreasing symptoms of re-experiencing and hyperarousal.

6. **a.** Use of prazosin, a centrally acting α_1-adrenoceptor antagonist more commonly used in hypertension and benign prostatic hypertrophy, has led to large reductions in nightmares and insomnia in a number of studies of patients with PTSD. Other treatment strategies that have shown some promise include the combination of SSRI and atypical antipsychotic medication.

7. **a.** The most common psychiatric comorbidity in women with PTSD is depression. In men, substance abuse is the most common comorbidity.

Summary

1. Epidemiology: It is particularly important and common in war veterans. Survivors and witnesses of terrorist attacks and other life-threatening events are at increased risk for PTSD. Lifetime prevalence rates as high as 30% in war veterans have been reported.

2. Definition: PTSD is defined as a specific constellation of symptoms that present as an immediate or delayed response to a catastrophic life event. Symptoms include recurrent or intrusive distressing recollections or dreams of the event, psychological distress at exposure to events that symbolize or resemble the event, and physiologic reactivity on exposure to internal or external cues. There is also persistent avoidance of stimuli associated with the trauma or numbing of general responsiveness and persistent symptoms of increased arousal (e.g., being unable to fall asleep or stay asleep).

3. Examples of typical traumatic events that can generate PTSD include the following: (a) combat or war experiences; (b) terrorist attacks; (c) serious accidents (automobile, bus, plane, or train crashes); (d) natural disasters (tornado, hurricane, flood, or earthquake);

(e) physical assault (rape, physical or sexual abuse, mugging, or torture); (f) other personal serious associations with danger, death, or severe injury; and (g) witnessing the mutilation, serious injury, or violent death of another person.

4. Treatment
   a. Nonpharmacologic therapy includes the following: (i) CBT, (ii) psychodynamic therapy, and (iii) hypnotherapy.
   b. Pharmacologic therapy: Drug classes that have been shown to be effective for various symptoms include SSRIs, other antidepressants, beta blockers, mood stabilizers, and buspirone. Long-term use of benzodiazepines is contraindicated when treating this disorder because of the increased association with substance dependence.

5. Risk factors for development of PTSD: The risk factors for development of PTSD include separation from parents during childhood, family history of anxiety, preexisting anxiety or depression, family history of antisocial behavior, and female sex.

Suggested Reading

American Psychiatric Association: *Diagnostic and Statistical Manual of Mental Disorders*, 4th ed., text revision. Washington, DC: American Psychiatric Association, 2000.

Davidson JR: Pharmacologic treatment of acute and chronic stress following trauma: 2006. *J Clin Psychiatry* 67(Suppl 2):34–39, 2006.

Foa EB: Psychosocial therapy for posttraumatic stress disorder. *J Clin Psychiatry* 67(Suppl 2):40–45, 2006.

Vieweg WV, Julius DA, Fernandez A, et al: Posttraumatic stress disorder: Clinical features, pathophysiology, and treatment. *Am J Med* 119(5):383–390, 2006.

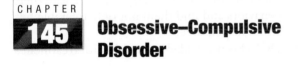

CHAPTER 145

Obsessive–Compulsive Disorder

CLINICAL CASE PROBLEM 1

A New 19-Year-Old Female Patient

A 19-year-old female comes to your office as a new patient to establish care. She has recently moved to the area to start school at a nearby university. As you examine her, you notice that the skin on her hands is quite dry and cracked in places. She says, "I have to wash them a lot. I can't stand leaving them dirty.' After you examine her, you notice that she is becoming increasingly restless. Suddenly, she stands up from the exam table and moves to the sink, where she washes her hands. "I'm so sorry … I know this seems weird, but I really can't stand having germs on my hands!"

As you begin to question her further, the patient tells you that although she has always been a "clean freak," she has recently started washing her hands countless times per day. "I wish I could stop but I just can't." She admits that the recent move away from home has been stressful. In her new apartment, her organizational prowess is beginning to affect her relationship with her new roommate. "I have to organize the spice rack alphabetically. My roommate never puts them back in the right place, but I feel like I always have to check and make sure they're in the right order before I leave the house." At the end of your visit with you, she says, "Please help me … I'm tired of this!"

SELECT THE BEST ANSWER TO THE FOLLOWING QUESTIONS

1. What is the most likely diagnosis in this patient?
   a. atypical depression
   b. schizophreniform disorder
   c. obsessive–compulsive disorder (OCD)
   d. generalized anxiety disorder
   e. specific phobia

2. Which of the following medications is the best initial choice for the treatment of this disorder?
   a. clomipramine
   b. phenelzine
   c. risperidone
   d. selective serotonin reuptake inhibitors (SSRIs)
   e. peroxide

3. Which of the following psychotherapies is most useful for treatment of this disorder?
   a. psychodynamic psychotherapy
   b. humanistic psychotherapy
   c. supportive psychotherapy
   d. crisis counseling
   e. cognitive–behavioral therapy (CBT)

4. Which of the following disorders is closely linked to patients with the disorder described in this case?
   a. Tourette's syndrome
   b. Huntington's disease
   c. Alzheimer's dementia
   d. Sjogren's syndrome
   e. CREST syndrome (calcinosis, Raynaud phenomenon, esophageal dysfunction, sclerodactyly, telangiectasia)

5. The patient asks you what are the chances of a first-degree relative having this disease. What is your answer?
   a. there is no evidence of a genetic link for this disorder
   b. this disorder is only more likely in those patients with a strong family history of depression.
   c. some studies indicate more than a five-fold increased risk in first-degree relatives of patients with this disorder
   d. there is a mosaic pattern of heritability associated with this disorder
   e. this disorder skips a generation, so she should look to her grandparents' history for clues to her own presentation

6. Which of the following statements about this disorder is incorrect?
   a. the prevalence of this disorder is between 2% and 3%
   b. the mean age of onset is the mid-20s
   c. the disorder rarely has an onset in people older than age 35 years
   d. it is associated with structural abnormalities in the caudate nucleus as seen on magnetic resonance imaging (MRI)
   e. this disorder often has spontaneous periods of complete remission

CLINICAL CASE PROBLEM 2

A Nervous Pizza Delivery Man

A 24-year-old male is chronically preoccupied by the fear that he has run someone over while delivering pizzas for a local eatery. His anxiety increases as he tries to convince himself that his concerns are unfounded. Finally, he returns to the "scene of the crime" and is relieved to see that no one is there.

7. This is an example of which of the following?
   a. a brief psychotic disorder
   b. an obsession with an overlaying delusion
   c. a compulsion with an overlaying hallucination
   d. both an obsession and a compulsion
   e. a persistent specific phobia

8. Which of the following is true regarding the association of this disorder with obsessive–compulsive personality disorder (OCPD)?
   a. they are identical except that OCPD is more often associated with a lifelong pattern of dysfunction
   b. OCPD is more often associated with frank hallucinations and delusions
   c. the treatment for both disorders is the same
   d. patients with OCPD are more at ease with their behaviors and find them not only tolerable but also indispensable
   e. OCPD is more likely to remit with treatment

Clinical Case Management Problem

List five common obsessions and five common compulsions associated with OCD.

Answers

1. **C.** This patient has OCD, which consists of recurrent obsessions, recurrent compulsions, or both. The recurrent obsessions include persistent thoughts, impulses, or images that the patient attempts to ignore

but cannot. In addition, the obsessions are not just excessive worries about real-life problems; the patient also recognizes that these obsessions are, in fact, the product of his or her own mind.

Common obsessions include obsessions regarding contamination or illness; violent images; fear of harming others or harming oneself; perverse or forbidden sexual thoughts, images, or impulses; symmetry or exactness; somatic situations; and religious thoughts.

Compulsions are repetitive behaviors or mental acts that the individual feels driven to perform in response to an obsession or according to rigid rules. The behavior or mental act is aimed at preventing or reducing distress or preventing a dreaded event or situation. These behaviors, however, are not connected in a realistic manner with what they are designed to neutralize or prevent and are clearly excessive.

The individual realizes that the compulsions are excessive and unreasonable. They cause marked distress in the person's life or significantly interfere with the person's normal routine, occupation, or social activities.

Common compulsions include checking things (e.g., door locks, water taps, and the oven), cleaning or washing articles or parts of the body, counting objects or things, hoarding or collecting articles or things, ordering or arranging articles or things, and repeating things (e.g., tapping).

2. **d.** SSRIs such as fluvoxamine have become the drugs of choice for treatment of OCD and have replaced clomipramine as the first-line medications for this indication. Importantly, the doses needed for treatment of OCD are often higher than what is needed to treat other disorders, such as anxiety or depression.

3. **e.** In addition to pharmacotherapy, CBT techniques are also often effective. There are several important components to this treatment. Informational interventions help educate the patient about the diagnosis and set the stage for treatment. Exposure and response prevention are implemented to break the chronic cycles of intrusive obsessions and the anxiety-reducing rituals that often follow. Cognitive interventions focus on enhancing the specific skills that patients can use to reframe cognition distortions such as fear of germs or other such obsessions. Studies have consistently shown that CBT is as effective as medication for OCD. However, for severe cases, the use of both CBT and medication may be the best approach.

4. **a.** Tourette's syndrome is defined as multiple motor tics and at least one vocal tic lasting more than 1 year and starting before the age of 18 years. Patients with OCD are very commonly diagnosed with Tourette's syndrome as a comorbid illness. None of the other disorders described have a link with OCD.

5. **c.** There is a clear genetic link in OCD that passes from one generation to the next. The risk to first-degree relatives of patients with OCD has been higher than the population prevalence in several studies. In one case–control family study, the risk was 10.3% compared with 1.9% in controls.

6. **e.** The prevalence of OCD is between 2% and 3%. The mean age of onset is the mid-20s, with a usual range from late childhood to early adulthood. Less than 5% of cases have an onset after age 35 years. Structural abnormalities of the caudate nucleus are very often seen on MRI in patients with this disorder. Although a minority of patients do remit spontaneously, the vast majority have continued symptoms and more than 60% of patients have a chronic course.

7. **d.** Recurrent obsessions or compulsions are the hallmark of this disorder. A patient need not present with both in order to be diagnosed. In this case, the patient demonstrates an obsession characterized by persistent thoughts that are experienced as intrusive and that increase his anxiety, as well as a compulsion to act in such a way as to alleviate the anxiety elicited by the obsession.

8. **d.** Because these two disorders share much in common, they are often confused. The major features of OCPD are perfectionism and lack of compromise. These patients maintain an inflexible adherence to their own strict and often unattainable standards. Patients with OCD, on the other hand, have true obsessions and/or compulsions that they experience as anxiety provoking, whereas those with OCPD find great pleasure despite (and often as a result of) their rigid standards and inflexibility.

Solution to the Clinical Case Management Problem

Some common obsessions are as follows: (1) contamination and illness; (2) fear of harming others or self; (3) perverse or forbidden sexual thoughts, images, or impulses; (4) violent images; (5) symmetry or exactness; (6) exaggerated health concerns; and (7) religious thoughts.

Some common compulsions are as follows: (1) checking things (e.g., doors, locks, and water taps); (2) cleaning or washing; (3) counting objects of various types; (4) hoarding or collecting objects of various types; (5) ordering or arranging articles of various types; (6) repeating things (speech and tapping); and (7) committing some unethical, immoral, or criminal acts.

Summary

1. Epidemiology: The measured prevalence rate has been estimated to be 2% to 3%.
2. Definition: OCD is a mental disorder in which obsessions (recurrent distressing thoughts, ideas, or impulses) are experienced as both unwanted and senseless but at the same time irresistible. Compulsions are repetitive, purposeful, intentional behaviors, usually performed in response to an obsession, and are recognized as unrealistic and unreasonable but instrumental in temporarily relieving anxiety.

   Common obsessions and compulsions are listed in the Solution to the Clinical Case Management Problem.

3. Treatment
   a. Nonpharmacologic: Prolonged exposure to ritual-eliciting stimuli together with prevention of the compulsive response resulting in desensitization.
   b. Pharmacologic: SSRIs are the drugs of choice; clomipramine is also effective, but it has more untoward effects. MAOIs and alprazolam or other high-potency benzodiazepines can also be used.
4. Coexisting disorders include the following: (1) other anxiety disorders, (2) eating disorders, (3) Tourette's syndrome, (4) schizophrenia, and (5) separation anxiety in childhood.

Suggested Reading

American Psychiatric Association: *Diagnostic and Statistical Manual of Mental Disorders*, 4th ed, text revision. Washington, DC: American Psychiatric Association, 2000.

Denys D: Pharmacotherapy of obsessive-compulsive disorder and obsessive-compulsive spectrum disorders. *Psychiatr Clin North Am* 29(2):553–584, 2006.

Heyman I, Mataix-Cols D, Fineberg NA: Obsessive-compulsive disorder. *BMJ* 333(7565):424–429, 2006.

Jenike MA: Obsessive-compulsive disorder. *N Engl J Med* 350:259–265, 2004.

CLINICAL CASE PROBLEM 1

*A 6-Year-Old Child Who Is "Always on
the Go," "Into Everything," and "Easily
Distractible"*

A mother brings her 6-year-old son to the office for
a complete assessment. She states that "there is
something very wrong with him." He just sprinkled
baby powder all over the house, and last night he
opened a bottle of ink and threw it on the floor. He
is unable to sit still at school, is easily distracted,
has difficulty waiting his turn in games, has
difficulty in sustaining attention in play situations,
talks all the time, always interrupts others, does
not listen when talked to, and is constantly shifting
from one activity to another.

As you enter the examining room, the child is
in the process of destroying it. On examination
(what examination you can manage), you
discover that there are no physical abnormalities
demonstrated.

SELECT THE BEST ANSWER TO THE FOLLOWING QUESTIONS

1. What is the most likely diagnosis in this patient?
   a. mental retardation
   b. childhood depression
   c. attention-deficit/hyperactivity disorder (ADHD)
   d. maternal deprivation
   e. childhood schizophrenia

2. Which of the following is (are) associated with the disorder described?
   a. feelings of low self-esteem
   b. feelings of depression
   c. impaired interpersonal relationships
   d. a reduction in life successes
   e. all of the above

3. Who is the person who usually makes this diagnosis?
   a. the child psychiatrist
   b. the family physician
   c. the mother or father
   d. the schoolteacher
   e. the grandparents

4. The differential diagnosis of this disorder includes which of the following?
   a. adjustment disorder
   b. bipolar disorder
   c. anxiety disorder
   d. childhood schizophrenia
   e. a, b, and c
   f. a, b, c, and d

5. Which of the following is (are) true regarding the prevalence of the disorder?
   a. prevalence rates are higher in preschool children than in school-age children
   b. affected boys outnumber girls in surveys of school-age children
   c. prevalence rates decline as a cohort of children ages into adulthood
   d. a, b, and c
   e. none of the above

6. Which of the following are pharmacologic treatment options in the disorder described?
   a. methylphenidate or its derivatives
   b. dextroamphetamine or amphetamine derivatives
   c. magnesium pemoline
   d. modafinil
   e. a or b

CLINICAL CASE PROBLEM 2

*A 9-Year-Old Male Who Is Being Treated
for ADHD*

A 9-year-old male comes in for follow-up of his
ADHD. In reviewing the chart, you note that the
patient is taking short-acting methylphenidate
twice daily, and his mother has noted significant
improvement with morning classes but a
significant problem with hyperactivity and
inattentiveness as the day progresses. As you
review the comments on his most recent report
card, you can clearly see that his academic
performance is stronger in his morning classes.
His mother is afraid that the treatment is not
working well enough. In talking to the patient, it
becomes apparent that he is unhappy with the
medication. He says, "I have to go to the nurse
and take my medication when all of the other kids
are playing. Everyone knows I'm different."

7. What is the next appropriate step in the management of this patient?
   a. increase the dose of his current medication
   b. stop the methylphenidate and begin dextroamphetamine (Dexedrine)
   c. do nothing and see the patient in 1 month
   d. add a selective serotonin reuptake inhibitor (SSRI) as an adjunctive treatment
   e. initiate treatment with a long-acting form of methylphenidate (Concerta)

8. One month later, the patient returns to you for follow-up. Now his parents report he is doing quite well throughout the school day. His teachers are reporting significant improvement in focus and attention. However, his parents note that his appetite has decreased and it is somewhat difficult for him to fall asleep. What is the most appropriate management at this stage?
   a. increase the dose of his current medication
   b. stop the methylphenidate and begin dextroamphetamine (Dexedrine)
   c. begin behavioral therapy
   d. reassure the parents and recheck the patient in 1 month
   e. add an SSRI as an adjunctive treatment

9. Which of the following is a pharmacologic treatment alternative for ADHD in patients who do not respond to stimulants?
   a. atomoxetine
   b. fluoxetine
   c. guanfacine
   d. clonidine
   e. pemoline

10. Which of the following disorders often appear together in the same individual at various life stages?
    a. mental retardation, ADHD, and learning disability
    b. childhood depression, ADHD, and early onset adult schizophrenia
    c. ADHD, conduct disorder, and antisocial personality disorder
    d. adjustment disorder, ADHD, and major depression
    e. ADHD, bipolar disorder, and conduct disorder

11. Which of the following statements regarding the effects of stimulants on children, adolescents, and adults is (are) correct?
    a. treatment with stimulants at an early age in children with ADHD increases their risk of substance abuse and dependence as adults

    b. normal and hyperactive children, adolescents, and adults have similar cognitive responses to comparable doses of stimulants
    c. normal and hyperactive children, adolescents, and adults have similar behavioral responses to comparable doses of stimulants
    d. b and c
    e. a, b, and c

CLINICAL CASE PROBLEM 3

A 19-Year-Old College Student Who Is Struggling to Succeed

A 19-year-old female comes in for a routine physical examination. She admits she has been under a lot of stress in her first year as a college freshman. She says that she earned outstanding grades in high school but admits that she resigned herself "to working twice as hard as everyone else" because, as she says, "I can't stand to do one thing for too long." She notes that since she can remember, she has always been "high energy" compared with her friends and siblings but believed she was just "a little weird." In her first year of college, she tells you she has been finding it difficult to choose her classes and organize her schedule. She says, "There's so much to do, it's overwhelming. It's not like in high school where they give you a schedule and you just go from one class to another."

As you examine her, you notice that she is fidgeting and her speech seems slightly pressured. Her vital signs are within normal limits, and her physical examination is unremarkable.

12. Which of the following statements regarding this case is true?
    a. this patient cannot have ADHD given her academic success while untreated in the past
    b. ADHD cannot be diagnosed in patients older than age 18 years
    c. because of her age, this patient would be unlikely to benefit from medication
    d. the vast majority of children with ADHD "outgrow" their diagnosis as they become adults
    e. the diagnosis of adults with ADHD is increasing in frequency

13. Which of the following statements regarding the treatment of this case is true?
    a. adult ADHD patients receive nearly one-third of all prescriptions written for this disorder
    b. the majority of prescriptions written for this disorder are for children 5 to 9 years old

c. the number of prescriptions written for the treatment of ADHD has declined in recent years

d. all patients with ADHD and school difficulties must be formally tested for learning disability prior to treatment with medication

e. although a genetic link has been established, there is no known prenatal environmental risk factor for ADHD

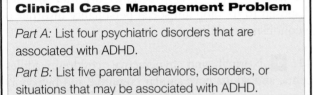

Clinical Case Management Problem

Part A: List four psychiatric disorders that are associated with ADHD.

Part B: List five parental behaviors, disorders, or situations that may be associated with ADHD.

Part C: Comment on the association between ADHD and schoolteachers.

Answers

1. c. This child has ADHD. Diagnostic criteria from the *Diagnostic and Statistical Manual of Mental Disorders*, 4th edition (*DSM-IV*), for ADHD require a pattern of behavior that appears no later than the age of 7 years, has been present for at least 6 months, and is excessive for age and intelligence. The symptoms of the disorder are divided into inattention and hyperactivity/impulsivity; either must be present often, although not necessarily all of the time or in every situation. Either six inattention symptoms or six hyperactivity symptoms are required for the diagnosis.

For a diagnosis of inattention, six or more of the following symptoms must be present: (1) does not pay attention to details or makes careless mistakes; (2) has difficulty sustaining attention; (3) does not seem to listen when spoken to; (4) does not follow through on instructions and fails to finish; (5) has difficulty organizing tasks or activities; (6) avoids, dislikes, or is reluctant to engage in tasks that require sustained mental effort; (7) loses things; (8) is easily distracted by stimuli; and (9) is forgetful.

For a diagnosis of hyperactivity–impulsivity, six or more of the following symptoms must be present: (1) fidgets or squirms; (2) leaves seat when staying put is expected; (3) inappropriately runs about or climbs; (4) has difficultly in quietly engaging in leisure activities; (5) seems "on the go" or "driven by a motor"; (6) talks excessively; (7) bursts out answers before questions are asked; (8) has difficulty waiting for his or her turn; and (9) interrupts or intrudes.

2. e. Commonly associated features of ADHD are low self-esteem, feelings of depression, feelings of demoralization, and lack of ability to take responsibility for one's actions. In social situations, these young children are immature, bossy, intrusive, loud, uncooperative, out of synchrony with situational expectations, and irritating to both adults and peers. Children with ADHD are more likely to sustain severe injuries than those without ADHD.

3. d. The most common person to make the diagnosis of ADHD is the schoolteacher. There is considerable controversy concerning the fact that many children who are hyperactive take medication because of the remarks or diagnosis of the schoolteacher. There may be some truth to this statement. Inexperienced or overly critical teachers may in fact confuse normal age-appropriate overactivity with ADHD.

4. e. The differential diagnosis of ADHD includes the following: (1) adjustment disorder (an identifiable stressor is identified at home and the duration of symptoms is less than 6 months); (2) an anxiety disorder (instead of or in addition to the diagnosis of ADHD); (3) bipolar disorder (bipolar disorder in children may manifest as a chronic mixed affective state marked by irritability, overactivity, and difficulty concentrating); (4) mental retardation; (5) a specific developmental disorder; (6) drugs (phenobarbital prescribed for children as an anticonvulsant and theophylline prescribed for asthma); (7) systemic disorders (hyperthyroidism); and (8) other disruptive behavioral disorders, including oppositional defiant disorder (ODD) and conduct disorder, but does not include childhood schizophrenia.

5. d. Some studies suggest that between 14% and 20% of preschool and kindergarten boys and approximately one-third as many girls have ADHD. In elementary school studies, 3% to 10% of students have ADHD symptoms. Affected boys outnumber girls until young adulthood, when women predominate.

6. e. The pharmacologic agents of choice for the management of ADHD are the stimulant medications (1) methylphenidate or derivatives or (2) dextroamphetamine or amphetamine derivatives.

As many as 96% of children with ADHD have at least some positive behavioral response to stimulants, of which methylphenidate and dextroamphetamine are the two tried and true medications. Both are available in various formulations, including longer acting derivatives. Methylphenidate is available in short- (Ritalin), intermediate- (Ritalin-SR), and long-acting (Concerta) preparations. Dextroamphetamine is also available as short- (6 to 8 hours; Dexedrine and Adderall) or long-acting (Dexedrine spansules and Adderall XR) formulations. Unfortunately, side effects may limit efficacy or require discontinuation of medication in some children. Both preschool children and adolescents may require lower weight-adjusted doses than school-aged children and manifest a greater likelihood of side effects and somewhat lower therapeutic efficacy. Pemoline was removed from the market because of liver toxicity and should not be used. Atomoxetine, an inhibitor of presynaptic norepinephrine, is also less effective than stimulants but is an option for some patients.

7. e. Although the dosing of short-acting stimulants may offer some flexibility in treatment, the long-acting stimulants tend to increase adherence. The administration of short-acting medications can be timed to correspond to certain of the child's activities. Long-acting medications obviate the need for doses during the school day while minimizing the decreased effect of the short-acting formulations at the end of the school day. Randomized trials directly comparing methylphenidate and dextroamphetamine have shown similar benefits from the two medications but more frequent mild side effects with dextroamphetamine.

8. d. Anorexia, mild weight loss, and early insomnia are all common side effects of the stimulants prescribed for ADHD. Whereas the short-acting agents can be timed to minimize the effect on sleep, the long-acting formulations are more difficult to adjust. As in this case, there is often a trade-off between ease of administration, which may increase adherence, and the common side effects that may occur. Alternative medication options are available, such as atomoxetine, clonidine, and antidepressant medication, but none have been shown to be as effective as stimulants. Reassurance and close follow-up may be all that is necessary in a case such as this, in which side effects are mild and symptoms have come under control.

9. a. Atomoxetine, a norepinephrine reuptake inhibitor, is approved for treatment of ADHD. Studies indicate that 58% to 64% of children treated during a 6- to 12-week period achieved 25% to 30% or greater improvement in symptoms. Reports of severe liver injury (which apparently reversed after drug cessation) have led to the addition of a bolded warning to the label indicating that atomoxetine should be discontinued in patients with jaundice or laboratory evidence of liver injury. Seizures and prolonged QT intervals corrected for heart rate are reported with overdoses of atomoxetine but not with therapeutic doses.

The tricyclic antidepressants imipramine and desipramine, and the α-adrenergic agonist clonidine, are not often used in the treatment of ADHD because of concerns about cardiac effects and the availability of safe, effective medications described previously. The stimulant pemoline remains available but is no longer recommended based on reports of fatal hepatotoxicity.

10. c. ADHD commonly leads to conduct disorder. Adolescents who develop conduct disorder are predisposed to develop antisocial personality disorder or alcoholism as adults.

11. d. Normal and hyperactive children, adolescents, and adults have similar cognitive and behavioral responses to comparable doses of stimulants. Stimulants do not have a paradoxical sedative action. Studies confirm that the use of stimulants in children with ADHD does not lead to substance abuse or dependence in adulthood. In fact, children with untreated ADHD have an increased risk of substance dependence into adulthood compared with children who have been treated with stimulants appropriately.

12. e. Once considered a disorder of the elementary school years that children "outgrew" during adolescence as their brains matured, ADHD is now thought to persist into adulthood, impairing functioning, in approximately 50% of cases. Adults often turn to psychiatrists or primary care physicians for help with difficulties at work or in personal relationships and are told for the first time that they have ADHD. At a clinic for adults with the disorder at Massachusetts General Hospital in Boston, the average age of patients receiving treatment is 40 years. ADHD can be diagnosed in adults older than age 18 years when there is evidence of behavior congruent with the diagnosis beginning before age 7 years. Medication is equally efficacious in children and adults for this disorder.

13. a. Prescriptions given to people 19 years of age or older for eight drugs commonly used in ADHD have increased 90% in recent years. Adults now receive approximately one-third of all prescriptions for these drugs. At least seven genes are thought to influence the susceptibility to ADHD, and neurotransmitters such as dopamine, norepinephrine, and serotonin are considered to play a role in the disorder. Prenatal environmental factors, such as pregnancy or delivery complications, prematurity, and fetal exposure to alcohol or tobacco, also appear to be risk factors.

Solution to the Clinical Case Management Problem

Part A
Four psychiatric disorders associated with ADHD are as follows: (1) childhood depression, (2) conduct disorder, (3) ODD, and (4) alcoholism.

Part B
Five parental behaviors, disorders, or situations that may be associated with ADHD are as follows: (1) providing attention to problem behavior and ignoring good behavior, (2) parental modeling (impulsivity and rule breaking), (3) parental marital conflict, (4) family poverty, and (5) inheritance (genetic predisposition).

Part C
The relationship between ADHD and schoolteacher input in many cases is that the diagnosis of ADHD is made by the teacher, not by the physician. Instead of carefully considering the diagnostic criteria elaborated in the *DSM-IV*, the physician may simply accept the word of the schoolteacher and begin treatment with stimulant medication. The basic problem is the inability, in some cases on the part of the schoolteacher and ultimately on the part of the physician, to distinguish between ADHD and normal appropriate-for-age overactivity. Most school systems in the United States by law provide for a comprehensive developmental assessment by a child study team of professionals. These evaluations provide important information for the physician, and they complement the medical assessment. Physicians and other clinicians must learn to work in tandem with school systems and parents to provide optimal diagnosis and care to patients with ADHD. High levels of communication among all parties are essential.

Summary

1. Prevalence: highest in preschoolers, 7% of school-age children; decreases with age; males predominate; between 18% and 35% of affected children have an additional psychiatric disorder.
2. Signs and symptoms: See the diagnostic criteria described in answer 1.
3. Treatment
   a. Nonpharmacologic: Behavior modification can improve both academic achievement and behavioral compliance if they are targeted specifically.
   b. Pharmacologic
      i. First choice: stimulants, such as methylphenidate, dextroamphetamine, or derivatives
      ii. Second choice: desipramine, clonidine, or guanfacine
   c. Stepwise therapy
      i. Begin first stimulant (usually methylphenidate).
      ii. Increase dose gradually.
      iii. End of dose failure: Consider another one of the two recommended stimulants.
      iv. Failure: Switch to nonstimulant.
   d. Length of time and dosing
      i. Consider early morning and noon dosing.
      ii. Consider "drug holidays" on weekends and vacations.
      iii. Use for as long as needed.

Suggested Reading

American Psychiatric Association: *Diagnostic and Statistical Manual of Mental Disorders*, 4th ed., text revision. Washington, DC: American Psychiatric Association, 2000.

Kirby K, Rutman LE, Bernstein H: Attention-deficit/hyperactivity disorder: A therapeutic update. *Curr Opin Pediatr* 14(2):236–246, 2002.

Okie S: ADHD in adults. *N Engl J Med* 354:2637–2641, 2006.

Rappley MD: Attention deficit–hyperactivity disorder. *N Engl J Med* 352:165–173, 2005.

Weiss M, Murray C: Assessment and management of attention-deficit hyperactivity disorder in adults. *Can Med Assoc J* 168(6):715–722, 2003.

Conduct Disorder and Oppositional Defiant Disorder

CLINICAL CASE PROBLEM 1

A 13-Year-Old Child with a "Rap Sheet" a Mile Long

A 13-year-old male is brought in by police officers to the emergency department, where his parents soon arrive. He was placed under arrest and charged with destruction of property as well as assault and battery after police arrived at the scene and found the patient beating the owner of a liquor store with a baseball bat. According to police, the patient cut his arm on a piece of glass while jumping through a store window in an attempt to evade arrest. The police officer tells you, "We know this one … he's a regular customer of ours. We've had him down at juvenile hall more times than I can count."

The patient's parents tell you that his aggressive behavior started in the past couple of years: "Sure he would argue and fight with us when he was younger, but he didn't start getting arrested until he was about eleven." His parents recount a number of disturbing instances of cruelty to animals, leading to the death or maiming of several neighborhood cats.

After an examination, you note that his wounds are not serious. His vitals sign are within normal limits. The patient appears cheerful and unconcerned. He is more worried about getting the blood off of his favorite baseball bat than about the fate of the man he injured.

SELECT THE BEST ANSWER TO THE FOLLOWING QUESTIONS

1. What is the most likely diagnosis in this case?
   a. conduct disorder
   b. childhood depression
   c. attention deficit disorder
   d. sociopathy, not otherwise specified
   e. bipolar disorder

2. The diagnosis of conduct disorder is made when which of the following criteria is (are) fulfilled?
   a. repetitive and persistent patterns of behavior that violate the rights of others
   b. stealing
   c. lying
   d. vandalism
   e. a and any two of b, c, and d

3. Which of the following disorders often appear together in the same individual at various life stages?
   a. mental retardation, attention-deficit/hyperactivity disorder (ADHD), and learning disability
   b. childhood depression, ADHD, and early onset adult schizophrenia
   c. ADHD, conduct disorder, and antisocial personality disorder
   d. adjustment disorder, ADHD, and major depression
   e. ADHD, bipolar disorder, and conduct disorder

4. Conduct disorder appears to result from an interaction of which of the following factors?
   a. temperament
   b. attention to problem behavior and ignoring good behavior
   c. association with a delinquent peer group
   d. a and c
   e. a, b, and c

5. What is the most common reason for referral to either a child psychiatry service or an adolescent psychiatry service?
   a. conduct disorder
   b. ADHD
   c. oppositional defiant disorder (ODD)
   d. childhood–adolescent depression
   e. childhood–adolescent schizophrenia

6. Which treatment(s) is (are) used to manage symptoms of this disorder?
   a. behavioral therapy
   b. mood stabilizers
   c. alpha agonists
   d. beta blockers
   e. all of the above

CLINICAL CASE PROBLEM 2

A 7-Year-Old Male with "Bad Behavior"

A 7-year-old male is brought in by his parents, who say, "Doctor, you have to help us … we're at our wit's end!" They tell you that their young son's "bad behavior" started after just 3 months in preschool at the age of 4 years. His teacher complained that he refused to follow directions and was unable to sustain attention to tasks. His parents tell you that during the past 2 years he has been increasingly oppositional at home, so much so that they have been unable to get any babysitter to return for a second time. He is regularly argumentative and disrespectful to his parents and seems to go out of his way to do the opposite of what his parents or teachers ask of him. His parents tell you that "he seems angry all the time and still throws temper tantrums like you wouldn't believe!"

7. What is the most likely diagnosis in this case?
   a. major depression
   b. childhood anxiety disorder
   c. ODD
   d. mental retardation
   e. antisocial personality disorder

8. Which of the following statements is false regarding the disorder described in this case?
   a. the prevalence of this disorder is between 2% and 16%
   b. males with the disorder are more prevalent than females prior to puberty; after puberty, the prevalence is similar between the sexes
   c. 25% of children diagnosed with this disorder no longer meet the criteria in adulthood
   d. aggressive treatment with medication is the mainstay of treatment
   e. all of the above are true

9. What is the best definition of the term *oppositional defiant disorder*?
   a. chronic behavior patterns in children and adolescents that are more severe than those in conduct disorder
   b. chronic behavior patterns in children and adolescents that result in serious violation of the law and incarceration
   c. chronic behavior patterns in children and adolescents that are less severe than those seen in conduct disorder
   d. a and b
   e. none of the above

Clinical Case Management Problem

Part A: List four categories of behavior that correspond to conduct disorder.

Part B: Describe the relationship between conduct disorder and antisocial personality disorder.

Answers

1. **a.** This patient has conduct disorder. The average age of onset is 10 to 12 years in boys and 16 years in girls, although the vast majority of children with this disorder are boys.

2. **e.** The diagnosis of conduct disorder requires a repetitive and persistent pattern of behavior that violates the basic rights of others or age-appropriate rules of society, manifested by at least three of the following behaviors: (1) stealing, (2) running away from home, (3) staying out after dark without permission, (4) lying so as to "con" people, (5) deliberately setting fires, (6) repeatedly being truant (beginning before age 13 years), (7) vandalizing, (8) being cruel to animals, (9) bullying, (10) being physically aggressive, and (11) forcing someone else into sexual activity.

Conduct disorder is a purely descriptive label for a heterogeneous group of children and adolescents. Many of these individuals also lack appropriate feelings of guilt or remorse, empathy for others, and a feeling of responsibility for their own behavior.

3. **c.** ADHD commonly leads to conduct disorder. Adolescents who develop conduct disorder are predisposed to develop antisocial personality disorder or alcoholism as adults.

4. **e.** Conduct disorder appears to result from an interaction among the following factors: (1) temperament, (2) parents who provide attention to problem behavior and ignore good behavior, (3) association with a delinquent peer group, (4) a parent "role model" of impulsivity and rule-breaking behavior, (5) genetic predisposition, (6) marital disharmony in the family, (7) placement outside of the home as an infant or toddler, (8) poverty, and (9) low intelligence quotient or brain damage.

5. **a.** The most common reason for referral to a child or adolescent psychiatry clinic or hospital is conduct disorder.

6. **e.** Although behavioral therapy is the mainstay of treatment for the core symptoms of conduct disorder, target symptoms such as aggression and agitation may be treated with medications such as alpha agonists, mood stabilizers, beta blockers, and antipsychotics. Of course, it is also crucial to identify and treat comorbid disorders.

7. **c.** This patient has ODD. This disorder is characterized by a pattern of negativistic, hostile, and defiant

behavior lasting at least 6 months, during which four (or more) of the following are present: (1) often loses temper, (2) often argues with adults, (3) often actively defies or refuses to comply with adults' requests or rules, (4) often deliberately annoys people, (5) often blames others for his or her mistakes or misbehavior, (6) is often touchy or easily annoyed by others, (7) is often angry and resentful, and (8) is often spiteful or vindictive. It is important to consider a criterion met only if the behavior occurs more frequently than is typically observed in individuals of comparable age and developmental level. Also, if the patient meets the criteria for conduct disorder, then the conduct disorder becomes the primary diagnosis.

8. **C.** In the case of ODD, behavioral therapy is the mainstay of treatment. Medications are rarely used for ODD. The prevalence of this disorder is between 2% and 16%. Males with the disorder are more prevalent than females prior to puberty; after puberty, prevalence is similar between the sexes. As mentioned previously, 25% of children diagnosed with this disorder no longer meet the criteria in adulthood.

9. **C.** ODD is often seen as a milder form of conduct disorder, but it is important to note that although many children who are diagnosed as having ODD are at risk for developing conduct disorder, 25% will resolve their symptoms of ODD as they become adults.

Solution to the Clinical Case Management Problem

Part A
The four categories of behavior that correspond to conduct disorder are as follows: (1) aggression toward people and/or animals, (2) destruction of property, (3) deceitfulness or theft, and (4) serious violations of rules.

Part B
Many of the symptoms of antisocial personality disorder overlap with those of conduct disorder.

Not surprisingly, some history of symptoms of conduct disorder occurring before the age of 15 years are required to establish the diagnosis of antisocial personality disorder. The two disorders are considered to be on a continuum of antisocial behavior.

Summary

CONDUCT DISORDER
1. Prevalence: It is estimated at 3% to 7%; males predominate.
2. Signs and symptoms: See the criteria listed in answer 7. Conduct disorder is the most common reason for referral to a child or adolescent psychiatry service.
3. Treatment
   a. Nonpharmacologic: Cognitive–behavior modification (when used together) is the most effective nonpharmacologic therapy.
   b. Pharmacologic: Lithium is used for severe impulse aggression. Carbamazepine is used for severe impulse aggression accompanied by emotional lability and irritability. Propranolol is used for uncontrollable rage reactions, especially when associated with impulse aggression. Neuroleptics (e.g., haloperidol) may reduce aggression, hostility, negativism, and explosiveness in severely aggressive children, and antidepressants may help if the conduct disorder is secondary to major depression.

ODD
1. Prevalence: It is 6% to 10%; males predominate.
2. Differential diagnosis: "stubbornness"
3. Signs and symptoms: It is best described simply as a less severe form of conduct disorder.
4. Treatment
   a. Nonpharmacologic: An operant approach using environmental positive and negative contingencies to increase or decrease the frequency of behaviors is most useful.
   b. Pharmacologic: If ADHD and ODD coexist, treat with stimulant medication.
5. Possible progression: ADHD to conduct disorder or ODD to antisocial personality disorder to alcoholism
6. Major differential diagnosis of disruptive behavior disorders includes the following: (1) major depressive illness, (2) bipolar affective disorder, (3) anxiety disorder, (4) mental retardation, (5) specific developmental disorder, (6) adjustment disorder, (7) pharmacotherapy (phenobarbital and theophylline), and (8) systemic disorders (hyperthyroidism).

Suggested Reading

American Psychiatric Association: *Diagnostic and Statistical Manual of Mental Disorders*, 4th ed, text revision. Washington, DC: American Psychiatric Association, 2000.

Guevara JP, Stein MT: Evidence-based management of attention deficit hyperactivity disorder. *BMJ* 323(7323):1232–1235, 2001.

Karnik NS, McMullin MA, Steiner H: Disruptive behaviors: Conduct and oppositional disorders in adolescents. *Adolesc Med Clin* 17(1): 97–114, 2006.

Turgay A: Aggression and disruptive behavior disorders in children and adolescents. *Expert Rev Neurother* 4(4):623–632, 2004.

CHAPTER

148 Diagnosis and Management of Schizophrenia

CLINICAL CASE PROBLEM 1

A 21-Year-Old Male Brought to the Emergency Room by the Paramedics

A 21-year-old male is brought to the emergency room by paramedics and accompanied by his parents. The patient's father tells you that up until approximately 1 year ago the patient was doing well in his studies at the local college. After suddenly dropping all of his classes, he returned home and has essentially locked himself in his room for the past year. He eats all of his meals there and rarely leaves. Approximately 1 week ago, the patient began telling his parents that aliens were planning to invade the planet. He said, "They're coming … they can read our thoughts and they know everything about us. They're just waiting for the right moment…. We have to protect ourselves!" This morning, after spending most of the evening lining the walls and ceiling of his bedroom with aluminum foil, he requested that his parents take him to the airport "to prove that the aliens have put transmitters in my brain, and yours too!" At the airport, he began shouting and insisting that he be let through the metal detector: "Once I show you what they've put in my brain, you have to take me to the hospital to cut it all out!"

In the emergency room, the patient stares straight ahead and refuses to answer any questions. The silence is only interrupted occasionally as the patient slowly repeats, "You must obtain a CT scan of my head. You must remove the hardware and decipher the alien code before they land, or the planet will be doomed. Heed this warning or ignore it at your peril."

The patient had a job at a local hardware store but was fired 6 months ago when he started to build "interstellar communication deflectors" out of roofing materials and PVC pipe, which he placed in various locations in the store parking lot. It was at that point that he locked himself in his room for good. He experienced episodes of major depression as a child. Other significant history includes enuresis, encopresis, and separation anxiety as a child. The father assures you that his son is taking no drugs, prescription or otherwise.

The mental status examination on this patient is difficult to complete because the patient is uncooperative with testing and is mute for prolonged periods. The patient's vitals signs are normal, as is the rest of the physical examination except for the aluminum foil the patient has layered under his clothing.

SELECT THE BEST ANSWER TO THE FOLLOWING QUESTIONS

1. What is the most likely diagnosis in this patient at this time?
   a. schizoaffective disorder
   b. schizophrenia
   c. schizophreniform disorder
   d. bipolar disorder
   e. delusional disorder

2. Of the following features, which one is most suggestive of the diagnosis?
   a. disorganized speech
   b. delusions
   c. hallucinations
   d. the presence of both positive and negative symptoms
   e. disorganized or catatonic behavior

3. Approximately what percentage of patients with the disorder described in this case eventually commit suicide?
   a. 1%
   b. 5%
   c. 10%
   d. 15%
   e. 20%

4. The differential diagnosis of this disorder includes which of the following?
   a. bipolar disorder
   b. schizoaffective disorder
   c. delusional disorder
   d. brief psychotic disorder
   e. all of the above

5. Which of the following is not considered a good prognostic factor in this disorder?
   a. good premorbid functioning
   b. age of onset between 20 and 25 years
   c. stable occupational record
   d. higher socioeconomic status
   e. male gender

6. Which of the following is not true regarding this disorder?
   a. 80% of patients do not have a parental history of the same disorder
   b. there is a lifetime risk of 13% in children who have one parent with this disorder
   c. there is a lifetime risk of 35% to 40% in children who have two parents with this disorder
   d. there is a concordance rate among monozygotic twins of 50%, and the rate is 9% for dizygotic twins and siblings
   e. there is a strong association between advanced maternal age and this disorder

7. A patient comes to the family physician's office with almost identical symptoms as those of the patient described in Clinical Case Problem 1. However, the time from the beginning of the illness (the onset of the first symptom) to the termination of all symptoms is only 4 months. What is the most likely diagnosis in this patient?
   a. schizophrenia
   b. schizoaffective disorder
   c. schizophreniform disorder
   d. bipolar disorder
   e. brief psychotic disorder

8. A patient develops acute psychiatric symptoms much like those described in Clinical Case Problem 1 but in whom the symptoms of depression or mania are more prominent than the psychotic symptoms. This patient has most likely developed which of the following conditions?
   a. schizophrenia
   b. schizoaffective disorder
   c. schizophreniform disorder
   d. bipolar disorder
   e. brief psychotic disorder

9. Disturbances in which of the following pairs of neurotransmitter systems are implicated most clearly in the pathogenesis of the condition described in Clinical Case Problem 1?
   a. serotonin/dopamine
   b. serotonin/norepinephrine
   c. serotonin/γ-aminobutyric acid (GABA)
   d. acetylcholine/dopamine
   e. acetylcholine/GABA

10. Which of the following drugs is the best choice for the patient presented in Clinical Case Problem 1?
    a. risperidone
    b. clozapine
    c. haloperidol
    d. lithium carbonate
    e. fluoxetine

11. Which of the following antipsychotic medications is least likely to lead to weight gain or an increased risk of metabolic syndrome?
    a. olanzapine
    b. risperidone
    c. clozapine
    d. aripiprazole
    e. quetiapine

12. Which test(s) is (are) indicated in the diagnostic workup of new-onset psychosis?
    a. complete blood count (CBC)
    b. complete chemistry profile
    c. thyroid function tests
    d. head computed tomography (CT) or magnetic resonance imaging (MRI) scan
    e. all of the above

13. Which of the following evidence-based psychosocial interventions integrated with psychopharmacological strategies has (have) been shown to most effectively help individuals with this disorder recover?
    a. supported employment
    b. assertive community treatment
    c. cognitive–behavioral therapy (CBT)
    d. family interventions
    e. all of the above

Clinical Case Management Problem

Describe the differential diagnosis of psychosis.

Answers

1. b. The most likely diagnosis in this patient is schizophrenia. The following features characterize schizophrenia:

1. Psychotic symptoms, including at least two of the following symptoms, present for at least 1 month: (a) hallucinations, (b) delusions, (c) disorganized speech (incoherence and evidence of a thought disorder), or (d) disorganized or catatonic behavior
2. Negative symptoms (flattening of affect and lack of motivation)
3. Impairment in social or occupational functioning
4. Duration of the illness for at least 6 months
5. Symptoms not primarily a result of a mood disorder or schizoaffective disorder
6. Symptoms not caused by a medical, neurologic, or substance-induced disorder

2. d. The most suggestive symptom of schizophrenia is the presence of both positive and negative symptoms.

Positive symptoms include the psychotic symptoms just described. The dramatic symptoms of hallucinations and delusions are the most reliably recognized symptoms of the illness.

Negative symptoms include the flattening of affect (emotional blunting), apathy, and the lack of motivation. Negative symptoms are sometimes called deficit symptoms.

3. c. Between 9% and 13% of patients with schizophrenia ultimately commit suicide. Often, this is related to a comorbid depression or anxiety, or patients may respond to command-type auditory hallucinations that tell them to harm themselves.

4. e. The differential diagnosis of schizophrenia includes the following:

1. Delusional disorder: A delusional disorder is a condition in which the patient has a delusion lasting for at least 1 month in the absence of prominent hallucinations or bizarre behaviors.
2. Brief psychotic disorder: A brief psychotic disorder is characterized by a relatively sudden onset of psychosis that lasts for a few hours to a month with a quick return to normal premorbid functioning thereafter.
3. Schizoaffective disorder: A schizoaffective disorder is a psychotic disorder that is differentiated from schizophrenia by either depressive symptoms or manic symptoms that are prominent and consistent features of a patient's long-term psychotic illness (see answer 7). In contrast, a schizophreniform disorder

is a disorder displaying the signs and symptoms of schizophrenia but lasting less than 6 months (see answer 6).
4. Bipolar disorder is distinguished from schizophrenia by a history of discreet mood disordered episodes (mania and depression). Psychosis is present only during the mood episodes. During periods of euthymia (normal mood), no psychotic symptoms are present.
5. Psychotic disorder caused by a general medical condition.
6. A substance-induced psychotic disorder: Substances commonly associated with this condition include amphetamines, cocaine, various "designer drugs," and hallucinogens.

5. e. Schizophrenia with an onset between ages 20 and 25 years, in a patient with a higher socioeconomic status, and in a patient with good premorbid function including a good work history all portend a better prognosis. Female gender is also considered a better prognostic factor compared to male gender.

6. e. Advanced paternal age is considered a risk factor for schizophrenia. There is an increasing lifetime risk directly related to the number of parents who also have the disorder. Twins studies clearly demonstrate the heritability of schizophrenia, and a child has a 9% lifetime risk if a sibling has schizophrenia.

7. c. A patient who meets the *Diagnostic and Statistical Manual of Mental Disorders*, 4th edition, criteria for schizophrenia but whose symptoms last for a period shorter than 6 months is classified as having schizophreniform disorder. Patients with schizophreniform disorder can be classified as those with or without good prognostic features. Good prognostic features include an acute onset, good premorbid functioning, and the absence of a flat affect. Patients without good prognostic features are more likely to have a condition that persists longer than 6 months. When symptoms persist past this point, the diagnosis is changed to schizophrenia.

8. b. This patient has a schizoaffective disorder. A schizoaffective disorder is usually diagnosed when depressive or manic symptoms are a prominent and consistent feature of a patient's long-term psychotic illness. The diagnosis can be substantiated if the longitudinal course is consistent with schizophrenia and if residual psychotic symptoms persist when the patient is not depressed or manic for a period of at least 2 weeks. If, however, the psychotic symptoms are present only when the patient is depressed or manic and the patient has a relatively good interim functioning between episodes, the patient should be considered to have a primary mood disorder (either a major depressive disorder with psychotic features or a bipolar disorder).

9. a. The neurochemical basis of schizophrenia is not understood. However, medications that block some dopamine receptors (D2 and D4) and some serotonin receptors (5-HT$_2$) ameliorate symptoms of the illness. Drugs that stimulate dopamine receptors (e.g., amphetamines) can produce psychotic symptoms. Drugs that stimulate serotonin receptors, such as lysergic acid (LSD), cause hallucinations.

10. a. Risperidone and newer antipsychotic medications, including olanzapine and quetiapine, present advantages over older agents and should be used as drugs of first choice. These medications have minimal or absent extrapyramidal movement side effects and may also be more effective for treatment of negative symptoms of schizophrenia. In addition to blockading dopamine receptors, newer antipsychotic medications block serotonin (5-HT$_2$) receptors. Like newer antipsychotic medications, clozapine blocks both dopamine and serotonin receptors, has no movement side effects, and may be effective for negative symptoms of schizophrenia. However, it has a 5% incidence of seizures and a 1% incidence of agranulocytosis. Therefore, it is not used as a first-line medication.

11. e. Compared with the general population, people with schizophrenia have up to a 20% shorter life span, with cardiovascular disease the leading cause of death. Results from the Clinical Antipsychotic Trials of Intervention Effectiveness provide further evidence of the metabolic risk associated with different atypical antipsychotics. Clozapine and olanzapine treatment can produce substantial weight gain and an increased risk of associated metabolic disturbances. Risperidone and quetiapine treatment can produce weight gain and appear to increase metabolic risk. Aripiprazole confers little or no weight gain or risk for adverse metabolic changes. It is crucial for primary care professionals to increase awareness of how to appropriately manage the metabolic risks associated with psychiatric medications.

12. e. Blood tests such as a CBC, a serum chemistry including electrolytes, glucose, blood urea nitrogen, creatinine, calcium, phosphate, and liver function tests, thyroid function tests, urinalysis, and a urine toxicology screen are obtained routinely. Sexually transmitted disease screening for syphilis and human immunodeficiency virus infection is strongly recommended. An electrocardiogram will rule out cardiac disorders. Imaging studies such as a CT or MRI of the head are useful in ruling out organic disease.

Other imaging techniques, including single photon emission computed tomography and positron emission tomography, can provide information on blood flow and metabolism in the brain but are not done routinely. Blood levels of therapeutic medications are obtained if appropriate. Occasionally, additional tests, such as sleep-deprived electroencephalogram or lumbar puncture, are indicated.

13. e. Although schizophrenia is categorized as a brain disease, and not a psychologic disorder, an approach integrating nonpharmacologic measures with drug therapy has been shown to be superior in preventing relapses. Recovery is the new goal for mental health services. Psychosocial interventions integrated with psychopharmacological strategies have been shown to most effectively help individuals recover. Effective interventions are those that are evidence based and include illness management, supported employment, assertive community treatment, services to families, and dually diagnosed services. However, in the majority of cases, patients with schizophrenia do not even receive routine psychiatric care with medication. Their access to primary care and preventive services is often severely curtailed because of either the patients' social situations or their impaired social and cognitive functioning. Although care coordination services for these patients are imperative, they are rarely available.

Solution to the Clinical Case Management Problem

A differential diagnosis of psychosis includes the following: (1) schizophrenia, (2) schizophreniform disorder, (3) schizoaffective disorder, (4) bipolar disorder (manic phase), (5) delusional disorder, (6) brief psychotic disorder, (7) psychotic disorder caused by a general medical condition, and (8) substance-induced psychotic disorder.

Summary

1. Prevalence: The lifetime incidence of schizophrenia is 1% to 2%. This figure is remarkably stable across racial, cultural, and national dimensions.

2. Characteristics of psychotic symptoms: (a) They are nonspecific and occur in a variety of medical, psychiatric, neurologic, and substance-induced disorders; (b) the onset of schizophrenia after the age of 45 years is rare; and (c) as a consequence, first-onset psychosis after the age of 45 years generally suggests a neurologic disorder, a medical condition, a substance-induced disorder, or a psychotic depression.

3. Main diagnostic clues to the diagnosis of schizophrenia are positive symptoms and negative symptoms. Positive symptoms include hallucinations, delusions, and bizarre behavior, whereas negative symptoms include emotional blunting, apathy, and avolition (lack of purposeful action).

4. Differential diagnosis of schizophrenia and clues to each one
   a. Delusion disorder: A disorder in which a delusion lasts at least 1 month. No other positive symptoms or negative symptoms of schizophrenia are present.
   b. Brief psychotic disorder: A disorder that is characterized by a relatively sudden onset of psychosis that lasts for a few hours to 1 month with a return to premorbid functioning thereafter. No other positive or negative symptoms are present.
   c. Bipolar I disorder: A disorder in which the psychotic symptoms are present only when the patient is depressed or manic; the patient has relatively good interim functioning between episodes.
   d. Major depressive disorder with psychotic features: A disorder in which the psychotic symptoms are present only when the patient is depressed; the patient has relatively good interim functioning between episodes.
   e. Schizophreniform disorder: Both the positive and the negative symptoms of schizophrenia are present, but the patient either recovers without residual symptoms within a 6-month period or has symptoms for less than 6 months.
   f. Schizoaffective disorder: If a patient has symptoms of depression or mania with psychosis and the depressive or manic symptoms are a prominent and consistent feature of the patient's long-term psychotic illness, schizoaffective disorder is the most likely diagnosis.
   g. Psychotic disorder caused by a general medical condition: A disorder that may produce psychotic symptoms including cerebral neoplasms, cerebrovascular disease, epilepsy, thyroid disorders, infections such as acquired immune deficiency syndrome, parathyroid disorders, hypoxia, hypoglycemia, hepatic disorders, renal disorders, and autoimmune disorders.
   h. Substance-induced psychotic disorder: This most commonly occurs with amphetamines.

5. Symptoms and signs of schizophrenia
   a. Psychotic symptoms are present for at least 1 month including two of the following: (i) delusions, (ii) disorganized speech (incoherence and evidence of a thought disorder), and (iii) disorganized or catatonic behavior.
   b. Negative symptoms are present (flattened affect and lack of motivation).
   c. There is impairment in social or occupational functioning.
   d. The illness is present for at least 6 months.
   e. Symptoms are not caused by a mood disorder or schizoaffective disorder.
   f. Symptoms are not caused by a medical, neurologic, or substance-induced disorder.

6. Subtypes of schizophrenia
   a. Catatonic: This subtype is dominated by motor abnormalities such as rigidity and posturing.
   b. Disorganized: This subtype is marked by flat affect and disorganized speech and behavior.
   c. Paranoid: This subtype is marked by paranoid symptoms in the absence of catatonic and disorganized features.
   d. Undifferentiated: None of the previously listed symptoms predominate.
   e. Residual: Only negative symptoms or attenuated symptoms remain after an active phase.

7. Causation
   a. Schizophrenia is believed to have a pathogenesis that results from an interaction between genetic influences and environmental variables.
   b. There are gross morphologic and cytoarchitectural abnormalities in the brains of some individuals with schizophrenia, but there are no pathognomonic findings. An increased prevalence of perceptual–motor and cognitive abnormalities is described in many studies.

8. Treatment
   a. Active phase includes the following: (i) hospitalization for severely disorganized or dangerous behavior; (ii) antipsychotic medications, with newer antipsychotic medications being the drugs of first choice; and (iii) reassurance and support for both patient and family members.
   b. Chronic phase includes the following: (i) continued antipsychotic medication at the lowest effective dose (often will prevent relapse for long periods) and (ii) psychosocial treatment. Underlying goals are treatment of symptoms, prevention of acute episodes through the management of stress, mobilization of social supports, and assistance with deficits in instrumental living skills caused by the illness. Comprehensive treatment aims to gradually rehabilitate the patient socially and occupationally to the most autonomous level of functioning possible for that individual.

Suggested Reading

American Psychiatric Association: *Diagnostic and Statistical Manual of Mental Disorders*, 4th ed, text revision. Washington, DC: American Psychiatric Association, 2000.

Corrigan PW: Recovery from schizophrenia and the role of evidence-based psychosocial interventions. *Expert Rev Neurother* 6(7): 993–1004, 2006.

Freedman R: Drug therapy: Schizophrenia. *N Engl J Med* 349(18): 1738–1749, 2003.

Lieberman JA: Effectiveness of antipsychotic drugs in patients with chronic schizophrenia: Efficacy, safety and cost outcomes of CATIE and other trials. *J Clin Psychiatry* 68(2):e04, 2007. Available at www.psychiatrist.com/toc.

Newcomer JW: Metabolic considerations in the use of antipsychotic medications: A review of recent evidence. *J Clin Psychiatry* 68 (Suppl 1):20–27, 2007.

CHAPTER

149 Drug Abuse

CLINICAL CASE PROBLEM 1

A 32-Year-Old Administrator with "Rapidly Swinging Moods"

A 32-year-old male is brought into the emergency room (ER) by his wife one evening. She tells you that "something is desperately wrong with my husband." She states that he used to be kind, even-keeled, and fun to be with, but during the past year he has "changed drastically."

He now exhibits behavior that can best be described as "very erratic." He will go from periods of extreme depression to short intervals of "being on top of the world," "extremely elated," with "extremely fast speech and restlessness." After a few hours, he goes back into a state of depression and often retreats to the bedroom to sleep for long stretches of time. His wife brought him into the ER tonight because he was in a period of elation and euphoria.

She also tells you that her husband has not been performing well at work lately and that "some of his colleagues have noticed some strange behavior." In addition, she tells you that "money seems to be disappearing from our bank account at a rate far faster than I can explain."

On examination, the patient is obviously euphoric and elated. When you ask him why he agreed to come tonight, he tells you that he feels so good that he would do anything to please his wife. His speech appears extremely pressured.

On physical examination, his blood pressure is 198/110 mmHg. His pulse is 128 beats/minute and regular. His pupils are widely dilated, and he is sweating profusely. The remainder of his physical examination is normal.

SELECT THE BEST ANSWER TO THE FOLLOWING QUESTIONS

1. What is the most likely diagnosis in this case?
   a. bipolar I disorder, rapid cycling
   b. heroine intoxication
   c. amphetamine intoxication
   d. cocaine intoxication
   e. schizophrenia: catatonic subtype

2. At this time, what would be the most appropriate course of action?
   a. call the family into the office right away for an intervention
   b. arrange for a social worker to see the patient and his wife now
   c. arrange for an immediate psychiatric consultation
   d. call the appropriate consultant and relate the history, your findings, and diagnosis and facilitate appropriate acute intervention
   e. prescribe diazepam and follow up as an outpatient in 1 week

3. The term *dual diagnosis* in psychiatry usually refers to which of the following?
   a. any two closely related psychiatric disorders in the same patient
   b. any two relatively unrelated psychiatric disorders in the same patient
   c. the manic and depressive episodes of bipolar disorder
   d. the existence of both a psychiatric disorder and a substance abuse disorder in the same patient
   e. the existence of both a chronic medical disorder and a psychiatric disorder in the same patient

4. What is the most effective interview strategy to motivate this patient to engage in treatment of his disorder?
   a. to focus on the precise details of the euphoria and the elation the patient is experiencing
   b. to focus on the precise details of the longer periods of the depression the patient is experiencing

c. to focus on the precise details of the negative consequences that have resulted from the patient's symptoms

d. to focus on the relationship between the patient's symptoms and the possible use or abuse of substances

e. to focus on the relationship between the patient's symptoms and the relationship with his wife

5. Which of the following substances has had the most dramatic epidemic increase in the past decade in the United States?
   a. anabolic steroids
   b. crack cocaine
   c. hallucinogens
   d. marijuana
   e. alcohol

6. Following informed consent, which of the following laboratory tests will yield the most significant information concerning the confirmation of the diagnosis made in this patient?
   a. serum cotinine level
   b. urine benzoylecgonine level
   c. urine opioid and serum opioid metabolite levels
   d. serum γ-glutamyl transferase
   e. serum barbiturate level

7. Which of the following medications should not be considered in the treatment of this patient's current hypertension and tachycardia?
   a. lidocaine
   b. verapamil
   c. sodium bicarbonate
   d. metoprolol
   e. nitroglycerin

8. Which of the following statements regarding opioid abuse in the United States is (are) true?
   a. the prevalence of human immunodeficiency virus (HIV) infection among intravenous (IV) drug abusers in the United States continues to increase
   b. opioid overdose should be suspected in any patient who is in a coma and has respiratory depression
   c. nausea, vomiting, cramps, and diarrhea are symptoms of opioid withdrawal
   d. b and c
   e. a, b, and c

9. Which of the following substances is responsible for the highest mortality rate in our society?
   a. nicotine
   b. alcohol

c. cocaine
d. heroin
e. cannabis

10. Which of the following drugs would not be used in cases of opiate detoxification?
    a. naloxone
    b. naltrexone
    c. clonidine
    d. buprenorphine
    e. methadone

11. Which of the following is a specific benzodiazepine antagonist?
    a. flumazenil
    b. naltrexone
    c. clonidine
    d. methadone
    e. sertraline

12. Which of the following drugs is least effective for alcohol and benzodiazepine detoxification?
    a. phenytoin
    b. oxazepam
    c. carbamazepine
    d. lorazepam
    e. chlordiazepoxide

Clinical Case Management Problem

Describe the general principles of interviewing a patient you suspect of having a substance abuse problem but who denies the problem.

Answers

1. **d.** This patient most likely has cocaine intoxication. Cocaine intoxication is characterized by elation, euphoria, excitement, pressured speech, restlessness, stereotyped movements, and bruxism. It causes sympathetic stimulation characterized by symptoms such as tachycardia, hypertension, mydriasis, and sweating. Paranoia, suspiciousness, and psychosis may occur with prolonged use. Overdose produces hyperpyrexia, hyperreflexia, seizures, coma, and respiratory arrest.

Amphetamines produce similar symptoms, but rapid changes in mood from elation to depression are less common because of a longer half-life. They are much less expensive than cocaine and less likely to rapidly deplete someone's savings.

2. **d.** Call the appropriate consultant and relate the history, your findings, and diagnosis and facilitate appropriate acute intervention, which ideally would provide detoxification and drug rehabilitation. The rehabilitation should include individual psychotherapy and group (family) psychotherapy.

3. **d.** The term dual diagnosis is used most often in psychiatry to denote the occurrence of substance abuse and another psychiatric illness. It is also used to refer to the co-occurrence of a developmental disorder (e.g., mental retardation) and another psychiatric illness.

4. **c.** The most effective strategy for engaging individuals in substance abuse treatment is to focus on the negative consequences resulting from drug abuse. This will produce the greatest likelihood of convincing the patient that he or she has a problem. Substance abuse treatment is rarely successful when patients do not believe that they actually have a problem. Often, the family needs to be engaged to confront the patient with the negative consequences of his or her behavior.

5. **b.** The most substantial increase has been in the use of crack cocaine. In the early 1970s, approximately 5 million people had tried cocaine at least once, whereas in the late 1980s, approximately 40 million people had tried it. Cocaine is used in either powder or crystallized ("rock" or "crack") forms; it can be injected, snorted, or smoked. Crack cocaine is generally inhaled as smoke. The drug has a very rapid onset of action and thus a very high addiction potential. It is the least expensive form of cocaine.

Amphetamines are sold as prescription medications (dextroamphetamine and methamphetamine), but the majority of the drug is manufactured illicitly as powder or crystallized ("ice") methamphetamine. Amphetamines are used orally or smoked, snorted, or injected. Marijuana is the most widely used illicit drug in the United States. Approximately two-thirds of the U.S. population has tried marijuana. According to the 1994 National Comorbidity Survey, 23% of Americans reported alcohol abuse or dependence. Men are two or three times more likely to be problem drinkers than women.

6. **b.** The metabolite of cocaine that can be detected in the urine is benzoylecgonine. A complete urine drug screen needs to be performed to check for possible combination drug abuse.

7. **d.** This patient presents with hypertension and tachycardia likely related to acute cocaine intoxication. However, in the absence of an electrocardiogram it is impossible to determine whether an arrhythmia, a common cardiac abnormality in this condition, is present. β-Adrenergic blocking agents such as metoprolol may exacerbate cocaine-induced coronary arterial vasoconstriction, thereby increasing the magnitude of myocardial ischemia. In contrast, nitroglycerin and verapamil reverse cocaine-induced hypertension and coronary arterial vasoconstriction; therefore, they are the agents of choice in treating patients with cocaine-associated chest pain. Sodium bicarbonate, benzodiazepines, and lidocaine are sometimes also used in the management of cocaine-induced arrhythmias.

8. **e.** Despite a number of local initiatives, the prevalence of HIV infection among IV drug abusers continues to increase because IV drug abusers frequently engage in needle sharing and unprotected sexual intercourse. Opioid overdose should be suspected in any patient who presents to the ER with coma, convulsions, and respiratory depression. Therefore, naloxone, an opioid antagonist, is often indicated even before the diagnosis of opioid intoxication can be confirmed. Nausea, vomiting, cramps, and diarrhea are common signs and symptoms of opioid withdrawal. Other signs and symptoms include generalized pain, dysphoria, lacrimation, yawning, rhinorrhea, and piloerection.

9. **a.** Nicotine addiction and tobacco use are legally sanctioned, although restrictions on exposure of others to secondhand smoke have increased. Tobacco accounts for more than 350,000 premature deaths per year in the United States, far more than any other recreational substance. Evaluation of smoking and, if present, counseling about tobacco cessation is an integral part of every primary care visit. Physicians' repeated questioning over time regarding the intention to quit has been shown to be an effective strategy. Using a combination of various counseling techniques, nicotine replacement products, and other medications such as bupropion may be helpful in the treatment of tobacco addiction and in managing nicotine withdrawal. Often, more than one attempt to quit is necessary before patients become permanently tobacco free.

10. **a.** Naloxone is generally reserved for acute opiate intoxication. Severe respiratory depression can be reversed rapidly with 0.4 mg of IV naloxone, although acute intoxication does not generally require any treatment. The remaining medications can play a role in opioid detoxification.

The α_2-adrenergic agonist clonidine may also be used to suppress some of the signs and symptoms of opioid withdrawal. Clonidine acts at presynaptic noradrenergic nerve endings in the locus coeruleus of the brain and blocks the adrenergic discharge produced by opioid withdrawal. Naltrexone is an opioid receptor antagonist. The addition of naltrexone can significantly shorten the time to detoxification. Methadone effectively treats the symptoms of heroin withdrawal and is often used acutely for this purpose. As a component of detoxification treatment, methadone is then gradually reduced to minimize withdrawal symptoms. Methadone maintenance programs help many addicts to lead productive lives and avoid most of the deleterious effects of heroin addiction. Buprenorphine is a partial μ-agonist analgesic that is very effective for detoxification from opiates.

11. **a.** Flumazenil (Romazicon) is a benzodiazepine antagonist that binds competitively and reversibly to the γ-aminobutyric acid/benzodiazepine receptor complex and inhibits the effects of the benzodiazepines. The drug is approved for the treatment of benzodiazepine overdose or the reversal of benzodiazepine sedation.

12. **a.** Tapering doses of lorazepam or other benzodiazepines are the most effective treatment for most serious alcohol and benzodiazepine withdrawals. For patients who may have active liver disease, a common result of chronic alcohol use, it is best to recall the benzodiazepines that are safe to use in these cases by remembering the following mnemonic: **O**utside **T**he **L**iver (oxazepam, temazepam, and lorazepam). Carbamazepine is used extensively in Europe for alcohol withdrawal and is still a mainstay of treatment in the United States, but studies have concluded that the evidence to support its use is less than the evidence to support the use of benzodiazepines. Also, the adverse effects of carbamazepine, including blood dyscrasias and hepatitis, make it less useful than benzodiazepines for this indication. There is no evidence of efficacy for phenytoin in the prevention and treatment of alcohol withdrawal seizures.

Solution to the Clinical Case Management Problem

The general principles of interviewing a patient who may be abusing drugs but who initially denies drug abuse (and that includes most patients) includes the following: (1) attempting to obtain a detailed history of any substance used (start with nicotine and alcohol); (2) asking about peer group use of these substances; (3) inquiring about physical and behavioral problems; (4) providing empathy and concern to encourage trust on the part of the patient; (5) avoiding judgmental attitudes and pejorative statements; (6) focusing on whether the patient has experienced negative consequences as a result of his or her use of psychoactive substances, has poor control of use, or has been criticized by others concerning his or her pattern of behavior or use of the substance (this can be the most effective interview strategy); (7) confronting the patient if you have solid evidence, including test results; and (8) including input from family members and significant others whenever possible.

Summary

Many ramifications that concern drug abuse are also outlined in Chapter 8. Others are as follows:

1. Individuals predisposed to substance abuse often first start to abuse alcohol and marijuana and then progress to cocaine, opioids, or other dangerous drugs.
2. The most destructive recreational substance in terms of morbidity and mortality worldwide is nicotine.
3. Stimulant abuse: Crack cocaine abuse is increasingly common in the United States, and amphetamine abuse is also escalating.
4. Opioid abuse: IV heroin users are now the second largest group of patients with acquired immunodeficiency syndrome in the United States.

5. Specific drugs
   a. Cocaine: Cocaine increases the sympathetic stimulation of the central nervous system (CNS) and produces initial euphoria as a high. Cocaine (crack) is potent and significantly less expensive than many other drugs.
   b. Caffeine: Caffeine and related methylxanthines are ubiquitous drugs in our society. These drugs produce sympathetic stimulation, diuresis, bronchodilatation, and CNS stimulation.
   c. Cannabis: Marijuana, although illegal, has been used at one time or another by 64.8% of adult Americans. Cannabis intoxication is characterized

by tachycardia, muscle relaxation, euphoria, and a sense of well-being. Tachycardia, time-sense alteration, and emotional lability are common.

d. Anabolic steroids: Some data suggest that 6.5% of adolescent boys and 1.9% of adolescent girls in the United States have used anabolic steroids. The medical complications of these drugs include myocardial infarction, stroke, and hepatic disease. Psychiatric symptoms associated with anabolic steroid use include severe depression, psychotic (paranoid) symptoms, aggressive behavior, homicidal impulses, euphoria, irritability, anxiety, racing thoughts, and hyperactivity. (All of these symptoms decline or are eliminated on discontinuation of the drug.)

e. Hallucinogens: The hallucinogens include lysergic acid diethylamide, mescaline, psilocybin, dimethyltryptamine, hallucinogenic amphetamines, and methylenedioxyamphetamine. The mechanism of action of these substances includes stimulation of CNS dopamine or serotonin.

f. Inhalants: Inhalants are volatile compounds that are inhaled for their intoxicating effects. Substances in this class include organic solvents (e.g., gasoline, toluene, and ethyl ether). Inhalants are ubiquitous and readily available in most households and can be lethal if used in overdose. These are drugs of choice for many disadvantaged youths in both urban and rural environments, along with crack cocaine.

g. Nicotine: More than 50 million Americans smoke cigarettes daily and another 10 million use other forms of tobacco. Nicotine addiction and tobacco use are generally legally sanctioned for adults. Tobacco accounts for more than 350,000 premature deaths per year, primarily as a result of cardiovascular disease and cancer.

h. Opioids: Opioid dependence remains a significant sociologic and medical problem in the United States. There are an estimated 500,000 opioid addicts. Opioid addicts are frequent users of medical and surgical services because of multiple medical sequelae of IV drug use and associated lifestyle.

6. Treatment

a. The general characteristics of drug abuse treatment have already been outlined; however, the most important principles include the following: (i) detoxification and elimination of withdrawal symptoms, (ii) initial admittance of a problem and alignment of social support systems (family and others), (iii) long-term intensive individual and group therapy, and (iv) inclusion of the family members in therapy.

b. Special treatments include the following:

   i. For opioid addiction, methadone; for short periods of opioid use, naltrexone (a long-acting orally active opioid antagonist also used for alcoholism); and for opioid withdrawal, clonidine, which blocks many symptoms.

   ii. For benzodiazepine sedation, flumazenil (Romazicon) is the first benzodiazepine antagonist approved by the Food and Drug Administration. Benzodiazepines are considered first-line medical management for alcohol withdrawal.

Suggested Reading

American Psychiatric Association: *Diagnostic and Statistical Manual of Mental Disorders*, 4th ed, text revision. Washington, DC: American Psychiatric Association, 2000.

Lange RA, et al: Cardiovascular complications of cocaine use. *N Engl J Med* 345(5):351–358, 2001.

Schneider RK, et al: Update in addiction medicine. *Ann Intern Med* 134(5):387–395, 2001.

Schuckit MA: *Drug and Alcohol Abuse: A Clinical Guide to Diagnosis and Treatment*. New York: Springer, 2006.

CLINICAL CASE PROBLEM 1

A 19-Year-Old Female with Rapid Weight Loss and an Intense Fear of Gaining Weight

A 19-year-old female comes to your office with a 30-pound weight loss during the past 6 months. She states that she has an intense fear of gaining weight. She has had no menstrual period during the past 4 months. When questioned about her perception of her weight, she states, "I still feel fat."

She denies episodes of binge eating and purging. She also denies the use of laxatives or diuretics.

On examination, the patient is approximately 25% below expected body weight. There is evidence of significant muscle wasting. Her blood pressure is 90/70 mmHg, and her heart rate is 52 beats/minute and regular. There appears to be significant fine hair growth over her entire body. The remainder of her physical examination is normal.

SELECT THE BEST ANSWER TO THE FOLLOWING QUESTIONS

1. What is the most likely diagnosis in this patient?
   a. borderline personality disorder
   b. bulimia nervosa
   c. anorexia nervosa
   d. generalized anxiety disorder
   e. masked depression

2. Which of the following is not true regarding the diagnosis?
   a. it has an annual mortality rate of 0.6%
   b. it is associated with an intense fear of weight gain
   c. patients have a body weight of less than 85% of that expected
   d. in postmenarcheal women, there is the presence of amenorrhea for three consecutive cycles
   e. 70% of patients fully recover from their illness

3. What percentage of individuals with the disorder described have an accompanying major depressive disorder or a coexisting anxiety disorder?
   a. 10%
   b. 20%
   c. 30%
   d. 50%
   e. 75%

4. Which of the following is the most important goal in the initial treatment of this disorder?
   a. provide family counseling and therapy
   b. restore and maintain a healthy weight
   c. address negative cognitive distortions regarding body image
   d. educate the patient about the diagnosis and its treatment
   e. encourage healthy eating and exercise habits

5. Which complication of this disorder has the greatest potential for precipitating a life-threatening circumstance?
   a. muscle wasting
   b. generalized fatigue and weakness
   c. hypokalemia
   d. bradycardia
   e. hypotension

6. Which of the following physical exam findings is least likely to be seen in patients with the disorder described in this case?
   a. hirsutism
   b. parotid gland enlargement
   c. Russell's sign
   d. lanugo
   e. peripheral neuropathy

CLINICAL CASE PROBLEM 2

A 23-Year-Old Female Who Binges and then Vomits to Prevent Weight Gain

A 23-year-old patient comes to your office with recurrent episodes of binge eating that last approximately 1 or 2 hours and occur approximately four times a week. After each episode, she vomits to prevent weight gain. She says she feels "out of control" during these episodes and becomes depressed because of her inability to control herself. These episodes have been occurring for the past 2 years. When you ask her about other methods she has used to compensate for her binging behavior, she tearfully admits to using self-induced vomiting, laxatives, diuretics, and exercise to lose weight, with most behaviors occurring directly after binge episodes.

On examination, the patient's blood pressure is 110/70 mmHg, and her pulse is 72 beats/minute and regular. She is in no apparent distress. Her physical examination is entirely normal.

7. What is the most likely diagnosis in this patient?
   a. borderline personality disorder
   b. anorexia nervosa
   c. bulimia nervosa
   d. major depression
   e. substance abuse

8. Regarding the suicide risk in the disorders described in the previous two clinical case problems, which of the following statements is true?
   a. the rate of completed suicide is equal in both disorders
   b. the rate of attempted suicide is higher in patients with the disorder described in Clinical Case Problem 1
   c. in both cases, only patients with comorbid anxiety or depression have an increased suicide rate
   d. all patients with these disorders should be assessed routinely for suicidal ideation
   e. suicide risk is clearly averted when patients sign a "contract for safety"

9. Regarding the prevalence of the disorders described in the previous two clinical case problems, which of the following statements is true?
   a. the prevalence of the disorder described in Clinical Case Problem 1 is increasing, whereas the prevalence of the disorder described in Clinical Case Problem 2 is decreasing
   b. the prevalence of the disorder described in Clinical Case Problem 1 is decreasing, whereas the prevalence of the disorder described in Clinical Case Problem 2 is increasing
   c. the prevalence of both disorders is increasing
   d. the prevalence of both disorders is decreasing
   e. the prevalence of both disorders has remained unchanged during the past decade

10. The patient described in Clinical Case Problem 1 should be treated in which manner?
    a. as an outpatient: treatment focused on pharmacotherapy, psychotherapy, and behavior modification
    b. as an inpatient: treatment focused on pharmacotherapy, psychotherapy, and behavior modification
    c. as an inpatient: treatment focused on psychotherapy and behavior modification
    d. as an outpatient: treatment focused on psychotherapy and behavior modification
    e. as an outpatient: treatment focused on pharmacotherapy

11. Which of the following drugs has (have) been shown to be of benefit in the treatment of the disorder described in Clinical Case Problem 2?
    a. monoamine oxidase inhibitors (MAOIs)
    b. tricyclic antidepressants (TCAs)
    c. selective serotonin reuptake inhibitors (SSRIs)
    d. b and c
    e. a, b, and c

12. Which of the following psychotherapies is (are) generally considered most effective for the treatment of the disorder described in Clinical Case Problem 2?
    a. supportive psychotherapy
    b. psychodynamic psychotherapy
    c. psychoanalytic psychotherapy
    d. cognitive–behavioral therapy (CBT)
    e. a, b, and d

Clinical Case Management Problem

List the psychiatric disorders and associated conditions that have been shown to be related to the conditions described in this chapter.

Answers

1. **c.** This patient has anorexia nervosa.

2. **e.** Anorexia nervosa is characterized by the following: (1) a patient who refuses to maintain her minimal normal body weight for age and height, leading to maintenance of body weight at least 15% below normal, or a patient who fails to gain weight as expected during growth, leading to body weight 15% below that which is expected; (2) although underweight, the patient displays an intense fear of gaining weight or becoming fat; (3) the patient experiences body weight, size, or shape in a disturbed manner, such as claiming to feel fat even when she is clearly underweight; and (4) in female patients, at least three menstrual periods that should otherwise have been expected to occur have not occurred. There is an annual mortality rate of 0.6%. Approximately 50% of patients with anorexia nervosa recover fully, whereas 30% partially recover and 20% follow a chronic course.

3. **e.** Up to 75% of patients with anorexia nervosa have a coexisting major depressive disorder or anxiety disorder. Although these are the most common comorbidities, it is important to note that of patients with anorexia nervosa, 25% also develop obsessive–compulsive disorder some time in their life. Patients being screened for any eating disorder should also be asked about symptoms of these common comorbidities.

4. **b.** Although all of the options are important in the management of anorexia nervosa, any treatment must begin with the restoration and maintenance of a healthy weight. Once the patient is at a safe weight, other considerations such as psychoeducation, personal and family therapy, and the initiation of medication can be introduced.

5. **c.** The medical complications of anorexia nervosa include muscle wasting, fatigue, depression of cardiovascular function leading to bradycardia and hypotension, and depression of body temperature mechanisms leading to hypothermia. Although all of these conditions can become life threatening, the abnormality of greatest medical concern is hypokalemia, caused by inadequate nutrition and sometimes exacerbated by the misuse of diuretics and laxatives. Hypokalemia can cause cardiac dysrhythmias and, if severe enough, sudden death.

6. **d.** There are several important characteristic findings to be mindful of during the physical exam of patients with eating disorders. Vital signs can offer an important immediate clue even before the patient is examined. Hypotension, bradycardia, and hypothermia are commonly seen in both anorexia nervosa and bulimia nervosa. The assessment for anorexia nervosa should include examination for lanugo (fine hair), hair loss, arrhythmia, dry skin, yellow skin (secondary to carotenemia), and peripheral neuropathy. Individuals engaging in binge/purge behavior may also present with dental carries, parotid or salivary gland enlargement, or skin excoriation on the hand or on the extensor surface of one digit (Russell's sign)—all from self-induced vomiting and the acidic environment that results in the mouth.

7. **c.** This patient has bulimia nervosa. Bulimia nervosa is characterized by a patient who (1) engages in repeated episodes of binge eating large amounts of food in brief periods; (2) regularly engages in severe compensatory behaviors to prevent weight gain, such as self-induced vomiting, misusing laxatives or diuretics, taking diet pills, fasting, eating very strict diets, and/or exercising very vigorously; (3) engages in at least two binge eating and purging/severe compensatory behaviors per week for a minimum of 3 months; and (4) is relentlessly overconcerned regarding weight and body shape.

Although bulimia nervosa certainly explains this patient's symptoms, it is important to note that mood disorders, substance abuse, and personality disorders are commonly seen in patients with this disorder.

8. **d.** Many studies have found high rates of completed suicide in patients with anorexia nervosa, whereas completed suicide rates do not appear to be elevated in bulimia nervosa. In contrast, suicide attempts occur in approximately 3% to 20% of patients with anorexia nervosa and in 25% to 35% of patients with bulimia nervosa. Important clinical risk factors for suicidality in eating disorders include purging behaviors, depression, substance abuse, and a history of childhood physical and/or sexual abuse. All patients with eating disorders should be assessed routinely for suicidal ideation, regardless of the severity of eating disorder or depressive symptoms.

9. **c.** Studies suggest that among adolescent and young adult women in high school and college settings, the prevalence of clinically significant eating disorders is approximately 4% and, for more broadly defined syndromes, may be as high as 8%. The prevalence of these disorders seems to have increased during the past several decades. The prevalence of eating disorders may be influenced by societal attitudes regarding beauty and fashion. During the past few years, so-called "pro-ana" Web sites have appeared where anorexics claim this condition is not a disease but a lifestyle choice. These sites, usually run by young patients who are anorexic, hold a dangerous fascination for patients with an already severely disturbed body image.

10. **c.** A 30-pound weight loss in 6 months suggests that this patient is at immediate risk for life-threatening complications. In this circumstance, most clinicians would suggest inpatient therapy with a focus on reestablishing a reasonable weight through calorie supplementation, CBT, and possibly other forms of psychotherapy. SSRI antidepressant medication would be indicated only for treatment of comorbid depression that commonly accompanies anorexia nervosa.

11. **c.** SSRI agents such as fluoxetine or sertraline have been shown to be successful in reducing binge eating and purging episodes, whether or not there is comorbid depression. MAOIs have no role in the treatment of bulimia. TCAs should be avoided in eating disorders because of their potential to cause dangerous arrhythmias.

12. **d.** CBT appears to be the most effective treatment for bulimia nervosa. This treatment includes several stages, each consisting of several weeks of biweekly individual or group sessions. The first stage emphasizes the patient's establishing control over eating using behavioral techniques such as self-monitoring. The second stage focuses on attempts to restructure the patient's unrealistic cognitions about eating and body image. It also instills more effective modes of problem solving.

The final stage emphasizes maintaining the gains and preventing relapse, often by providing 6 months to 1 year of weekly sessions, with close follow-up during times when relapse is common. Self-help groups, especially Overeaters Anonymous, may also be useful for individuals with bulimia nervosa.

Solution to the Clinical Case Management Problem

The psychiatric disorders related to the eating disorders described include the following: (1) major depressive disorder (MDD), (2) anxiety disorders (75% of patients with an eating disorder have either MDD or an anxiety disorder at the same time), (3) chemical dependency and substance abuse, and (4) personality disorders.

Summary

1. Prevalence: (a) The prevalence of eating disorders is 4%; (b) the prevalence of abnormal eating behaviors not classified strictly as eating disorders may be as high as 8%; (c) the prevalence of these disorders has increased significantly during the past several decades; and (d) these diseases are more common in females than in males (9:1).
2. Symptoms: The symptoms of both anorexia nervosa and bulimia nervosa have been described previously. The major diagnostic clues are as follows:
   a. Anorexia nervosa: (i) failure to maintain normal weight (less than 85% of ideal weight), (ii) having an intense fear of gaining weight, (iii) having a distorted body image (feeling fat despite being grossly underweight), and (iv) having amenorrhea.
   b. Bulimia nervosa: (i) repeated episodes of rapid binge eating, (ii) severe compensatory behaviors to lose weight, and (iii) an unrelenting overconcern with weight and body image.
3. Relationships between the two disorders: (a) Both disorders involve abnormal eating behaviors and concern with body image; (b) of individuals with anorexia nervosa, 50% have binge eating and purging behavior;
and (c) a diagnosis of bulimia nervosa is not made if the criteria for diagnosis of anorexia nervosa are present.
4. Complications
   a. Anorexia nervosa: the physical complications of starvation, namely (i) depletion of fat, (ii) muscle wasting (including cardiac muscle in severe wasting), (iii) bradycardia, (iv) cardiac arrhythmias (sudden death may follow), (v) leucopenia, (vi) amenorrhea, (vii) osteoporosis, (viii) cachexia, and (ix) lanugo (fine body hair).
   b. Bulimia nervosa: (i) dental caries and dental disease from vomiting; (ii) metabolic abnormalities (hypokalemia secondary to vomiting); (iii) black stools from laxative abuse; and (iv) if significant weight loss occurs, physical symptoms as listed previously for anorexia nervosa may develop.
5. Treatment
   a. Anorexia nervosa: (i) for severe cases, hospitalization to reestablish weight and correct metabolic abnormalities; (ii) CBT and often family therapy focusing on dynamics related to issues of control; and (iii) SSRIs for coexisting depression.
   b. Bulimia nervosa: (i) CBT and (ii) SSRIs to treat the binge eating component.

Suggested Reading

American Psychiatric Association: *Diagnostic and Statistical Manual of Mental Disorders*, 4th ed, text revision. Washington, DC: American Psychiatric Association, 2000.

Bergh C, Ejderhamn J, and Södersten P: What is the evidence basis for existing treatments of eating disorders? *Curr Opin Pediatr* 15(3): 344–345, 2003.

Franko DL, Keel PK: Suicidality in eating disorders: Occurrence, correlates, and clinical implications. *Clin Psychol Rev* 26(6):769–782, 2006.

Lamberg L: Advances in eating disorders offer food for thought. *JAMA* 290(11):1437–1442, 2003.

Pritts SD, et al: Diagnosis of eating disorders in primary care. *Am Fam Physician* 67(2):297–304, 2003.

Yager J, et al: Anorexia nervosa. *N Engl J Med* 353:1481–1488, 2005.

Somatoform Disorders

CLINICAL CASE PROBLEM 1

A 29-Year-Old Female with 22 Different Symptoms

A 29-year-old female comes to your office for an evaluation of multiple complaints. She has seen several other physicians but has not been satisfied with her treatment to date. She has heard from her best friend that "you are the best doctor for complicated medical problems." She tells you that she has been "sickly" for most of her adult life and describes the following chronic but intermittent complaints: chest pain, palpitations, shortness of breath, muscle weakness, nausea with periodic vomiting, difficulty swallowing, abdominal pain, diarrhea, dizziness, double vision, occasional numbness of the hands and feet, dysuria, back pain, abdominal pain, joint pain, headaches, dyspareunia, intolerance to fatty foods, intolerance to high-fiber foods, heartburn, and "constant gas." She notes that she is sleeping well and denies feeling depressed or anxious.

Her vital signs are within normal limits and a thorough physical examination reveals no physical cause for any of her complaints.

SELECT THE BEST ANSWER TO THE FOLLOWING QUESTIONS

1. What is the most likely diagnosis in this patient?
   a. somatization disorder
   b. conversion disorder
   c. thyroid cancer
   d. hypochondriasis
   e. masked depression

2. At this first visit, what is the next step in the initial management of this patient?
   a. order a computed tomography scan of the head and abdomen
   b. start a selective serotonin reuptake inhibitor (SSRI) and explain the importance of patient insight in the treatment of this disorder
   c. prescribe a benzodiazepine and explain the importance of patient insight in the treatment of this disorder

   d. make another appointment with the patient to establish a more trusting relationship and perform a thorough history and physical
   e. refer her to a psychotherapist specializing in this disorder

3. What is the pharmacologic treatment of choice for the disorder described?
   a. a benzodiazepine
   b. divalproex
   c. an SSRI
   d. a monoamine oxidase inhibitor
   e. none of the above

CLINICAL CASE PROBLEM 2

A 23-Year-Old Female Complaining of Having "a Peculiarly Prominent Jaw"

A 23-year-old female comes to your office with a chief complaint of having "a peculiarly prominent jaw." She tells you that she has seen a number of plastic surgeons about this problem, but "every one has refused to do anything."

On examination, there is no protrusion that you can see, and it appears to you that she has a completely normal jaw and face. Although the physical examination is completely normal, she appears depressed.

4. What is the most likely diagnosis in this patient?
   a. dysthymia
   b. major depressive disorder (MDD) with somatic concerns
   c. somatization disorder
   d. body dysmorphic disorder
   e. hypochondriasis

5. Therapies that reportedly have produced successful results in this disorder include which of the following?
   a. cognitive–behavioral therapy (CBT)
   b. SSRIs
   c. tricyclic antidepressants (TCAs)
   d. individual or group psychotherapies
   e. all of the above

CLINICAL CASE PROBLEM 3

A Mother of Five with a Constant Headache

A 29-year-old mother of five comes to your office with a "constant headache." She states that she is unable to ambulate without assistance because of her neck, abdominal, pelvic, and rib pain. She goes on to say that she has been diagnosed as having fibromyalgia. After performing a complete history, physical examination, and laboratory and radiologic workup, you make a diagnosis of tension headache. She then tells you that she has seen a number of other physicians about the same problem and that they have come to the same conclusion (which she believes is totally incorrect). You ask her to return for a further discussion about this problem next week, shake hands, and are about to leave. However, she continues to discuss the details of her pain and the difficulties that the pain causes her.

You tell her that you will continue discussion of these problems with her when you see her next week. You again attempt to leave the office.

6. What is the most likely diagnosis in this patient?
   a. schizophrenia
   b. conversion disorder
   c. chronic pain syndrome
   d. somatization disorder
   e. none of the above

7. What is the preferred treatment for this patient?
   a. weekly (daily, if needed) visits with you
   b. group psychotherapy
   c. CBT
   d. supportive psychotherapy
   e. treatment in a multidisciplinary pain clinic

CLINICAL CASE PROBLEM 4

A 23-Year-Old Woman Suddenly Becomes Blind

A 23-year-old patient is brought by her husband to the emergency room with a complaint of "having suddenly gone blind." She tells you that she was walking down the street trying to "cool off" after an argument on the phone with her mother and suddenly she could not see. The visual impairment that she describes is bilateral, complete (no vision), and associated with "numbness, tingling, and weakness" in both lower extremities.

The physical examination of the patient suggests a significant difference between the subjective symptoms and the objective complaints. Specifically, both the knee jerks and the ankle jerks are present and brisk; however, motor strength and sensation in both lower extremities appear diminished, not following anatomic pathways.

8. Based on the information provided, what is the most likely diagnosis?
   a. factitious disorder
   b. conversion disorder
   c. bilateral ophthalmic artery occlusion and spinal artery occlusion
   d. somatization disorder
   e. malingering

9. What is the most appropriate next step at this time?
   a. call an ophthalmologist immediately (stat)
   b. call a neurologist stat
   c. call a psychiatrist stat
   d. call a social worker stat
   e. reassure the patient and initiate discussion about stressors

CLINICAL CASE PROBLEM 5

A 41-Year-Old Male Requesting a Cancer Checkup

A 41-year-old male comes to you for his first visit, requesting a "complete cancer checkup." You learn that this patient has had six complete cancer checkups already this year. He has had two of the six done at "executive checkup centers." He is the chief executive officer (CEO) of a large company and thus has the opportunity to take advantage of some "health perks." He provides a list of the tests he wishes to have done, including a complete history, a complete physical examination, a complete laboratory profile, a colonoscopy, an upper endoscopy, a skeletal x-ray survey, and a "head-to-toe" magnetic resonance imaging scan.

You learn that this patient is afraid that he has cancer, specifically colon cancer, because a close relative was diagnosed with colon cancer 2 years earlier and advised him to get checked as often as possible.

You are amazed that he actually has time to function as the CEO of his company. The truth is, however, that he does not. He admits that this fear is greatly interfering with his work and social life.

10. What is the most likely diagnosis in this patient?
    a. somatization disorder
    b. hypochondriasis
    c. factitious disorder
    d. obsessive–compulsive disorder (OCD)
    e. MDD

11. What is the treatment of choice for the patient described?
    a. cognitive–educational group therapy
    b. SSRI medication
    c. collaboration between the primary care physician and a psychiatrist to develop a plan for regularly seeing this patient, managing his condition, alleviating his anxiety, and providing coping skills training
    d. a and c
    e. a, b, and c

12. Of the following choices, which is a negative prognostic factor in patients with the disorder described in this case?
    a. an acute onset
    b. high levels of general medical comorbidity
    c. absence of secondary gain
    d. absence of a comorbid personality disorder
    e. lower socioeconomic status

Clinical Case Management Problem

Describe the most important factors in the assessment of pain complaints.

Answers

1. a. This patient has somatization disorder. Somatization disorder is characterized by the following symptoms: (1) multiple physical complaints of long-standing occurrence; (2) these symptoms usually have resulted in significant medical diagnostic testing, medical interventions, and invasive procedures often causing iatrogenic sequelae; (3) the illness has resulted in significant occupational or social malfunction; (4) the patient's complaints include symptoms that are not fully explained by a known medical condition or by clinical findings; (5) pain is experienced in at least four different sites, including headache or related pain, abdominal pain, back pain, joint pain, extremity pain, chest pain, rectal pain, or dyspareunia; (6) the symptoms include two or more gastrointestinal (GI) symptoms including nausea, diarrhea, bloating, vomiting, and food intolerance; (7) also included are one or more sexual symptoms, including erectile or ejaculatory dysfunction, menstrual irregularities, or decreased libido or indifference; (8) the symptoms include one or more pseudoneurologic symptoms, including a conversion symptom or a dissociative symptom; and (9) these symptoms are not produced consciously.

The patient has no volitional control over these manifestations, which are believed to be expressions of underlying unacceptable emotion.

2. d. For this patient, another visit is reasonable to establish a more trusting relationship and perform a thorough history and physical examination. The goal of treatment is to provide care for the patient without focusing on "curing" the disease. The best treatment hinges on the long-term relationship between the patient and an empathic primary care provider. The physician must allow the patient to play the "sick role." Also important is the scheduling of regular visits with a defined length and a set agenda. Limits should be set regarding contacts outside of the visit time. Diagnostic procedures and therapeutic interventions must be chosen carefully to minimize adverse reactions and problems with indeterminate results fueling the disease. The dialogue that occurs between the doctor and the patient must address symptoms and signs from both a somatic and a psychosocial viewpoint, including the emotional precipitants and consequences of the symptoms. Once the patient has gained insight into the psychological nature of the condition, a referral to a therapist may be indicated.

3. e. Pharmacologic treatment is not helpful in the treatment of somatoform disorders. However, sometimes pharmacologic treatment of symptoms is helpful in establishing the therapeutic alliance. Concomitant psychiatric conditions may be treated with appropriate medications.

4. d. This patient has body dysmorphic disorder, a condition characterized by the following: (1) a preoccupation with an imagined or grossly exaggerated body defect; (2) clinically apparent distress associated with social, occupational, or functional impairment; and (3) psychiatric conditions such as OCD, anorexia nervosa, psychosis, or other psychiatric disorders cannot account for the preoccupation and the impairment.

In addition, the differential diagnosis of body dysmorphic disorder includes the following: (1) anxiety disorders, (2) MDD, (3) hypochondriasis, (4) other somatoform disorders, (5) factitious disorders, and (6) malingering.

5. e. General principles for somatization disorders discussed in the previous question apply to management of body dysmorphic disorder; however, the somatic preoccupations are often persistent. Individual or group psychotherapy is sometimes useful. CBT is used increasingly for the treatment of this condition. SSRIs or TCAs have been used for some patients, especially in cases with coexisting depression. Overall, however, pharmacologic approaches are not the mainstay of therapy for this condition.

6. c. The diagnosis for this patient is chronic pain syndrome, sometimes called "pain disorder associated with psychological factors." The criteria for this diagnosis are as follows: (1) Pain is the central clinical feature and is of sufficient severity to require assessment; (2) the pain results in social, occupational, or functional impairment or clinically significant distress; (3) psychological factors precipitate, exacerbate, or maintain the pain or contribute to the severity of the pain; and (4) the pain is not a component of somatization disorder or other psychiatric disorders including sexual dysfunction.

The differential diagnosis of chronic pain syndrome must take into consideration other psychiatric disorders, such as psychological factors affecting a general medical condition, somatization disorder, hypochondriasis, depressive disorders, generalized anxiety disorder, factitious disorder, and malingering.

Sometimes, it is very difficult to differentiate this somatoform disorder from established medical conditions such as degenerative disc disease. In addition, pain disorders often develop after an initial injury or illness.

Chronic pain syndrome is more common in women than in men and may occur at any age. Often, patients have severe functional impairment and use pain medications extensively.

7. e. The treatment of choice for this patient is treatment in a multidisciplinary pain clinic. Such treatment has several objectives. Often, patients first must be detoxified from analgesics and sedative hypnotics. Other nonpharmacologic treatments for pain control, including transcutaneous nerve stimulation, biofeedback, and other forms of behavioral psychotherapy, are substituted. The therapeutic emphasis must be shifted from elimination of all pain to management of pain and its consequences. Both psychological and physical therapies are used to minimize the functional limitations caused by the pain. Patients are encouraged to increase their social, occupational, and physical activities. These techniques are similar to those used in the management of patients with chronic pain caused by general medical conditions. Specialized pain clinics are often the optimal treatment setting.

Depressive symptoms must also be addressed in pain management. Antidepressants are indicated when depressive disorders are present in these patients.

8. b. This patient has conversion disorder. Conversion disorders represent a type of somatoform disorder in which there is a loss or alteration in physical functioning during a period of psychological stress that suggests a physical disorder but that cannot be explained on the basis of known physiologic mechanisms. Often, symptoms are brought on by stressful and overwhelming events. Contrary to malingering or factitious disorder, conversion disorder is not volitional. The disorder occurs more frequently in women, with its highest prevalence in rural areas and among underserved and undereducated patients.

The *Diagnostic and Statistical Manual of Mental Disorders*, 4th edition (*DSM-IV*), criteria for conversion disorder are as follows: (1) The symptom(s) or deficit(s) is not consciously or intentionally produced; (2) the symptom(s) or deficit(s) is not medically explained after clinical assessment; (3) the initiation or exacerbation of the symptom(s) or deficit(s) is usually preceded by conflicts or stressors; psychological factors are prominent; (4) the symptom(s) or deficit(s) impairs social or occupational functioning, creates significant distress, or requires medical intervention; and (5) the symptom(s) or deficit(s) is not limited to pain or sexual dysfunction and is not a component of somatization disorder or other psychiatric syndrome.

Common examples of conversion symptoms include paralysis, abnormal movements, aphonia, blindness, deafness, or pseudoseizures.

9. e. A wide variety of treatment techniques have been used successfully for the treatment of conversion disorder. The initial step in the management of acute symptoms is to quickly decrease the psychological stress. Brief psychotherapy focusing on stress and coping and suggestive therapy and sometimes hypnosis may be extremely effective. Pharmacologic interventions, including the acute use of benzodiazepines, may also be useful. Brief hospitalization may sometimes be indicated, particularly when symptoms are disabling or alarming. Hospitalization may serve to remove the patient from the stressful situation and to assess for possible underlying general medical conditions.

10. b. This patient has the disorder known as hypochondriasis, which is defined as a preoccupation with having a serious illness based on misinterpretation of physical symptoms that does not respond to physician reassurance after an appropriate evaluation. Individuals with hypochondriasis often have a profound fear of disease and an intense focus on multiple physical complaints and are hypervigilant to transient symptoms. On presentation, the medical history is often related in great detail. There is commonly a history of assessment by multiple physicians, deteriorating doctor–patient relationships, and associated feelings of frustration and anger. The clinical course is chronic, with waxing and waning of symptoms.

The *DSM-IV* diagnostic criteria for hypochondriasis include the following: (1) The patient is preoccupied or afraid of serious disease with misinterpretation of bodily symptoms for 6 months or longer; (2) medical evaluation and reassurance are not effective in allaying the preoccupation; (3) the preoccupation is not delusional, is not consistent with body dysmorphic disorder, and is not a component of another psychiatric disorder; and (4) significant social, occupational, and functional impairment occurs together with clinically significant distress.

The differential diagnosis of hypochondriasis includes somatization disorder, anxiety disorders, MDD, factitious disorders, malingering, and psychotic disorders manifesting hypochondriacal delusions.

Hypochondriasis may be distinguished from somatization disorder by the patient's source of concern. In hypochondriasis, the concern is that the symptoms imply a serious illness. In somatization disorder, the concern is with discomfort of the symptoms. The patient's anxiety regarding the experience of the symptoms is real and should not be discounted.

Factitious disorder is another important differential diagnosis. It is less likely in this case because there is no evidence of pathologic lying or recurrent, feigned, or simulated illness.

11. e. The primary care physician should consult with a psychiatrist about this patient and subsequently manage his condition. The patient should be seen on a regular basis to assure him that he will be followed closely and that any disease will be caught and treated at an early stage.

During these regular visits, attention must be paid to the psychosocial aspects of the patient's life. Coping skills training is useful. Psychological stress is often associated with the onset and maintenance of hypochondriasis.

Regular visits are essential to monitor symptoms, monitor anxiety or depression associated with the hypochondriacal symptoms, and help the patient come to terms with the condition. The use of cognitive-based educational group treatment has been shown to be an effective component of comprehensive treatment. A comprehensive review of the literature published from 1970 to 2003 indicates that hypochondriasis responds well to SSRIs, and these medications should certainly be part of any comprehensive treatment plan after a firm therapeutic alliance has been established.

12. d. In cases of hypochondriasis, good prognostic factors include acute onset, high levels of general medical comorbidity, the absence of personality disorder or secondary gain, high socioeconomic status, and less conviction of having a specific disease.

Solution to the Clinical Case Management Problem

Pain is a prominent symptom in somatoform disorders and must be evaluated carefully. The experience of pain is real. Pain must be considered as a signal of a dysfunction in the physiologic, social, and/or psychological realms. The physician needs to determine whether the symptom of pain is caused primarily by a physical condition or is mediated predominantly by psychological factors. An assessment of the severity of impairment to the patient's functioning must also be made.

Summary

1. Somatization disorder
Diagnostic clues include multiple physical complaints with onset before the age of 30 years. The tendency of these complaints is to be both chronic and long-standing. The complaints involve each of the following: pain symptoms, GI symptoms, sexual dysfunction symptoms, and pseudoneurologic symptoms. There is impairment of social or occupational functioning associated with these symptoms.

2. Conversion disorder
Diagnostic clues include physical symptoms primarily involving loss of motor or sensory function that are produced because of psychological conflicts or stressors. They cannot be fully explained on an anatomic basis and result in impairment of social or occupational functioning. Conversion disorder is more common among medically unsophisticated groups; it may also be a manifestation of a disturbed family or marital situation.

3. Chronic pain syndrome

Diagnostic clues include pain as the prominent clinical presentation, and it results in social, occupational, or functional impairment. This diagnosis is made when psychological factors are believed by the physician to have a significant role in the outset, severity, exacerbation, or perpetuation of the pain syndrome. Major depression or anxiety are often present and may be a component of the pain syndrome. The best therapeutic strategy is to limit inappropriate use of analgesics and other medical resources and to modify the patient's therapeutic expectations from cure to management of the pain while attempting to appreciate the role of psychosocial or psychological factors and stress. A multidisciplinary pain clinic is the treatment of choice in most cases.

4. Hypochondriasis

Hypochondriasis is characterized by a worry about having a serious disease that is based on hypervigilance and a misinterpretation of physical symptoms. It is not alleviated with appropriate physician reassurance. As with pain, the possibility of comorbid anxiety or depression should be strongly considered, and physical disease should be excluded. Treatment is most effective when there is collaboration between a primary care physician who continues regular appointments and a consulting psychiatrist. Again, the diagnosis requires significant social, occupational, or functional impairment.

5. Body dysmorphic disorder

The fundamental diagnostic feature is a pervasive feeling of ugliness or physical defect based on a grossly exaggerated perception of a minor (or even absent) physical anomaly. Patients frequently consult multiple primary care physicians, dermatologists, and plastic surgeons. Depressive symptoms, anxiety symptoms, social phobia, obsessive personality traits, and psychosocial distress frequently coexist. Intervention includes group or family therapy and, occasionally, the use of SSRIs or other medication to decrease obsessive concerns and depression.

6. Malingering

The essential feature of malingering is the intentional production of illness consciously motivated by external incentives, such as avoiding military duty, obtaining financial compensation through litigation or disability, evading criminal prosecution, obtaining drugs, or securing better living conditions. Malingering is more likely when medical and legal context overshadows the presentation, marked discrepancy exists between the clinical presentation and objective findings, and a lack of cooperation is experienced with the patient. Confrontation in a confidential and empathic but firm manner that allows an opportunity for constructive dialogue and appreciation of any psychological or psychosocial problems is imperative.

Suggested Reading

Allen LA, Escobar JI, Lehrer PM, et al: Psychosocial treatments for multiple unexplained physical symptoms: A review of the literature. *Psychosom Med* 64(6):939–950, 2002.

American Psychiatric Association: *Diagnostic and Statistical Manual of Mental Disorders*, 4th ed, text revision. Washington, DC: American Psychiatric Association, 2000.

Fallon BA: Pharmacotherapy of somatoform disorders. *J Psychosom Res* 56(4):455–460, 2004.

Fischhoff B, Wessely S: Managing patients with inexplicable health problems. *BMJ* 326(7389):595–597, 2003.

Kaplan HI, Sadock BJ: Somatoform disorders. In: Kaplan HI, Sadock BJ, eds, *Kaplan and Sadock's Synopsis of Psychiatry: Behavioral Sciences/ Clinical Psychiatry*, 8th ed. Baltimore: Williams & Wilkins, 1998.

Smith RC, Lein C, Collins C, et al: Treating patients with medically unexplained symptoms in primary care. *J Gen Intern Med* 18(6): 478–489, 2003.

Stuart MR, Lieberman JA: *The Fifteen-Minute Hour: Practical Therapeutic Interventions in Primary Care*, 3rd ed. Philadelphia: Saunders, 2002.

CLINICAL CASE PROBLEM 1

A 65-Year-Old Male with Hypertension and Erectile Dysfunction

A 65-year-old male with hypertension, congestive heart failure, and peptic ulcer disease comes to your office for his regular blood pressure check. Although his blood pressure is now under control, he complains of an inability to maintain an erection. He is currently taking β-methyldopa, propranolol, verapamil, hydrochlorothiazide, and cimetidine.

On examination, his blood pressure is 125/76 mmHg. His pulse is 56 beats/minute and regular. The rest of the cardiovascular examination and the rest of the physical examination are normal.

SELECT THE BEST ANSWER TO THE FOLLOWING QUESTIONS

1. Which of the following medications is the least likely to be the cause of this patient's erectile dysfunction (ED)?
   a. α-methyldopa
   b. propranolol
   c. verapamil
   d. hydrochlorothiazide
   e. cimetidine

2. Which of the following is generally considered to be the most common cause of sexual dysfunction in both males and females?
   a. pharmacologic agents
   b. panic disorder
   c. generalized anxiety disorder (GAD)
   d. major depressive disorder (MDD)
   e. dysthymic disorder

3. Which of the following is considered a normal change in sexual functioning in the aging male?
   a. the length of time needed to achieve erection increases
   b. decreased need for direct tactile stimulation to promote erection
   c. the inability to maintain erection between ejaculations
   d. increased forcefulness of ejaculation
   e. the increasing presence of hemospermia

4. Which of the following is the most common sexual complaint in younger males?
   a. hypoactive sexual desire disorder
   b. male erectile disorder
   c. orgasmic disorder
   d. premature ejaculation
   e. none of the above

5. Which of the following is the most common sexual complaint in older males?
   a. hypoactive sexual desire disorder
   b. ED
   c. orgasmic disorder
   d. premature ejaculation
   e. none of the above

6. Which of the following statements regarding male sexual dysfunction is most accurate?
   a. there is a strong association between increased exercise and sexual dysfunction
   b. the estimated prevalence of ED in the United States is 18%
   c. it is usually the treatment for cardiovascular disease rather than the disease itself that leads to sexual dysfunction
   d. male sexual dysfunction in a younger patient tends to be organic in origin
   e. male sexual dysfunction in an older patient tends to be psychologically based

7. Which of the following organic disorders is the most common cause of organic male sexual dysfunction?
   a. benign prostatic hypertrophy
   b. hyperthyroidism
   c. Parkinson's disease
   d. diabetes mellitus
   e. atherosclerosis of the abdominal aorta

8. What is the most important aspect of the evaluation of male sexual dysfunction?
   a. the history
   b. the physical examination
   c. nocturnal penile tumescence measurement
   d. ratio of penile/brachial blood pressure
   e. serum testosterone measurement

9. Which of the following laboratory tests may be indicated in a male patient with sexual dysfunction?
   a. complete blood count (CBC)
   b. blood urea nitrogen (BUN) and serum creatinine
   c. thyroid function studies
   d. serum testosterone level
   e. all of the above

10. Which of the following is an important coun-
    seling aspect in the treatment of male sexual
    dysfunction?
    a. reducing performance anxiety by prohibiting
       intercourse
    b. reducing anxiety by identification and
       verbalization
    c. instructing in "sensate focus" techniques
    d. instructing in interpersonal communication
       skills
    e. all of the above

11. Which of the following treatments should be con-
    sidered in the initial management of male sexual
    dysfunction?
    a. sildenafil
    b. a vacuum assist device
    c. penile prosthesis
    d. intracavernous injections of alprostadil
    e. all of the above

12. Which of the following is specifically indicated as
    a treatment for premature ejaculation?
    a. the penile squeeze technique
    b. the injection of testosterone
    c. structured behavior modification programs
    d. the intermittent injection of medroxyprogesterone
    e. intraarterial penile injection of local
       vasoconstrictors

CLINICAL CASE PROBLEM 2

*A 24-Year-Old Female Who Is Unable to
Have Sexual Intercourse*

A 24-year-old female who has been married for
6 months comes to your office in tears. She and
her husband have been unable to have sexual
intercourse. She says that when he tries to
penetrate her, she "tenses up" and is "unable to
go any further."

   Her significant history includes being raped at the
age of 12 years. The patient has vivid memories of
this event.

   Her general physical examination is normal. At this
time, you do not attempt a vaginal examination.

13. Which of the following statements regarding vag-
    inismus is true?
    a. vaginismus is under voluntary control
    b. there is no association between vaginismus and
       traumatic sexual experiences
    c. most women with vaginismus also have diffi-
       culty with sexual arousal

d. vaginismus is a condition of involuntary spasm
   or constriction of the musculature surrounding
   the vaginal outlet
e. by definition, vaginismus only occurs during
   attempted sexual intercourse

14. Regarding the diagnosis and treatment of vaginis-
    mus, which of the following statements is false?
    a. throughout the diagnostic examination, the
       woman must feel that she is in control and may
       terminate the examination at any time
    b. the diagnosis of vaginismus can often be made
       without inserting a speculum
    c. it is helpful if the sexual partner is involved in
       all aspects of the treatment process
    d. the insertion of vaginal dilators is not a recog-
       nized part of the treatment protocol
    e. "sensate focus" techniques are an important
       part of the treatment protocol

15. Which of the following is the most common
    female sexual dysfunction disorder?
    a. anorgasmy
    b. delayed orgasm
    c. hypoactive sexual desire disorder
    d. sexual aversion disorder
    e. none of the above

16. Which of the following statements regarding
    female sexual arousal disorder is false?
    a. it is more common in women than in men
    b. the diagnosis takes into account the focus,
       intensity, and duration of the sexual activity
    c. if sexual stimulation is inadequate in focus,
       intensity, or duration, the diagnosis cannot be
       made
    d. in women it is not associated with inadequate
       vaginal lubrication
    e. in women it is often associated with inhibited
       female orgasm

17. Of the following causes, which is the most com-
    mon cause of hypoactive sexual desire disorder in
    women?
    a. major psychiatric illness
    b. major psychiatric illness in the woman's partner
    c. exhaustion from work and family responsibilities
    d. major physical illness in the woman
    e. alcoholism in the woman's partner

18. Which of the following statements regarding
    inhibited female orgasm is false?
    a. it is the most common female sexual dysfunction
    b. primary anorgasmia is more common among
       unmarried women than among married women

c. women older than age 35 years have increased orgasm potential

d. women may have more than one orgasm without a refractory period

e. fear of impregnation is a common cause

19. Which of the following statements regarding dyspareunia is (are) true?
    a. it may be caused by endometriosis
    b. it may be caused by vaginitis or cervicitis
    c. it may be caused by an episiotomy scar
    d. all of the above
    e. none of the above

20. Which of the following methods is (are) useful in the treatment of female sexual dysfunction?
    a. sexual anatomy and physiology education
    b. "sensate focus" exercises
    c. treatment of underlying anxiety and depression
    d. none of the above methods are useful
    e. all of the above methods are useful

21. Which of the following major psychiatric conditions is linked most closely to sexual dysfunction?
    a. panic attacks/panic disorder
    b. GAD
    c. MDD
    d. schizoaffective disorder
    e. schizophrenia

Clinical Case Management Problem

Describe the goal, selection, types, and duration of sexual dysfunction psychotherapies most commonly practiced today.

Answers

1. c. Of the medications described for the patient in Clinical Case Problem 1, the only antihypertensive agent that has not been associated with sexual dysfunction is verapamil (a calcium channel blocker).

2. a. Recreational and medicinal drugs are the most common cause of sexual dysfunction. As discussed later in this chapter, arousal disorders, ED, and others have been described. This problem affects patients of both genders and all ages.

3. a. As men age, the length of time needed to achieve erection increases and there is an increased need for direct tactile stimulation to promote erection.

There is also a decrease in the forcefulness of ejaculation. An inability to maintain erection between ejaculations or the presence of blood in the semen are not considered a normal part of the aging process.

4. d. The most common sexual complaint in younger males is premature ejaculation. Estimated prevalence rates for sexual dysfunctions vary greatly, depending on the surveyed population and the survey method. Although this condition tends to lessen with age, counseling is important to avoid long-term consequences for the patient's intimate relationships.

5. b. The most common sexual complaint in older males is ED. This condition is associated with an increase in chronic medical problems, the concomitant increased use of medications that interfere with erection, and aging. The incidence of ED increases steadily with age, but it is not an inevitable consequence of aging. In one study, one-third of 70-year-old men surveyed reported no erectile difficulty. Although by the age of 80 years only 8% of men still reported no difficulty, another 40% claimed only to have mild difficulty and are likely to respond favorably to treatment.

6. b. The overall prevalence of ED in men is 18.4%, indicating that ED affects 18 million men in the United States. The prevalence of ED is positively related to age but is also particularly high among men with one or more cardiovascular risk factors, men with hypertension, and men with a history of cardiovascular disease. Erectile dysfunction is significantly and independently associated with diabetes, lower attained education, and lack of physical activity. In young men, most cases of male sexual dysfunction are psychological in origin. In older men, as the incidence of concurrent disease and use of medication increases, so does the prevalence of organic sexual dysfunction.

7. d. Among men with diabetes, the crude prevalence of ED is 51.3%, making diabetes mellitus the most common organic cause of male sexual dysfunction. Patients with diabetes mellitus experience high rates of ED as a result of vascular disease and autonomic dysfunction.

Other common causes of organic male sexual dysfunction include (1) atherosclerotic vascular disease; (2) congestive heart failure; (3) renal failure; (4) hepatic failure; (5) respiratory failure; (6) genetic causes (Klinefelter's syndrome); (7) hypothyroidism; (8) hyperthyroidism; (9) multiple sclerosis; (10) Parkinson's disease; (11) surgical procedures, including radical prostatectomy, orchiectomy, and abdominal–perineal colon resection; and (12) radiation therapy.

8. **a.** The most important aspect in the evaluation of male (and female) sexual dysfunction is the patient's history. For example, in a patient with ED, if erections are achieved under certain conditions but not others, the likelihood is high that the dysfunction is psychogenic. Normal erectile function during masturbation and extramarital sex and in response to erotic material suggests a psychological cause. Similarly, if a normal erection is lost during vaginal insertion, a psychological cause is suspected. A complete drug history is also essential.

The history should include present and previous birth control methods, a complete past medical and psychiatric history, a family history, a history of surgical procedures, a history of the marital relationship, and an assessment of current job satisfaction and other stressors. A complete physical examination including a genital examination should be performed. The physical examination will determine whether there is any evidence of organic pathology associated with the sexual dysfunction.

Measurement of nocturnal penile tumescence (most simply done using a strain gauge), the ratio of penile/brachial blood pressure, and serum testosterone levels are investigations that may have a role in the overall evaluation of sexual dysfunction but are not always indicated. Vascular impairment as a potential cause of impotence essentially can be ruled out if an injection of alprostadil (see answer 11) induces an erection.

9. **e.** If the family physician suspects an organic cause, baseline screening blood work is indicated. This should include a CBC, BUN and serum creatinine, fasting blood sugar, fasting cholesterol, thyroid function studies, liver function tests, and (if indicated) a serum testosterone level.

10. **e.** Most cases of sexual dysfunction have, as discussed previously, a significant psychological component. The psychological treatment of male sexual dysfunction is composed of several important steps: (1) reduction or, it is hoped, elimination of performance anxiety by prohibiting intercourse during the initial treatment period; (2) anxiety reduction by identification and verbalization of the problem and relaxation and visualization techniques; (3) introduction of the process of "sensate focus" (semistructured touching that will permit focus on sensory awareness without any need to perform sexually); and (4) improvement of interpersonal communication skills.

11. **e.** Several treatment options are available today, most of which are associated with high efficacy rates and favorable safety profiles. A patient-centered approach that involves both the patient and his partner is encouraged. The clinician must educate the patient and provide a supportive environment for shared decision making.

Phosphodiesterase type 5 (PDE-5) inhibitors such as sildenafil (Viagra), tadalafil (Cialis), and vardenafil (Levitra) are currently the first choice of most physicians and patients for the treatment of ED. PDE-5 inhibitors have differences in their pharmacological profiles, the most obvious being the long duration of action of tadalafil, but there are no data supporting superiority for any one of them in terms of efficacy or safety. Many PDE-5 inhibitors are available over the Internet to patients without a doctor's prescription. Physicians should warn their patients against procuring their ED treatment in this way because serious side effects have been described, especially in patients who are taking nitrates for coronary artery disease. A fourth oral medication, sublingual apomorphine (Uprima), works via the central nervous system. Apomorphine has limited efficacy compared with the PDE-5 inhibitors, and its use is limited to patients with mild ED.

Treatment failures with oral drugs may be due to medication, clinician, and patient issues. The physician needs to address all of these issues in order to identify true treatment failures. Patients who are truly unresponsive to oral drugs may be offered other treatment options. Intracavernous injections of alprostadil alone, or in combination with other vasoactive agents (papaverine and phentolamine), remain an excellent treatment option with proven efficacy and safety over time. Vacuum constriction devices may be offered mainly to elderly patients with occasional intercourse attempts; younger patients show limited preference because of the unnatural erection that is associated with this treatment modality. Penile prostheses are generally the last treatment option offered because of invasiveness, cost, and nonreversibility; however, they are associated with high satisfaction rates in properly selected patients. All treatment options are associated with particular advantages and disadvantages.

12. **a.** The initial treatment of premature ejaculation is the same as other therapies described here. In addition, an exercise known as the "penile squeeze technique" is used to raise the threshold of penile excitability. The penis is stimulated until impending ejaculation is perceived. At this time, the partner squeezes the coronal ridge of the glans penis, resulting in diminished erection and inhibited ejaculation. Eventually, with repeated practice, the threshold for ejaculation is raised. Pharmacologically, premature ejaculation may be ameliorated with SSRIs.

13. **a.** Vaginismus is a recurrent or persistent involuntary spasm of the musculature of the outer third of the vagina that can interfere with coitus. There is an association between vaginismus and an intense childhood or adolescent exposure to strong condemnation of sexual behavior based on some religious beliefs. Most women with vaginismus have normal sexual arousal. The spasm can occur with any attempt to penetrate the introitus, including routine pelvic examination.

In this patient, the cause of vaginismus is most likely from the traumatic sexual experience that took place during her childhood.

14. **d.** The evaluation and treatment of vaginismus begins with a carefully performed physical examination in which the patient is always in full control. She may terminate the examination at any time.

On inspection of the external genitalia, spasm and rigidity of the perineal muscles are often felt. In this case, the diagnosis can be made even without inserting a speculum. From inspection, the examination may proceed to the insertion of one or more of the examiner's fingers.

The use of vaginal dilators in gradually increasing sizes has proved helpful in the treatment of vaginismus. Beginning with the smallest size, the woman inserts these herself until she becomes both comfortable and relaxed with their insertion. When the largest plastic dilator can be inserted, the couple can proceed to intercourse.

The partner should be involved in all aspects of assessment and treatment. Ideally, the partner should be present to observe the entire evaluation and treatment. Together with anatomy and physiology education, the couple learns the concept of sensate focus exercises, which plays a major part in the therapy of any sexual dysfunction.

15. **c.** The most commonly reported female sexual dysfunction disorder is hypoactive sexual desire disorder, present in up to one-third of women in some studies. Orgasmic disorder, however, is present in 5% to 10%. The prevalence of the other forms of female sexual dysfunction is less clear.

16. **d.** Female sexual arousal disorder is defined as persistent or recurrent partial or complete failure to attain or maintain the lubrication-swelling response of sexual excitement until completion of the sexual activity. The diagnosis includes the subjective sense of sexual excitement and pleasure and requires the focus, intensity, and duration of stimulation to be adequate. Sexual arousal disorder is often associated with inhibited female orgasm.

17. **c.** Hypoactive sexual desire disorder is defined as persistent or recurrent deficient or absent desire for sexual activity. The definition includes a lack of sexual fantasies. The major reasons for hypoactive sexual desire disorder are marital dysfunction, mismatched activity schedules, and exhaustion from work and family responsibilities.

18. **a.** Inhibited female orgasm is defined as persistent or recurrent delay in, or absence of, orgasm in a female following a normal sexual excitement phase during sexual activity. The definition takes into account the adequacy of focus, intensity, and duration of the sexual activity.

Inhibited female orgasm (as one of the orgasmic disorders) is not the most common disorder of female sexual dysfunction (5% to 10%). It is surpassed by hypoactive sexual desire disorder (33%).

Primary anorgasmia (never having had an orgasm) is more common in unmarried women than in married women. Women older than age 35 years appear to have an increased orgasmic potential.

Women may have more than one orgasm without a refractory period.

Causes for inhibited female orgasm include fear of impregnation, rejection by the woman's sexual partner, hostility, and feelings of guilt regarding sexual impulses.

19. **d.** Dyspareunia is defined as recurrent or persistent genital pain before, during, or after sexual intercourse. This dyspareunia cannot be caused exclusively by lack of lubrication or by vaginismus.

In many cases, however, vaginismus and dyspareunia are closely associated. Other causes of dyspareunia include episiotomy scars, vaginitis, cervicitis, endometriosis, postmenopausal vaginal atrophy, and anxiety regarding the sexual act.

20. **e.** For a woman with sexual dysfunction, it is imperative that she and her partner become knowledgeable about sexual anatomy and physiology. "Sensate focus" exercises are useful. Possible underlying anxiety and depression need to be addressed and treated. If life and marital stressors are present, marital and stress management counseling are indicated. Because side effects of medication can cause sexual dysfunction in women as well as in men, reviewing the patient's medication is very important. As mentioned previously, antidepressants, particularly SSRIs, often cause significant sexual dysfunction, which often leads to poor acceptance of the drug. Changing the patient to a different class of antidepressant may be indicated.

21. **C.** The most common psychiatric condition associated with sexual dysfunction is major depressive illness in one or both mates.

In the absence of a psychiatric pathologic condition, dual sex therapy is the most accepted approach to the treatment of sexual dysfunction. One approach often used in the therapy of sexual dysfunction in couples is called the LEDO approach. The LEDO approach centers on the following:

Lowering stress, tension, and anxiety levels through discussion, examination, and observation

Ensuring that both parties understand each other's desires, pleasures, and difficulties

Determining the partners' genuine awareness and knowledge of their own and each other's sexual anatomy and the process of intercourse

Outlining, drawing, and explaining alternative approaches to arousal and excitation and intercourse techniques

The sexual problem often reflects other areas of disharmony or partner misunderstanding. The marital relationship as a whole is treated, with emphasis on sexual functioning as a part of that relationship. When a referral for sex therapy is necessary, both a female and a male therapist should be involved in the treatment of the couple's sexual problem. The therapy is short term and behaviorally oriented. The goal is to reestablish communication within the marital unit. Information regarding anatomy and physiology is given. Specific sensate focus exercises are prescribed. The couple proceeds from nongenital touching and sensory awareness to genital touching and sensory awareness, to genital touching, and, finally, to intercourse. The couple learns to communicate with each other through these graded exercises.

If underlying MDD, dysthymic disorder, GAD, or other anxiety disorders are present, they must be treated concurrently.

Solution to the Clinical Case Management Problem

The description of the goal, selection, types, and duration of sexual dysfunction psychotherapies most commonly practiced today is a refinement, reinforcement, and expansion of the LEDO approach to sexual dysfunction psychotherapies, as described as follows:

Goal: The goal is resolution of specific sexual dysfunctions.

Selection: (a) All sexual dysfunction psychotherapy ideally should be performed with both partners; and (b) sexual dysfunctions most suited for psychotherapy

include male erectile disorder, premature ejaculation, vaginismus, and orgasmic dysfunction.

Treatment: (a) Make sure all medical causes are ruled out; (b) psychotherapy (types of psychotherapies used include behavior modification techniques including systemic desensitization, homework, and education); and (c) psychodynamic approaches, such as hypnotherapy, group therapy, and couples therapy as needed to deal with system dynamics.

Duration: The length of treatment is weeks to months.

Summary

1. Prevalence: It is extremely difficult to estimate the prevalence of sexual dysfunction disorders. However, it is estimated that 40% of U.S. couples at one time or another have had a sexual dysfunction of some type. The estimated prevalence of certain disorders is as follows:
   a. Males: (i) premature ejaculation, 37%; (ii) hypoactive sexual desire disorder, 16%; (iii) orgasmic disorder, 6%; and (iv) male erectile disorder, 7%
   b. Females: (i) hypoactive sexual desire disorder, 33%; (ii) dyspareunia or vaginismus, not known; and (iii) orgasmic disorder, 7%
2. Most common causes are as follows: (a) Pharmaceutical agents appear to be the most common cause of sexual

dysfunction (antihypertensives and antidepressant drugs are especially important); (b) diabetes mellitus is the most common organic disorder responsible for sexual dysfunction; and (c) psychological factors, even if not the predominant cause, accompany most sexual dysfunction disorders.

3. Nonpharmacologic approaches to sexual dysfunction in couples: (a) Always begin by treating the relationship in reference to the couple; (b) get complete histories from both partners; (c) do complete physical examinations; (d) perform laboratory testing, which may include CBC, renal function, liver function, thyroid function, blood glucose, serum cholesterol, and hormone levels

(testosterone, follicle-stimulating hormone, luteinizing hormone, estrogen, and progesterone); (e) remember that there is an association between dyspareunia or vaginismus and previous sexual abuse; (f) consider the possibility of family violence in the present (e.g., spousal abuse leading to rape); and (g) use the LEDO approach (guidelines described in the Solution to the Clinical Case Management Problem).

4. Pharmacologic treatment of male sexual dysfunction: (a) Erectile dysfunction may be treated with sildenafil, vardenafil, or tadalafil; (b) premature ejaculation may

be ameliorated with SSRIs; and (c) although no reliable aphrodisiacs exist, some patients with hypoactive sexual desire disorder may respond to androgenic steroids or yohimbine. If a medication causes side effects that cannot be controlled, a change to a different medication class should be considered.

5. Pharmacologic treatment of female sexual dysfunction is under investigation.

6. Other treatments: ED can also be treated with nonprescription vacuum devices or with surgical implants.

Suggested Reading

American Psychiatric Association: *Diagnostic and Statistical Manual of Mental Disorders*, 4th ed, text revision. Washington, DC: American Psychiatric Association, 2000.

Hatzimouratidis K, Hatzichristou DG: A comparative review of the options for treatment of erectile dysfunction: Which treatment for which patient? *Drugs* 65(12):1621–1650, 2005.

Miller TA: Diagnostic evaluation of erectile dysfunction. *Am Fam Physician* 61(1):95–111, 2000.

Selvin E, Burnett AL, Platz EA: Prevalence and risk factors for erectile dysfunction in the US. *Am J Med* 120(2):151–157, 2007.

Tomb DA: *Psychiatry*, 6th ed. Baltimore: Williams & Wilkins, 1999.

CHAPTER

153 Psychotherapy in Family Medicine

CLINICAL CASE PROBLEM 1

A 29-Year-Old Working Mother with Two Young Children Who Is Unable to Cope

A 29-year-old mother who holds a full-time out-of-the-home job has just gone back to work after the birth of her second child. The child is currently 8 weeks old. She works as an accountant in a large company. Her company is restructuring, and she worries that her job is not secure. Her husband has been laid off from his job as an assembly line worker at an automobile assembly plant.

After her maternity leave, she fears that the management was unhappy with her for "taking so much time off to have a baby." She is staying up late every night to get the housework done. She wakes up often during the night in order to feed the baby. She is too tired to spend quality time with the older child and feels guilty about that. She is crying, fatigued, and absolutely exhausted after 10 days back on the job.

She finds herself becoming "very sleepy every day at work," and the management has commented on that. She tells you, "I just can't take it any longer. I have to work to pay the mortgage and put food on the table. There are no other jobs available. What am I going to do? I just can't go on this way."

She has no history of psychiatric problems or sleep disorders. She has no family history of psychiatric disorders or personal or family history of drug or alcohol use. She is not taking any drugs at present.

SELECT THE BEST ANSWER TO THE FOLLOWING QUESTIONS

1. What is the most likely diagnosis in this patient at this time?
   a. major depressive disorder (MDD)
   b. generalized anxiety disorder
   c. adjustment disorder
   d. dysthymic disorder
   e. panic disorder

2. Which of the following would be the next therapeutic step in the care of this patient?
   a. schedule regular follow-up in order to allow the patient to "vent" her concerns

  b. if the patient is not nursing, start fluoxetine for 1 week with the addition of zolpidem as needed for sleep
  c. refer this patient and her husband to social services such as vocational rehabilitation in order to facilitate a more ordered entry into the workforce
  d. none of the above
  e. all of the above

3. You decide to initiate psychotherapy. At this time, in this patient and given this diagnosis, what is the best psychotherapy to initiate in a primary care setting?
  a. cognitive psychotherapy
  b. brief psychodynamic psychotherapy
  c. behavioral psychotherapy (behavior modification)
  d. supportive psychotherapy
  e. intensive psychoanalytically oriented psychotherapy

4. What is the major goal of the psychotherapy in this patient's situation?
  a. to identify and alter cognitive distortions
  b. to understand the conflict area and the particular defense mechanisms used
  c. to maintain or reestablish the best level of functioning
  d. to eliminate involuntary disruptive behavior patterns and substitute appropriate behaviors
  e. to resolve symptoms and rework major personality structures related to childhood conflicts

5. What is the first priority at this time?
  a. foster a good working relationship with the patient
  b. approach the patient as a "blank screen"
  c. develop a "therapeutic alliance" with the patient
  d. begin the assignment of tasks for the patient to complete
  e. develop "free association" with the patient

6. What is the therapeutic method at this time?
  a. validate and explore the patient's concerns, provide direction for problem solving, and help her deal with the situation
  b. have the patient express her anger in the "here and now"
  c. prescribe a sedative to "get things under control"
  d. have the patient "intellectualize" her concerns
  e. have the patient discuss her dreams and free associations

7. Which of the following is (are) a technique(s) of supportive psychotherapy?
  a. support problem-solving techniques and behaviors
  b. develop a short-term "mentoring" relationship
  c. develop a short-term "guiding" relationship
  d. suggest, reinforce, advise, and reality test
  e. all of the above

8. Depression is the most frequent psychiatric condition seen in the primary care setting. Which of the following psychotherapies has been shown to be most efficacious in the treatment of psychiatric conditions encountered in primary health care settings?
  a. intensive analytically oriented psychotherapy
  b. psychoanalysis
  c. cognitive–behavioral therapy (CBT)
  d. brief psychodynamic psychotherapy
  e. Gestalt psychotherapy

CLINICAL CASE PROBLEM 2

A 39-Year-Old Female with a 4-Month History of Depression

A 39-year-old female comes to your office with a 4-month history of depression. She meets the *Diagnostic and Statistical Manual of Mental Disorders*, 4th edition, criteria for MDD. She was started on an antidepressant 6 weeks ago, and it appears to be helping significantly.

9. Which of the following statements is (are) true regarding the therapeutic approach to this disorder?
  a. the combination of cognitive therapy and antidepressants has been shown to effectively manage severe or chronic depression
  b. supportive psychotherapy is the ideal psychotherapy for this patient
  c. there is little evidence to support a combination of medication and psychotherapy in preference to psychotherapy alone
  d. brief psychodynamic psychotherapy has been shown to be the most effective psychotherapy when used in combination with a selective serotonin reuptake inhibitor (SSRI)
  e. all of the above statements are true

10. Which of the following statements regarding CBT is (are) true?
  a. cognitive therapy is a treatment process that enables patients to correct false self-beliefs that can lead to negative moods and behaviors

b. CBT has proved beneficial in treating patients who have only a partial response to adequate antidepressant therapy

c. formal CBT is generally conducted over a period of 15 to 25 weeks in weekly sessions

d. CBT is best suited to patients who have depressive disorders without psychotic features

e. all of the above statements are true

11. What is the major goal of CBT?

a. to help patients "pick themselves up by the bootstraps" and change their lives

b. to reestablish their previous best level of functioning

c. to understand the major conflict area and the particular defense mechanisms they are using

d. to identify and alter cognitive distortions

e. to clarify and resolve the focal area of conflict that interferes with current functioning

---

Clinical Case Management Problem

Describe the forms of psychotherapy that are useful in the family practice setting.

Answers

1. c. This patient has an adjustment disorder. Although this condition is detailed in Chapter 141, the basic characteristics of adjustment disorder are provided here again: (1) the development of a psychological reaction to identifiable stressors or events, (2) the reaction reflects a change in the individual's normal personality and is different from the person's usual style of functioning, (3) the psychological reaction is either "maladaptive" in that normal functioning (including social and occupational functioning) is impaired or greater than normally expected of others in similar circumstances, and (4) the psychological reaction does not represent an exacerbation of another psychiatric disorder.

2. d. Although it is important to address target symptoms such as sleep, the first-line treatment of adjustment disorder does not involve medication. Rather, a supportive and empathic approach is applied with a strong development of the therapeutic alliance in order to facilitate therapy. Allowing patients to "vent" may be helpful in the short term, but this approach lacks the structured guidance that is required to promote change in the patient's thinking, feeling, or behavior necessary to lead to clinical improvement. Furthermore, this patient would likely feel overwhelmed in any work environment, making a "job change" an unlikely therapeutic intervention.

3. d. The type of psychotherapy that best fits treatment of this patient's life situation in a primary care setting is supportive psychotherapy. Supportive psychotherapy is discussed in detail in answers 4 through 7.

4. c. The major goal of supportive psychotherapy is to reestablish the best possible level of functioning given the patient's current circumstances, personality, and previous coping style. In general, this distinguishes supportive psychotherapy from the change-oriented psychotherapies that aim to modify primary disease processes, adjust thinking style, change behavior, or restructure personality.

5. a. The first priority of supportive psychotherapy is to foster a good working relationship with the patient. This will make the patient feel competent and connected, which are the two basic social needs of any human being. When people feel overwhelmed, they lose the sense of being competent and connected.

6. a. Once a working relationship is established between patient and physician, the physician encourages the patient to explore his or her concerns and validates the patient's feelings. In this clinical case problem, enlisting the husband's practical support, exploring options for temporary part-time employment, and validating the patient's need to take care of herself are important. It is extremely useful to elicit her stories about overcoming previous difficult times.

The prescription of a sedative risks compounding her problem and is contraindicated.

7. e. Specific techniques used in supportive psychotherapy include the following: (1) regular sessions in which therapy for the patient is consistently available; (2) the support by the therapist of problem solving by the patient; (3) guiding or mentoring on the part of the therapist; (4) the concomitant use of medication (especially antidepressant medication) if indicated; and (5) depending on the physician's level of expertise, specific techniques such as suggestion, reinforcement, advice, teaching, reality testing, cognitive restructuring, reassurance, the encouragement of alternate behavior, and the discussion of social and interpersonal skills.

8. c. There is an increasing amount of literature that supports the efficacy of CBT in primary care settings. Studies examining the outcome of CBT have found it to be an effective treatment in ambulatory patients with mild to moderate degrees of depression. One advantage of CBT is that the therapeutic techniques can often be learned more easily and integrated into primary care treatment than can psychodynamic techniques. Cognitive techniques include the questioning of maladaptive assumptions about problems, provision of information, and assignments for dealing with specific situations. There is a trend to combine these techniques with behavioral techniques such as relaxation training and desensitization, which are also very useful in the family practice setting.

9. a. Family physicians are usually the first to diagnose and treat patients with depression. Studies have shown that the best treatment for MDD is a combination of antidepressant medications with CBT, not supportive psychotherapy. Physicians should inform patients that psychotherapy and pharmacotherapy are valid options, and that cognitive therapy, and therefore CBT, is the most studied psychotherapy. If the patient and physician initially elect to use pharmacotherapy and the patient does not respond adequately, the physician should again suggest adding psychotherapy or CBT. A combination of psychotherapy and pharmacotherapy is more effective than either method alone in patients with MDD without psychotic features. Some qualitative studies have suggested that full implementation of the CBT model by primary care physicians can be difficult in the context of visit and time constraints of a primary care practice, even with adequate training. If the family physician is unable to provide the psychotherapy because of either lack of training or lack of time, a referral to a psychotherapist is indicated.

10. e. The process of CBT helps patients to reinterpret their views about their lives. It helps them to edit their stories. Although formal CBT is generally conducted over a period of 15 to 25 weeks in weekly sessions, family physicians can make very effective interventions during brief visits. CBT can also be used in patients who refuse to take antidepressant medication, fail to respond to antidepressant medication, or are unable to tolerate antidepressant medications.

11. d. CBT is a method of brief psychotherapy developed during the past 25 years primarily for the treatment of mild to moderate depression and other psychiatric conditions encountered in the primary care setting.

People who are depressed tend to have negative interpretations of the world, themselves, and the future. Also, patients who are depressed interpret events as reflecting defeat, deprivation, or disparagement and view their lives as being filled with obstacles and burdens. They also view themselves as unworthy, deficient, undesirable, or worthless and see the future as bringing a continuation of the miseries of the past.

The major goal of cognitive psychotherapy is to identify and alter cognitive distortions and thoughts. CBT helps patients to identify and alter these cognitive distortions (negative stories). The techniques that are used include behavioral assignments, reading materials, and teaching that helps these patients recognize the difference between positively and negatively biased automatic thoughts. At first glance, it may seem completely straightforward, but it is sometimes difficult for the patient to tell the difference between the two. It also helps patients identify negative schemas, beliefs, and attitudes.

Solution to the Clinical Case Management Problem

Family physicians can incorporate effective psychotherapeutic interventions into a brief office visit. Supportive psychotherapy and CBT are the two most appropriate psychotherapeutic approaches for use in a family physician's practice.

CBT is useful in the treatment of nonpsychotic depressive disorders and in stress management. Supportive psychotherapy is useful in the treatment of adjustment disorders, family and marital conflicts, and any condition to which importance is attached by the patient.

Family physicians should be familiar with some of the differences in goals among popular forms of psychotherapy: (1) Psychoanalysis aims to resolve symptoms and perform major reworking of personality structures related to childhood conflicts; (2) psychoanalytically oriented psychotherapy aims to understand a conflict area and the particular defense mechanisms used to defend it; (3) brief psychodynamic psychotherapy is used to clarify and resolve focal areas of conflict that interfere with current functioning; (4) cognitive psychotherapy primarily identifies and alters cognitive distortions; (5) supportive psychotherapy aims to reestablish the optimal level of functioning possible for the patient; and (6) behavioral therapy (behavioral modification) aims to change disruptive behavior patterns through reinforcing positive responses and ignoring negative ones; relaxation approaches, rewards systems, and breathing techniques can be used for the patient's benefit.

Many of these psychotherapeutic modalities can be used in a group setting. This approach provides significant support to groups of patients dealing with serious general medical conditions, smoking cessation, and stress disorders.

Summary

1. Consider the use of supportive psychotherapy in any condition, recognizing the biopsychosocial model of illness.
2. Consider the increased efficacy of treating depressive disorders with a combination of SSRIs and cognitive psychotherapy.
3. Although formal CBT is generally conducted over a period of 15 to 25 weeks in weekly sessions, family physicians can make very effective interventions during brief visits.
4. Some studies indicate significant cost-effectiveness of psychotherapy in relationship to other interventions.
5. Therapeutic intervention in family medicine is a skill that can be acquired with some additional training.
6. A referral to a qualified mental health professional is indicated when long-standing and complex problems are uncovered.
7. Supportive psychotherapy and CBT are the two most appropriate psychotherapeutic approaches for use in a family physician's practice.

Suggested Reading

American Psychiatric Association: *Diagnostic and Statistical Manual of Mental Disorders*, 4th ed, text revision. Washington, DC: American Psychiatric Association, 2000.

Kaplan HI, Sadock BJ: Psychotherapies. In: Kaplan HI, Sadock BJ, eds, *Kaplan and Sadock's Synopsis of Psychiatry: Behavioral Sciences/Clinical Psychiatry*, 8th ed. Baltimore: Williams & Wilkins, 1998.

Rupke SJ, Blecke D, Renfrow M: Cognitive therapy for depression. *Am Fam Physician* 73(1):83–86, 2006.

Stuart MR, Lieberman JA: *The Fifteen-Minute Hour. Practical Therapeutic Interventions in Primary Care*, 3rd ed. Philadelphia: Saunders, 2002.

EMERGENCY MEDICINE

CHAPTER

154 Cardiac Arrest

CLINICAL CASE PROBLEM 1

A 55-Year-Old Male Found Collapsed in the Street

A 55-year-old male is found collapsed in the street by a passerby. The passerby begins cardiopulmonary resuscitation (CPR) and is soon joined by another citizen. Someone calls 911, and CPR is continued until the paramedics arrive and initiate advanced cardiac life support (ACLS). Despite complete ACLS maneuvers, the patient remains pulseless and breathless as the paramedics hand over care to the emergency room doctor on duty at the nearest hospital.

SELECT THE BEST ANSWER TO THE FOLLOWING QUESTIONS

1. Which of the following rhythms is not one of the most commonly associated with pulseless cardiac arrest?
   a. ventricular fibrillation (VF)
   b. asystole
   c. rapid ventricular tachycardia (VT)
   d. pulseless electrical activity
   e. Mobitz II second-degree heart block

2. Components of good basic life support care include all of the following except
   a. high-quality bystander CPR
   b. early defibrillation within minutes of collapse if pulseless VT or VF
   c. await ACLS trained personnel to begin CPR
   d. focus on CPR rather than getting medications and intravenous (IV) access in the field
   e. early contact of the emergency medical services (EMS) system

3. Which of the following statements about delivering medications during cardiac arrest is true?
   a. the only drugs that can be given through the endotracheal tube are epinephrine and lidocaine
   b. there is strong evidence for the effectiveness of all drugs used in ACLS
   c. central lines are critical in the success of ACLS
   d. if a drug is given through a peripheral IV, follow it with a 500-mL bolus of IV fluid
   e. intraosseous access is useful for fluid resuscitation but not drug delivery or blood sampling

4. Which of the following is incorrect with regard to the management of witnessed arrest with a defibrillator on-site?
   a. defibrillation should be done first, without starting CPR
   b. after the delivery of two rescue breaths, the pulse should be checked
   c. if no pulse is felt within 10 seconds, the defibrillator should be turned on and then adhesive pads or paddles should be placed and the rhythm checked
   d. The automatic defibrillator will analyze the rhythm and provide instructions about whether and how to administer shocks

5. A "quick look" with paddles is performed on the patient in Clinical Case Problem 1. You diagnose VF. What should be your first step?
   a. defibrillate with 200 J
   b. defibrillate with 360 J
   c. administer epinephrine 1 mg IV push
   d. administer vasopressin 40 units IV bolus
   e. intubate the trachea

6. What is the antiarrhythmic of choice in the management of VF?
   a. bretylium
   b. lidocaine
   c. procainamide
   d. magnesium
   e. amiodarone

7. The patient is successfully converted to sinus rhythm. Unfortunately, on the way to the coronary care unit he arrests again. The rhythm strip reveals asystole. CPR is restarted. Which of the following is the next logical step in treatment?
   a. administer epinephrine 1 mg IV push
   b. administer calcium chloride 10 mL of a 10% solution IV push
   c. administer sodium bicarbonate 1 mEq/kg IV push
   d. administer isoproterenol 2 to 20 μg
   e. administer lidocaine 75 mg IV push

8. With appropriate treatment, the patient again converts to sinus rhythm. He is stabilized in the coronary care unit. Unfortunately, 2 hours later he develops VT. His blood pressure is 100/60 mmHg, and he has a palpable pulse. Your next step should be to administer which of the following?
   a. lidocaine 1 to 1.5 mg/kg IV
   b. procainamide 20 to 30 mg/minute up to a maximum of 50 mg/minute
   c. bretylium 5 mg IV bolus
   d. verapamil 5 mg IV bolus
   e. none of the above

9. Sinus rhythm is restored again, and his condition returns to satisfactory. Unfortunately, he develops a second-degree atrioventricular (AV) block (Mobitz type II). His pulse is 40 beats/minute, and his blood pressure drops to 70/40 mmHg. Given this change, what would you do now?
   a. observe the patient only
   b. administer isoproterenol 2 to 10 mg/minute
   c. administer atropine 0.5 to 1 mg
   d. administer epinephrine 0.5 to 1 mg
   e. none of the above

10. What is the definitive therapy for the dysrhythmia described in the previous question?
    a. a constant infusion of isoproterenol 2 to 20 mg/minute
    b. a constant infusion of lidocaine 2 to 4 mg/minute
    c. a constant infusion of procainamide 2 to 4 mg/minute
    d. a transvenous pacemaker
    e. none of the above

CLINICAL CASE PROBLEM 2

A Witnessed Cardiac Arrest

CPR is in progress on a 70-kg male who collapsed in the street (witnessed arrest). Basic life support (BLS) was begun, as was ACLS when the paramedics arrived. He was brought immediately to the emergency room and a blood gas sample was drawn. The results were as follows: pH, 7.1; P_{CO_2}, 60 mmHg; P_{O_2}, 75 mmHg; and HCO_3^-, 15 mEq/L.

11. These results represent which of the following?
    a. metabolic acidosis with respiratory alkalosis
    b. respiratory acidosis with metabolic alkalosis
    c. pure metabolic acidosis
    d. pure respiratory acidosis
    e. mixed respiratory and metabolic acidosis

12. What is the most appropriate treatment of this patient?
    a. sodium bicarbonate 1 mEq/kg
    b. sodium bicarbonate 0.5 mEq/kg
    c. increased ventilation
    d. a and c
    e. b and c

13. Which of the following should be treated first in this patient?
    a. respiratory acidosis
    b. metabolic acidosis
    c. respiratory alkalosis
    d. metabolic alkalosis
    e. all of the above

14. A 53-year-old male presents to your emergency room with a 2-hour history of a "rapid heartbeat," nausea, and dizziness. A 12-lead electrocardiogram shows atrial flutter with variable AV conduction. As you are taking his history, he becomes disoriented. You are only able to obtain his systolic blood pressure (40 mmHg). At this time, what should you do?
    a. administer epinephrine 1 mg IV
    b. administer isoproterenol 2 to 20 mg/minute IV
    c. defibrillate with 300 J
    d. Cardiovert with 300 J
    e. Cardiovert with 100 J

15. What is the first step in initiation of resuscitation following a witnessed or unwitnessed cardiac arrest in the community?
    a. begin rescue breathing
    b. begin chest compressions
    c. initiate a call to 911
    d. check pulse
    e. go for help

16. Which of the following statements concerning BLS is false?
    a. the prompt administration of BLS is the key to success

b. mouth-to-mouth resuscitation is the recommended method of respiratory exchange in performing BLS

c. BLS is used most commonly in family situations—one family member resuscitating another

d. BLS succeeds no more frequently than in 15% of out-of-hospital attempts

e. infectious diseases such as acquired immune deficiency syndrome and serum hepatitis pose little, if any, risk to rescuers

17. What is the recommended BLS compression/ventilation rescue sequence in one- or two-person CPR?
   a. 15/2
   b. 15/1
   c. 20/4
   d. 10/1
   e. 10/3

Answers

1. **e.** According to the 2005 American Heart Association guidelines on the management of cardiac arrest, the four rhythms that produce pulseless cardiac arrest are VF, rapid VT, pulseless electrical activity (PEA), and asystole. Patients with one of these arrest rhythms must have both BLS and ACLS in order to survive. Mobitz II second-degree heart block can be associated with hypotension, chest pain, and other cardiac symptoms, but it is not usually found when the patient is in pulseless cardiac arrest.

2. **c.** Good BLS should precede ACLS when pulseless cardiac arrest has occurred. High-quality bystander CPR should begin promptly, and early defibrillation, with either an available automatic defibrillator or ambulance equipment if EMS arrives very early, should follow within minutes of collapse. Good CPR is more likely to lead to survival than are medications and IV access in the field. Awaiting ACLS-trained personnel and delaying CPR is associated with worse outcomes.

3. **b.** See answer 4.

4. **d.** The most common initial rhythm diagnosed in patients who suffer a cardiac arrest is VF. The usual course of events is as follows: coarse VF to fine VF to asystole. If CPR is started within 4 minutes after collapse, the likelihood of survival to hospital discharge doubles. Early defibrillation is essential. An out-of-hospital goal of defibrillation within 5 minutes

of a telephone call is recommended. An in-hospital goal of defibrillation within 3 minutes of collapse is recommended. Communities report survival rates for out-of-hospital cardiac arrest ranging from 4% to 34%. Once ventricular asystole develops, the probability of successful resuscitation is virtually zero. Thus, although VF is the most common initial rhythm, ventricular asystole is the most common arrhythmia leading directly to death.

5. **a.** The first step in the treatment of VF is defibrillation with an energy level of 200 J. If the first attempt is unsuccessful, two further defibrillations (200 to 300 and 360 J) should follow immediately. If defibrillation is not successful, the trachea is intubated, IV access is established, and epinephrine or vasopressin is administered. Defibrillation may also be performed via biphasic nonescalating shocks at 150 to 200 J.

6. **e.** Amiodarone is a class IIb intervention (supported by "fair to good" scientific evidence) for VF/pulseless VT after defibrillation and after epinephrine or vasopressin have failed to restore a perfusing rhythm. Amiodarone is administered in a dosage of 300 mg IV push and repeated doses of 150 mg may be given if required. Bretylium is not recommended as an antidysrhythmic agent in CPR because of a lack of demonstrated efficacy and its high side effect profile. Lidocaine is classified as an indeterminate intervention because of little evidence supporting its use. Procainamide is given for recurrent or intermittent VF or pulseless VT. Patients who convert from VF to a perfusing rhythm and then revert back to VF may benefit. Procainamide is administered in a dose of 20 to 30 mg/minute until one of the following is observed: (1) The arrhythmia is suppressed, (2) hypotension ensues, (3) the QRS complex is widened by 50% of its original width, or (4) a total of 17 mg/kg of drug has been administered. Magnesium is given for VF or VT only if an underlying rhythm is caused by hypomagnesemia.

7. **a.** The next step in the management of the original patient is the administration of epinephrine 10.0 mg IV push. This should be repeated every 3 to 5 minutes. If intubation has not been performed, it should be done. Atropine in a dose of 1 mg IV push should be given as well and repeated every 3 to 5 minutes to a total of 3 mg. Transcutaneous cardiac pacing, if available, should be performed early. Termination of resuscitation efforts should be considered if asystole lasts more than 10 minutes and no treatable condition exists. The rate of survival in patients with asystole is close to zero.

8. a. The treatment of choice for patients with VT who are hemodynamically stable is lidocaine 1 to 1.5 mg/kg. This can be repeated until a total of 3 mg/kg has been given. The second-line drug in this case is procainamide in a dose of 20 to 30 mg/minute until the VT resolves or a total of 17 mg/kg has been given. Bretylium is no longer recommended for use in CPR. Verapamil, a calcium channel blocker, may be used in the treatment of stable narrow complex tachycardia.

9. c. See answer 8.

10. d. Second-degree heart block (Mobitz type II) occurs below the level of the AV node either at the bundle of His (uncommon) or bundle branch level (more common). It is usually associated with an organic lesion in the conduction pathway. Its usual progression is to a third-degree (complete) heart block. Initial treatment is aimed at increasing the heart rate in an attempt to increase cardiac output. Thus, atropine in a dose of 0.5 to 1 mg is the drug of choice. The maximum dose of atropine is 0.04 mg/kg. Transcutaneous pacing should be used early if available. Dopamine and epinephrine can be given if signs or symptoms persist. The definitive treatment in this patient is a transvenous pacemaker.

11. e. See answer 13.

12. c. See answer 13.

13. a. Most patients who have arrested and who are undergoing CPR have a mixed respiratory and metabolic acidosis. The normal P_{CO_2} is 40 mmHg. The patient in this case has a markedly elevated P_{CO_2} of 60 mmHg and thus is being hypoventilated. The patient's bicarbonate level of 15 mEq/L is below the normal range of 21 to 28 mEq/L; thus, he has a metabolic acidosis as well. Recommendations are that bicarbonate should be used with caution. Although cardiac function is depressed by acidosis, the determining factor is intracellular pH, not extracellular pH, as is measured by arterial pH. Hypoxia, not acidosis, accounts for most of the cardiac depression. Respiratory acidosis, however, produces immediate and profound depression. Thus, increasing ventilation should be used as the primary means of correcting acidosis, and respiratory acidosis should be treated first.

By contrast, the use of bicarbonate has long been known to present risks that are not limited to alkalosis but include hypernatremia and hyperosmolarity. The accumulation of metabolic by-products, not bicarbonate deficits, produces the acidosis. Giving bicarbonate to buffer the arterial pH will not benefit the patient.

14. e. The treatment of choice for acute unstable atrial flutter is synchronized cardioversion. The initial energy chosen should be 100 J. If unsuccessful, this should be followed by cardioversion at 200, 300, and 360 J. If the patient is stable, vagal maneuvers can be attempted, followed by medications (calcium channel blockers and beta blockers).

15. c. When witnessing a collapse or seeing an unresponsive victim, the first step in cardiac resuscitation is to access the EMS system by dialing 911 or the emergency number in your area. In children younger than age 8 years, however, before calling EMS, 1 minute of CPR should follow the initial assessment.

16. b. Previously, the recommended method of BLS ventilation was mouth-to-mouth. Current American Heart Association guidelines call for use of mouth-to-mask ventilation if a mask is available. The risk of contracting an infectious disease through mouth-to-mouth resuscitation is remote.

17. a. For one or two rescuers providing CPR, the recommended compression/ventilation ratio is 15/2. The compression rate should be approximately 100/minute.

Summary

IN THE SITUATION OF PULSELESS ARREST

1. Follow the BLS algorithm: Call for help and give CPR. Give oxygen when available. If a monitor/defibrillator is available, attach the leads and/or pads.
2. Check the rhythm. If it is a shockable rhythm (VF or VT), follow these steps (if it is not a shockable rhythm, go to step 5):
   a. Give one shock (manual biphasic—this is device specific, typically 120 to 200 J; if unknown, use 200 J;
   or automated electronic defibrillator, device-specific energy level; or monophasic device, use 360 J).
   b. Resume CPR immediately for five cycles.
3. Check the rhythm. If it is a shockable rhythm, follow these steps (if it is not a shockable rhythm, go to step 5):
   a. Continue CPR while defibrillator is charging.
   b. Give one shock as above.
   c. Resume CPR immediately after shock.

d. When IV/intraosseous (IO) access is available, give either epinephrine 1 mg IV/IO every 3 to 5 minutes or vasopressin 40 U IV/IO to replace the first or second dose of epinephrine.

e. Give five more cycles of CPR.

4. Check the rhythm. If it is a shockable rhythm, follow these steps (if it is not a shockable rhythm, go to step 5):

a. Continue CPR while defibrillator is charging.

b. Give one shock as above.

c. Resume CPR immediately after shock.

d. Consider antiarrhythmics; give during CPR, before or after the shock.

   i. Amiodarone (300 mg IV/IO once, then consider additional 150 mg IV/IO once) or

   ii. Lidocaine (1 to 15 mg/kg first dose, then 0.5 to 0.75 mg/kg IV/IO; maximum three doses or 3 mg/kg)

e. Consider magnesium, loading dose 1 or 2 g IV/IO for torsades de pointes.

f. After five cycles of CPR, go back to step 3.

5. If it is not a shockable rhythm (if it is asystole or PEA):

a. Resume CPR immediately for five cycles.

b. When IV/IO access is available, give vasopressor.

   i. Epinephrine 1 mg IV/IO every 3 to 5 minutes or

   ii. May give one dose of vasopressin 40 U IV/IO to replace first or second dose of epinephrine

c. Consider atropine 1 mg IV/IO for asystole or slow PEA rate

d. Repeat every 3 to 5 minutes up to three doses.

e. Give five cycles of CPR.

6. Check rhythm. If it is a shockable rhythm, go to steps 1 through 4; if it is not shockable:

a. If asystole, repeat step 5.

b. If there is electrical activity, check pulse; if there is no pulse, go back to step 5.

c. If pulse is present, begin postresuscitation care.

DURING CPR

1. Compress hard and fast (100/minute).
2. Ensure full chest recoil.
3. Minimize interruptions in chest compressions.
4. One cycle of CPR: 30 compressions and then 2 breaths; 5 cycles = 2 minutes.
5. Do not hyperventilate.
6. Secure airway and confirm placement.
7. After an advanced airway is in place and secured, do not give "cycles" of CPR; instead, give chest compressions continuously, without pausing for ventilation. Ventilate at a rate of 8 to 10/minute. Check rhythm every 2 minutes.
8. Search for and treat possible contributing factors:

a. Seven H's: hypovolemia, hypoxia, hydrogen ion (acidosis), hypokalemia, hyperkalemia, hypoglycemia, and hypothermia

b. Six T's: toxins (salicylate overdose, narcotics, tricyclic antidepressants, and others), cardiac tamponade, tension pneumothorax, coronary thrombosis (myocardial infarction), pulmonary thrombosis (embolism), and trauma.

Suggested Reading

American Heart Association: Part 7.2 Management of cardiac arrest. *Circulation* 112:58–66. 2005.

Bunch TJ, West CP, Packer DL, et al: Admission predictors of in-hospital mortality and subsequent long-term outcome in survivors of ventricular fibrillation out-of-hospital cardiac arrest: A population-based study. *Cardiology* 102:41–47, 2004.

Moretti MA, Cesar LA, Nusbacher A, et al: Advanced cardiac life support training improves long-term survival from in-hospital cardiac arrest. *Resuscitation* 72:458–465, 2007.

O'Neill JE, Deakin CD: Do we hyperventilate cardiac arrest patients? *Resuscitation* 73:82–85, 2007.

Sunde K, Kramer-Johanse J, Pytte M, Steen PA: Predicting survival with good neurologic recovery at hospital admission after successful resuscitation of out-of-hospital cardiac arrest: The OHCA score. *Eur Heart J* 21:2840–2845, 2007.

155 Advanced Trauma Life Support

CLINICAL CASE PROBLEM 1

A 27-Year-Old Male Injured in a Motor Vehicle Accident

Paramedics wheel a 27-year-old male, in a C-collar and strapped to a stretcher, into the emergency room of a small, rural hospital. The nearest trauma center is 180 miles away. He was extracted from the driver's seat of a midsized sedan after a head-on collision with a similar-sized car. Airbags deployed; the patient was not wearing a seat belt.

The cervical spine appears to be adequately immobilized, and the patient is in acute respiratory distress, with a respiratory rate of 32 breaths/minute. Breath sounds are absent in the right lung field. There is blood and pink-tinged fluid leaking from his nose, and a large scalp laceration is present.

SELECT THE BEST ANSWER TO THE FOLLOWING QUESTIONS

1. At this time, what should be your first priority?
   a. carry on with the rest of the complete assessment
   b. establish an intravenous (IV) infusion
   c. send the patient to x-ray for a stat chest x-ray
   d. send the patient to x-ray for a lateral x-ray of the cervical spine
   e. none of the above

2. What is the most likely cause of this patient's respiratory distress?
   a. flail chest
   b. tension pneumothorax
   c. acute pulmonary embolus
   d. pericardial tamponade
   e. none of the above

3. After establishing an airway and dealing with the patient's respiratory status, what should you do?
   a. complete the neurologic examination
   b. perform a Glasgow Coma Scale
   c. establish a central venous pressure (CVP) line or two large peripheral IVs
   d. perform a diagnostic paracentesis
   e. perform a stat electrocardiogram (ECG)

4. What is the most likely cause of this patient's dilated right pupil?
   a. a middle meningeal artery tear
   b. a chronic subdural hematoma
   c. an acute subdural hematoma
   d. a or c
   e. none of the above

5. The patient's neurologic status changes are as follows: (1) eyes: closed, no response to verbal commands but eyes open in response to pain; (2) best verbal response: none; and (3) best motor response: flexion withdrawal to pressure on the brachial plexus. What is the patient's Glasgow Coma Scale?
   a. 12
   b. 8
   c. 7
   d. 4
   e. 2

6. The indications for an immediate computed tomography (CT) scan include which of the following?
   a. a Glasgow Coma Scale of less than 13/15 at any time since the injury
   b. a posttraumatic seizure
   c. sign of basal skull fracture
   d. more than one episode of vomiting post injury
   e. all of the above

7. A diagnostic peritoneal lavage is performed and draws bloody fluid. On examination, pain is maximal in the left upper quadrant. What is the most likely cause of this patient's abdominal pain?
   a. liver laceration
   b. duodenal rupture
   c. renal hematoma
   d. splenic rupture
   e. pancreatic tear

8. Following blunt abdominal trauma, physical examination is
   a. less important than including the abdomen in the CT scan
   b. able to predict with better than 90% effectiveness surgically significant intraabdominal injury
   c. minimally predictive unless paired with significant hematologic and blood chemistry results
   d. only important for the hemodynamically unstable patient
   e. none of the above

CLINICAL CASE PROBLEM 2

A 51-Year-Old Male Involved in a Car–Motorcycle Collision

A 51-year-old male is brought to the emergency room after having been involved in a car–motorcycle collision.

On examination, he is drowsy but conscious. His respiratory rate is 40 breaths/minute. His blood pressure is 70/50 mmHg. His heart sounds are muffled. He has significant elevation of the jugular venous pressure (JVP) and a large contusion over the sternal area. There is a laceration seen over the precordial region. No other significant abnormalities are noted on primary survey.

9. What is the most likely diagnosis in this patient?
   a. myocardial contusion
   b. pericardial tamponade
   c. aortic rupture
   d. pulmonary contusion
   e. pneumothorax

10. What is the treatment of choice for the patient's diagnosis from question 9?
    a. pericardiocentesis
    b. increased rate of crystalloid infusion
    c. crystalloid infusion plus blood
    d. urgent thoracotomy
    e. chest tube insertion

11. What is the minimal gauge of a peripheral IV catheter that should be inserted in a patient in shock?
    a. #25 gauge
    b. #22 gauge
    c. #18 gauge
    d. #16 gauge
    e. #12 gauge

Clinical Case Management Problem

What is a reasonable probable problem list for the patient in Clinical Case Problem 1?

Answers

1. **e.** Your first priority is to attend to the ABCs (airway, breathing, and circulation) of resuscitation. Thus, the establishment of an airway is first. Following that, breathing should be assessed (this includes assessment of breath sounds in both lung fields and respiratory rate). Finally, the patient's circulatory status must be attended to with the establishment of either a CVP line or two large-bore IV lines.

2. **b.** The most likely cause of this patient's respiratory distress is a tension pneumothorax. Tension pneumothorax occurs from air in the pleural space under pressure. It is a common life-threatening injury that needs to be assessed and treated immediately. Clues to the high probability of a tension pneumothorax include complete absence of breath sounds in a lung field and hypotension in the presence of distended neck veins. The most common error in this situation would be to transport the patient to x-ray without a physician. In fact, with the history and physical findings it would be entirely appropriate to treat the patient on the basis of your presumed diagnosis without an x-ray. A needle can be inserted into the chest wall cavity to decompress the potentially life-threatening tension pneumothorax. A "rush of air" will confirm the diagnosis. Subsequent management requires a chest tube thoracostomy.

3. **c.** As mentioned previously, the priority following A and B is C, which is circulation. A CVP line or two large-bore (#16 gauge IV catheters) should be inserted to maximize the ability to replace intravascular volume.

4. **d.** The dilated right pupil is most likely caused by an initial skull fracture producing tearing of either veins (subdural hematoma) or the middle meningeal artery (epidural hematoma). If CT scanning is unavailable and the patient is comatose with decerebrate or decorticate posturing that is unresponsive to mannitol or hyperventilation, a burr hole should be placed. The burr hole is placed in the temporal region on the ipsilateral side of the dilated pupil.

5. **c.** This patient's Glasgow Coma Scale is 7. The Glasgow Coma Scale rating is as follows:

1. Eyes opening: spontaneously, 4; in response to verbal command, 3; in response to pain, 2; no response (stay closed), 1
2. Best verbal response: oriented and converses, 5; disorientated and converses, 4; inappropriate words, 3; incomprehensible sounds, 2; no response, 1
3. Best motor response: obeys verbal command, 6; localizes pain in response to painful stimulus, 5; flexion withdrawal, 4; abnormal flexion, 3; (decorticate rigidity) extension, 2; (decerebrate rigidity) no response, 1.

Total 2 + 1 + 4 = 7

6. **e.** All of the these are indicators of potential head injury and should lead to immediately requesting a CT of the head, which is the assessment of choice to evaluate closed head injury.

7. **d.** A diagnostic peritoneal lavage that draws bloody fluid suggests an intraabdominal bleed most likely resulting from organ laceration or organ rupture. Pain maximal in the left upper quadrant suggests that this is most likely the result of splenic rupture. Splenic rupture is one of the most common abdominal injuries seen in multiple trauma victims. In many trauma centers, ultrasound has replaced diagnostic peritoneal lavage for the emergency evaluation of trauma patients. The technique known as the FAST (focused assessment with sonography for trauma) examination is rapid and accurate for detection of intraabdominal fluid or blood. In addition to the peritoneal cavity, the FAST examination can also scan the pericardium and pleural space.

8. **b.** Physical examination has been found to be predictive of surgically significant injury in blunt abdominal trauma. Although CT occasionally identifies additional injuries, they are often not surgically significant. Most hematologic and blood chemistries serve only as adjuvants in the management of patients with abdominal injuries.

9. **b.** See answer 7.

10. **d.** This patient has a pericardial tamponade. Pericardial tamponade is an injury that is often missed. It is also a frequent injury in motor vehicle accidents in which multiple injuries are sustained. It is particularly common in car–motorcycle accidents, in which the motorcyclist is often thrown a significant distance. In stable patients, diagnosis can be confirmed by echocardiography. Pericardiocentesis (the removal of fluid from around the heart) is the treatment. Unstable patients require urgent thoracotomy.

11. **d.** The minimum gauge of an IV catheter that should be inserted in a patient in shock is #16 gauge. It is recommended that two #16 gauge catheters be inserted, one in each arm.

Solution to the Clinical Case Management Problem

A probable problem list for the patient in Clinical Case Problem 1 is as follows: (1) motor vehicle accident—patient in critical condition; (2) cervical spine injury until proved otherwise; (3) hypovolemic shock; (4) tension pneumothorax; (5) pericardial tamponade; (6) skull fracture, with acute epidural or subdural hematoma; (7) cerebrospinal fluid leak secondary to item 6; (8) probable splenic rupture or tear; (9) probable pelvic fracture; (10) probable femoral fracture; (11) probable urethral tear secondary to item 9; and (12) scalp laceration.

Summary

The major interventions that should be undertaken when a patient presents with traumatic shock are as follows:

1. ABCs: airway, breathing, circulation
   Airway: Airway management with protection of the cervical spine. Techniques to maintain an airway include chin lift, jaw thrust, artificial airway placement, and suctioning. Supplemental oxygen should be provided to patients with multiple trauma. Intubation is often necessary.
   Breathing: Ensure breath sounds are heard on both sides of the chest. Evaluate for degree of chest expansion, tachypnea, crepitus from rib fractures, subcutaneous emphysema, and the presence of penetrating or open wounds. Acute life-threatening pulmonary conditions are tension pneumothorax, open pneumothorax, flail chest, and, in some cases, massive hemothorax.
   Circulation: Establish CVP line or two large-bore IV lines. Continuous monitoring of vital signs is necessary. Fluid resuscitation should begin with Ringer's lactate or normal saline. Type and cross-match for blood transfusion early.
   Deficits of neurologic function: Perform a neurologic examination. Assess the level of consciousness, pupil size and reactivity, and motor and sensory function.
   Exposure: Completely undress all trauma patients for examination of all surfaces for injury.

2. Monitor input and output: urinary catheter and naso-gastric tube.
3. Perform primary survey of all systems, and pay particular attention to the following:
   a. Neurologic status: the Glasgow Coma Scale. Is there any sign of increased intracranial pressure? Consider IV mannitol and hyperventilation, and also maintain Po_2 greater than 80 mmHg and control blood pressure. Burr holes should be used in dire circumstances when indicated.
   b. Cardiovascular system: Low blood pressure, elevated JVP, and muffled heart sounds suggest pericardial tamponade; consider other myocardial injuries, such as contusion.
   c. Respiratory system: Is there any evidence of pneumothorax? Is a flail chest present? Are there any other injuries?
   d. Abdomen: Is there any abdominal tenderness or bruising? Is there any tenderness in the right upper quadrant (possible liver laceration) or left upper quadrant (splenic laceration or rupture)? Is there any other injury? Is CT or ultrasound available in the emergency room?
   e. Reassess ABCs at regular intervals.
   f. Musculoskeletal: Are there any obvious fractures, especially open? Is there any evidence of pelvic fracture? Is there blood at the urethral meatus?
   g. Maxillary–facial trauma: Do not let injuries that look worse than they are detract your attention from more serious injuries.
   h. Perform secondary survey.
   i. Contact tertiary care facility and arrange transfer if this has not already been done.
   j. Order investigations: complete blood count, electrolytes, chest x-ray, C-spine x-ray, skull x-ray, ECG, amylase, urinalysis, x-rays of abdomen, abdominal ultrasound, and any other appropriate investigations deemed necessary for the individual patient (x-rays of long bones, etc.). If CT or magnetic resonance imaging facilities are available, other investigations may be ordered.
   k. Treat non-life-threatening injuries when the patient has been stabilized.

The major mistakes (in order of frequency) in treating patients with trauma are as follows:

1. Inadequate airway management
2. Inadequate shock management: includes delay in surgical or angiographic control of intraabdominal and pelvic bleeding (often due to performance of nonurgent tests or procedures) and delay in treating intrathoracic hemorrhage
3. Inadequate C-spine immobilization
4. Failure to recognize and decompress pneumothorax
5. Distracting visually impressive but not life-threatening injuries (maxillofacial trauma and open fractures)
6. Delay in transfer to tertiary care facility
7. Failure to transfer patient to tertiary care facility at all

A 2% or 3% error-related death rate continues to be considered the absolute baseline in complex trauma systems. Initial assessment, resuscitation, and initial intervention phases are the most error-prone phases of trauma care. Poor management decisions, such as failure to transfer appropriately and failure to accompany an unstable patient to imaging studies, as well as lengthy surgeries rather than "damage-control" procedures in unstable patients also contribute to error-related deaths.

Suggested Reading

American College of Surgeons: *Advanced Trauma Life Support Student Manual*, 7th ed. Chicago: American College of Surgeons, 2006.

Driscoll P, Wardrope J: ATLS: Past, present, and future. *Emerg Med J* 22:2–3, 2005.

Gruen RL, Jurkovich GJ, McIntyre LK, et al: Patterns of errors contributing to trauma mortality: Lessons learned from 2594 deaths. *Ann Surg* 244(3):371–380, 2006.

Isenhour JL, Marx J: Advances in abdominal trauma. *Emerg Med Clin North Am* 25(3):713–733, 2007.

O'Higgins N, Gillen P, Walsh TN, et al: *Initial Management of the Severely Injured Patient. Clinical Guidelines*. Dublin: Royal College of Surgeons in Ireland, 2003.

Parks JK, Elliott AC, Gentilello LM, Shafi S: Systemic hypotension is a late marker of shock after trauma: A validation study of Advanced Trauma Life Support principles in a large national sample. *Am J Surg* 192(6):727–731, 2006.

CHAPTER

156 **Diabetic Ketoacidosis**

CLINICAL CASE PROBLEM 1

A 60-Year-Old Diabetic Female with
Vomiting and Abdominal Pain

A 60-year-old female with a history of diabetes presents to the emergency room with progressive nausea, vomiting, and weakness. During the past 3 days, she has also had some burning on urination and mild abdominal pain. On examination, the patient appears somewhat confused and dehydrated. The mucous membranes are dry, and the skin is doughy. Her temperature is 100°F, respiratory rate 30 breaths/minute, pulse 100 beats/minute, and blood pressure 100/70 mmHg. The lungs are clear. The heart sounds normal. Abdominal exam reveals some generalized tenderness, no rebound, and no CVA tenderness. Rectal exam is normal, with negative guaiac test.

SELECT THE BEST ANSWER TO THE FOLLOWING QUESTIONS

1. The lab tests that you should perform at this time include all of the following except
    a. complete blood count (CBC)
    b. urinalysis
    c. serum electrolytes
    d. cardiac enzymes
    e. B-type natriuretic peptide

    The laboratory investigations ordered give the following results: potassium, 5.9 mEq/L; chloride, 76 mEq/L; sodium, 130 mEq/L; bicarbonate, 10 mEq/L; creatinine, 1.5; blood pH, 7.1; glucose, 450 mg/dL; and white blood cell (WBC) count, 17,500 with 10% bands. Urinalysis: pH is 4.5; >50 WBCs, positive leukocyte esterase, positive nitrites, positive ketones, and positive glucose. Cardiac enzymes are normal. B-type natriuretic peptide is pending.

2. What is the most likely diagnosis at this time?
    a. diabetic ketoacidosis secondary to infection
    b. uremia secondary to infection
    c. meningitis
    d. hyperosmolar hyperglycemic state secondary to infection
    e. lactic acidosis secondary to ischemic bowel

3. At this time, what should you do with the patient?
    a. rehydrate patient with oral fluids, give antibiotics, and discharge home
    b. rehydrate patient with IV fluids, give one dose of IV antibiotics and a loading dose of insulin, and discharge home
    c. admit the patient for active treatment and observation
    d. rehydrate patient with IV fluids and arrange for home health to administer IV antibiotics
    e. discuss options with husband and decide on disposition based on home situation

4. In this patient's situation, which fluid replacement would you begin with?
    a. dextrose 5% normal saline
    b. one-half normal saline
    c. Ringer's lactate
    d. normal saline
    e. hypertonic saline

5. In the condition described, which one of the following situations regarding the serum/body potassium is usually true?
    a. serum potassium is low; total body potassium is low
    b. serum potassium is elevated; total body potassium is low
    c. serum potassium is low; total body potassium is high
    d. serum potassium is elevated; total body potassium is high
    e. serum and total body potassium are usually unaltered

6. The preferred method of insulin administration in this condition is:
    a. regular insulin 0.15 U/kg intramuscular (IM) loading dose followed by 0.1 U/kg/hour IV infusion
    b. regular insulin 0.15 U/kg IV loading dose followed by 0.1 U/kg/hour IV infusion
    c. lispro 0.15 U/kg IV loading dose followed by hourly administration of 0.1 U/kg IV
    d. lispro 0.15 U/kg subcutaneous (SQ) loading dose followed by hourly administration of 0.1 U/kg SQ
    e. lispro 0.15 U/kg IM loading dose followed by hourly administration of 0.1 U/kg IM

7. At what pH must bicarbonate therapy be initiated?
    a. 6.9
    b. 7.0
    c. 7.1

d. 7.2

e. there is no pH at which bicarbonate therapy must be initiated

The patient responds to treatment and her nausea begins to lessen. She is hungry, alert, and asking about going home.

8. In this condition, when would you add glucose to the IV solution?
   a. when anion gap normalizes
   b. when serum glucose decreases to 250 mg/dL
   c. after the first liter of normal saline has been administered
   d. when it appears that the patient is no longer clinically dehydrated
   e. when the serum glucose normalizes

9. In this condition, when should one consider discontinuing the IV insulin infusion and switching to subcutaneous insulin administration?
   a. when the patient is able to eat
   b. when glucose normalizes
   c. when serum glucose decreases to 250 mg/dL
   d. when anion gap normalizes
   e. when fluid deficit has been corrected

10. On average, what is the expected total fluid deficit in patients with this condition?
    a. 1 or 2 L
    b. 3 or 4 L
    c. 5 to 8 L
    d. 10 to 12 L
    e. 15 L

Answers

1. **e.** This patient presented to the emergency room with nausea, vomiting, abdominal pain, dysuria, and fever. This should prompt the physician to order a CBC with differential, electrolytes, serum glucose, lipase, amylase, blood urea nitrogen, creatinine, and urinalysis. Blood and urine cultures should be ordered to determine the source of infection. Elderly patients with diabetes can also have atypical presentations of myocardial ischemia; therefore, cardiac enzymes and electrocardiogram should also be ordered. The B-type natriuretic peptide is a test used to diagnose heart failure and would not be helpful in this patient, who has no symptoms of heart failure.

2. **a.** The most likely diagnosis in this patient is diabetic ketoacidosis (DKA) secondary to a urinary tract infection. Patients with DKA often present with symp-

toms of nausea, weakness, and abdominal pain. They may also complain of polyuria and polydypsia. The classic physical exam also includes tachycardia, hypotension, altered sensorium, and Kussmaul's respirations. Common lab abnormalities include elevated glucose, but often not as elevated as that in a patient with hyperosmolar hyperglycemia. In the latter case, blood glucose is usually greater than 600 mg/dL. Acidosis is also more profound in DKA. Lactic acidosis and uremia can produce an anion gap acidosis, although this patient's creatinine is only 1.5 and she does not have evidence of ischemic bowel (guaiac negative and mild abdominal pain). Although meningitis can precipitate DKA, this patient did not complain of headache or neck stiffness.

3. **c.** This patient needs to be admitted for active treatment and very close observation. This can be done on the medical floor or intensive care unit, depending on the institution and the available nursing staff on the medical floors. The patient's age and severity of acidosis, dehydration, and electrolyte imbalances are important factors to consider when trying to decide the best treatment option. Patients may be considered for same-day treatment and discharge home if they have mild DKA, are alert, are able to drink fluids, and can be relied on to follow instructions and return if the condition worsens.

4. **d.** Normal saline is the best solution to begin with to replace intravascular volume. This can be started with a 1 to 1.5 L bolus in most adult patients. In children, 10 to 20 mL/kg/hour in the first 2 hours should be used. The subsequent rate is calculated from the estimated deficit and replaced during the next 24 hours in adults and 48 hours in children. Remember that adding potassium to a normal saline solution creates a hypertonic solution, so you should consider switching to half-normal saline if adding large amounts of potassium. This is especially important in children.

5. **b.** The serum potassium in a patient with DKA is often significantly elevated. However, this is deceptive. Although the serum potassium is usually elevated, total body potassium is usually low and the patient needs potassium added to the IV fluids. This is true for two basic reasons. First, there exists a general total body potassium deficit because of urinary losses; however, since the vast majority of the body's potassium is intracellular, this loss is not reflected in the extracellular compartment. Second, acidosis causes a spurious elevation in the serum potassium because much of the excess extracellular hydrogen ion is exchanged by the cells for potassium; that is, hydrogen ions flow into cells and potassium flows out.

6. b. The preferred method of insulin administration is regular insulin 0.15 U/kg IV loading dose followed by 0.1 U/kg/hour IV infusion. If an IV infusion pump is not available, it may be acceptable to administer the loading dose of regular insulin intramuscularly. Lispro is more expensive and, if given intravenously, does not work any faster than regular insulin given intravenously. Lispro administered subcutaneously every hour may be a safe alternative to intravenous regular insulin infusion in adults with DKA, but the dose should be 0.3 U/kg loading dose followed by 0.1 U/kg/hour SQ.

7. e. There is no pH at which bicarbonate therapy must be initiated. Hydration and correction of hyperglycemia usually correct acidosis. There are potential complications to bicarbonate therapy, including worsening hypokalemia and production of paradoxical central nervous system acidosis. Bicarbonate therapy may be considered in patients with a pH lower than 6.9 since there are no studies guiding therapy in this patient group.

8. b. When serum glucose decreases to approximately 250 mg/dL, solution should be changed to either D5 normal saline or D5 half-normal saline, and the rate of insulin should be decreased slightly.

9. d. IV insulin therapy should not be stopped until the anion gap normalizes. IV insulin should be continued for approximately 1 hour after the administration of subcutaneous regular insulin to ensure that there is no insulin-free period.

10. c. The average fluid deficit in adult patients with DKA is 5 to 8 L.

Summary

See Figure 156-1 for diagnosis and treatment algorithm.

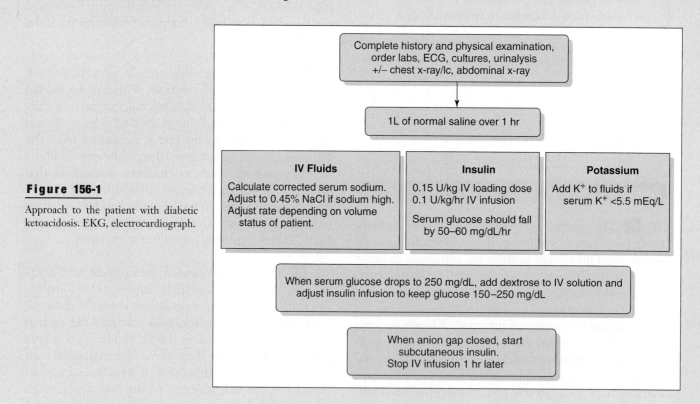

Figure 156-1

Approach to the patient with diabetic ketoacidosis. EKG, electrocardiograph.

Suggested Reading

Charfen M, Fernandez-Frackelton M: Diabetic ketoacidosis. *Emerg Med Clin North Am* 23(3):609–628, 2005.

Trachtenbarg D: Diabetic ketoacidosis. *Am Fam Physician* 71(9): 1705–1714, 1721–1722, 2005.

157 Acute and Chronic Poisoning

CLINICAL CASE PROBLEM 1

An Antidepressant Overdose

A 20-year-old female ingested 30 amitripyline 150-mg tablets 2 hours ago.

SELECT THE BEST ANSWER TO THE FOLLOWING QUESTIONS

1. She exhibits all of the follow symptoms except
   a. mydriasis
   b. dry mucous membranes
   c. bradycardia
   d. hyperthermia
   e. seizures

2. Which of the following is the most important treatment for tricyclic antidepressant overdose?
   a. calcium gluconate
   b. alkalinization of the urine
   c. cardioversion
   d. quinidine
   e. procainamide

3. A 3-year-old male swallows a bottle of acetaminophen elixir "cause it tastes good." For optimal treatment, how soon does he need treatment with *N*-acetylcysteine?
   a. 2 hours
   b. 4 hours
   c. 8 hours
   d. 24 hours
   e. 48 hours

4. Which of the following is the most common cause of poison mortality in the United States?
   a. carbon monoxide
   b. acetaminophen
   c. narcotics
   d. amphetamines
   e. salicylates

5. Which of the following is a symptom of carbon monoxide overdose?
   a. bradycardia
   b. agitation
   c. skin vesicles
   d. angioedema
   e. blurred vision

6. Peak age range for completed suicide by poisoning is:
   a. 15 to 19 years
   b. 20 to 24 years
   c. 25 to 34 years
   d. 35 to 44 years
   e. 45 to 49 years

7. Approximately what percentage of poisonings in the United States are intentional?
   a. 10%
   b. 20%
   c. 30%
   d. 40%
   e. 50%

8. Which of the following is the peak exposure age for any poisoning?
   a. 1 or 2 years
   b. 3 to 5 years
   c. 6 to 10 years
   d. 11 to 19 years
   e. 20 to 25 years

9. The American Academy of Pediatrics recommends prevention of poisonings by incorporating all of the following guidelines except
   a. dispose of unused medicines
   b. keep medicines in the original containers
   c. use child-resistant closures
   d. keep poisons out of sight and reach
   e. tell the child that the medicine is candy to improve cooperation

CLINICAL CASE PROBLEM 2

Unexplained Unconsciousness

A 57-year-old male is found unresponsive by his daughter, who last saw him 6 hours ago before he retired to bed. By the bedside, multiple medicine bottles are empty. Emergency medical services (EMS) is activated. Vitals on arrival are heart rate 36 beats/minute, respiratory rate 6 breaths/minute, blood pressure 82/30 mmHg, and clammy skin. EMS begins assisting respirations with an ambubag. For stabilization, EMS is instructed to proceed immediately to the emergency room (ER) two blocks away.

10. On arrival in the ER, what is the first step in treating this patient?
    a. order a urine drug screen

b. give intravenous (IV) thiamine
c. intubate
d. apply external pacemaker
e. order cardiac enzymes

11. His daughter brings in his bottles of medicine, which include Xanax, metoprolol, glyburide, potassium chloride, and Lasix. She notes that he drinks and uses street drugs occasionally. The ER physician orders a drug screen, chemistry panel, complete blood count, cardiac enzymes, chest x-ray, electrocardiogram (ECG), and blood gas. While waiting for data, he gives the patient
    a. IV glucose two ampules, if his glucose finger-stick is elevated
    b. flumazenil
    c. thiamine 100 mg
    d. naloxone
    e. all the above

12. The patient still has a low heart rate and blood pressure. What is the next recommended treatment?
    a. atropine
    b. IV fluids and glucagon
    c. external pacer
    d. internal pacer
    e. calcium gluconate

13. The patient is waking up and his vitals have normalized. He has an abnormal ECG with peaked T waves. His potassium is 7, verified twice. What is the first-line treatment for this condition?
    a. glucose and insulin
    b. IV normal saline
    c. magnesium sulfate
    d. magnesium chloride
    e. hemodialysis

14. Which of the following is the most common cause of poison fatalities in adults?
    a. amphetamines
    b. benzodiazepines
    c. alcohol
    d. cleaning substances
    e. analgesics

15. Tanya swallows a bottle of unknown chemical in the garage. She becomes ill and is taken to the ER by her family. In the ER, she has a pH of 7 and an increased anion gap. Which of the following did she likely swallow?
    a. gasoline
    b. turpentine

c. vinegar
d. ethylene glycol
e. dish soap

Answers

1. **c.** Tricyclic antidepressants cause tachycardia plus mydriasis, flushing, dry membranes, hyperthermia, delirium, seizures, hallucination, and coma.

2. **b.** Alkalinization of the urine with sodium bicarbonate with an initial bolus of 1 or 2 mEq/kg is the standard therapy. Hypertonic saline is used for pH greater than 7.5. Quinidine and procainamide adversely affect sodium channels and are not used. Intensive care unit admission is required for monitoring.

3. **c.** Referring to the Rumack–Mathew treatment nomogram, *N*-acetylcysteine should be given ideally in the first 8 hours. Treatment can be given after this time but with decreasing effectiveness. Dosing is 140 mg/kg bolus orally and then 70 mg/kg every 4 hours for 17 doses. IV dosing is now available. Nausea and vomiting are common side effects. Bronchospasm, angioedema, and hypotension also occur.

4. **a.** Carbon monoxide poisoning kills approximately 5000 people annually, 70% intentionally. The poisoning mechanism is a combination of direct hemoglobin binding due to increased CO_2 affinity plus cellular toxicity and nitric oxide vasodilation, leading to vascular collapse.

5. **e.** Symptoms include headache, nausea, dizziness, blurred vision, and confusion followed by tachypnea, tachycardia, hypotension, and seizures.

6. **e.** The peak age for suicide is 45 to 49 years. Peak age for attempt with survival is 15 to 19 years.

7. **b.** The 2004 Annual Report of American Association of Poison Control Centers reported 2.2 to 2.5 million exposures to poisoning annually in the United States. Approximately 20% were intentional.

8. **a.** This age group has the highest incidence due to accidental ingestions by toddlers. Children younger than age 4 years comprise 46% of the poisonings. A total of 99.4% of exposures to children younger than age 6 years are unintentional. Only 10% of the exposures in this age group are ultimately seen in the emergency department for care.

9. e. Medicines should not be referred to as candy. In addition, posting the poison control number, 800-222-1222, is recommended.

10. c. This patient is hemodynamically unstable and in respiratory failure. The first step in treating the possible poison patient is to follow ABC (airway, breathing, and circulation).

11. e. Standard treatment of a patient who is confused and may have overdosed, while waiting for more definitive diagnosis, is to treat the most common offenders—hypoglycemia in diabetics or alcoholics, benzodiazepines, alcohol use, and narcotics, in addition to giving IV fluids and oxygen.

12. b. Initial therapy should be IV fluids and glucagon. Vasopressors may be necessary. Calcium is used for calcium channel blocker overdose.

13. a. Glucose and insulin will shift potassium intracellularly. Magnesium may increase potassium levels. Hemodialysis takes hours. Kayexalate orally or by enema can be used to decrease persistently elevated levels of potassium.

14. e. Analgesics are the most frequent, including acetaminophen and its combination with opioids. Following analgesics are sedative/hypnotics, antidepressants, and street drugs (cocaine, methamphetamine, and heroin).

15. d. Gasoline and turpentine are organic solvents and do not affect acid–base. Vinegar is a mild acid. Dish soap will cause diarrhea but is not absorbed. Increased anion gap metabolic acidosis can occur with ethylene glycol, among others: anion gap = (sodium + potassium) – (chloride + bicarbonate).

Summary

Poisonings are quite common, affecting approximately 2.5 million people in the United States yearly. The majority are nonintentional, with half occurring in those younger than age 6 years. Fifty percent of fatalities involve multiple drugs.

Basic principles of caring for acute and chronic poisonings involve first responder evaluation of the ABCs (airway, breathing, and cardiac), with subsequent use of advanced cardiac life support criteria and treatment.

Following the ABCs, the mentally altered patient may need immediate treatment with glucose, naloxone, thiamine, and flumazenil until a definitive diagnosis is available.

Testing with complete blood count, chemistry panel, cardiac enzymes, drug screens, specific toxin screens (lead, digoxin, arsenic, etc.), ECG, and computed tomography scan is common in the poisoned or toxic patient.

History of prior medication or illicit drug use is paramount, including any medicines other family members may be taking. Chemicals in the home or garage should be considered, as well as industrial exposure. Search pockets, purses, and the household. Decontamination of the person and clothing for industrial chemicals may be necessary. The physician should consider combinations of toxins, such as medicines plus street drugs or home cleaners.

For all poisoning cases, the poison control center should be called for treatment assistance and statistics.

Physical exam will help in the following overdose cases:

Amphetamines: tachycardia, mydriasis, agitation, paranoia, and seizures
Opiates: respiratory depression, mental depression, and miosis
anticholinergics: red as a beet, dry as a bone, blind as a bat, hot as a hare, and mad as a hatter
Cholinergics: SLUDGE—**s**alivation, **l**acrimation, **u**rination, **d**efecation, **g**astrointestinal upset, and **e**mesis
Carbon dioxide: bright red flushing
Cyanide: almond odor

MUD PILES is a mnemonic for some common causes of increased anion gap metabolic acidosis:

Methanol
Uremia
Diabetic ketoacidosis
Paraldehyde
Iron, isoniazid
Lactic acidosis
Ethylene glycol
Salicylates

For treatment, the plan should be specific to the problem. No longer are ipecac syrup and activated charcoal given routinely. Prolonged gastric exposure generally precludes gastric decontamination with lavage or other intestinal decontamination techniques.

For certain chemicals, hemodialysis, plasmapheresis, exchange transfusion, or hemoperfusion can be considered.

Table 157-1 Treatments for Specific Toxins

Toxin	Treatment
Acetaminophen	N-acetylcysteine
Amphetamines	Benzodiazepines
Beta blockers	Glucagon, vasopressors
Calcium blockers	Calcium, vasopressors
Digoxin	Digoxin-specific antibody fragments
Cyclic antidepressants	Alkalinization up to pH 7.5
Methanol	Ethanol or fomepizole
Lithium	IV fluids, oral polyethylene glycol solution, hemodialysis
Opioids	Naloxone
Organophosphates	Atropine
Salicylates	Activated charcoal, urine alkalinization

Adapted from Goldman L, Ausiello D: *Cecil Textbook of Medicine*, 22nd ed. Philadelphia: Saunders, 2003.

Suggested Reading

Ford M, Delaney KA, Ling L, Erickson T: *Clinical Toxicology.* Philadelphia: Saunders, 2000.

Goldman L, Ausiello D: *Cecil Textbook of Medicine*, 22nd ed. Philadelphia: Saunders, 2004.

Marx JA: *Rosen's Emergency Medicine: Concepts and Clinical Practice*, 6th ed. St. Louis: Mosby, 2006.

See Table 157-1 for specific treatments adapted from *Cecil Textbook of Medicine*, 22nd edition.

Drug screens typically include PCP, cocaine, opiates, benzodiazepines, tricyclic antidepressants, amphetamines, THC, and barbiturates. Drug screens do not include anticoagulants, caustics, cardiac or hypertensive meds, digoxin, ethylene glycol, fentanyl, LSD, herbicides, hypoglycemics, lithium, nonsteroidal anti-inflammatory drugs, and pesticides.

Rakel RE, Bope ET: *Conn's Current Therapy*. Philadelphia: Saunders, 2006.

Watson WA, Litovitz TL, Rodgers GC, et al: 2004 Annual report of the American Association of Poison Control Centers Toxic Exposure Surveillance System. *Am J Emerg Med* 23(5):589–666, 2005.

CHAPTER 158

Urticaria and Angioneurotic Edema

CLINICAL CASE PROBLEM 1

"Doctor, I Have a Fat Lip"

A 37-year-old woman has been taking an angiotensin receptor blocker medication for the treatment of hypertension for 2 weeks. She has taken the medication as prescribed, and she reports during a follow-up visit that her home blood pressure readings have been 110 to 130 systolic and 60 to 70 diastolic, a marked improvement from her readings prior to beginning therapy. She also reports two episodes of transient lip swelling (both lasting 2 hours), and during the second episode her eyelids also swelled.

CLINICAL CASE PROBLEM 2

Extremity Swelling and Gastrointestinal Symptoms

An 18-year-old woman recently diagnosed with systemic lupus erythematosis is in the office for follow-up after an emergency room visit for face, hand, and foot swelling along with abdominal pain and diarrhea. She reports that her symptoms improved after treatment with epinephrine and prednisone, and she notes that the emergency room physician recommended that she talk with you about danazol therapy.

SELECT THE BEST ANSWER TO THE FOLLOWING QUESTIONS

1. Angioedema has been reported to be associated with which of the following medications?
   a. angiotensin-converting enzyme (ACE) inhibitors

b. angiotensin receptor blockers

c. cyclooxygenase-2 (COX-2) inhibitors

d. clozapine

e. all of the above

2. Which of the following pairs of etiology and mechanism of initiation of angioedema is (are) correct?

a. angiotensin receptor blocker medication: stimulation of angiotensin II AT2 receptors, which leads to an increase in tissue bradykinin

b. COX-2 inhibitors: release of stored tissue bradykinin

c. systemic lupus erythematosis: consumption of complement C4

d. a and c

e. all of the above

3. How long after beginning an ACE inhibitor should a clinician be concerned about the development of angioedema?

a. 1 week

b. 1 month

c. 1 year

d. 10 years

4. Hereditary angioedema (HAE) differs from acquired angioedema due to collagen vascular diseases or medications in which of the following ways?

a. patients with HAE have a defect on chromosome 11

b. patients with HAE have high complement C1 inhibitor levels

c. patients with acquired angioedema due to collagen vascular diseases do not have involvement of bradykinin in the production of angioedema

d. angioedema is in the epidermal layer in HAE, but it is in the subdermal and deep dermal layers when associated with medications

e. a and d

5. Regarding treatment of acute episodes of HAE, which of the following statements is false?

a. epinephrine is of no help and should not be used

b. antihistamines and steroids do not work as well as they do for allergic urticaria but are still of some help

c. fresh frozen plasma (FFP) is thought to supply complement inhibitor proteins and can shorten attack duration

d. some patients worsen with FFP, possibly due to an increase in substrate for inflammatory mediators; as a result, FFP is not recommended when laryngeal edema is life threatening

e. medications may be needed over a 1- or 2-day period during an acute episode

6. Danazol is commonly used to reduce frequency and severity of angioedema episodes. Which of the following is (are) a common side effect(s) of danazol?

a. virilization

b. hepatitis

c. anovulation

d. acne

e. all of the above

7. Which of the following is (are) the most common site(s) for angioedema?

a. face and lips

b. larynx

c. gastrointestinal (GI) tract (leading to diarrhea and abdominal cramps)

d. genitals

e. all of the above

Answers

1. **e.** Angioedema is a recognized side effect of ACE inhibitor medications, and until recently it was thought that angiotensin receptor blocker (ARB) medications would not lead to this potentially life-threatening side effect. However, case reports of ARB-associated angioedema have appeared in the literature. The mechanism is thought to be secondary stimulation of angiotensin II AT2 receptors that produces an increase in tissue bradykinin, which causes the angioedema. This has occurred even in patients who have never taken an ACE inhibitor. Cases have also been reported after treatment with nonsteroidal anti-inflammatory drugs (NSAIDs), especially those with more COX-2 inhibition, and after treatment with clozapine. Many NSAIDs inhibit COX-2. Patients in a Japanese study who had NSAID-induced angioedema were found to have the most problems with loxoprofen, acetylsalicylic acid, etodolac, diclofenac, and acetaminophen. Meloxicam was better tolerated. Urticaria often accompanies the angioedema in these patients. Patients whose angioedema is due to ACE inhibitors have normal C1 inhibitor function because their angiotensin converting is blocked and therefore unable to contribute to degradation of bradykinin and substance P, allowing progression to angioedema.

2. **e.** ARB medications stimulate the angiotensin II AT2 receptors, leading to an increase in tissue bradykinin, which in turn leads to localized angioedema. NSAIDs with COX-2 inhibition cause the release of stored tissue bradykinin with similar effect. Collagen vascular disease and other autoimmune conditions are associated with consumption of complement C4. This leads to a decrease in phagocytic activity by cells that

normally bind and remove products of normal cell death, leaving these products, which stimulate inflammatory mediator production and cascades.

3. **b.** On average, patients who develop angioedema due to ACE inhibitors and ARBs develop symptoms 1.8 years after starting the medication, but one-fourth of patients have symptoms in the first month of exposure to the drug.

4. **e.** Angioedema can be inherited (HAE) or acquired. Acquired forms associated with lymphoproliferative disease or autoimmune disease are the result of C1 inhibitor deficiency. Lupus erythematosus and HAE are thought to share a common feature: consumption of C4 complement with resultant impairment in the clearance of apoptotic cells (cells disintegrate into membrane-bound particles that can be cleared by phagocytosis). Patients with lupus and low C4 levels are at elevated risk of angioedema symptoms.

Lymphosarcoma, leukemia, lymphoma, and paraproteinemias may develop circulating or cellular factors that activate C1 and deplete serum C1 inhibitor. In patients with immune complex diseases, activation of the complement cascade and then depletion of C1 inhibitor can occur, with angioedema resulting. These patients differ from HAE patients (who have normal C1 levels) in that they have low C1, C2, and C4 levels. Glucocorticoid therapy as well as cytotoxic therapies have been shown to be helpful.

5. **a.** Episodes of angioedema usually peak in minutes to hours and fade over 1 or 2 days. The edema fluid is in the deep dermal and subdermal layers, unlike in urticaria, in which the fluid is more superficial. Angioedema is brawny and nonpitting, and it is not always associated with itching. Thirty percent of patients have a flat, nonpruritic erythema marginatum-like rash at the onset of episodes. Swelling of the face, eyelids, lips, GI tract, genitals, hands, and feet is uncomfortable, but laryngeal edema, another common symptom, is life threatening. Although the standard of care in the United States of a combination of epinephrine, antihistamines, and steroids usually prevents airway closure, laryngeal edema and other symptoms are much more responsive to C1 inhibitor concentrate, which is used as first-line therapy in other countries. Medications should be continued over 1 or 2 days to prevent relapse. Danazol is of no use in acute episodes.

6. **e.** Treatment with danazol increases liver synthesis of C1 inhibitor and decreases episodes of angioedema, but virilization and hepatitis can result. Danazol is used primarily as a treatment for endometriosis and it suppresses ovarian function, leading to anovulation. Acne is a common side effect associated with the androgenic activity of the medication. The hepatitis that can result is called peliosis hepatitis, and it may be associated with liver adenoma formation.

7. **e.** See answer 6.

Summary

Angioedema can be hereditary (HAE) or acquired, and it results from a deficiency of circulating complement C1 inhibitor. The hereditary form, believed to be inherited in an autosomal dominant manner, has an estimated prevalence of 1/10,000 to 1/50,000. It is usually due to a defect on chromosome 11 leading to inadequate synthesis of complement C1 inhibitor. However, rarer forms are caused by deficiency of complement factor I or interleukin-2. The acquired form can result from lymphoproliferative disease, autoimmune diseases, or some medications, all of which are associated with C1 inhibitor deficiency. C1 inhibitor is a protein that controls several pathways—complement, kinin generation, fibrinolysis, and the intrinsic clotting pathway. This C1 inhibitor deficiency leads to an inability to control local inflammatory responses so that when a physical or emotional stress occurs, the patient's complement system is activated and bradykinin is synthesized and released.

The bradykinin release leads to localized edema. The edema occurs when intravascular fluid leaks from postcapillary venules in response to the vasodilation caused by inflammatory mediators such as bradykinin in a localized area. Measured C1 levels do not predict disease or attack severity, but low C2 and C4 levels are found. When C1 is not inhibited, the C1 then cleaves C2 and C4, leading to the inflammatory cascade. This constant elevation in complement cascade activity is thought to lead to autoimmune disease, which is more common in patients with HAE.

Puberty usually marks the onset of significant symptoms, but clinical onset late in life has been described. With regard to treatment, epinephrine, antihistamines, and steroids do not work as well as they do in urticaria, but they are still used for treatment of acute angioedema episodes. Epinephrine 1:1000, 0.2 or 0.3 mL given every 20 minutes for three doses is used, along with standard doses of diphenhydramine and prednisone or methylprednisolone. Chronic suppressive therapies with artificial androgens such as danazol cause C1 inhibitor levels to increase and C2 and C4 levels to fall; therefore, symptoms are generally less frequent and less severe. Danazol is given at doses of 200 to 600 mg/day, or stanozolol is given at 2 to 6 mg/day. Because these drugs are synthetic androgens and cause masculinization, doses as low as possible should be used. Hepatitis is also a common side effect of danazol. Men can be treated with methyltestosterone (which is less expensive than danazol and stanozolol) at 10 to 30 mg/day. Some patients do no respond to androgens or cannot tolerate them; for these patients, aminocaproic acid or other plasmin inhibitors can be tried. In patients with angioedema due to leukemia, lymphoma, and paraproteinemias, plasmin inhibitors can be effective in preventing episodes of angioedema.

Emergent treatment with C1 inhibitor concentrate is being used successfully in Europe, South America, and Japan. Tibolone is a synthetic steroid with estrogenic, androgenic, and progestational effect. It has been shown to be as effective as danazol in reducing the number and severity of attacks but with fewer androgenic side effects. Used in Europe for 20 years, it is unlikely to be approved by the Food and Drug Administration.

Suggested Reading

Davis AE: The pathophysiology of hereditary angioedema. *Clin Immunol* 114:3–9, 2005.

Frank MM: Urticaria and angioedema. In: Goldman L, Ausiello D, eds: *Cecil Textbook of Medicine*, 22nd ed. Philadelphia: Saunders, 2004.

Longhurst HJ: Emergency treatment of acute attacks in hereditary angioedema due to C1 inhibitor deficiency: What is the evidence? *Int J Clin Pract* 59:594–599, 2005.

CHAPTER

159   Heat and Cold Illness

CLINICAL CASE PROBLEM 1

A 51-Year-Old Alcoholic Male Brought to the Emergency Room

A 51-year-old alcoholic male is brought into the emergency room (ER) after having been found in a snow bank. He is unconscious, and no history can be obtained. No family is known. On physical examination, his blood pressure is 90/60 mmHg. His pulse is 36 beats/minute and regular. His core body temperature is 28°C (82.4°F). His electrocardiogram (ECG) reveals sinus bradycardia and a J wave after each QRS complex.

SELECT THE BEST ANSWER TO THE FOLLOWING QUESTIONS

1. Which of the following statements regarding the hypothermia in this patient is true?
   a. body temperatures between 32°C and 35°C constitute mild hypothermia
   b. the Osborne J wave on the ECG is characteristic of hypothermia
   c. arrhythmias and dysrhythmias are common when the core body temperature drops below 30°C (86°F)
   d. intravascular volume is usually not maintained in patients with hypothermia
   e. all of the above

2. What is the treatment of choice for this patient?
   a. passive rewarming
   b. active external rewarming
   c. active core rewarming
   d. a and b
   e. none of the above

CLINICAL CASE PROBLEM 2

A 46-Year-Old Male with Blanched Feet

A 46-year-old male is brought to the ER from his worksite with numbness of both feet after working in 0°C (32°F) weather for 6 hours. On examination, both feet are blanched. Sensation is decreased in both feet to the level of the ankles. Both feet are cold to touch and are bloodless. You suspect frostbite.

3. What is the most appropriate treatment of this patient at this time?
   a. passive rewarming
   b. vigorous rubbing
   c. immersion in water at 42°C (107.6°F)
   d. placement close to a radiant heater
   e. immersion in water at 30°C (86°F)

d. b or c

e. none of the above

CLINICAL CASE PROBLEM 3

A 4-Year-Old Male with a Core Temperature of 28°C

A 4-year-old male is brought to the ER after having fallen through the ice into a lake. He was rescued approximately 15 minutes later. Cardiopulmonary resuscitation (CPR) was begun at the scene and is in progress on arrival. On examination, you note no spontaneous breathing or cardiac activity. The core temperature is 28°C (82.4°F).

4. At this time, what is the most appropriate action?
   a. stop CPR
   b. continue CPR while rewarming the patient with active external rewarming
   c. continue CPR while rewarming the patient with inhalation warming therapy
   d. continue CPR while rewarming the patient with peritoneal dialysis
   e. activate the advanced cardiac life support (ACLS) protocol

5. Following the initial treatment just selected, what would be your next step?
   a. stop CPR
   b. continue CPR while rewarming the patient with active external rewarming
   c. continue CPR while rewarming the patient with inhalation warming therapy
   d. continue CPR while rewarming the patient with active core rewarming
   e. none of the above

CLINICAL CASE PROBLEM 4

An Overheated 34-Year-Old Male

A 34-year-old male soldier is brought to the ER after having been outdoors on patrol all day in temperatures exceeding 42°C (107.6°F). He complains of painful spasms of the skeletal muscles, which are worse in the legs and in the abdomen. He denies other symptoms. He is alert and cooperative, with a blood pressure of 120/80 mmHg and a pulse of 108 beats/minute. The temperature is 38°C (100.4°F). The remainder of the physical exam is normal.

6. Which of the following conditions does this patient have?
   a. heat cramps
   b. heatstroke
   c. heat exhaustion

7. What is the treatment of choice for this patient at this time?
   a. oral electrolyte replacement therapy
   b. core body cooling
   c. warm intravenous (IV) fluids
   d. intensive care monitoring and Swan–Ganz catheter insertion
   e. none of the above

CLINICAL CASE PROBLEM 5

An Exhausted 23-Year-Old Female Marathon Runner

A 23-year-old female marathon runner presents to the ER after she completed a marathon. During the last mile, she became lightheaded and experienced nausea, vomiting, headache, tachycardia, and tachypnea. Her blood pressure is 90/70 mmHg, and the pulse is 120 beats/minute and regular. She is orthostatic. Her temperature is 37.5°C (99.5°F). The rest of the physical exam is normal.

8. Which of the following conditions does she have?
   a. heat cramps
   b. heatstroke
   c. heat exhaustion
   d. b or c
   e. none of the above

9. Which of the following statements regarding this patient's condition is true?
   a. rapid IV volume and electrolyte replacement are indicated
   b. she can be safely discharged without any active treatment; oral fluids will suffice
   c. her temperature will likely increase significantly in the next few hours
   d. serum potassium and sodium levels are likely to be normal
   e. none of the above

CLINICAL CASE PROBLEM 6

A 34-Year-Old Male Marathon Runner Who Collapsed

While running a marathon, a 34-year-old male collapsed at mile 18. He is unconscious, with a blood pressure of 90/60 mmHg. His pulse is 128 beats/minute, and his respiratory rate is 45 breaths/minute. His temperature is 41°C (105.8°F).

10. Which of the following statements about this patient is true?
   a. he has heatstroke
   b. hepatic and renal abnormalities are common in this condition
   c. treatment should be directed at lowering the core temperature as quickly as possible
   d. all of the above
   e. none of the above

Answers

1. **e.** Hypothermia is defined as mild if the body temperature is between 32°C and 35°C, moderate if the temperature is between 28°C and 32°C, and severe if the temperature is less than 28°C. Shivering stops at 31°C. Characteristic ECG changes in hypothermia include the Osborne (J) wave, which is a slow, positive deflection at the end of the QRS. Hypothermia increases the risk of ventricular fibrillation and asystole. Extravascular fluid shifts lead to intravascular volume depletion. Depression of central nervous system (CNS) function from confusion to coma can occur.

2. **c.** Active core rewarming is recommended in moderate to severe hypothermia; this will correct temperature rapidly but decrease the risk of sudden release of cold blood into circulation as peripheral vasoconstriction is relieved.

3. **c.** Frostnip is a superficial and reversible injury, characterized by blanching and numbness of the skin and then a sudden cessation of cold and pain. Impending frostbite is characterized by the loss of pain and cold sensation. Rapid rewarming is recommended, and the best method is immersion in 40°C water. Slow rewarming is less effective and is associated with increased risk of tissue damage. Rubbing is contraindicated. Placement next to a radiant heater increases the risk of focal burns.

4. **e.** Since basic life support has begun, the next step is ACLS. While these resuscitative measures are being performed, rewarming measures should continue until the core temperature is 32°C (89.6°F); then, continuation of ACLS should be evaluated.

5. **d.** The old adage "a patient is not dead until he is warm and dead" is still true. Continuation of resuscitative efforts should be a priority while active core rewarming is pursued.

6. **a.** This patient has the classic symptoms of heat cramps.

7. **a.** Heat cramps usually occur when strenuous physical activity occurs in a very hot environment. Skeletal muscles have painful spasms, and patients may experience weakness, fatigue, nausea, vomiting, and tachycardia. Body temperature is normal. The muscle cramps are caused by total body salt deficiency, and the treatment is oral repletion of electrolytes and mild cooling.

8. **c.** See answer 9.

9. **a.** This patient has heat exhaustion. Heat exhaustion is characterized by volume depletion with resultant tissue hypoperfusion and also fluid and electrolyte losses from sweating. Heat exhaustion usually presents with fatigue, lightheadedness, nausea and/or vomiting, and headache. Tachycardia, hyperventilation, and hypotension are common. Body temperature is usually normal or only slightly elevated. Patients normally are sweating profusely. Treatment includes IV saline or Ringer's lactate infusion, removal to a cool environment, spraying with tepid water (40°C, 104°F), and cooling with fans.

10. **d.** This patient has heatstroke, defined as core temperature higher than 40°C and associated neurologic symptoms. When heatstroke occurs in the elderly, patients are "hot and dry"; sweating is not present, and they are not losing body heat through evaporation or convection. In young patients who experience heatstroke during vigorous exercise, sweating is profuse. In both cases, tachycardia and hyperventilation are present. Liver and kidney function is often impaired, and disseminated intravascular coagulation can occur. Dehydration and volume depletion are not a given, as they are in heat exhaustion. Fluid replacement must be judicious, and central venous pressure must be monitored either clinically or invasively to avoid pulmonary edema. Treatment includes removal of clothing, application of tepid water or mist to entire skin, fanning of air, ice packs to groins and axillae, and possibly cold water gastric/bladder lavage or even peritoneal lavage. Throughout the course of treatment, the ABCs of resuscitation and monitoring should be attended to (airway, breathing, and circulation).

Summary

Heat illness is common in outdoor laborers, athletes, children, and the elderly. The incidence in the United States is 20/100,000 during summer, with approximately 240 deaths per year.

HEATSTROKE

Defined as core hyperthermia, with core temperature higher than 40°C (104°F).

Heat injury proceeds to heatstroke more commonly in the elderly and in patients with chronic illness.

Present with delirium, convulsions, coma, anhydrosis, arrhythmias, disseminated intravascular coagulation, hepatic failure, renal failure, rhabdomyolysis, and shock.

Mortality rate is 10%.

Elderly or chronically ill patients are "hot and dry," while young, athletic patients are sweating profusely.

Monitoring: Rectal or bladder/esophageal temperature probe is recommended because peripheral temperatures are 1°C lower than core.

Treatment
  Cooling is primary: external—evaporative, immersion (15°C/59°F water sprayed on skin, 45°C/113°F air fanned over the body).
  Can immerse with cooling blanket/ice packs to axilla, groin, neck, and head.
  Watch for shivering.
  Internal—gastric, bladder, and rectal coldwater lavage
  Goal: Obtain a core temperature of 38°C (100.4°F).
  Lab: Check renal and liver functions, blood glucose, CPK, and electrolytes.

HEAT EXHAUSTION

Heat exhaustion is more common than heatstoke.

Temperature is 37°C to 40°C; dizziness, thirst, weakness, headache, and malaise

No CNS impairment

Resolution with hydration and cooling

Present with nausea/malaise, anxiety, confusion, hypotension, oliguria, and tachycardia

Hot and sweaty

Stabilize in cool area

Hydrate, remove from heat source, and monitor. If resolved in 20 to 30 minutes, educate; if symptoms persist, treat as for heatstroke. If symptoms persist for 2 or 3 hours, look for underlying medical illness/drugs.

If hyponatremic heat exhaustion, patients can have CNS symptoms and seizures; this can be fatal.

Treat with normal saline; raise serum sodium no faster than 2.5 mEq/L/hour to prevent central pontine myelinolysis.

Heat regulation in healthy adults:
  Conduction—direct contact with cooler object
  Convection—cool air passes over exposed skin
  Radiation—release of heat from body into environment
  Evaporation—perspiration (most effective)

The hypothalamus is activated at a core temperature elevation of 1°C, leading to peripheral vasodilation and thermal sweating in normal individuals.

COLD INJURIES AND SYNDROMES

Hypothermia causes approximately 700 deaths per year in the United States; more than half of these patients are older than age 65 years, and the male:female ratio is 2.5 :1. Risk factors include alcohol intoxication, extremes of age, and chronic illness. Already compromised patients may respond to infection with hypothermia rather than fever.

Monitoring: Standard thermometers read only to 34.4°C (94°F), so temperature may be lower than first thought.

Complications include renal failure due to rhabdomyolysis, electrolyte shifts, and coagulopathies (which are usually self-limited). Many patients have ventricular dysrhythmias.

Treatment: Remove wet clothing, warm with blankets, and administer warm IV fluids (saline). Passive rewarming with blankets alone is sufficient if the hypothermia is mild and the patient is otherwise healthy. In severe hypothermia, warm gastric and bladder lavage, inhaled humidified oxygen at 40°C, or even peritoneal dialysis or cardiopulmonary bypass can be used. If a Doppler confirms pulselessness, CPR/ACLS should ensue. If the patient has ventricular fibrillation and the first defibrillation is unsuccessful, the next shock should not be done until the core temperature is up to 30°C (86°F). Then, if the ventricular fibrillation persists, amiodarone is recommended. Thiamine should be given if alcohol abuse is known or suspected.

Suggested Reading

Fulcher W, White W, Rodney WM: Thermal and environmental injuries. In: Rakel R, ed, *Textbook of Family Practice*, 6th ed. Philadelphia: Saunders, 2002.

Glazer JL. Management of heatstroke and heat exhaustion. *Am Fam Physician* 71(11):2133–2140, 2005.

Jurkovich GJ: Environmental cold-induced injury. *Surg Clin North Am* 87(1):247–267, viii, 2007.

McCullough L, Arora S: Diagnosis and treatment of hypothermia. *Am Fam Physician* 70:2325–2332, 2004.

Sanchez LD, Corwell B, Berkoff D: Medical problems of marathon runners. *Am J Emerg Med* 24(5):608–615, 2006.

CLINICAL CASE PROBLEM 1

"Oh, My Head Hurts!"

A high school senior class group has decided to spend spring break skiing in Colorado. Two students develop headache and malaise after spending their first night at the ski lodge.

SELECT THE BEST ANSWER TO THE FOLLOWING QUESTIONS

1. What are the students most likely experiencing?
   a. the symptoms meet clinical criteria of sinus pressure headache
   b. the symptoms meet clinical criteria of acute mountain sickness (AMS)
   c. these symptoms suggest they are not enjoying their vacation
   d. these symptoms meet criteria for high-altitude pulmonary edema (HAPE)
   e. these symptoms suggest high-altitude cerebral edema (HACE)

2. After 72 hours, one of the sick students feels fine and the other seems confused and has trouble putting on his socks. What treatment should be instituted?
   a. the well student should be evacuated and treated with acetazolamide
   b. the confused student should be evacuated and treated with dexamethazone
   c. both students should be evacuated and treated with oxygen
   d. neither needs treatment; the confused student needs ski instruction
   e. both students should be evacuated to lower altitude

3. What is the underlying cause of HACE?
   a. overexertion at high altitude
   b. it is an extension of AMS
   c. cell phone use at high altitude
   d. overhydration at high altitude
   e. underhydration at high altitude

4. After 72 hours, two other students begin having trouble keeping up and tire easily. High-altitude-related pulmonary edema requires at least two of four symptoms for diagnosis. They are which of the following?
   a. dyspnea at rest, cough, weakness, abdominal pain
   b. dyspnea at rest, cough, weakness, chest congestion or tightness
   c. dyspnea at rest, cough, retractions with breathing, abdominal pain
   d. dyspnea at rest, cough, retractions with breathing, costochondritis
   e. sneezing, stuffy head, fever, cough

5. Factors that can be modified to prevent AMS, HACE, and HAPE include all of the following except
   a. rate of ascent
   b. time for acclimatization
   c. use of preventive medication
   d. types of fluids consumed
   e. altitude at which one sleeps

6. The Lake Louise scoring system is a standardized diagnostic system to help with diagnosing high-altitude illness. It includes all of the following criteria except
   a. headache
   b. malaise
   c. gastrointestinal complaints (nausea and fatigue)
   d. lightheadedness
   e. vertigo

7. Chronic mountain sickness (CMS) occurs in people adapted to high altitude who eventually succumb to problems from life in a hypoxic environment. All of the following commonly occur except
   a. polycythemia
   b. fatigue
   c. adult respiratory distress syndrome (ARDS)
   d. right heart failure
   e. pulmonary hypertension

CLINICAL CASE PROBLEM 2

Coming Up Too Quick

Another group from the same senior class decided to go to Mexico and take scuba classes. After 3 days of shallow diving, two students do a 100-foot dive. After 5 minutes on their second dive, one of the student's equipment fails. The two students share the working breathing equipment and quickly rise to the surface in a panic for air.

8. Which of the following is (are) the most frequent symptom(s) of arterial gas embolism and pulmonary barotrauma?
   a. paresthesias and/or paralysis
   b. unconsciousness
   c. headache
   d. visual disturbances
   e. all of the above

9. One of the students develops joint pain in the elbows, hips, and knees, and during transport to an emergency room the student develops swelling in the lower extremities. What treatment should be given in the emergency room if available?
   a. conservative care with pain relievers and dismissal
   b. oxygen should be given with narcotic pain reliever
   c. hyperbaric treatment to 100 feet, the same as dive depth
   d. hyperbaric treatment to 60 feet
   e. pack extremities in ice for 30 minutes to relieve pain

10. The other student experiences the same symptoms but with no feeling in his legs and with difficulty breathing. All of the following should be considered in his care except
    a. recompression
    b. continuous oxygen
    c. intermittent intervals of oxygen
    d. advanced cardiac life support (ACLS) protocols
    e. careful exam

Answers

1. **b.** AMS is a clinical diagnosis; diagnostics and physical findings are not necessary. Diagnosis is based on headache and one or more of the following symptoms: nausea, vomiting, fatigue, lightheadedness, anorexia, and insomnia at high altitude. Sinus infection can cause similar symptoms and should be considered.

2. **b.** This student is suffering from HACE. This is an extension of AMS. Brain herniation from edema is of great concern. Immediate decent, oxygen treatment, and dexamethasone are needed as soon as possible. Consider magnetic resonance imaging if available.

The healthy student does not require intervention and is likely acclimatizing well.

3. **b.** See answer 2.

4. **b.** Symptoms should include two of those listed and at least two signs (crackles, wheezing, central cyanosis, tachypnea, or tachycardia) per the Lake Louise Consensus Committee for a diagnosis of HAPE.

5. **d.** The type of fluid consumed does not appear to relate to the possibility of disease occurrence. Dehydration is a controversial factor in the cause of AMS.

6. **e.** Vertigo is not a symptom of high-altitude sickness but one of labyrinthitis. The Lake Louise Consensus Committee defines AMS as headache and an additional symptom of nausea, vomiting, fatigue, weakness, dizziness, lightheadedness, insomnia, or anorexia. These all have to relate to a recent ascent to high altitude.

7. **c.** An estimated 140 million people live at high altitude and suffer specific illness from chronic hypoxia. Low birth weight, chronic right heart failure from hypoxic pulmonary hypertension, polycythemia, and fatigue can be expected. ARDS could be expected in HAPE but not in CMS.

8. **e.** The most frequent symptoms of arterial gas embolism and pulmonary barotraumas include unconsciousness, paresthesias and/or paralysis, dizziness, nausea and/or vertigo, visual disturbances, convulsions, and headache. Risk factors for barotraumas include incorrect ascent technique and previous pulmonary scarring or lesions.

9. **c.** The student is suffering from decompression sickness (DCS). Treatment should be with recompression to 60 feet or deeper with hyperbaric oxygen breathing as per the U.S. Navy treatment table.

10. **b.** This student is suffering from type II DCS with neurologic symptoms. These deficits could include hemiplegia, paresthesias, and peripheral neuropathies. Type II DCS includes those with cardiopulmonary symptoms as well. Treatment should include careful exam, recompression with slow ascent and intermittent oxygen breathing periods to prevent toxicity, and ACLS as needed.

Summary

AMS

1. AMS can occur as early as 6 hours and up to 72 hours upon rapid accent to high altitude.
2. Symptoms are headache plus one of the following: nausea, vomiting, fatigue, lightheadedness, anorexia, and insomnia.
3. Treatment: Stop ascent for 1 or 2 days or start descent. Use of acetazolamide to speed acclimatization or analgesics and antiemetics as needed. If severe, descend and consider use of dexamethasone. Use oxygen 1 or 2 L for a few hours.
4. Prevention: Slow ascent for acclimatization, use of acetazolamide to hasten acclimatization, or use of dexamethasone to prevent swelling.

HAPE

1. Severe altitude illness
2. Pathophysiology: noncardiogenic pulmonary edema associated with pulmonary hypertension and elevated capillary pressure
3. Risk factors: rate of ascent, high altitudes, individual susceptibility, exertion, cold temperatures, and usually higher altitudes than those at which AMS occurs
4. Symptoms: dry cough; shortness of breath; decreased exercise tolerance; can progress to severe dyspnea, pink or bloody sputum, coma, and death
5. Treatment: immediate descent, supplemental oxygen, nifedipine, and hyperbaric chamber
6. Prevention: slow and gradual ascent; avoid overexertion; consider acetazolamide beginning 1 day prior to ascent and continuing for 2 days at the new altitudes; treat symptoms of AMS early

HACE

1. Most severe form of altitude illness
2. Symptoms: confusion or ataxia in a person with AMS
3. Treatment: immediate descent, oxygen, hyperbaric chamber, and dexamethasone. Acetazolamide should be used if descent is delayed.
4. Prevention: same as that for HAPE

DECOMPRESSION SICKNESS

1. Can develop in scuba divers after ascent from depth
2. Factors increasing risk of developing decompression sickness: (a) rate of ascent, (b) hypothermia, (c) fatigue, (d) older age, (e) dehydration, (f) alcohol use, (g) female sex, (h) obesity, and (i) patent foramen ovale
3. Cause: inert gas bubbles, usually nitrogen, released into bloodstream and tissues
4. Signs/symptoms: (a) itching, (b) rash, (c) headache, (d) joint and muscle pain, (e) extreme fatigue, (f) sensory loss and paresthesias (severe cases), and (g) loss of bowel and/or bladder control (severe cases)
5. Treatment: hyperbaric chamber, supplemental oxygen, and intravenous hydration

PULMONARY BAROTRAUMA

1. Can occur in scuba divers during ascent.
2. Cause: (a) most common cause in recreational divers is breath holding, (b) rapid ascent, (c) strenuous exertion while diving, and (d) pulmonary obstructive disease
3. Arterial gas embolism (most serious form of pulmonary barotraumas), signs and symptoms: focal weakness, visual loss, confusion, seizures, and coma
4. Treatment: cardiac life support, supplemental oxygen, hydration, and transport to a facility with a hyperbaric chamber

Suggested Reading

Campbell ES: Decompression illness in sports divers: Part I. *Medscape Orthopaedics Sports Med eJournal* 1(5): 1997.

Gallagher SA: Images in emergency medicine. *Ann Emerg Med* 44(2):177, 2004.

Gallagher SA, Hackett PH: High-altitude illness. *Emerg Med Clin North Am* 22(2):329–355, 2004.

Levitzky MG: *Pulmonary Physiology*, Lange Physiology Series, 6th ed. New York, McGraw–Hill, 2003.

Maloney JP, Broeckel U: Epidemiology, risk factors, and genetics of high altitude related pulmonary disease. *Clin Chest Med* 26(3): 395–404, 2005.

Schoene RB: Limits of respiration at high altitude. *Clin Chest Med* 26(3):405–414, 2005.

Telzlaff K, Thorsen E. Breathing at depth: Physiologic and clinical aspects of diving while breathing compressed gas. *Clin Chest Med* 26(3):355–380, 2005.

SPORTS MEDICINE

CLINICAL CASE PROBLEM 1

The First-Year Team Physician's Dilemma

This is your first year as team physician for the local high school. All the talk in the community is about the school's football team, which is expected to win the state championship this season. The coach of the football team "doesn't like to lose" and was known to put pressure on the previous team physician to give medical clearance to players before games.

SELECT THE BEST ANSWER TO THE FOLLOWING QUESTIONS

1. Which of the following is a contraindication to participation in contact sports?
   a. sickle cell trait
   b. human immunodeficiency virus (HIV) infection
   c. solitary testicle
   d. fever of 102°F
   e. convulsive disorder, well-controlled

2. Which of the following is the most common cause of sudden death in an athlete younger than age 35 years?
   a. coronary artery anomaly
   b. premature coronary artery disease
   c. myocarditis
   d. hypertrophic cardiomyopathy
   e. rupture of the aorta

3. Which of the following tests is recommended for routine screening of athletes during the preparticipation evaluation (PPE)?
   a. electrocardiography
   b. echocardiography
   c. exercise stress testing
   d. vision screen
   e. urinalysis

4. During the PPE, you note that the 17-year-old star quarterback of the high school football team has a blood pressure of 148/95 mmHg. His past medical history is negative, and he has never been told that he has high blood pressure. He is 6 foot 2 inches tall and weighs 175 pounds. As the team physician, you tell him that
   a. he cannot play any contact sports
   b. he cannot play football until his blood pressure is under control
   c. he is cleared to play but must have his blood pressure measured twice during the next month
   d. if he begins taking antihypertensive medication immediately, then he is cleared to play
   e. he must lose 10 pounds before he will be cleared to play football

5. The school's wrestling team has had an unusually high amount of injuries this season. Which of the following conditions is reason to disqualify a wrestler from competition?
   a. herpes simplex
   b. HIV
   c. hepatitis C
   d. inguinal hernia
   e. diabetes mellitus

6. When performing a PPE on a female athlete, certain considerations should be taken for gender-specific predispositions. Which of the following conditions

are more common in female athletes than in male athletes?
a. eating disorders
b. stress fractures in runners
c. anterior cruciate ligament injuries in basketball players
d. osteoporosis
e. all of the above

7. Which of the following statements concerning the PPE is true?
a. approximately 10% of athletes are denied clearance during the PPE
b. the PPE ideally should be performed 6 months prior to preseason practice
c. a primary objective of the PPE is to detect conditions that may predispose an athlete to injury
d. a primary objective of the PPE is to counsel athletes on health-related issues, such as tobacco and drug use
e. a complete history will identify approximately 95% of problems affecting athletes

8. Which of the following sports is considered limited contact?
a. downhill skiing
b. basketball
c. soccer
d. diving
e. lacrosse

9. You are the physician for the town's football league and are performing PPEs for the senior division (13- to 15-year-old boys). You note that one of the players is much smaller than the rest. He is 4 foot 10 inches tall, weighs 100 pounds, and is Tanner stage 1. Regarding clearance to play, which of the following is recommended?
a. clearance only after evaluation by an endocrinologist
b. may play but limited to only certain positions on the field
c. no clearance until he has grown in size and weight and is at Tanner stage 2
d. recommend he plays this season with the younger division
e. full clearance to play

10. When performing a PPE on an athlete with a spinal cord injury, which of the following is important to ask about in the history?
a. use of adaptive equipment
b. heat illness
c. autonomic dysreflexia
d. medication use
e. all of the above

Answers

1. **d.** Fever of 102°F. A fever in an athlete or exercising individual can have negative effects, including increased cardiopulmonary effort, reduced maximum exercise capacity, orthostatic hypotension, and increased risk for heat illness and myocarditis (especially if the fever is caused by the coxsackievirus).

Athletes with sickle cell trait can participate in all sports. These athletes have an increased risk of developing exertional rhabdomyolysis and should be counseled regarding proper conditioning, hydration, and acclimatization.

There have been no known cases of transmission of HIV infection during sports. The risk of transmission of HIV in football has been estimated to be less than one transmission per 1 million games.

An athlete with a solitary testicle may be cleared for contact sports. The athlete should be informed of the risk of injury and should wear a protective cup.

Athletes with well-controlled convulsive disorders may be cleared for most school-sponsored sports. Neurologic consultation is recommended for high-risk sports such as skiing, gymnastics, and high diving.

2. **d.** The most common cause of sudden death in an athlete younger than age 35 years is hypertrophic cardiomyopathy. Coronary artery disease is the most common cause of sudden death in athletes 35 years of age or older. Coronary artery anomalies, premature coronary artery disease, myocarditis, and rupture of the aorta can all cause sudden death in an athlete.

3. **d.** A vision screen should be performed in all athletes and should be 20/40 or better in each eye with or without corrective lenses. Athletes with only one eye or corrected vision worse than 20/40 in either eye should wear protective eye gear when playing in sports with a high risk of eye injury.

Routine electrocardiography is not recommended as a screening tool for the PPE.

Echocardiography and exercise stress testing are not cost-effective in large screening programs of athletes.

Urinalysis is not recommended. This test has a low yield in an asymptomatic, healthy population.

4. **c.** He is cleared to play but must have his blood pressure measured twice during the next month. Athletes with severe hypertension (i.e., adolescents 16 to 18 years old with systolic blood pressure of 150 mmHg and diastolic blood pressure of 98 mmHg) need to have their blood pressure controlled before being allowed to participate in sports. When measuring an athlete's blood pressure, be certain that the cuff fits properly.

5. **a.** A wrestler could be disqualified for having herpes simplex. While an athlete is contagious with such conditions as herpes simplex, scabies, impetigo, or molluscum contagiosum, he or she is disqualified from certain contact/collision sports. HIV, hepatitis C, inguinal hernia, and diabetes mellitus are not reasons to disqualify an athlete from sports.

6. **e.** Anorexia nervosa, bulimia nervosa, and other eating disorders are more common in female athletes. Disordered eating is reported in 15% to 62% of college female athletes. All athletes should be questioned about a desire to lose weight or displeasure with body habitus.

Stress fractures are more common in female runners. The reason is probably multifactorial and includes such factors as muscle strength and balance, limb alignment, and medical factors such as nutrition, eating habits, menstrual dysfunction, and osteopenia or osteoporosis.

Noncontact anterior cruciate ligament injury rates are higher in female athletes. Risk factors probably include anatomic, biomechanical, and neuromuscular differences. These injuries occur commonly during deceleration, landing, or pivoting.

Osteoporosis is more common in female athletes and, along with osteopenia, can exist in the young female athlete. Disordered eating and menstrual dysfunction are risk factors that should be screened for during the PPE.

7. **c.** A primary objective of the PPE is to detect conditions that may predispose an athlete for injury. Other primary objectives are to detect conditions that may be life threatening or disabling and to meet legal and insurance requirements.

Approximately 0.3% to 1.3% of athletes are denied clearance during the PPE.

The best time to perform the PPE is 6 weeks prior to the start of preseason practice. This gives enough time to rehabilitate any injuries or workup and treat other conditions.

Counseling athletes on health-related issues, such as tobacco and drug use, is not a primary objective of the PPE. This is because of time constraints. When time permits, physicians should counsel athletes on such health-related topics.

A complete history identifies approximately 75% of problems affecting athletes. It is a very important part of the PPE. To obtain a more accurate history, the athlete and parents should complete a history form prior to the examination.

8. **a.** Downhill skiing is considered limited contact. Sports are classified as noncontact, limited contact, and full contact/collision. The categories are based on the potential for injury from collision. In some cases, athletes may not be able to safely participate in some sports but may be able to participate in others. The classifications can help the physician make return-to-play decisions.

Noncontact sports include golf, running, swimming, and tennis.

Limited contact sports include baseball, bicycling, volleyball, in-line skating, and downhill skiing.

Contact/collision sports include basketball, soccer, diving, lacrosse, football, wrestling, and ice hockey.

9. **e.** The patient should be given full clearance to play. There is no evidence that assessing physical maturity and separating athletes according to stage of development decreases the rate of injuries. Therefore, Tanner staging is not a recommended part of the PPE.

10. **e.** Athletes with spinal cord injuries are at risk of injury from adaptive equipment such as wheelchairs and prostheses.

Heat illness is a concern in athletes with a spinal cord injury, especially when lesions are above T8. These athletes are more susceptible to heat illness because of abnormal sweating below the lesion level; venous pooling and decreased venous return in the lower limbs; and certain medications that they may be taking, such as sympathomimetics and anticholinergics. Athletes with spinal cord injuries are also more susceptible to hypothermia.

Autonomic dysreflexia is a serious condition that can occur in athletes with spinal cord injuries. It occurs more commonly in athletes with lesions above T6. An uncontrolled sympathetic response leads to cardiac dysrhythmias, sweating above the lesion, chest tightness, headache, an acute increase in blood pressure, hyperthermia, and gastrointestinal disturbances. Autonomic dysreflexia can be triggered from such things as urinary tract infection, bladder or bowel distension, pressure sores, and exercising in hot or cold weather. At the first sign of symptoms, athletes should be removed from the sports activity, potential triggers should be treated, and athletes should be transported to the nearest hospital.

It is important to know all the medications, prescription and over-the-counter, and nutritional supplements that an athlete is taking. Athletes with a spinal cord injury may be taking medications that make them more susceptible to heat and cold injuries, dehydration, sedation, and cardiovascular events. Also, be aware of potential drug side effects and drug interactions.

Summary

1. Primary objectives are as follows:
   a. Detect conditions that may predispose to injury.
   b. Detect conditions that may be life threatening or disabling.
   c. Meet legal and insurance requirements.
2. Only approximately 0.3% to 1.3% of athletes are denied clearance during the PPE.
3. The best time to perform the PPE is 6 weeks before the start of preseason practice.
4. The most common causes of sudden death in athletes are as follows:
   a. Hypertrophic cardiomyopathy (younger than age 35 years)
   b. Coronary artery disease (35 years or older)
5. Contraindications to participation in sports include the following (partial list):
   a. Fever
   b. Acute myocarditis or pericarditis
   c. Hypertrophic cardiomyopathy
   d. Long QT interval syndrome
   e. History of recent concussion and symptoms of postconcussion syndrome

   f. Acute enlargement of spleen or liver (e.g., splenomegaly seen in infectious mononucleosis)
   g. Contagious skin infections such as herpes simplex, impetigo, and molluscum contagiosum
6. The PPE should include vision screen, height, weight, blood pressure, and pulse.
7. Tanner staging is not a recommended part of the PPE.
8. Physicians should be aware of certain conditions that are more common in female athletes:
   a. Eating disorders
   b. Noncontact anterior cruciate ligament injuries
   c. Stress fractures in runners
   d. Osteopenia and osteoporosis
9. When performing a PPE on an athlete with a spinal cord injury, it is important to ask about the following:
   a. Use of adaptive equipment
   b. History of heat or cold illness
   c. History of autonomic hyperreflexia
   d. Medications (prescription and over-the-counter) and nutritional supplements

Suggested Reading

Giese EA, O'Conner FG, Brennan FH, et al: The athletic preparticipation evaluation: Cardiovascular assessment. *Am Fam Physician* 75:1008–1014, 2007.

Kurowski K, Chandran S: The preparticipation athletic evaluation. *Am Fam Physician* 61:2683–2690, 2696–2698, 2000.

Patel DR, Greydanus DE: The pediatric athlete with disabilities. *Pediatr Clin North Am* 49(4):803–827, 2002.

Smith DM, Kovan JR, Rich BSE, Tanner SM: *Preparticipation Physical Examination*, 2nd ed. Minneapolis, MN: Physician and Sports Medicine, 1997.

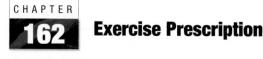

CHAPTER
162 Exercise Prescription

CLINICAL CASE PROBLEM 1

A 48-Year-Old Woman Wanting to Start an Exercise Program

A 48-year-old woman comes into the office with questions and concerns about starting an exercise program. Although she has been sedentary most of her life, she is very determined to change. She has heard about all the benefits of exercise. Her past medical history is positive for hypertension that is well controlled by taking a low dose of hydrochlorothiazide, and she has a history of irregular heavy menses now controlled by low-dose oral contraceptives.

On physical examination, her blood pressure is 125/85 mmHg and her pulse is 82 beats/minute. Her cardiovascular examination reveals regular rhythm and rate with a midsystolic click. Her lungs are clear and her abdomen is benign. The rest of the examination is normal.

SELECT THE BEST ANSWER TO THE FOLLOWING QUESTIONS

1. Which of the following would be an appropriate intervention prior to this patient's commencement of an exercise program?
   a. echocardiography
   b. complete blood count
   c. ferritin level
   d. exercise stress test
   e. no testing is indicated

2. Exercise improves outcomes for which of the following conditions?
   a. type 2 diabetes mellitus
   b. depression
   c. obesity
   d. hypertension
   e. all of the above

3. Which one of the following statements regarding exercise is true?
   a. approximately 40% of adults in the United Stated exercise enough to derive health benefits from physical activity
   b. previous athletic performance or exercise provides lasting protection
   c. increased levels of physical activity are inversely proportional to long-term cardiovascular mortality
   d. approximately 70% of physicians counsel their patients about exercise
   e. there is no evidence to support exercise as a primary intervention to promote health

4. The cardiovascular benefits of exercise include which of the following?
   a. reduced systolic and diastolic blood pressure
   b. reduced serum triglyceride level
   c. increased serum high-density lipoprotein (HDL) level
   d. reduced arterial stiffness
   e. all of the above

5. Which one of the following statements about exercise, heart rate, and autonomic function is true?
   a. regular exercise does not lower resting heart rates
   b. exercise increases heart rate variability
   c. endurance training results in decreased parasympathetic (vagal) tone
   d. endurance training results in a less rapid decrease in heart rate after exercise
   e. all of the above

6. The exercise prescription should include which of the following?
   a. flexibility training
   b. resistance or weight training
   c. duration of exercise
   d. intensity of exercise
   e. all of the above

7. Which one of the following statements about the exercise prescription is true?
   a. exercise should be performed 2 days every week
   b. exercise should be performed continuously for 90 minutes to gain any health benefits
   c. resistance training is not recommended for people older than age 60 years
   d. increasing the intensity of exercise does not reduce the risk of coronary heart disease
   e. there is a lack of evidence regarding the benefit of flexibility exercises in the prevention and treatment of musculoskeletal injuries

8. Which one of the following statements about exercise intensity is true?
   a. high-intensity exercise is defined as 65% of an individual's maximum heart rate
   b. exercise intensity can be measured in metabolic equivalents (METs); a MET is the amount of oxygen consumed during low-intensity exercise
   c. low-intensity exercise has no health benefits
   d. the formula, 220 minus the age of the patient, underestimates the maximum heart rate, especially in people older than age 55 years
   e. if a person can hold a conversation while exercising, he or she is exercising at an intensity too low to derive any health benefits

9. Approximately 50% of people stop an exercise program within 6 to 12 months. Which of the following has been shown to increase adherence to an exercise program?
   a. a high-intensity exercise program
   b. exercising alone
   c. increasing the intensity and duration of an exercise program by 40% each week
   d. alternating activities
   e. exercising just before bedtime

10. Which of the following is (are) a normal response(s) during exercise?
    a. the diastolic blood pressure remains the same or decreases
    b. the systolic blood pressure increases
    c. heart rate decreases by 12 beats or more during the first minute after peak exercise
    d. heart rate increases with exercise secondary to a withdrawal of vagal tone and increasing sympathetic tone
    e. all of the above

Answers

1. e. No testing is indicated. According to the American College of Sports Medicine guidelines, a woman younger than age 55 years who is asymptomatic and has only one risk factor for coronary artery disease does not need an exercise stress test prior to the start of an exercise program. Unless an individual is at high risk for coronary artery disease, an exercise stress test is not necessary before beginning a moderate exercise program. Moderate exercise is defined as an intensity well within the individual's capacity and one that can be sustained for a prolonged period (45 minutes). There is no evidence that an exercise stress test or echocardiogram at this age will predict increased mortality or morbidity. An exercise stress test can have false-positive results. Despite the history of heavy menses, there is no need to check for anemia because she is taking an oral contraceptive.

2. e. Exercise improves outcomes for many conditions, including atherosclerosis; ischemic heart disease; hypertension; type 2 diabetes mellitus; osteoarthritis; obesity; asthma; chronic obstructive pulmonary disease; osteoporosis; depression; anxiety; and cancer of the colon, breast, prostate, and rectum.

3. c. Increased levels of physical activity are inversely proportional to long-term cardiovascular mortality. Only 20% to 25% of adults exercise enough to derive health benefits from physical activity. Vigorous exercise early in life does not provide lasting protection. A physically active lifestyle throughout life confers significant health benefits. Less than 35% of physicians counsel their patients about exercise. Evidence supports exercise as a primary intervention to promote health.

4. e. The cardiovascular benefits of exercise include reduced systolic and diastolic blood pressure, decreased low-density lipoprotein levels, increased HDL levels, reduced triglyceride levels, reduced obesity, increased maximal volume of oxygen utilization (Vo$_2$ max), increased insulin sensitivity, improved fibrinolysis and lowered levels of fibrinogen, reduced arterial stiffness and improved arterial compliance, and increased heart rate variability. It also improves myocardial function, including increased contractility, faster relaxation rates, enzymatic alterations, increased calcium availability, and improved autonomic and hormonal function.

5. b. Exercise increases heart rate variability. A delayed recovery of heart rate after exercise significantly increases mortality. Regular exercise lowers resting and submaximal heart rates. Endurance training results in an increased parasympathetic (vagal) tone and a more rapid decrease in heart rate after exercise.

6. e. An exercise prescription should include mention of the following:
1. The type of activity: This should take into account a patient's medical status, level of fitness, interests, available exercise facilities, climate, and geographic location.
2. The frequency of exercise: The current recommendation is for people to exercise on most, preferably all, days of the week.
3. The duration of exercise: People should engage in 20 to 60 minutes of continuous or intermittent aerobic activity throughout the day.
4. The intensity of exercise: Moderate-intensity exercise, exercising at a level equal to 65% to 75% of a person's maximum heart rate, is recommended. Several methods are used to calculate the proper intensity. These include the following:
   a. The commonly used formula "220 minus age" to measure the maximal heart rate. This formula, however, underestimates the maximum heart rate, especially in people older than age 55 years.
   b. The Karvonen method to calculate exercise intensity is as follows: Training heart rate = $(HR_{max} - RHR) \times 0.7 + RHR$, where HR_{max} is the maximum heart rate, and RHR is the resting heart rate.
   c. The "talk test" can be used to avoid exercising at too high an intensity. People should exercise at an intensity not to exceed that of being able to carry on a conversation.
   d. Exercise intensity can also be measured in METs. A MET is the resting metabolic rate or the amount of oxygen consumed at rest, which is approximately 3.5 ml O$_2$/kg/minute. Metabolic equivalents are determined by treadmill testing.
5. Resistance training or weight lifting: Resistance training results in lower heart rate and blood pressure response to any given load and can improve aerobic endurance. Weight training reduces risk of coronary heart disease. Recommendation is a minimum of 8 to 10 exercises involving major muscle groups performed 2 or 3 days per week using a minimum of one set of 8 to 12 repetitions. For older people, 10 to 15 repetitions at lower resistance is more desirable because muscle strength declines by 15% per decade after age 50 years and 30% per decade after age 70 years. The goal is to lift weight that is 70% to 80% of one maximum lift.

Contraindications to resistance training are unstable angina, uncontrolled hypertension, uncontrolled dysrhythmias, uncontrolled chronic heart failure, severe stenotic or regurgitant valvular disease, and hypertrophic cardiomyopathy.

6. Flexibility training: Although there is a lack of evidence regarding benefit of flexibility exercises in the prevention and treatment of musculoskeletal injuries, it is still recommended to stretch major muscle/tendon groups, four repetitions per muscle group, a minimum of 2 or 3 days per week. Static stretches should be held for 10 to 30 seconds.

7. Warm-up and cool-down periods: Before and after exercise there should be a 5- to 10-minute period of stretching and low-level aerobic exercise.

7. **e.** As stated previously, there is a lack of evidence regarding the benefit of flexibility exercises in the prevention and treatment of musculoskeletal injuries. Exercise should be performed on all or most days of the week. Exercise does not have to be continuous to gain health benefits. Short bouts of exercise throughout the day are just as beneficial as continuous exercise. Resistance training is recommended for all adult age groups. Increasing the intensity of exercise does reduce the risk of coronary artery disease.

8. **d.** As stated previously, the formula "220 minus age" underestimates the maximum heart rate, especially in people older than age 55 years. High-intensity exercise is defined as 75% to 90% of a person's maximum heart rate. A MET is the amount of oxygen consumed at rest. Low-intensity exercise has health benefits. Exercising at an intensity still permitting one to hold a conversation has health benefits and prevents exercising at too high an intensity.

9. **d.** Alternating activities has been shown to increase adherence to an exercise program. Other interventions to increase adherence to an exercise program include the following: setting specific goals, physician's active interest, repeated counseling and educating patients about health benefits of exercise, encouragement of family and friends, limiting increases in duration and intensity to 5% to 10% per week to reduce risk of injury, and exercising with others. Patients are also more likely to adhere to a moderate-intensity program than a high-intensity one.

10. **e.** All of the responses are part of normal exercise.

Summary

1. Exercise is a primary intervention to promote health and is as powerful as smoking cessation, blood pressure control, and lipid management in lowering mortality from coronary artery disease.
2. Exercise has a favorable influence on multiple body systems and improves outcomes for many chronic diseases, including diabetes, hypertension, obesity, and depression.
3. Exercise training results in increased parasympathetic (vagal) tone and a subsequent more rapid decrease in heart rate after exercise, lower resting and submaximal heart rates, and increased heart rate variability.
4. Components of exercise prescription include the following: (a) type of activity, (b) frequency, (c) duration, (e) intensity, (f) resistance training, (g) flexibility training, (h) and warm-up and cool-down.
5. Encourage adherence to an exercise program.
6. Increasing physical activity is a major goal in the health initiative *Healthy People 2010* by the U.S. Department of Health and Human Services.

Suggested Reading

Andersen RE, Blair SN, Cheskin LJ, Bartlett SJ: Encouraging patients to become more physically active: The physician's role. *Ann Intern Med* 127(5):395–400, 1997.

Dustan D, Daly RM, Owen N, et al: High intensity resistance training improves glycemic control in older patients with type 2 diabetes. *Diabetes Care* 25(10):1729–1736, 2002.

Haskell WL, Lee IM, Pate RR, et al: Physical activity and public health: Updated recommendations from the American College of Sports Medicine and the American Heart Association. *Circulation* 116:1081–1093, 2007.

Heyward VH: *Advanced Fitness Assessment and Exercise Prescription.* Champaign, IL: Human Kinetics, 2006.

Manson JE, Greenland P, LaCroix AZ, et al: Walking compared with vigorous exercise for the prevention of cardiovascular events in women. *N Engl J Med* 347(10):716–725, 2002.

Rosenwinkel ET, Bloomfield DM, Arwady MA, Goldsmith RL: Exercise and autonomic function in health and cardiovascular disease. *Cardiol Clin* 19(3):369–387, 2001.

Stein PK, Ehsani AA, Domitrovich PP, et al: Effect of exercise training on heart rate variability in healthy older adults. *Am Heart J* 138(3):567–576, 1999.

Tanasescu M, Leitzmann MF, Rimm EB, et al: Exercise type and intensity in relation to coronary heart disease in men. *JAMA* 288(16):1994–2000, 2002.

U.S. Department of Health and Human Services: *Healthy People 2010: Understanding and Improving Health,* 2nd ed. Washington, DC: U.S. Government Printing Office, 2000.

U.S. Preventive Services Task Force: Behavioral counseling in primary care to promote physical activity: Recommendations and rationale. *Am Fam Physician* 66(10):1931–1936, 2002.

An Unconscious Football Player

As team physician for a high school football team, you are standing on the sideline during a game when you note that one player does not rise after a play. When you reach him, he is lying on his back with his eyes closed. He is not moving.

SELECT THE BEST ANSWER TO THE FOLLOWING QUESTIONS

1. Which of the following should you do first?
   a. establish that the patient has a patent airway and is breathing
   b. place a roll under the patient's neck for support
   c. check the pupils
   d. take off the patient's helmet and pads
   e. place an intravenous line

2. After approximately 10 seconds, the patient awakens. He is disoriented and confused but can tell you his name and what he had for breakfast. He does not, however, remember anything about the game. He denies any neck pain or radiating symptoms and is allowed to sit up. With help, he walks to the sideline and sits down again for your evaluation. He says that he feels perfectly fine and wants to go back into the game. Your evaluation should include:
   a. a complete neurologic evaluation
   b. immediate and long-term memory recall
   c. balance testing
   d. using the Sport Concussion Assessment Tool (SCAT) card
   e. all of the above

3. After a few moments of evaluation, the athlete begins to complain of a severe right-sided headache. He becomes lethargic and lapses again into unconsciousness. He is immediately taken to the emergency room by the ambulance on the sideline. What injury is most likely to account for his second collapse?
   a. subdural hematoma
   b. epidural hematoma
   c. diffuse axonal injury
   d. second-impact syndrome
   e. subarachnoid hemorrhage

A Confused Football Player

You are covering a college football game as a team physician. A player sustains a hard hit to the head while being tackled by two other players. He stands up directly after the play, shakes his head for a moment, and then joins the huddle for the next play. He appears confused and runs to the wrong spot. After a few more plays, one of his teammates tells the trainer that he is not remembering the plays.

4. When the trainer tells you this information, you
   a. allow him to continue play because he had no loss of consciousness and the game is almost over
   b. have the trainer check to make sure that there is enough air in his helmet
   c. watch him more carefully on the next play
   d. remove him immediately from play for evaluation
   e. remind the trainer that this particular player failed most of his classes the previous semester

5. When you speak to the athlete, he states that he feels fine and wants to go back to play. He denies headache or dizziness and has a normal neurologic examination. He cannot recall three objects 2 minutes after being told them. He also cannot subtract serial 7s accurately. You now should
   a. allow him to return to play because he has a normal neurologic examination
   b. send him directly to the hospital for a computed tomography (CT) scan of the head
   c. have the athlete sit down quietly and retest him in 15 minutes
   d. send him to the showers
   e. send him home with his parents

6. The most important reason for not allowing an athlete with symptoms of a concussion to play is
   a. he has not been checked for a neck injury
   b. the athlete may experience headache and dizziness with exertion
   c. if the athlete is injured, the physician is likely to be sued
   d. if the patient cannot remember the plays, the team is likely to lose the game
   e. the athlete is at risk for much more severe injury if he sustains another hit

7. Which of the following statements is false?
   a. in high school football players, there is a 15% to 20% risk of a head injury per season
   b. multiple concussions can result in cumulative brain damage

c. there does not have to be a loss of consciousness for there to be a diagnosis of concussion

d. athletes readily admit to symptoms of a concussion

e. close observation of the athlete is of critical importance after a head injury

8. Warning signs for which an athlete who has sustained a concussion should seek immediate medical evaluation include which of the following?
   a. difficulty in staying awake
   b. seizures
   c. urinary or bowel incontinence
   d. weakness or numbness of any part of the body
   e. all of the above

CLINICAL CASE PROBLEM 3

A Gymnast Who Fell and Hit Her Head

A gymnast fell off the uneven bars during a competition and hit her head on the ground. She had a 2-minute loss of consciousness and had posttraumatic amnesia for 2 hours, which completely resolved. She was sent to the emergency room and had a CT scan of the head, which was negative for any intracranial bleeding. She was discharged home. Two days later, she comes to your office complaining of headache and the inability to concentrate in class.

9. This patient has signs and symptoms of which of the following?
   a. postconcussive syndrome
   b. continuing symptoms of a concussion
   c. second-impact syndrome
   d. epidural hematoma
   e. malingering

10. This athlete has an important competition in 2 days. She should be
    a. allowed to participate because her CT scan was negative for any bleeding
    b. allowed to do any event except for the uneven bars
    c. restricted from any activity until she has been asymptomatic for at least 1 week and has no symptoms on exertion
    d. restricted until her headache goes away at rest
    e. readmitted to the hospital for another CT scan of the head

11. This athlete recovers and returns to competition after 2 weeks. Three weeks later, she receives a glancing blow to the head and sustains another loss of consciousness, this time of less than 30 seconds. She has no amnesia and recovers quickly with no symptoms of headache or difficulty concentrating. She should do which of the following?
    a. return to competition as soon as she is asymptomatic
    b. return to competition when she has been asymptomatic for 1 week
    c. be restricted from activity for at least 2 weeks
    d. return to competition but wear a helmet
    e. exercise on a stationary bicycle for 2 weeks even if she has symptoms to retain conditioning

12. According to the *Summary and Agreement Statement of the 2nd International Conference of Concussion in Sport, Prague 2004*, which one of the following statements is false?
    a. concussions are classified as simple or complex
    b. concussion severity can only be determined in retrospect after all symptoms resolve and neurological and cognitive exams are normal
    c. "cognitive rest" may be one consideration for children recovering from concussion
    d. neuropsychological testing can be the sole basis for return to play decisions
    e. the SCAT is useful for sideline physicians in evaluating and educating athletes who sustain a concussion

13. Which one of the following statements is false?
    a. the Glasgow Coma Scale is a useful adjunct for evaluating an athlete after a head injury
    b. despite the different guidelines for return to play, the final decision should be based on the individual situation and the best clinical judgment
    c. types of intracranial injuries that can be encountered in the athlete include epidural hematomas, subdural hematomas, subarachnoid hemorrhages, diffuse axonal injury, and intracerebral hematomas
    d. concussions can have long-lasting effects on cognitive abilities and concentration
    e. concussions can be prevented by proper helmet use

Answers

1. **a.** No matter what the situation, the ABCs of airway, breathing, and circulation should be the clinician's first concern. Once these are established, other concerns can be addressed. An unconscious football player cannot tell the physician if his neck is hurting; therefore, any unconscious player is assumed to have a cervical spine injury until proven otherwise. The spine should be immobilized, and if the patient is prone, experienced

team members can help to logroll the patient. Football pads and helmets are specially designed to keep the head and neck in a proper position, so they should not be removed until the patient is under controlled circumstances in which the entire head and spine can be stabilized. The face mask of the helmet can be removed if the athlete's airway is an issue. A roll should not be placed under the patient's neck. Checking the pupils will be a part of the later assessment.

2. e. Evaluation after a head injury should include a complete neurologic examination. Sports concussion is defined by the *Summary and Agreement Statement of the 2nd International Conference on Concussion in Sport, Prague 2004* as "a complex pathophysiological process affecting the brain, induced by traumatic biomechanical forces." Concussion can result from direct force to the head or to anywhere on the body with resultant forces transmitted to the head. Any loss or alteration of consciousness requires a complete examination. Neuropsychological testing can aid in determining the athlete's cognitive function and coordination. Athletes can be apparently asymptomatic after a concussion and still have severe problems with memory, concentration, and coordination. Asking patients to recall what they had for breakfast tests long-term memory. Giving the athlete several items to remember and then asking for them a few moments later tests immediate recall. Asking the athlete to subtract serial 7s from 100 assesses figuring and concentration. Balancing on one foot with the eyes closed tests coordination. The SCAT is useful to the physician in assessing the athlete on the sideline.

3. b. This case shows a common presentation of an epidural hematoma. The typical scenario is that of an athlete sustaining a head injury, commonly on the temple. The athlete has a brief period of confusion or unconsciousness and then has a "lucid period," during which the athlete feels fine. Rapid deterioration, lethargy, and unconsciousness occur in the next stage. This is caused by a high-pressure arterial bleed into the epidural space, often from rupture of the middle meningeal artery as it passes behind the temporal bone. Prompt neurosurgical evacuation of the hematoma is critical and must be done emergently. If the hematoma can be recognized and evacuated in a timely manner, the prognosis is good for these patients because there is usually little underlying brain damage. Failure to recognize and evacuate this hematoma can lead to coma and death.

4. d. The player should be immediately removed from play for evaluation. Despite having no loss of consciousness, he is symptomatic with amnesia and has sustained at least a grade I concussion. He must be evaluated and protected from subsequent hits, which could worsen his condition. Hits such as the one that this athlete sustained are often referred to as "dings" or having one's "bell rung." Safety equipment such as helmets should be checked regularly, but in this situation the athlete has already sustained the hit. The athlete's academic performance has no bearing on whether he can remember his regular plays.

There are several different systems of scoring concussions and determining subsequent return-to-play decisions. One was developed by the American Academy of Neurology (AAN) and another was developed by Dr. Robert C. Cantu. In both systems, concussions are graded from I to III. According to AAN guidelines, grade I concussion consists of transient confusion, no loss of consciousness, and symptoms less than 15 minutes. Grade II concussion consists of transient confusion, no loss of consciousness, and symptoms more than 15 minutes. Grade III concussion consists of any loss of consciousness. According to the Cantu guidelines, a grade I concussion consists of no loss of consciousness and posttraumatic amnesia or symptoms lasting less than 30 minutes. Grade II concussion consists of a loss of consciousness of less than 1 minute and/or posttraumatic amnesia or symptoms lasting more than 30 minutes but less than 24 hours. Grade III concussion consists of a loss of consciousness of 1 minute or more and/or posttraumatic amnesia or symptoms lasting 24 hours or more.

5. c. The athlete is still experiencing posttraumatic amnesia and must continue to be evaluated. There are no focal deficits on neurologic examination to cause concern. The athlete should sit quietly on the bench (and not exert himself on the sideline) under close observation. In approximately 15 to 20 minutes, he can be reevaluated for amnesia. He should not go home with his parents until his symptoms have resolved, and he should definitely not go to the showers, where he will be unobserved. At this time, there is no indication for a CT scan of the head; however, if there is any neurological decline, emergent CT scan of the head should be performed.

6. e. Athletes still suffering symptoms from a concussion should not be allowed to play. Concussion symptoms include cognitive defects (e.g., confusion and unaware of score of game), physical signs (e.g., poor balance, vomiting, vacant stare, and significant decrease in playing ability), and typical symptoms (e.g., headache, nausea, dizziness, and vision disturbance). The effects of multiple head injuries have been found to be cumulative. Also, after an athlete sustains one concussion, he or she is more likely to sustain another concussion, often with a milder hit. The most significant cause for concern is the so-called "second-impact syndrome." Although widely known, the existence of this entity has been questioned because there were only 17 reported cases between 1984 and 1997. It is theorized to occur when an athlete sustains a second hit while still recovering from the first. When this occurs, the autoregulation of the brain is lost, and there is an intense reaction of brain swelling and edema. There is a greater than 50% mortality rate with this condition. This catastrophic possibility is the reasoning behind limiting the activity of all athletes who continue to be symptomatic after a head injury.

7. d. Often, athletes are so enthusiastic about their sport that they wish to participate even after a significant head injury. Athletes may not understand the dangers of participation and may lie about their symptoms so as to return to play. This is where accurate neuropsychological testing is critical; if an athlete has amnesia, he or she cannot "fake" memory. If hand–eye coordination or balance have not yet recovered, this will also be obvious on testing.

Prevalence studies have shown an approximately 10% rate of concussion per season for college football players and 15% to 20% risk of head injury per season for high school football players. Other risky sports include ice hockey, soccer, boxing, wrestling, and rugby.

As discussed previously, there does not need to be a loss of consciousness for a diagnosis of concussion. Multiple head injuries can cause cumulative brain damage. Close observation is of critical importance for any athlete with any type of head injury.

8. e. Any athlete who develops the following symptoms should seek immediate medical attention, even if he or she has been asymptomatic after a head injury: lethargy or difficulty in staying awake, loss of bowel or bladder function, vomiting, severe or worsening headache, neck pain, seizures, weakness or numbness, or difficulties with vision. Any of these symptoms could indicate a more serious injury.

9. a. This patient has signs and symptoms of postconcussive syndrome. These symptoms include headache, dizziness, inability to concentrate, irritability, tinnitus, problems with balance, fatigue, or difficulty sleeping. These symptoms can last for days to weeks after a concussion.

Because this patient recovered her memory within 2 hours of the injury, she is no longer experiencing the actual concussion. The patient, by history, has not sustained another head injury, so second-impact syndrome would be highly unlikely.

10. c. The athlete should be restricted from activity until she has been asymptomatic for at least 1 week. When she has been asymptomatic, she may begin light exercise. If the headache or other symptoms recur, she should cease the activity and rest. Symptoms may recur with exertion, even when the athlete feels normal at rest. Allowing her to participate puts her at risk for another head injury, especially in a sport such as gymnastics, in which precision and balance are critical for safety.

Even without bleeding on CT scan, the athlete may have sustained significant shearing injury or diffuse axonal injury. These injuries can cause disability and place the athlete at risk for further head injuries.

It is relatively common for an athlete to experience symptoms such as this after a significant concussion as described. If the symptoms do not improve over the following days, however, a repeat CT or magnetic resonance imaging of the head may be warranted to rule out any further injury, such as cerebral contusion or slow bleeding subdural hematoma.

11. c. Separate systems exist for return-to-play guidelines after multiple concussions. All exertional physical activity, including stationary bicycling, should be restricted while the patient is experiencing symptoms. Many different guidelines have been proposed for grading concussions, including the AAN and Cantu guidelines. However, the *Summary and Agreement Statement of the 2nd International Conference on Concussion in Sport, Prague 2004* suggested abandoning them and classified concussions as simple or complex. In this case, a more conservative return-to-play approach is warranted because this is the second concussion sustained with loss of consciousness.

12. d. Neuropsychological testing is one tool, but not the only tool, in making return-to-play decisions. Best clinical judgment, taking into account various factors including, but not limited to, patient's concussion history, physical findings, cognitive defects, and type of sport played, should be the basis for making these decisions. As stated previously, according to the Prague guidelines, concussions were classified as simple or complex. A simple concussion "progressively resolves without complication in 7 to 10 days." An athlete who suffers a simple concussion should rest until all symptoms resolve and then start on a graduated exertional program. Complex concussion involves "persistent symptoms, specific sequelae, prolonged loss of consciousness (>1 minute), or prolonged cognitive impairment following the injury." Concussions for athletes who have suffered multiple prior concussions are also labeled as complex. Athletes with complex concussions should be managed with a multidisciplinary approach by a physician experienced in managing sport concussions. Formal neuropsychological testing should also be considered in patients with complex concussions. Also, according to the Prague guidelines, concussion severity can only be determined in retrospect after all symptoms resolve. SCAT was developed as a standardized tool to aid the sideline physician in evaluating and educating athletes who sustain a concussion.

13. **e.** Proper helmet and other safety equipment use can decrease the likelihood of concussion, but no helmets or safety measures have been found to eliminate risk altogether. In fact, it has been proposed that protective equipment including helmets, although designed to prevent injuries, may prompt the user to act more aggressively and take more risk leading to more injuries. This is known as the risk compensation theory. Certain sports carry a small but definite risk of serious, even fatal, injury. Athletes and parents should be aware of this. The Glasgow Coma Scale should be used as a helpful tool in evaluating an athlete with a head injury. Intracranial injuries that may be encountered in the athlete include epidural hematomas, subdural hematomas, subarachnoid hemorrhages, diffuse axonal injury, and intracerebral hematomas. Cognitive deficits and impaired concentration can linger for weeks after a concussion, as described as a part of the postconcussion syndrome. It must be remembered that the guidelines for return to play are comprehensive and of great use, but they are only guidelines. Each athlete is an individual, and clinical judgment must be the deciding factor in decisions to return to play safely.

Summary

Sports concussion is defined by the *Summary and Agreement Statement of the 2nd International Conference on Concussion in Sport, Prague 2004* as "a complex pathophysiological process affecting the brain, induced by traumatic biomechanical forces." Participation in certain sports, especially contact sports, places the athlete at risk for concussion. Several grading systems have been developed for evaluating the severity of a concussion. These guidelines grade concussions from grade I to grade III or as simplex or complex.

Concussion can represent different types of brain injury, and the clinician must be considering epidural hematomas, subdural hematomas, subarachnoid hemorrhages, diffuse axonal injury, and intracerebral hematomas in the differential examination. Suspicion of intracranial bleeding, lethargy, emesis, worsening headaches, neck injury, bowel or bladder incontinence, and focal neurologic signs should elicit prompt referral to a hospital with a neurosurgical service.

Postconcussion syndrome is characterized by continuing headache, dizziness, inability to concentrate, impaired balance or cognitive ability, irritability, fatigue, and difficulties sleeping. Patients should be followed closely by the physician and/or responsible party and kept at rest because exercise may exacerbate the symptoms.

Return-to-play guidelines were listed previously in the chapter and are very useful to the clinician, but individual clinical judgment should be the deciding factor. Athletes who have sustained one concussion are more likely than others to sustain another concussion. In addition, the "second-impact syndrome" is a catastrophic syndrome of sudden brain edema after a second head injury, in which the athlete had not yet recovered from the first head injury. This carries a high mortality rate and is the basis for keeping an athlete out of activity until completely recovered.

Suggested Reading

McCrory P, Johnston K, Meeuwisse W, et al: Summary and agreement statement of the 2nd International Conference on Concussion in Sport, Prague 2004. *Br J Sports Med* 39:196–204, 2005.

Ropper AH, Gorson KC: Concussion. *N Engl J Med* 356:166–172, 2007.
Whiteside JW: Management of head and neck injuries by the sideline physician. *Am Fam Physician* 74(8):1357–1362, 2006.

CHAPTER 164

Acceleration and Deceleration Neck Injuries

CLINICAL CASE PROBLEM 1

A 32-Year-Old Female with Very Severe Neck Pain

A 32-year-old female comes into your office complaining of "very severe" neck pain that radiates to the region of the left shoulder. She was involved in a motor vehicle accident 1 day ago. Her car was struck from behind while stopped at a traffic light. The pain did not start until this morning and has gotten progressively worse. Over-the-counter analgesics have given no relief. Past medical history is negative, including no previous history of neck pain.

On examination, there is significantly decreased range of motion of the neck in all planes. There is tenderness to palpation in the cervical paraspinal muscles bilaterally. There is no bony tenderness. You try to perform a Spurling's test, but the patient has too much pain when you attempt to put the neck into the provocative position. There are no neurologic deficits.

SELECT THE BEST ANSWER TO THE FOLLOWING QUESTIONS

1. Which of the following statements regarding whip-lash injury is correct?
   a. symptoms are often out of proportion to physical findings
   b. only approximately 1% of patients will have an abnormality on magnetic resonance imaging (MRI) scan related to the trauma
   c. x-rays often show a slight flattening of the normal lordotic curvature of the cervical spine
   d. the annual economic cost in the United States related to whiplash injury is in the billions of dollars
   e. all of the above

2. Which of the following statements regarding the mechanism of whiplash injury is correct?
   a. most commonly results from motor vehicle accident
   b. after a rear impact, the lower cervical vertebrae appear to move into extension and the upper cervical vertebrae appear to move into relative flexion
   c. the cervical paraspinal muscles are not involved

   d. a and b
   e. a, b, and c

3. Which of the following is the best treatment option for this patient?
   a. soft cervical collar
   b. hard cervical collar
   c. early exercise therapy
   d. bed rest
   e. none of the above

4. Which of the following is a predictor of delayed recovery from a whiplash injury?
   a. older age
   b. severe pain
   c. radicular symptoms
   d. a and c
   e. a, b, and c

5. Which of the following is a correct statement regarding whiplash injury?
   a. insurance and compensation systems have no impact on prognosis
   b. without any treatment, a large number of patients will get better within 6 months
   c. patients rarely have loss of neck motion
   d. all of the above
   e. none of the above

Answers

1. **e.** The symptoms of whiplash injury are often out of proportion to the findings on examination. Only approximately 1% of patients with a whiplash injury will have an abnormality related to trauma, such as prevertebral edema, on MRI. After an acceleration–deceleration injury, radiographs often show a slight flattening of the normal lordotic curve of the cervical spine. Whiplash injuries pose a tremendous economic cost, in the billions of dollars, in the United States.

2. **d.** Whiplash injuries most commonly result when a person in a stopped car is struck from behind. Studies have demonstrated that with a rear impact the cervical spine moves into an abnormal S-shaped pattern, with the lower cervical vertebrae moving into an extended position and the upper cervical vertebrae moving into a flexed position. The cervical paraspinal muscles respond by contracting.

3. **c.** The best treatment is early exercise therapy. This has been shown to reduce pain and increase motion of the cervical spine. Bed rest and cervical collars have been shown to slow healing.

4. **e.** Predictors of delayed recovery from a whiplash injury include older age, radicular symptoms, poor coping style, depressed mood, and severe neck or head pain.

5. **b.** Insurance and compensation systems significantly influence the prognosis of whiplash injuries.

Even without any treatment, a large number of patients will get better within 6 months after sustaining a whiplash injury. Patients commonly have restricted motion of the cervical spine after sustaining an acceleration–deceleration type neck injury.

Summary

1. The neck injury most commonly results when the patient is in a stopped car that is struck from behind by another vehicle. There is a resultant hyperflexion and hyperextension of the neck.
2. Such injuries have a major economic cost (billions of dollars).
3. Radiographs frequently show a slight flattening of the normal lordotic curve of the cervical spine.
4. MRI usually shows no abnormality related to the trauma sustained in an acceleration–deceleration injury.
5. The cervical spine assumes an S-shaped pattern immediately on impact, with the lower cervical vertebrae

moving into an extended position and the upper cervical vertebrae moving into a flexed position.
6. Predictors of delayed recovery include older age, radicular symptoms, severe neck or head pain, poor coping style, and depressed mood.
7. Insurance and compensation systems influence the prognosis of these injuries.
8. Exercise therapy is recommended early on in the treatment.
9. Even without treatment, most people will get better within 6 months. Nonetheless, evidence suggests that 50% of those who sustain whiplash will report symptoms of neck pain 1 year later.

Suggested Reading

Bagley LJ: Imaging of spinal trauma. *Radiol Clin North Am* 44(1):1–12, vii, 2006.

Carroll LJ, Holm LW, Hogg-Johnson S, et al: Course and prognostic factors for neck pain in whiplash-associated disorders: Results of the

Bone and Joint Decade 2000–2010 Task Force on Neck Pain and Its Associated Disorders. *Spine* 33(4 Suppl):s83–s92, 2008.

Eck JC, Hodges SD, Humphreys SC: Whiplash: A review of a commonly misunderstood injury. *Am J Med* 110(8):651–656, 2001.

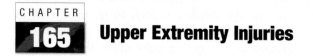

CHAPTER

165 Upper Extremity Injuries

CLINICAL CASE PROBLEM 1

A 42-Year-Old Male with Right Shoulder Pain

A 42-year-old male comes to your office with complaints of right shoulder pain. He does not remember any specific injury but has been playing a lot of tennis during the past 4 months. He tells you that "opposing players no longer fear my serve." It has become difficult and painful for him to reach overhead and behind him. Even rolling onto his shoulder in bed is painful.

On examination of the right shoulder, there is full range of motion in all planes with obvious discomfort at end ranges of flexion, abduction, and internal

rotation. There is significant pain when you place the shoulder in a position of 90 degrees flexion and then internally rotate. There is also moderate weakness with abduction and external rotation of the shoulder. The rest of the musculoskeletal examination is normal.

SELECT THE BEST ANSWER TO THE FOLLOWING QUESTIONS

1. Which of the following is the most likely diagnosis?
   a. acromioclavicular sprain
   b. rotator cuff tear
   c. adhesive capsulitis
   d. impingement syndrome
   e. cervical radiculopathy

2. Which of the following is the the best initial treatment?
   a. corticosteroid injection
   b. arthroscopic subacromial decompression

c. strengthening and range-of-motion exercises
d. elbow sling
e. cervical collar

3. Predisposing factors for this problem include which of the following?
   a. repetitive motion of the shoulder above the horizontal plane
   b. hooked acromion
   c. acromioclavicular spurring
   d. shoulder instability
   e. all of the above

CLINICAL CASE PROBLEM 2

A 37-Year-Old Male with Right Elbow Pain

A 37-year-old male comes to the office complaining of right elbow pain. He has been painting the walls of his kitchen for the past 5 days. He tells you that the colors came out beautiful, his wife is very happy, but he is "really paying the price." He has pain with lifting, shaking hands, and elbow extension.

On examination, he has full range of motion of the elbow but pain when the elbow is fully extended. There is also pain and weakness with wrist extension and supination against resistance. Palpation reveals tenderness over the dorsum of the forearm extending proximally to the elbow. The rest of the musculoskeletal examination is normal.

4. Which of the following is the most likely diagnosis?
   a. lateral epicondylitis
   b. olecranon bursitis
   c. wrist strain
   d. cubital tunnel syndrome
   e. olecranon stress fracture

5. What is the the primary muscle involved in this condition?
   a. triceps
   b. extensor carpi radialis brevis
   c. extensor carpi ulnaris
   d. flexor digitorum profundus
   e. pronator teres

6. Which of the following is the best initial treatment?
   a. corticosteroid injection
   b. surgical debridement
   c. short arm cast
   d. rest and a progressive stretching and strengthening program
   e. elbow sling

CLINICAL CASE PROBLEM 3

A 29-Year-Old Woman with Severe Wrist Pain

A 29-year-old woman comes to the office with severe wrist pain. She has had the pain for a few months, but during the past month it has worsened significantly. She denies any trauma, and other than having a cesarean section 4 months ago, her past medical and surgical histories are unremarkable.

On examination, there is tenderness just distal to the radial styloid. Finkelstein's test is positive. Phalen's test is negative. There is full range of motion of the wrist.

7. Which of the following is the most likely diagnosis?
   a. carpal tunnel syndrome
   b. scaphoid fracture
   c. ulnar nerve entrapment
   d. Kienböck's disease
   e. De Quervain's tenosynovitis

8. What is the best initial treatment?
   a. thumb spica splint
   b. surgical release
   c. long arm cast
   d. volar wrist splint
   e. low-dose amitriptyline

CLINICAL CASE PROBLEM 4

A 23-Year-Old Female with a Painful Thumb

A 23-year-old female injured her hand while skiing 1 day ago. She "caught an edge" and fell onto her right ski pole. She notices swelling at the base of her thumb and has pain when she moves or bangs the thumb.

On examination, there is tenderness over the medial aspect of the first metacarpophalangeal joint. When you stress test the ulnar collateral ligament, you note laxity compared to the opposite hand, but there is a firm endpoint. There is no tenderness to palpation of the anatomic snuffbox.

9. Which of the following is the most likely diagnosis?
   a. grade I sprain of the ulnar collateral ligament
   b. grade II sprain of the ulnar collateral ligament
   c. grade III sprain of the ulnar collateral ligament
   d. fracture of the head of the first metacarpal
   e. fracture of the scaphoid

10. What is the best initial treatment?
   a. surgical repair
   b. physical therapy
   c. corticosteroid injection
   d. nonsteroidal anti-inflammatory drugs (NSAIDs)
   e. cast immobilization

Answers

1. d. Shoulder impingement, also known as "painful arc syndrome," is a common shoulder disorder. It is often the result of the supraspinatus tendon and the subacromial bursa impinging between the greater tubercle of the humeral head and the lateral edge of the acromion process. This may be the result of a curved or hooked acromion, acromioclavicular spurring, repetitive motion of the shoulder above the horizontal plane, or instability of the glenohumeral joint leading to a functional loss of the subacromial space. Physical examination often reveals a limitation in shoulder range of motion and pain with provocative tests. In the Neer's maneuver, the shoulder is passively flexed to 180 degrees and internally rotated with the examiner holding the scapula stable. With Hawkin's maneuver, the shoulder is forward flexed to 90 degrees with forearm parallel to the floor, and the examiner passively internally rotates the shoulder while keeping the arm in the forward flexed position.

2. c. Strengthening and range-of-motion exercises are essential in the treatment of rotator cuff impingement syndrome and are prescribed early in the course of treatment. Corticosteroid injection into the subacromial bursa is typically given later in the course of treatment, if more conservative therapeutic modalities have failed. Arthroscopic subacromial decompression is considered if conservative treatment fails after 3 to 6 months. An elbow sling is not indicated. If the shoulder is immobilized for an extended period, the patient is at risk for developing adhesive capsulitis.

3. e. All are predisposing factors for rotator cuff impingement syndrome.

4. a. Lateral epicondylitis, an injury to the wrist extensor and supinator muscles, results from either repetitive strain or a single traumatic event. Patients typically complain of pain in the elbow or dorsum of the forearm that is aggravated with activity. Physical examination reveals tenderness on the lateral epicondyle, pain with passive wrist flexion, and pain with resisted wrist extension and supination.

5. b. The primary muscles involved in this condition are the extensor carpi radialis brevis and longus.

6. d. The best initial treatment is rest and a progressive stretching and strengthening program. Other treatments include NSAIDs, a compression strap or counterforce bracing, and modifying aggravating activities. Corticosteroid injection may be given later in the course of treatment. Surgical debridement is reserved for patients who have failed all conservative therapy. Immobilization of the elbow and a short arm cast are not part of the treatment for lateral epicondylitis; however, splinting the wrist may provide some relief for patients suffering from a chronic condition.

7. e. De Quervain's disease is a stenosing tenosynovitis of the first dorsal compartment of the wrist. The abductor pollicis longus and the extensor pollicis brevis tendons traverse a thick sheath at the radial styloid that can become thick and fibrous with repetitive or unaccustomed use of the thumb. On physical examination, there is tenderness to palpation in the region of the radial styloid and pain with Finkelstein's test. This test is performed by having the patient make a fist with the thumb tucked inside the fingers and the wrist is ulnar deviated.

8. a. The best initial treatment is a thumb spica splint for 3 or 4 weeks. Additional treatment includes NSAIDs, modifying aggravating activities, and stretching exercises when pain-free. For resistant cases, a corticosteroid injection may be beneficial. Surgery is indicated when all conservative management fails.

9. b. The most likely diagnosis is a grade II sprain of the ulnar collateral ligament. This injury is commonly referred to as "skier's thumb" or "gamekeeper's thumb." Patients present with pain and swelling along the ulnar aspect of the metacarpophalangeal joint of the thumb. It is important to stress test the ulnar collateral ligament to grade the degree of injury after x-rays are completed and show no bony involvement. Compared to a grade II sprain, a grade I sprain has no laxity when stress testing and a grade III sprain does not have a firm endpoint when stress testing.

10. e. The best initial treatment is cast immobilization for at least 3 weeks. A grade III sprain of the ulnar collateral ligament or bony involvement may require surgical treatment.

Summary

1. Rotator cuff impingement is a common shoulder disorder caused by the supraspinatus tendon being pinched between the greater tubercle of the humerus and the acromion process
   a. Predisposing factors: curved or hooked acromion, acromioclavicular spurring, repetitive motion of the shoulder above the horizontal plane, and instability of the glenohumeral joint
   b. Clues on examination: painful arc, decreased range of motion, and Neer's and Hawkin's maneuvers produce pain
   c. Treatment: strengthening and range-of-motion exercises, avoidance of aggravating activities, NSAIDs, corticosteroid injection, and arthroscopic subacromial decompression if conservative treatment fails
2. Lateral epicondylitis is caused by injury to wrist extensor and supinator muscles as the result of repetitive strain or a single traumatic event. The extensor carpi radialis brevis and longus are most commonly involved.
   a. Clues on examination: tenderness over lateral epicondyle, pain with passive wrist flexion, and pain with resisted wrist extension and supination

   b. Treatment: rest, progressive stretching and strengthening program, counterforce bracing, modifying aggravating activities, and corticosteroid injection if necessary
3. De Quervain's tenosynovitis is stenosing tenosynovitis of the first dorsal compartment of the wrist and is caused by repetitive grasping or repetitive use of the thumb.
   a. Clues on examination: tenderness in the region of radial styloid and a positive Finkelstein's test
   b. Treatment: thumb spica splint, NSAIDs, modifying aggravating activities, physical therapy, corticosteroid injection if necessary, and surgery if conservative treatment fails
4. Ulnar collateral ligament sprain of thumb (skier's thumb or gamekeeper's thumb) is caused by a traumatic injury to the thumb in abduction.
   a. Clues on examination: tenderness at insertion of ulnar collateral ligament and stress testing on the ulnar collateral ligament to check for laxity and severity of injury
   b. Treatment: thumb spica splint or cast immobilization, and surgery sometimes necessary in grade III injuries or when an avulsion fracture is present

Suggested Reading

Mellion MB, Walsh, WM, Madden, C, et al, eds: *Team Physician's Handbook*, 3rd ed. Philadelphia: Hanley & Belfus, 2002.

Sallis RE, Massimino F, eds: *ACSM's Essentials of Sports Medicine.* St. Louis: Mosby, 1997.
Wilson JJ, Best TM: Common overuse tendon problems: A review and recommendations for treatment. *Am Fam Physician* 72:811–818, 2005.

CHAPTER 166 — Low Back Pain

CLINICAL CASE PROBLEM 1

A 28-Year-Old Male with Chronic Low Back Pain

A 28-year-old male with chronic low back pain (LBP) comes to your office for renewal of his medication. He was injured at work 5 years ago while attempting to lift a box of very heavy tools. Since that time, he has been off work, living on compensation insurance payments, and has not been able to find a job that does not aggravate his back.

On physical examination, the patient demonstrates some vague tenderness in the paravertebral area around L3 to L5. He has some limitations on both flexion and extension.

SELECT THE BEST ANSWER TO THE FOLLOWING QUESTIONS

1. Which of the following statements regarding chronic LBP is false?
   a. approximately 35% of patients with acute LBP will develop chronic LBP
   b. patients who develop chronic LBP account for up to 85% of workers' compensation cost
   c. patients older than age 50 years are more likely to develop chronic LBP
   d. patients who miss work for up to 2 years are unlikely to return to work in any capacity, regardless of treatment
   e. there are multiple psychosocial factors that can lead to developing chronic LBP

2. Regarding the pathogenesis of LBP, which of the following statements is true?
   a. in up to 90% of cases of LBP, a definite anatomic or pathophysiologic diagnosis cannot be made
   b. approximately 10% of patients with acute LBP will eventually require surgery
   c. patients with acute LBP and no previous surgical procedures have a 20% to 25% chance of recovering after 6 weeks, regardless of the treatment used
   d. the anatomic structures causing LBP are identified clearly
   e. none of the above statements are true

3. Regarding the treatment of chronic LBP, which of the following statements is false?
   a. cognitive–behavioral therapy has been shown to decrease pain intensity
   b. studies have shown that treatment at back schools has no long-term effectiveness after 1 year
   c. of all the antidepressant classes, the tricyclic and tetracyclic classes have been shown to be of most benefit in the treatment of chronic LBP
   d. spinal decompression is a valid recommendation for the treatment of chronic LBP
   e. none of the above

4. Which of the following is the most common cause of LBP?
   a. metastatic bone disease
   b. inflammatory back pain
   c. lumbosacral sprain or strain
   d. posterior facet strain
   e. none of the above

5. Which of the following treatments has little support for its effectiveness in the treatment of chronic LBP?
   a. physical therapy
   b. acupuncture
   c. osteopathic manipulation
   d. prolotherapy
   e. massage therapy

CLINICAL CASE PROBLEM 2

A 64-Year-Old Male with Back and Leg Pain Aggravated by Walking

A 64-year-old male comes to the office complaining of back and leg pain that is aggravated by walking. He tells you that the pain starts after walking two blocks. He gets relief when sitting or when walking and leaning forward. Physical examination reveals

pain and decreased motion with backward bending of the lumbosacral spine. There is a negative straight leg raise test, and there are no neurologic deficits.

6. What is the most likely diagnosis?
   a. vascular claudication
   b. Reiter syndrome
   c. spinal stenosis
   d. herniated disc L5
   e. mechanical LBP

7. Which of the following is not indicative of inflammatory back pain such as ankylosing spondylitis?
   a. insidious onset
   b. onset before age 40 years
   c. pain for more than 3 months
   d. morning stiffness
   e. aggravation of pain with activity

8. Which of the following statements regarding the history and physical examination of a patient with LBP is true?
   a. the positive predictive value of the history in LBP is high
   b. the positive predictive value of the physical examination in LBP is high
   c. the positive predictive value of the radiographic investigations for patients with LBP is high
   d. the positive predictive value of serum blood and chemistry for LBP is high
   e. none of the above statements are true

9. Which of the following is (are) characteristic of a history of mechanical LBP?
   a. relatively acute onset
   b. a history of overuse or a precipitating injury
   c. pain worse during the day
   d. a and b
   e. a, b, and c

10. Which of the following is (are) a "red flag(s)" or danger signal(s) relative to the diagnosis of LBP?
    a. bowel or bladder dysfunction
    b. impotence
    c. weight loss
    d. significant night pain
    e. all of the above

11. Which of the following statements regarding plain spinal x-rays of patients with LBP is false?
    a. osteophyte formation in the intervertebral space is predictive of discogenic disease
    b. there is little justification for the extensive use of radiography in LBP
    c. there is a poor relationship between most radiographic abnormalities and symptoms of LBP

d. x-rays of the lumbar spine are associated with gonadal radiation exposure

e. there is a low yield of findings on plain x-rays that alter management of LBP

12. Which of the following statements regarding the use of computed tomography (CT) or magnetic resonance imaging (MRI) scanning in the diagnosis of disc herniation and spinal stenosis is false?
   a. CT and MRI scanning have largely replaced myelography in the diagnosis of disc herniation
   b. as many as 25% of asymptomatic people will have findings of a herniated disc on MRI
   c. CT scanning is better than MRI scanning with regard to imaging soft tissues
   d. if CT or MRI scanning is to be used in the diagnosis of a disc herniation and/or spinal stenosis, then surgery should be a serious pretest consideration
   e. none of the above statements are false

13. What is the most cost-effective and crucial aspect of the treatment of chronic LBP?
   a. patient education
   b. physiotherapy
   c. bed rest
   d. muscle relaxants
   e. nonsteroidal anti-inflammatory drugs (NSAIDs)

14. Regarding the use of exercises in the treatment of chronic LBP, which of the following statements is true?
   a. exercises allow patients to participate in their treatment program
   b. exercises should follow a graduated progression
   c. following the beginning of an exercise program for LBP, a temporary increase in pain may occur
   d. stretching exercises are recommended in the initial exercise program; isometric strengthening exercises follow
   e. all of the above

15. Which of the following statements regarding the treatment of acute LBP is true?
   a. bed rest for 7 days is recommended
   b. acupuncture is not an effective treatment for acute LBP
   c. specific exercises are effective for the treatment of acute LBP
   d. NSAIDs are effective for short-term symptomatic relief in acute LBP
   e. osteopathic manipulation has not been shown to be effective for the treatment of acute LBP

Answers

1. **a.** Up to 90% of patients will improve within 3 months; the 10% who develop chronic LBP (lasting more than 3 months) account for up to 85% of the cost of workers' compensation. There are many psychosocial factors that contribute to developing chronic LBP, including depression, job dissatisfaction, education level, and having the case be a workers' compensation case. Patients older than age 50 years are more likely to develop chronic LBP. Those who miss work for up to 2 years are unlikely to return to work in any capacity.

2. **a.** For up to 90% of cases of LBP, a definite anatomic or pathophysiologic diagnosis cannot be made. Only 1% of patients with acute LBP eventually require surgery. Patients with acute LBP and no previous surgical procedure have an 80% to 90% chance of recovering after 6 weeks, no matter what treatment is prescribed.

3. **d.** Because of limited or conflicting evidence, lumbar decompression cannot be recommended in the treatment of nonspecific LBP. Cognitive–behavioral therapy has been shown to decrease pain intensity. Although back schools integrate education and exercise, studies have shown that this type of rehabilitation does not improve pain and function after 1 year. Tricyclic and tetracyclic antidepressants appear to produce moderate reductions in symptoms among patients with chronic LBP, but SSRIs do not appear to be of any benefit.

4. **c.** The most common diagnosis in LBP is lumbosacral sprain or strain, or mechanical LBP. Injury is thought to result from abnormal stress on normal tissues or normal stress on damaged or degenerated tissues.

5. **d.** With the exception of prolotherapy, several studies have shown that physical therapy, acupuncture, osteopathic manipulation, and massage therapy have some benefit in the treatment of LBP.

6. **c.** The most likely diagnosis is spinal stenosis. Back pain that is associated with exertional leg pain (claudication) often represents spinal stenosis. On examination, there is usually pain with backward bending or extension of the lumbosacral spine. To differentiate from vascular claudication, symptoms often occur when standing up, and to relieve symptoms patients need to sit down (simply stopping walking usually will not relieve symptoms).

7. e. Inflammatory back pain (ankylosing spondylitis) is an important subset of chronic LBP, although it accounts for very few cases of acute or chronic LBP. Diagnostic clues to inflammatory LBP include the following: (1) insidious onset of back pain; (2) onset before the age of 40 years; (3) pain 3 months in duration; (4) morning stiffness (longer than 30 minutes); (5) pain relief with activity; (6) pain forcing patient from bed; (7) a history of psoriasis, Reiter's disease, colitis, or ankylosing spondylitis; (8) limitation of lumbar spine in sagittal and frontal planes; (9) chest inspiratory expansion less than 2 cm; (10) evidence of sacroiliitis during physical examination; and (11) evidence of peripheral inflammatory joint disease. However, activity does not increase the pain.

8. e. One of the problems with the diagnosis, physical examination, laboratory investigation, and radiographic investigation of chronic LBP is that the sensitivity, specificity, and positive predictive value of the assessments, procedures, and other diagnostic modalities produce false-positive results and many false-negative results. From this, it follows that the patient ends up with misinformation that actually may "create" disease (anxiety, worry, and increased pain) where none existed before.

9. e. The history of mechanical back pain is typically one of relatively acute onset of pain, often with known precipitating injury or history of overuse. The pain is worse during the day, is relieved by rest (although the pain might worsen with prolonged rest), and is worse with activity.

In contrast, the history of inflammatory back pain classically presents with an insidious onset of pain and stiffness, worse at rest and improved with activity, and often worse at night and in the morning. Many patients need to get up at night to find a comfortable position to partially relieve the pain and stiffness.

10. e. Danger signals in patients with acute or chronic LBP include the following: (1) bowel or bladder dysfunction, (2) impotence, (3) ankle clonus, (4) color change in extremities, (5) considerable night pain, (6) constant and progressive symptoms, (7) fever and chills, (8) weight loss, (9) lymphadenopathy, (10) distended abdominal veins, (11) buttock claudication, and (12) new-onset LBP in children/adolescents and individuals older than age 50 years.

11. a. Plain x-rays of the lumbar spine are frequently ordered for LBP. However, there is little justification for such extensive use of radiography. A much more cost-effective and selective approach should be undertaken.

Apart from the cost factor, routine radiographs of the lumbar spine have three important drawbacks: a very low yield of findings that do not alter management in any way, a poor relationship between most radiographic abnormalities and signs and symptoms of LBP, and the potential of gonadal irradiation. Abnormalities seen on x-ray, particularly changes such as degenerative osteoarthritis, spondylosis, and congenital abnormalities, are often as common in asymptomatic individuals as they are in symptomatic individuals. Also, many patients who present with chronic LBP have normal x-ray examination results. There is no direct correlation between intervertebral osteophyte formation and discogenic disease. Most important, radiographs rarely alter treatment plans.

Specific indications for radiographic studies include the following: (1) ruling out an infectious or malignant process; (2) assessing a patient with objective evidence of neurologic abnormalities in the lower extremities, with loss of bowel or bladder control, or with loss of sexual function unexplained by another cause; (3) identifying a compression fracture; and (4) chronic sacroiliitis.

12. c. CT scanning and MRI have largely replaced myelography and are valuable for diagnosing disc disease and spinal stenosis. If the test is to influence management, then surgery must be considered a serious option before the test is performed. Consider obtaining an MRI or CT scan in patients with intractable pain or progressive neurologic deficits or if a systemic cause of back pain, such as infection or neoplasm, is suspected. MRI scans will reveal herniated discs in up to 25% of asymptomatic people. The presence of abnormal findings on MRI scan does not correlate well with clinical symptoms.

13. a. Patient education is the most crucial and cost-effective aspect of the treatment protocol for LBP. Many patients are very worried that they have a "serious illness" that is causing their pain and are dissatisfied by what they perceive as an inadequate explanation of their symptoms.

Most patients with mild to moderate LBP do not even consult physicians, and many symptomatic patients are more interested in seeking information and reassurance (the diagnosis and prognosis) than they are in "finding a cure." It is extremely important to reassure patients that "hurt is not equal to harm" in almost all cases. Older treatment regimens recommended bed rest, but studies have shown that early activity as tolerated leads to a better outcome.

14. e. A cornerstone of treating LBP is physical exercise. The Cochrane Review of exercise for LBP concluded that there was no evidence to indicate that specific exercises are effective for the treatment of acute LBP, but exercises may be helpful for chronic LBP. Scientific information about the method of action exerted by physical exercise is limited, which reflects the uncertainty regarding the pathophysiology of LBP. Exercises allow patients to participate in the treatment program and serve to prevent contractures, deconditioning, and weakness. Contrary to popular belief, exercise programs can safely begin within hours of developing LBP or an exacerbation of chronic LBP, even with the persisting muscle spasm.

The exercise programs that have been developed tend to emphasize repeated flexion and extension exercises and abdominal and lumbar strengthening exercises.

Any exercise program that is developed and begun should follow a graduated course. Patients need to be warned about a temporary increase in pain; otherwise, they will tend to stop the program when the increased

pain occurs. Stretching exercises are recommended first, followed by isometric strengthening exercises. One of the most important aspects of any exercise program is regularity.

15. **d.** In the treatment of acute LBP and sciatica, there is no good evidence to support the recommendation of bed rest or exercise therapy. Transcutaneous electrical nerve stimulation has not been shown to be effective in the treatment of chronic LBP. Although muscle relaxants are effective in managing LBP, they have not been shown to be more effective than NSAIDs. NSAIDs are effective for short-term relief of symptoms from acute LBP.

Physical therapy and spinal manipulation are other modalities used in the treatment of LBP. At 6 months, the functional status of patients with LBP demonstrates no difference regardless of the type of therapy that has been used. Patient satisfaction, however, is higher with hands-on types of therapy.

Summary

1. Incidence: 5% per year. Lifetime prevalence is approximately 90%. LBP is considered one of the most expensive ailments in advanced industrial societies. LBP in industrialized countries can be labeled an epidemic.
2. History/physical examination: Both the history and the physical examination lack both sensitivity and specificity.
3. Pathophysiology: LBP has been described as "an illness in search of a disease." Specific medical diagnosis and specific medical therapy are seldom possible. It is very difficult to specifically identify if chronic LBP is muscular, ligamentous/tendinous, facet joint, or discogenic in origin.
4. Common diagnoses
   a. Mechanical LBP or back strain: pain in low back, buttock, or posterior thigh increased with activity or bending. Examination: localized tenderness, limited spinal motion
   b. Acute disc herniation: usually acute onset of sharp, burning, radiating pain. Pain aggravated with coughing, sneezing, straining, sitting, and forward bending. Examination: positive straight leg raise test in seated and supine positions, possible weakness or asymmetric reflexes
   c. Spinal stenosis: pain aggravated with standing and walking and relieved with sitting, spinal flexion, or walking uphill. Examination: limited and/or painful spinal extension
   d. Spondylolysis: stress fracture of the pars interarticularis, seen mostly in athletes who perform repetitive spinal extension movements (e.g., gymnasts and football offensive linemen). Examination: pain with extension (single leg hyperextension test)

Suggested Reading

Assendelft WJ, Morton, SC, Yu, EI, et al: Spinal manipulative therapy for low back pain. A meta-analysis of effectiveness relative to other therapies. *Ann Intern Med* 138:871–881, 2003.

Cherkin DC, Sherman KJ, Deyo RA, Shekelle PG: A review of the evidence for the effectiveness, safety, and cost of acupuncture, massage therapy, and spinal manipulation for back pain. *Ann Intern Med* 138:898–906, 2003.

Cochrane Database of Systematic Reviews: *The Cochrane Collaboration*, vol. 3, 2003.

Kinkade S: Evaluation and treatment of acute low back pain. *Am Fam Physician* 75(8):1181–1188, 2007.

Manheimer E, White A, Berman B, et al: Meta-analysis: Acupuncture for low back pain. *Ann Intern Med* 142:651–663, 2005.

Nguyen TH, Randolph DC: Nonspecific low back pain and return to work. *Am Fam Physician* 76(10):1497–1502, 2007.

Patel AT, Ogle AA: Diagnosis and management of acute low back pain. *Am Fam Physician* 61:1779–1786, 1789–1790, 2000.

Shaughnessy AF, Spinal manipulation, other treatments for low back pain. Available at www.aafp.org/afp/20031201/tips/1.html.

Sierpina VS, Curtis P, Doering J: An integrative approach to low back pain. *Clin Fam Pract* 4(4):817–831, 2002.

Staiger TO, Gaster B, Sullivan MD, Deyo RA: Systematic review of antidepressants in the treatment of chronic low back pain. *Spine* 28:2540–2545, 2003.

Hicks, SG, Duddleston DN, Russell LD, et al: Low back pain symposium. *Am J Med Sci* 324(4):207–211, 2002.

CHAPTER 167

Lower Extremity Strains and Sprains

A 26-Year-Old Football Player Hit on the Lateral Side of the Knee

A 26-year-old professional football player is brought to the ER after being hit on the lateral side of the left knee. His knee buckled, and he is now in severe pain.

On examination, there is swelling over the medial aspect of the left knee. There is laxity when a valgus stress test is performed on the knee. There is a negative Lachman's test and McMurray's test.

4. What is the most likely injury in this patient?
   a. lateral meniscus tear
   b. medial meniscus tear
   c. lateral collateral ligament sprain
   d. medial collateral ligament sprain
   e. tibial plateau fracture

5. Based on your diagnosis in question 4, what is the initial treatment of choice?
   a. corticosteroid injection
   b. knee brace
   c. fiberglass cast
   d. complete bed rest
   e. surgical repair

CLINICAL CASE PROBLEM 1

A 21-Year-Old Female with a Swollen Ankle

A 21-year-old female comes to the emergency room (ER) after "twisting" her ankle while playing lacrosse. She tells you her ankle "rolled in" at the time of injury, and she says she has pain at her right ankle. She is able to walk without any assistance.

On examination, there is minimal ecchymosis and swelling on the lateral side of her right ankle. There is pain with inversion of the right ankle. Ankle tenderness is maximal just anterior to the tip of the lateral malleolus. There is no actual bone tenderness. There is no ligamentous laxity.

SELECT THE BEST ANSWER TO THE FOLLOWING QUESTIONS

1. The injury in this patient is most likely which of the following?
   a. a grade I sprain of the ligament complex on the medial side of the right ankle
   b. a grade III sprain of the ligament complex on the lateral side of the right ankle
   c. a grade I sprain of the ligament complex on the lateral side of the right ankle
   d. a strain of the peroneus brevis tendon
   e. a fracture of the distal fibula

2. What is the most likely ligament involved in this injury?
   a. anterior inferior tibiofibular ligament
   b. calcaneofibular ligament
   c. anterior talofibular ligament
   d. dorsal calcaneocuboid ligament
   e. interosseous talocalcaneal ligament

3. What is the treatment of choice in this patient?
   a. a fiberglass cast
   b. weight bearing as tolerated with active range-of-motion exercises
   c. non-weight bearing and a posterior splint
   d. a corticosteroid injection
   e. surgical repair of the ligament

CLINICAL CASE PROBLEM 3

A 22-Year-Old Male Who Twisted His Right Knee

A 22-year-old male is brought to the ER 8 hours after twisting his right knee while playing in a soccer match. At the time of injury, he felt a sharp pain on the "inner" part of his right knee. He has been unable to straighten his knee fully and had to be carried off the field by his teammates.

On examination, there is a moderate joint effusion, tenderness at the medial joint line, and limitation of the last 20 degrees of extension by a springy resistance. There is sharp anteromedial knee pain when passive extension is forced.

6. What is the most likely diagnosis in this patient?
   a. medial meniscus tear
   b. lateral meniscus tear
   c. medial collateral ligament sprain
   d. anterior cruciate ligament sprain
   e. fractured patella

7. The radiologic procedure of choice to confirm the diagnosis in this patient is which of the following?
a. a plain anterior–posterior and lateral x-ray of the right knee
b. a cone-view c-ray of the right knee
c. an arthrogram
d. a computed tomography scan
e. a magnetic resonance imaging (MRI) scan

8. What is the treatment of choice for the injury to this patient?
a. non-weight bearing and a knee immobilizer
b. non-weight bearing and a full cast
c. ice, elevation, and an elastic bandage
d. arthroscopic surgery
e. physical therapy

CLINICAL CASE PROBLEM 4

A 23-Year-Old Female with Right Posterior Thigh Pain

A 23-year-old female comes to your office with right posterior thigh pain. She was running in a 100-meter race when she felt a "pop" in her thigh.

On examination, there is tenderness over the midportion of the right hamstring muscles and pain with resisted stress testing. There is mild swelling and discoloration. There is no bony tenderness and no palpable defect.

9. What is the most likely diagnosis in this patient?
a. right hamstring strain
b. right hamstring sprain
c. popliteus artery hemorrhage
d. right hamstring avulsion
e. none of the above

10. What is the initial treatment of choice for this patient?
a. surgical repair
b. splint
c. a full cast
d. ice, rest, elevation, and compression
e. none of the above

CLINICAL CASE PROBLEM 5

A 16-Year-Old Female Who Injured Her Knee while Pivoting

A 16-year-old female, the star on her high school basketball team, sustains a knee injury after pivoting on her right knee during a game. She

collapses to the floor in pain and is immediately taken to the ER.

She arrives at the ER approximately 45 minutes after the injury, and her right knee is already very swollen. Laxity is noted with the anterior drawer test and Lachman's test.

11. What three structures are involved in the "unhappy triad"?
a. anterior cruciate ligament, posterior cruciate ligament, medial meniscus
b. anterior cruciate ligament, medial collateral ligament, lateral meniscus
c. anterior cruciate ligament, lateral collateral ligament, medial meniscus
d. anterior cruciate ligament, medial collateral ligament, medial meniscus
e. anterior cruciate ligament, lateral collateral ligament, lateral meniscus

12. The diagnosis of an anterior cruciate ligament injury is best confirmed by which of the following?
a. anterior drawer test
b. posterior drawer
c. Lachman's test
d. McMurray's test
e. Apley's compression/distraction test

13. What is the definitive treatment of choice in this patient?
a. ice, elevation, compression
b. a long leg cast
c. corticosteroid injection
d. reconstruction surgery
e. none of the above

Clinical Case Management Problem

Differentiate a collateral ligament tear from a meniscus tear.

Answers

1. **c.** This patient most likely has a grade I sprain of the ligament complex on the lateral side of the ankle.

A sprain is defined as a complete or partial tear of a ligament (intrasubstance or at origin/insertion). Swelling and tenderness over a ligament and pain when it is stretched suggest a sprain. Note that when a ligament is completely torn, as in a grade III injury, there may be no pain when the involved ligament is passively stretched. Excessive motion of the joint when the ligament is stretched confirms the diagnosis of a grade III sprain. Sprains are graded according to the following criteria:

Grade I: A tear of a few ligament fibers. The joint is tender and painful, but there is no laxity. Swelling and ecchymosis are usually minimal.

Grade II: A tear of a moderate number of ligament fibers. On physical examination, there is a moderate amount of swelling and pain. There is little or no instability of joint.

Grade III: Total disruption or tear of the ligament involved. No endpoint is felt when the joint is stressed. Swelling and ecchymosis are prominent.

The most common ankle injury is an inversion-type injury with partial or complete disruption of the lateral ligament complex.

2. c. Most ankle sprains are caused by inversion-type injuries. The lateral ligaments are most commonly involved. Specifically, the anterior talofibular ligament is the most commonly injured ligament. Tenderness is maximal anterior to the tip of the lateral malleolus.

3. b. The treatment of choice in this patient is ice, elevation, weight bearing as tolerated, active range-of-motion exercises, and an ankle support brace. Early weight bearing hastens healing and return to activity.

A cast is inappropriate and can lead to complications if the swelling worsens. Surgical intervention is not indicated in most ankle sprains. Corticosteroid injection is also not indicated in the acute management of ankle sprains.

4. d. The most likely injury in this patient is a sprain of the medial collateral ligament. The mechanism of injury (a blow to the lateral side of the knee), the swelling demonstrated on the medial side of the knee, and the laxity with valgus stress testing suggest a sprain of the medial collateral ligament complex. Lachman's test is used to diagnose injuries to the anterior cruciate ligament. McMurray's test is used to diagnose tears of the menisci.

5. b. Initial treatment consists of a knee brace, ice, elevation, and straight leg raise exercises in the brace. The patient may ambulate as tolerated in the brace. It is not necessary to apply a cast. Surgery and corticosteroid injection are not indicated. The patient does not need to be on bed rest.

6. a. This patient has a torn right medial meniscus. The history of the injury is quite characteristic. Often, a torn meniscus is the result of a twisting- or squatting-type injury. The patient then has pain along the affected joint line. The knee usually swells during the first 12 hours, and there is sometimes a sensation of "locking." This locking can be from a displaced meniscal fragment or from hamstring spasm ("pseudolocking").

On physical examination, there is joint line tenderness and an effusion may be present. There is a positive McMurray's test and Apley's test. For McMurray's test, with the patient in a supine position, the clinician holds the lower leg, flexing and extending the knee while simultaneously internally and externally rotating the tibia on the femur. A positive test is a "clicking" sensation felt with the other hand along the joint line with the patient experiencing pain. For Apley's compression test, the patient lies prone with the knee flexed 90 degrees. The leg is internally and externally rotated with pressure applied to the heel. Pain with downward pressure is a positive test for meniscal disease. In addition to meniscal tears, twisting injuries may also give rise to anterior cruciate ligament tears.

7. e. The diagnostic test of choice for a suspected medial meniscal tear and locking is an MRI scan.

8. d. The treatment of choice is arthroscopic surgery. With the use of an arthroscope, the torn fragment can either be removed or be repaired.

9. a. This patient most likely has a right hamstring muscle strain. A strain is defined as an "overstretching" of some portion of muscle or tendon. As with sprains, every degree of strain, ranging from the overstretching of just a few muscle fibers to the complete rupture of a muscle or tendon, may occur.

10. d. The initial treatment of choice is ice, rest, elevation, and compression bandage. This is followed by a gradually progressive stretching and strengthening program.

11. d. Although this triad was originally described by O'Donoghue in 1950, the existence of damage to all three structures after one injury event has not been documented.

12. c. The mechanism of injury to the anterior cruciate ligament is usually noncontact: a deceleration, hyperextension, or marked internal rotation of the involved knee. It may also be associated with a medial meniscus tear. Because the anterior cruciate ligament is a very vascular structure, a tear will cause an immediate knee effusion.

Injury to the anterior cruciate ligament is diagnosed by performing the Lachman test, the anterior drawer test, and the pivot shift test. Although the anterior drawer test is a time-honored test, it is not very sensitive. The Lachman test is much more sensitive. In this test, the examiner places the knee in 20 to 30 degrees of flexion by resting it on a pillow and stabilizes the femur, just above the knee, with his or her nondominant hand. The dominant hand of the examiner is placed behind the leg at the level of the tibial tubercle, and the examiner introduces an anterior force, attempting to displace the tibia forward. If there is excessive anterior translation of the tibia and lack of a firm endpoint, a tear in the anterior cruciate ligament has occurred.

13. **d.** The initial treatment includes a knee brace, ice packs, and elevation, followed by isometric and range-of-motion exercises. The definitive treatment in young active patients is most often reconstruction. Surgery is usually delayed 3 weeks postinjury to allow for increased range-of-motion and strength and decreased swelling.

Solution to the Clinical Case Management Problem

To help differentiate a collateral ligament tear from a meniscus tear, note the following: A positive varus or valgus stress test present on clinical examination is consistent with a collateral ligament injury, whereas joint line tenderness is consistent with a meniscus tear.

Summary

1. Definitions
   a. Sprain: a ligament injury. Sprains are classified as follows: first-degree: tear of only a few ligament fibers with no joint instability; second-degree: tear of a moderate number of ligament fibers with little or no joint instability; and third-degree: complete rupture of ligament with joint instability.
   b. Strain: a muscle–tendon injury. Strain injuries are classified as follows, ranging from tearing only a few fibers to a complete rupture of the muscle–tendon unit: first degree, second degree, and third degree.
2. Common sites
   a. Ankle sprain: lateral ligament complex injured more frequently than medial ligament complex (tenderness is usually maximal anterior to the tip of lateral malleolus over the anterior talofibular ligament)
   b. Knee sprain: (1) medial and lateral collateral ligaments: varus and valgus stress testing; (2) anterior cruciate ligament: Lachman's test

3. Other significant injury: medial and lateral meniscal injuries of the knee
   a. Clinical clue: joint line tenderness, positive McMurray's test, and Apley's test (see answer 6)
   b. Diagnosis: if further diagnostic procedure needed, MRI is radiologic test of choice
4. Treatments: sprain (ankle)—conservative; use the mnemonic RICE:

   Rest: Stop physical activity; protected weight bearing as tolerated
   Ice: Apply ice to the injury for 15 to 20 minutes each hour while awake for the first 24 hours. Wrap the ice in a wet towel or other buffer to prevent skin damage. Ice reduces swelling and pain. To prevent nerve injuries, do not leave ice on longer than 20 minutes.
   Compression: Use an elastic bandage or air-filled splint to apply pressure to an injury. Wear it all day. Compression helps control swelling.
   Elevation: keep the injured area elevated. This allows fluid to drain from the injury site, reducing swelling.

Suggested Reading

Barber FA: What is the terrible triad? *Arthroscopy* 8(1):19–22, 1992.

Hoppenfeld S: *Physical Examination of the Spine and Extremities.* New York: Prentice Hall, 1976.

Ivins D: Acute ankle sprain: An update. *Am Fam Physician* 74(10): 1714–1720, 2006.

Jackson JL, O'Malley PG, Kroenke K: Evaluation of acute knee pain in primary care. *Ann Intern Med* 139:575–588, 2003.

Mellion MB, Walsh WM, Madden C, et al, eds: *Team Physician's Handbook,* 3rd ed. Philadelphia: Hanley & Belfus, 2002.

CLINICAL CASE PROBLEM 1

A Landscaper with a Sore Shoulder

A 34-year-old male presents to your office requesting soft tissue injection of painful trigger points in his right shoulder. He read about this therapy on the Internet. He works as a laborer at a local landscaping business and has tried a variety of treatments, including acupuncture and chiropractic manipulation, for chronic intermittent pain in his right shoulder. There is no history of trauma or arthritides. On examination, he is a muscular white male with several tender points along the anterior border of his right trapezius muscle. The rest of his examination is normal.

SELECT THE BEST ANSWER TO THE FOLLOWING QUESTIONS

1. All of the following are reasonable and acceptable reasons for use of diagnostic and therapeutic injections except
   a. to aspirate fluid from a joint for diagnosis
   b. to deliver an antibiotic into an infected joint space
   c. to relieve pain and inflammation at a trigger point
   d. to confirm a presumptive diagnosis through pain relief
   e. to deliver an anti-inflammatory medication to an affected joint space

2. Which of the following aspects of history, if present, is not an absolute contraindication to therapeutic injection of a corticosteroid?
   a. the presence of a history of allergy to local anesthetic
   b. type 2 diabetes mellitus
   c. evidence of an infected joint space
   d. high possibility of a fracture involving the targeted joint
   e. the presence of a local cellulitis

3. Possible complications of therapeutic corticosteroid injection include all of the following except
   a. local infection caused by the injection
   b. a steroid flare after injection of corticosteroids
   c. local swelling and redness
   d. local depigmentation
   e. induction of coagulopathy

4. Postinjection instructions should pay particular attention to which of the following?
   a. proper dressing of the site
   b. signs of complications
   c. mobility restrictions, if any
   d. use of medications
   e. all of the above

CLINICAL CASE PROBLEM 2

A Woman with a Hot Knee

A 58-year-old female presents to your office with acute onset of a painful, swollen, hot knee. This is the first episode of this illness in this patient, which began 24 hours ago. There is no history of trauma, hyperurecemia, fever, chills, or other recent infections. Her only medication is hydrochlorothiazide for hypertension. On examination, vital signs are normal, and the left knee is as described with an obvious effusion. The rest of the examination is normal.

5. Reasonable management at this time includes which of the following?
   a. discontinuation of the hydrochlorothiazide
   b. aspiration of the affected joint
   c. instituting physical therapy
   d. beginning a nonsteroidal anti-inflammatory
   e. all of the above

6. Laboratory analysis of joint fluid is obtained and reveals gram-negative cocci seen in pairs. What is the most appropriate therapy at this time?
   a. intraarticular fluroquinolone
   b. oral dicloxacillin
   c. intravenous ceftriaxone
   d. a or c
   e. none of the above

CLINICAL CASE PROBLEM 3

A Man with a Painful Shoulder

A 42-year-old male comes to your office with left shoulder pain of several months' duration, not responsive to nonsteroidal anti-inflammatory medications and physical therapy. The Hawkin's test elicits pain with the shoulder passively flexed to 90 degrees and internally rotated. A magnetic resonance imaging scan confirms your diagnosis of a rotator cuff tendonosis and reveals no tear. At this point, you decide to inject a corticosteroid.

7. The most appropriate technique for delivery of the corticosteroid includes which of the following?
 a. preparation of pharmaceuticals and equipment
 b. proper positioning of the patient
 c. palpation of landmarks and use of sterile technique
 d. appropriate needle approach and entry
 e. all of the above

Answers

1. b. Reasonable and acceptable reasons for use of diagnostic and therapeutic injections include aspiration of fluid from a joint for diagnosis, delivery of pharmaceuticals to relieve pain and inflammation at trigger points, confirmation of a presumptive diagnosis through pain relief by delivery of a local anesthetic at an anatomical site, and delivery of an anti-inflammatory medication to an affected joint space.

2. b. Absolute contraindications to therapeutic injection of a corticosteroid include the presence of a history of allergy to the local anesthetic to be used, evidence of an infected joint space, a high possibility of a fracture involving the targeted joint, and the presence of a local cellulitis at the injection site.

3. e. Possible complications of therapeutic corticosteroid injection include local infection caused by the injection, a steroid flare after injection of corticosteroids (pain due to crystallization of pharmaceuticals used), local swelling and redness, and local depigmentation due to steroid effect. Also possible is subcutaneous fat atrophy that can result in skin puckering.

4. e. Postinjection instructions should pay particular attention to proper dressing and care of the injection site; signs of complications; mobility restrictions, if any; and use of other medications. Keeping the area injected clean and dry is a reasonable operating procedure. Some physicians like to immobilize the area injected, but there are no controlled trial data of outcomes on this recommendation. Analgesics are often prescribed to handle any discomfort from steroid flares. Refraining from overuse of the area is generally recommended for the first 48 hours.

5. b. This case is a classic presentation for the need for joint aspiration for diagnostic purposes. None of the other options are reasonable until a diagnosis has been established.

6. c. Joint aspiration should be performed in a swollen, red, hot joint to rule out infection or other causes of inflammation. Synovial fluid analysis should include the following: cell count—usually greater than 50,000 white blood cells/µL in infection (typically >90% polymorphonuclear cells); appearance—synovial fluid in infectious situations may appear purulent; analysis for crystals—key for assessment of the presence of crystalloid arthropathies; Gram stain—gram-positive or -negative intracellular organisms may be demonstrated; and culture—to determine infectious organisms and, if present, susceptibility to antimicrobials.

7. e. The most appropriate technique for delivery of the corticosteroid includes attention to all of the following: (a) preparation of pharmaceuticals and equipment—appropriate syringe size, needle, anesthetic, and costicosteroid should be prepared; (b) proper positioning of the patient—for a subacromial injection as in this case, the patient should be seated comfortably; (c) palpation of landmarks and use of sterile technique—sterile technique is a must for injection into any joint space and a good idea elsewhere; landmarks should be identified through palpation; and (d) appropriate needle approach and entry—in this case, a subacromial injection is used. Using aseptic technique, the needle is inserted just inferior to the posterolateral or lateral edge of the acromion. The needle is directed toward the opposite nipple. The pharmaceutical material should flow freely into the space without any resistance or significant discomfort from the patient. The Suggested Reading section at the end of this chapter provides articles that detail directions for a variety of injection sites and that include pictures to aid technique.

Summary

1. Injection techniques are helpful for diagnosis and therapy in a wide range of musculoskeletal conditions.
2. Diagnostic indications include the aspiration of fluid for analysis and the assessment of pain relief and increased range of motion as a tool to confirm diagnosis.
3. Therapeutic indications include the delivery of local anesthetics for pain relief, the delivery of corticosteroids for inflammation suppression, and the delivery of other pharmaceuticals to improve joint functioning.
4. Soft tissue indications include bursitis, tendinitis/tendinosis, trigger points, ganglions, neuromas,

entrapment syndromes, and fasciitis. Joint condition indications include effusion of unknown origin or suspected infection (only diagnostic), crystalloid arthropathies, synovitis, inflammatory arthritis, and advanced osteoarthritis.

5. Drug allergies, infection, fracture, and tendinous sites at high risk of rupture are absolute contraindications to joint/soft tissue therapeutic injection.

6. Suspected septic arthritis is a contraindication for therapeutic injection but an indication for joint aspiration.

7. Side effects of therapeutic injection are few but include the potential of tendon rupture, infection, steroid flare, hypopigmentation, and soft tissue atrophy.

8. Injection technique requires careful knowledge of the anatomy of the targeted area and a thorough understanding of the pharmacotherapeutic agents utilized.

Suggested Reading

Cardone DA, Tallia AF: Diagnostic and therapeutic injections of the elbow. *Am Fam Physician* 66(11):2097–2100, 2002.
Cardone DA, Tallia AF: Joint and soft tissue injection. *Am Fam Physician* 66:283–289, 2002.
Cardone DA, Tallia AF: Diagnostic and therapeutic injections of the hip and knee. *Am Fam Physician* 67(10):2147–2156, 2003.

Tallia AF, Cardone DA: Diagnostic and therapeutic injection of the shoulder region. *Am Fam Physician* 67:1271–1278, 2003.
Tallia AF, Cardone DA: Diagnostic and therapeutic injection of the wrist and hand region. *Am Fam Physician* 67(4):745–750, 2003.
Tallia AF, Cardone DA: Diagnostic and therapeutic injection of the ankle and foot. *Am Fam Physician* 68(7):1356–1364, 2003.

CHAPTER
169 Fracture Management

CLINICAL CASE PROBLEM 1

A 75-Year-Old Female Who Slipped and Fell on Her Outstretched Hand

A 75-year-old female is brought to the emergency room (ER) after having fallen on her outstretched hand. She complains of pain in the area of the right wrist.

On examination, there is a deformity in the area of the right wrist. The wrist has the appearance of a dinner fork. There is significant tenderness over the distal radius. Both pulses and sensation distally to the injury are completely normal.

SELECT THE BEST ANSWER TO THE FOLLOWING QUESTIONS

1. What is the most likely diagnosis in this patient?
   a. fracture of the distal ulna with dislocation of the radial head
   b. fracture of the carpal scaphoid
   c. fracture of the carpal lumate
   d. Colles' fracture
   e. fracture of the shaft of the radius with dislocation of the ulnar head

2. What is the treatment of choice for this patient?
   a. internal reduction and immobilization
   b. internal reduction and fixation
   c. external reduction and immobilization
   d. external reduction and fixation
   e. none of the above

CLINICAL CASE PROBLEM 2

The Team's Top Scorer Fell and Hurt His Hand

An 18-year-old basketball player is brought to the ER after having fallen on his outstretched hand. He is the league's leading scorer, and his coach directs you to "fix it and fix it fast."

On examination, there is slight tenderness and swelling just distal to the radius, in the snuffbox. No other abnormalities are found. X-ray examination of the wrist and hand is normal.

3. What is the most likely diagnosis in this patient?
   a. second-degree wrist sprain
   b. avulsion fracture of the distal radius
   c. fractured scaphoid
   d. fractured triquetrum
   e. none of the above

4. What is the treatment of choice for this patient?
   a. active physiotherapy
   b. passive physiotherapy

c. nonsteroidal anti-inflammatory drugs

d. surgical exploration of the wrist

e. none of the above

5. What is the major complication of the injury described in this case?

a. peripheral nerve injury

b. local muscle damage

c. peripheral arterial injury

d. avascular necrosis of the bone

e. septic arthritis of the joint

CLINICAL CASE PROBLEM 3

A 25-Year-Old Male with Pain in His Ankle

A 25-year-old male is brought to the ER after having been thrown from his motorcycle. He complains of severe pain in the area of the right ankle and is unable to bear weight on the foot.

On examination, there is swelling of the entire right ankle, with more prominent swelling on the lateral side. There is point tenderness over the lateral malleolus. There does not appear to be any other deformity or abnormality.

6. What is the most likely diagnosis in this patient?

a. second-degree ankle sprain

b. third-degree ankle sprain

c. fractured distal tibia

d. fractured distal fibula

e. fractured talus

7. What is the treatment of choice for this patient?

a. internal reduction and fixation

b. external reduction and fixation

c. active physiotherapy

d. ice, compression, and elevation

e. immobilization of the ankle

8. Which of the following statements regarding acute compartment syndrome is (are) true?

a. acute compartment syndrome is caused by increasing pressure within a closed fascial space as a result of effects of the injury

b. acute compartment syndrome is found primarily in the lower leg and the forearm

c. acute compartment syndrome may lead to muscle and nerve ischemia

d. acute compartment syndrome may lead to muscle and nerve death

e. all of the above

9. The emergency treatment of orthopedic injuries includes which of the following?

a. assessment of all injuries, many of which are multiple

b. assessment of vascular and neurologic injury in the involved region

c. correction of deformities

d. splinting or immobilization of all injured areas

e. all of the above

10. Which of the following is (are) part of the Ottawa ankle rules for determining the need for x-rays when evaluating ankle injuries?

a. bone tenderness at the distal lateral malleolus

b. bone tenderness at the distal medial malleolus

c. inability to bear weight both immediately at the time of injury and at the time of assessment

d. patient is age 18 years or older

e. all of the above

Answers

1. **d.** This patient has a Colles' fracture—a fracture of the distal radius. It occurs most commonly in elderly patients, especially women, after falling onto an outstretched hand. It is most often associated with osteoporosis. The typical displacement is reflected in a characteristic appearance that has been termed the dinner fork deformity. The clinical history and deformity are not compatible with any of the other choices listed.

2. **c.** The treatment of choice for the patient described is external reduction under a regional block or a local hematoma block, followed by immobilization in a splint or bivalve cast. Because of the age of the patient, the cast will probably have to remain for 6 weeks to ensure complete healing. Follow-up within 1 week is necessary to ensure no skin or vascular complications from the immobilization or significant loss of angulation correction. Osteoporosis is a risk factor for poor healing.

3. **c.** This young man most likely has a fractured scaphoid bone. This is an injury that is significantly more common in younger adults. The most common cause of a scaphoid fracture is a fall on an outstretched hand.

Fracture of the scaphoid bone should be suspected if there is tenderness in the anatomical snuffbox and/or at the scaphoid tubercle. Radiographs may be negative initially. If a fracture is suspected, despite negative x-rays, the region should be immobilized in a thumb spica cast or long arm splint. After 2 weeks, reevaluate the injured area and repeat x-rays. If there is a fracture of the scaphoid, x-rays will be positive at 2 weeks (a bone scan will be positive within 72 hours of a scaphoid fracture). A nondisplaced fracture of the scaphoid requires 8 to 12 weeks of cast immobilization. Bone scan (positive 72 hours postinjury), computed tomography, or magnetic resonance imaging may allow for more rapid and accurate diagnosis. Confirmed fracture of the waist or proximal aspect of the scaphoid often requires surgical consultation.

4. **e.** See answer 5.

5. **d.** Failure to properly treat a scaphoid fracture will likely lead to complications. The major complication is avascular necrosis.

6. **d.** The history of trauma, the symptoms elicited, and the signs present suggest a fracture of the lateral malleolus. Although the physical findings of a major (second- or third-degree) ankle sprain may be somewhat similar, the injury (being thrown from a motorcycle) and his inability to bear weight are definitely more suggestive of a fracture injury than a sprain injury.

7. **e.** The treatment of choice for this patient is immobilization. Initially, it should be in a posterior splint, and then, after swelling adequately diminished, a walking cast or boot is to be applied for 4 to 6 weeks. Weight bearing is allowed as tolerated by patient. In the absence of significant deformity and confirmation on x-ray of a nondisplaced fracture to the lateral malleolus, no other treatment is indicated. An x-ray should be repeated 1 or 2 weeks after the injury to check for any displacement of the fracture.

8. **e.** Acute compartment syndromes are caused by increasing tissue pressure in a closed fascial space. The fascial compartments of the leg and forearm are most frequently involved. Acute compartment syndromes are usually the result of a fracture with subsequent hemorrhage, limb compression, or a crushing injury. In an acute compartment syndrome, fluid pressure is increased. This leads to muscle and tissue ischemia. Severe ischemia for a period of 6 to 8 hours results in subsequent muscle and nerve death.

Physical examination reveals swelling and definitive palpable tenseness over the muscle compartment. The signs on physical examination include paresis in the involved area and a sensory deficit over the involved area. Acute compartment syndrome should be treated with immediate fasciotomy.

9. **e.** In treating orthopedic injuries in a patient who has been involved in a traumatic event, it is very important to remember that these injuries must be seen and treated within the overall context of the patient's condition. Thus, the ABCs of resuscitation (airway, breathing, and circulation), which are discussed in other chapters, must take first priority. Associated cardiac dysrhythmias must be treated according to basic cardiac life support and advanced cardiac life support protocols. Traumatic injuries must be treated according to basic trauma life support and advanced trauma life support (ATLS) protocols.

First, the trauma patient must be suspected of having multiple injuries rather than a single injury. Cervical spine injuries should be assumed to be present until they have been excluded. Primary and secondary surveys must be performed as per ATLS protocol.

Second, with any injured extremity, arterial injury must be suspected and pulses must be assessed quickly. Acute compartment syndromes must be ruled out.

Third, deformities should be corrected as soon as possible under local (hematoma block), regional, or general anesthesia. Ideally, the injured limb(s) should be splinted before the patient arrives in the ER. Open fractures and surrounding tissue must be thoroughly debrided and cleaned as quickly as possible.

Fourth, after stabilization is complete, tetanus prophylaxis should be given and antibiotics active against coagulase-positive staphylococcus must be started.

10. **e.** The Ottawa ankle rules are guidelines to determine the need for ankle radiographs in patients who have sustained an ankle injury. If there is boney tenderness on the tip or posterior aspect of the lateral or medial malleolus, or an inability to bear weight both immediately at the time of injury and at the time of assessment, x-rays should be obtained. The Ottawa ankle rules do not apply to patients younger than age 18 years. It is important to also use clinical judgment when deciding when to obtain x-rays.

Summary

1. Fall on an outstretched hand
   a. Elderly: possible Colles' fracture
   b. Young adult: possible scaphoid fracture
2. Colles' fracture
   a. Fracture of distal metaphysis of radius, which is dorsally displaced and angulated

   b. "Dinner fork" deformity: requires immediate reduction (closed reduction usually adequate) and immobilization
3. Scaphoid fracture: tenderness in snuffbox
   a. Radiographs may take more than 2 weeks to reveal fracture.

b. If scaphoid fracture is suspected, must immobilize even if initial x-rays are negative.

c. Bone scan or magnetic resonance imaging studies will show scaphoid fractures earlier than x-rays.

d. Must immobilize for a period of 8 to 12 weeks; some scaphoid fractures require internal fixation.

e. Possible complications include avascular necrosis and nonunion of fracture.

4. Nondisplaced lateral ankle fracture

a. Immobilize in posterior splint until swelling adequately diminished, then place in short leg cast or walking cast boot for 4 to 6 weeks.

b. Advance weight bearing as tolerated.

5. The basics of fracture management and other orthopedic and trauma injuries are as follows:

a. Remember the ABCs of resuscitation: **a**irway, **b**reathing, and **c**irculation

b. Suspect and search for multiple injuries.

c. Suspect and prevent potential spine injuries. Immobilize cervical spine in trauma patients.

d. Rule out arterial injury in the affected limb.

e. Rule out a compartment syndrome.

f. Recognize and treat open fractures with copious irrigation, debridement, and initiation of intravenous antibiotics.

g. Correct deformities whenever possible.

h. Splint each injured area.

i. If there is significant swelling in a limb, consider either a bivalve cast or splint until swelling has decreased significantly. A full cast can lead to complications such as compartment syndrome if applied too soon after injury when there is significant swelling.

j. If one fracture is found, always check the joint above and the joint below for additional fractures, dislocations, or other injuries.

Suggested Reading

DeLee JC, Drez D, Miller MD, eds: *DeLee and Drez's Orthopaedic Sports Medicine: Principles and Practice*. Philadelphia: Saunders, 2003.

Eiff MP, Hatch RL, Calmbach WL: *Fracture Management for Primary Care*. Philadelphia: Saunders, 2003.

Mellion MB, Walsh WM, Madden C, et al, eds: *Team Physician's Handbook*, 3rd ed. Philadelphia: Hanley & Belfus, 2002.

CHAPTER 170 — Infectious Disease and Sports

CLINICAL CASE PROBLEM 1

A 17-Year-Old Soccer Player with Aches, Pains, and Fever

A 17-year-old high school student comes into the office complaining of having generalized body aches, feeling "feverish," and having a dry cough for the past 2 days. She has been taking acetaminophen to help relieve symptoms. She tells you that she is the leading scorer on the school's soccer team and that there is a big game against a rival school in 3 days.

On examination, her blood pressure is 100/70 mmHg, pulse is 94 beats/minute, respiration is 20 breaths/minute, and temperature is 101°F. Examination of her head, ears, eyes, nose, and throat shows a mild pharyngeal erythema. Her neck is supple, with no adenopathy; cardiovascular regular rhythm and rate is S1, S2, with no murmurs.

Her lungs are clear, her abdomen is soft and not tender, there is no organomegaly, and bowel sounds are active.

SELECT THE BEST ANSWER TO THE FOLLOWING QUESTIONS

1. Which of the following statements regarding exercise and viral upper respiratory tract infections is true?

a. exercising during a viral illness can decrease the duration and severity of illness

b. all over-the-counter cold medications are approved by sports governing bodies for use during competition

c. a fever decreases strength and endurance

d. athletes with a fever less than 103°F can safely participate in sports

e. none of the above

2. After you complete your examination, she asks if she can practice with the soccer team later that day. Which of the following is the best response?

a. she should not exercise until the fever has resolved

b. she may exercise but only at a moderate intensity

c. to decrease the duration of illness, she should exercise at a high intensity
d. she may play only noncontact sports until her symptoms resolve
e. none of the above

3. Which of the following statements regarding exercising during a febrile viral illness is true?
   a. the athlete is at an increased risk for myocarditis
   b. the athlete is at an increased risk for heat illness
   c. recovery from the illness is quickest for the athlete who allows for adequate rest
   d. all of the above
   e. none of the above

4. Which of the following statements regarding exercise and the immune system is true?
   a. white blood cells decrease during exercise
   b. salivary and nasal immunoglobulin A (IgA) is increased for 24 hours after strenuous exercise
   c. exercising at moderate intensity appears to enhance immune function
   d. lymphocytes decrease during exercise
   e. none of the above

CLINICAL CASE PROBLEM 2

A 20-Year-Old Football Player with Mononucleosis

A 20-year-old male with mononucleosis follows up in your office 3 weeks after the start of symptoms. He tells you that he "feels fine." The examination is normal. The spleen does not feel enlarged, and all lab tests are normal. He plays on his college football team and wants to immediately start practicing with the team.

5. Regarding return to play, which of the following is recommended in athletes with mononucleosis (assuming the spleen is not enlarged, the athlete is afebrile, and liver function tests [LFTs] are normal)?
   a. the athlete may return to contact and strenuous activity at 8 weeks after the onset of illness
   b. the athlete may return to contact and strenuous activity at 12 weeks after the onset of illness
   c. the athlete may return to noncontact practice and nonstrenuous activity at 3 weeks after the onset of illness
   d. the athlete may return to noncontact practice and nonstrenuous activity at 6 weeks after the onset of illness
   e. none of the above

CLINICAL CASE PROBLEM 3

Three Wrestlers with Herpes Gladiatorum

Three members of the college wrestling team have herpes gladiatorum. The coach is concerned that the breakout is going to "ruin the season" and his chance to get into the coaches hall of fame.

6. Which of the following statements regarding herpes gladiatorum is true?
   a. athletes with a history of recurrent herpes gladiatorum may benefit from prophylactic acyclovir
   b. wrestlers may continue to compete as long as the lesions are covered with a gauze dressing
   c. a Tzanck smear of scrapings from the wound will always be negative
   d. herpes gladiatorum is caused only by herpes simplex virus 1
   e. none of the above

7. Which of the following is true regarding exercise and human immunodeficiency virus (HIV) infection?
   a. exercise is a safe and beneficial activity for people with HIV
   b. there have been no documented cases of HIV transmission in sports
   c. exercise can increase the number of CD4 cells in people with HIV
   d. mild to moderate exercise has been shown to limit or decelerate the body wasting seen in people with acquired immune deficiency syndrome (AIDS)
   e. all of the above

8. Which of the following statements regarding hepatitis B infection (HBV) and sports is true?
   a. there have been no documented cases of HBV transmission in sports
   b. the risk of HBV transmission in sports is greater than that for HIV
   c. an athlete who is asymptomatic and is a chronic HBV carrier with the e-antigen present should be restricted from strenuous activity
   d. the hepatitis B vaccine should not be given to elite athletes
   e. all of the above

9. Which of the following statements regarding the athlete and myocarditis is true?
   a. the most common cause of myocarditis is a virus
   b. myocarditis can cause sudden death in athletes
   c. according to the 26th Bethesda Conference, athletes suspected of having myocarditis should be kept out of sports for 6 months

d. the coxsackievirus appears to have a predilection for the heart in exercising individuals

e. all of the above

10. A 15-year-old comes to your office complaining of vomiting and diarrhea for the past 2 days. You diagnose viral gastroenteritis. Which of the following statements regarding viral gastroenteritis and sports is true?

a. athletes with viral gastroenteritis are at an increased risk for heat injuries

b. athletes should not be allowed to return to play until they are well hydrated and afebrile

c. the most common agents are the rotavirus and Norwalk virus

d. antimotility drugs may prolong the gastrointestinal infection

e. all of the above

Answers

1. **c.** During the course of a viral upper respiratory infection, an athlete's performance is adversely affected. Muscle strength, aerobic power, and endurance are decreased. Exercising during a viral illness can prolong and increase the severity of the illness. Certain over-the-counter medications are banned by sports governing bodies and, if taken during competition, can lead to disqualification of an athlete. Certain medications can also impair athletic performance and increase the risk of injury. Athletes with a temperature of 100.8°F or higher should not participate in sports.

2. **a.** As discussed previously, she should not exercise until the fever has resolved.

3. **d.** Exercising during a febrile viral illness increases an athlete's risk of developing heat illness, injury, and myocarditis. Performance will also be impaired.

4. **c.** Exercising at moderate intensity appears to enhance immune function. When exercising at moderate levels, athletes tend to experience fewer viral infections. Elite or high-level athletes, however, complain of frequent viral infections when training hard or after competitions. There is a transient increase in white blood cells and lymphocytes during exercise. Salivary and nasal IgA levels decrease after strenuous exercise and return to normal within 24 hours of rest. This may explain the increased susceptibility to viral illness after strenuous exercise.

5. **c.** The current return-to-play recommendations for athletes with mononucleosis are that if an athlete is afebrile, the spleen is not enlarged, lab tests including LFTs are normal, and there are no other complications, the athlete may return to noncontact and nonstrenuous sports at 3 weeks after the onset of symptoms. The athlete may return to full-contact sports and strenuous activity at 4 weeks after the onset of symptoms.

6. **a.** Herpes gladiatorum is a herpes infection of the skin caused by herpes simplex virus 1 and 2. The skin lesions are usually found on the face and body and are transmitted via direct skin-to-skin contact as seen in such sports as wrestling and rugby. Wrestlers and other athletes with herpes gladiatorum are prohibited from competition until skin lesions have resolved. Treatment includes antiviral agents, such as acyclovir, famciclovir, and valacyclovir. Prophylactic therapy should be considered if recurrences are frequent and before any important competition.

7. **e.** Exercise is safe and beneficial for people with HIV. In addition to psychological benefits, exercise can increase the number of CD4 cells and can limit or slow down the body wasting seen in AIDS. There have been no documented cases of HIV transmission in sports.

8. **b.** Like HIV, HBV is transmitted via direct contact with infected blood and body fluids. The risk of transmission is much greater for HBV than for HIV. HBV transmission in sports has been reported in the literature. People who are chronic HBV carriers with e-antigen present may fully participate in all levels of activity. Hepatitis B vaccine should be considered in all athletes who participate in contact sports.

9. **e.** Myocarditis is most commonly the result of a virus and can cause sudden death in athletes. The coxsackievirus has been shown to have a predilection for the heart in exercising individuals. The 26th Bethesda Conference recommends that athletes with myocarditis not be allowed to return to sports for 6 months. Before returning to sports, the athlete needs to have normal ventricular function, normal cardiac size, and no arrhythmias.

10. **e.** Viral gastroenteritis most commonly is caused by the rotavirus and Norwalk virus. There is an increased risk of heat injuries in athletes with viral gastroenteritis because of dehydration from fever, diarrhea, or vomiting and an impaired thirst drive because of nausea. Antimotility drugs have the potential to prolong the infection because of resulting decreased bowel motility and transit time. Athletes with viral gastroenteritis should be afebrile and well hydrated before returning to sports.

Summary

1. Effects of exercise on the immune system
   a. Transient increase in white blood cells and lymphocytes during exercise (lymphocytes may decrease for a short time after exercise to below preexercise levels).
   b. Salivary and nasal IgA are decreased for 24 hours after strenuous activity.
   c. Exercising at moderate levels enhances immune function.
   d. Strenuous exercise can increase susceptibility to upper respiratory infections.
2. Exercise and viral respiratory infections
   a. Exercise during a viral illness can increase the duration and severity of illness.
   b. Fever decreases the strength and performance of athletes.
   c. Athletes with a fever of 100.8°F or higher or myalgias should not participate in sports. There is an increased risk for heat illness, injury, and myocarditis.
3. Mononucleosis and return-to-play decisions (assuming there is no spleen enlargement, no fever, normal LFTs, and no complications)
   a. Athletes may return to noncontact and nonstrenuous activity at 3 weeks after the onset of symptoms.
   b. Athletes may return to contact and strenuous activities at 4 weeks after the onset of symptoms.
4. Herpes gladiatorum
   a. This is caused by herpes simplex virus 1 and 2.
   b. Transmission is a result of direct skin-to-skin contact.
   c. The virus is seen in sports such as wrestling and rugby.
   d. Skin lesions are seen on the face and body.
   e. Tzanck smear can confirm diagnosis.
   f. Treat with an antiviral medication such as acyclovir.
   g. Consider prophylactic treatment if recurrences are frequent or before important matches.
5. HIV infection and sports
   a. Exercise is safe and has many health benefits.
   b. Exercise can increase the number of CD4 cells and limit or slow down body wasting seen in AIDS.
   c. There are no documented cases of HIV transmission in sports.
6. HBV infection and sports
   a. The risk of transmission in sports is greater than that for HIV.
   b. Consider giving vaccine to all athletes participating in contact sports.
7. Viral gastroenteritis and sports
   a. The most common agents are rotavirus and Norwalk virus.
   b. Athletes with viral gastroenteritis are at increased risk of heat illness.
   c. Athletes should not be allowed to return to sports until they are afebrile and well hydrated.
   d. Antimotility drugs may prolong the illness.

Suggested Reading

Bamberger DM, Boyd SE: Management of *Staphylococcus aureus* infections. *Am Fam Physician* 72:2474–2481, 2005.

Mellion MB, Walsh WM, Madden C, et al, eds, Philadelphia: Hanley & Belfus, 2002.

Wilckens JH, Glorioso JE: Viral disease. In: DeLee JC, Drez D, Miller MD, eds, *DeLee and Drez's Orthopaedic Sports Medicine: Principles and Practice*. Philadelphia: Saunders, 2002.

Female Athlete Triad

CLINICAL CASE PROBLEM 1

A 20-Year-Old Female Runner with "Shin Splints"

A 20-year-old cross-country runner presents for evaluation of "shin splints." She is a very competitive runner, averaging approximately 50 to 60 miles per week. On examination, the patient is a small, thin female with very well-defined musculature. She has some tenderness over both medial tibias but has one discrete area of increased point tenderness 3 cm proximal to the medial malleolus. Her coach is waiting outside to find out when she will be able to return to running because they have an important meet next weekend.

SELECT THE BEST ANSWER TO THE FOLLOWING QUESTIONS

1. What is the most important piece of history to obtain from this patient when suspecting a stress fracture?
   a. whether she has been icing the painful areas
   b. complete menstrual history
   c. how much she stretches before exercise
   d. medications that she is taking
   e. types of surfaces on which she runs

2. The female athlete triad consists of which of the following?
   a. anorexia, oligomenorrhea, calcium deficiency
   b. osteoporosis, stress fractures, calcium deficiency
   c. disordered eating, amenorrhea, osteoporosis
   d. disordered eating, use of laxatives, osteoporosis
   e. metamenorrhagia, hypothalamic dysfunction, osteoporosis

3. When is the best time to screen female athletes for risk factors for the female athlete triad?
   a. at the preparticipation physical examination
   b. when the patient presents with an injury
   c. when the clinician notices that the patient is underweight or losing weight
   d. when the patient presents for a routine Pap test and pelvic examination
   e. after competition is complete for the season

4. What critical questions should be asked when obtaining a history from a female athlete?
   a. age of menarche, regularity, and date of last menstrual period
   b. whether the patient is happy with her weight and the patient's idea of her ideal body weight
   c. maximum and minimum weights that the patient has achieved
   d. history of any stress injuries or stress fractures
   e. all of the above

CLINICAL CASE PROBLEM 2

An 18-Year-Old Female with Amenorrhea

An 18-year-old female comes to the office with a complaint of amenorrhea. She experienced menarche at age 14 years, and since that time she has been having approximately four to six menses per year. However, her last menstrual period was 9 months ago. She is a competitive gymnast and travels a great deal with her team and coaches. She says that she knows that it is "normal" for athletes to miss their periods but that her mother had wanted her to come in. She wants to know if there is any medication that you can give her that "won't make me fat."

5. Amenorrhea in the athlete is most specifically associated with which of the following?
   a. decreased levels of estrogen
   b. increased levels of progesterone
   c. calcium deficiency
   d. use of laxatives to lose weight
   e. exercise

6. Workup for amenorrhea for more than 6 months' duration in a female athlete could include all of the following except
   a. dual-energy x-ray absorptiometry (DEXA) bone mineral density scan
   b. serum electrolytes, complete blood count, thyroid panel, and hormonal evaluation
   c. pelvic examination
   d. ultrasound of the abdomen and pelvis
   e. psychological evaluation

7. All of the following are characteristics of anorexia nervosa except
   a. distorted body image and excessive fear of gaining weight
   b. amenorrhea
   c. complete recovery in 50% of patients with counseling

d. weight less than the 85th percentile for age and height

e. severe restriction of calories

8. Which of the following statements is true?
   a. there are optimal body fat percentages specific for each sport
   b. athletes with disordered eating habits often disclose this information on the first visit
   c. teammates are almost always aware of another athlete's disordered eating behaviors
   d. coaches and parents may promote and perpetuate disordered eating by emphasizing the importance of winning and slim physiques
   e. caloric needs are the same for each athlete

9. Which of the following statements is true?
   a. the primary care provider is usually able to care for a patient with the female athlete triad without the involvement of others
   b. treatment should include a multidisciplinary team including the primary care physician, a nutritionist, a psychologist or psychiatrist, coaches, trainers, and parents
   c. for a diagnosis of the female athlete triad, the patient must meet the *Diagnostic and Statistical Manual of Mental Disorders*, 4th edition (*DSM-IV*), criteria for either anorexia or bulimia
   d. societal pressures concerning the importance of thinness have no effect on athletes
   e. continuing to vigorously exercise through illness and injury demonstrates toughness and a healthy attitude

10. Which of the following is the most important intervention for an athlete diagnosed with female athlete triad?
    a. hormone replacement therapy
    b. psychologic counseling
    c. calcium and vitamin D replacement
    d. monthly x-rays
    e. changes in eating behaviors and training regimens

Answers

1. b. The most important piece of history from the choices listed is a complete menstrual history. The patient's thin physique, high running mileage, and obvious competitive nature place her at risk for the female athlete triad. The coach's active involvement in the waiting room suggests pressure for success. The menstrual history should include age at menarche, frequency and duration of periods, dysmenorrhea or associated symptoms with menses, last menstrual period, longest gap between menses, and any birth control pills or other hormonal therapy taken previously.

Shoe type, running surfaces, preseason conditioning, icing, and stretching are all important questions to ask when evaluating a patient for stress injury. In the female patient with so many red flags, however, the menstrual history is the most critical.

2. c. The female athlete triad consists of disordered eating, amenorrhea, and osteoporosis.

3. a. The optimal time to screen female patients for the female athlete triad is during the preparticipation physical examination, before the season has begun. At this time, athletes at risk can be identified for further evaluation and treatment. The sports that place athletes at most risk are those that place pressure on athletes to maintain a slim physique, especially gymnastics, dance, figure skating, track, and cross-country. However, studies have shown that all female athletes may be at risk, and the prevalence of disordered eating behaviors has been reported to be between 15% and 62% of female college athletes.

After a stress injury, it is obviously too late to screen a patient for the female athlete triad. However, if a patient was missed, a stress injury gives a very opportune time for an evaluation. A stress fracture can be a very serious injury, and this may convince the patient that disordered eating and excessive exercise place her body at risk.

4. e. All of the choices provided are crucial to ask during a complete evaluation of a female athlete. A complete menstrual history, as described previously, cannot be emphasized enough. A weight history is also critical. Obtaining the athlete's perception of her own weight is critical for diagnosis. Minimum and maximum weights achieved and perceived ideal body weight also are important. An attempt to elicit weight loss techniques should be made, although many patients are initially reluctant to answer honestly. An exercise history should include training schedule, extracurricular activity, and time commitment. A history of previous stress injury, including "shin splints," stress fractures, compartment syndromes, and other overuse injuries, should be elicited.

5. a. Amenorrhea in the athlete is associated most specifically with decreased levels of estrogen. Changes in the hypothalamus cause decreased secretion of estrogen. Researchers are still trying to delineate the causative factors of decreased estrogen production. Caloric restriction and excessive exercise training regimens have been associated with low estrogen levels, but the exact mechanism of this disruption has yet to be elucidated.

6. **d.** Workup for a patient with suspected female athlete triad could include a DEXA bone scan. This will delineate areas of osteopenia and can be compared to age-related norms. X-rays will show old fractures and may show acute stress fractures. A three-phase bone scan can also find areas of stress injury where the athlete is at risk for frank stress fractures. Serum electrolytes and complete blood count are critical, especially in a patient suspected of restricting calories and/or fluids. A thyroid panel and hormonal panel (follicle-stimulating hormone, luteinizing hormone, and prolactin) will help with the diagnosis of amenorrhea. A complete pelvic examination is also part of the workup. A complete psychological evaluation is also indicated at this time to delineate harmful eating and exercise behaviors and to explore the reasoning behind this behavior. An ultrasound of the abdomen and pelvis is not indicated at this time unless the clinician has other diagnostic suspicions.

7. **c.** Anorexia is characterized by the *DSM-IV* as a refusal to maintain body weight more than 85% of expected weight for age and height. It is also characterized by an intense fear of gaining weight, a distorted body image, and amenorrhea (in postmenarcheal females). Unfortunately, the prognosis for anorexia nervosa is generally poor. Approximately 25% of patients may recover fully, with approximately 50% having some improvement over time but still suffering symptoms and approximately 25% with chronic symptoms. Researchers have estimated between 2% and 10% mortality for the disease. This is a long-term disease, and recovery can take 5 to 10 years. These numbers are elusive, and further studies may show more specific outcomes.

8. **d.** There is no such thing as an ideal body weight percentage specific for each sport. Individual athletes can excel in the same sport with widely different body types. Caloric needs are different for each individual and depend on activity level, percentage lean body mass, and individual metabolism. Teammates are often not aware of an athlete's eating disorder. Behaviors associated with eating disorders are often secretive, and

athletes may eat normally in public and then perform purging behaviors later in private. Coaches and parents are sometimes not aware of the pressures that they are placing on athletes. Constant reminders of the need to succeed and win at all costs may make eating disorder behaviors seem necessary and almost normal to an athlete. The concentration on thinness in many sports and in society in general puts further pressure on athletes to achieve success by any method necessary.

9. **b.** Treatment for a patient diagnosed with the female athlete triad should include a multidisciplinary team. The primary care or team physician must act as a coordinator for all services. The nutritionist is critical to advise the patient on meal plans and eating techniques that will work with the athlete's desires and also maintain a healthy diet. A psychiatrist/psychologist is also critical to explore eating behavior issues and other stressors that may contribute to pathology. Coaches, trainers, and parents should be involved as much as the patient wishes for them to be involved. Usually, however, open communication and education produce the best results.

Disordered eating behaviors for the female athlete triad do not have to specifically meet the *DSM-IV* criteria for anorexia nervosa or bulimia nervosa. Any type of disordered eating behavior will qualify and usually can be referred to as an eating disorder not otherwise specified.

Another critical myth to debunk is that of "no pain, no gain." Continuing to exercise vigorously through serious illness or injury demonstrates pathology, not "mental toughness." Athletes need to understand that discomfort is common in exercise and can be overcome. Actual pain, however, is a sign that there is something wrong—something that requires stopping the activity and seeking medical attention.

10. **e.** The most important intervention to make for an athlete with female athlete triad is to convince the athlete to make significant changes in her eating behaviors and exercise regimens. This is often the most difficult intervention to achieve but clearly the most critical and long-lasting. Hormone replacement therapy is an important adjunct and is commonly used to allow patients to resume normal menses. A balanced diet with calcium supplementation and vitamin D is also important for general bone health. Psychological counseling can be an important "lifeline" for these patients. X-rays should be performed according to specific complaints and diagnostic suspicions, not as a screening tool.

Summary

1. The female athlete triad consists of disordered eating, amenorrhea, and osteoporosis. Disordered eating can refer to a wide range of eating behaviors and can include restricting, binging, purging, and the use of laxatives and diuretics. The key factors for these athletes are lower energy intake and higher energy expenditures through exercise.

2. Amenorrhea can be common among female athletes, but this does not make it "normal." Amenorrhea can be primary (patient has never had menarche) or secondary (patient has had menarche but now has stopped having menses for more than 6 months). In the general female population, studies estimate a prevalence of 2% to 5% for amenorrhea. Among athletes, this percentage increases to 34% to 66%. Accurate prevalence data are very difficult to obtain because of the secretive nature of eating disorders. Studies have tried to determine the exact cause of amenorrhea. Athletes whose energy expenditure is significantly greater than their energy intake have lower estrogen levels and also fail to have appropriate release of follicle-stimulating hormone and luteinizing hormone. Lower body fat percentages also contribute to lower levels of estrogen. Some studies have estimated the lowest body fat percentage that would allow an athlete to have menses to be approximately 18%. Although other studies have shown that the percentage of body fat necessary for menses is different in different patients, it is an important indicator of normal menstrual and reproductive function.

3. Osteoporosis is the third component of the female athlete triad. Amenorrhea and low levels of gonadal hormones have been shown to be associated with low bone mass. Decreased bone mass results in cortical thinning, increased fragility, and increased risk of fractures. One area of study is trying to determine if these bone losses are reversible. Some studies have shown that resumption of menses does cause an increase in bone mineral density but that values may still remain below age-matched norms.

4. Prevalence is difficult to determine because of the secretive nature of disordered behavior and athletes' intense desire to continue to compete.

5. For screening, clinicians must remember to question the athlete, especially during the preparticipation examination. A complete menstrual history, a history of previous stress injuries, and the presence or history of eating behaviors should be asked.

6. For diagnosis, patients with amenorrhea should have complete histories taken, as mentioned previously. Athletes with suspected female athlete triad should have x-rays and/or bone scans to delineate current symptomatic fractures. A DEXA scan can also be used to determine overall bone mineral density. A complete blood count, metabolic panel, thyroid panel, and hormone levels should be checked. A complete pelvic examination should be performed. A history of eating behaviors and sample daily intake should be elicited.

7. Treatment should involve a multidisciplinary team composed of a primary care doctor, a nutritionist, a psychologist or psychiatrist, coaches, trainers, and parents. The most important intervention is to convince the athlete to modify her eating and exercise behavior. Other interventions can include hormonal therapy to induce menses, calcium supplements and vitamin D for better bone health, close work with a nutritionist, and work with a psychologist/psychiatrist. Agreeing on a goal weight or body fat percentage with the athlete can be one method, but this can be controversial because it encourages the athlete to concentrate excessively on the "numbers" instead of general good nutrition and reasonable exercise goals. Dispelling myths about the importance of thinness and excessive exercise is critical. Eating disorders in general represent long-term pathology, and constant and close supervision will be necessary to ensure the best outcomes.

Suggested Reading

Hobart JA, Smucker DR: The female athlete triad. *Am Fam Physician* 61(11):3357–3364, 2000.

Master-Hunter T, Heiman DL: Amenorrhea: Evaluation and treatment. *Am Fam Physician* 73:1374–1382, 2006.

Otis CL, Drinkwater B, Johnson M, et al: American College of Sports Medicine position stand. The female athlete triad. *Med Sci Sports Exer* 29:i–ix, 1997.

Sanborn CF, Horea M, Siemers BJ, Dieringer KI: Disordered eating and the female athlete triad. *Clin Sports Med* 19(2):199–213, 2000.

ILLUSTRATED REVIEW

172 Illustrated Review

Each picture in this section is accompanied by a brief clinical vignette. For each picture, determine the diagnosis. Wherever a figure relates directly to a previously discussed topic in an earlier chapter, that chapter and page are cross-referenced for you. Answers are at the end of this section.

PRIMARY DERMATOLOGICAL CONDITIONS

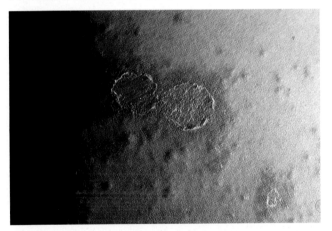

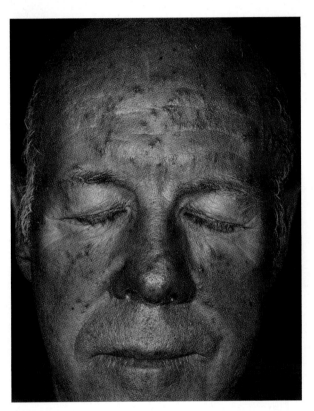

2. This 57-year-old man presents to your office with a many-year history of this facial eruption that has never been treated.

1. A 26-year-old man presents with this rash, which subsequently spreads in a Christmas-tree fashion over his entire back and resolves with conservative treatment in approximately 6 to 8 weeks.

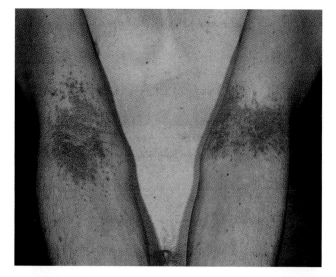

3. This 15-year-old teenager has a history of mild persistent asthma.

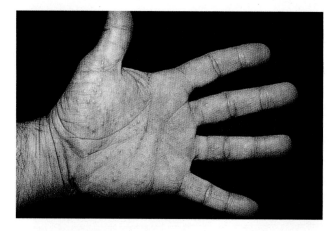

4. This 29-year-old auto mechanic has had this outbreak for several years. He finds mild over-the-counter topical steroid creams somewhat effective.

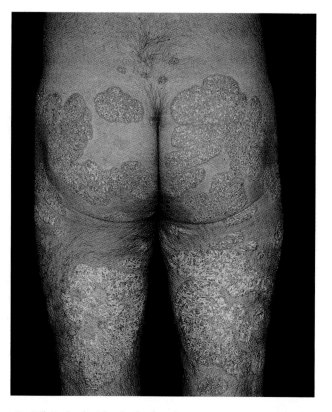

5. This individual finds these eruptions improve somewhat in the summertime.

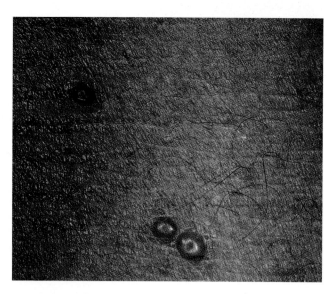

6. This painless rash presents on a 16-year-old high school wrestler.

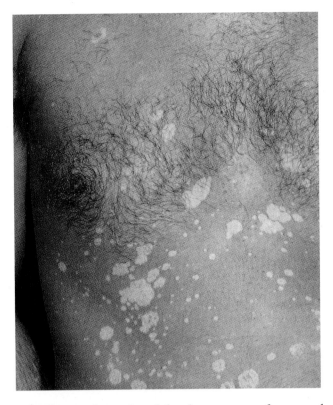

7. This gentleman's rash has been present for several months, is slowly spreading, and has worsened with over-the-counter steroids.

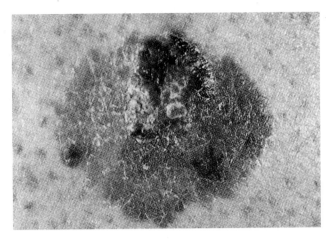

9. This lesion recently changed color in this 48-year-old lifeguard.

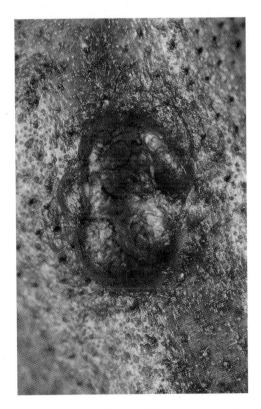

8. This lesion on a chronically sun-exposed area has been slowly enlarging for 9 months.

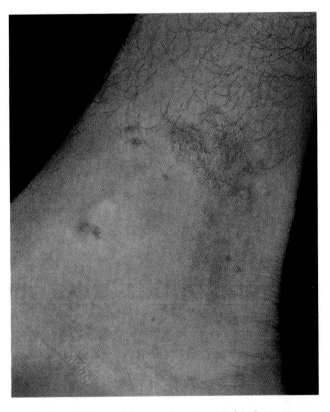

10. This 40-year-old man developed this lesion once before, but it went away. This lesion is characterized by five P's: pruritic, planar (flat-topped), polyangulat, purple papules.

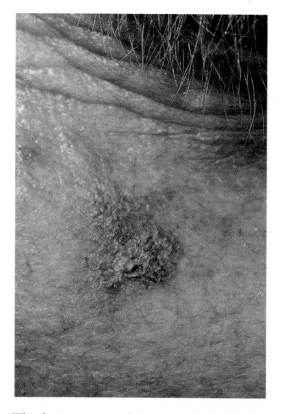

11. This lesion, on a yachting captain's neck, is one of many in sun-exposed areas of his head and neck.

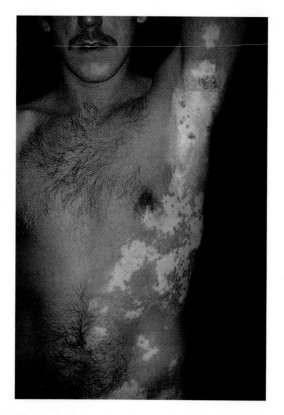

12. This condition has been slowly worsening and affects all areas of his skin.

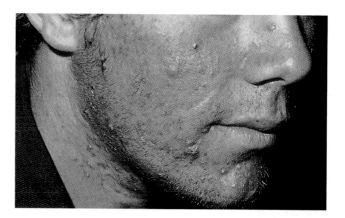

13. This teenager was told by his grandmother to avoid chocolate and wash his face more often to alleviate this condition.

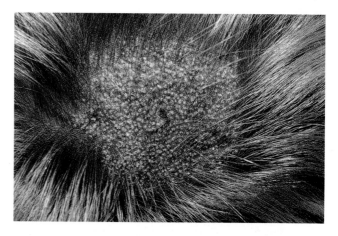

14. This third-grade student was sent home by the school nurse and told to seek treatment for the condition, which is pruritic.

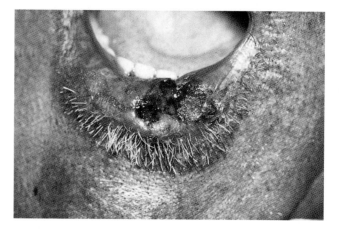

15. This smoker noticed this growing lesion approximately 5 months ago.

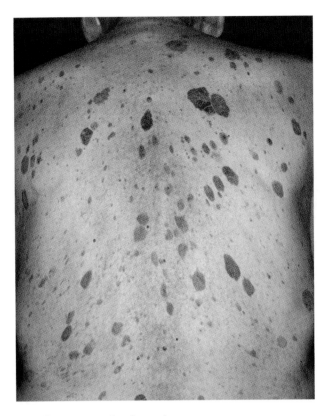

16. These growths have become more common as this patient ages.

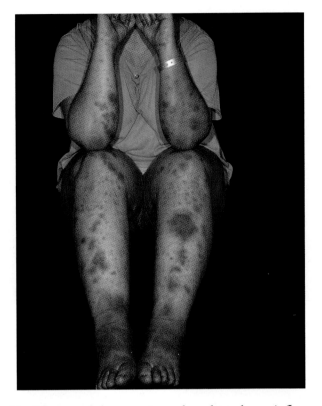

18. These nodular eruptions, thought to be an inflammatory hypersensitivity reaction in subcutaneous fat, began after a course of sulfonamide antibiotics.

DERMATOLOGIC MANIFESTATIONS OF UNDERLYING DISEASE

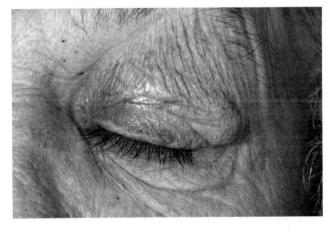

17. This patient had a total cholesterol level of 450 mg/dL and a family history of premature cardiovascular mortality.

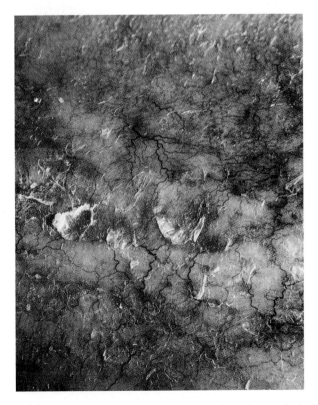

19. This chronic eruption is on the shin of this 24-year-old woman with type 1 diabetes.

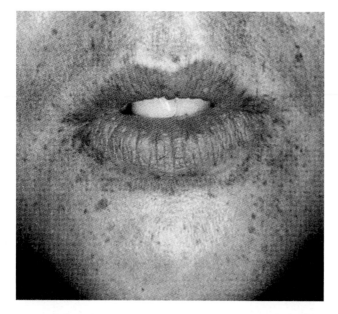

20. This patient has multiple hamartomatous polyps throughout the gastrointestinal tract, from the stomach to the rectum, and an iron deficiency anemia.

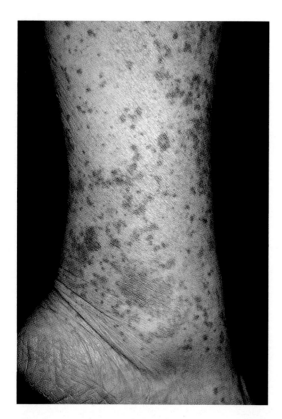

21. This eruption is palpable in a 35-year-old with leukemia.

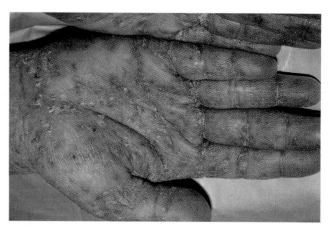

22. This intensely pruritic eruption is also present in a close contact of this patient.

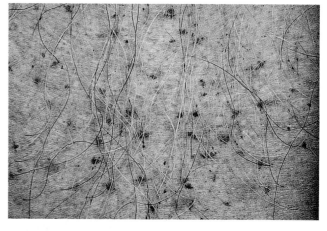

23. This patient's pubic area shown here has been the source of constant irritation and itching for several weeks.

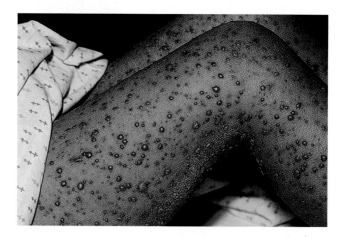

24. The pruritic lesions of this disease erupted initially on the face and trunk and then spread to the extremities.

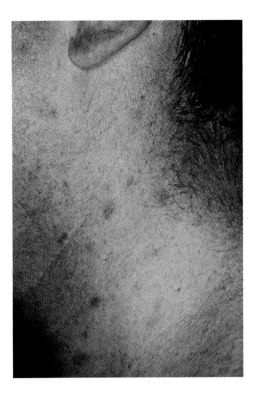

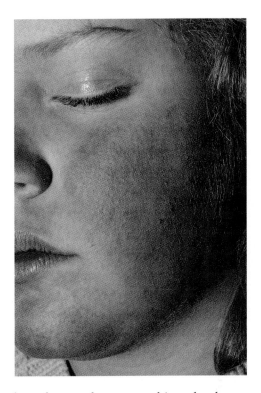

25. This infection is spread by aerosolized particles from respiratory secretions of infected individuals. Patients with this disease are most infectious from the prodrome (days 7 to 10 postexposure) through the fourth day after rash onset.

27. The infection that causes this rash, characterized by a slapped face appearance, is parvovirus B19. The prodrome to the rash is usually mild with low-grade fever, headache, and mild upper respiratory tract infection symptoms.

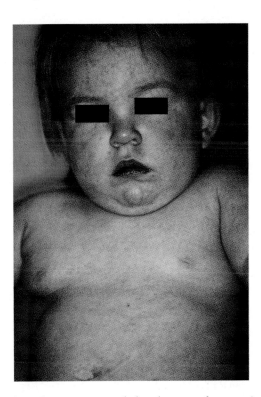

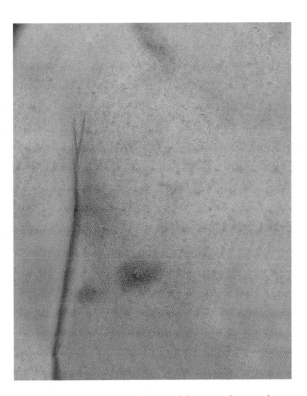

26. This disease, caused by human herpesvirus 6 and 7, is characterized by high fever (37.9°C to 40°C [101°F to 106°F]) that ends abruptly and is followed by onset of the rash depicted.

28. The variable rash of this mild to moderate disease, which usually begins on the face and spreads cephalocaudal over 24 hours, belies the serious complications the underlying virus can cause to the fetus of a pregnant woman. Characteristic findings include lymphadenopathy, particularly posterior auricular and suboccipital.

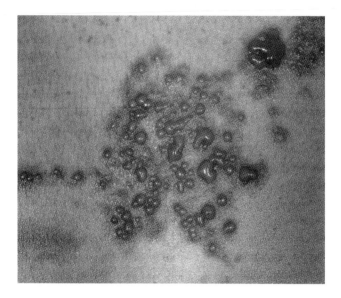

29. This rash, which occurs in a dermatomal distribution, is usually preceded by paresthesias of the affected area. Pain can be quite intense and last long after the rash has resolved.

OPHTHALMOSCOPY

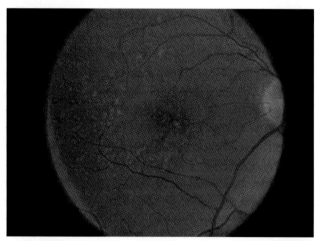

30. The condition seen here is now the main cause of blindness in the United States. Decreased central vision is the hallmark of this condition, whose prevalence increases with age. Yellowish deposits on the retina shown here are characteristic.

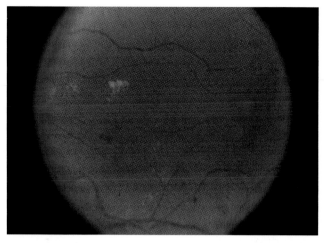

31. These eye grounds are of a 54-year-old woman with a long-standing chronic disease that has compromised her vision.

MICROSCOPY

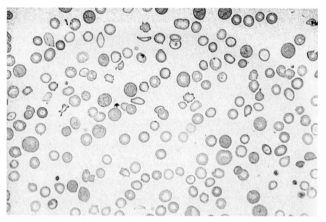

32. This smear was obtained on a 36-year-old woman who has been having heavy menstrual bleeding for years.

Answers

1. Herald patch, pityriasis rosea (see Chapter 112, Answer 28).

Figure from Miller RG, Sisson SD, Ashar B: *The Johns Hopkins Internal Medicine Board Review*. Philadelphia: Mosby, 2004, Fig. 63-9.

2. Rosacea (see Chapter 52, Answers 16 to 19).

Figure from Miller RG, Sisson SD, Ashar B: *The Johns Hopkins Internal Medicine Board Review*. Philadelphia: Mosby, 2004, Fig. 63-1.

3. Atopic dermatitis (see Chapter 103, Answers 1 to 5). Note that although 90% of children resolve their symptoms by adolescence, people with asthma often have a persistent history of atopy.

Figure from Miller RG, Sisson SD, Ashar B: *The Johns Hopkins Internal Medicine Board Review*. Philadelphia: Mosby, 2004, Fig. 63-2.

4. Dyshidrotic eczema, pictured here, is a vesicular pattern of eczema generally affecting the hands and occasionally the feet. Affected individuals may have a history of contact dermatitis, often induced by nickel. However, in many cases no specific allergen can be identified and a history of atopic dermatitis is rare. The condition tends to be aggravated by sweating and may arise secondary to a fungal infection.

Figure from Miller RG, Sisson SD, Ashar B: *The Johns Hopkins Internal Medicine Board Review*. Philadelphia: Mosby, 2004, Fig. 63-4.

5. Chronic plaque psoriasis. This is a chronic autoimmune condition with a strong genetic component. The skin lesions are caused by dermal hyperproliferation causing the skin to literally "pile up." It affects more than 4 million Americans and has a wide range of symptoms. Most individuals have the relatively mild plaque type similar to that pictured, which tends to localize to the elbows and knees. However, some individuals have severe cases covering most of the body, and gross open lesions may occur. Psoriatic arthritis, a condition similar to rheumatic arthritis, develops in approximately 23% of the cases.

Figure from Miller RG, Sisson SD, Ashar B: *The Johns Hopkins Internal Medicine Board Review*. Philadelphia: Mosby, 2004, Fig. 63-6.

6. Molluscum (see Chapter 112, Answer 29).

Figure from Miller RG, Sisson SD, Ashar B: *The Johns Hopkins Internal Medicine Board Review*. Philadelphia: Mosby, 2004, Fig. 63-12.

7. Tinea versicolor (see Chapter 112, Answer 26).

Figure from Miller RG, Sisson SD, Ashar B: *The Johns Hopkins Internal Medicine Board Review*. Philadelphia: Mosby, 2004, Fig. 62-13.

8. Basal cell carcinoma (see Chapter 53, Answers 1 and 2).

Figure from Miller RG, Sisson SD, Ashar B: *The Johns Hopkins Internal Medicine Board Review*. Philadelphia: Mosby, 2004, Fig. 63-15.

9. Melanoma (see Chapter 53, Answers 8 to 10).

Figure from Miller RG, Sisson SD, Ashar B: *The Johns Hopkins Internal Medicine Board Review*. Philadelphia: Mosby, 2004, Fig. 63-14B.

10. Lichen planus. A pruritic, papular skin eruption usually found on the genitalia, mucous membranes, or flexor surfaces of the extremities, lichen planus occurs most commonly between the ages of 30 and 60 years. Diagnosis may be confirmed by biopsy. The cause is unknown, although some eruptions have been associated with antibiotic use, and spontaneous remissions occur in up to 65% of cases within 1 year. Topical steroids are often used for cutaneous lesions, although no randomized controlled trials have been performed to demonstrate efficacy.

Figure from Miller RG, Sisson SD, Ashar B: *The Johns Hopkins Internal Medicine Board Review*. Philadelphia: Mosby, 2004, Fig. 63-18.

11. Actinic keratosis (see Chapter 53, Answers 3 to 5).

Figure from Miller RG, Sisson SD, Ashar B: *The Johns Hopkins Internal Medicine Board Review*. Philadelphia: Mosby, 2004, Fig. 63-16.

12. Vitiligo. A probable autoimmune disease related to destruction of melanocytes, vitiligo is a disease of hypopigmentation. Approximately 1% of the population is affected, with half of cases beginning before adulthood. Thyroid disease is seen in approximately 30% of patients with vitiligo. Oral photochemotherapy and topical steroids have been used for treatment with some success.

Figure from Miller RG, Sisson SD, Ashar B: *The Johns Hopkins Internal Medicine Board Review*. Philadelphia: Mosby, 2004, Fig. 63-24.

13. Acne vulgaris (see Chapter 52, Answers 1 to 14).

Figure from Hooper BJ, Goldman MP: *Primary Dermatologic Care*. St. Louis: Mosby, 1999, p. 12.

14. Tinea capitis. Scalp ringworm is a common occurrence in grade school children. It may resemble seborrheic dermatitis but more often presents with broken off hair shafts and smooth plaques. They may be surrounded with inflammation, and secondary lymphadenitis is common. Oral antifungals are generally required for successful treatment.

Figure from White G, Cox N: *Diseases of the Skin: Color Atlas and Text*. St. Louis: Mosby, p. 371, Fig. 23-12.b.

15. Squamous cell carcinoma (see Chapter 53, Answers 6 and 7).

Figure from Lawrence CM, Cox NH: *Physical Signs in Dermatology*. St. Louis: Mosby, 2002, p. 184, Fig. 9-96.

16. Seborrheic keratosis. These, the most common of benign skin neoplasms, have a characteristic stuck-on appearance with a well-circumscribed border. They are typically tan-brown to dark brown in color, and increasing numbers often appear with aging. Sudden appearance of large numbers has been associated with the presence of internal malignancy (mostly adenocarcinoma of the stomach) in some case reports, although this observation has not been substantiated in other epidemiologic studies.

Figure from Miller RG, Sisson SD, Ashar B: *The Johns Hopkins Internal Medicine Board Review*. Philadelphia: Mosby, 2004, Fig. 63-8.

17. Xanthoma. These yellowish nodular skin lesions are typically seen in patients with type I or type V hyperlipoproteinemia.

Figure from Miller RG, Sisson SD, Ashar B: *The Johns Hopkins Internal Medicine Board Review*. Philadelphia: Mosby, 2004, Fig. 2-1.

18. Erythema nodosum. An acute, nodular, and tender skin eruption that results from inflammation of subcutaneous fat, erythema nodosum is the result of a cell-mediated immune reaction to a variety of stimuli, including various infectious agents (bacteria, fungi, and viruses), drugs (antibiotics, aspirin, oral contraceptives, and antihypertensives), and diseases (sarcoidosis, lymphomas, and reactive arthropathies). Nodules usually resolve within 8 weeks.

Figure from Miller RG, Sisson SD, Ashar B: *The Johns Hopkins Internal Medicine Board Review*. Philadelphia: Mosby, 2004, Fig. 63-10.

19. Necrobiosis lipoidica. These plaque-like reddened areas that fade over time and take on a mottled yellowish appearance are found on the anterior surfaces of the legs of diabetics, and they may ulcerate with very little trauma to the area.

Figure from Miller RG, Sisson SD, Ashar B: *The Johns Hopkins Internal Medicine Board Review*. Philadelphia: Mosby, 2004, Fig. 63-23.

20. Peutz–Jeghers syndrome. An autosomal dominant genetically transmitted disease with incomplete penetrance. In addition to the polyposis, these patients have pigmented lesions of the lips, buccal mucosa, nose, hands, feet, and genital area. They are at high risk for gastrointestinal, breast, pancreatic, ovarian, and Sertoli cell malignancies.

Figure from Gawkrodger DJ: *An Illustrated Colour Text: Dermatology*. Edinburgh, UK: Churchill-Livingstone, 1992, p. 67, Fig. 4.

21. Palpable purpura. A circumscribed collection of blood greater than 0.5 cm. Diagnostic considerations for palpable purpura are numerous and include malignancies, infection, drug reactions, disseminated intravascular coagulation, collagen–vascular diseases, trauma, cryoglobulinemias, and embolization.

Figure from Miller RG, Sisson SD, Ashar B: *The Johns Hopkins Internal Medicine Board Review*. Philadelphia: Mosby, 2004, Fig. 63-29.

22. Scabies. This eruption is caused by a mite that burrows under the skin surface and travels through the stratum corneum depositing eggs and feces. Contagious, it is commonly spread among close contacts, especially through infested bedding. Primary lesions are intensely pruritic and are common in the web spaces of the hands and feet, genitals, wrists, and buttocks. It is treated with topical insecticide applied as a cream (lindane in adults or permethrin in children and pregnant women). Itching may last for weeks after mites are successfully treated and may also require treatment.

Figure from White G, Cox N: *Diseases of the Skin: Color Atlas and Text*. St. Louis: Mosby, p. 371, Fig. 23-12.b.

23. Pediculosis pubis. Pubic lice are a common infestation frequently spread between sexual partners. Patients complain about itching, and the infection is apparent upon inspection. Live nits fluoresce white or gray with a Wood's lamp. Permethrin or lindane are effective as treatments.

Figure from Callen JP, Greer KE, Paller AS, Swinyer LJ: *Color Atlas of Dermatology*, 2nd ed. Philadelphia: Saunders, 2000, p. 309, Fig. 20-28.

24. Chickenpox (varicella) (see Chapter 112, Answers 1 to 3).

Figure from Callen JP, Greer KE, Paller AS, Swinyer LJ: *Color Atlas of Dermatology*, 2nd ed. Philadelphia: Saunders, 2000, p. 143, Fig. 5-43.

25. Measles (rubeola) (see Chapter 112, Answers 8 to 13).

Figure from Hooper BJ, Goldman MP: *Primary Dermatologic Care*. St. Louis: Mosby, 1999, p. 166, Fig. 4-26.

26. Roseola (exanthema subitum; sixth disease), exanthem subitum (roseola infantum) (see Chapter 103). Note: Antibiotics have essentially eliminated scarlet fever, one of the earlier major exanthemas, leaving roseola (the sixth disease) as one of the big five exanthems.

Figure from Hooper BJ, Goldman MP: *Primary Dermatologic Care*. St. Louis: Mosby, 1999, p. 173, Fig. 4-34.

27. Erythema infectiosum (fifth disease) (see Chapter 112, Answers 14 to 18).

Figure from Hooper BJ, Goldman MP: *Primary Dermatologic Care*. St. Louis: Mosby, 1999, p. 157, Fig. 4-13.

28. Rubella (see Chapter 112, "Summary" and Chapter 85, Answer 1). Fetuses exposed during gestation may develop congenital rubella syndrome. Common abnormalities include deafness, eye defects, central nervous system anomalies, cardiac malformations (patent ductus arteriosis and pulmonic stenosis), and mental retardation.

Figure from Hooper BJ, Goldman MP: *Primary Dermatologic Care*. St. Louis: Mosby, 1999, p. 57, Fig. 2-7.

29. Herpes zoster (see Chapter 112, Answers 4 and 5).

Figure from Miller RG, Sisson SD, Ashar B: *The Johns Hopkins Internal Medicine Board Review*. Philadelphia: Mosby, 2004, Fig. 63-11.

30. Macular degeneration. Two forms exist: wet and dry. Degenerative changes occur with aging in the vascular neural and pigmented layers of the macula. The wet form is more common and is associated with fluid leakage from the blood vessels. The dry form is thought to be ischemic in origin. Laser treatment slows the course of the disease somewhat, but in most cases progression occurs.

Figure from Miller RG, Sisson SD, Ashar B: *The Johns Hopkins Internal Medicine Board Review*. Philadelphia: Mosby, 2004, Fig. 65-2.

31. Nonproliferative diabetic retinopathy. Diabetic retinopathy is an eye disorder manifested by microaneurysms, hemorrhages, exudates, and neovascularity. Found in 80% of those who have had diabetes for 15 or more years, it is a leading cause of blindness. Treatment is by laser photocoagulation.

Figure from Miller RG, Sisson SD, Ashar B: *The Johns Hopkins Internal Medicine Board Review*. Philadelphia: Mosby, 2004, Fig. 65-3.

32. Hypochromic, microcytic red cells characteristic of iron deficiency anemia (see Chapter 63, Answers 1 to 11).

Figure from Miller RG, Sisson SD, Ashar B: *The Johns Hopkins Internal Medicine Board Review*. Philadelphia: Mosby, 2004, Plate 2.

INDEX

Note: Page numbers followed by f indicate figures; those followed by t indicate tables; and those followed by b indicate boxed material.